Nursing Foundation for BSc Nursing-II

As per the Revised Nursing Syllabus

Shiv Shankar Tyagi
PhD (N) MSc (N)
Director
RK Institute of Medical Sciences
Bareilly, Uttar Pradesh, India
Vice President
Nursing Scholar Society (NSS, UP Chapter)
President
Rohilkhand Nursing Association

Richa Gangwar
MSc (N)
Nursing Faculty
Government College of Nursing
Azamgarh, Uttar Pradesh, India
Formerly Vice Principal
RK Institute of Medical Sciences
College of Nursing
Bareilly, Uttar Pradesh, India

Foreword
C Vasantha Kalyani

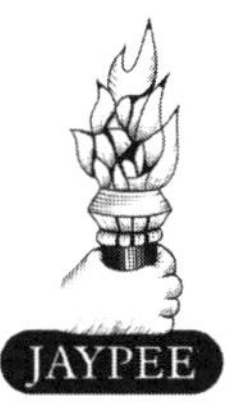

JAYPEE BROTHERS MEDICAL PUBLISHERS
The Health Sciences Publisher
New Delhi | London

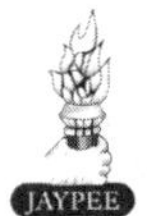 **Jaypee Brothers Medical Publishers (P) Ltd**

Headquarters

Jaypee Brothers Medical Publishers (P) Ltd
EMCA House, 23/23-B
Ansari Road, Daryaganj
New Delhi 110 002, India
Landline: +91-11-23272143, +91-11-23272703
+91-11-23282021, +91-11-23245672
Email: jaypee@jaypeebrothers.com

Corporate Office

Jaypee Brothers Medical Publishers (P) Ltd
4838/24, Ansari Road, Daryaganj
New Delhi 110 002, India
Phone: +91-11-43574357
Fax: +91-11-43574314
Email: jaypee@jaypeebrothers.com

Overseas Office

J.P. Medical Ltd
83 Victoria Street, London
SW1H 0HW (UK)
Phone: +44 20 3170 8910
Fax: +44 (0)20 3008 6180
Email: info@jpmedpub.com

Website: www.jaypeebrothers.com
Website: www.jaypeedigital.com

Inquiries for bulk sales may be solicited at: jaypee@jaypeebrothers.com

Nursing Foundation for BSc Nursing-II

First Edition: **2024**

ISBN: 978-93-5696-487-7

Printed in India at Rajkamal Electric Press, Kundli, Haryana.

Nursing Foundation for BSc Nursing-II

Dedicated to

Swami Vivekanand Ji

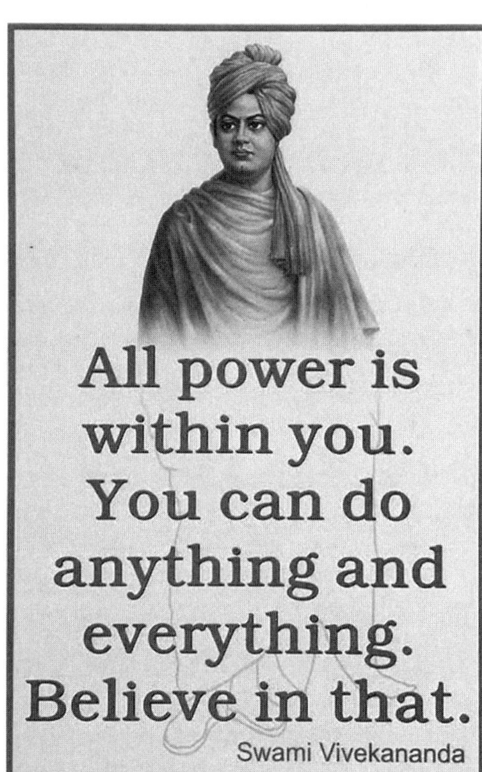

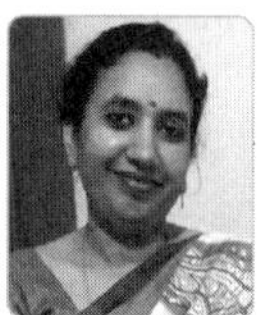

Abha
MSc Nursing (Community Health Nursing)
PHN Tutor
Rural Health Training Centre
New Delhi, India

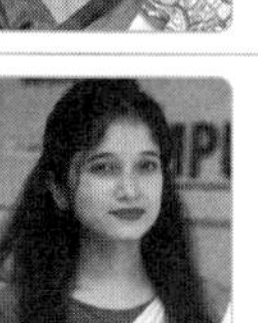

Akansha
MSc Nursing (Medical Surgical Nursing)
Assistant Professor
MIET Kumaon College of Nursing
Nainital, Uttarakhand, India

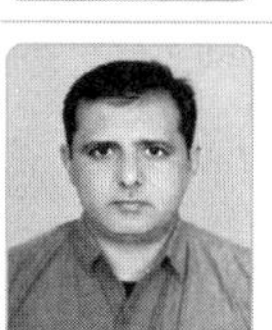

Anil Kumar Gurjar
MSc Nursing (Mental Health Nursing)
Vice Principal
College of Nursing Government
Medical College
Budaun, Uttar Pradesh, India

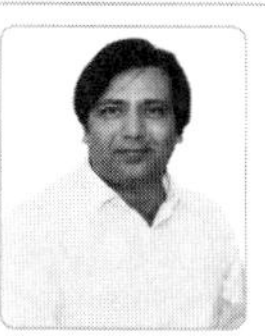

Arjun Yadav
MSc Nursing (Medical Surgical Nursing)
Principal
Barala Nursing College
Jaipur, Rajasthan, India

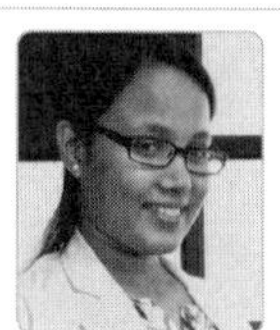

Ashmita
PBBSc Nursing
Nursing Officer
GMC College of Nursing
Azamgarh, Uttar Pradesh, India

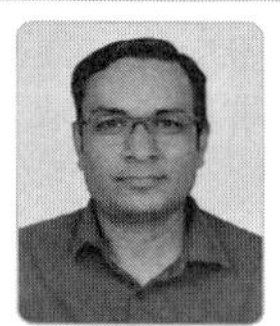

Aslam Abbas
MSc Nursing (Community Health
Nursing)
Associate Professor
Rama College of Nursing
Rama University
Kanpur, Uttar Pradesh, India

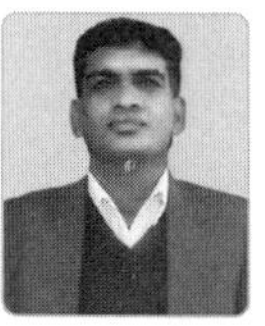

Banwari Lal Bhaira
MSc Nursing (Community Health
Nursing)
Principal
Sikar Nursing College
Sikar, Rajasthan, India

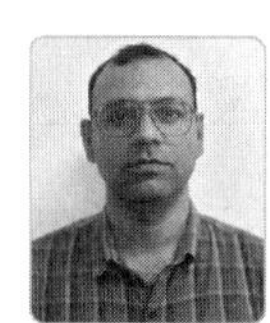

Deepak Suwalka
MSc Nursing (Mental Health Nursing)
Associate Professor
(Mental Health Nursing)
Rama College of Nursing
Rama University
Kanpur, Uttar Pradesh, India

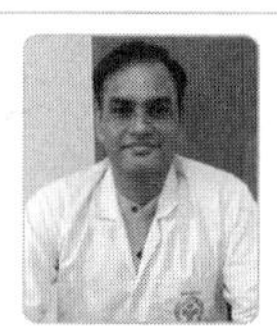

Gajendra Singh
MSc Nursing (Medical Surgical Nursing)
Associate Professor
Shree Dev Bhoomi College of Nursing
Dehradun, Uttarakhand, India

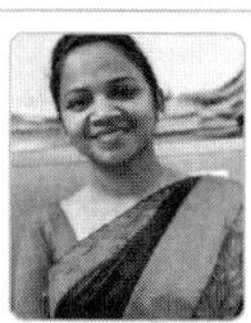

Ganga Potai
MSc Nursing (Medical Surgical Nursing)
Associate Professor
Vivekananda College of Nursing
Lucknow, Uttar Pradesh, India

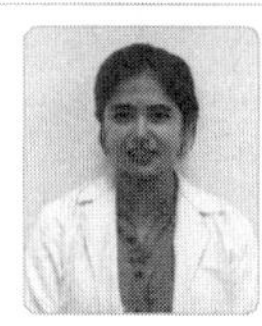

Geetanjali Sah
MSc Nursing (Obstetrics and
Gynecological Nursing)
Nursing Tutor
Government Nursing College
Nainital, Uttarakhand, India

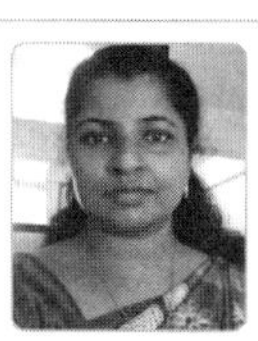

Hemalatha M
MSc Nursing (Obstetrics and
Gynecological Nursing)
Associate Professor
SN College of Nursing
SN Medical College
Agra, Uttar Pradesh, India

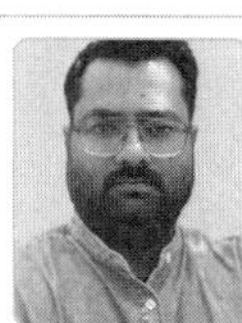

Hemant Tyagi
MSc Nursing (Medical Surgical Nursing)
Professor-cum-Principal
Imperial College of Nursing
Jaipur, Rajasthan, India

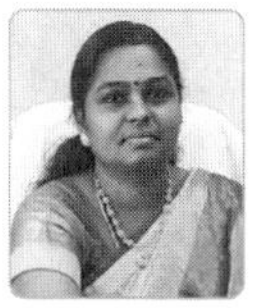

Jasline M
PhD MSc Nursing
Vice Principal
Teerthanker Mahaveer College of
Nursing
Teerthanker Mahaveer University
Moradabad, Uttar Pradesh, India

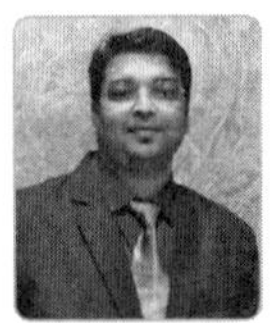

Jitendra Kumar Jain
MSc Nursing (Medical Surgical Nursing)
Principal
Aayushman Institute of Medical
Science and College of Nursing
Jaipur, Rajasthan, India

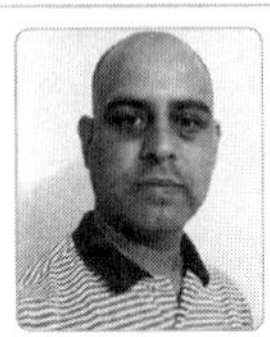

Jitendra Prasad Yadav
MSc Nursing (Child Health Nursing)
Nursing Officer
ESIC Model Hospital
Andheri, Mumbai, India

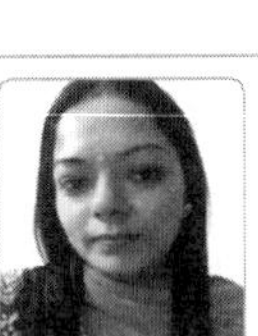

Kuljeet Kaur
MSc Nursing (Child Health Nursing)
Assistant Professor
Maharaja Agrasen Nursing College
Bahadurgarh, Haryana, India

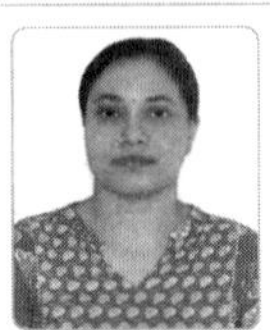

Kumkum Yadav
MSc Nursing (Obstetrics and
Gynecological Nursing)
Assistant Professor
Government Medical College
College of Nursing
Azamgarh, Uttar Pradesh, India

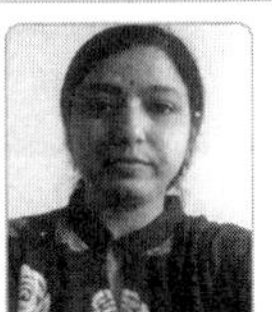

Meena Soni
MSc (Obstetric and Gynecological
Nursing)
Associate Professor
Government College of Nursing
Ajmer, Rajasthan, India

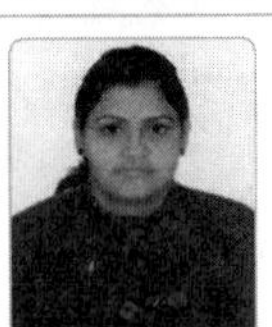

Mishri Aechra
MSc Nursing (Child Health Nursing)
Nursing Officer
AIIMS
Patna, Bihar, India

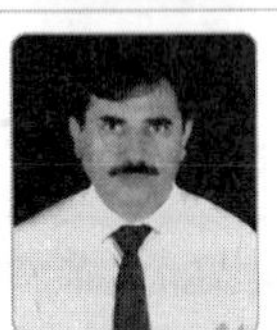

Narsimha Prasad
MSc Nursing (Community Health Nursing)
Principal
RBMI College of Nursing
Bareilly, Uttar Pradesh, India

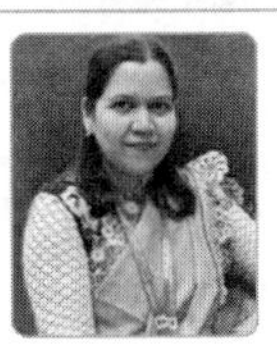

Nilam Victoria Dayal
MSc Nursing (Child Health Nursing)
Tutor
College of Nursing
Indira Gandhi Institute of Medical
Sciences
Patna, Bihar, India

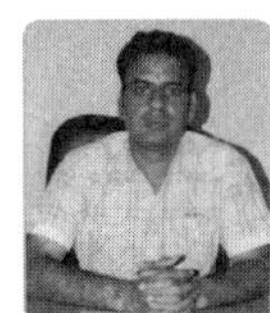

Nitesh Kumar Sharma
PhD MSc Nursing (Child Health Nursing)
Principal
Marudhar College of Nursing
Kuchaman City, Rajasthan, India

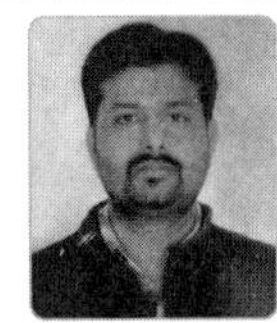

Pankaj Singhal
MSc Nursing (Community Health Nursing)
Faculty
Government College of Nursing
Uttar Pradesh University of Medical
Sciences
Saifai, Uttar Pradesh, India

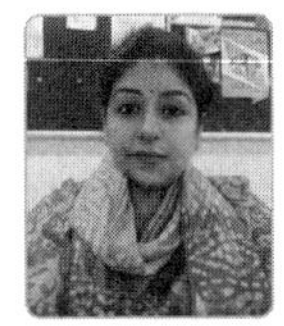

Prachi Awasthi
PhD MSc Nursing (Obstetrics and
Gynecological Nursing)
Professor and Head
Choithram College of Nursing
Indore, Madhya Pradesh, India

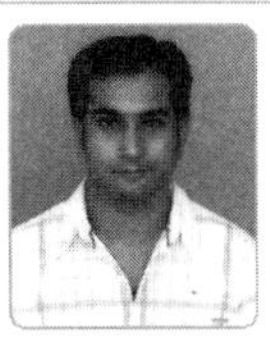

Prakash Sheshma
MSc Nursing (Medical Surgical Nursing)
Associate Professor
RK Instititute of Medical Sciences
Bareilly, Uttar Pradesh, India

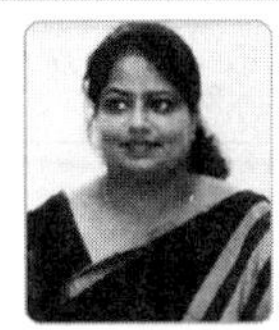

Priyanka A Masih
PhD MSc Nursing
Principal
Rohilkhand College of Nursing
Bareilly International University
Bareilly, Uttar Pradesh, India

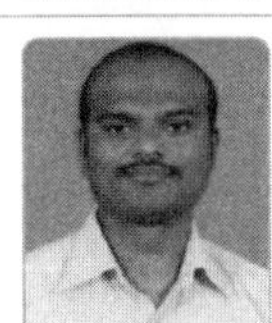

Ranganath MG
MSc Nursing (Mental Health Nursing)
Principal
Vivek College of Education
Bijnor, Uttar Pradesh, India

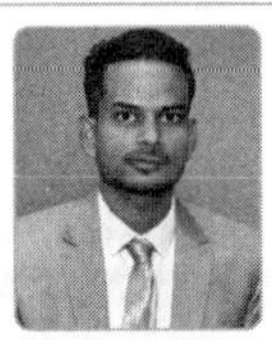

Rohit Singh
NPCC
Assistant Professor
RK Institute of Medical Sciences
Bareilly, Uttar Pradesh, India

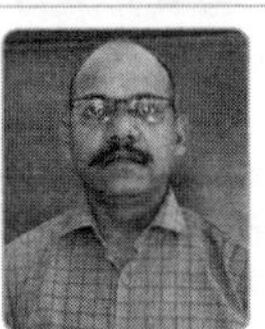

Rohitash Jogi
MSc (Child Health Nursing)
Associate Professor
Government College of Nursing
Ajmer, Rajasthan, India

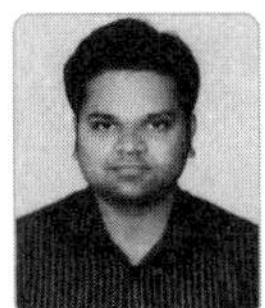

Saurabh Kumar Gupta
MSc Nursing (Mental Health Nursing)
Professor
Government College of Nursing
Ajmer, Rajasthan, India

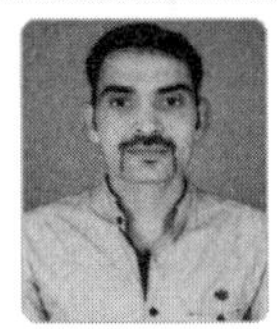

Sharwan Choudhary
MSc Nursing (Medical Surgical Nursing)
Assistant Nursing Superintendent
AIIMS
Patna, Bihar, India

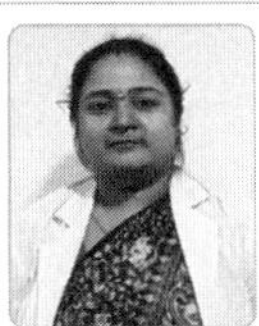

Shirish Upadhyay
MSc Nursing (Obstetrics and Gynecological Nursing)
Vice Principal
Ashirvad Nursing and Paramedical Institute
Varanasi, Uttar Pradesh, India

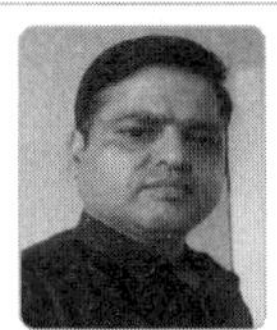

Shivraj Singh Tyagi
MSc Nursing (Medical Surgical Nursing)
Principal
Kanti Devi College of Nursing and Paramedical Sciences
Mathura, Uttar Pradesh, India

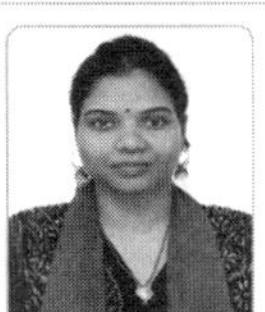

Shweta Singh
MSc Nursing (Mental Health Nursing)
Lecturer
GMC College of Nursing
Azamgarh, Uttar Pradesh, India

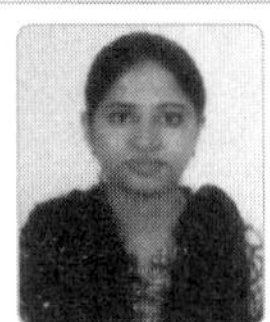

Sijo N Sam
MSc Nursing (Child Health Nursing)
Associate Professor
Upchar College of Nursing
Jaipur, Rajasthan, India

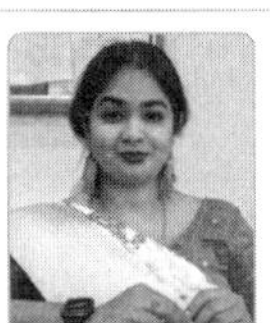

Smriti Nand
MSc Nursing (Medical Surgical Nursing)
Associate Professor
Maitri College of Nursing
Anjora, Chhattisgarh, India

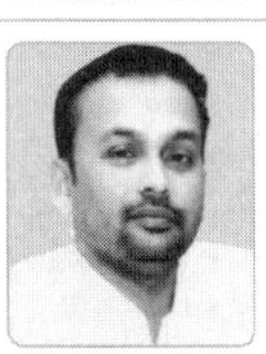

Sreejith S
MSc Nursing (Mental Health Nursing)
Vice Principal
Ch. Sughar Singh Nursing and Paramedical College
Jaswant Nagar, Uttar Pradesh, India

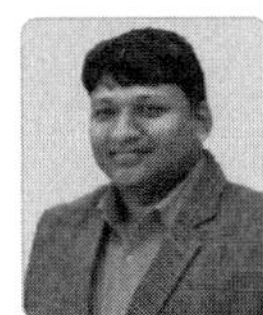

Sunil Kumar Garg
MSc Nursing (Community Health Nursing)
Principal
University Institute of Nursing
Jalalabad, Punjab, India
Baba Farid University of Health Sciences
Faridkot, Punjab, India

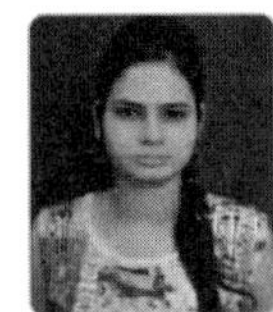

Swati
MSc Nursing (Child Health Nursing)
Lecturer
Prakash Institute of Physiotherapy and Allied of Medical Sciences
Greater Noida, Uttar Pradesh, India

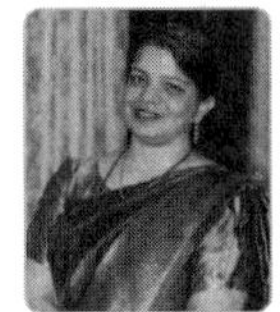

Swati Ompal Patanwal
PhD MSc Nursing (Child Health Nursing)
Assistant Professor
Rajkiya Medical College
Jalaun, Uttar Pradesh, India

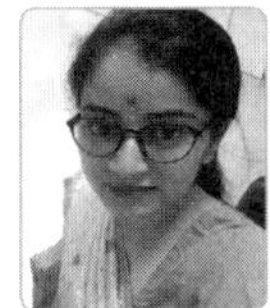

Uma Negi
MSc Nursing (Child Health Nursing)
Assistant Professor
PAL College of Nursing and Medical Sciences
Haldwani, Uttarakhand, India

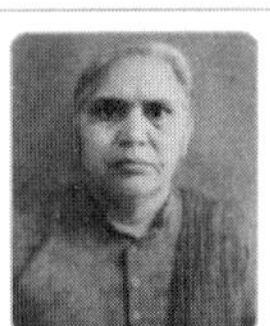

Vijender Kaur
PhD MSc Nursing (Community Health Nursing)
Nursing Lecturer
College of Nursing
VMMC and Safdarjung Hospital
New Delhi, India

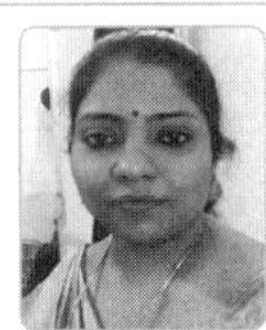

Vineeta Satya Kumar
MSc Nursing (Mental Health Nursing)
Vice Principal and Head
Shankaracharya Swami Swaroopanand College of Nursing
Bhilai, Chhattisgarh, India

Foreword

I am very much pleased to write the Foreword to *Nursing Foundation for BSc Nursing-II* based on the semester-wise curriculum authored by one of my students Dr Shiv Shankar Tyagi with his co-author Ms Richa Gangwar.

I would like to congratulate Jaypee Brothers Medical Publishers and authors for their efforts to write this title as per the need of students. I applaud the publication of this wonderful book on the basic foundation of nursing profession.

This book is based on semester system curriculum prescribed by Indian Nursing Council. This book is divided into two volumes for semesters I and II. This book also has special Procedure Boxes and Table, and Diagrams as per curriculum. It provides step-by-step guides to performing basic clinical nursing skills on emphasizing the application of nursing process.

Study, share, and discuss this book with your colleagues and students.

I wish the book and authors great success.

C Vasantha Kalyani
Principal
College of Nursing
All India Institute of Medical Sciences
Deoghar, Jharkhand, India

Preface

This book aims to provide nurses with the appropriate knowledge to meet the challenge of caring for patients. It is designed to be an easy-to-use guide and not as an exhaustive textbook. Additional sources will need to be accessed to provide any further required information.

This book has arisen primarily in response to the increasing concern expressed about the perceived lack of ability in both students and newly qualified staff nurses to perform clinical skills.

Innovations in nursing such as the nursing process, nursing models, and new methods of organizing care delivery each lays emphasis on providing individualized nursing care. Consequently, nurses and the increasing number of healthcare workers in new roles such as cadet nurses, health care assistants, and generic ward practitioners no longer have an easily accessible source of reference in the nursing profession's arena.

Charts, tables, diagrams, and pictures have been used to highlight important points and make the book an easy read.

This book has a practical approach for medical and nursing staff and offers a step-by-step guide to caring for patients in a variety of clinical settings. It follows a patient's path of care from management in the outpatient clinic to the hospital ward, operation theater, recovery room, and back to the follow-up outpatient clinic. A clear, concise format is used throughout the book with reference to evidence-based interventions and the physiology underpinning them, and simple line diagrams and treatment flowcharts have been used to illustrate the essential aspects of care.

The book reflects the multidisciplinary nature of patient care and will be a valuable resource for nurses, surgeons, and other healthcare professionals involved in caring for this patient group.

Special attention has been given to provide a clear, concise presentation of content that is realistic for the beginning nursing student. This text is timely in its approach to content, recognizing the inherent changes affecting the healthcare delivery system and the nursing curriculum. We recognize the student as an active participant who assumes a collaborative role in the learning process. Content is presented to challenge the student to develop critical thinking skills.

The book is the first of a series which aims to promote professional and personal development from a novice to an expert in sequential stages. We have retained in a concise and readable format the content is basic to a textbook that has the nursing profession as its focus.

While every attempt has been made throughout the text to reflect contemporary practices, the reader is reminded that practice will continue to develop in the light of new evidence and changing policy. A commitment to lifelong learning is therefore essential.

Shiv Shankar Tyagi
Richa Gangwar

Acknowledgments

With the blessing of God Ganesha, this title has become possible. We would like to express our gratitude to the entire team of M/s Jaypee Brothers Medical Publishers (P) Ltd, specially Mr Rishi Sharma (Regional Business Development Manager—North), Dr Madhu Choudhary (Director-Educational Publishing), Ms Samina Khan (Executive Assistant to Director-Educational Publishing), and Ms Alisha Talwar (Team Lead–Nursing) for publishing this book. We also acknowledge encouragement by Mr Nilamber Kumar (Sr Executive E-Accounts) of Jaypee Brothers Medical Publishers. We are grateful to Mr Om Prakash Mishra (Typesetter) for his hard work and timely completion of assigned work associated with this title. We also acknowledge the work of research scholars and reputed authors of different titles of Nursing Foundation. We are very much grateful to our family members for their continuous support and motivation.

Contents

NURSING FOUNDATION - II (INCLUDING HEALTH ASSESSMENT MODULE)

Placement: II Semester

Theory: 6 Credits (120 hours)

Practicum: Skill Lab: 3 Credits (120 hours), Clinical: 4 Credits (320 hours)

Description: This course is designed to help novice nursing students develop knowledge and competencies required to provide evidence-based, comprehensive basic nursing care for adult patients, using nursing process approach.

Competencies: On completion of the course, the students will be able to:
1. Develop understanding about fundamentals of health assessment and perform health assessment in supervised clinical settings.
2. Demonstrate fundamental skills of assessment, planning, implementation and evaluation of nursing care using nursing process approach in supervised clinical settings.
3. Assess the Nutritional needs of patients and provide relevant care under supervision.
4. Identify and meet the hygienic needs of patients.
5. Identify and meet the elimination needs of patient.
6. Interpret findings of specimen testing applying the knowledge of normal values.
7. Promote oxygenation based on identified oxygenation needs of patients under supervision.
8. Review the concept of fluid, electrolyte balance integrating the knowledge of applied physiology.
9. Apply the knowledge of the principles, routes, effects of administration of medications in administering medication.
10. Calculate conversions of drugs and dosages within and between systems of measurements.
11. Demonstrate knowledge and understanding in caring for patients with altered functioning of sense organs and unconsciousness.
12. Explain loss, death and grief.
13. Describe sexual development and sexuality.
14. Identify stressors and stress adaptation modes.
15. Integrate the knowledge of culture and cultural differences in meeting the spiritual needs.
16. Explain the introductory concepts relevant to models of health and illness in patient care.

***Mandatory Module Used in Teaching/Learning:**

Health Assessment Module: 40 hours

COURSE OUTLINE

T – Theory, SL – Skill Lab

Unit	Time (Hrs)	Learning outcomes	Content	Teaching/ learning activities	Assessment methods

I	20 (T) 20 (SL)	Describe the purpose and process of health assessment and perform assessment under supervised clinical practice	**Health Assessment**
			• Interview techniques
			• Observation techniques
			• Purposes of health assessment
			• Process of health assessment
			  ➤ Health history
			  ➤ Physical examination:
			    ◆ Methods: inspection, palpation, percussion, auscultation, olfaction
			    ◆ Preparation for examination: patient and unit
			    ◆ General assessment
			    ◆ Assessment of each body system
			    ◆ Documenting health assessment findings
				• Modular learning
				***Health Assessment Module**
				• Lecture cum discussion
				• Demonstration
					• Essay
					• Short answer
					• Objective type
					• OSCE

II	13 (T) 8 (SL)	Describe assessment, planning, implementation and evaluation of nursing care using nursing process approach	**The Nursing Process**
			• Critical thinking competencies, attitudes for critical thinking, levels of critical thinking in nursing
			• Nursing process overview
			  ➤ *Assessment*
			    ◆ Collection of data: types, sources, methods
			    ◆ Organizing data
			    ◆ Validating data
			    ◆ Documenting data
			  ➤ *Nursing diagnosis*
			    ◆ Identification of client problems, risks and strengths
			    ◆ Nursing diagnosis statement – parts, types, formulating, guidelines for formulating nursing diagnosis
			    ◆ NANDA approved diagnoses
			    ◆ Difference between medical and nursing diagnosis
				• Lecture
				• Discussion
				• Demonstration
				• Supervised clinical practice
					• Essay
					• Short answer
					• Objective type
					• Evaluation of care plan

Unit	Time (Hrs)	Learning outcomes	Content	Teaching/ learning activities	Assessment methods

			➢ *Planning*
			   ◆ Types of planning
			   ◆ Establishing priorities
			   ◆ Establishing goals and expected outcomes – purposes, types, guidelines, components of goals and outcome statements
			   ◆ Types of nursing interventions, selecting interventions: protocols and standing orders
			   ◆ Introduction to nursing intervention classification and nursing outcome classification
			   ◆ Guidelines for writing care plan
			 ➢ *Implementation*
			   ◆ Process of implementing the plan of care
			   ◆ Types of care – direct and indirect
			 ➢ *Evaluation*
			   ◆ Evaluation process, documentation and reporting		

III	5 (T)
	 5 (SL)
		Identify and meet the nutritional needs of patients	**Nutritional Needs**
			 • Importance
			 • Factors affecting nutritional needs
			 • Assessment of nutritional status
			 • *Review:* Special diets – solid, liquid, soft
			 • *Review* on therapeutic diets
			 • Care of patient with dysphagia, anorexia, nausea, vomiting
			 • Meeting nutritional needs: principles, equipment, procedure, indications
			   ➢ Oral
			   ➢ Enteral: Nasogastric/orogastric
			   ➢ Introduction to other enteral feeds – types, indications, gastrostomy, jejunostomy
			   ➢ Parenteral – TPN (total parenteral nutrition)
				• Lecture
				 • Discussion
				 • Demonstration
				 • Exercise
				 • Supervised clinical practice
					• Essay
					 • Short answer
					 • Objective type
					 • Evaluation of nutritional assessment and diet planning

Unit	Time (Hrs)	Learning outcomes	Content	Teaching/ learning activities	Assessment methods

IV	5 (T)
	15 (SL)
		Identify and meet the hygienic needs of patients	**Hygiene**
			• Factors influencing hygienic practice
			• Hygienic care: indications and purposes, effects of neglected care
			  ➢ Care of the skin – (bath, feet and nail, hair care)
			  ➢ Care of pressure points
			  ➢ Assessment of pressure ulcers using braden scale and norton scale
			  ➢ Pressure ulcers – causes, stages and manifestations, care and prevention
			  ➢ Perineal care/meatal care
			  ➢ Oral care, care of eyes, ears and nose including assistive devices (eye glasses, contact lens, dentures, hearing aid)
				• Lecture
				• Discussion
				• Demonstration
					• Essay
					• Short answer
					• Objective type
					• OSCE

V	10 (T)
	10 (SL)
		Identify and meet the elimination needs of patient	**Elimination Needs**
			• Urinary elimination
			  ➢ Review of physiology of urine elimination, composition and characteristics of urine
			  ➢ Factors influencing urination
			  ➢ Alteration in urinary elimination
			  ➢ Facilitating urine elimination: assessment, types, equipment, procedures and special considerations
			  ➢ Providing urinal/bed pan
			  ➢ Care of patients with
			    ♦ Condom drainage
			    ♦ Intermittent catheterization
			    ♦ Indwelling urinary catheter and urinary drainage
			    ♦ Urinary diversions
			    ♦ Bladder irrigation
				• Lecture
				• Discussion
				• Demonstration
					• Essay
					• Short answer
					• Objective type
					• OSCE

Unit	Time (Hrs)	Learning outcomes	Content	Teaching/ learning activities	Assessment methods

			• Bowel elimination
			  ➢ Review of physiology of bowel elimination, composition and characteristics of feces
			  ➢ Factors affecting bowel elimination
			  ➢ Alteration in bowel elimination
			  ➢ Facilitating bowel elimination: assessment, equipment, procedures
			    ♦ Enemas
			    ♦ Suppository
			    ♦ Bowel wash
			    ♦ Digital evacuation of impacted feces
			    ♦ Care of patients with ostomies (bowel diversion procedures)		

VI	3 (T)
	4 (SL)
		Explain various types of specimens and identify normal values of tests
		
		Develop skill in specimen collection, handling and transport
			Diagnostic Testing
			• Phases of diagnostic testing (pre-test, intra-test and post-test) in common investigations and clinical implications
			  ➢ Complete blood count
			  ➢ Serum electrolytes
			  ➢ LFT
			  ➢ Lipid/lipoprotein profile
			  ➢ Serum glucose – AC, PC, HbA1c
			  ➢ Monitoring capillary blood glucose (glucometer random blood sugar – GRBS)
			  ➢ Stool routine examination
			  ➢ Urine testing – albumin, Acetone, pH, specific gravity
			  ➢ Urine culture, routine, timed urine specimen
			  ➢ Sputum culture
			  ➢ Overview of radiologic and endoscopic procedures
				• Lecture
				• Discussion
				• Demonstration
					• Essay
					• Short answer
					• Objective type

Unit	Time (Hrs)	Learning outcomes	Content	Teaching/ learning activities	Assessment methods

VII	11 (T) 10 (SL)	Assess patients for oxygenation needs, promote oxygenation and provide care during oxygen therapy	**Oxygenation Needs**
			• Review of cardiovascular and respiratory physiology
			• Factors affecting respiratory functioning
			• Alterations in respiratory functioning
			• Conditions affecting
			  ➢ Airway
			  ➢ Movement of air
			  ➢ Diffusion
			  ➢ Oxygen transport
			• Alterations in oxygenation
			• Nursing interventions to promote oxygenation: assessment, types, equipment used and procedure
			  ➢ Maintenance of patent airway
			  ➢ Oxygen administration
			  ➢ Suctioning – oral, tracheal
			  ➢ Chest physiotherapy – Percussion, Vibration and Postural drainage
			  ➢ Care of chest drainage – principles and purposes
			  ➢ Pulse oximetry – factors affecting measurement of oxygen saturation using pulse oximeter, interpretation
			• Restorative and continuing care
			  ➢ Hydration
			  ➢ Humidification
			  ➢ Coughing techniques
			  ➢ Breathing exercises
			  ➢ Incentive spirometry
				• Lecture
				• Discussion
				• Demonstration and re-demonstration
					• Essay
					• Short answer
					• Objective type

VIII	5 (T) 10 (SL)	Describe the concept of fluid, electrolyte balance	**Fluid, Electrolyte, and Acid-base Balances** • Review of physiological regulation of fluid, electrolyte and acid-base balances • Factors affecting fluid, electrolyte and acid-base balances	• Lecture • Discussion • Demonstration	• Essay • Short answer • Objective type • Problem solving – calculations

Unit	Time (Hrs)	Learning outcomes	Content	Teaching/ learning activities	Assessment methods

			• Disturbances in fluid volume:
			  ➢ Deficit
			    ♦ Hypovolemia
			    ♦ Dehydration
			  ➢ Excess
			    ♦ Fluid overload
			    ♦ Edema
			• Electrolyte imbalances (hypo and hyper)
			  ➢ Acid-base imbalances
			    ♦ Metabolic – acidosis and alkalosis
			    ♦ Respiratory – acidosis and alkalosis
			  ➢ Intravenous therapy
			    ♦ Peripheral venipuncture sites
			    ♦ Types of IV fluids
			    ♦ Calculation for making IV fluid plan
			    ♦ Complications of IV fluid therapy
			    ♦ Measuring fluid intake and output
			    ♦ Administering blood and blood components
			    ♦ Restricting fluid intake
			    ♦ Enhancing fluid intake		

IX	20 (T) 22 (SL)	Explain the principles, routes, effects of administration of medications Calculate conversions of drugs and dosages within and between systems of measurements Administer oral and topical medication and document accurately under supervision	**Administration of Medications** • Introduction – definition of medication, administration of medication, drug nomenclature, effects of drugs, forms of medications, purposes, pharmacodynamics and pharmacokinetics • Factors influencing medication action • Medication orders and prescriptions • Systems of measurement • Medication dose calculation • Principles, 10 rights of medication administration • Errors in medication administration	• Lecture • Discussion • Demonstration and re-demonstration	• Essay • Short answer • Objective type • OSCE

Unit	Time (Hrs)	Learning outcomes	Content	Teaching/ learning activities	Assessment methods

			• Routes of administration
			• Storage and maintenance of drugs and nurses responsibility
			• Terminologies and abbreviations used in prescriptions and medications orders
			• Developmental considerations
			• Oral, sublingual and buccal routes: equipment, procedure
			• Introduction to parenteral administration of drugs – intramuscular, intravenous, subcutaneous, intradermal: location of site, advantages and disadvantages of the specific sites, indication and contraindications for the different routes and sites.
			• Equipment – syringes and needles, cannulas, infusion sets – parts, types, sizes
			• Types of vials and ampoules, preparing injectable medicines from vials and ampoules
			  ➢ Care of equipment: decontamination and disposal of syringes, needles, infusion sets
			  ➢ Prevention of needle-stick injuries
			• Topical administration: types, purposes, site, equipment, procedure
			  ➢ Application to skin and mucous membrane
			  ➢ Direct application of liquids, gargle and swabbing the throat
			  ➢ Insertion of drug into body cavity: suppository/ medicated packing in rectum/vagina		

Unit	Time (Hrs)	Learning outcomes	Content	Teaching/ learning activities	Assessment methods
			➤ Instillations: ear, eye, nasal, bladder, and rectal ➤ Irrigations: eye, ear, bladder, vaginal and rectal ➤ Spraying: nose and throat • Inhalation: nasal, oral, endotracheal/tracheal (steam, oxygen and medications) – purposes, types, equipment, procedure, recording and reporting of medications administered • Other parenteral routes: meaning of epidural, intrathecal, intraosseous, intraperitoneal, intra-pleural, intra-arterial		
X	5 (T) 6 (SL)	Provide care to patients with altered functioning of sense organs and unconsciousness in supervised clinical practice	**Sensory Needs** • Introduction • Components of sensory experience – Reception, Perception and Reaction • Arousal Mechanism • Factors affecting sensory function • Assessment of Sensory alterations – sensory deficit, deprivation, overload and sensory poverty • Management • Promoting meaningful communication (patients with aphasia, artificial airway and visual and hearing impairment) **Care of Unconscious Patients** • Unconsciousness: definition, causes and risk factors, pathophysiology, stages of unconsciousness, clinical manifestations • Assessment and nursing management of patient with unconsciousness, complications	• Lecture • Discussion • Demonstration	• Essay • Short answer • Objective type

Unit	Time (Hrs)	Learning outcomes	Content	Teaching/ learning activities	Assessment methods
XI	4 (T) 6 (SL)	Explain loss, death and grief	**Care of Terminally ill, Death and Dying** • Loss – types • Grief, bereavement and mourning • Types of grief responses • Manifestations of grief • Factors influencing loss and grief responses • Theories of grief and loss – kubler ross • Five Stages of dying • The R process model (rando's) • Death – definition, meaning, types (brain and circulatory deaths) • Signs of impending death • Dying patient's bill of rights • Care of dying patient • Physiological changes occurring after death • Death declaration, certification • Autopsy • Embalming • Last office/death care • Counseling and supporting grieving relatives • Placing body in the mortuary • Releasing body from mortuary • Overview – medico-legal cases, advance directives, DNI/DNR, organ donation, euthanasia	• Lecture • Discussion • Case discussions • Death care/last office	• Essay • Short answer • Objective type
			PSYCHOSOCIAL NEEDS (A–D)		
XII	3 (T)	Develop basic understanding of self-concept	**A. Self-concept** • Introduction • Components (personal identity, body image, role performance, self-esteem) • Factors affecting self-concept • Nursing management	• Lecture • Discussion • Demonstration • Case Discussion/ Role play	• Essay • Short answer • Objective type
XIII	2 (T)	Describe sexual development and sexuality	**B. Sexuality** • Sexual development throughout life • Sexual health • Sexual orientation	• Lecture • Discussion	• Essay • Short answer • Objective type

Unit	Time (Hrs)	Learning outcomes	Content	Teaching/ learning activities	Assessment methods
			• Factors affecting sexuality • Prevention of STIs, unwanted pregnancy, avoiding sexual harassment and abuse • Dealing with inappropriate sexual behavior		
XIV	2 (T) 4 (SL)	Describe stress and adaptation	**C. Stress and Adaptation – Introductory Concepts** • Introduction • Sources, effects, indicators and types of stress • Types of stressors • Stress adaptation – general adaptation syndrome (GAS), local adaptation syndrome (LAS) • Manifestation of stress – Physical and psychological • Coping strategies/mechanisms • Stress management ➢ Assist with coping and adaptation ➢ Creating therapeutic environment • Recreational and diversion therapies	• Lecture • Discussion	• Essay • Short answer • Objective type
XV	6 (T)	Explain culture and cultural norms Integrate cultural differences and spiritual needs in providing care to patients under supervision	**D. Concepts of Cultural Diversity and Spirituality** • Cultural diversity ➢ Cultural concepts – culture, subculture, multicultural, diversity, race, acculturation, assimilation ➢ Transcultural nursing ➢ Cultural competence ➢ Providing culturally responsive care • Spirituality ➢ Concepts – faith, hope, religion, spirituality, spiritual wellbeing ➢ Factors affecting spirituality ➢ Spiritual problems in acute, chronic, terminal illnesses and near-death experience ➢ Dealing with spiritual distress/problems	• Lecture • Discussion	• Essay • Short answer • Objective type

Unit	Time (Hrs)	Learning outcomes	Content	Teaching/ learning activities	Assessment methods
XVI	6 (T)	Explain the significance of nursing theories	**Nursing Theories: Introduction** • Meaning and definition, purposes, types of theories with examples, overview of selected nursing theories – Nightingale, Orem, Roy • Use of theories in nursing practice	• Lecture • Discussion	• Essay • Short answer • Objective type

<table><tr><td>

Health Assessment

</td><td>

UNIT

1

</td></tr></table>

UNIT OUTLINE

- Health assessment
- Process of health assessment
- Health history
- Physical examination: methods—inspection, palpation, percussion, auscultation, olfaction
- Preparation for examination of patient and unit
- General assessment
- Assessment of each body system
- Documenting health assessment findings

LEARNING OBJECTIVES

At the end of this unit, the reader will be able to:
- Define concept of health assessment.
- Explain purposes of health assessment.
- Identify principles of health assessment.
- Describe methods of health assessment.
- List down steps of data collection.
- Categorize types and methods of data collection.
- Define health history.
- Explain physical examination and its methods.
- Interpret general assessment.

Health: According to the World Health Organization, is "a state of complete physical, mental and social well-being and not merely the absence of disease and infirmity".

Nursing: "The unique function of the nurse is to assist the individual, sick or well, in the performance of those activities contributing to health or its recovery (or to peaceful death) that he would perform unaided if he had the necessary strength, will or knowledge".

Health assessment is the assessment of a person's health state in relation to the health continuum.

A health assessment is a plan of care that identifies the specific needs of a person and how those needs will be addressed by the healthcare system or skilled nursing facility. Health assessment is the evaluation of the health status by performing a physical exam after taking a health history. It is done to detect diseases early in people that may look and feel well.

Preventing health issues is always preferable than waiting for them to arise before treating them. But, many a times people come to the health professionals with health problems that have already occurred. They require their medical issues to be examined, identified, and addressed. In both cases, whether for preventative or for treatment, we need to be aware of the individual's real state of health. We may start by posing the question, "What has happened?" When did it occur? "How has it happened?" and more questions follow. The responses to these questions aid in the planning of health care initiatives that may be educational, preventative, curative, restorative, or rehabilitative. "Health assessment" refers to all of these actions taken to determine a person's health requirements and concerns.

CONCEPTS OF HEALTH ASSESSMENT

Meaning of Health Assessment

The term "health assessment" refers to a two-step procedure that aids the nurse in determining the patient's medical requirements and medical issues. 'Data collecting' is the first phase, and 'nursing diagnosis' is the second step, which is when the data are analyzed.

The term "health" refers to a person's physical, mental, and spiritual well-being, i.e., the body organs, which in normal condition help the person to perform his day-to-day activities without any difficulty. It also refers to the individual's ability to cope psychologically or emotionally with daily stressors. Faith on God or other principles that provide guidance for all aspects of life is referred to as having a healthy spiritual life.

Assessment means to measure or find out the functioning capacity of the person's body organs or systems and his/her ability to maintain emotional balance in all life situations. If there is any difficulty or deficiency in these abilities, a systematic examination can identify the cause and thus help in making a suitable plan of treatment and nursing care.

Purposes of Health Assessment

The following are the reasons for our requirement to gather data about the client's state of health:
- Prepare a database.
- Comprehend how the client's health is improving while the therapy continues.
- Based on the client's changing health status, determine the nursing care's efficacy.
- Determine the client's health issue or requirement, which may vary over time.
- Develop nursing diagnoses.
- Aid in developing and validating medical diagnosis.

Principles of Health Assessment

Principles are verifiable scientific truths. We follow these principles in all of our work at health assessment. The guidelines are:
- Each person has unique health issues and requirements that must be met.
- Every person needs privacy if they are conscious of their surroundings.
- Assessing health is a methodical, sequential procedure.
- An individual's physical, mental, and spiritual health are all interconnected.
- An individual's level of healthiness is always changing.

A full health exam (head-to-toe assessment) may be carried out by beginning at the top and working your way down methodically. However, the process may differ depending on the patient's age, the severity of their sickness, the nurse's preferences, the location during the examination, and the agency's goals and protocols. Whatever method is used, the client's time and efforts must be taken into account. As a consequence, the health evaluation is carried out in a systematic and effective way with the client in the fewest number of positions possible. Instead of evaluating the complete body, nurses often focus on a single bodily part. These precise evaluations are based on patient complaints, the nurse's personal observations of issues, the client's presenting issue, nursing interventions given, and medical treatments. Some of the objectives of the physical assessment include:

❖ To get initial information about the client's functional capacities.
❖ To supplement, confirm, or refute data obtained in the nursing history.
❖ To gather information that will aid in developing nurse diagnoses and treatment regimens.
❖ To assess the physiological effects of medical treatment and the development of a client's health issue.
❖ To assess a client's health using professional judgment.
❖ To identify areas for health promotion and disease prevention.

Steps of Health Assessment

Step One

Data Collection or Data Gathering

Data collecting is the gathering the collection of details regarding a client's physical and mental health, social situation, community and family life, his capacity for daily functioning, habits, and hobbies, etc.

Step Two

Nursing Diagnosis

Nursing diagnosis is a statement showing the cause and effect relationship of a person's health problem.

The cause of a health condition is one of the contributing factors.

Effect is the person's present and future health problems, e.g., alteration in comfort, abdominal pain, related to indigestion and gas formation.

Here,

'Indigestion and gas formation' is the cause, 'alteration in comfort' is the effect, and abdominal discomfort serves as evidence for the causal link between cause and consequence.

In nursing diagnoses, the impacts of sickness on the patient, his family, and the community are identified and described. For example, alterations in comfort, body temperature, or breathing.

Database

The particular fundamental data, or facts, are organized in a meaningful way, create a database. In order to properly arrange nursing care, it is helpful to recognize the client's significant health issues and medical requirements.

With the database, data collection is a continual process that never ends. Because a person's health situation changes constantly, so do their demands for health care.

Remember that data-gathering does not include interpretation or analysis of the information gathered. That is done in the second step of health assessment.

What is there in a database?

The following is a typical database or basic client's information:

A description of the person himself (Identification Data):

- Name
- Gender
- Age
- Address
- Observed physical and mental condition (e.g., thin man, looks anxious).
- Education
- Occupation
- Family members
- Other important people in his life
- His involvement in sociocultural activities.
- His current state of health and, if any, any difficulties, as recommended by him.
- His prior medical history will reveal any small discomforts, serious health issues, treatments received, hospitalizations, etc.
- Information regarding the health and causes of death of the family members is included in the family health history.
- His interactions with his friends, family, and other individuals. the manner in which he interacts with everyone.

His capacity for daily living activities, or ADLs:

- Personal cleanliness
- Wearing dresses
- Sleep pattern
- Safety practices
- Movement
- Working
- The capacity to provide nutritional needs
- Maintaining elimination.

His mental and emotional condition:

- How he reacts to stressful situations.
- Mood changes
- Views he has about his physical self, intellect, and personality
- Mental maturity
- Thought process (organized, meaningful)
- Special interests, motivations
- Willingness to take risk
- Nonverbal behavior (posture, limb movements)
- He is aware of his sentiments of joy, sorrow, fear, dread, wrath, and jealousy as well as how he controls these emotions.

Awareness to environment:

- Understands what is going on around him
- Keeps environment clean
- Reacts normally to bodily discomforts such as severe heat, cold, noise, etc.
- What he believes about his condition? What he wants and expects from the medical staff?

A child's data collection is similar to an adult's. The further details will include:

- ❖ Parent-child interaction
- ❖ The kid's school adaptation
- ❖ The nature of his friendships
- ❖ Data about his physical development and growth
- ❖ Data regarding his mental development and evolution.

Types of Data

There are two categories of data gathered/collected:

1. **Subjective data:** The client's own self-reporting. The client's statements regarding his feelings, sights, sounds, thoughts, and sensations concerning himself and his surroundings are referred to as "subjective data," for example, "I feel pain here."

   "I can't see the writings clearly," "I don't feel hungry," "I'm afraid of the dark," "I hear strange noises," etc.

   Subjective information also includes what the client's friends and family say about them, for example, "He is not returning our calls."

   He claims to be in agony. She consumes poorly.

   The measuring of subjective data is challenging since they are not visible.

   When a customer first interacts with a health practitioner, subjective data are often obtained. Additionally, it is acquired by regular interactions with him.

2. **Objective data:** What the healthcare professional notices about the patient constitutes objective data.

   "Objective data" are the details about the patient that health care professionals learn by the use of their senses, such as visual observations, stethoscope listening, touching bodily parts, feeling the skin and warmth or dryness, smelling the breath for odor, etc. The objective information might be noted as:

   "He opens his eyes when called" "His speech is slurred"

   "His body temperature is 38°C "His pulse is bounding."

   Objective data are observable and measurable, and are gathered during the physical examination or functional assessment. However, objective data gathering is also a process. It requires daily, sometimes hourly or even minute-to-minute assessment, depending on the client's health condition.

Sources of Data

There are two major sources of data as described:

1. The primary source is the client himself/herself.
2. The secondary sources are the following:
   - ◆ The client's family, friends, colleagues and other close persons.
   - ◆ Hospital and clinic records
   - ◆ Admission history
   - ◆ Progress record
   - ◆ Discharge summary, etc.
   - ◆ Laboratory reports
   - ◆ Other members of the health team—the doctor, other nurses, physiotherapist, etc.

   Books and journals on health care matters. Two points must be considered about data sources:

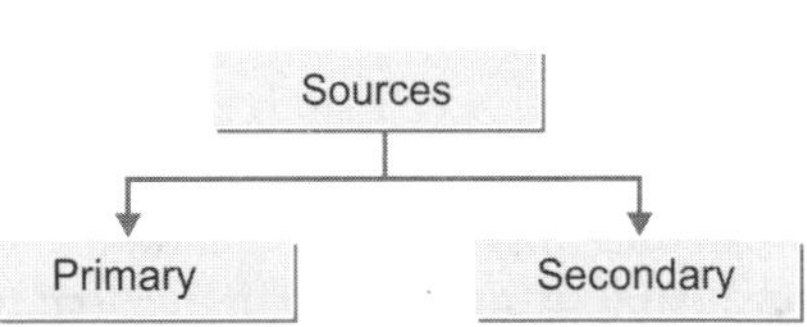

1. First, most people will give information about themselves frankly, if they are convinced that the information will be kept confidential. So, we must guarantee that his privacy will be respected.
2. Second, we must constantly take human prejudice into account. The objectivity of the client's knowledge may be influenced by his emotions, such as fear, worry, etc. Additionally, the emotions, experiences, and knowledge that a health professional has of a client "may affect their assessment of the client's health state.

METHODS OF DATA GATHERING

The methods of data gathering are the following:
- ❖ The interview
- ❖ The nursing history
- ❖ Questioning technique
- ❖ The physical examination
- ❖ Observation and measurement
- ❖ The psychologic and mental health examination
- ❖ Psychosocial measurement
- ❖ Laboratory data

The Interview

Definition

It is a purposeful and goal-directed interaction between two persons, one acting as an interviewer and the other as interviewee.

Purposes

- ❖ To establish and maintain a positive and open relationship between client and nurse.
- ❖ To create an opportunity for the nurse to observe the client's behavior and nonverbal communication.
- ❖ To provide information to the client.
- ❖ To gather information from the client.
- ❖ To counsel to the client regarding his problems.
- ❖ To teach the client and his relatives regarding his condition and treatment.

Types

Interview method can be classified as:
- ❖ **Problem seeking:** To get data to find out client's problems.
- ❖ **Problem solving:** To help client to solve his problems. To find out whether the procedures have helped to solve his problems.

Interviews can be classified as:
1. **Directive:** The interviewer directs the conversation by asking a sequence of pre-planned questions. 'Yes' or 'no' or a few sentences might be used as the response. This technique is used to gather data from the customer, such as his age, employment, the number of children he has, his habits, his interests, etc.

2. **Non-directive open-ended interview:** It leads to an open ended discussion between interviewer and interviewee. The interviewer directs the talks and the interviewee is made to talk much. For example, asking for client's past medical history, present conditions, etc.

Phases of Interview

The phases of interview are:

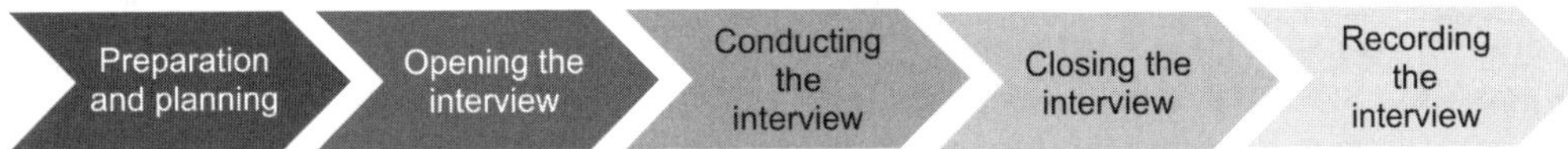

❖ **Preparation and planning:**
  • Before starting the interview, you should review the client's past history chart, and care plan to learn about his past illnesses and treatments.
  • Review the client's most recent hospitalization and admission records. Discuss the client's condition, symptoms, and issues with the doctor.
  • Write out the interview's goals and some of the inquiries you want to ask the patient.
  • After that, get ready for the interview by getting the patient and the surroundings ready. The location should be comfortable and pleasant so that the patient may relax.
  • There shouldn't be any music playing, TV on, or presence of other people.
  • For privacy, close doors and draw the drapes. During the interview, avoid disruptions. When he is scheduled to obtain therapy or during visitation, avoid conducting interviews.
  • Remove the client's discomfort such as by giving him a drink if he is thirsty, and make him comfortable. His discomfort will cause him to stop talking.
  • Nurse also should be mentally and physically at ease. A comfortable chair, good lighting for taking notes. You should not be thinking of other matters and problems. You should concentrate on the interview.
❖ **Opening the conversation:** Start the interview with a smile and good friendly way. Otherwise, the client could hide information. You need to act with regard and care. Use the client's name when addressing them. You greet yourself and explain the reason for the interview as well as how the data acquired will be helpful for his treatment. This may begin by asking, "How are you right now?"
❖ **Conducting the interview:** Pay attention to the questions, as well as the verbal and nonverbal communication patterns, during the interview.
  Questions
  The types of questions to be asked:
  • Open questions, e.g., What reduces your pain?
  • Closed questions, e.g., Have you taken food?
  • Direct questions, e.g., Did you sleep well last night?
  • Indirect questions, e.g., Did sleep come to you last night?
    ◊ Questions should be simple and short.
    ◊ Ask one question at a time and give sufficient time for him to answer before asking the next question.
    ◊ Use broad, indirect and open questions to begin with and then later on can ask closed questions.

◊ Use words which he/she can understand. Use language according to age, education and background of the patient.

◊ Use his own terms when wording questions.

◊ Do not use words which will be of suggestive type, e.g., too many.

◊ Avoid using 'How' and 'Why' questions as far as possible. If at all asked they should not sound as a threat.

* **Closing the interview:** Close the interview in a warm and friendly manner. Summarize the content of the interview at the closing time.

* **Recording the interview:** Inform the client that you are going to write down information which will be needed to plan his care. Write only points. Your writing should not interfere with your listening. Can use a prepared assessment form for recording.

THE NURSING HISTORY OR HEALTH HISTORY

Definition

A nursing history describes the client's total health condition and his physical, mental and emotional reactions to illness and the changes in his daily life activities and lifestyle as a result of the illness.

Whereas, a medical history focuses on the client's symptoms and process of the disease.

Thus, while medical and nursing histories are based upon similar content, they focus upon different aspects of the client's life.

Purposes

The nursing history is a valuable assessment tool. Because it:

* Is the first stage of identifying health problems and needs of client and planning for immediate and long-term patient care.

* Establishes a basis of information on which nursing diagnosis and plans for treatment can be made.

* Helps to establish rapport and interrelationship with the client and his family.

* Allows us to observe the client's ability to communicate and his general behavior.

* Gives the client an opportunity to express all his health problems and health needs, doubts, worries, feelings, etc.

* Is a written document about client's health condition, treatment and care process.

* Includes clients past and present health condition.

* Helps to measure the progress of client's health condition.

It is easy to gather all information if we have a structured outline or format for collecting client's health history. A format is suggested here.

NURSING HISTORY FORMAT

1. **Demographic data**
   a. Date and time of History Collection   Source of information
   b. To be given by faculty   : ....
      i. Client's name   : ....
      ii. If in hospital, Hospital No.   : ....

    iii. If hospitalized (admitted to hospital) : ....
        Date and time of hospitalization : ....
    iv. Medical diagnosis : ....
    v. Surgery done (if any) : ....
    vi. Date of surgery : ....

c. Client profile
    i.   Age : ....
    ii.   Gender : ....
    iii. Religion : ....
    iv. Marital status : ....
    v.   Education : ....
    vi. Occupation : ....
    vii. Monthly/weekly/daily income : ....
    viii. Home address : ....
                         ....

    ix. Any special habits:
        Interests (reading, cinema, etc.) : ....
        Hobbies (gardening, fishing, etc.) : ....
        Habits (chewing pan, drinking alcohol, : ....
        smoking tobacco, etc.).

2. **Client's health condition**
  a. Present health condition:
    i. Does s/he feel healthy?
    ii. If s/he feels healthy, is he aware of the need for prevention of illnesses and ways to maintain optimum health?
    iii. If he is feeling ill
      – What is his present health problem?
      – Is his ability to carry out ADL affected because of ill health?
      – Factors which increase the problem
      – Factors which reduce the problem
      – Treatment taken and result
      – What does he understand about his present health problem and what is his opinion about it?
  b. Past health condition:
    i.   Health condition from infancy
    ii.   Health condition in the immediate past, as for the last 5 years.
    iii. If any history of illness
      – What was it?
      – When was it?
      – How had it occurred?
      – What treatment was taken?
      – Duration of illness
    iv.   What is the client's understanding and opinion about his past health condition?

FAMILY HEALTH HISTORY

	i	ii	iii		iv	v	vi	vii
Sl. no.	**Client's position in the family**	**Family members and their relationship with the client**	**Healthy**		**If 'No' what is the illness?**	**Duration of illness**	**What treatment taken?**	**Their present condition**
			Yes	**No**				
1								
2								
3								
4								
5								
6								

   viii. Any blood relatives, who have died because of cancer, heart disease, diabetes, hypertension, stroke, mental disorder, etc.
   ix. Approximate monthly expenditure towards family's health maintenance.
   x. What is the client's understanding and opinion about his family's health condition? You may ask questions like:
   - Do you think your family's general health condition is good?
   - If not, how do the illnesses of your family members affect your life and vice versa?

3. **Review of body systems:** For an understanding of the client's health situation, subjective data from each of the bodily functions is important. Start by asking generic inquiries, such as "Do you come from such a far-off place?" or "Are you experiencing too tired to talk?" to gather facts. Next, inquire about particular symptoms, such as "Do you have any hearing problems?"
"If yes, in which ear?"
"Have you taken any treatment for that?"
Similarly cover each body system

4. **Activities of daily living (ADLs):** You may ask questions as, "Which way your health condition has affected your activities and daily routine?"
Such activities are—eating, drinking, brushing teeth, bathing, wearing clothes, using toilets for urination and defecation, sleeping/resting, all types of movements, talking, writing, working, participating in some form of recreation, learning, etc. Also questions on his ability to avoid danger in environment, need to be asked.
ADLs can be taken as data observed.

Socioeconomic and Environmental Condition

a. *Socioeconomic Condition*
   You may ask the following questions to get information in these areas:
   i. Is your, or your family's income enough to meet the family's day-to-day needs adequately?
   ii. What type of house you live in? Do you get enough sunlight and air in your home?

   iii. How far are the nearest hospital/clinic/other health care facilities from your home?

   iv. If you fall sick, who will take care of you at home or in the hospital? (Relatives, friends, neighbors, etc.)

   v. In any urgent need, on whom can you depend on? (Relatives, friends, neighbors, etc.)

   vi. Can you/your family meet the expenditure of your treatment?

b. ***Environmental Conditions***

You may ask the following questions (or pick up the relevant questions) to get information in this area:

   i.   Is there any factory or big market near to your home?

   ii. Does anyone in your home smoke tobacco?

   iii. From where you get your drinking water?

   iv. Are the surroundings of your home clean?

   v.   Where do you throw the household wastes?

   vi. What is the source of water?

   vii. How congested is your leaving accommodation?

Recording of the Nursing History

Nursing history has to be written in such a way that the information can be used whenever necessary. For that a few suggestions are given:

1. Write the information **Accurately** by writing accurate grammar, spelling and tense.
2. Writing the information **Briefly**. Sentences do not have to be complete as long as they are giving correct and clear meaning.
3. Write **Clear** information. Avoid long sentences, technical phrases and uncommon words. Use only standard medical abbreviations. Never use a word unless you understand its meaning. Handwriting must be legible.
4. **Descriptions** must be to-the-point. Avoid the use of words which need interpretation, e.g., good, bad, thin, fat, etc.
5. Do not give your **Explanation** of client's behavior as, he is "depressed", "uncooperative", or "overanxious". That may be misleading. Only describe his behavior, as, "he is not talking to anyone, turning his face towards the wall and crying silently".
6. Write only the **Factual** information, which can be checked if necessary.
7. **Gentle** probing type of communication helps to bring our specific information.

Physical Examination

Meaning

Lot of health-related information may be obtained by looking thoroughly at all parts of the client's body. A systematic way of doing that is called 'physical examination'.

Preparation

Before starting physical examination, the client, environment, equipment and the nurse must be prepared.

a. ***The Client Preparation***

   i. Explain to the client what you are planning to do and why.

   ii. Make sure that his/her clothing do not interfere with physical examination.

   iii. Make sure that he empties his bladder and bowel (if necessary) before examination.

iv. Help the client to relax as much as possible.

v. Put him/her in a position in which the patient feels comfortable.

b. ***Environmental Preparation***

i. Make sure that the place used for physical examination is clean quiet, warm and well lighted. Direct sunlight is better than artificial light.

ii. One of the close relatives or friends must be with the client to give him/her support. Because the first time physical examination may be a frightening experience to the client.

iii. Provide adequate privacy by putting screen around the client. Also do not expose the body parts unless it is necessary for physical examination use draping.

c. ***Preparation of Equipment or Articles***

For a systematic physical examination you need to collect the following articles:

A medium size steel/enamel tray, containing the following articles:

1. BP apparatus
2. Stethoscope
3. TPR tray
4. Inch tape—to measure height, abdominal girth
5. Weighing machine
6. Otoscope
7. Tongue depressor
8. Nasal speculum
9. Ophthalmoscope
10. Knee hammer—to check nervous system reflexes
11. Test tubes with hot and cold water—for testing the ability to differentiate temperature variation
12. A feather or a cotton ball—to check the touch sensation
13. Small amount of sugar and salt—to check his ability to differentiate taste
14. Torch—to see inside any body cavity
15. Sample specimen containers for blood, urine, sputum, etc.

d. ***Preparation of the Nurse***

i. Wash your hands in presence of the client even if your hands are clean. This simple act will increase his confidence in you as a conscientious professional.

ii. Wear gloves and mask.

iii. You must learn to perform basic skills of physical examination. These are:

◊ Measurement
◊ Inspection
◊ Palpation
◊ Percussion
◊ Auscultation
◊ Detection of odors.

These skills require training in the use of your eyes, ears, hands and nose. Now let us discuss each of these skills briefly.

Measurement: It is an activity to calculate the magnitude of the body's structure and function and record the findings in numbers and symbols.

The data obtained by measurement are blood pressure, temperature, pulse rate, respiratory rate, height, weight, circumference of body parts (e.g., abdomen, leg). Length and diameter of bony structures (e.g., pelvic outlet in prenatal examination).

Inspection or observation: It is a detail visual examination of the client's general physical appearance and specific body parts, noting its size, color, position, symmetry and degree of movement.

Inspection can be done while talking to the client and while performing other skills of physical examination.

Palpation or touch: A client's body can be examined by touch or palpation. By this method nurse can feel any hardness, size, texture, swelling and movability of an internal organ or part. The pads of the fingers, the most sensitive area of the fingers, are used for palpation.

Percussion or tapping: This technique involves touching the body with the fingertips to examine it. The method that is most often used is to put one hand on the surface of the body and place the middle finger, or "pleximeter," over the spot to be percussion. To hit quickly and forcefully immediately proximal to the terminal interphalangeal joint, use the middle fingertip of the opposite hand. The pleximeter-adjacent bodily structures vibrate, which creates the sound.

You will be able to find out the following points by percussion:
❖ The amount of air, liquid or solid materials.
❖ The positions and boundaries of organs such as the heart and liver.
❖ The excursion of the diaphragm.

Auscultation: is listening for noises the body produces. The noises of the abdominal and thoracic viscera as well as the circulation of blood in the arteries and veins are those that are most commonly heard. Rarely is direct auscultation performed using just the ear. Usually, a stethoscope is used for indirect auscultation.

The detection of abnormal odors: It is a very important diagnostic skill. Odor of blood, rotten fruit odor and foul odor in breath, alcoholic odor, odor of some poisonous chemicals, ammonia odor of urine, odor of decomposed tissue, etc. are very helpful in detecting the cause of the ailments.

Approaches/Ways of Doing Physical Examination

Experts have suggested many approaches/ways of doing physical examination systematically. These are:
1. **Body system approach:** In this approach, examination is done for each of the body systems, namely, nervous system, respiratory system, cardiovascular system, etc.
   The review of system in nursing history is based on this system.
2. **Head-to-foot examination**

Systematic Physical Assessment

A systematic physical assessment includes assessment of the following:
❖ Vital signs
❖ Height and weight
❖ Head to be examination
❖ Examination of extremities
❖ Reflex examination
❖ Neurologic, mental and emotional examination
❖ **Vital signs:** The vital or cardinal signs are body temperature, pulse, respirations, and blood pressure. These signs, which should be looked at in total, monitor the functions of the body; the signs reflect changes in function that otherwise might not be observed.

❖ **Height and weight:** Use proper scales to measure height and weights and record the findings.
❖ **Head-to-toe assessment criteria**

General Appearance

❖ Observations—age, race, nutritional status, general health status, development
❖ Color—pink, pale, red, jaundiced, mottled, blanched, cyanotic
❖ Skin—pigmentation, vascularity, temperature, texture, turgor, lesions (type, color, size shape, distribution), bruises, bleeding, scars, edema.

Vital Signs

❖ Temperature
❖ Pulses—apical, radial (others when appropriate)
❖ Respirations
❖ Blood pressure—supine, sitting, right and left arms
❖ Height and weight

Head and Face

Size—contour, symmetry, color, pain, tenderness, lesions, edema
Scalp—color, texture, scales, lumps, lesions, inflammation
Face—movement, expression, pigmentation, acne, tics, tremors, scars

Eyes

Acuity—visual loss, glasses, contacts, prosthesis, diplopia, photophobia, color vision, pain burning
Eyelids—color, ptosis, edema, styes, exophthalmos
Extra ocular movement—position and alignment of eyes, strabismus, nystagmus
Conjunctiva—color, discharge, vascular changes
Iris—color, markings
Sclera—color, vascularity, jaundice
Pupils—size, shape, equality, reaction to light

Ears

Acuity—hearing loss, aid, pain, tinnitus, sensitivity to sound
External ear—lobe, auricle, canal
Inner ear—vertigo
Smell, nasal size, symmetry, flaring sneezing, deformities
Mucosa—color edema, exudate, bleeding, pain tenderness
Sinus tenderness, pain

Mouth and Throat

Odor, pain, ability to speak, chew, swallow, taste
Lips—color, symmetry, hydration, lesions, crusting, fever blisters, cracking swelling, numbness, drooling

Gums—color, edema, bleeding, retraction, pain
Teeth—number, missing, caries, caps, dentures, sensitivity to heat, cold
Tongue—symmetry, color, size, hydration, markings, protrusion, ulcers, burning, swelling, coating
Throat—gag reflex, soreness, cough, sputum, hemoptysis
Voice—hoarseness, loss, change in pitch.

Neck

Symmetry, movement, range of motion, masses, scars, pain stiffness
Trachea—deviation, scars
Thyroid—size, shape, symmetry, tenderness, enlargement, nodules, scars
Vessels (carotid, jugular)—quality, strength and symmetry of pulsations bruits, venous distention
Lymph nodes—size, shape, mobility, tenderness, enlargement

Chest

Size, shape, symmetry, deformities, pain, tenderness
Skin—color, rashes, scars, hair distribution, turgor, temperature, edema, crepitation
Breasts—contour, symmetry color, size shape, inflammation, scars, masses (location, sizeshape, mobility, tenderness) pain, dimpling swelling.
Nipples—color, discharge, ulceration, bleeding, inversion, pain
Axillae—nodes, enlargement, tenderness, rash, inflammation
Breathing patterns—rate, regularity, depth, case, normal or adventitious, fremitus, use of accessory muscles.
Sounds—normal, adventitious, intensity, pitch, quality, duration, equality, vocal resonance.

Heart

Cardiac patterns—rate, rhythm, intensity, regularity, skipped or extra beats, point of maximum impulse.
Right and left cardiac borders, implanted pacemaker.

Abdomen

Size, color, counter, symmetry, fat, muscle tone, turgor, hair distribution, scars, umbilicus, stretch marks, fetus, rashes, distention, abnormal pulsations.
Sounds—absent, hypoactive, hyperactive, normal, bruits
   Liver border, gastric air bubble, splenic dullness, air fluid, muscle spasm, rigidity, masses, guarding, tenderness, pain, rebound, bladder distention.

Kidney

Urinary output (amount, color odor, sediment), frequency, urgency, hesitancy, burning, pain, dribbling, incontinence, hematuria, nocturia, oliguria.

Genitalia

Female—labia majora and minora, urethral and vaginal orifices, discharge, swelling, ulceration, nodules, masses, tenderness, pain.

Male—penis, discharge, ulceration, pain, scrotum, color, size, modules, swelling, ulcerations, tenderness; tests, size, shape, swelling, masses, absence.

Rectum

Pigmentation, hemorrhoids, excoriation, rashes, abscess, pilonidal cyst, masses, lesions, tenderness, pain, itching, burning.

Back—scars, edema, spatial abnormality, pain, tenderness.

Extremities

General Assessment

Joints: The extremities (the arms and legs) are inspected, palpated, and moved. First the skin is observed. The limb is assessed for any unusual joint angle, which could indicate a current or old bone fracture. The joints are next moved to assess range of motion. The joints are also assessed for size and redness. Note complaints of pain by the patient.

Muscles: Muscles are observed for tremors or unsteadiness. A fine tremor can sometimes be observed by asking the patient to extend the arms toward the front for a few minutes. Each extremity is observed.

Extremities for Edema

The feet and legs are also observed for shape, color, and edema (excess fluid). The swelling may be tense and hard, stretching the skin, or it may be possible to press the skin and produce an indentation that disappears in a few minutes. The latter is called *pitting edema.* Inspect the legs for varicose veins-distended, bluish veins, which may be tortuous and lumpy and tender to the touch.

Reflexes

A *reflex* is an automatic response of the body to a stimulus. Reflexes are tested using a percussion hammer. They are described on a scale of 0 to ++++. 0 means no reflex, + is minimal activity (hypoactive), ++ is a normal reflex, +++ is more active, and ++++ means maximum activity (hyperactive). It is important to compare one side of the body with the other when assessing reflexes.

Several reflexes are normally tested during a physical examination. These are (a) *the biceps and triceps reflex.* (b) *the patellar reflex,* (c) *the Achilles reflex.* and (d) *the plantar reflex.*

Biceps and Triceps Reflexes

The biceps reflex is tested with your thumb on the biceps tendon while the patient's arm is supported. When your thumb is tapped with the hammer, the biceps muscle normally contracts noticeably.

In the triceps reflex test, the patient relaxes the arm, which is supported. Tap the patient's arm with the hammer just above the olecranon process. Normally, the forearm will straighten.

Patellar Reflex

To test this reflex, make the patient sit on the edge of a table so that the legs hang freely. The hammer strikes the area just below the patella, and normally the lower leg kicks forward.

Achilles Reflex

The patient must assume the position for the patellar reflex test. Support the toes slightly and tap the Achilles tendon. The normal response is a downward jerk of the foot.

Plantar Reflex

To test the plantar or Babinski reflex, stroke the sole of the foot with a thumb nail or the sharp end of a percussion hammer. Normally, all five toes bend downward; this reaction is negative Babinski. In an abnormal response, positive Babinski, the toes spread outward and the big toe moves upward. Positive Babinski is abnormal after age 1.

Neurologic, Mental and Emotional Assessment

Neurologic assessment includes examination of the reflexes and the cranial nerves and the functions of the cerebrum, the cerebellum, and the sensory and motor systems.

Psychological and Mental Health Examination

The psychological and mental health assessment is as important as the physical examination. It has to be done along with the interview and physical examination.

The following are the specific observations to be made and recorded:

General Appearance and Posture

Note the client's physical cleanliness, appropriateness of the dress, manner of his standing, sitting and walking.

Motor Activity

Observe for unnecessary movements, signs of agitation and hyperactivity.

Facial Expression

Watch for changes in facial expression appropriate to the conversation.

Speech Pattern

Listen for clarity, loudness, speed, voice modulation and organization.

General Mood and Manner

Observe for sudden mood changes, easy to talk or withdrawn.

Memory

Test for memory of past and recent events.

Orientation

Awareness of date, day, time, place and person (own name, names of the relatives and friends).

Thought Content

The thoughts which are disturbing his daily activities and life.

Thought Process

Are the thoughts organized in normal sequence?

Methods of Examining

Four primary techniques are used in the physical examination:
1. Inspection,
2. Palpation,
3. Percussion, and
4. Auscultation.

These techniques are:

INSPECTION

Inspection is the process of visually examining something to make an assessment. It ought to be attentive, systematic, and purposeful. The nurse examines with only their eyes as well as a lit device like an otoscope, which is used to observe the ear. In addition to visual observations, olfactory (smell) and auditory (hearing) cues are noted. Visual examination is a common technique used by nurses to evaluate the location, size, color, or symmetry of the body as well as the moisture, color, and smoothness of the body's surfaces. The nurse must have access to enough lighting, which may be either artificial or natural lighting. For correct hearing while employing the auditory senses, a calm environment is essential. Inspection may be used in combination with other evaluation methods.

PALPATION

Palpation is the examination of the body using the sense of touch. The pads of the fingers are used because their concentration of nerve endings makes them highly sensitive to tactile discrimination. Palpation is used to determine:

- Texture (e.g., of the hair);
- Temperature (e.g., of a skin area);
- Vibration (e.g., of a joint);
- Position, size, consistency, and mobility of organs or masses;
- Distension (e.g., of the urinary bladder);
- Pulsation; and
- Tenderness or pain.

Types

There are two types of palpation:
1. **Superficial palpation:** Light (superficial) palpation should always precede deep palpation because heavy pressure on the fingertips can dull the sense of touch. The healthcare professional extends the fingers of the dominant hand parallel to the skin's surface and

softly pushes while circling the hand. The skin seems somewhat depressed when softly palpated. The nurse softly pushes numerous times rather than applying sustained pressure if it is important to get information about a mass.

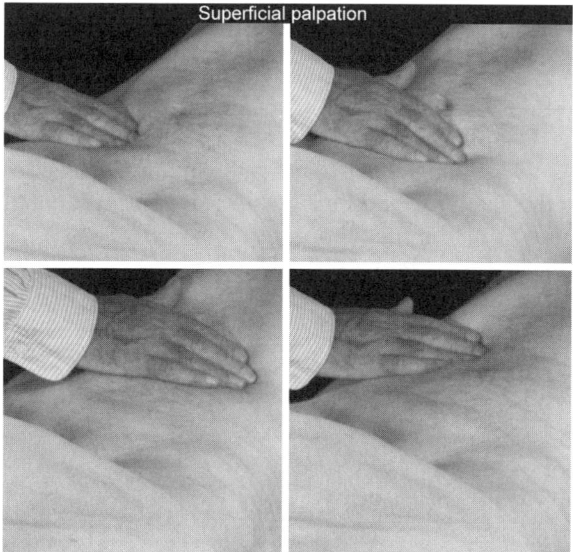

2. **Deep palpation:** Deep palpation needs great practitioner experience and is often not performed during a routine examination. Due to the possibility of internal organ injury from pressure, it is done with the utmost care. It is usually not indicated in clients who have acute abdominal pain or pain that is not yet diagnosed. One hand may be used for deep palpation or two hands (bimanually). In deep bimanual palpation, the nurse extends the dominant hand as for light palpation, and then places the finger pads of the nondominant hand on the dorsal surface of the distal interphalangeal joint of the middle three fingers of the dominant hand.

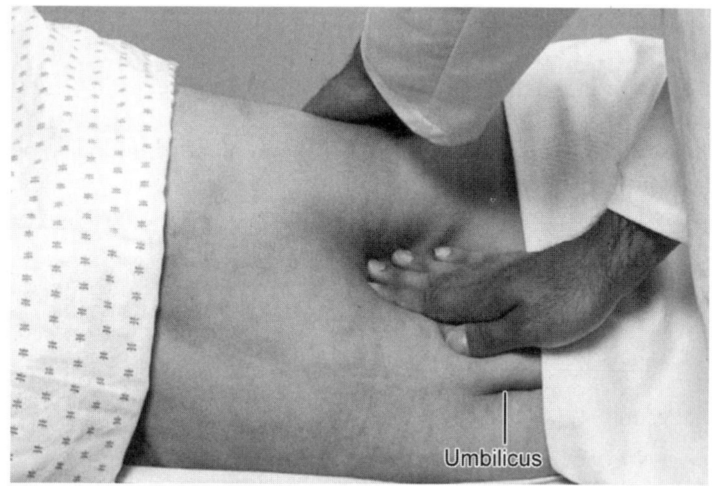

To feel the tactile sensations, the upper hand exerts pressure while the bottom hand is relaxed. When palpating deeply with one hand, push the finger pads in the dominant hand over the target location. Frequently, the opposite hand is used for lateral support. The back of the hand and the fingers, where the examiner's skin is the thinnest, are the finest places to check the temperature of the skin. The palmar area of the nurse's hand should be used to check for vibration. The following are general recommendations for palpation:

* The nurse's hands should be clean and warm, and the fingernails short.
* Areas of tenderness should be palpated last.
* Deep palpation should be done after superficial palpation. The effectiveness of palpation depends largely on the client's relaxation. Nurses can assist a client to relax by:
  * Gowning and/or draping the client appropriately,
  * Positioning the client comfortably, and
  * Ensuring that their own hands are warm before beginning. During palpation, the nurse should be sensitive to the client's verbal and facial expressions indicating discomfort.

PERCUSSION

Percussion is the act of striking the body surface to elicit sounds that can be heard or vibrations that can be felt.

There are two types of percussion: Direct and indirect.

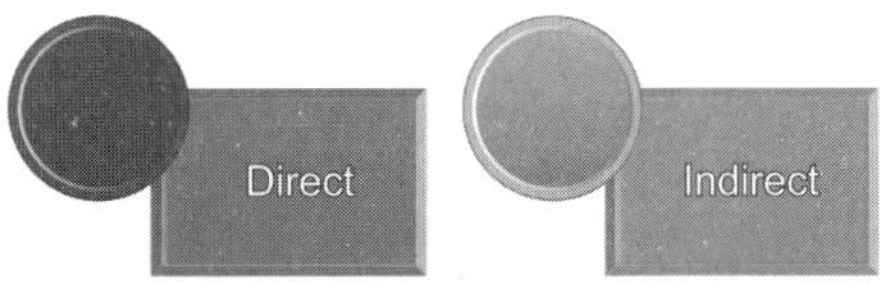

Direct percussion: In direct a percussion the nurse strike the area to be percussed by using the pads of all four of the fingers or the pad of her center finger to hit the target region directly. The strikes are rapid, and the movement is from the wrist. Although the thorax is not often percussed with this method, it is effective for percussing an adult's sinuses.

Indirect percussion: The act of hitting anything (such a finger) that is being held against the bodily part to be examined is known as indirect percussion. In this technique, the middle finger of the nondominant hand, referred to as the pleximeter, is placed firmly on the client's skin. This finger should only have its distal phalanx or joint in touch with the skin. The nurse presses on the pleximeter with the flexed thumb of the opposite hand, known as the plexor, often at the interphalangeal joint on the distal end or a position between the distally and proximal joints. The striking motion comes from the wrist; the forearm remains stationary.

The angle between the plexor and the pleximeter should be 90°, and the blows must be firm, rapid, and short to obtain a clear sound.

Percussion is used to determine the size and shape of internal organs by establishing their borders. It indicates whether tissue is fluid filled, air filled, or solid.

Percussion elicits five types of sound:
1. Flatness,
2. Dullness,
3. Resonance,
4. Hyperresonance, and
5. Tympany.

Flatness: Flatness is an extremely dull sound produced by very dense tissue, such as muscle or bone.

Dullness: Dullness is a thud-like sound produced by dense tissue such as the liver, spleen, or heart.

Resonance: Resonance is a hollow sound such as that produced by lungs filled with air.

Hyperresonance: Hyperresonance is not produced in the normal body. It is described as booming and can be heard over an emphysematous lung.

Tympany: Tympany is a musical or drum like sound produced from an air-filled stomach. On a continuum, flatness reflects the most dense tissue (the least amount of air) and tympany the least dense tissue (the greatest amount of air). A percussion sound is described according to its intensity, pitch, duration, and quality.

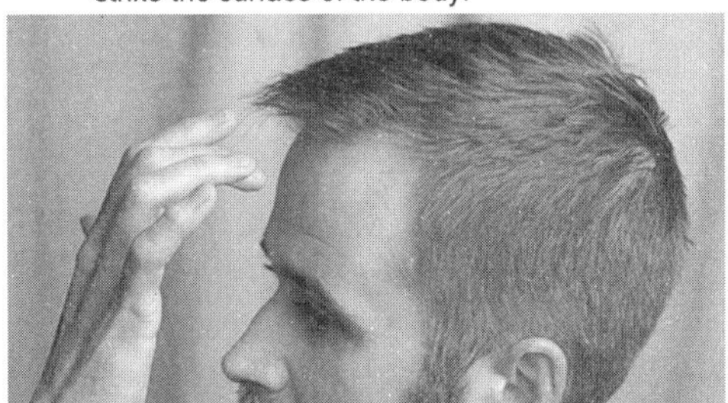

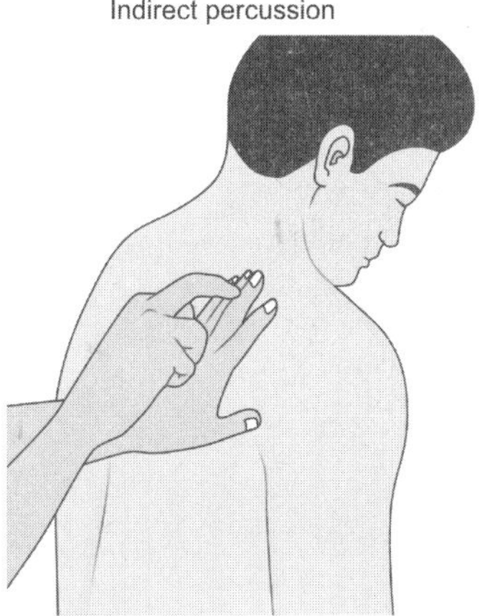

AUSCULTATION

Auscultation is the process of listening to sounds produced within the body. There may be two types of auscultation are direct or indirect. Direct auscultation is done using the unassisted ear. For example, to listen to a pulmonary wheeze or the noise of a moving joint, a stethoscope is used for indirect auscultation, which sends noises to the nurse's ears. A stethoscope is generally used to listen to internal body noises, such as bowel sounds, heart valve sounds, and blood pressure.

The internal diameter of the stethoscope tube should be around 0.3 cm (1/8 in.), and its length should range from 30 to 35 cm (12 to 14 in.). It should feature a bell-shaped amplifier and a flat-disk diaphragm. High-pitched noises, like certain bronchial sounds, are better sent by the diaphragm, whereas low-pitched sounds, like some heart sounds, are best transmitted by the bell. The stethoscope's earpieces should fit snuggly into the nurse's ears and face forward. The client's skin is softly yet firmly touched by the stethoscope's amplifier. If the client has excessive hair, it may be necessary to dampen the hairs with a moist cloth so that they will lie flat against the skin and not interfere with clear sound transmission.

According to their pitch, duration, strength, and quality, auscultated sounds are classified. The pitch is the frequency of the vibrations (the number of vibrations per second). There are fewer vibrations per second in low-pitched sounds like certain heartbeats than high-pitched ones like bronchial sounds. The loudness as well as the softness of a sound may be described by its intensity (amplitude). Some bodily noises are loud, like the tracheal bronchial sounds, while others are soft, like the regular breath sounds in the lungs. The length (long or short) of a sound is its duration. The quality of sound is a subjective description of a sound, for example, whistling, gurgling, or snapping.

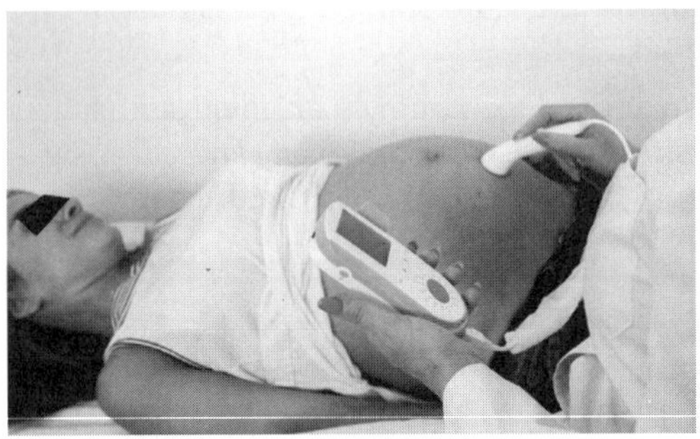 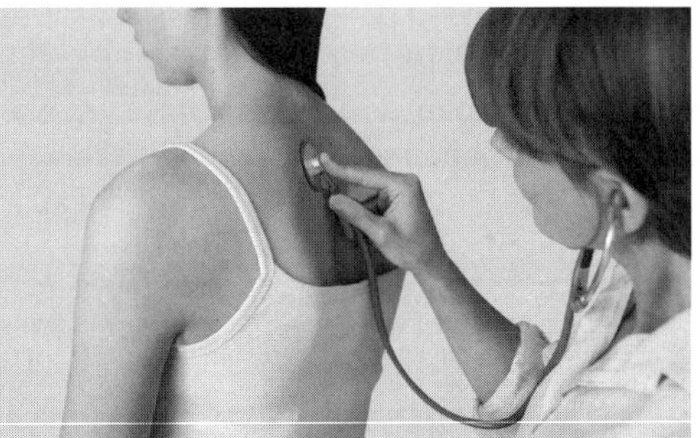

Equipment and supplies used for a health examination.		
Supplies		**Purpose**
Flashlight or penlight		To assist viewing of the pharynx or to determine the reactions of the pupils of the eye
Ophthalmoscope		A lighted instrument to visualize the interior of the eye
Otoscope		A lighted instrument to visualize the eardrum and external auditory canal (a nasal speculum may be attached to the otoscope to inspect the nasal cavities)
Percussion (reflex) hammer		An instrument with a rubber head to test reflexes
Tuning fork		A two-pronged metal instrument used to test hearing acuity and vibratory sense
Cotton applicators		To obtain specimens

Contd...

Contd...

Gloves	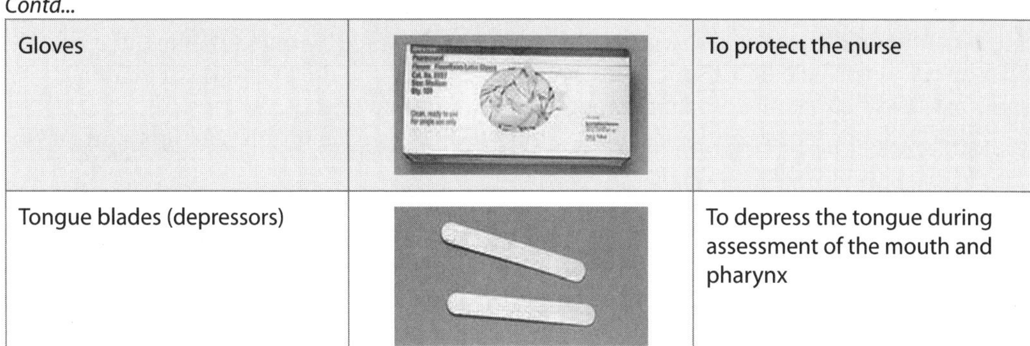	To protect the nurse
Tongue blades (depressors)		To depress the tongue during assessment of the mouth and pharynx

GENERAL ASSESSMENT

Integument

The integument includes the skin, hair, and nails. The examination begins with a generalized inspection using a good source of lighting, preferably indirect natural daylight.

Skin

Assessment of the skin involves inspection and palpation. The entire skin surface may be assessed at one time or as each aspect of the body is assessed. In some instances, the nurse may also use the olfactory sense to detect unusual skin odors; these are usually most evident in the skinfolds or in the axillae. Pungent body odor is frequently related to poor hygiene, hyperhidrosis (excessive perspiration), or bromhidrosis (foul-smelling perspiration).

Pallor is the result of inadequate circulating blood or hemoglobin and subsequent reduction in tissue oxygenation. In clients with dark skin, it is usually characterized by the absence of underlying red tones in the skin and may be most readily seen in the buccal mucosa. In brown-skinned clients, pallor may appear as a yellowish-brown tinge; in black-skinned clients, the skin may appear ashen grey. Pallor in all people is usually most evident in areas with the least pigmentation such as the conjunctiva, oral mucous membranes, nail beds, palms of the hand, and soles of thefeet.

Cyanosis (a bluish tinge) is most evident in the nail beds, lips, and buccal mucosa. In dark-skinned clients, close inspection of the palpebral conjunctiva (the lining of the eyelids) and palms and soles may also show evidence of cyanosis.

Jaundice (a yellowish tinge) may first be evident in the sclera of the eyes and then in the mucous membranes and the skin. Nurses should take care not to confuse jaundice with the normal yellow pigmentation in the sclera of a dark-skinned client. If jaundice is suspected, the posterior part of the hard palate should also be inspected for a yellowish color tone.

Erythema is skin redness associated with a variety of rashes and other conditions. Localized areas of hyperpigmentation (increased pigmentation) and hypopigmentation (decreased pigmentation) may occur as a result of changes in the distribution of melanin (the dark pigment) or in the function of the melanocytes in the epidermis. An example of hyperpigmentation in a defined area is a birthmark; an example of hypopigmentation is vitiligo.

Vitiligo, seen as patches of hypopigmented skin, is caused by the destruction of melanocytes in the area. Albinism is the complete or partial lack of melanin in the skin, hair, and eyes. Other localized color changes may indicate a problem such as oedema or a localized infection. Dark-skinned clients normally have areas of lighter pigmentation, such as the palms, lips, and nail beds.

Edema is the presence of excess interstitial fluid. An area of oedema appears swollen, shiny, and taut and tends to blanch the skin color or, if accompanied by inflammation, may redden the skin. Generalized edema is most often an indication of impaired venous circulation and in some cases reflects cardiac dysfunction or venous abnormalities.

A change in a client's natural skin look is referred to as a skin lesion. The first skin lesions occur that develop in reaction to a change in the skin's internal or external environment. Secondary skin lesions are ones that develop later after the main lesion has changed due to factors including chronicity, trauma, or infection. A vesicle or blister, for instance, may burst and result in a chipping (secondary lesion). Nurses are liable for accurately describing skin lesions in terms of location (for example, the face), distribution (for example, the body regions involved), configuration (for example, how to organize or position of a few lesions), as well as the color, shape, size, stiffness, texture, as well as features of individual lesions.

Macule, Patch: Flat, unelevated change in color. Macules are 1 mm to 1 cm (0.04 to 0.4 in.) in size and circumscribed. Examples: freckles, measles, petechiae, flat moles. Patches are larger than 1 cm (0.4 in.) and may have an irregular shape. Examples: port wine birthmark, vitiligo (white patches), and rubella.

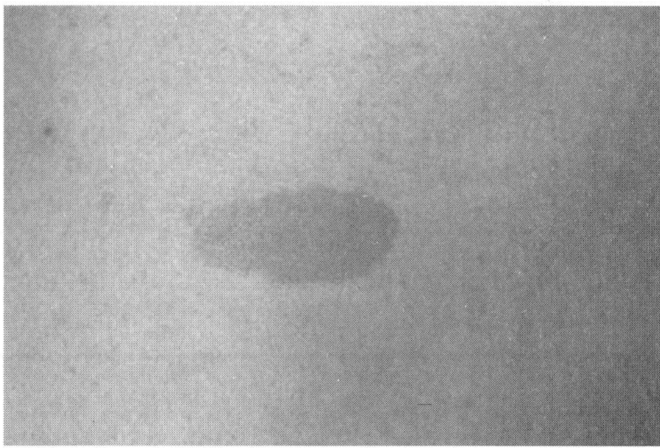

Cafe-au-lait macules (CALMs).

Nodule, Tumor: Elevated, solid, hard mass that extends deeper into the dermis than a papule. Nodules have a circumscribed border and are 0.5 to 2 cm (0.2 to 0.8 in.). Examples: squamous cell carcinoma, fibroma. Tumors are larger than 2 cm (0.8 in.) and may have an irregular border. Examples: malignant melanoma, hemangioma.

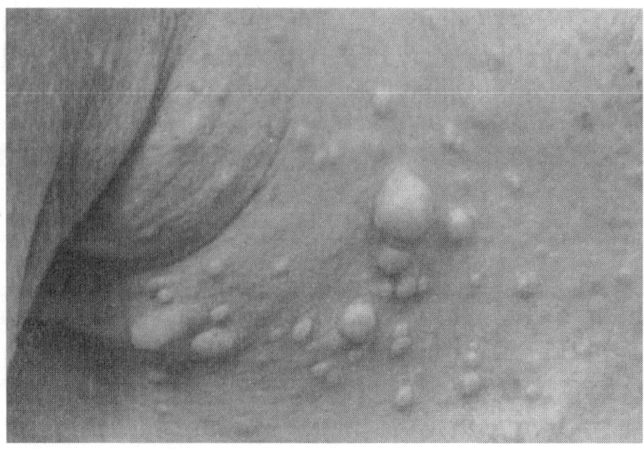

Papule: Circumscribed, solid elevation of skin. Papules are less than 1 cm (0.4 in.). Examples: warts, acne, pimples, elevated moles.

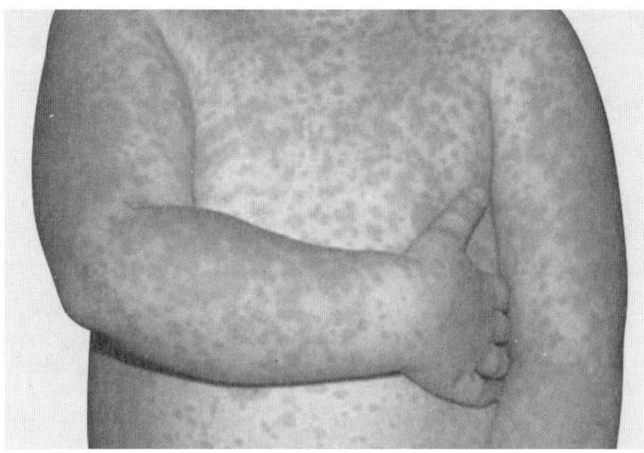

Papular lesions drug eruption.

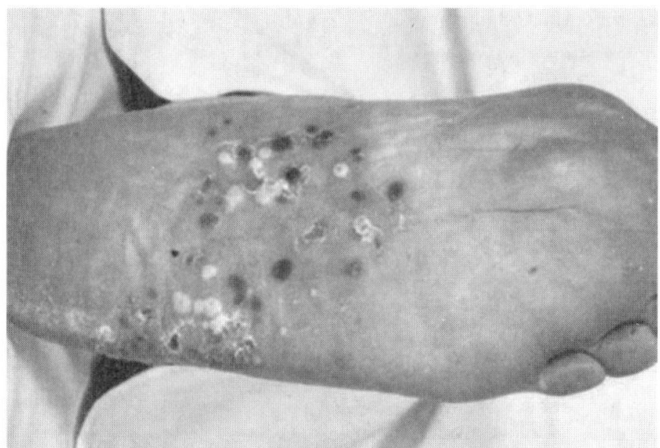

Pustule: Vesicle or bulla filled with pus. Examples: acne vulgaris, impetigo.

Plaque: Plaques are larger than 1 cm (0.4 in.). Examples: psoriasis, rubella.

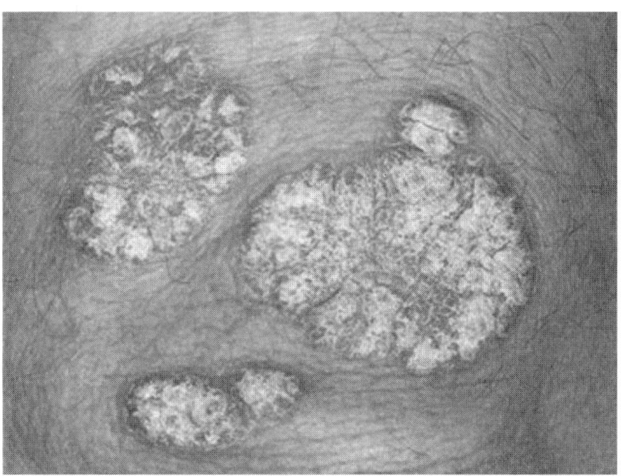

Wheal: A reddened, localized collection of edema fluid; irregular in shape. Size varies.

Examples: hives, mosquito bites.

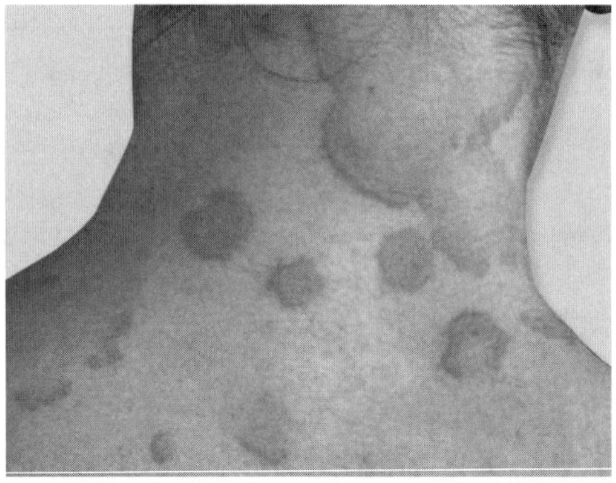

Atrophy

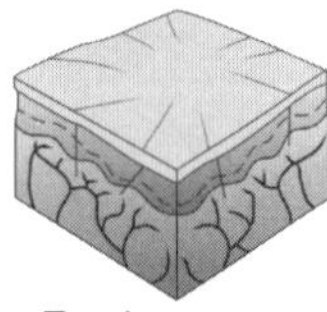

A translucent, dry, paper-like, sometimes wrinkled skin surface resulting from thinning or wasting of the skin due to loss of collagen and elastin.

Examples: striae, aged skin

Erosion

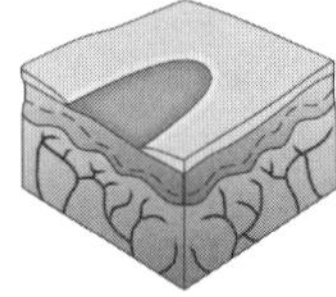

Wearing away of the superficial epidermis causing a moist, shallow depression. Because erosions do not extend into the dermis, they heal without scarring.

Examples: scratch marks, ruptured vesicles

Lichenification

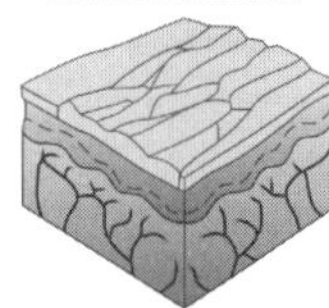

Rough, thickened, hardened area of epidermis resulting from chronic irritation such as scratching or rubbing.

Examples: chronic dermatitis

Scales

Shedding flakes of greasy, keratinized skin tissue. Color may be white, gray, or silver. Texture may vary from fine to thick.

Examples: dry skin, dandruff, psoriasis, and eczema

Crust

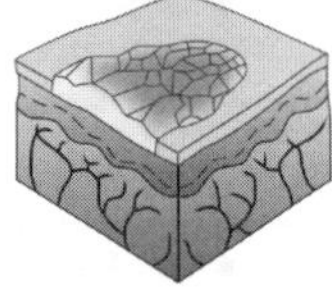

Dry blood, serum, or pus left on the skin surface when vesicles or pustules burst. Can be red-brown, orange, or yellow. Large crusts that adhere to the skin surface are called scabs.

Examples: eczema, impetigo, herpes, or scabs following abrasion

Ulcer

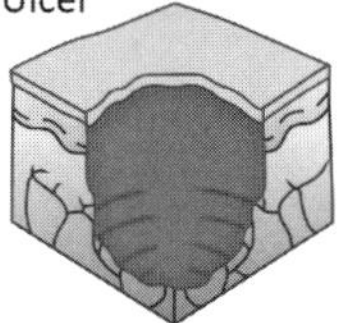

Deep, irregularly shaped area of skin loss extending into the dermis or subcutaneous tissue. May bleed. May leave scar.

Examples: pressure ulcers, stasis ulcers, chancres

Fissure

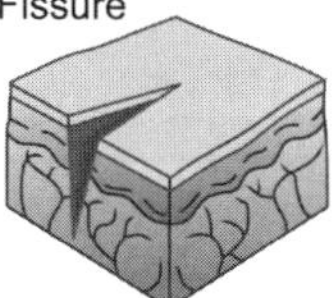

Linear crack with sharp edges, extending into the dermis.

Examples: cracks at the corners of the mouth or in the hands, athlete's foot

Scar

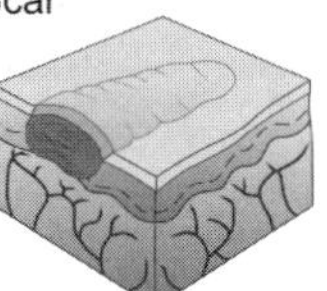

Flat, irregular area of connective tissue left after a lesion or wound has healed. New scars may be red or purple; older scars may be silvery or white.

Examples: healed surgical wound or injury, healed acne

Keloid

Elevated, irregular, darkened area of excess scar tissue caused by excessive collagen formation during healing.
Extends beyond the site of the original injury. Higher incidence in people of African descent.

Examples: keloid from ear piercing or surgery.
Linear erosion.

Excoriation

Examples: scratches, some chemical burns

Identification of different skin lesions.

Hair

Assessing a client's hair includes inspecting the hair, considering developmental changes and ethnic differences, and determining the individual's hair care practices and factors influencing them. Much of the information about hair can be obtained by questioning the client.

Normal hair is resilient and evenly distributed. In people with severe protein deficiency (kwashiorkor), the hair color is faded and appears reddish or bleached, and the texture is coarse and dry. Some therapies cause **alopecia** (hair loss), and some disease conditions and medications affect the coarseness of hair.

For example, hypothyroidism can cause very thin and brittle hair.

Nails

Nails are inspected for nail plate shape, angle between the fingernail and the nail bed, nail texture, nail bed color, and the intactness of the tissues around the nails.

The nail plate is normally colorless and has a convex curve. The angle between the fingernail and the nail bed is normally 160 degrees. One nail abnormality is the spoon shape, in which the nail curves upward from the nail bed.

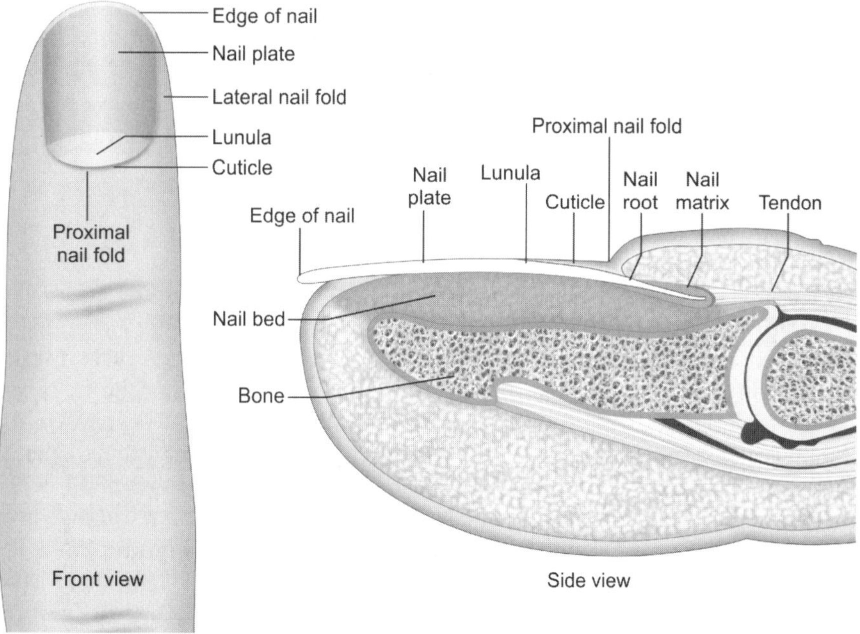

This condition, called koilonychia, may be seen in clients with iron deficiency anemia. **Clubbing** is a condition in which the angle between the nail and the nail bed is 180 degrees, or greater. Clubbing may be caused by a long-term lack of oxygen.

Nail texture is normally smooth. Excessively thick nails can appear in older adults, in the presence of poor circulation, or in relation to a chronic fungal infection. Excessively thin nails or the presence of grooves or furrows can reflect prolonged iron deficiency anemia. Beau's lines are horizontal depressions in the nail that can result from injury or severe illness. The nail bed is highly vascular, a characteristic that accounts for its color. A bluish or purplish tint to the nail bed may reflect cyanosis, and pallor may reflect poor arterial circulation. Should the client report a history of nail fungus (onychomycosis), a referral to a podiatrist or dermatologist for treatment of nail fungus may be appropriate. Symptoms of nail fungus include brittleness, discoloration, thickening, distortion of nail shape, crumbling of the nail, and loosening (detaching) of the nail.

The tissue surrounding the nails is normally intact epidermis. Paronychia is an inflammation of the tissues surrounding a nail. The tissues appear inflamed and swollen, and tenderness is usually present.

A **blanch test** can be carried out to test the capillary refill, that is, peripheral circulation. Normal nail bed capillaries blanch when pressed, but quickly turn pink or their usual color when pressure is released. A slow rate of capillary refill may indicate circulatory problems.

HEAD

During assessment of the head, the nurse inspects and palpates simultaneously and also auscultates. The nurse examines the skull, face, eyes, ears, nose, sinuses, mouth, and pharynx.

Skull and Face

There is a large range of normal shapes of skulls. A normal head size is referred to as **normocephalic**. If head size appears to be outside of the normal range, the circumference can be compared to standard size tables. Measurements more than two standard deviations from the norm for the age, sex, and race of the client are abnormal and should be reported to the primary care provider. Names of areas of the head are derived from names of the underlying bones: mastoid process, mandible, maxilla, and frontal, parietal, occipital.

Eyes and Vision

To maintain optimum vision, people need to have their eyes examined regularly throughout life. It is recommended that people under age 40 have their eyes tested every 3 to 5 years or more frequently if there is a family history of diabetes, hypertension, blood dyscrasia, or eye disease (e.g., glaucoma). After age 40, an eye examination is recommended every 2 years.

Examination of the eyes includes assessment of the external structures, **visual acuity** (the degree of detail the eye can discern in an image), ocular movement, and **visual fields** (the area an individual can see when looking straight ahead). Most eye assessment procedures involve inspection. Consideration is also given to developmental changes and to individual hygienic practices, if the client wears contact lenses or has an artificial eye. For the anatomic structures of the eye.

Many people wear eyeglasses or contact lenses to correct common refractive errors of the lens of the eye. These errors include **myopia** (near-sightedness), **hyperopia** (farsightedness), and **presbyopia** (loss of elasticity of the lens and thus loss of ability to see close objects). Presbyopia begins at about 45 years of age. People notice that they have difficulty reading newsprint. When both far structures.

Conjunctivitis (inflammation of the bulbar and palpebral conjunctiva) may result from foreign bodies, chemicals, allergenic agents, bacteria, or viruses. Redness, itching, tearing, and mucopurulent discharge occur. During sleep, the eyelids may become encrusted and matted together.

Dacryocystitis (inflammation of the lacrimal sac) is manifested by tearing and a discharge from the nasolacrimal duct.

Hordeolum (stye) is a redness, swelling, and tenderness of the hair follicle and glands that empty at the edge of the eyelids. *Iritis* (inflammation of the iris) may be caused by local or systemic infections and results in pain, tearing, and photophobia (sensitivity to light). Contusions or hematomas are "black eyes" resulting from injury.

Cataracts tend to occur in individuals over 65 years old although they may be present at any age. This opacity of the lens or its capsule, which blocks light rays, is frequently removed and replaced by a lens implant. Cataracts may also occur in infants due to a malformation of the lens if the mother contracted rubella in the first trimester of pregnancy.

Glaucoma (a disturbance in the circulation of aqueous fluid, which causes an increase in intraocular pressure) is the most frequent cause of blindness in people over age 40 although it can occur at younger ages. It can be controlled if diagnosed early. Danger signs of glaucoma include blurred or foggy vision, loss of peripheral vision, difficulty focusing on close objects, difficulty adjusting to dark rooms, and seeing rainbow-colored rings around lights.

Upper eyelids that lie at or below the pupil margin are referred to as ptosis and are usually associated with aging, edema from drug allergy or systemic disease (e.g., kidney disease), congenital lid muscle dysfunction, neuromuscular disease (e.g., myasthenia gravis), and third cranial nerve impairment. Eversion, an out turning of the eyelid, is called ectropion; inversion, an in turning of the lid, is called entropion. These abnormalities are often associated with scarring injuries or the aging process.

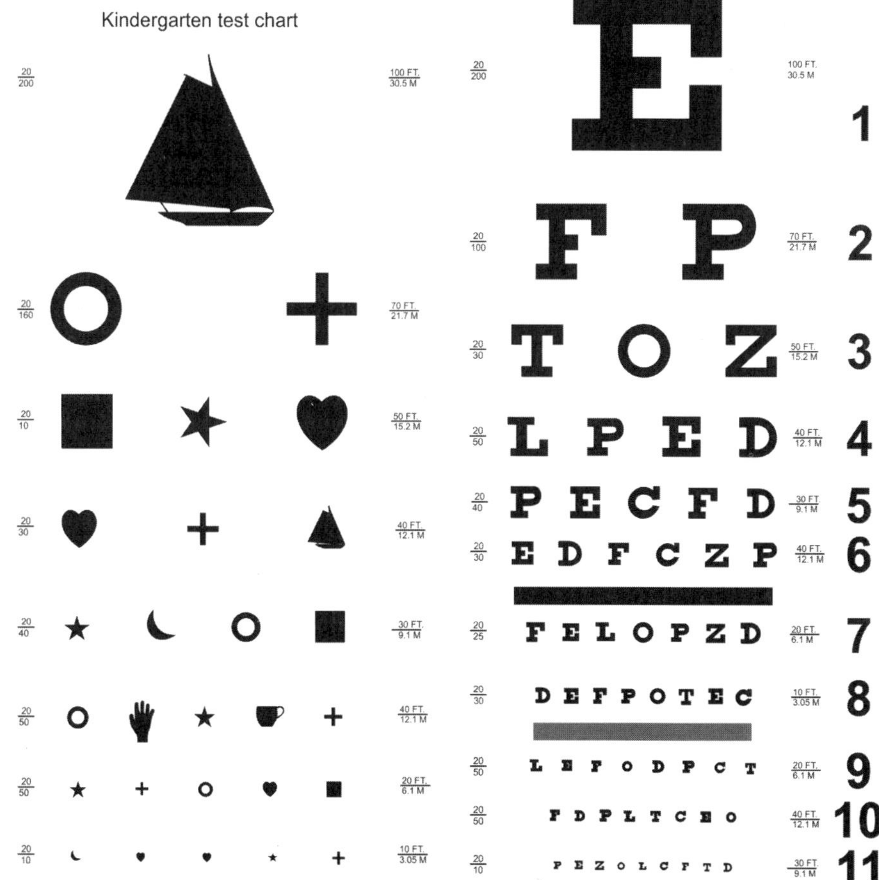

Pupils are normally black, are equal in size (about 3 to 7 mm in diameter), and have round, smooth borders. Cloudy pupils are often indicative of cataracts.

Mydriasis (enlarged pupils) may indicate injury or glaucoma, or result from certain drugs (e.g., atropine, cocaine, amphetamines). **Miosis** (constricted pupils) may indicate an inflammation of the iris or result from such drugs as morphine/heroin and other narcotics, barbiturates, or pilocarpine. It is also an age-related change in older adults. *Anisocoria* (unequal pupils) may result from a central nervous system disorder; however, slight variations may be normal.

The iris is normally flat and round. A bulging toward the cornea can indicate increased intraocular pressure.

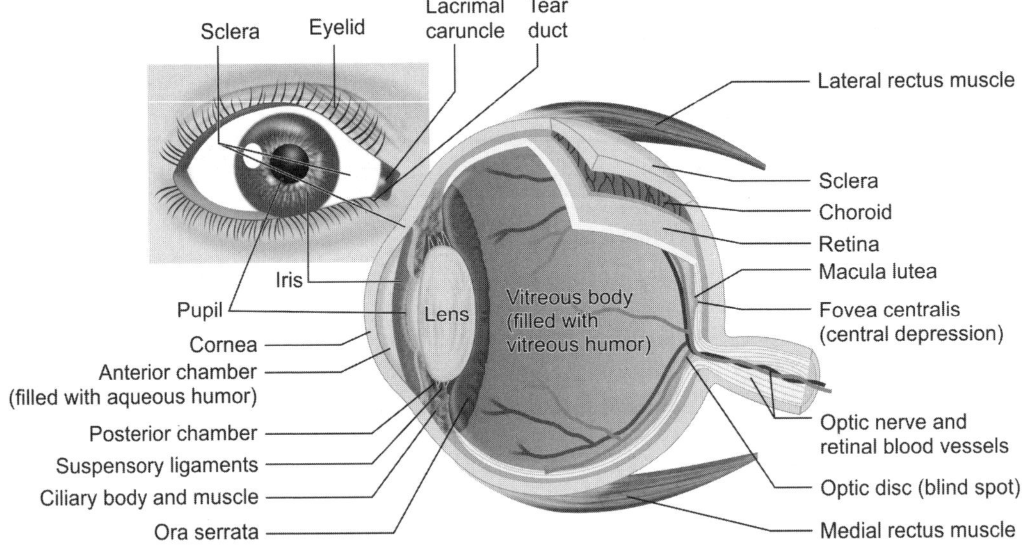

Ears and Hearing

The evaluation of the ear involves direct examination and palpation of the external ear, examination of the internal components of the ear using an otoscope, which is a (instrument for examining the interior of the ear, particularly the eardrum, consisting primarily of a telescope and a light), and determination of auditory acuity. The ear is often examined at a first physical examination; long-term patients or those with difficulty hearing may need frequent reassessments. Only experienced nurses are permitted to do otoscopic evaluations in particular in medical settings.

The ear is divided into three parts: external ear, middle ear, and inner ear. The external ear includes the **auricle** or **pinna**, the external auditory canal, and the **tympanic membrane**, or eardrum. Landmarks of the auricle include the **lobule** (earlobe), **helix** (the posterior curve of the auricle's upper aspect), **antihelix** (the anterior curve of the auricle's upper aspect), **tragus** (the cartilaginous protrusion at the entrance to the ear canal), **triangular fossa** (a depression of the antihelix), and **external auditory meatus** (the entrance to the ear canal). Although not part of the ear, the **mastoid**, a bony prominence behind the ear, is another important landmark. The external ear canal is curved, is about 2.5 cm (1 in.) long in the adult, and ends at the tympanic membrane. It is covered with skin that has many fine hairs, glands, and nerve endings. The glands secrete **cerumen** (earwax), which lubricates and protects the canal.

The curvature of the external ear canal differs with age. In the infant and toddler, the canal has an upward curvature. By age 3, the ear canal assumes the more downward curvature of adulthood.

The middle ear is an air-filled cavity that starts at the tympanic membrane and contains three **ossicles** (bones of sound transmission): the **malleus** (hammer), the **incus** (anvil), and the **stapes** (stirrups). The **eustachian tube**, another part of the middle ear, connects the middle ear to the nasopharynx. The tube stabilizes the air pressure between the external atmosphere and the middle ear, thus preventing rupture of the tympanic membrane and discomfort produced by marked pressure differences.

The inner ear contains the **cochlea**, a seashell-shaped structure essential for sound transmission and hearing, and the **vestibule** and **semi-circular canals**, which contain the organs of equilibrium.

Sound transmission and hearing are complex processes. In brief, sound can be transmitted by air conduction or bone conduction. Air- conducted transmission occurs by this process:

- The sound waves vibrate the tympanic membrane and reach the ossicles.
- The sound waves travel from the ossicles to the opening in the inner ear (oval window).
- The cochlea receives the sound vibrations.
- The stimulus travels to the auditory nerve (the eighth cranial nerve) and the cerebral cortex.
- A sound stimulus enters the external canal and reaches the tympanic membrane

Bone-conducted sound transmission occurs when skull bones transport the sound directly to the auditory nerve.

Audiometric evaluations, which measure hearing at various decibels, are recommended for children and older adults. A common hearing deficit with age is loss of ability to hear high-frequency sounds, such as *f, s, sh,* and *ph.* This neurosensory hearing deficit does not respond well to use of a hearing aid.

Conductive hearing loss is the result of interrupted transmission of sound waves through the outer and middle ear structures. Possible causes are a tear in the tympanic membrane or an obstruction, due to swelling or other causes, in the auditory canal. **Sensorineural hearing loss** is the result of damage to the inner ear, the auditory nerve, or the hearing center in the brain. **Mixed hearing loss** is a combination of conduction and sensorineural loss.

Nose and Sinuses

A nurse can inspect the nasal passages very simply with a flashlight. However, a nasal speculum and a penlight or an otoscope with a nasal attachment facilitates examination of the nasal cavity.

Assessment of the nose includes inspection and palpation of the external nose (the upper third of the nose is bone; the remainder is cartilage); patency of the nasal cavities; and inspection of the nasal cavities.

If the client reports difficulty or abnormality in smell, the nurse may test the client's olfactory sense by asking the client to identify common odors such as coffee or mint. This is done by asking the client to close the eyes and placing vials containing the scent under the client's nose.

Mouth and Oropharynx

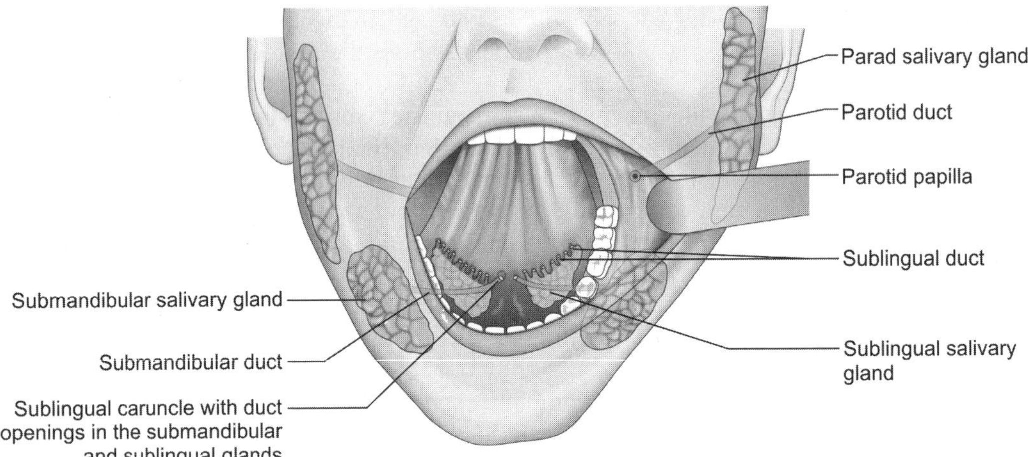

Lips, the oral mucosa, the oral cavity and floor of the mouths, teeth and gums, the hard and soft palate, the uvula, the glands that produce saliva, the tonsillar foundations, and tonsils are among the components that make up the mouth and oropharynx. Most individuals get all of their permanent teeth by the tender age of 25. To learn more about the dental structures, The parotid gland, the submandibular are three of the pairs of glands that secrete saliva that normally drain into the mouth cavity. The biggest gland, the parotid, discharges via Stensen's duct, which is located next to the second molar. Wharton's duct, which is located on each side of the frenulum along the floor of the mouth, is where the submandibular gland drains. There are multiple openings in the sublingual salivary gland, which is located at the floor of the mouth.

Dental **caries** (cavities) and **periodontal disease** (or **pyorrhea**) are the two problems that most frequently affect the teeth. Both problems are commonly associated with plaque and tartar deposits. **Plaque** is an invisible soft film that adheres to the enamel surface of teeth; it consists of bacteria, molecules of saliva, and remnants of epithelial cells and leukocytes. When plaque is unchecked, tartar (dental calculus) forms. **Tartar** is a visible, hard deposit of plaque and dead bacteria that forms at the gum lines. Tartar buildup can alter the fibers that attach the teeth to the gum and eventually disrupt bone tissue. Periodontal disease is characterized by **gingivitis** (red, swollen gingiva [gum]), bleeding, receding gum lines, and the formation of pockets between the teeth and gums. In advanced periodontal disease, the teeth are loose and pus is evident when the gums are pressed.

Other problems nurses may see are **glossitis** (inflammation of the tongue), **stomatitis** (inflammation of the oral mucosa), and **parotitis** (inflammation of the parotid salivary gland). The accumulation of foul matter (food, microorganisms, and epithelial elements) on the teeth and gums is referred to as **sordes**.

The Nursing Process

UNIT OUTLINE

- Critical thinking
- Nursing process: assessment, nursing diagnosis, planning, implementation, evaluation
- Collection of data
- Nursing diagnosis statement: parts, types, formulating, guidelines for formulating nursing diagnosis
- NANDA approved diagnoses
- Establishing goals and expected outcomes: purposes, types, guidelines, components of goals and outcome statements
- Process of implementing the plan of care
- Evaluation process

LEARNING OBJECTIVES

At the end of this unit, the reader will be able to:
- Define critical thinking.
- Categorize stages of critical thinking.
- Classify the levels of critical thinking.
- Outline use of critical thinking in nursing.
- Explain nursing process.
- Illustrate historical development of nursing process.
- Define characteristics of nursing process.
- Outline steps of nursing process.
- Define nursing assessment and its types.
- Define nursing diagnosis.
- Formulate NANDA nursing diagnosis.
- Describe the types of nursing diagnosis.
- Distinguish nursing and medical diagnosis.
- Interpret guidelines for formulating nursing diagnosis.
- Explain planning.
- Define intervention.
- Describe implementation.
- Explain evaluation.

CRITICAL THINKING

Introduction

Nurses deal with a wide range of circumstances including patients, family members, medical professionals, and colleagues. Each circumstance brings with it fresh client care challenges and experiences. In order to provide the greatest nursing care to clients, it is vital for nurses to exercise critical thinking and make wise decisions. Thinking critically is not a straightforward, linear technique that can be picked up in a single day. It is a skill that can only be attained with perseverance, dedication, and a keen interest in learning.

Critical thinking involves thinking about the 'why' question, or the set of assumptions and biases that influence any thought or action.

Definitions

According to Parse:

- ❖ "Carefully choosing a direction in light of personal tacit and explicit knowing" describes critical thinking as "the art of thinking about thinking."
- ❖ "Critical thinking problem solving and decision making can enhances the effectiveness of the solutions or decisions made, thus critical thinking problem process with creativity enhancing the result."
- ❖ "Critical thinking is an active, organized, cognitive process used to carefully examine one's thinking and the thinking of others."

Characteristics

- ❖ **Rationality and reflection:** It is based on reasons and evidence rather than on preference or self-interest. Critical thinkers do not "Jump to conclusions." They take the time to collect data fact and think the matter through."
  Examples:
  - ◆ Rahul decided to become a nurse after watching a film in which nurses were shown as attractive and heroic.
  - ◆ Rahul asked a counselor about the job opportunities available for nurses and also talked several nurses then decided to go to nursing college.
- ❖ **Healthy, constructive sceptic:** Critical thinkers do not accept or reject ideas unless they understand them they do not mindlessly follow rules but seek to understand the rationale behind them—Following those that make sense and working to improve those that do not.
  Examples: When a salesperson insisted that new IV tubing was better than being used on nurses then nurse asked "what information do you have to show that this is so?
- ❖ **Autonomy:** Critical thinkers are not easily manipulated, they think for themselves rather than being led by their peer group or passively accepting the beliefs of others.
  Examples: When, without being asked, a nurse responds to this concern and evaluates the patient's vital signs and symptoms is example of Clinical Autonomy.
- ❖ **Creative thinking:** Critical thinkers create original ideas by finding connections among thoughts and concepts.

Examples: Nurses remembered a song his mother used to him and sang it to help comport a frightened child in the hospital.

❖ **Fair thinking:** Critical thinking is not biased or one sided, critical thinkers recognize the bias and prejudice of others thinking and seek information from all points of view before taking a standard or active decision.

Examples: Nurse—the unit manager needed to make the schedule for the Christmas and New Year's holidays. Before requesting to a nurses request to be off for Christmas, then she asked all staff members to submit their preferences then she was able to determine that staffing was adequate for both holidays.

❖ **Focus on what to believe and do:** Critical thinking is used to decide on a course of action, make reliable observations, draw sound conclusions, solve problems, and evaluate policies and action.

Stages of Creative Thinking

According to Strader 1992, he gives four steps of creative thinking:

1. **Preparation stage:** The creative thinker gathers information related to the problem or concern.
2. **Incubation:** The creative thinker unconsciously considers and consciously works on possible solutions or decisions, all possibilities—both old and new are considered during this phase.
3. **Insight stage:** Appropriate solutions emerge and are developed and the solution believed to be most appropriate is implemented.
4. **Verification stage:** The implemented solution is evaluated for its effectiveness.

Levels of Critical Thinking in Nursing

The ability to critically think expands as a nurse gains new knowledge and experience and matures into a competent professional.

According to Kataoka–Yahiro and Saylor 1994, that includes three levels of critical thinking:

1. **Basic critical thinking:** At the basic level of critical thinking a learner trusts that experts have the right answers for every problem. Thinking is concrete and based on a set of rules or principles.

   Examples: A nurse uses an institutions procedure manual to confirm how to insert a Foley catheter, the student nurse follows procedure step-by-step without adjusting the procedure to meet a clients unique needs.

2. **Complex critical thinking:** A person begins to detach from authorities and analyze and examine alternatives more at the complex level of critical thinking. They note that the nurse's best answer to a problem at this level is "It depends the persons thinking abilities", the nurse realizes that alternative solutions do exist.

   Examples: A 36-year-old man who underwent hip surgery, the client is having pain but refusing his ordered analgesics then the nurse learns that the client practices medication.

3. **Commitment critical thinking:** The third level of critical thinking is commitment, the individual anticipates the need to others at this level the nurse does more than just consider

the complex alternatives a problem poses more than just consider the complex alternatives a problem poses.

Critical Thinking Model

This model helps to explain concepts because critical thinking in nursing is complex. A model can help to explain all of the factors involved in making decisions judgements about clients.

Kataoka-Yahiro and Saylor have developed a model of critical thinking for nursing. The model defines the outcome of critical thinking. Nursing judgement that is relevant to nursing problems in a variety of settings.

According to this model—there are five components of critical thinking:
1. Knowledge base
2. Experience
3. Competence
4. Attitudes
5. Standards

The element of the model combines to explain how nurses make clinical judgment that is necessary for safe, effective, nursing care.

❖ **Specific knowledge base:** The first component of critical thinking is a nurse's specific knowledge base.
  - This varies according to a nurses educational experience, including—basic nursing education, continuing education course and additional college degrees.
  - It includes the initiative a nurse shows in reading the nursing literature so as to remain current in nursing science
  - A nurse's knowledge base includes information and theory from the basics science, humanities, behavioral sciences and nursing.
  - Nurse use their knowledge base in a different way from other health care disciplines.
  - **Examples:** A nurse's broad knowledge base gives the nurse a more holistic view of clients and their health care needs, the depth and extent of knowledge influence the nurse's ability to think critically about nursing problems.

❖ **Experience:** The second component of the critical thinking model is experience in nursing unless a nurse has the opportunity to practice and make decisions about client care; critical thinking in clinical decision making will not develop.
  - In clinical situation the nurse learns from observing sensing, talking with clients and families.
  - Clinical experience is the laboratory for testing nursing knowledge.
  - The experience gained nurse from using the approaches from previous clients with experiences; the nurse begins to understand clinical situations, recognize cues of client's health pattern.

❖ **Attitudes for critical thinking:** The 4th component of the critical thinking model is attitudes has identified 11 attitudes that are central features of a critical thinker.
  Example: When a client complains of anxiety before undergoing a diagnostic procedure the nurse will be the client's concerns.

Critical thinking attitudes offer guidelines for how to approach a problem or decision making situation.

The attitudes for critical thinking are:

A. Confidence
B. Independence
C. Fairness
D. Responsibility
E. Risk taking
F. Discipline
G. Perseverance
H. Creativity
I. Curiosity
J. Integrity
K. Humility

Confidence

- To be confident is to feel certain in one's ability to accomplish a task or goal.
- Confidence grows with experience and the maturity to recognize ones strengths and limitations.
- Confident critical thinkers remain aware of the balance between what they know and what they do not know.
- When a nurse shows confidence, clients recognize it in the manner in which the nurse communicates and performs nursing care.

Thinking independently

- As persons mature and gain new knowledge they learn to consider a wide range of ideas and concepts before forming an making judgment.
- A critical thinker does not customarily accept another person's ideas with ought to question.
- Independent thinking and reasoning are essential to the improvement and expansion of nursing practice.

Fairness

- Critical thinkers deal with situations in a just manner, this means that they recognize their own biases and prejudices.
- Example, how a nurse feels about obesity he or she should not allow personal attitudes to influence the way care is delivered to an obese patient.
- Developing a sense of imagination aids in the development of fairness.

Responsibility and accountability: When caring for client as a nurse has a responsibility to correctly perform nursing care activities based upon standards of practice.

Examples: The nurse does not take short cuts when administering medications a professional nurse must be competent in performing nursing therapies and in making decision about clients.

Risk taking

- When a person takes a risk in acting or decision making.

- Risk taking does not have to cause injury without intellectual risk taking, knowledge cannot advance.
- A critical thinker is willing to take risks in trying different approaches to solving problems, willing to be wrong.
- Nurse in the past event taken risk in taking different approaches to skin and wound care pulmonary hygiene, pain management.

Discipline

- A disciplined thinker misses few details and follows an orderly approach when making decisions or taking action.
- Disciplined thinking ensures that decisions are made systematically and in a compressive manner.

Examples: Assessment of client's pain includes more than just the location, the nurse also assesses the severity of pain, its duration, factors that aggravate or relieve the pain.

Perseverance

- A critical thinker will take on a problem with determination.
- Perseverance helps critical thinkers finds effective solution to client care problems.
- This is especially important when problems remain unresolved or when they reoccur.

Examples: A client who is unable to speak following the throat surgery—often possess challenges for the nurse—to be able to communicate effectively.

- Perseverance leads the nurse to try different communication approaches, e.g., massage boards, or alarm bells.

Creativity

- It involves the use of imaginative and innovative skills in problem solving this means finding new or innovative solutions to client problems of practice.
- Creativity is a great motivator that enables one to generate options.

Examples: a home health nurse must find a way to help an older client with arthritis gain greater mobility in the home

Curiosity

- A critical thinker always has the desire to know or to seek knowledge.
- Curiosity is what drives a critical thinker to ask the question why.
- As the nurse analyzes client information, data, patterns emerge that are not always clear.

Integrity

- A person of integrity acts on the basis of a sound moral and ethical position.
- Personal integrity builds trust from peers and subordinates.

Humility

- It is important to be humble and admit to one's own limitations in knowledge and skills, critical thinkers admit what they do not know and try to acquire the knowledge needed to make proper decisions.
- The nurse must rethink a situation, acquire additional knowledge then use new information to form opinions.

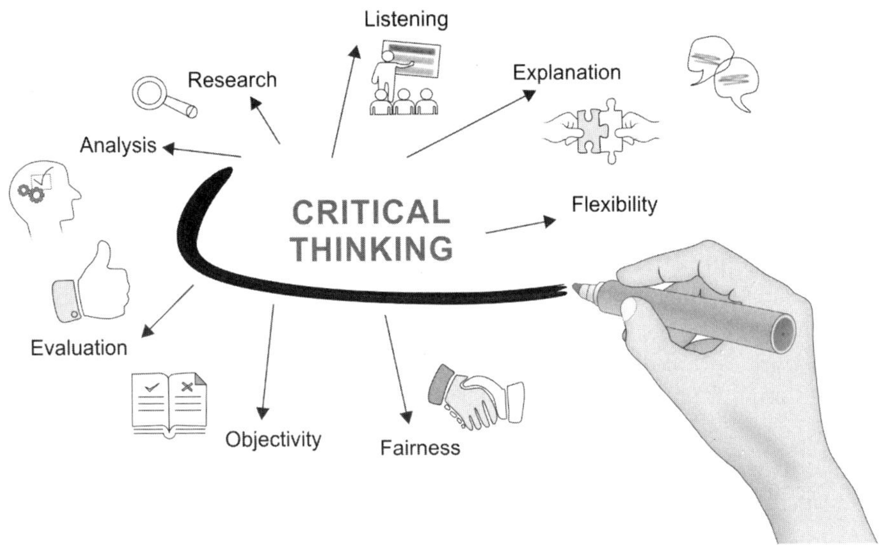

❖ **Standards for critical thinking:** It includes intellectual and professional standards.
  ♦ Intellectual standards—Paul 1993 identified 14 intellectual standards:
     1. Clear
     2. Logical
     3. Precise
     4. Deep
     5. Specific
     6. Broad
     7. Accurate
     8. Complete
     9. Relevant
     10. Significant
     11. Plausible
     12. Adequate
     13. Consistent
     14. Logical
  ♦ Professional standards: These standards are commonly applied when a nurse conducts the nursing.
     ◊ Professional standards for critical thinking refer to ethical criteria for nursing judgments, scientific and practice-based criteria used for evolution.
     ◊ Professional standards ensure that the highest level of quality nursing care is promoted.
     ◊ It includes—ethical criteria for nursing judgment.
     ◊ Criteria for evaluation.
     ◊ Professional responsibility.

Use of Critical Thinking for Nurse

- ❖ Nurse use knowledge from other subjects and fields
    - ◆ Using insight from one subject to shed light on another subject requires critical thinking skills.
    - ◆ Nurses deal holistically with human responses; they must draw meaningful information from other subject's areas.
    - ◆ Nursing students are required to take course in the biologic and social sciences and in the humanities so that they can acquire a strong foundation.

    Examples: The nurse might use knowledge from nutrition, physiology and physics to promote wound healing and prevent further injury to a client with a pressure ulcer.

- ❖ Nurses deals with change in stressful environments
    - ◆ Nurses work in rapidly changing situations, treatments, medications and technology change from minute to minute.

    Examples:
    - ◆ Familiarity with routine for giving medications.
    - ◆ Does not help the nurse deal with a client who is frightened of injections or with one who does not wish to take a medication, when expected situations arise. Critical thinking enables the nurse to recognize important to meet specific client needs.

- ❖ Nurse make's important decisions:
    - ◆ During the course of a work in a day, a nurse makes vital decisions of many kinds.
    - ◆ These decisions often determine the well being of clients and even their very survival.
    - ◆ Nurse use critical thinking skills to collect and interpret the information needed to make decisions.

    Examples: Use good judgement to decide which observations must be reported to the physician immediately which can be noted in the client record for the physician to address later.

    - ◆ Need to make accurate and appropriate clinical decisions.
    - ◆ Need to solve problems and find solutions.
    - ◆ Need to plan care for each unique client and client problem.
    - ◆ Need to seek knowledge and use it to make clinical decisions and solving problems.
    - ◆ Need to be able to think creatively when planning care for clients.

Critical Thinking Competencies

Kataoka-Yahiro and Saylor (1994) describe critical thinking competencies as the cognitive processes a nurse uses to make judgments about the clinical care of patients. These include general critical thinking, specific critical thinking in clinical situations, and specific critical thinking in nursing. General critical thinking processes are not unique to nursing. They include the scientific method, problem solving, and decision making. Specific critical thinking competencies in clinical health care situations include diagnostic reasoning, clinical inference, and clinical decision making. The specific critical thinking competency in nursing involves use of the nursing process. Each of the competencies is discussed in the following paragraphs.

Scientific Method

The scientific method is a way to solve problems using reasoning. It is a systematic, ordered approach to gathering data and solving problems used by nurses, physicians, and a variety of other health care professionals. This approach looks for the truth or verifies that a set of facts agrees with reality. Nurse researchers use the **scientific method** when testing research questions in nursing practice situations. The scientific method has five steps:

1. Identifying the problem
2. Collecting data
3. Formulating a question or hypothesis
4. Testing the question or hypothesis
5. Evaluating results of the test or study

Consider the following example of the scientific method in nursing practice.

A nurse caring for patients who receive large doses of chemotherapy for ovarian cancer sees a pattern of patients developing severe inflammation in the mouth (mucositis) (identifies problem). The nurse reads research articles (collects data) about mucositis and learns that there is evidence to show that having patients keep ice in their mouths (cryotherapy) during the chemotherapy infusion reduces severity of mucositis after treatment. He or she asks (forms question), "Do patients with ovarian cancer who receive chemotherapy have less severe mucositis when given cryotherapy versus standard mouth rinse in the oral cavity?" The nurse then collaborates with colleagues to develop a nursing protocol for using ice with certain chemotherapy infusions. The nurses on the oncology unit collect information that allows them to compare the incidence and severity of mucositis for a group of patients who use cryotherapy versus those who use standard-practice mouth rinse (tests the question). They analyze the results of their project and find that the use of cryotherapy reduced the frequency and severity of mucositis in their patients (evaluating the results). They decide to continue the protocol for all patients with ovarian cancer.

Problem Solving

Every day, you deal with issues like a computer software that isn't working correctly or an elderly relative who passed away a beloved pet. When an issue occurs, you gather knowledge and combine it with what you are already familiar with to come up with a solution. In the clinic, patients often come with issues. For instance, a nurse who works in home care may discover that a patient struggles to take her pills on time. The person receiving treatment is unable to recall the three days' worth of prescriptions she has taken. The pill bottles have labels and are full with medicine. The patient's failure to adhere to or follow her medication regimen is an issue that the nurse must address. The nurse is aware that the client was released from the hospital after receiving a prescription for five drugs. The patient discloses to the caregiver that she also frequently uses two over-the-counter drugs. The nurse notes that she has trouble reading the prescription labels when she asks her to exhibit the pills she uses in the morning. The patient can explain the meds she needs to take, but she is unsure of when to take them. The nurse advises that the pharmacist relabel the patient's prescriptions with bigger letters. Additionally, the nurse gives the patient samples of pill planners that will enable her to arrange her prescriptions according to the time of day throughout the course of seven days.

Effective issue resolution also entails periodically assessing the efficacy of the proposed solution. If an issue persists, other approaches must be tried. In the above scenario, the nurse observes that the individual has appropriately arranged her prescriptions during a subsequent visit and can easily read the labels. The nurse gathered details that accurately identified the patient's problem's root cause and tried an effective treatment. A nurse's practice experience increases with each difficulty they have handled, enabling them to apply their skills to new patient circumstances.

Decision Making

Nurses make decisions when they must choose a course to follow from a range of possibilities in response to a problem or circumstance. Critical thinking that prioritizes issue solving results in decision-making. Making a comprehensive and considered choice is made easier by adhering to a set of criteria. The standards may be based on personal preferences, corporate policies, or, as is commonly the case in the field of nursing, professional standards. For instance, decision-making takes place when a person selects a healthcare provider. A person must identify and describe the issue or circumstance (the requirement for a certain kind of healthcare provider to offer medical treatment) before evaluating all available possibilities (such as taking into account suggested healthcare providers or selecting one that is near to home). The individual must evaluate each option in light of a set of personal standards (experience, friendliness, or reputation), test potential choices by speaking with various healthcare providers, take into account the results of the decision (examine advantages and disadvantages of choosing one healthcare provider over another), then make a final choice. Even if the criteria are organized into phases, decision-making entails switching back and forth between all of the criteria. It results in well-informed decisions that are backed by logic and proof. Choosing a type of wearing clothes for a patient with a wound caused by surgery, deciding which teaching strategy is best for the caregiver helping a patient whose is returning their homes after a stroke, and choosing which patient care first requires an immediate response are a few examples of clinical decision making.

Specific Critical Thinking

Diagnostic Reasoning and Inference

Once nurse receive information about a patient in a clinical situation, **diagnostic reasoning** begins. It is the analytical process for determining a patient's health problems. Accurate recognition of a patient's problems is necessary before she decide on solutions and implement action. It requires you to assign meaning to the behaviors and physical signs and symptoms presented by a patient. Diagnostic reasoning begins when you interact with a patient or make physical or behavioral observations. An expert nurse sees the context of a patient situation (e.g., a patient who is feeling light-headed with blurred vision and who has a history of diabetes is possibly experiencing a problem with blood glucose levels), observes patterns and themes (e.g., symptoms that include weakness, hunger, and visual disturbances suggest hypoglycemia), and makes decisions quickly (e.g., offers a food source containing glucose). The information a nurse collects and analyzes leads to a diagnosis of a patient's condition. Nurses do not make medical diagnoses, but they do assess and monitor patients closely and compare the patients' signs and symptoms with those that are common to a medical diagnosis. This type of diagnostic reasoning helps health care providers pinpoint the nature of a problem more quickly and select proper therapies.

Clinical inference, the procedure of deriving inferences from linked bits of data and prior experience with the evidence, is a component of diagnostic thinking. Before establishing a diagnosis, an inference entails constructing informational patterns from data. The nurse assumes there is a dietary issue when she notices that the individual has decreased her appetite and weight during the last month. Making a nursing diagnosis like unbalanced nutrition: less than body requirement is an example of medical reasoning in action.

Utilize patient information that you receive or collect through diagnostic reasoning to rationally identify the issue. For instance, after rotating a patient, you see a red spot on the hip to the right. The person in question complains of soreness, and when you palpate the region you see that it is pleasant to the touch. When you release pressure after applying pressure with your finger, the region does not blanch or become white. You come to the diagnosis that the person in question has pressure ulcers after considering what you consider to be normal skin resilience and the consequences of pressure. Verify your conclusions as a student with knowledgeable nurses. Although there may be occasions when you are incorrect, speaking with nursing professionals may help you improve for next clinical scenarios.

Frequently, you cannot provide an accurate diagnosis on the first consultation with a patient. There are occasions when you feel there is an issue but lack the information to diagnose it specifically. Some patient's physical problems make it difficult for them to describe their symptoms to you. Some people decide not to provide critical or crucial information during your first evaluation. Some patient's actions and bodily reactions can only be seen in circumstances that weren't present during your first exam. Continue gathering data even if you're unsure about the diagnosis. Until you can identify the patient's particular circumstance, you must critically study shifting clinical scenarios. In nursing practice, clinical reasoning is a consistent habit. Any conclusions you get from your diagnostic work will aid the medical professional in promptly determining the source of a disease and deciding on the best course of treatment.

Clinical Decision Making

Clinical choices are an activity involving solving problems that focuses on describing a problem and choosing an acceptable course of action, much like general decision making. A nurse decides on a nursing intervention after determining the patient's issue via clinical decision-making. When you near a clinical issue, such as someone who is less mobile or develops a red spot over the hip, you decide on the most effective nursing approaches (skin care and a changing schedule) and identify the issue (impaired skin integrity as the appearance of a pressure ulcer). Every day, nurses make clinical judgments to preserve or enhance the health of their patients. This entails lessening the problem's intensity or fixing it entirely. Making clinical decisions takes thorough consideration (i.e., selecting the alternatives that will result in the greatest results for the patient based on the patient's state and the urgency of the issue).

Improve your clinical decision making by knowing your patients. Nurse researchers found that expert nurses develop a level of knowledge that leads to pattern recognition of patient symptoms and responses. For example, an experienced nurse who has been working on a general surgical unit for a lengthy period is more likely than a novice nurse to be able to recognize symptoms of internal bleeding, such as a drop in blood pressure, a fast heartbeat, or a change in awareness. Expert nurses may get familiar with clinical circumstances and swiftly predict and choose the best course of action over time thanks to a mix of expertise, dedication in a particular clinical field, or the quality of connections created with patients. To have a better understanding of your patients, take additional time during first patient evaluations to monitor patient behavior and evaluate physical findings. Additionally, continuously evaluating and keeping track of patients when issues arise enables you to see whether clinical changes alter over time. Nursing remedies are chosen based on both clinical expertise and unique patient information, such as:

- ❖ The identified status and situation you assessed about the patient, including data collected by actively listening to the patient regarding his or her health care needs.
- ❖ Knowledge about the clinical variables (e.g., age, seriousness of the problem, pathology of the problem, patient's pre-existing disease conditions) involved in the situation, and how the variables are linked together.
- ❖ A judgment about the likely course of events and outcome of the diagnosed problem, considering any health risks the patient has; includes knowledge about usual patterns of any diagnosed problem or prognosis.
- ❖ Any additional relevant data about requirements in the patient's daily living, functional capacity, and social resources.
- ❖ Knowledge about the nursing therapy options available and the way in which specific interventions will predictably affect the patient's situation.

NURSING PROCESS

Introduction

A nursing process is an accredited nurse's method for choosing, planning, and providing a patient with the best possible nursing care. Identification, diagnosis, and treatment of human reactions to health and sickness are done via the nursing process. Assessment, diagnosis in nursing, planning, implementation, and evaluation are the first five phases of the procedure. The nursing approach will be regularly used in practice, enabling nurses to adapt as the patient's requirements change. Individualized nursing care is promoted by using the nursing process. Whether the individual receiving treatment is a person, a family, or a society, it still applies.

Definitions

- ❖ The nursing process is a systematic, patient-centered, goal-oriented method of caring that provides a framework for nursing practice.
- ❖ The nursing process is used to identify, diagnose, and treat human responses to health and illness.
- ❖ The nursing process is an orderly, systematic manner of determining the client's health status, specifying problems defined as alterations in human need fulfillment, making plans to solve them, initiating and implementing the plan, and evaluating the extent to which the plan was effective in promoting optimum wellness and resolving the problems identified.
- ❖ Nursing process is a method of problem identification and problem solving. Although derived from the supposedly objective scientific method, nursing process is not applied in and objective, value-free way human values influence both problem identification and problem solving. The components of nursing process discussed in textbooks vary but generally include assessment and diagnosis. These are the problem-identification components. Outcome projection, intervention, and outcome evaluation are the problem-solving components.

The cornerstone of clinical nursing, the nursing process is a systematic method for taking independent nursing action. Steps in the nursing process include:

- Assessing the patient's problems.
- Forming a diagnostic statement.
- Identifying expected outcomes.
- Creating a plan to achieve expected outcomes and to solve the patient's problems.
- Implementing the plan or assigning others to implement it.
- Evaluating the plan's effectiveness.

These phases of the nursing process—assessment, nursing diagnosis, outcome identification, planning, implementation, and evaluation—are dynamic and flexible; they commonly overlap".

❖ The nursing process generally is defined as a systematic problem-solving approach toward giving individualized nursing care.

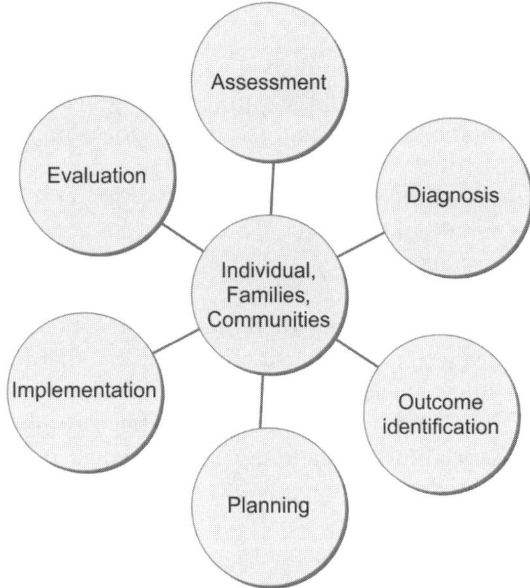

Historical Development of the Nursing Process

The problem-solving method for determining the clients' requirements for medical and nursing care is known as the nursing process. Nurses provided care for patients within a loosely organized framework centered around the medical model before the term "nursing process" became widely used in the late 1960s. Since then, several leaders in nursing have contributed to the development of the nursing method that is used today, and numerous nursing process models have been developed.

Although Lydia Hall has been associated with coining the phrase "nursing process" in 1955, it wasn't until the 1960s that nursing magazines began to use it often. A three-step nursing procedure was reported a few years later by Dorothy Johnson (1959), Ida Jean Orlando (1961), and Ernestine Wiedenbach (1963). In 1967, Lois Knowles wrote "the five D's"—discover, delve, decide, do, and discriminate—as a five-step nursing procedure. Discover and Delve represent the assessment phase, Decide represents the planning phase, Do represents the implementation phase, and Discriminate represents the assessment of client reactions to nursing interventions.

Several articles established and outlined the phases of the nursing process in 1967. The Western Interstate Commission for Higher Education (WICHE) and the faculty at the Catholic University of America were instrumental in moving the nursing process forward. The nursing process is described as "The nursing process is that which goes on between a client and a nurse in a given setting; it records the behaviors of client and nurse and the resulting interaction. The steps of the process are perception, communication, interpretation, and evaluation" (WICHE, 1967). Although it was never universally adopted, this definition served as a catalyst for the advancement of the process of nursing.

The phases of the nursing process were established by Helen Yura and Mary B Walsh and the nursing faculty from the Catholic University of America in 1973 as assessment, planning, implementation, and evaluation. The nursing process idea has been developed and improved upon by Yura and Walsh ever since 1967.

In its standards of nursing practice published in 1973, the American Nurses Association (ANA) identified diagnosis as a distinct nursing process stage. The five phases of the process of nursing were used to organize the standards. Around this time, nursing instructors and providers started using the five-step nursing model.

Further support for establishing diagnosis a discrete nursing role and a different phase of the nursing method emerged in the 1980s. The ANA once again recognized diagnosis of current and future health issues as a crucial component of nursing practice in its A Social Policy Statements (ANA, 1980; 1995).

The six-step nursing process paradigm, which the ANA presented in its updated Standards for Clinical Nursing Practice (1991), is the most recent advancement in nursing practice. The ANA designated outcome identification being the final phase of the nursing process in their six-step model. Recently, the ANA model's six stages have been employed.

The American Nurses Association (ANA) produced a new social policy statement for nursing in the new century that defined nursing in a larger framework to satisfy society's demands, but the evaluation and therapy of people's reactions still forms a crucial aspect of the nursing profession. The nursing process is still referred to as the cornerstone of decision-making and competent nursing care in the 2004 publication nursing: Scope and Standards of Practice by the American Nurses Association (ANA).

Theoretical foundations for use of the nursing process concepts: An understating of the theoretical foundations of the nursing process is necessary to apply it effectively. Systems theory, problem-solving process, decision-making process, information-processing theory, and diagnostic reasoning process are the basic structural units of the nursing process.

Systems Theory

Systems theory, one conceptual foundation on which nursing process is built, illustrates how the steps of the nursing process interact with each other, forming a unique blend that is greater than the sum of its parts. Systems terminology provides a common language for the members of the healthcare team.

A system is composed of a set of subsystems, and each higher level is made up of systems of the lower levels. All systems, including the nursing process, have cyclical patterns. Six subsystems make up the nursing process: assessment, diagnosis, outcome identification, planning, implementation, and evaluation. These subsystems interact with one another and have an impact on the others.

Input, the information that enters a system, is the data collected during the assessment step (observation, nursing interview, and physical examination). Input includes assessment data about the client and his or her immediate environment.

Throughput is the process by which a system transforms, creates and organizes input, resulting in a reorganization of the input. After the nurse identifies nursing diagnoses and outcomes and plans and implements nursing care, throughout takes place.

Output, the end product of a system, is the client's health status (i.e., whether the client's health has been maintained or improved). Evaluating goal attainment and the need for modification provides feedback for revising the plan, thereby completing the cycle.

Problem-Solving Process

Nurses run across issues, from straightforward inquiries to challenging clinical conditions that call for remedies. Nurses deal with issues including tools, patients, families, and other heath team members. Issue-solving methods (complex or simple): the experience, expertise, and mental capacity of the issue solver; the alternative or viewpoint selected to solve the problem.

The nursing method is built on the concept of problem resolution. The technique of problem-solving is a modified version of scientific problem-solving. The scientific approach concentrates on a single issue, is completed in a lab, involves a lengthy period of time, and attempts to control every one of the factors or aspects as feasible. In contrast, the technique of problem-solving includes individuals who have a variety of issues and takes place in a therapeutic context. It happens more quickly and usually involves unanticipated elements and occurrences. In the "real world" of clinical nursing practice, flexibility is necessary, and the process of problem-solving allows for this.

Solving problems is not something that happens alone. Nurses communicate and collaborate with patients, families, and other care team members to find solutions to issues. It is a social strategy that might include one, two, or more persons. When feasible, the patient is engaged in problem-solving.

Decision-Making Process

The core of nursing practice is making decisions about client care. Making decisions is a important part of the procedure of nursing at every stage. Identifying the issue, identifying the options, and choosing the best option are the three steps that make up decision-making in its most basic form. People continuously make choices, including what to dress, when to eat, and what time to study. All of these judgments are influenced by prior encounters and exposure to diverse life situations.

In clinical settings, nurses must make decisions on which patients should get treatment first, when it is appropriate to delegate care to other members of the healthcare team, as well as which client care tasks are necessary. Depending on the current situation, each choice is followed through with or modified. Decisions taken at the start of the day may not cause issues on certain days, but more often than not, priorities must shift to deal with emergencies, forcing nurses to cope with ambiguity and develop their clinical decision-making skills.

The stages of the nursing procedure may be compared to the processes utilized in this technique. Information gathering is comparable to evaluation, pinpointing the issue area is to diagnosing, weighing the pros and drawbacks of different courses of action is to planning. This procedure includes evaluating the available data and the recommended course of action.

Information-Processing Theory

After completing the interview, reviewing the chart, and examining the client, nurses must synthesize the data. In this complex task, the processing of information requires the cognitive skills of logical and inductive-deductive thinking and the decision-making and diagnostic processes.

Data must be arranged in a framework or outline as the brain can only process five to seven bits of information at once. The functional health framework model is used here. Nurses may then see how each component fits together to form the total. According to studies, experienced nurses may diagnose patients more accurately with less clues. Either inductive or deductive methods may be used to gather and analyze information. Both methods are used by nurses to identify and resolve the issues. A method of thinking called induction moves from the particular to the general.

Diagnostic Reasoning Process

The diagnostic reasoning process is used to make accurate clinical diagnosis about client problems. A number of interconnected processes make up the complex procedure, which is influenced by factors including the client's and diagnostician's backgrounds. The practitioners must follow the diagnostic' recommendations:

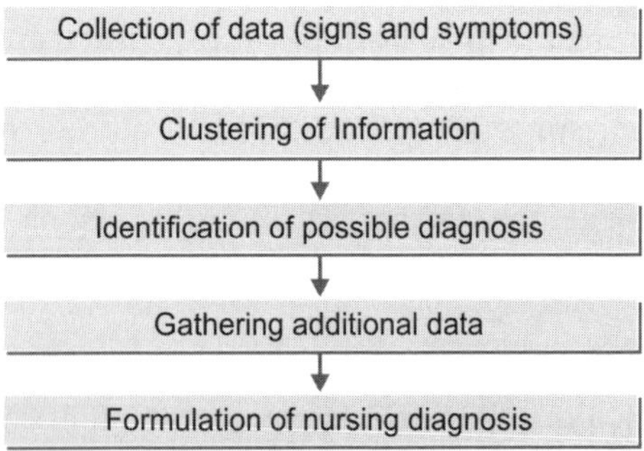

1. Acquire a good working knowledge of the relevant structures and their function
2. Be able to comprehend the meaning of that knowledge
3. Know when and how to apply the knowledge
4. Be able to analyze the relationships among different pieces of information
5. Be able to synthesize pieces of information and their relationships into a meaningful whole
6. Cross-check the processing of the entire information to evaluate whether their conclusions are defensible.

Although the steps are discussed sequentially, in practice there is much overlap until the diagnosis is made and confirmed. The steps include the following:
* Considering the background of the diagnostician and client
* Collecting pre-encounter data about the client
* Entering into the assessment situation
* Collecting the database
* Gathering and coalescing cues and cue clusters
* Selecting priority sign clusters
* Identifying possible diagnoses
* Confirming or refuting the diagnosis
* Selecting the diagnosis or making the clinical judgment.

Purpose of the Nursing Process

The primary goal of the nursing process is to provide a systematic framework for nursing practice. It regulates, coordinates, and integrates nursing practice. The nurse's roles and responsibilities, communication, cooperation, and synchronization may promote maintenance, restoration, or enhancement of a peaceful death depending on the client's condition. The nursing process also has the following other goals:
* Facilitate documentation of data, diagnosis, plans client responses and evaluation.
* Evaluate the efficiency and effectiveness of care.
* Give direction, guidance and meaning to nursing and nursing care.
* Provide for continuity of care and a reduce errors in care. Individualize client participation.
* Promote creatively and flexibility in nursing practice.

Characteristics of Nursing Process

* **Systematic approach:** Nursing process is a systematic methods that directs the nurse and client as together determine the need for nursing care plan and implements the care and evaluate the result. It is a client centered process and is interrelated.
* **Dynamic:** The nursing process is dynamic, because it involves continuous change. It is an ongoing process focused on the changing responses of the client identified throughout the nurse-client relationship.
* **Interpersonal and collaborative:** The nursing process is interpersonal and collaborative. It is interactive nature based on the reciprocal relationship that occurs between nurse and the client, family and other health professionals.
* **Open and flexible:** The flexibility of the process may be adapted to nursing practice and any setting or area of specializations dealing with individuals, groups or communities. It may be used sequentially and concurrently, the nurse may use more than one step one step at a time.
* **Client centered:** Through nursing process, the client becomes your partners in determining the goals for care. You focus on meeting individualized client needs rather than on performing specific skills or tasks. Nursing thus becomes client-oriented rather than task-oriented.
* **Planned and goal oriented:** In nursing process all activities and goals may be planned or should be set and met in nursing care goals are ranked according clients priority needs. Short-term goals are achieved with in hours and long-term goals take weeks or months to achieve.

❖ **Theoretically based:** The process is devised from a broad based knowledge including the science and humanities and can be applied to any other theoretical models of nursing. Nursing process is universally applicable it is a valuable tool that can be used in any type of practice setting or with case in any nursing situation.

Steps of Nursing Process

The nursing process has define steps as:

❖ **Assessment:** Is the deliberate systematic and logical collection of data that are helpful to identify and define the problems of the patient before the nurse proceeds to plan his care.

❖ **Nursing diagnosis:** Is a clinical judgment about individual, family or community responses to actual or potential problems/life process. Nursing diagnosis provides the base for selection of nursing inter actions to achieve for which the nursing is accountable.

❖ **Outcome identification/objective or goal:** According to the ANA's scope and standards of practice (2004). Outcome identification refers to formulating and documenting measurable, realistic, client-focused goals. Identification of outcomes, including client goals and outcome criteria, is an integral part of the nursing process.

❖ **Planning:** There is planning of activities to promote healthy client response to prevent, correct or reduce unhealthy client response.

❖ **Implementation:** This phase consists of giving actual nursing care to assist client to achieve desired goals carrying out the plan of care, continuing data collection and modifying the plan of care as needed for documenting care.

❖ **Evaluation:** The nurse is responsible for evaluating the care that has been provided by making a judgment about the effectiveness of the nursing care.

Elements of Nursing Process

Basic knowledge of the discipline of nursing and its distinct qualities appear to fall into five elements:

1. The first element is the continuous the mastery of human relation, including the mastery of teaching and managerial skills needed to take care of patients.

2. The second element is the ability to observe and report with clarity, signs, symptoms, and would include the mastery of basic communication skills.

3. The third element is the ability to interpret the signs and symptoms which comprise the deviation from health and constitute nursing problems. The deviation from health usually is identified from one more signs and symptoms, which the nurse has observed. They involve nursing problems. Thus a nursing problem exists in a situation involving patient care, a possible solution to which is found through the services which are the function of nursing.

4. Fourth element requires the analysis of nursing problems which will guide the nurse in carrying out nursing function, and the selection of the necessary course of action which will help the patient to attain a goal that is realistic for him, as she plans for total patient care.

5. The fifth is the organization of her efforts to assure the desired outcome. Effective patient care would thus result when the nurse is able to help the patient to return to help or what can be approximate normal health for him. This process may be referred to as nursing diagnosis and treatment.

The nursing process is really not as complicated as it seems. It consists of basically five steps. Originally, Ms. Orlando had four, but through practical application over the past 40 years, one step evolved into two and now there are five. All nursing personnel take part in the nursing process. The RN has the primary responsibility however.

The five steps:
1. Assessment
2. Diagnosis
3. Planning
4. Implementation
5. Evaluation

Nursing assessment and the formulation of nursing diagnosis initiate the planning step of the nursing process. Planning is a category of nursing behavior in which client-centered goals are established and strategies are designed to achieve the goals.

Setting goals to improve the outcomes for the patient is a primary focus of the nursing process. Based on the nursing diagnoses, what are the expectations for this patient? *This not about nursing goals.* They are patient goals. This is about improving the health status and quality of life for your patient. This is about what your patient needs to do to improve his health status and/or better cope with his illness.

Assessment

Assessment is the first step of the nursing process (and the first *Standard of Practice* set by the American Nurses Association). This standard is defined as, "The registered nurse collects pertinent data and information relative to the health care consumer's health or the situation." This includes collecting "pertinent data related to the health and quality of life in a systematic, ongoing manner, with compassion and respect for the wholeness, inherent dignity, worth, and unique attributes of every person, including but not limited to, demographics, environmental and occupational exposures, social determinants of health, health disparities, physical, functional, psychosocial, emotional, cognitive, spiritual/transpersonal, sexual, sociocultural, age-related, environmental, and lifestyle/economic assessments."

A nursing assessment is a process of gathering relevant patient information by a registered nurse. The information can describe the patient's physical, psychological, sociological and spiritual situation and is usually the first step in the nursing process. The process consists of collecting the data and applying medical and critical thinking skills to create a care plan for the respective patient, based on their exact needs.
The nursing assessment is the first step of the nursing process.

Nurses assess patients to gather clues, make generalizations, and diagnose human responses to health conditions and life processes. Patient data is considered either subjective or objective, and it can be collected from multiple sources.

Sources of Assessment Data

There are three sources of assessment data: interview, physical examination, and review of laboratory or diagnostic test results.
1. **Interviewing:** Interviewing includes asking the patient questions, listening, and observing verbal and nonverbal communication. Reviewing the chart prior to interviewing the patient

may eliminate redundancy in the interview process and allows the nurse to hone in on the most significant areas of concern or need for clarification. However, if information in the chart does not make sense or is incomplete, the nurse should use the interview process to verify data with the patient.

After performing patient identification, the best way to initiate a caring relationship is to introduce yourself to the patient and explain your role.

Share the purpose of your interview and the approximate time it will take. When beginning an interview, it may be helpful to start with questions related to the patient's **medical diagnoses** to gather information about how they have affected the patient's functioning, relationships, and lifestyle.

Listen carefully and ask for clarification when something isn't clear to you. Patients may not volunteer important information because they don't realize it is important for their care. By using critical thinking and active listening, you may discover valuable cues that are important to provide safe, quality nursing care.

Sometimes nursing students can feel uncomfortable having difficult conversations or asking personal questions due to generational or other cultural differences. Don't shy away from asking about information that is important to know for safe patient care. Most patients will be grateful that you cared enough to ask and listen.

Be alert and attentive to how the patient answers questions, as well as when they do not answer a question. Nonverbal communication and body language can be cues to important information that requires further investigation. A keen sense of observation is important. To avoid making inappropriate **inferences**, the nurse should validate any cues. For example, a nurse may make an inference that a patient is depressed when the patient avoids making eye contact during an interview. However, upon further questioning, the nurse may discover that the patient's cultural background believes direct eye contact to be disrespectful and this is why they are avoiding eye contact.

2. **Physical examination:** A physical examination is a systematic data collection method of the body that uses the techniques of inspection, auscultation, palpation, and percussion. Inspection is the observation of a patient's anatomical structures. Auscultation is listening to sounds, such as heart, lung, and bowel sounds, created by organs using a stethoscope. Palpation is the use of touch to evaluate organs for size, location, or tenderness. Percussion is an advanced physical examination technique typically performed by providers where body parts are tapped with fingers to determine their size and if fluid is present. Physical examination also includes the collection and analysis of vital signs.

   Registered Nurses (RNs) complete the initial physical examination and analyze the findings as part of the nursing process. Collection of follow-up physical examination data can be delegated to Licensed Practical Nurses/Licensed Vocational Nurses (LPNs/LVNs), or measurements such as vital signs and weight may be delegated to trained Unlicensed Assistive Personnel (UAP) when appropriate to do so. However, the RN remains responsible for supervising these tasks, analyzing the findings, and ensuring they are documented.

   A physical examination can be performed as a comprehensive, head-to-toe assessment or as a focused assessment related to a particular condition or problem. Assessment data is documented in the patient's Electronic Medical Record (EMR), an electronic version of the patient's medical chart.

3. **Reviewing laboratory and diagnostic test results:** Reviewing laboratory and diagnostic test results provides relevant and useful information related to the needs of the patient.

Understanding how normal and abnormal results affect patient care is important when implementing the nursing care plan and administering provider prescriptions. If results cause concern, it is the nurse's responsibility to notify the provider and verify the appropriateness of prescriptions based on the patient's current status before implementing them.

Types of Nursing Assessment

* **Initial assessment/survey:** Used during every patient encounter to briefly evaluate level of consciousness, airway, breathing, and circulation and implement emergency care if needed.
  * **Admission assessment:** A comprehensive assessment completed when a patient is admitted to a facility that involves assessing a large amount of information using an organized approach.
  * **Ongoing assessment:** In acute care agencies such as hospitals, a head-to-toe assessment is completed and documented at least once every shift. Any changes in patient condition are reported to the health care provider.
* **Focus assessment:** Focused assessments are used to reevaluate the status of a previously diagnosed problem.
* **Time lapsed assessment:** Time-lapsed reassessments are used in long-term care facilities when three or more months have elapsed since the previous assessment to evaluate progress on previously identified outcomes.
* **Emergency assessment:** The emergency assessment is performed during emergency procedures, when it is crucial to evaluate the patient's airway, breathing and circulation, as well as the exact cause of the problem. Emergency assessments can take place outside typical healthcare settings and in these situations the registered nurse must also make sure that no other people are negatively affected by the emergency rescue process. If the emergency assessment is a success and the patient's vital signs are stabilized, the next step is usually a focused assessment.

Nursing Diagnosis

* Nursing diagnosis are judgements or conclusions reached by nurses after analyzing the data base that indicate a potential or actual human need that you as a nurse can address.
* It is a description of current and potential problems of client that can be alleviated by nursing interventions.
* Actual problem or potential problem and factors that produced the problem. It is a statement of a client's actual potentials and factors that produced the problems.

NANDA International, originally known as the North American Nursing Diagnosis Association, was founded in 1982. The purpose of NANDA is to develop standardized terminology so nurses can have a common language to communicate the needs of their patients and more easily understand what needs to be done for patients.

NANDA members perform research, refining and setting criteria for each diagnosis and placing each in its proper place with the taxonomy of nursing diagnoses. Once the new terminology is finalized, NANDA distributes the new information to nurses worldwide.

A nursing diagnosis is a part of the nursing process and is a clinical judgment that helps nurses determine the plan of care for their patients. These diagnoses drive possible interventions for the patient, family, and community. They are developed with thoughtful consideration of a patient's physical assessment and can help measure outcomes for the nursing care plan. Here, we'll explore the NANDA nursing diagnosis list, examples of nursing diagnoses, and the four types.

Some nurses may see nursing diagnoses as outdated and arduous. However, it is an essential tool that promotes patient safety by utilizing evidence-based nursing research.

According to NANDA-I, the official definition of the nursing diagnosis is:

"Nursing diagnosis is a clinical judgment about individual, family, or community responses to actual or potential health problems/life processes. A nursing diagnosis provides the basis for selection of nursing interventions to achieve outcomes for which the nurse is accountable."

Nursing Diagnosis Components

The three main components of a nursing diagnosis are as follows:
1. Problem and its definition
2. Etiology
3. Defining characteristics or risk factors

Examples of proper nursing diagnoses may include:

"Ineffective breathing patterns related to pulmonary hypoplasia as evidenced by intermittent subcostal and intercostal retractions, tachypnea, abdominal breathing, and the need for ongoing oxygen support."

or

"Ineffective airway clearance related to gastroesophageal reflux as evidenced by retching, upper airway congestion, and persistent coughing."

Purpose of a Nursing Diagnosis

According to NANDA International, a nursing diagnosis is "a judgment based on a comprehensive nursing assessment." The nursing diagnosis is based on the patient's current situation and health assessment, allowing nurses and other healthcare providers to see a patient's care from a holistic perspective.

NANDA Diagnosis

NANDA diagnoses help strengthen a nurse's awareness, professional role, and professional abilities.

Formed in 1982, NANDA is a professional organization that develops research, disseminates, and refines the nursing terminology of nursing diagnosis. Originally an acronym for the North American Nursing Diagnosis Association, NANDA was renamed to NANDA International in 2002 as a response to its broadening worldwide membership.

NANDA International's mission is to:
- Provide the world's leading evidence-based nursing diagnoses for use in practice and to determine interventions and outcomes
- Contribute to patient safety through the integration of evidence-based terminology into clinical practice and clinical decision-making
- Fund research through the NANDA-I Foundation
- Be a supportive and energetic global network of nurses, who are committed to improving the quality of nursing care and improvement of patient safety through evidence-based practice.

The Four Types of Nursing Diagnoses

According to NANDA-I, there are four types of nursing diagnoses. They are:

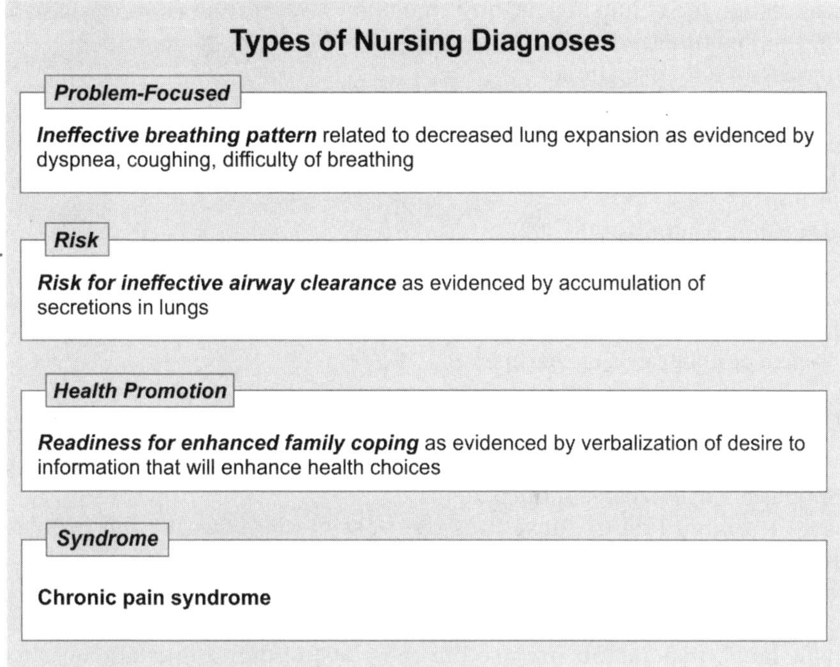

1. **Problem-focused diagnosis:** A patient problem present during a nursing assessment is known as a problem-focused diagnosis. Generally, the problem is seen throughout several shifts or a patient's entire hospitalization. However, it may be resolved during a shift depending on the nursing and medical care.
   Problem-focused diagnoses have three components:
   a. Nursing diagnosis
   b. Related factors
   c. Defining characteristics
   Examples of this type of nursing diagnosis include:
   - Decreased cardiac output
   - Chronic functional constipation
   - Impaired gas exchange
   Problem-focused nursing diagnoses are typically based on signs and symptoms present in the patient. They are the most common nursing diagnoses and the easiest to identify.
2. **Risk nursing diagnosis:** A risk nursing diagnosis applies when risk factors require intervention from the nurse and healthcare team prior to a real problem developing.
   Examples of this type of nursing diagnosis include:
   - Risk for imbalanced fluid volume
   - Risk for ineffective childbearing process
   - Risk for impaired oral mucous membrane integrity

This type of diagnosis often requires clinical reasoning and nursing judgment.

3. **Health promotion diagnosis:** The goal of a health promotion nursing diagnosis is to improve the overall well-being of an individual, family, or community.

   Examples of this type of nursing diagnosis include:
   - Readiness for enhanced family processes
   - Readiness for enhanced hope
   - Sedentary lifestyle

4. **Syndrome diagnosis:** A syndrome diagnosis refers to a cluster of nursing diagnoses that occur in a pattern or can all be addressed through the same or similar nursing interventions.

   Examples of this diagnosis include:
   - Decreased cardiac output
   - Decreased cardiac tissue perfusion
   - Ineffective cerebral tissue perfusion
   - Ineffective peripheral tissue perfusion

Defining Characteristics or Risk Factors

- ❖ The problem statement explains the patient's current health problem and the nursing interventions needed to care for the patient.
- ❖ Etiology, or related factors, describes the possible reasons for the problem or the conditions in which it developed. These related factors guide the appropriate nursing interventions.
- ❖ Finally, defining characteristics are signs and symptoms that allow for applying a specific diagnostic label. Risk factors are used in the place of defining characteristics for risk nursing diagnosis. They refer to factors that increase the patient's vulnerability to health problems.

Writing a Nursing Diagnosis

Problem-focused and risk diagnoses are the most difficult nursing diagnoses to write because they have multiple parts. According to NANDA-I, the simplest ways to write these nursing diagnoses are as follows:

Problem-Focused Diagnosis

Problem-Focused Diagnosis related to _________________________ (Related Factors) as evidenced by _________________________ (Defining Characteristics).

Risk Diagnosis

The correct statement for a NANDA-I nursing diagnosis would be: Risk for _____________ as evidenced by _________________________ (Risk Factors).

Classification of nursing diagnoses

NANDA-I adopted the Taxonomy II after consideration and collaboration with the National Library of Medicine (NLM) in regards to healthcare terminology codes. Taxonomy II has three levels: domains, classes, and nursing diagnoses.

There are currently 13 domains and 47 classes:

Domain 1: Health promotion
1. Health awareness
2. Health management

Domain 2: Nutrition
3. Ingestion
4. Digestion
5. Absorption
6. Metabolism
7. Hydration

Domain 3: Elimination/exchange
8. Urinary function
9. Gastrointestinal function
10. Integumentary function
11. Respiratory function

Domain 4: Activity/rest
12. Sleep/rest
13. Activity/exercise
14. Energy balance
15. Cardiovascular—pulmonary responses
16. Self-care

Domain 5: Perception/cognition
17. Attention
18. Orientation
19. Sensation/perception
20. Cognition
21. Communication

Domain 6: Self-perception
22. Self-concept
23. Self-esteem
24. Body image

Domain 7: Role relationship
25. Caregiving roles
26. Family relationships
27. Role performance

Domain 8: Sexuality
28. Sexual identity
29. Sexual function
30. Reproduction

Domain 9: Coping/stress tolerance
31. Post-trauma responses
32. Coping response
33. Neuro-behavioral stress

Classification of Nursing Diagnoses

Domain	Health promotion	Nutrition	Elimination/ exchange	Activity/ rest	Perception/ cognition	Self-perception	Role relationship	Sexuality	Coping/stress tolerance	Life principles	Safety/ protection	Comfort	Growth/ development
Class 1	Health awareness	Ingestion	Urinary/ function	Sleep/rest	Attention	Self-concept	Caregiving roles	Sexual identity	Post-trauma responses	Values	Infection	Physical comfort	Growth
Class 2	Health management	Digestion	Gastrointestinal function	Activity/ exercise	Orientation	Self-esteem	Family relationships	Sexual function	Coping responses	Beliefs	Physical injury	Environmental comfort	Development
Class 3		Absorption	Integumentary function	Energy balance	Sensation/ perception	Body image	Role performance	Reproduction	Neuro-behavioral stress	Value/belief/ action congruence	Violence	Social comfort	
Class 4		Metabolism	Respiratory function	Cardio-vascular/ pulmonary responses	Cognition						Environmental hazards		
Class 5		Hydration		Self-care	Communi-cation						Defensive processes		
Class 6											Thermo-regulation		

Domain 10: Life principles
34. Values
35. Beliefs
36. Value/belief action congruence

Domain 11: Safety/protection
37. Infection
38. Physical injury
39. Violence
40. Environmental hazards
41. Defensive processes
42. Thermoregulation

Domain 12: Comfort
43. Physical comfort
44. Environmental comfort
45. Social comfort

Domain 13: Growth/development
46. Growth
47. Development

NANDA-I nursing diagnoses and Taxonomy II comply with the International Standards Organization (ISO) terminology model for a nursing diagnosis.

The terminology is also registered with Health Level Seven International (HL7), an international healthcare informatics standard that allows for nursing diagnoses to be identified in specific electronic messages among different clinical information systems.

Nursing Diagnosis vs Medical Diagnosis vs Collaborative Problems

While all important, the nursing diagnosis is primarily handled through specific nursing interventions while a medical diagnosis is made by a physician or advanced healthcare practitioner.

The nursing diagnosis can be mental, spiritual, psychosocial, and/or physical. It focuses on the overall care of the patient while the medical diagnosis involves the medical aspect of the patient's condition.

A medical diagnosis does not change if the condition is resolved, and it remains part of the patient's health history forever. A nursing diagnosis, however, generally refers to a specific period of time.

Examples of medical diagnosis include:
❖ Arthritis
❖ Congestive heart failure
❖ Diabetes insipidus
❖ Meningitis
❖ Scoliosis
❖ Stroke

Collaborative problems are ones that can be resolved or worked on through both nursing and medical interventions. Oftentimes, nurses will monitor the problems while the medical providers prescribe medications or obtain diagnostic tests.

History of Nursing Diagnosis

1973: The first conference to identify nursing knowledge and a classification system; NANDA was founded

1977: First Canadian Conference takes place in Toronto

1982: NANDA formed with members from the United States and Canada

1984: NANDA established a Diagnosis Review Committee

1987: American Nurses Association (ANA) officially recognizes NANDA to govern the development of a classification system for nursing diagnosis

1987: International Nursing Conference held in Alberta, Canada

1990: 9th NANDA conference and the official definition of the nursing diagnosis established

1997: Official journal renamed from "Nursing Diagnosis" to "Nursing Diagnosis: The International Journal of Nursing Terminologies and Classifications"

2002: NANDA changes to NANDA International (NANDA-I) and Taxonomy II released

2020: 244 NANDA-I approved diagnosis

American Nursing Diagnosis vs International Nursing Diagnosis

There is currently no difference between American nursing diagnoses and international nursing diagnoses. Because NANDA-I is an international organization, the approved nursing diagnoses are the same.

Discrepancies may occur when the translation of a nursing diagnosis into another language alters the syntax and structure. However, since there are NANDA-I offices around the world, the non-English nursing diagnoses are essentially the same.

Nursing Diagnosis List

Additional examples include:
- Dysfunctional ventilatory weaning response
- Impaired transferability
- Activity intolerance
- Situational low self-esteem
- Risk for disturbed maternal-fetal dyad
- Impaired emancipated decision-making
- Risk for impaired skin integrity
- Risk for metabolic imbalance syndrome
- Urge urinary incontinence
- Risk for unstable blood pressure
- Impaired verbal communication
- Acute confusion
- Disturbed body image
- Relocation stress syndrome
- Ineffective role performance
- Readiness for enhanced sleep

Guidelines for Formulating Nursing Diagnosis

In writing nursing diagnostic statements, describe an individual's health status and the factors that have contributed to the status.

Each diagnostic label has **three components:**

Title (label): Offers a concise description of the health problem.

Defining characteristics: Cluster of signs and symptoms that are often seen with that particular diagnosis.

Etiological and contributive factors: Identifies those situational, pathophysiological and maturational factors that can cause or contribute to the problem.

Writing diagnostic statements for actual nursing diagnosis
Three part statement that includes problem, cause or etiology and signs and symptoms (defining characteristics).

Rule: Link the problem and its etiology using "related to" add "as manifested by" or "as evidenced by" and state major signs and symptoms (that validate that diagnosis exist).
   Example: Fluid volume excess related to inability of kidney to excrete waste products as manifested by edema, weight gain, decreased urine output, SOB, abnormal breath sounds, JVD.

Writing diagnostic statement for potential nursing diagnosis
Two part statement, high risk factors present but there are no signs and symptoms.
   Example: Potential for impaired skin integrity related to prolong immobility.

Rule: State potential problem adding 'related to' to link problem with contributing factors.

Writing diagnostic statement for possible nursing diagnosis
Two part statement
❖ You suspect a nursing diagnosis but here is no adequate information
❖ Label it as a possible nursing diagnosis.

Rule: State possible problem adding 'related to' to link it with possible contributive factors.
   Example: Possible spiritual distress related to terminal/chronic illness (cancer).

Plan of care: Gather more data to determine whether diagnosis is actually present.

Nursing Diagnosis vs Medical Diagnosis

A nursing diagnosis is a diagnosis that is based upon the response of the patient to the medical condition. This is why it is called a 'nursing diagnosis' because these are things that have a specific action that is related to what nurses have autonomy to take action about. Nurses treat the patient with everything that is related to human response to a specific disease. This includes anything that is a physical, mental, and spiritual type of response. Simply put, a nursing diagnosis is care focused.

A medical diagnosis, on the other hand, deals more with the medical condition. Any diagnosis or finding made by the doctor is based on the physiologic state of the patient, or his medical condition. Moreover, the diagnosis of a doctor focuses on the illness itself. As much as possible, through experience and know-how, the exact and precise clinical entity that might be the possible cause of the illness will then be tackled by the doctor, hence, giving the proper medication that would cure the illness.

Writing Diagnostic Statements

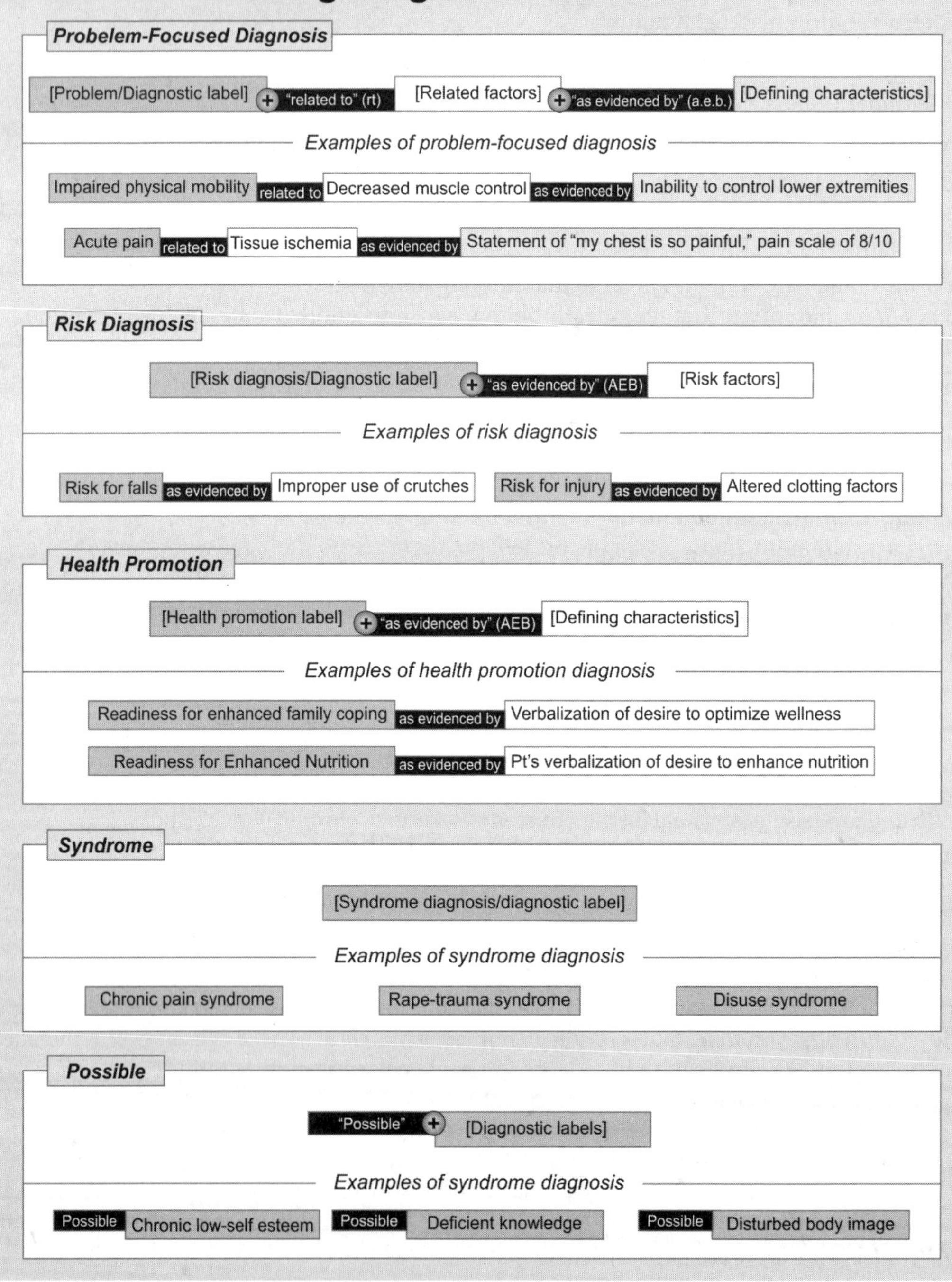

Steps	Nursing diagnosis	Collaborative problem and medical diagnosis
Focus of assessment activities	Main focus is upon monitoring **human responses** to actual and potential health problems	Main focus is on monitoring for **pathophysiological response** of body organs or systems
Problem identification	Nurse identifies and validates that problem exists independently	• Nurse may identify problem but is **required to refer** to physician for validation that problem exists • Nurse may not be qualified to diagnose exact nature of problems, but **refers abnormal data** to the physician
Treatment	Nurse initiates interventions for treatment independently	• Nurse **collaborates with the physician** to initiate intervention for treatment • Nurse may have **standing orders to initiate diagnostic studies** or treatment for the problem without physician order

PLANNING

Definition

Planning is the deliberate and systematic phase of the nursing process that involves decision making and problem solving.

In planning the nurse refers to the client's assessment data and diagnostic statements for direction in formulating client goals and designing the nursing strategies required to prevent, reduce, or eliminate the client's health problems. During planning, priorities are set, goals are determined, expected outcomes are developed and a nursing care plan is formulated.

Although planning is basically the nurse's responsibility, input from the client and support persons is essential if a plan is to be effective. In addition to collaborating with the client and family, the nurse consults with other members of the health care team, reviews pertinent literature, modifies care, and records relevant information about the client's health care needs and clinical management.

Type of Planning

Planning begins with the first client contact and continues until the nurse-client relationship ends, usually when the client is discharged from the health care agency.

The types of planning include:
❖ Initial planning
❖ Ongoing planning, and
❖ Discharge planning

Initial Planning

The nurse who performs the admission assessment usually develops the initial comprehensive plan of care. This nurse has the benefit of the client's body language as well as some intuitive kinds of information that are not available solely from the written database.

Planning should be initiated as soon as possible after the initial assessment, especially because of the trend toward shorter hospital stays.

Ongoing Planning

Ongoing planning is done by all nurses who work with the client. As nurses obtain new information and evaluate the client's response to care, they can individualize the initial care plan further. Ongoing planning also occurs at the beginning of a shift as the nurse plans the care to be given that day. Using ongoing assessment data, the nurse carries out daily planning for the following purposes:

❖ To determine whether the client's health status has changed.
❖ To set priorities for the client's care during the shift.
❖ To decide which problems to focus on during the shift.
❖ To coordinate the nurse's activities so that more than one problem can be addressed at each client contact.

Discharge Planning

Discharge planning, the process of anticipating and planning for needs after discharge, is a crucial part of comprehensive health care and should be addresses in each client's care plan. Because the average stay of clients in acute care hospitals has become shorter, people are sometimes discharged still needing care. Although, many clients are discharged to other agencies (e.g., Nursing homes), such care is increasingly being delivered in the home.

Effective discharge planning begins at first client contact and involves comprehensive and ongoing assessment to obtain information about the client's ongoing needs.

The Planning Process

In the process of developing client care plans, the nurse engages in the following activities:

❖ Setting priorities
❖ Establishing client's goals/desired outcomes
❖ Selecting nursing interventions
❖ Write the plan of care

Setting Priorities

After formulating specific nursing diagnosis, the nurse establishes the priorities of the diagnoses by ranking them in order of importance. Priorities of care are established so that the nurse can best direct health care resources when a client has multiple problems or alterations.

Establishing priorities is not merely a matter of numbering the nursing diagnosis on the basis of severity or physiological importance. Rather, it is a method by which the nurse and the client mutually rank the diagnoses in order of importance based on the client's desires, needs, and safety.

Because clients have multiple diagnoses, the nurse is not able to treat all of them when they are identified. The nurse selects mutually agreed priorities based on the urgency of the problem, the nature of the treatment indicated, and the interaction among the diagnoses. Priorities are classified as high, intermediate or medium, and low.

Nursing diagnoses that, if untreated, could result in harm to the client or others have the *highest priorities*. For example, Life threatening problems, such as loss of respiratory or cardiac function. High priorities occur in the psychological dimensions, and the nurse should avoid classifying only physiological nursing diagnoses as high priority.

Intermediate or medium priority nursing diagnoses involve the nonemergency, non-life-threatening needs of the client. Or else we can call it as the health threatening problems, such as acute illness and decreased coping ability because they may result in delayed development or cause destructive physical or emotional changes.

Low- priority nursing diagnoses are client needs that may not be directly related to a specific illness or prognosis but may affect their future well-being. A Low- priority problem is one that arises from normal developmental needs or that requires only minimal nursing support.

Whenever possible, the client should be involved in priority setting and subsequent goal setting. In some situations the client and nurse assign different priority ranking to the nursing diagnoses.

It is not necessary to resolve all high priority diagnoses before addressing others. The nurse may partially address a high priority diagnosis and then deal with a diagnosis of lesser priority. Furthermore, because clients usually have several problems, the nurse often deals with more than one diagnosis at a time.

Priorities change as the client's responses, problems, and therapies change. The nurse must consider a variety of factors when assigning priorities. These include the following:

1. ***Client's health values and beliefs:*** Values concerning health may be more important to the nurse than to the client. For example, a client may believe being home for the children to be more urgent than a health problem. When there is such a difference of opinion, the client and nurse should discuss it openly to resolve any conflict. However, in a life-threatening situation the nurse usually must take the initiative.

2. ***Client's priorities:*** Involving the client in prioritizing and care planning enhances cooperation. Sometimes, however, the client's perception of what is important conflicts with the nurse's knowledge of potential problems or complications. For example, an elderly client may not regard turning and repositioning in bed as important, preferring to be undisturbed. The nurse, however, aware of the potential complications of prolonged bed rest (e.g., muscle weakness and decubitus ulcers), needs to inform the client and carry out these necessary interventions.

3. ***Resources available to the nurses and client:*** If money, equipment, or personnel are scarce in a health care agency, then problem may be given a lower priority than usual. Nurses in a home setting, for example, do not have the resources of a hospital. If the necessary resources are not available, the solution of the problem might need to be postponed, or the client may need referral. Client resources, such as finances or coping ability, may also influence the setting of priorities. For example, a client who is unemployed may defer dental treatment; a client whose husband is terminally ill and dependent on her may feel unable to cope with nutritional guidance directed toward losing weight.

4. ***Urgency of the health problem:*** Regardless of the framework used, life-threatening situations require that the nurse assign them high priority. For example, for an anxious child ineffective airway clearance may be the higher priority. Situations that affect the integrity of the client, that is, those that could have a negative or destructive effect on the client, also have high priority. Such health problems as drug abuse and radical alteration of self-concept due to amputation can be destructive both to the individual and to the family.

5. ***Medical treatment plan:*** The priorities for treating health problems must be congruent with treatment by other health professionals. For example, a high priority for the client might be to become ambulatory; however, if the physician's therapeutic regimen calls for extended bed rest, then ambulation must assume a lower priority or teach exercises to facilitate ambulation later, provided the client's health permits. The nursing diagnosis related to ambulation is not ignored; it is merely deferred.

Guidelines for setting priorities:

❖ Those problems that involve actual or life-threatening concerns are considered prior to actual or potential health-threatening concerns.

❖ Consideration must be given to time constraints and to the human and material resources available.

❖ Those diagnosis that the client identifies as important must be given high priority and consideration by the nurse.

❖ Priority setting is guided by theories, models, and principles that provide the standard of comparison for evaluating the list of nursing diagnosis.

Establishing Client's Goals/Desired Outcomes

After establishing priorities, the nurse and client set goals for each nursing diagnosis. Goals and expected outcomes are specific statements of client behaviors or responses that the nurse anticipates from nursing care. The term goal and desired outcome are used interchangeably.

Some nursing literature differentiates the terms by defining *goals* as broad statements about the client's status and *desired outcomes* as the more specific, observable criteria used to evaluate whether the goals have been met, e.g.:

Goal (broad)   : Improve nutritional status
Desired outcome (specific)   : Gain 2 kg by April 25

When goals are stated broadly, as in this example, the care plan must include both goals and desired outcomes. They are sometimes combined into one statement linked by the words "as evidenced by", as follows:

"Improved nutritional status as evidenced by weight gain of 2 kg by April 25."

Writing the broad, general goal first may help students to think of the specific outcomes that are needed, but the goal is just a starting point for planning. It is the specific, observable outcomes that must be written on the care plan and used to evaluate client progress.

Goals of care: Individual nursing diagnosis and priority setting help determine the goals of care. Goals are defining as "guideposts to the selection of nursing interventions and criteria in the evaluation of nursing interventions". Setting goals in an activity that includes the client and family or significant others.

Nursing goals are established according to nursing diagnosis and priority setting established by the client and nurse. The nursing diagnosis formulated are based on the client's response and perception of changes in level of wellness , activities of daily living, life style patterns and role performance. Because each person responds uniquely to a situation, the nursing diagnoses and client goals of health care are also unique.

Role of the client in goal setting: A client centered goal is a specific and measurable objective designed to reflect the client's highest level of wellness and independence in function. Client centered goals are mutually set between the nurse and client. When developing goals, the nurse can act as an advocate for the client to ensure that the goals are realistic and to prevent further deterioration in the level of wellbeing or of the cognitive and physical functioning.

Short-term goals: A short-term goal is an objective that is expected to be achieved in a short period of time, usually less than a week. With the present health care system and shorter hospital stays, short-term goals are the direction for a client with ineffective airway clearance, for example may be "return of normal lung sounds within 2 days".

Long-term goals: A long-term goal is an objective that is expected to be achieved over a longer period of time, usually over weeks or months. Long-term goals are appropriate for some clients in rehabilitation, mental health, ambulatory care, and community nursing settings. For example, a long-term goal for a client with an ineffective airway clearance may be to "remain free of upper respiratory infection for 6 months".

Expected outcomes: Expected outcomes should be specified before an intervention is selected. An expected outcome is the specific, step-by-step objective that leads to attainment of the goal and the resolution of the etiology for the nursing diagnosis. An outcome is the measurable criterion against which to judge the success of a nursing intervention. The outcome represents the observable or measurable client response to nursing care. Outcomes are the desired responses of client condition in the physiological, social, emotional, developmental, or spiritual dimensions.

In addition, expected outcomes have other functions. Projected before nursing actions are formulated, expected outcomes provide a direction for nursing activities. Second, they also provide a projected time span for goal attainment. Finally, the nurse uses expected outcomes as criteria to evaluate the effectiveness of nursing activities.

Characteristics of outcome statements:
- ❖ Be focused on the client, for it is the client who must achieve the designated outcome.
- ❖ Be concise and explicit. The statement should be clear to the members of the health care team.
- ❖ Reflect a mutual agreement between the client and the nurse. The desired outcome should be decided by both the client and the nurse, if possible.
- ❖ Be observable and measurable. Effectiveness of the nursing care plan is determined by the evaluation of the client's responses after care is rendered.
- ❖ Be realistic. Consideration must be given to the client's physical abilities, growth and development, mental status, and usual coping abilities.
- ❖ Have a specified time limit. The outcome statement should contain the time frame for achievement of the objective.

Components of outcomes:
- ❖ **Subject:** Who is the person expected to achieve the outcome?
- ❖ **Verb:** What actions must the person take to achieve the outcome?
- ❖ **Condition:** Under what circumstances is the person to perform the actions?
- ❖ **Performance criteria:** How well is the person to perform the actions?
- ❖ **Target time:** By when is the person expected to be able to perform the actions?

Guidelines for writing goals and expected outcomes: The goal should be written as a positive measure that indicates the absence of the problem. There are seven guidelines for writing goals and expected outcome:
1. Client centered
2. Singular factors
3. Observable factors
4. Measurable factors

5. Time limited factors
6. Mutual factors
7. Realistic factors

Selecting Nursing Interventions

A nursing intervention are those action performed by the nurse that helps the client achieve the results specified by the goals and expected outcomes. The specific strategies chosen should focus on eliminating or reducing the etiology (cause) of the nursing diagnosis, which is the second clause of the diagnostic statement.

When it is not possible to change the etiologic factors, the nurse chooses interventions to treat the signs and symptoms or the defining characteristics in NANDA terminology. Example for this situation would be ***Pain*** related to surgical incision and ***Anxiety*** related to unknown etiology.

Strategies for potential (risk) nursing diagnosis should focus on measures to reduce the client's risk factors, which are also found in the second clause.

Correct identification of the etiology during the diagnosis phase provides the framework for choosing successful nursing interventions. For example, the diagnostic label ***Activity intolerance*** may have several etiologies—pain, weakness, sedentary lifestyle, anxiety, or cardiac arrhythmias. Intervention will vary according to the cause of the problem.

Types of nursing interventions: A nursing intervention is "any treatment, based upon clinical judgment and knowledge that the nurse performs to enhance patient/client outcomes". Nursing interventions includes both direct and indirect care, as well as nurse-initiated, physician-initiated, and other provider-initiated treatments. *Direct care* is an intervention performed through interaction with the client. *Indirect care* is an intervention performed away from but on behalf of the client such as interdisciplinary collaboration or management of the care environment.

❖ ***Independent:*** Actions initiated by nurse that do not require direction or an order from another health care professional. They include physical care, ongoing assessment, emotional support and comfort, teaching, counseling, environmental management, and making referrals to other health care professionals.

❖ ***Interdependent:*** Actions implemented in collaborative manner by nurse in conjunction with other health care professionals such as physical therapists, social workers, dietitians, and physicians. Collaborative nursing activities reflect the overlapping responsibilities of, and collegial relationships between, health personnel. For example, the physician might order physical therapy to teach the client crutch walking. The nurse would be responsible for informing the physical therapy department and for coordinating the client's care to include the physical therapy sessions.

❖ ***Dependent:*** Actions that require an order from a physician or other health care professional. Usually call it as physician-initiated treatments. For example, medical orders commonly include orders for medications, intravenous therapy, diagnostic tests, treatments, diet, and activity.

Criteria for choosing nursing interventions: The following criteria can help the nurse choose the best nursing strategy. The planned action must be:

❖ Safe and appropriate for the individual's age, health, and condition.

❖ Achievable with the resources available.

❖ Congruent with the client's values, beliefs, and culture.

* Congruent with other therapies (e.g., if the client is not permitted food, the strategy of an evening snack must be deferred until health permits).
* Based on nursing knowledge and experience or knowledge from relevant sciences (i.e., based on a rationale).
* Within established standards of care as determined by state laws, professional associations and the policies of the institutions.

Write the Plan of Care

After choosing the appropriate nursing interventions, the nurse writes them on the care plan as nursing orders. A nursing care plan is a written guide that organizes data about a client's care into a formal statement of the strategies that will be implemented to help the client achieve optimal health.

Nursing orders are the instructions for the interventions prescribed to help achieve the stated goals and objectives.

The components of nursing orders:
* *Date:* Nursing orders are dated when they are written and reviewed regularly at intervals that depend on the individual's needs. In an intensive care unit, for example, the plan of care may be continually monitored and revised.
* *Action verb:* The verb starts the order and must be precise. For example, "Explain (to the client) the actions of insulin" is a more precise statement than "Teach (the client) about insulin".
* *Content area:* The content is the where and the what of the order. In the preceding order, "spiral bandage" and "left leg" state that what and where of the order. The content area in this example would also clarify whether the foot or toes are to be left exposed.
* *Time element:* The time element answers when, how long, or how often the nursing action is to occur. **Examples:** "Assist client with tub bath at 07.00 am daily"; or "Immense client's left arm in sterile saline soak for 1 hour."
* *Signature:* The signature of the nurse prescribing the order shows the nurse's accountability and has legal significance.

Guidelines for writing nursing orders:
* There should be a separate list of nursing orders for each nursing diagnosis and client outcome.
* There should be a sufficient number of nursing orders to address each nursing diagnosis.
* Nursing orders should be dated and signed by the nurse to indicate when the orders were written and to verify the accountability of the nurse.
* Nursing orders should be documented in ink.
* Nursing orders should include specific actions that are to be implemented and should indicate the individual who is to carry out the action.
* Nursing orders should be revised and updated as the client's health status changes.
* Nursing orders should incorporate the physician's orders and identify all nursing actions related to the implementation of physician's orders.
* The nursing plan of care should be part of the client's permanent record to document the provision of nursing interventions and the achievement of client outcomes.
* All entries on the nursing care plan of care should be done using appropriate and acceptable terminology and abbreviations.

Documentation: Documentation of the nursing plan of care in a formal record provides a clear and concise method for ensuring continuity of care. A written plan keeps all members of the health care team informed about the identified client outcomes or goals, the selected nursing interventions, and the client's progress toward achieving those outcomes. The documentation should be:

- ❖ Clear and concise
- ❖ **Appropriate terminology:** Usually on a designated form
- ❖ **Physical assessment:** Usually by review of systems
  - ◆ Overview of symptoms
  - ◆ Diet
  - ◆ Each body system
- ❖ Use patient's own words in subjective data—enclose in " ___ " (quotation marks)
- ❖ Avoid generalizations—be specific
- ❖ Don't make summative statements—describe, e.g., *patient is being ornery* should be patient resists instruction or patient states "Don't talk to me, I don't care about that".

Implementation

The planned goals and strategies are translated into nursing intervention by means of the nursing care plan. It is essential that the client and family participate in nursing care to alleviate or correct the problems and to prevent potential problems. This phase of nursing process ends when the Pursing strategies have been completed and the client's responses have been recorded.

Implementation is the initiation/carrying out of the nursing care plan to achieve specific outcomes. Specific nursing interventions are implemented to modify factors contributing to client's problems

Prerequisites

- ❖ Positive attitude and acceptance of client's observation skills
- ❖ Technical skills, ability to use resources
- ❖ Communication abilities
- ❖ Teaching learning skills
- ❖ Counselling skills

Steps

- ❖ Preparation
- ❖ Action/intervention
- ❖ Documentation

Preparation

- ❖ Review the nursing interventions identified in the planning phase.
- ❖ Analyze the client's potentials/abilities and how much nursing assistance would be required.
- ❖ Recognize the potential complications associated with specific nursing activities.
- ❖ Determine and provide necessary resources: Personnel, material/equipment. Identify the level of knowledge and type of skills required by personnel to perform.
- ❖ Prepare an environment conducive to the types of activities required.
- ❖ Identify the ethical and legal concerns associated with intervention. Follow hospital policy.

❖ Use appropriate nursing care approach/care delivery system to achieve outcomes, e.g., functional nursing, team nursing, primary nursing, case management; individualized critical care/progressive patient care, etc.

Action/Intervention

❖ Make a quick assessment of the client and environment just before the intervention. **Example:** Nursing intervention required ambulation of post-operative client. You notice that the client is short of breath and diaphoretic based on this observation. You must check the vital signs and postpone ambulation at that time.
❖ Carry out preventive/promotive/corrective (curative) rehabilitative or palliative nursing actions to eliminate the related factors in nursing diagnosis.
❖ Recognize independent; inter dependent and dependent nursing actions. Collaborate with other nursing team members (nurse specialist) doctors, dietitian, physiotherapist, anesthetist, technician, psychologist, medical social worker and others associated with care of client.
❖ Use various opportunities for communicating teaching and supporting client.
❖ Refer to nursing prescriptions/hospital or unit protocols/procedure manual/nursing standards for carrying out appropriate nursing interventions. Select standard protocols from a computerized menu.

These recordings must be related to:
❖ Nursing diagnosis
❖ Nursing actions
❖ Clients responses
❖ Additional important information
Recording is done in an objective and concise manner as it is the basis for evaluation of the nursing care plan.

NURSING PROCESS: EVALUATION

Introduction

Evaluation is a fifth and last phase of nursing process. It is on-going and occurs when the nurse has contact with the client. The emphasis on client outcomes which are set in the planning phase of nursing process. Evaluation is an important aspect in the nursing process because conclusions drawn from the evaluation determine whether the nursing interventions should terminate, continued or changed.

Evaluation is continuous. Evaluation is done while or immediately after implementing a nursing order or nursing interventions enables the nurse to make spot modifications in an interventions. Evaluation reformed at specified intervals (e.g., after one week for the home care client) shows the extent of progress towards goal achievement and enables the nurse to correct any deficiencies and modify care plan as needed.

Another aspect of evaluation involves measurement of the quality of nursing care provided in a health care setting. It ensures quality professional nursing practice.

I. **Historical perspective of evaluation:** In the last two decades, evaluation of health care delivery has changed. Previously client evaluation was formally the prerogative (control or right) of physician. With new legislation and interest among all health care providers, evaluations are now performed by each profession.

Traditionally nurses were evaluated by their supervisors in terms of skills, organization, leadership, dependability and punctuality. Later on these evaluations did not consider the effectiveness of nursing care or improvement in the client's health status. Nurses recognized the need to change their focus and improve their methods.

In 1990, the JCAHO (Joint Commission on Accreditation of Health Care Organization) suggested to document the evaluation, currently professional nurses use established standards of clinical nursing practice on JCAHO Standards to deliver quality care and to evaluate their ability to provide high quality care.

II. **Meaning of evaluation:** Evaluation means to judge or appraise, in nursing process evaluation means to identify whether or to what degree the client goals have been met.

III. **Definition of evaluation:**

- **According to JCAHO, 1990:** Evaluation is defined as "Analysis of collected completed and organized data pertaining to important aspects of care or service. Data are compared with threshold (a pre-established level of performance) for evaluation and variations are judged and problems or opportunities to improve care identified.

- **According to Kenny, 1996:** "Evaluation is a planned, systematic, continuous process that compares the client's health status with the desired expected outcomes".

IV. **Purposes of evaluation:** The purposes of evaluation, as described by the Open University Publication (1984) are:

- To determine whether the patient goals/expected outcomes have been achieved.
- To measure the standards of nursing care.
- To measure the quality of care.
- To discover which nursing care actions are most consistently effective in solving patient problem.
- To measure staff performance.
- Evaluation also helps to determine the effectiveness of the nursing care plan:
  ◊ Whether the patient is making positive or negative progress.
  ◊ Whether the patient is able to understand and participate in his care.
  ◊ Whether changes have to be made in care plan.
  ◊ Whether new problems have been identified and new priorities have to be set for care.
  ◊ Whether there is any change in the patient's condition
  ◊ Whether there is need to revise care plans.
  ◊ Whether the outcome of nursing care has been documented.

The process of evaluation also serves as a tool for discovering the effective nursing actions to solve particular problem in future.

V. **Characteristics of evaluation:** Evaluation always involves judgments based on knowledge and experience.

The quality of care is based on:

- *Who participates in the evaluation?*
  According to ANA (1974) Standard of Nursing Practice, the client nurse and health team members may also participate but the nurse is responsible for documenting evaluation data in client's chart.

- *What should be evaluated?*
  The client's health behaviors, which indicate progress or lack of progress towards goal attainment, are evaluated.

This broad comprehensive evaluation process includes judging the adequacy, appropriateness, effectiveness, and efficiency of each component of nursing process.

- *When should evaluation occur?*

  As evaluation is an ongoing process so it could be continuous evaluation or summative evaluation.

VI. **Types of evaluation:** The types of evaluation are of two types:

1. *Formative evaluation:* It is also called as continuous evaluation or concurrent process evaluation. It is nothing but judging or evaluating the each component of nursing process.

   Example: In assessment to evaluate is—were sufficient data collected to formulate diagnosis and plan of care?

   It may be performed by the nurse as frequently as every few minutes in critical situation, every hour, during every change of shift, daily or weekly. Formative evaluation compares the client's response with the action and the client's progress towards objectives.

   Example: An unconscious client in an acute care unit may need to be checked every 15 min whereas a chronic disability may be evaluated on a weekly schedule.

2. *Summative evaluation:* It is also called retrospective evaluation. It occurs after the client has met several objectives. The nurse judges the client's progress or lack of progress towards goal attainment.

   Sometimes objectives or resources are insufficient to attain a goal or the timetable for achieving goal is unrealistic. Occasionally the objectives may be met, but the client has not achieved the goal.

   Example: The goal may state "The client will modify his diet to lose weight" after achieving several objectives toward goal, the nurses summative evaluation may read, " The client can explain the reason for weight loss and plan appropriate menus, but lacks motivation to stay on the diet. Further counselling is needed.

VII. **Forms of evaluation:** Evaluation has been categorized according to what is to be judged and when. Three major types of evaluation describe what is to be evaluated. They are:

1. **Structure evaluation:** It focuses on the physical facilities, equipment, organizational pattern, service provided, and staffing pattern. It is the determination of health care agencies ability to provide the service offered to the client. This type of evaluation assesses the system by which nursing care is delivered. The purpose of structure evaluation is to identify any system errors in the agency, which can be corrected.

2. **Process evaluation:** It focuses on the nurses activities. The activities are judged by:

   ◊ Observing the nurses performance.

   ◊ Asking the client, what the nurse did.

   ◊ Reviewing the nurses note in the chart.

   It mainly determines whether nursing care was adequate, appropriate, effective, and efficient. There are two forms of process evaluation. Those are:

   a. **Concurrent process evaluation:** It judges nurses performance as it takes place. The nurse is observed during the interaction with client or client may be asked what the nursing action was? **Example:** A nurse may be evaluated while giving an injection on use of appropriate technique, or after client a nurse may be evaluated to determine whether specific topic were covered.

The Standard Nursing Competences Rating Scale (1975) and quality patient care (1974) are examples of tools used for concurrent process evaluation; also the clients chart may be reviewed while client receiving service in order to determine whether appropriate nursing actions are charted.

Examples of Questions are:

- Does the nurse identify the client before giving medications?
- Is the consent form signed before surgery?
- Are all procedures adequately explained to client, before procedure?
- Are all nursing actions properly performed?

b. **Retrospective process evaluation:** It judges nursing performance after service to the client have been discontinue. This evaluation can also be called as "Nursing Audit" or "Chart Review". It examines any aspect of nursing that should be documented in client's chart and determines whether specific nursing action were performed and documented.

Examples of Questions are:

- Were the client's intake and output accurately recorded?
- Were client's history and nursing physical examination recorded?
- Were all medications and treatments are signed?

3. **Outcome evaluation:** Outcome evaluation focuses on changes in client health status and response after the nursing action. There are two forms of process evaluation. Those are:

a. **Concurrent outcome evaluation:** Concurrent outcome evaluation judges the client's present status, skills, knowledge and abilities before services are discontinued. The nurse measures the client's progress by comparing the initial database with current health status in relation to goals and objectives.

The Wisconsin system, as reported by Hover and Zimer (1978) illustrated a concurrent and retrospective outcome evaluation.

Examples of Questions are:

- Can the client demonstrate crutch walking correctly?
- Can the client prepare and administer insulin accurately?
- Are the client's vital signs stable?
- Does the client relate to others appropriately?

b. **Retrospective Outcome Evaluation:** It judges the client's health status and behavior as documented in the chart after service to the client has been discontinued.

The JCAH (1985) incorporated some aspects of retrospective outcome evaluation in their guidelines.

Examples of questions are:

- Was the client's attitude positive upon discharge?
- Did the client demonstrate appropriate bonding behaviors?
- Was the client's care giver able to perform physical care activities?
- Was the client able to plan a diabetic daily menu?

VIII. Elements in each type of evaluation:

Structure	*Process*	*Outcome*
Purpose: Measure the adequacy of facility to meet client needs **Data sources:** • Policy and procedure manuals • Job descriptions • Staffing pattern • Written care plan **Sample evaluation questions:** • Does the orientation program provide nurses with information relevant to the needs of their assigned areas? • Do the nursing policies adhere to legal requirements? • Are nursing policies easily accessed by staff?	**Purpose:** Measure the adequacy of nursing activities implementing the nursing process **Data sources:** Documentation in client's record about nursing action performed **Sample evaluation questions:** Is the plan of care individualized? • Is every client assessed by a nurse upon admission to the agency? • Is the nursing care based on identified client's needs? • Is the client's response to the nursing action documented?	**Purpose:** Compare client's progress towards expected outcome **Data sources:** • Observation of client • Client interview • Chart audit • Written discharge plan **Sample evaluation questions:** Does client demonstrates new knowledge or skills? • Is there documented evidence of client progress toward achievement of expected outcome? • Is there documentation of the client abilities to cope the problem after discharge?

IX. **Methods or process of evaluation:** The evaluation has five components:

1. **Collecting data related to the desired outcomes:** Using measurable desired outcomes as a guide, the nurse collects objective and subjective data. Data must be recorded concisely and accurately to facilitate the next part of the evaluation process and to determine the extent of goal achievement.

2. **Comparing the date with outcomes:** After collecting the desired data according to expected outcome. The data must be compared with desired outcome. Both the nurse and client play an active role in comparing the client's actual response with desired outcomes. After comparing the desired outcomes the nurse can draw one of the three possible conclusions:

    a. The goal was met, i.e. client response is same as the desired outcome.

    b. The was partially met, i.e., either the short-term goal achieved but long-term goal was not, or desired outcome partially attained.

    c. The goal was not met.

    After determining whether a goal has been met, the nurse writes an evaluative statement which includes two parts, i.e., a conclusion and supporting data.

    Example: Oral intake 3,000 mL more than output; skin turgor good; mucous membrane moist.

3. **Relating nursing activities to outcomes:** The next aspect of evaluation process is determine whether the nursing activities had any to the outcome.

4. **Drawing conclusions about problem status:** The nurse uses a judgment about goal achievement to determine whether the care plan was effective in resolving the problem or preventing client's problem.

    When goal have been achieved the nurse can draw following conclusions about status of the client's problem:

    ◊ The actual problem stated in nursing diagnosis has been resolved; or potential problem is prevented and risk factor no longer exists. In these instances the nurse documents that the goals have been met and discontinued the care for the problem.

◊ The potential problem stated in nursing diagnosis has been prevented, but risk factors are present. In that case, the nurse keeps problem on the care plan.

◊ The actual problem still exists even though some goals being met. **Example:** A desired outcome on client's plan is "Will drink 3,000 mL of fluid daily". Even though data may show this outcome has been achieved but dry mucous (Oral) membrane indicate that there is a insufficient fluid volume therefore, the nursing intervention must be continued even though goal was met.

When goals have been partially met or when goals have not been met, two conclusions may be drawn:

a. The care plan needs to be revised, since the problem is partially resolved. **OR**

b. The care plan does not need revision, because client merely need more time to achieve the previously established goal.

5. **Continuing, modifying, or terminating the nursing care plan:** In this phase the nursing care plan will be either continued as it is or modified and then continued, also if the goals and criteria are met the care plan can be terminated or discontinued.

If the goals have not been met, when care plan needs modification, it can be carried out by repeating the nursing process steps to reassess, rediagnose, replan and implement replanned measures and then finally reassess the expected outcomes.

X. **Relationship of evaluation to other phases of nursing process:** Successful evaluation depends on the effectiveness of the steps which are followed before it. Assessment data must be accurate and complete so that nursing diagnosis and desired outcomes can be formulated accurately. The desired outcomes must be stated firmly in behavioral terms if they are to be useful for evaluating client's responses. Without the implementation phase evaluation is not possible.

- The evaluation and assessing are overlapping, i.e., performing a complete assessment to determine whether there are any changes in the client's status and make sure you are not missing any data.
- The evaluation in diagnoses ensures the diagnoses are accurate and complete.
- The evaluation in planning makes sure that effective plan of care, goals and interventions are appropriately set.
- The evaluation determines whether the plan of care was actually implemented and identifying factors that helped or hindered progress.
- Evaluation helps to modify or terminate the plan as indicated depending on the results of the above activities.

XI. **Guidelines for evaluation:**

- The nurse continuously monitors, appraises and reassesses the client's response to nursing actions.
- The client's response to nursing implementation is compared with the client's objectives to determine the extent to which the objectives have been achieved (Formative evaluation).
- The client's progress or lack of progress toward goal attainment is determined (Summative evaluation).
- The nursing care plan is revised to reflect changes in the client's condition or when the goals or objectives have not been adequately met.
- Documentation is an important part of evaluation.

XII. **Nursing audit:** The nursing audit means examination or review of records. It is also called as retrospective audit or chart review; these audits are usually performed by trained clerks.

The nursing audit or chart review focuses on evaluating nursing care through review of records. The success of these audits depends on accurate documentation; auditors assume that if the data have not be recorded the care has not been given.

XIII. **Evaluation and quality improvement:** Evaluation of health care is a process used to improve the quality care and service to clients. It is also known as continuous quality improvement (CQI), total quality management (TQM), performance improvement (PI) or persistent quality improvement (PQI).

According to Schroeder (1994) quality improvement is "the commitment and approach used to improve every process in every part of an organization with the intent of meeting and exceeding customer expectations and outcomes".

Quality improvement focuses on identifying and correcting a system error, such as duplication of services in a hospital setting.

The staff nurse plays an important role in quality improvement because the nurse is involved in majority of client care activities. Quality is a daily expectation of all staff nurses.

JCAHO'S (1991) 10 steps approach for quality improvement process within an organization:

1. Establish responsibility and accountability for a quality improvement program.
2. Define the scope of service for a clinical area.
3. Define the key aspects of service for clinical area.
4. Develop quality indicators to monitor the outcomes and appropriateness of care delivered.
5. Establish thresh hold for evaluation of indicators.
6. Collect and analyze data from monitoring activities.
7. Evaluate results of monitoring activities to determine the need for change in practice.
8. Resolve problems through development of action plans.
9. reevaluate to determine if the action plan was unsuccessful.
10. Communicate results of quality improvement to members of organization.

XIV. **Peer evaluation:** Peer evaluation means look closely or searchingly by the coworker. It can be used as a method of evaluating quality care. It is also referred as peer review.

- *Definitions:*
  - ◊ The process by which professionals provide to their peers critical performance appraisal and feedback that are geared toward corrective action.
  - ◊ According to ANA (1988): "Peer review in nursing is the process by which practicing registered nurses, systematically assess, ,monitor and make judgment about the quality of nursing care provided by peer. As measured against professional standards of practice".
  - ◊ According to Wakefield, Helms, 1995: "Peer review is a mechanical for evaluating the judgment of clinical care providers".
  - ◊ According to Lucille Joel, 1984: "Peer review is the basis of nursing autonomy and self-guidance".

- *Principles of effective peer evaluation:*
    - ◊ Improve quality of client care
    - ◊ Promotes professional growth
    - ◊ Is timely frequent and ongoing
    - ◊ May be verbal or written, formal or informal
    - ◊ Is not anonymous (Unidentified)
    - ◊ Is objective, i.e., addresses specific behavior
    - ◊ Is not linked to financial rewards (Salary raises) or promotional opportunities
    - ◊ Need to be documented.

UNIT

Nutritional Needs

3

UNIT OUTLINE

- Importance
- Factors affecting nutritional needs
- Assessment of nutritional status
- Review: special diets—solid, liquid, soft
- Review on therapeutic diets

- Care of patient with dysphagia
- Nutritional needs
- Enteral feeds
- TPN (Total parenteral nutrition)

LEARNING OBJECTIVES

At the end of this unit, the reader will be able to:

- Explain nutritional needs.
- Define importance and assessment of nutritional needs.
- Enumerate factors influencing nutritional needs.
- List out factors affecting nutritional needs.
- Describe special diet.
- Define therapeutic die.
- Categorize types of therapeutic diet.
- Explain care of patients with dysphagia.
- Interpret guidelines to minimize nausea.
- Explain enteral feeding.
- Define indications for enteral feeding.
- Practice assessment of nasogastric/orogastric tube.
- Administration of feeds.
- Explain jejunostomy feeding.
- Describe total parenteral nutrition.

Nutritional needs are defined as the amount and chemical form of a nutrient needed to support normal health, growth and development without disturbing the metabolism of other nutrients. Nutrient intake recommendations are based on the estimated average requirement (EAR) of a population group. Enteral and parenteral needs differ for many nutrients because of differences in bioavailability and utilization. Assuming a near-normal distribution of nutrient needs, the reference nutrient intake (RNI—also called population reference intake or recommended dietary allowance) is equal to the EAR plus two standard deviations of the distribution, with the exception of energy intake where the reference intake is equal to the EAR. The upper level (UL) is the highest level of intake where no untoward effects can be detected in virtually all individuals in a specific population group. The acceptable range of intakes (AR) is the range from the EAR to the UL that is considered safe, however preterm infants are not a homogeneous population thus intake often needs to be individualized based on clinical condition and developmental stage.

IMPORTANCE

Food and nutrition are basic indispensable needs of humans. Nutrition plays a critical role in maintaining the health and well-being of individuals and is also an essential component of the healthcare delivery system. The nutritional status of individuals affects the clinical outcomes. Essential nutrients are classified into six groups, namely carbohydrates, proteins, lipids, minerals, vitamins, and water.

Nutritional requirements of healthy individuals depend on various factors, such as age, sex, and activity. Hence, recommended values of dietary intakes vary for each group of individuals. In the United States, the Food and Nutrition Board of the Institutes of Medicine (IOM) under the National Academy of Sciences issues nutrition recommendations for populations throughout the life span called Dietary Reference Intakes.

ASSESSMENT

While performing nutritional assessment, information should be collected systematically, and an evaluation of nutritional status should be done based on the overall data collected. As per the American Society for Parenteral and Enteral Nutrition (ASPEN) guidelines, a comprehensive nutritional assessment involves a thorough clinical examination (history and physical examination), anthropometric measurements, diagnostic tests, and dietary assessments.

Additional clinical examinations or diagnostic tests may be necessary for different groups of populations and individuals with specific underlying pathology. As per the International Consensus guidelines committee, the diagnosis of malnutrition in adults can be categorized as (i) starvation-related malnutrition (chronic, non-inflammatory), (ii) acute disease or injury-related malnutrition (mild to severe inflammation), or (iii) chronic disease-related malnutrition (chronic mild to moderate inflammation).

Given below are the components of a comprehensive nutritional assessment that need to be performed while evaluating the nutritional status of individuals.

Clinical history: Patients' clinical history is a crucial component of nutritional assessment. Clinical history aims to look for indications of malnutrition and identify underlying factors that may lead to malnutrition or increase the risk of malnutrition.

❖ Once patient identification markers (name, age, sex) are noted, take a detailed history of chief complaints.

❖ If not mentioned in chief complaints, ask for other constitutional symptoms, such as fever, fatigue, malaise, loss of appetite, or sleep disturbances. The presence of these symptoms can be an indication of underlying pathologies. For example, fever suggests active infection or inflammation.

❖ Inquire about the patient's usual weight and ask if there have been any weight changes. Weight loss of >10% of body weight can signify underlying pathology. Weight gain can be suggestive of various underlying endocrine pathologies. Weight gain can also lead to insulin resistance contributing to metabolic syndrome.

❖ Ask if there are any symptoms suggestive of malnutrition other than weight changes, such as rashes, sores in the mouth, dryness of skin and eyes, loss of night vision, hair loss, bleeding gums, poor healing of wounds, swelling of extremities, tingling, or numbness.

❖ Ask about eating habits and dietary preferences. For example, ask about the number of meals eaten in a day, approximate portion sizes, whether they are following any restrictive diets, whether they are vegan or vegetarian, or if they are allergic to any food items. This can help in diagnosing a possible nutritional deficiency. For example, a vegan diet may be associated with vitamin B12 (cobalamin) deficiency. If patients are on parenteral or enteral diets, they should be interviewed accordingly.

❖ Ask about any factors affecting food intake, such as poor dentition, ulceration in the oral cavity, difficulty in swallowing, loss of appetite, heartburn, nausea, and/or vomiting. Further, inquire about bowel habits, which help assess the general functioning of the gastrointestinal system. Also, ask if there is any abdominal pain, abdominal distention, diarrhea, flatulence, or constipation, which can indicate underlying gastrointestinal pathologies that affect nutritional status.

❖ Ask about any current major clinical or surgical illnesses, including mental illnesses. Also, ask if they are taking any medications, either prescribed or over the counter. Ask if there is any history of chronic illnesses, hospitalization, trauma, or malignancies. The impact of current or past illnesses on nutritional status is discussed below.

❖ In female patients, detailed menstrual history should be taken. Amenorrhea in child-bearing aged women can indicate pregnancy, chronic infection, chronic illness, eating disorder, etc., which can affect the nutritional status of patients. History suggestive of menorrhagia can reveal the presence of anemia. Also, a history of contraceptive use is essential. Women on oral contraceptive pills have different nutritional requirements. Oral contraceptive pills have been shown to deplete B vitamins, vitamin C, and some minerals, such as magnesium, selenium, and zinc.

❖ Next, ask questions related to lifestyle habits (active vs. sedentary), daily physical activities, and exercise routine.

❖ History about social habits, such as drinking, smoking, tobacco consumption, or other non-prescription drugs should also be taken.

❖ Since socioeconomic conditions can affect nutritional status, request information related to this as well.

❖ Finally, family history can also be useful for the early diagnosis of conditions that can affect a patient's nutritional status or help identify underlying predisposing conditions.

Dietary assessment: Dietary assessment is necessary to ensure adequate nutrition and hydration intake. It is advised to consult a qualified registered dietitian-nutritionist (RDN), if available, to obtain a thorough dietary assessment.

❖ The information can be collected from various sources, such as the patients themselves, family members, caregivers, or medical records.

❖ History about dietary habits, frequency of meals, and serving sizes needs to be collected. As mentioned earlier, details about food preferences, restrictive diets, and allergies should be noted.

❖ Current nutrient and fluid intake should be recorded. Methods, such as the 24-hour recall method, food frequency questionnaire (FFQ), diet charts, observation, etc., can be used. Wearable monitoring devices, phone apps, or nutrition analysis software can be used as aids.

❖ If patients are on any nutritional supplements, care must be taken to record the frequency and dosage to limit the risk of nutrient insufficiency and toxicity.

❖ If patients are on parenteral or enteral diets, information on feeding regimens (quantity and frequency) should be noted. Factors affecting these feedings, such as displacement of feeding tubes, site irritation, or infections, should be considered.

Physical examination: The next component of the nutritional assessment is physical examination. The physical examination aims to identify signs of malnutrition and factors affecting nutritional status.

❖ **General condition:** General condition and appearance of the patient should be observed. Look for any signs of emaciation. Note whether the patient is conscious, alert, and ambulatory. Make a note of whether a patient is being examined in a hospital or outpatient setting. An initial observation of the patient's cognitive, mental, and emotional status should be noted. Also, note any parenteral or enteral feeding devices being used. A patient's general condition can help determine whether a patient can meet their nutritional needs and/or whether their condition is causing their malnutrition or putting them at a higher risk of nutrition deficiencies.

❖ **Vital signs:** Vital signs (body temperature, pulse, blood pressure, and respiratory rate) should be checked. Temperature >100.4°F or 38°C can signify active inflammation/infection. Hypothermia (temperature <95°F or 35°C) can be associated with conditions causing impaired nutritional status, such as sepsis, trauma, burns, stroke, alcohol intoxication, and metabolic disorders, such as hypothyroidism, adrenal insufficiency, and Wernicke encephalopathy. High pulse rates, apart from cardiac conditions, can indicate hyperdynamic circulation. Some causes of hyperdynamic circulation that are associated with altered nutritional status are fever, anemia, pregnancy, hyperthyroidism, septic shock, Beriberi, and anxiety. High blood pressure or hypertension is one of the risk criteria for metabolic syndrome. Abnormal rate and patterns of respiration can be indicative of various pathologies. For example, Kussmaul's breathing is associated with diabetic ketoacidosis (DKA).

❖ **Height and weight:** Measure the height and weight of the patient. Body mass index (BMI) calculated from these variables can help determine whether an individual is undernourished or over nourished. Details about BMI and other anthropometric measurements are discussed later.

❖ **Eyes:** Look for pallor, which may be indicative of various nutrient deficiencies (iron, vitamin B12, folic acid, vitamin B6, vitamin C, or protein deficiency), as well as various chronic illnesses. Look for icterus, suggesting metabolic disturbances associated with the hepatobiliary system. The presence of Bitot's spots and xerosis is indicative of vitamin A deficiency. Xanthelasmas, yellow-colored plaques on eyelids, can suggest obesity, hypercholesterolemia, or diabetes mellitus.

❖ **Oral cavity and perioral region:** Assess the general health of the oral cavity and look for pathologies that can affect the adequate intake of nutrients. Also, look for glossitis, angular stomatitis, and cheilosis, which can indicate vitamin B complex deficiency. Bleeding gums and gingivitis are suggestive of vitamin C deficiency. Again, look for pallor. If an eating disorder is suspected, look for vomiting-related oral damage, for example, discoloration of teeth, loss of enamel, cavities, and enlarged salivary glands. A consultation with a dentist may be helpful. Look for loss of buccal fat pads or sunken facial appearance. This can be associated with various conditions, such as eating disorders, marasmus, tuberculosis (TB), or HIV/AIDS.

❖ **Skin:** Assess the general health of the skin. Xeroderma (extremely dry skin) can signify vitamin A and/or essential fatty acid deficiencies. Petechia, purpura, and ecchymosis may be associated with vitamin C and vitamin K deficiencies. Vitamin C deficiency can also present with perifollicular hemorrhage. Poorly healed wounds indicate vitamin C, protein, and/or zinc deficiencies. Pigmentation and rashes in sun-exposed areas (around the neck and on extremities in glove and stocking patterns) can be due to niacin deficiency. The yellow-orange discoloration of the skin can be detected in cases of excessive consumption of carotenoids (pigments found in carrots, pumpkin, tomatoes, etc.). Xanthomas, which are localized lipid deposits, can be seen in individuals with obesity, hypercholesterolemia, or diabetes mellitus. Look for loss of subcutaneous adipose tissue in axillary folds, buttocks, and extremities. This can be associated with energy-deficient states like marasmus, TB, HIV, and eating disorders.

- **Hair:** Various nutrients are required to maintain the health of hair and hair follicles. Dry hair can be a sign of vitamin A or vitamin E deficiency. Biotin deficiency can make hair brittle. Severe under nutrition, especially protein deficiency, can lead to discolored and easily pluckable hair, eventually resulting in hair loss. Rapid hair loss can also be indicative of underlying systemic illnesses.

- **Nails:** Assess the general health of nails and nail beds. Dry and brittle nails can be associated with various nutritional deficiencies, such as deficiencies in biotin, zinc, and proteins. Discoloration of nails is another sign of poor nutrition. Koilonychia can be a sign of iron deficiency anemia. While clubbing is associated with much pathology, it may also be observed with malnutrition, chronic alcohol use disorder, and chronic laxative use, often seen in individuals with eating disorders.

- **Extremities:** Examine all extremities carefully. Protein or thiamine deficiency can lead to edema. Vitamin B12, thiamine, vitamin E, and vitamin B6 deficiencies can present with paresthesia and muscle weakness. Loss of vibration and position sensation can also be observed in individuals with vitamin B12 and/or vitamin E deficiencies. Patients with diabetes mellitus may also show signs of peripheral neuropathy, foot ulceration, or gangrene. Severe under nutrition, as well as chronic illnesses, can lead to muscle atrophy and wasting. Bowing of lower limbs can be seen in children with vitamin D deficiency rickets.

- **Odors:** Certain odors can be suggestive of specific disorders or substance use. Detection of fruity acetone odor in patients with ketoacidosis, musty odor in patients with phenylketonuria, sweet burnt sugary odor in patients with Maple syrup disorder, or the smell of alcohol can also be helpful during the examination of patients.

- **Functional assessment**: It is essential to do a functional assessment of patients. Observe whether patients are ambulatory and whether they can eat and drink with/without assistance. Examine the strength of extremities to determine whether they can perform activities of daily living (ADLs) or other physical activities. Mental assessment is also crucial, along with physical assessment. For example, elderly patients with severe malnutrition may be physically (due to weakness) and mentally (due to dementia) incapable of maintaining healthy nutritional status. Similarly, patients with thiamine deficiency may develop Wernicke encephalopathy and Korsakoff psychosis and may become incapable of meeting their own dietary needs.

- **Systemic evaluation:** An appropriate systemic examination should be performed based on the history and general examination findings.

ANTHROPOMETRIC MEASUREMENTS

- **Height, weight, and BMI:** Measure the weight and height of the patient, as mentioned above. Patients should be advised to avoid wearing heavy garments or shoes while these measurements are taken. Bed or chair scales may be needed if patients are not ambulatory or cannot stand. In pediatric age groups, these parameters are plotted on growth charts to assess growth and nutritional status. BMI (weight in kilograms divided by height in meters squared) is also calculated using these parameters, and the state of nutrition can be assessed. In adults, BMI <18.5 kg/m^2: underweight; BMI = 18.5 to 24.9 kg/m^2: within normal range; BMI >24.9 to 29.9 kg/m^2: overweight; and BMI ≥30 kg/m^2: obesity.

❖ Factors, such as edema and hydration should be considered while making these determinations, as they can affect the weight and BMI values. BMI cannot differentiate between muscle mass and adipose tissue/fat mass. And finally, BMI does not take into account micronutrient deficiencies.

❖ **Other anthropometric measurements:** Circumference (arm, abdomen, and thigh) measurements and skinfold (biceps skinfold, triceps skinfold, subscapular skinfold, and suprailiac skinfold) thickness measurements can also help with the evaluation of nutritional status. Skinfold thickness measurements are considered indicators of energy stores (mainly lipid stores). Circumference measurement, namely mid arm circumference (MAC), can be used to derive mid arm muscle circumference (MAMC = MAC – 3.1414 X triceps skinfold thickness), which is an indicator of protein stores. While these tests can quickly be done at the bedside without additional cost, subjectivity in terms of measurements and the applicability of results across various populations can make these tests less reliable.

❖ A complete anthropometric assessment may also involve body composition measurements, which are discussed in diagnostic tests.

Measurement	Equation/method	Interpretation of results
Weight and % weight change	% weight change = (previous weight – current weight/previous weight) x 100	A patient is indicated for nutrition support if they have: BMI <18.5 kg/m^2 Unintentional weight loss of >10% in the previous 3–6 months BMI <20 kg/m^2 and unintentional weight loss >5% in the previous 3–6 months *(NICE, 2006)*
Body mass index (BMI)	BMI (kg/m^2) = weight (kg)/height^2 (m^2)	If BMI <18.5 kg/m^2 patient is underweight If BMI 18.5–25 kg/m^2 patient is in normal BMI range If BMI >25 kg/m^2 patient is overweight *(WHO, 2016)*
Mid upper arm circumference (MUAC)	Involves measuring the circumference of the mid-point on upper arm using a tape measure. This is a surrogate measure of both fat mass and fat free mass. It is a useful measure when a person cannot be weighed or if their weight is not likely to be a true reflection of the persons' actual weight, e.g., if the patient has edema or ascites	If MUAC is >23.5 cm the patient is likely to have a healthy BMI and is at low risk of malnutrition If MUAC is <23.5 cm the patient is likely to have a BMI <20 kg/m^2 and may be at risk of malnutrition *(BAPEN, 2011)*

Contd...

Contd...

Measurement	Equation/method	Interpretation of results
Skin-fold thickness	Measurement requires a trained person using skin-fold callipers which have been calibrated. Skin-fold measurements can be taken at four different sites: suprailliac, suprailiac, biceps, triceps (TSF; most commonly used). Measurement should be repeated three times and the mean result recorded. This is a surrogate measure of total fat mass. Longitudinal measurements can be used to identify any changes in fat mass	Centile tables can be used to interpret skin-fold thickness measurements
Mid arm muscle circumference (MAMC)	MAMC is a surrogate measure of fat free mass and is calculated using MUAC and TSF MAMC (cm) = MUAC (cm) − 3.14 × TSF (cm)	Centile tables allow assessment of changes in total body muscle mass over time

Diagnostic tests: The next component of the nutritional assessment is diagnostic tests, which are done to validate the results of the clinical presentation.

Laboratory Tests

❖ **Routine clinical tests:** Routine clinical tests can help evaluate the patient's overall status (as well as nutritional status). These include serum electrolytes, blood urea nitrogen (BUN), creatinine, blood glucose levels, lipid profile, liver enzymes, and complete blood count. Serum electrolytes and hydration status may be deranged in malnourished individuals. BUN and serum creatinine are also predictors of nitrogen balance along with being indicators of renal function, and lower levels of these can be seen in malnourished patients. Low levels of serum creatinine can be indicative of lower muscle mass. Both BUN and creatinine levels, however, can be affected by hydration levels and kidney function. Elevated blood glucose levels and lipid profile (triglycerides and cholesterol) levels are indicators of metabolic syndrome. Hyperglycemia can also be a nonspecific indicator of the inflammatory response.

❖ Low cholesterol levels can be seen in undernourished individuals. Low hemoglobin is suggestive of anemia. Lymphocyte functioning and proliferation are affected in chronic malnutrition and may manifest as decreased lymphocyte count. Undernutrition and protein deficiency, in general, lead to impaired immune response. Taken together, an impaired, delayed hypersensitivity response (anergic or no reaction) may be seen in undernourished individuals. For example, malnourished individuals with TB may show an anergic tuberculin skin test.

❖ **Visceral proteins:** Levels of visceral proteins, such as albumin, prealbumin, transferrin, and retinol-binding protein can help evaluate nutritional status. However, none of these tests alone are specific for detecting malnutrition, and their levels can be affected by multiple factors. For example, low serum albumin levels suggest protein deficiency due to malnutrition and other pathologies that affect the protein status, such as liver cirrhosis or nephrotic syndrome. High levels of serum albumin could be associated with dehydration. Albumin has a long half-life (up to 20 days) and, hence, cannot be used for monitoring frequent changes in nutritional status during refeeding. Prealbumin (or transthyretin), a thyroid hormone carrier, is preferred in such cases as it has a shorter half-life (2 to 3 days), which allows for the detection of acute alterations in nutritional status. Retinol-binding protein is another protein with a very short half-life (12 hours) and can be used for monitoring changes in nutritional status. However, its levels are affected by vitamin A levels. Transferrin, an iron transport protein, is another nutritional indicator as well as an acute phase reactant. It has a half-life of approximately ten days, and its levels are affected by serum iron levels.

❖ **Micronutrient levels:** If specific micronutrient deficiencies are suspected, individual micronutrient levels can be measured. For example, levels of B vitamins (thiamine, riboflavin, niacin, pyridoxine, folic acid, B12), vitamins A, C, D, E, and K, iron, zinc, selenium, homocysteine, etc., can be measured. More specific tests, such as the Schilling test for B12 deficiency or iron panel to differentiate between different types of anemia can also be performed based on clinical presentation.

❖ Other non-nutrition-specific markers can also be used; for example, C-reactive protein (CRP) can be used to indicate inflammation.

Measurement	Rationale	Normal range (note that different laboratories may use different reference ranges)
Hemoglobin (Hb)	Assess for iron status or indicate anemia	Women = 12.0 to 15.5 g/dL Men = 13.5 to 17.5 g/dL
Albumin (Alb)	A low level may indicate inflammation or infection is present, therefore should not be used to determine nutritional status	35–50 g/L (3.5–5.0 g/dL)
C-reactive protein (CRP)	This is an inflammatory marker which is raised when infection or inflammation is present	Ideally <10 mg/L
White cell count (WCC)	Immune system marker; is raised if infection is present	$4-11 \times 10^9$/L (4000–11,000 per cubic millimeter of blood)
Glycated Hemoglobin (HbA1c)	Indicates an average blood sugar level over a period of months	Ideally <48 mmol/mol or <6.5% (diabetes UK)
Sodium (Na)	This is an indication of hydration status and kidney function. A raised sodium level may indicate dehydration	135–145 mmol/L
Urea (Ur)	Used to assess kidney function. High urea and other markers levels in combination may indicate dehydration	2.5–7.1 mmol/L
Calcium and phosphate	Used as a baseline when assessing risk of refeeding syndrome. Calcium is adjusted for albumin level	Adjusted Ca 2.0–2.6 mmol/L Phosphate 0.7–1.4 mmol/L
Magnesium	Likely to be low if there are large GI losses	0.7–1.0 mmol/L
Micronutrients	Include vitamins and trace elements. These are affected by the acute phase response if inflammation or infection is present and so best measured when CRP is low	

Body Composition Studies

Apart from laboratory tests, body composition studies can be performed to estimate the body's composition in terms of water, air, muscle, bones, and fat mass.

❖ **Bioelectrical impedance analysis (BIA):** This helps to analyze the body composition based on the ability of different body tissues to conduct electricity. Conductance is higher in tissues with more water and electrolytes (for example, blood) and less in adipose and bone tissues. This is an easy, non-invasive test that can be done at the bedside using low-cost equipment. However, in patients with extremely high BMI or fluid overload, the results may be less accurate.

❖ **Dual-energy X-ray absorptiometry (DEXA or DXA):** This is a standard method used to determine body composition and is also used as a reference to compare other body composition tests. However, it is expensive, requires a specialized machine, and involves exposure to X-rays. It is more commonly used in clinical research than in routine clinical practice.

❖ Other tests, such as computed tomography (CT) scan and magnetic resonance imaging (MRI), can also be used to determine body composition but are expensive options for routine nutritional assessment. Body composition, however, can be determined when imaging is done for other diagnostic purposes.

FACTORS INFLUENCING NUTRITIONAL NEEDS

❖ Lack of knowledge in the family and community about the importance of nutrition during adolescence.
❖ Lack of food because of socio-economic circumstances.
❖ Inequitable distribution of food in the family wherein girls being denied nutritious food.
❖ Poor dietary intake of food and vegetables rich in iron.
❖ Poor bioavailability of iron in the diet.
❖ Hookworm infestation.
❖ Diseases, such as malaria.
❖ Bad cooking habits (over boiling vegetables and straining water, removing husk from wheat, eating polished rice and straining rice water, etc.)
❖ Perpetuation of a vicious cycle of malnutrition and infection, which might begin, even before birth and may have more serious consequences for the girl child.

Factors Affecting Nutritional Status

It is important to consider the following factors affecting the nutritional status of individuals while performing a comprehensive nutritional assessment. It is also crucial to remember that these factors can be interdependent. The factors can be classified as physiological, pathological, and psychosocial factors.

Physiological factors: Physiological factors, such as age, sex, growth, pregnancy, and lactation can influence nutritional needs and should be considered while performing a nutritional assessment. For example, as a child grows, its nutritional requirements will increase. The recommended nutritional requirements for male and female children of the same age are equal early in life, but as they approach adolescence, males require additional nutritional intake. On reaching adulthood, the rise in nutritional requirements of individuals plateaus off in their respective ranges. However, the caloric and nutritional needs of females increase during pregnancy and lactation. Hence, along with a balanced diet, a pregnant or lactating mother may also require additional supplementation of micronutrients, such as iron, folic acid, calcium, and vitamin D. Maternal age at the time of pregnancy can further affect these requirements. For example, the calcium requirements of pregnant teens are higher than those of pregnant adults. Physical activity also determines the recommended macronutrient (carbohydrate, protein, and/or fat) nutritional requirements. Individuals with an active lifestyle require higher nutritional needs than individuals with a sedentary lifestyle. Failure to meet the additional nutritional needs in any of the situations mentioned above increases the risk of malnutrition, especially if other health conditions coexist. On the other hand, as age advances, the energy needs of elderly individuals decrease due to less mobility and loss of lean tissue leading to decreased appetite. Factors, such as poor dentition, increased prevalence of chronic conditions, and adverse effects of polypharmacy combined with psychosocial factors, such as poor socioeconomic conditions or dementia, can further decrease intake of nutritious food, thus leading to impairment of nutritional status.

Pathological factors: While performing nutritional assessment, it is important to understand how underlying pathologies can affect nutritional status. Some of these factors are discussed below.

* **Genetics:** Genetics play a significant role in maintaining an individual's nutritional status. Genetic predisposition combined with lack of physical activity and a high-energy diet can lead to obesity and metabolic syndrome, thus putting individuals at higher risk of developing cardio metabolic diseases. In various genetic disorders, multiple factors could be responsible for the pathogenesis of malnutrition. For example, in cystic fibrosis, malabsorption of nutrients results from decreased uptake by the intestines and reduced secretion of pancreatic enzymes. This, coupled with increased energy needs, can contribute to malnutrition in these patients. Similarly, many other genetic disorders, such as phenylketonuria, Prader-Willi syndrome, maple syrup urine disease, abetalipoproteinemia, and lysosomal storage disorders, significantly affect the nutritional status of individuals.

* **Infections:** Malnourished individuals are more susceptible to infections and related complications. Interestingly, both acute and chronic infections adversely affect the nutritional status of individuals and can precipitate malnutrition. For example, in measles, an acute viral infection, severe deterioration of the nutritional status of children is observed due to acute inflammatory response, increased energy needs, and decreased intake of nutrients due to sore throat or oral lesions. The coexistence of malnutrition increases the severity of measles infection, susceptibility to secondary infections, and mortality rate. Measles is also associated with vitamin A deficiency, which can lead to xerosis, keratomalacia, and corneal ulceration, contributing to ophthalmological complications. Chronic infections, such as tuberculosis (TB) and human immunodeficiency virus (HIV) infection, are associated with anorexia and cachexia. The underlying proinflammatory cytokine response and metabolic alterations are mainly responsible for this. Other factors, such as the adverse effects of drugs, can also contribute to this, thus aggravating malnutrition. Malnutrition, on the other hand, increases the severity of the infection, leading to a bidirectional relationship between infection and malnutrition. Parasitic infestations also severely affect the nutritional status of individuals. For example, intestinal parasite infestation, such as ascariasis, leads to a deficiency of macronutrients and micronutrients.

* **Medical and surgical illnesses:** Various medical and surgical illnesses affect the nutritional status of individuals through multiple mechanisms and may lead to malnutrition. An important mechanism that leads to malnutrition in patients with systemic disorders is the underlying inflammatory response.
  Many conditions like cardiovascular diseases, chronic obstructive pulmonary disorders, rheumatoid arthritis, chronic pancreatitis, neuromuscular disorders, etc., have some underlying chronic inflammatory response, which leads to an altered metabolic state.

Another mechanism that could lead to nutritional disturbances is malabsorption. Many gastrointestinal pathologies, such as inflammatory bowel disease, pernicious anemia, celiac disease, gastrointestinal obstruction, pancreatitis, and liver cirrhosis can lead to malnutrition through this mechanism.

Malabsorption can also occur because of conditions affecting other organ systems. For example, right-sided congestive cardiac failure may be associated with intestinal edema, resulting in malabsorption and malnutrition in these patients. The next mechanism is metabolic disturbances observed in conditions characterized by dysfunction of the liver, gallbladder, and pancreas and endocrine disorders, such as diabetes mellitus, Cushing syndrome, and hyperthyroidism.

Malnutrition also occurs due to decreased nutrient intake or loss of nutrients. Poor intake of nutrients can be seen in local pathologies affecting ingestion of food, as well as diseases that have dementia as one of the clinical features, such as Parkinson and Alzheimer diseases. Recurrent nausea or vomiting, which leads to either decrease in the nutrient intake or loss of nutrients, can be seen in gastrointestinal pathologies, cyclic vomiting syndrome, brain tumors, Meniere disease, allergies, migraines, and motion sickness. Similarly, conditions characterized by recurrent diarrhea or steatorrhea can also be associated with malnutrition due to loss of nutrients. Mental illnesses (also discussed in psychosocial factors) affect nutritional status too. The mental status of these patients, adverse reactions to prescription drugs, loss of appetite as part of the disease process, etc., can all lead to malnutrition in these individuals.

❖ **Surgery:** Malnutrition before surgery can increase the risk of complications, including increased need for ICU admission, longer recovery time, infections, and higher rates of morbidity and mortality. Hence, a nutritional assessment before surgery is crucial. Surgery alone can be a risk factor for malnutrition due to various factors, such as pre- and post-operative fasting, hypermetabolism, adverse effects due to drugs, pain, and other factors specific to the type of surgery.

❖ **Trauma:** Severe trauma cases, including head injuries, burns, and multiple fractures, can put patients at high risk of malnutrition. The initial acute inflammatory response and increased energy needs following trauma lead to a hypermetabolic phase. This, followed by a prolonged period of immobility, leads to muscle atrophy and protein breakdown, causing additional metabolic disturbances. The severe condition of these patients also affects food intake. Altogether, these factors often lead to malnutrition. Furthermore, malnutrition can adversely affect the recovery phase and increase the risk of complications, thus worsening clinical outcomes.

❖ **Malignancies:** Malnutrition in malignancies is multifactorial. Inflammatory mediators, increased energy needs, adverse effects of drugs/therapy (such as mouth ulceration, nausea, and vomiting), mental stress, anxiety, and depression can lead to deterioration of nutritional status. Furthermore, malnutrition can inhibit the effectiveness of therapy and worsen the prognosis of the disease.

❖ **Medications:** Adverse effects of various drugs, such as nausea, gastric irritation, or loss of appetite, can contribute to decreased food/nutrient intake. Commonly taken over-the-counter (OTC) drugs, such as NSAIDs, can lead to gastrointestinal irritation. Similarly, iron tablets can also cause gastrointestinal irritation and constipation as side effects. Some medications can lead to specific deficiencies, such as the drug isoniazid, which can lead to vitamin B6 (pyridoxine) deficiency. Hence, detailed drug-related history is needed as some drugs can cause drug-nutrient interactions.

Psychosocial factors: Often, the above-mentioned physiological and pathological factors may coexist with psychosocial elements, resulting in further deterioration of nutritional status and eventually leading to malnutrition.

❖ Factors, such as socioeconomic conditions, natural and man-made calamities, cultural norms, religious beliefs, etc., can affect nutritional intake. Undernutrition is the major concern in impoverished areas, famine-stricken, war zones, or refugee camps. Though it may seem obvious that overnutrition is mainly observed in affluent groups due to access to resources, the relationship between obesity and socioeconomic status is complicated. While undernutrition is one of the outcomes of lower socioeconomic status, paradoxically, individuals from these groups are also susceptible to developing obesity. This is due to limited access to fresh, nutrient-dense, and relatively more expensive food on the one hand and easy availability of less expensive, energy-dense food on the other hand. Malnutrition with dual manifestation may especially be seen in these groups of individuals.

❖ Other factors, such as eating disorders, mental illnesses, and unhealthy diet trends can also drastically affect nutritional status and increase the risk of malnutrition.

❖ Alcohol and substance use are other major factors that need to be considered. Excessive alcohol consumption affects macronutrient and micronutrient metabolism, leading to nutritional deficiencies. Excessive alcohol consumption is associated with multi-organ tissue injury, which leads to inflammation. Alcohol consumption can also affect fluid balance. Furthermore, patients' food habits with chronic alcohol use disorder may further contribute to malnutrition. Similarly, illicit drugs affect the metabolism of nutrients as well. Substance use also affects patients' food habits and emotional and mental status, potentially contributing to malnutrition.

SPECIAL DIET

Soft Diet

A large number of foods qualify as soft foods:

❖ Mush or porridge-type hot cereals, such as oatmeal, grits and Cream-of-Wheat

❖ Cereals that soften easily in milk, such as Rice Krispies and Corn Flakes

❖ Soft breads and muffins

❖ Pasta cooked to a soft consistency

❖ Potatoes and sweet potatoes without skin

❖ Soft fruits, such as ripe bananas and melon

❖ Pureed berries put through a strainer to remove skins and seeds

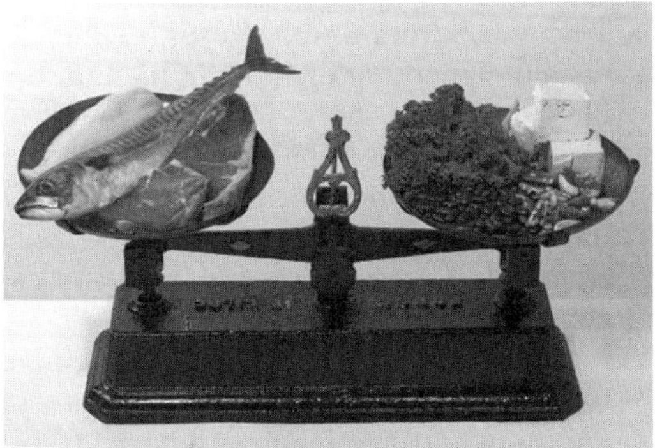

❖ Cooked fruits without seeds or skins, such as apples and pears

❖ Fruit juice

❖ Avocados

❖ Vegetable juice

❖ Skinless vegetables that cook to a soft consistency or can be mashed, such as carrots, cauliflower

❖ Soft fish carefully de-boned

❖ Canned tuna or chicken

❖ Scrambled or soft-boiled eggs
❖ Tender meats and ground meats that have been well-cooked—braised meats or meats cooked in a crock-pot are especially good for this purpose
❖ Tofu
❖ Well-cooked legumes with soft skins like baked beans
❖ Pureed or blended soups
❖ Pureed or blended sauces
❖ Yogurt
❖ Cottage cheese or ricotta cheese
❖ Finely grated/melted cheese
❖ Ice cream
❖ Pudding or custard
❖ Protein powders

THERAPEUTIC DIET

A therapeutic diet is a meal plan that controls the intake of certain foods or nutrients. It is part of the treatment of a medical condition and are normally prescribed by a physician and planned by a dietician.

A therapeutic diet is usually a modification of a regular diet. It is modified or tailored to fit the nutrition needs of a particular person.

Therapeutic diets are modified for:
1. Nutrients,
2. Texture, and/or
3. Food allergies or food intolerances.

Common reasons therapeutic diets may be ordered:
❖ To maintain nutritional status
❖ To restore nutritional status
❖ To correct nutritional status
❖ To decrease calories for weight control
❖ To provide extra calories for weight gain
❖ To balance amounts of carbohydrates, fat and protein for control of diabetes
❖ To provide a greater amount of a nutrient, such as protein
❖ To decrease the amount of a nutrient, such as sodium
❖ To exclude foods due to allergies or food intolerance
❖ To provide texture modifications due to problems with chewing and/or swallowing

Common Therapeutic Diets Include

1. Nutrient modifications:
   ◆ No concentrated sweets diet
   ◆ Diabetic diets
   ◆ No added salt diet
   ◆ Low sodium diet
   ◆ Low fat diet and/or low cholesterol diet
   ◆ High fiber diet
   ◆ Renal diet

2. **Texture modification:**
   - Mechanical soft diet
   - Puree diet
3. **Food allergy or food intolerance modification:**
   - Food allergy
   - Food intolerance
4. **Tube feedings:**
   - Liquid tube feedings in place of meals
   - Liquid tube feedings in addition to meals
5. **Additional feedings—in addition to meal, extra nutrition may be ordered as:**
   - Supplements—usually ordered as liquid nutritional shakes once, twice or three times per day; given either with meals or between meals
   - Nourishments—ordered as a snack food or beverage items to be given between meals mid-morning and/or mid-afternoon
   - HS snack—ordered as a snack food or beverage items to be given at the hour of sleep.

The following list includes brief descriptions of common therapeutic diets:
1. **Clear liquid diet:**
   - Includes minimum residue fluids that can be seen through.
   - Examples are juices without pulp, broth, and Jell-O.
   - Is often used as the first step to restarting oral feeding after surgery or an abdominal procedure.
   - Can also be used for fluid and electrolyte replacement in people with severe diarrhea.
   - Should not be used for an extended period as it does not provide enough calories and nutrients.
2. **Full liquid diet:**
   - Includes fluids that are creamy.
   - Some examples of food allowed are ice cream, pudding, thinned hot cereal, custard, strained cream soups, and juices with pulp.
   - Used as the second step to restarting oral feeding once clear liquids are tolerated.
   - Used for people who cannot tolerate a mechanical soft diet.
   - Should not be used for extended periods.
3. **No concentrated sweets (NCS) diet:**
   - Is considered a liberalized diet for diabetics when their weight and blood sugar levels are under control.
   - It includes regular foods without the addition of sugar.
   - Calories are not counted as in ADA calorie controlled diets.
4. **Diabetic or calorie controlled diet (ADA):**
   - These diets control calories, carbohydrates, protein, and fat intake in balanced amounts to meet nutritional needs, control blood sugar levels, and control weight.
   - Portion control is used at mealtimes as outlined in the ADA "Exchange List for Meal Planning."
   - Most commonly used calorie levels are: 1,200, 1,500, 1,800 and 2,000. No Added Salt (NAS) diet
   - Is a regular diet with no salt packet on the tray.
   - Food is seasoned as regular food. Low sodium (LS) diet
   - May also be called a 2 g sodium diet.

- Limits salt and salty foods, such as bacon, sausage, cured meats, canned soups, salty seasonings, pickled foods, salted crackers, etc.
- Is used for people who may be "holding water" (edema) or who have high blood pressure, heart disease, liver disease, or first stages of kidney disease.

5. **Low fat/low cholesterol diet:**
   - Is used to reduce fat levels and/or treat medical conditions that interfere with how the body uses fat, such as diseases of the liver, gallbladder, or pancreas.
   - Limits fat to 50 g or no >30% calories derived from fat.
   - Is low in total fat and saturated fats and contains approximately 250–300 mg cholesterol.

6. **High fiber diet:**
   - Is prescribed in the prevention or treatment of a number of gastrointestinal, cardiovascular, and metabolic diseases.
   - Increased fiber should come from a variety of sources including fruits, legumes, vegetables, whole breads, and cereals.

7. **Renal diet:**
   - Is for renal/kidney people.
   - The diet plan is individualized depending on if the person is on dialysis.
   - The diet restricts sodium, potassium, fluid, and protein specified levels.

8. **Mechanically altered or soft diet:**
   - Is used when there are problems with chewing and swallowing.
   - Changes the consistency of the regular diet to a softer texture.
   - Includes chopped or ground meats as well as chopped or ground raw fruits and vegetables.
   - Is for people with poor dental conditions, missing teeth, no teeth, or a condition known as dysphasia.

9. **Pureed diet:**
   - Changes the regular diet by pureeing it to a smooth liquid consistency.
   - Indicated for those with wired jaws extremely poor dentition in which chewing is inadequate.
   - Often thinned down so it can pass through a straw.
   - Is for people with chewing or swallowing difficulties or with the condition of dysphasia.
   - Foods should be pureed separately.
   - Avoid nuts, seeds, raw vegetables, and raw fruits.
   - Is nutritionally adequate when offering all food groups.

Food Allergy Modification

- Food allergies are due to an abnormal immune response to an otherwise harmless food.
- Foods implicated with allergies are strictly eliminated from the diet.
- Appropriate substitutions are made to ensure the meal is adequate.
- The most common food allergens are milk, egg, soy, wheat, peanuts, tree nuts, fish, and shellfish.
- A gluten free diet would include the elimination of wheat, rye, and barley. Replaced with potato, corn, and rice products.

Food Intolerance Modification

- The most common food intolerance is intolerance to lactose (milk sugar) because of a decreased amount of an enzyme in the body.

❖ Other common types of food intolerance include adverse reactions to certain products added to food to enhance taste, color, or protect against bacterial growth.

❖ Common symptoms involving food intolerances are vomiting, diarrhea, abdominal pain, and headaches.

Tube Feedings

❖ Tube feedings are used for people who cannot take adequate food or fluids by mouth.

❖ All or parts of nutritional needs are met through tube feedings.

❖ Some people may receive food by mouth if they can swallow safely and are working to be weaned off the tube feeding.

CARE OF PATIENT WITH DYSPHAGIA

❖ **Providing adequate rest periods prior to mealtime:** Fatigue can further add to swallowing impairment so providing the patient with rest periods prior to eating will assist in being able to properly eat as they will be more alert.

❖ **Eliminating distractions:** Turning the television and radio off will help the patient focus on eating and promote swallowing.

❖ **Providing oral care prior to eating:** Research has shown evidence of oral care prior to meals aiding in appetite and feeding. It will help clear any debris in the mouth that may get in the way of eating and swallowing.

❖ **Ensure the patient is sitting upright at ninety degrees:** This will aid in choking and aspiration prevention.

❖ **Stay near patient during mealtimes:** Nursing homes and other long-term care facilities usually require a nurse be present in the dining areas during the duration of the entire mealtime. This is important in case there is an emergency with a dysphagic patient or other health emergency with other patients; this will allow the nurse to assist the patient quickly.

❖ **Observe for signs of aspiration and pneumonia:** Listen to lung sounds after meals and note any new crackles or wheezes. Note the patient's temperature and notify the physician as needed of any new concerns or changes in health status.

❖ **Keeping suction equipment at the beside of dysphagic patients:** Secretions can rapidly accumulate in the pharynx and upper trachea which increases aspiration risk. Keeping suction equipment at the bedside will aid in the faster clearing of these secretions and prevent the patient from aspirating.

❖ **Educate family on the importance of following a patient's diet:** Dysphagic patients are usually on specialized diets to aid them in swallowing and getting the nutrients they need. If a family does not understand the importance of diet restrictions, they may give them something they should not have; this increases their aspiration and choking risk.

General Guidelines for Minimizing Nausea

❖ Smaller portions of foods that are low in fat seem to work best. These foods are easier to digest and move through the stomach faster. If patient is eating smaller portions of low-fat foods, be sure to give more often to meet calorie and protein needs.

❖ Eat salty foods and avoid overly sweet ones, especially if patient have been vomiting.

❖ If there are specific times when you know you are going to be nauseated or vomiting, do not eat foods that you really like. You may get turned off from these favorite foods by associating them with the nausea and vomiting.

❖ Clear, cool beverages are recommended. Take whatever you feel you can tolerate. Examples include clear soups, flavored gelatin, carbonated beverages, popsicles and ice cubes made of frozen drinks. (Note: when drinking with a straw, sip slowly to avoid swallowing air that can cause gas.)

❖ Sometimes the smell of foods cooking, especially greasy foods, can cause feeling of nausea. If you have problems with this, cold foods, such as dairy products, sandwiches and fruits may help.

Minimizing Nausea When Eating

❖ Avoid liquids at mealtimes. Take them 30 to 60 minutes before and after eating.

❖ Do not lie down flat for at least two hours after eating.

❖ If the smell of food makes you nauseated, let someone else do the cooking or use prepared food from the freezer.

❖ Do not consume food in a room filled with cooking odors or in a warm, stuffy room.

❖ Eat meals slowly.

Management Strategies

Effective management of nausea and vomiting not only influences a patient's symptom response; it also improves patient compliance with therapeutic treatments. However, because there is a vast array of possible management strategies, depending on the quality of the assessment and the resources available, it is essential that health professionals involve the patient in the decision process, and use a multimodal approach that incorporates both pharmacological and non-pharmacological management methods.

Pharmacological Management

The most common intervention used in today's healthcare system is the administration of medication because it is often a safe and effective way of managing many signs and symptoms of diseases [National Institute for Health and Care Excellence (NICE), 2015].

Concerning the nausea and vomiting, antiemetics (anti-sickness) medication should be prescribed only when the specific cause of nausea and vomiting are known, because antiemetics vary in their mechanism(s) of action and will depend on the cause and which receptor has initiated the emetic response For example, an antiemetic medication that is effective in the management of chemotherapy-induced nausea and vomiting may have no role in the prevention and treatment of emetic symptoms due to other causes, e.g., motion sickness.

Types of antiemetic drugs and uses.	
Types of antiemetics and examples of medications	**Uses**
Antihistamines • Cinnarizine • Cyclizine • Promethazine	Wide variety of uses, including motion sickness and vertigo

Contd...

Contd...

Types of antiemetics and examples of medications	Uses
Phenothiazines and related drugs • Perphenazine • Prochlorperazine • Trifluoperazine • Chlorpromazine • Levomepromazine • Droperidol • Haloperidol	Phenothiazines are dopamine antagonists that act centrally by blocking the chemoreceptor trigger zone. • Perphenazine, prochlorperazine and trifluoperazine are used in severe nausea and vomiting due to a variety of causes • Droperidol is used to prevent or treat nausea and vomiting following surgery • Haloperidol and levomepromazine are used in palliative care, and chlorpromazine is often prescribed as a last resort for patients who have a terminal illness
Domperidone and metoclopramide	• Domperidone is used to treat emetic symptoms, and it acts at the chemoreceptor trigger zone. It has the advantage of being less likely to cause drowsiness and dystonic reactions because it does not readily cross the blood-brain barrier • Metoclopramide hydrochloride is used to prevent postoperative nausea and vomiting, and to treat a variety of nausea and vomiting causes, such as migraine and radiotherapy. It acts directly on the gastrointestinal tract, thus it may be more beneficial than phenothiazine for treating nausea and vomiting associated with gastroduodenal, hepatic and biliary disease
Dexamethasone	A steroid used to manage nausea and vomiting during chemotherapy
5HT3-receptor antagonists • Granisetron • Ondansetron • Palonosetron	Therapy to prevent postoperative nausea and vomiting include 5HT3-receptor antagonists. A combination of these medications can be used with choice based on the assessed risk of postoperative nausea and vomiting in each patient. 5HT3-receptor antagonists are often used with dexamethasone
Neurokinin 1-receptor antagonists • Aprepitant • Fosaprepitant	Administered alongside 5HT3-receptor antagonist to prevent chemotherapy-induced nausea and vomiting
Nabilone	Nabilone is a synthetic cannabinoid that can be considered as an add-on for treating nausea and vomiting. Cannabinoids are used as a last resort when other antiemetics have failed to control nausea and vomiting caused by chemotherapy
Hyoscine	Hyoscine should be given to prevent motion sickness and should, therefore, be administered before vomiting has started

Antiemetic medication can also be administered via multiple routes (i.e., intravascular, oral, rectal), so it is important to consider which is the most appropriate approach for each patient. Additionally, because there may be more than one cause, individuals may require two or more antiemetics to achieve adequate symptom control.

Non-pharmacological

Although antiemetics are used worldwide to manage nausea and vomiting, pharmacological management is only partially effective, and for some individuals can cause side-effects (i.e., sedation, headache, constipation, and fatigue). Alternative strategies may therefore also need to be employed.

Acupressure

Acupoints are located at specific places on imaginary lines 'meridians' throughout the human body and acupressure of the P6 point, which lies 4 cm proximal (three fingers) to the wrist crease of the dominant arm, has proven helpful to some patients in controlling nausea and vomiting, with, minimal side-effects.

Ginger

Ginger is a herb belonging to the Zingiberaceae family, which has been shown to block the actions of serotonin and acetylcholine that stimulate the vomiting reflex and trigger involuntary stomach contractions in the body.

Its use as an adjuvant therapy or as a complementary natural alternative for alleviating symptoms of nausea and vomiting has been researched extensively within pregnancy, chemotherapy, postoperative nausea and vomiting, and motion sickness it is now regarded as just as effective as pharmacological therapies, with fewer potential side-effects.

Nursing Care

As well as the use of complementary therapies, to ensure adequate holistic management, there are additional nursing considerations that need to be addressed when caring for patients experiencing nausea and vomiting (below table), especially in relation to assisting patients with activities of living and biopsychosocial wellbeing:

Nursing considerations when caring for patients experiencing nausea and vomiting.	
• Nurse in a safe position to protect the airway and remove dentures • Assist with mouth care and personal hygiene (change of clothes, etc.) • Use appropriate infection control measures • Maintain adequate ventilation and comfortable environmental temperature • Observe for signs of dehydration • Restrict or provide oral fluids and diet, as instructed • Maintain an accurate fluid balance chart; measure and assess vomit • Administer antiemetics as prescribed, evaluate effectiveness and monitor for side-effects • Provide vomit bowls and tissues, and replace promptly when used	• Consider use of other strategies, e.g., acupressure, ginger, aromatherapy • Referral to another professional may be required, e.g., clinical psychologist • Administer intravenous fluid and electrolytes, as prescribed • Provide psychological support and education for the patient and family • Insert a nasogastric tube, if instructed • Identify any other strategies that the patient finds helpful • Monitor observations, inform the doctor and request a review, as appropriate • Maintain privacy and dignity and provide physical comfort. Hold vomit bowl and wipe mouth • Assist with the avoidance of food smells and strong odors

Mouth Care

Following episodes of vomiting, bile and acids from the stomach can cause damage to teeth, gums and throat, and result skin irritation around the mouth. To ensure that the structures and tissues of the mouth remain healthy it is essential to assist patients with oral mouth care and ensure that they have access to equipment to perform oral hygiene. Removing the taste through oral hygiene can also help with reducing nausea.

Privacy and Dignity

Close curtains to provide privacy and promote comfort by keeping clothes clean and ensure that tissues and vomit bowls are easily accessible.

Fluid Balance

Vomiting and nausea can change a patient's hydration status, putting them at risk of dehydration. It is therefore important to keep an accurate record of the patient's fluid balance and, if possible, encourage oral intake or administer intravenous fluids .

Environment

Following episodes of vomiting, it is important to consider the stimulation of the vomiting center via the cerebral cortex, because smells can trigger further episode. To reduce the stimulus, strong odors should be avoided by moving the patient or opening windows because fresh cool air can help alleviate symptoms of nausea.

Diet and Nutrition

Nausea and vomiting can lead to a reduction in appetite and/or cause a patient to stop eating. Consequently, food charts should be used and patients should be encouraged to eat small, frequent meals, consisting of bland, non-spicy, non-fatty foods.

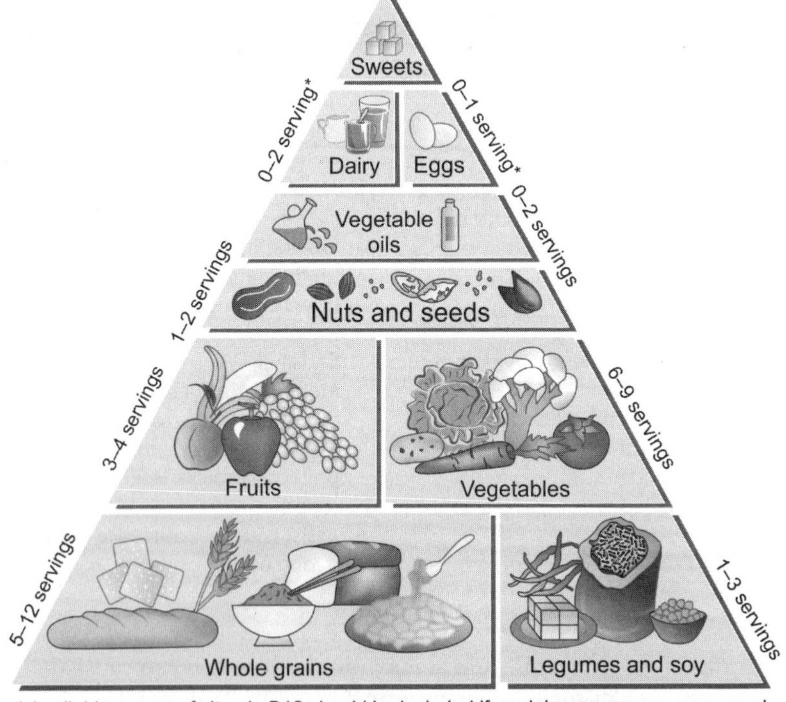

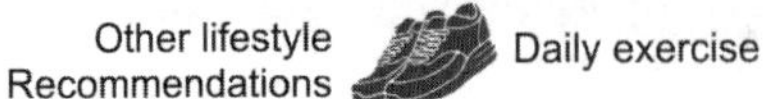

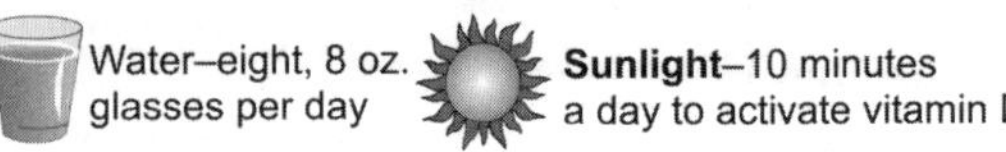

Enteral Feeding and Medication Administration

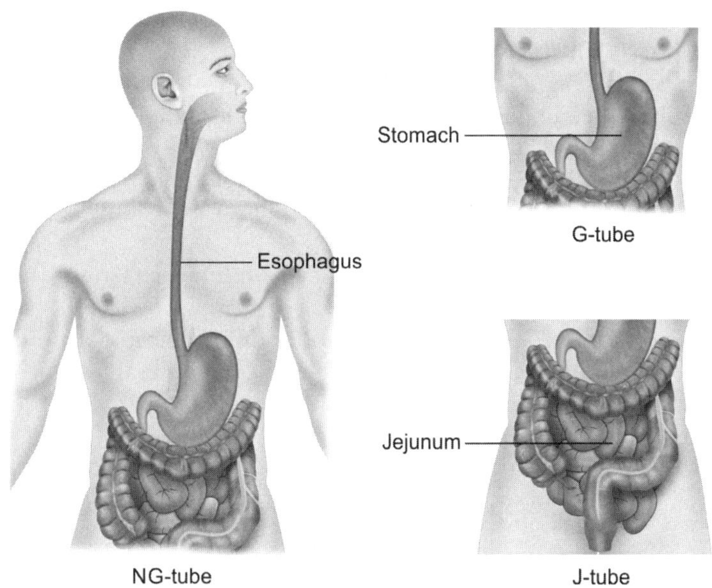

Introduction

Enteral feeding is a method of supplying nutrients directly into the gastrointestinal tract. This term describe orogastric, nasogastric and gastrostomy tube feeding.

Reasons for Enteral Tube Feeding

- ❖ Unable to consume adequate nutrients
- ❖ Impaired swallowing/sucking (children)
- ❖ Facial or esophageal structural abnormalities
- ❖ Anorexia related to a chronic illness
- ❖ Eating disorders
- ❖ Increased nutritional requirements
- ❖ Congenital anomalies
- ❖ Primary disease management

Enteral feeding tubes can be used to:
- ❖ Administer bolus, intermittent feeds and continuous feeds
- ❖ Medication administration
- ❖ Facilitate free drainage and aspiration of the stomach contents
- ❖ Facilitate venting/decompression of the stomach

Aim

This aims to support caregivers in administering feeds and medications via a nasogastric, orogastric or gastrostomy tube in a safe and appropriate manner.

Definition of Terms

- ❖ **Orogastric tube (OGT):** Thin soft tube passed through a client's mouth, through the oropharynx, through the esophagus and into the stomach.
- ❖ **Nasogastric tube (NGT):** Thin soft tube passed through a client's nose, down the back of the throat, through the esophagus and into the stomach.
- ❖ **Gastrostomy tube:** A feeding tube which is inserted endoscopically or surgically through the abdominal wall and directly into the stomach.
- ❖ **Temporary balloon device (G-tube):** A gastrostomy tube.
- ❖ **Percutaneous endoscopic gastrostomy tube (PEG):** A gastrostomy tube which is held in place with an internal fixator.
- ❖ **Gastrostomy-Button (Mickey-Button™):** Skin level button gastrostomy tube inserted into a pre-formed stoma.
- ❖ **Gastric residual volume (GRV's):** The amount of fluid aspirated from the stomach via an enteral tube to monitor gastric emptying, tolerance to enteral feeding and abdominal decompression. Once removed it may be returned to the patient or discarded.

Trans-Anastomotic Tube (TAT Tube)

Utilized after surgery to repair esophageal atresia inserted by surgeons in the neonatal patient population.

ASSESSMENT NASOGASTRIC TUBE/OROGASTRIC TUBE-CHECKING THE POSITION

Prior to accessing a NGT/OGT for any reason, caregivers must ensure that the tube is located in the stomach. Coughing, vomiting and movement can move the tube out of the correct position. The position of the tube must be checked:

- ❖ Prior to each feed
- ❖ Before each medication
- ❖ Before putting anything down the tube
- ❖ If the client has vomited
- ❖ Four hourly if receiving continuous feeds

Caregivers should perform the following observations and obtain a gastric aspirate to establish tube position.

- ❖ Ensure taping is secure
- ❖ Observe and document the position marker on NGT/OGT
- ❖ Observe client for any signs of respiratory distress.

Please note: Patients who have a history of liver failure and known/or suspected esophageal varices should not have a gastric aspirate removed from the NGT. Instead tube position should be initially confirmed via X-ray with clear documentation of NGT position marker. The medical team should document rationale for not obtaining gastric aspirate in the patient's progress note as well as an alternative plan to confirm NGT placement.

Obtain Gastric Aspirate

To check the position of the tube nursing staff members need to have prepared the following equipment:

❖ pH test indicators;
❖ Enteral/oral syringe—5 mL–20 mL for aspiration;
❖ Gloves

Procedure

❖ Attach a 10–20 mL oral/enteral syringe to the enteral tube in the infant/child
❖ Attach a 5–10 mL oral/enteral syringe to the enteral tube in a neonate
❖ Aspirate minimum 0.5–1 mL of gastric content (or sufficient amount to enable pH testing). Consider the "dead space" in the tubing.
❖ Utilising pH indicator strips a reading of between 0–5 should be obtained and documented.
❖ Some medications and formulas may affect the pH reading. If the patient is receiving a medication which is known to alter pH readings notify medical team, pharmacy and senior nursing staff, a clear plan for confirming the tubes position should be documented in the progress notes. If a reading >5 is obtained, placement of the tube is questionable and it should not be used until the position of the tube is confirmed. If a reading >5 is obtained leave for up to 1 hour and try aspirating again. Small-bore tubes can be difficult to aspirate therefore the following are suggested techniques to try enhance the ability to obtain aspirate:
❖ Turn the patient onto their side. This will allow the tip of the tube to move to a position where fluid has accumulate
❖ Using a 10–20 mL oral/enteral syringe (5–10 mL in neonates) insufflate 1–5 mL of air (1–2 mL in neonates) into the tube. This may move the tube away from the wall of the stomach. It will also clear the tube of any residual fluid. If a child belches immediately following air insufflation, the tip of the tube may be in the esophagus
❖ Wait for 15–30 minutes. This will allow fluid to accumulate in the stomach and try aspirating again.
❖ If it is safe to do so and the child is able to tolerate oral intake consider providing them with a drink and attempt aspirate in 15–30 minutes.
❖ If no aspirate obtained, advance the tube by 1–2 cm and try aspirating again.
❖ If aspirate not obtained discuss with senior nursing staff or medical staff and consider removing the tube or checking position by X-ray.

Gastrostomy Tube

Correct placement of the tube should be confirmed prior to administration of an enteral feed by checking insertion site at the abdominal wall and observing the client for abdominal pain or discomfort. If the nurse is unsure regarding the position of the gastrostomy or jejunostomy tube contact the medical team immediately.

Ongoing Assessment during Continuous Feeds

Nasogastric/Orogastric Tube

1. **The position of the tube needs to be checked 4 hourly with change of feeds:**
   ◆ It is recommended that the feed be ceased, withdraw aspirate and test pH.
   ◆ If reading >5, cease the feed for 30 minutes, aspirate and test pH
   ◆ Should there be any dispute as to the position of the tube, do not recommence feeds. Discuss with senior nursing staff or medical staff.

2. **The following needs to be checked two hourly during the feed:**
    - Taping
    - Marker on NGT
    - Observe client for signs of respiratory distress.
    - Check infusion hourly and document intake.

Feeds should hang for **no longer** than four hours to reduce the risk of bacterial growth.

Other Assessment Considerations for the Client Receiving Enteral Feeds

- ❖ Regular weights (at least twice weekly or as clinically indicated)
- ❖ Blood tests
- ❖ Referral to dietician to review feeding plan
- ❖ Referrals to speech therapy and/or occupational therapy.

Management Flushing Enteral Tubes

The purpose of flushing is to check for tube patency and prevent clogging of enteral tubes. Flushing is not routine on the unit and flushing with air is the preferred method. Enteral feeding tubes should be flushed regularly with water (or sterile water if appropriate):

- ❖ Prior to and after feeding
- ❖ Prior to, in-between and after medications
- ❖ Regularly in between tube use
- ❖ Modify flush volumes throughout as needed for infants and children with fluid restrictions—these patients may require minimal volume (0.5 mL) flushing and/or flushing with air to push feed or medication to the end of the tube Nurses should prepare an enteral/oral syringe, enteral tube connector and water for a flush.
- ❖ Tap water is suitable for most children with OGT or NGT
- ❖ Boiled/sterile water may be necessary for children under six months of age or as clinically indicated, e.g., immune compromised patients

Flushing

Enteral tubes should be flushed with between 5–20 mL of water depending on the viscosity of the feed/medication, the child's fluid status balance and the child's size. (The minimum volume required to clear the tube is 2 mL. However in shorter tubes 1.5 mL would be sufficient).

Venting

- ❖ Feeding tubes may be used to facilitate venting or decompression of the stomach from the accumulation of air during such interventions as high-flow nasal prongs, non-Invasive or invasive ventilation.
- ❖ Enteral feeding or administration of medication may proceed in this case dependent on the individual client's condition.
- ❖ The tube may be clamped for 30 minutes to an hour post-administration to prevent loss of feed or medication.
- ❖ Continuous venting may be facilitated following administration by securing the distal end of the tube above the head of the client. This may be attached to the end of a 5 or 10 mL enteral/oral syringe with the plunger removed to create a reservoir should gastric contents reflux.

Feeds

Feeds can be administered via syringe, gravity feeding set or feeding pump. The method selected is dependent of the nature of the feed and clinical status of the child. There is limited evidence available to support one method of feeding over the other.

Do not administer feeds through enteral tubes that are being used for aspiration or are on free drainage.

Administration of Feeds

When preparing to administer feeds caregivers must confirm the position of the enteral tube. Prior to and after feeds caregivers should adequately flush the enteral tube.

Position

❖ Lying prone/supine during feeding increases the risk of aspiration and therefore where clinically possible the client should be placed in an upright position.

❖ If unable to sit up for a bolus feed or if receiving continuous feeding, the head of the bed should be elevated 30–45° during feeding and for at least 30 minutes after the feed to reduce the risk of aspiration.

Using a Syringe for a Bolus Feed

❖ Remove the plunger from the syringe and place the tip of the syringe into the enteral tube connector at end of the enteral tube.

❖ Holding the syringe and enteral tube straight, pour the prescribed amount of feed into the syringe. Let it flow slowly through the tube, e.g., 250 mL over 20 minutes.

❖ Pour the prescribed amount of water into the syringe and allow to flow through to flush the feeding tube appropriately.

Using Gravity Feeding for Bolus, Intermittent Feeds and Continuous Feeds

❖ Using a gravity feeding set with the roller clamp closed, attach the set to the feeding container with the correct prescribed amount of feed and hang the container on the pole.

❖ Squeeze the drip chamber until it is one third full of the feeding solution.

❖ Remove the protective cap from the end of the giving set and open the roller clamp, allowing the feed to run down to the end of the giving set (to prime the line), then close the roller clamp.

❖ Connect the giving set to the enteral tube connector at the end of the enteral tube.

❖ Open the roller clamp and set the flow rate by counting the drops per minute. As a guide, 20 drops of standard feed is approximately 1 mL. Use the following equation to calculate the drip rate: (mL/hour)/3 = drops/minute

❖ Open and close the roller clamp until the desired drip rate is set correctly. Check the drip rate regularly to ensure the feed is still running at the required rate.

Using an Enteral Feeding Pump for Bolus or Intermittent Enteral Feeding

An enteral feeding pump can be used intermittent, bolus or continuous administration of feeds, but is best suited for continuous feeding when tolerance to rate of feeding is an issue. Enteral feeding pumps can be obtained via CARPS if the ward area does not have its own supply.

Infinity pumps are now in use throughout RCH and the giving set can be primed by pushing the fill set button.

Please note: In most situations, an IV syringe pump is not recommended for administration of enteral feeds and should not be used on the ward. If very small rates are required, consider using frequent syringe bolus feeding techniques as an alternative.

Temperature of the Feed

Bolus Feeds

For older children feeds given as a bolus should be removed from the fridge 15–20 minutes before administration to bring them to room temperature. Feeds given as a bolus may be warmed in an approved bottle warmer. This would be appropriate for all infants and older children who experience discomfort with cooler feeds.

Continuous Feeds

Continuous feeds should NOT be warmed. They may be removed from the fridge 15–20 minutes prior to administration to bring it to room temperature and should not hang for >4 hours—use the dose limit function on the feed pump to ensure this occurs.

Please Note: Feeds should NOT be warmed in a microwave or in jugs of boiling water.

Completion of Feed

The tube must be flushed with water (air in neonates) to prevent tube from blocking

Giving sets:
* Rinsed out with warm water (tap or sterile).
* Ensure tip of giving set is covered between uses.
* Only prime the giving set with formula immediately prior to feeding time.
* The set should be changed every 24 hours or as per manufactures instructions.

Titrating Feeds

* Nursing staff may need to titrate the rate/volume of an enteral feed up or downdepending on the clinical status, nutritional needs, size and ability to tolerate feeds.
* When titrating feeds up nurses should have a goal rate/volume of feed ordered by dietician or the medical team. Feeds should be titrated up in a slow but steady manner, which may need to be adjusted if the client is not able to tolerate the rate/volume of feed.
* Caution should be taken if titrating feeds up and down in patients with a metabolic condition.
* When titrating a feed down nursing staff should document why the feed was titrated down, notify dietician and/or medical team to inform them that the client is not tolerating feeds and make a plan to ensure the client is still receiving adequate nutrition and hydration.

Types of Feeds

The decision for which type of enteral feed a patient should receive should be made in consultation with the dietician, medical team, nursing staff and family, taking into account the nutritional needs, clinical status and tolerance of feeds. If a patient who receives regular enteral feeds at home is admitted to hospital, nursing staff can order and commence their regular feeding regime as the patient's clinical status allows.

Enteral feeds can be ordered from the hospital's formula room. The family should be offered a dietician review while they are an inpatient to ensure the current feeding regime meets the on-going nutritional needs of the patient.

Medication Administration

Nurses who are preparing and administrating medication via an enteral tube must adhere to the Medication Management Procedure.

❖ Do not administer drugs through tubes used for aspiration or on free drainage unless specifically directed by medical staff.
❖ Confirm that the enteral feeding tube is the intended route for a medication before administration.
❖ Confirm the position of the enteral tube prior to medication administration.
❖ Adequately flush the enteral tube before, in-between and after medication administration.

Choice of Drug Preparation

Consult your ward pharmacist or call medicines information for advice on how to prepare a drug for enteral administration.

❖ Liquid formulations are usually preferred for enteral tube administration; unless the formulation contains other ingredients that could cause unwanted side-effects (e.g., sorbitol can cause diarrhea). Liquid formulations may inappropriate in some patients (e.g., the carbohydrate content may be too high for patients on a ketogenic diet).
❖ Viscous liquid medications may require dilution to prevent clogging of the enteral tube.
❖ If a liquid formulation is not available consult a pharmacist to confirm if the tablet form can be crushed to a fine powder and then dispersed in water, or whether a capsules can be opened to disperse the contents in water.
❖ Do not mix medications with feeds.
❖ Do not crush enteric coated or sustained/controlled release medications.

Unblocking Tubes

Blocking of tubes can occur due to:
❖ Interaction between gastric acid, formula and medications
❖ Interactions between medications if tube is not flushed between medications
❖ Inappropriately prepared medications, e.g., inadequately crushed tablets
❖ Small internal diameter of the tubes and longer tubes
❖ Binding of medication to the tube
❖ Viscosity of some liquid preparation
❖ Poor flushing technique
❖ Bacterial colonization of the nasogastric tube.

Flushing is the single most effective action that prolongs the life of nasogastric tubes. It is recommended that flushing occur *before, during,* and *after* administration of enteral medications and feeds. To unblock enteral tubes, flush the tube in a pulsating manner (push/pull) with 10–20 mL with warm water; if it is safe to do so taking into account the child's age, size and clinical status. It may be appropriate to allow the warm water to soak, by clamping/capping the tube, in the tube to assist with unblocking.

Feed Intolerance

Nurses should monitor and observe the patient to assess if the patient is tolerating enteral feeds.

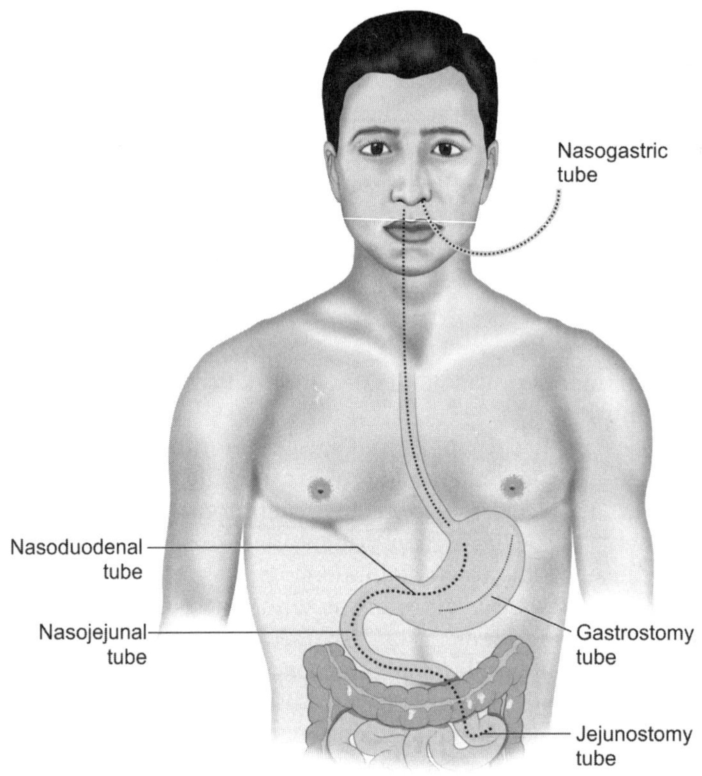

JEJUNOSTOMY FEEDING

Jejunostomy is a surgical procedure by which a tube is situated in the lumen of the proximal jejunum, primarily to administer nutrition. There are many techniques used for jejunostomy: longitudinal Witzel, transverse Witzel, open gastrojejunostomy, needle catheter technique, percutaneous endoscopy, and laparoscopy. The principal indication for a jejunostomy is as an additional procedure during major surgery of the upper digestive tract, where irrespective of the pathology or surgical procedures of the esophagus, stomach, duodenum, pancreas, liver, and biliary tracts, nutrition can be infused at the level of the jejunum. It is also used in laparotomy patients in whom a complicated postoperative recovery is expected, those with a prolonged fasting period, those in a hypercatabolic state, or those who will subsequently need chemotherapy or radiotherapy. As a sole procedure it is advised for neurologic and congenital illnesses, in geriatric patients who pose difficult care demands, and for patients with tumors of the head and neck. The complications seen with jejunostomy can be mechanical, infectious, gastrointestinal, or metabolic. The complications are moderate and severe—tube dislocation, obstruction or migration of the tube, cutaneous or intra-abdominal abscesses, enterocutaneous fistulas, pneumatosis, occlusion, and intestinal ischemia. The infectious complications are aspiration pneumonia and contamination of the diet. The gastrointestinal complications are diarrhea 2.3% to 6.8%, abdominal distension, colic, constipation, nausea, and vomiting. The metabolic complications are hyperglycemia 29%, hypokalemia 50%, water and electrolyte imbalance, hypophosphatemia, and hypomagnesemia. These complications are

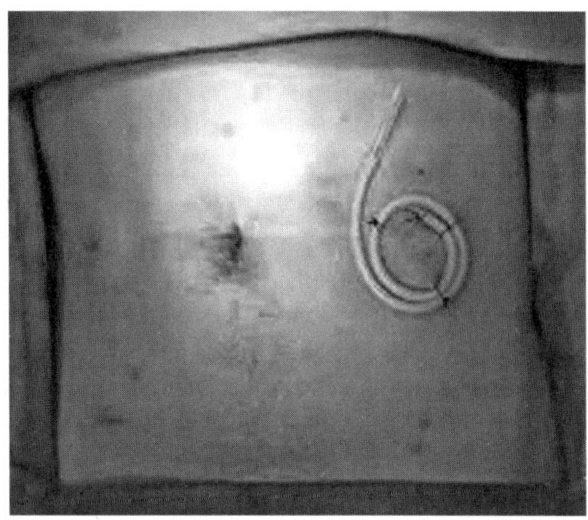

secondary to inadequate selection of nutrition relative to the characteristics of the patient, to inadequate management of the mixture, and to deficient clinical care.

Feeding jejunostomy refers to a surgically inserted tube, preferably in the proximal jejunum, to provide enteral nutrition or administer medications. This is different from a definitive jejunostomy, which is commonly done as part of gastric resection by a Roux-en-Y technique.

A jejunostomy tube (J-tube) is a soft, plastic tube placed through the skin of the abdomen into the midsection of the small intestine. The tube delivers food and medicine until the person is healthy enough to eat by mouth.

Indications

Feeding jejunostomy is a surgical route of enteral access. Indications for the placement of a feeding jejunostomy is:

❖ When the oral route cannot be accessed for nutrition,

❖ When nasoenteral access is impossible

❖ When the time duration of artificial nutrition is more than six weeks and as an additional procedure after major gastrointestinal surgery with prolonged recovery time.

Although the most common type of surgical enteral access is a gastrostomy, feeding jejunostomies are indicated when the GI tract is functioning, but there is an obstruction in the proximal part of the gut precluding placement of a gastrostomy tube.

One of the major group of candidates for jejunostomy feeding are patients with major gastrointestinal resection of the esophagus, stomach, pancreas, and duodenum.

Myers et al. reviewed 2022 consecutive cases if needle catheter jejunostomies and reported that 89.7% (1939) was performed as an adjunct to laparotomies. Regardless of the pathology, many of these major surgical procedures are associated with prolonged recovery times, concern for the anastomosis including dysfunction or dehiscence, enteroenteral or enterocutaneous fistulas, and gastric atony. Jejunostomy feeding is also employed in patients as an adjunct to trauma laparotomies involving duodenal and pancreatic resection.

Jejunostomy feeding is indicated in patients with gastroparesis, which is characterized by decreased gastric motor function in the absence of mechanical obstruction.

Strijbos et al. showed that 19 of 86 patients with gastroparesis ultimately required enteral nutrition through the placement of a PEG-Jejunostomy tube. The remaining responded to prokinetics and bowel rest. Jejunostomy feeding is also indicated in gastric outlet obstruction (GOO) caused by a mechanical cause, such as an inoperable tumor, refractory peptic ulcer, or Bouveret syndrome. Jejunostomy feeding may, at times, be the last resort in inoperable duodenal tumors or strictures, and when the duodenum is compromised in conditions, such as pancreatitis. Palliative stenting may be considered for symptomatic improvement oral feeding in inoperative tumors.

A feeding jejunostomy tube may be used for the delivery of drugs, such as levodopa-carbidopa for the treatment of Parkinson disease. Continuous jejunal infusion of levodopa and carbidopa was associated with reduced motor fluctuations compared to oral delivery of the drug in patients with Parkinson disease.

The selection of a candidate for placement of a feeding jejunostomy involves multiple factors. The general condition of the patient, risk for aspiration, institutional facilities, and surgeons' experience must all be evaluated when determining the route for enteral nutrition.

Contraindications

Often, a feeding jejunostomy may be the only option for enteral access for a patient. It then becomes a potentially life-saving procedure, eliminating the need for parenteral nutrition and its associated risks. The only absolute contraindication to a feeding jejunostomy is bowel obstruction distal to the site of tube implantation. Relative contraindications can be classified as follows:

Local

- ❖ Abdominal wall infection at the placement site
- ❖ Severe ascites
- ❖ Peritonitis
- ❖ History of bowel necrosis from the previous jejunostomy

Systemic

- ❖ Severe coagulopathy (INR >1.5, a PTT >50 seconds, PLT <50,000/mm^3)
- ❖ Hemodynamic instability requiring the use of vasopressors
- ❖ Ventilatory dependence preventing transport to the operating room

Equipment

The equipment required depends on the techniques being used for the placement of the jejunostomy tube.
- ❖ Skin preparation with alcohol swabs/povidone-iodine swabs
- ❖ No. 11 surgical blade
- ❖ Lidocaine for local sedation
- ❖ Sterile gown and gloves
- ❖ 14- to18-gauge needle, a guidewire, sheath, feeding jejunostomy tube
- ❖ Sutures for creation of Witzel tunnel
- ❖ Dressing with 2 × 2 or 4 × 4 gauze, adhesive tape
- ❖ Basic laparoscopic equipment in case of laparoscopic J-tube insertion

Preparation

❖ Informed consent regarding the procedure, type of anesthesia, and potential complications must be obtained.
❖ The patient should be nil per os (NPO) for at least six hours before the procedure.
❖ Antibiotic presurgical prophylaxis should be given as per institutional guidelines.
❖ Reliable bedside suction should be present.
❖ Intravenous sedation should be provided and administered at the bedside.

Technique or Treatment

There are four techniques for jejunostomy placement:
1. Open surgical technique (longitudinal or transverse Witzel),
2. Laparoscopic technique,
3. Needle catheter technique, and
4. Percutaneous technique.

Although the preferred technique depends on the type of patient and expertise of the surgeon, the minimally invasive techniques are standard of care.

Open Surgical Technique

The patient is prepped and draped with sterility. An exit site is chosen in the LUQ, preferable a few centimeters away from the midline. A stab incision is made and dissected with tonsil forceps. A loop of proximal jejunum is delivered into the wound. A diamond-shaped purse-string suture is tied to the antimesenteric border of the jejunal loop, and a small incision is given in the center of the suture, large enough to accommodate the jejunostomy tube. The tube is inserted into the jejunum with care to ensure enough length of tube into the jejunum to prevent the backflow of tube feeds. The purse-string suture is secured tightly without kinking the tube.

The Witzel technique is used to prevent extravasation of enteric contents at the exit site of the jejunostomy tube. This involves placing the tube along the length of the bowel for about 5 cm proximally and creating a serosal tunnel to imbricate the tube into position. The serosal tunnel is created by taking perpendicular Lambert sutures with 3–0 silk on either side of the tube. Once the tube is delivered through the abdominal wall, the jejunal loop is attached to the abdominal wall with seromuscular sutures. This is done to prevent bowel obstruction or volvulus.

Laparoscopic Technique

It is a minimally invasive approach and preferred modality with the current advancement of technology. The patient is placed in a supine position initially, and after the creation of pneumoperitoneum and visual entry into the abdomen, the ligament of Treitz is visualized by upward retraction of the bowel and removal of omentum. The patient is kept in a reverse Trendelenburg position to allow the bowel to be traced. The jejunum is traced from the ligament of Treitz for 1–2 ft, and a site is chosen, which may be adhered to the abdominal wall. Four seromuscular sutures in the shape of a diamond are placed on the antimesenteric border of the jejunum. The loose ends of the sutures are used to pull the jejunum to the corresponding site over the abdominal wall. A percutaneous needle is used to enter the jejunum, and a guidewire is passed into the jejunum. The opposite side of the abdominal wall is inspected to make sure the guidewire has not passed through. Using serial dilators, the skin and subcutaneous tissue are dilated to make a track for the passage of the jejunostomy tube with a stent. Once the tube is in position, the stent is removed, and the balloon is inflated. The tube is secured in position, and laparoscopic incisions are closed with sutures and glue.

Needle Catheter Technique

This technique is often used as part of laparotomy with major gastrointestinal resection. A submucosal tunnel is created through the antimesenteric well of the jejunum with a needle catheter after its introduction into the abdominal cavity. The tunnel should be about 4–5 cm. This prevents the development of fistula after the placement of the tube. The catheter is introduced through the needle and sutured to the jejunal wall with a purse-string suture. Finally, the jejunum is attached to the peritoneal lining with sutures. Tube feeds can be started soon after surgery, within 6–12 hours.

Percutaneous Technique (Direct Percutaneous Endoscopic Jejunostomy)

Percutaneous insertion is done with the help of endoscopy. An enteroscope or colonoscope is passed into the jejunum. Transillumination of the tip of the scope is used to identify the position of the endoscope over the abdominal wall. A trocar is inserted through the abdominal wall into the jejunum, and a guidewire is passed distally into the jejunum. The tips of an awaiting snare or forceps are used to grasp the wire. A dilator is subsequently passed to create the track for the tube, and the tube is secured similarly to a 'pull-PEG' technique.

Complications

There is no evidence suggesting the type of jejunostomy tube with the lowest rate of complications; however, all techniques are associated with complications. Complications may be classified into mechanical, infectious, gastrointestinal, and metabolic complications.

Mechanical

Intestinal obstruction is a frequent complication and can be caused by over-inflation of the balloon; deflation of the balloon is both diagnostic and therapeutic. Transverse Witzel technique has been associated with the reflux of intestinal contents from intestinal ischemia and erosion of mucosa by the tube. Needle catheterization has been associated with withdrawal or blockage of the catheter, enterocutaneous fistulas, intestinal pneumatosis, and intestinal abscesses within the tunneled tube site. A laparoscopic jejunostomy is associated with inherent complications of laparoscopic surgery, such as problems arising from increased intra-abdominal pressure and anesthetics.

Infectious

Pneumonia from aspiration and contamination of feeds are the two common infectious complications. Aspiration may result from improper placement of the jejunostomy tube. A tube placed proximally may be associated with reflux. Some studies have shown that continuous enteral nutrition is associated with aspiration pneumonia in critically-ill patients.

Gastrointestinal

Nausea, vomiting, diarrhea, abdominal distension, and colic are some of the frequently observed complications. The type of feed being used plays an essential role in the severity of complications.

Metabolic

Hypokalemia, hyperglycemia, and acid-base balance disturbances are frequently observed. Some causes are the improper placement of the jejunostomy tube, the use of incorrect feeds, and failure to correct resulting biochemical abnormalities. As the stomach and duodenum are bypassed, there is the possibility of deficiencies of vitamin B12 and iron, absorbed through these two organs, respectively. Initiation of tube feeding after a period of starvation may lead to the development of refeeding syndrome characterized by hypokalemia, hypophosphatemia, and hypomagnesemia. The pathophysiology is believed to be related to the release of insulin from the pancreas when feeding is initiated. It often manifests in ICU patients as hemodynamic instability, respiratory failure, and other non-specific features.

TOTAL PARENTERAL NUTRITION

Parenteral nutrition (PN) refers to the provision of nutrients by the intravenous route. In general, PN should only be used when it is not possible to supply nutrition using the GI tract, i.e., when intestinal failure is present.

Total parenteral nutrition (TPN) implies that all macronutrient (carbohydrate, proteins and lipid) and micronutrient (vitamins, trace elements and minerals) and fluid requirements are met by an intravenous nutrient solution and no significant nutrition is obtained from other sources. Some patients treated with PN can absorb some fluid and nutrition taken orally and in these patients PN is a supplement to their oral intake.

Total parenteral nutrition (TPN), also known as parenteral nutrition (PN) is a form of nutritional support given completely via the bloodstream, intravenously with an IV pump. TPN administers proteins, carbohydrates, fats, vitamins, and minerals. It aims to prevent and restore nutritional deficits, allowing bowel rest while supplying adequate caloric intake and essential nutrients, and removing antigenic mucosal stimuli.

TPN may be short-term or long-term nutritional therapy.

Indications

❖ Patients with paralyzed or nonfunctional GI tract, or conditions that require bowel rest, such as small bowel obstruction, ulcerative colitis, or pancreatitis.
❖ Patients who have had nothing by mouth (NPO) for seven days or longer.
❖ Critically-ill patients.
❖ Babies with an immature gastrointestinal system or congenital malformations.
❖ Patients with chronic or extreme malnutrition, or chronic diarrhea or vomiting with a need for surgery or chemotherapy.
❖ Patients in hyperbolic states, such as burns, sepsis, or trauma.

Specific conditions that may require TPN include:
❖ Abdominal surgery.
❖ Chemotherapy.
❖ Intestinal ischemia.
❖ Small or large intestinal obstructions.
❖ Intestinal pseudo-obstruction.
❖ Prolonged ileus.
❖ Gastrointestinal bleeding.
❖ Radiation enteritis.

* Extremely premature birth.
* Necrotizing enterocolitis.
* Prolonged diarrhea.
* Inflammatory bowel diseases.
* Short bowel syndrome.
* Persistent chyle leak.
* Graft-versus-host disease of the gut

Parenteral Nutrition Formulation

Modern parenteral nutrition (PN) solutions are referred to as All-in-One (AIO) or multi-chamber bags (MCB) containing all the required nutritional components. Standardized fixed feeding regimens or individually compounded mixtures are available. Vitamins, trace elements, minerals and water may be added to both regimens but must only be done under controlled aseptic pharmaceutical conditions. Individually compounded solutions are manufactured under strictly controlled aseptic conditions in a suitable pharmacy manufacturing unit.

In certain clinical conditions, e.g., patients with chronic intestinal failure requiring long-term home PN (HPN), the compounding of individualized parenteral nutrition is often required. This gives the possibility of meeting the particular nutritional and fluid requirements of these patients, particularly where parenteral nutrition is a supplement to their oral intake.

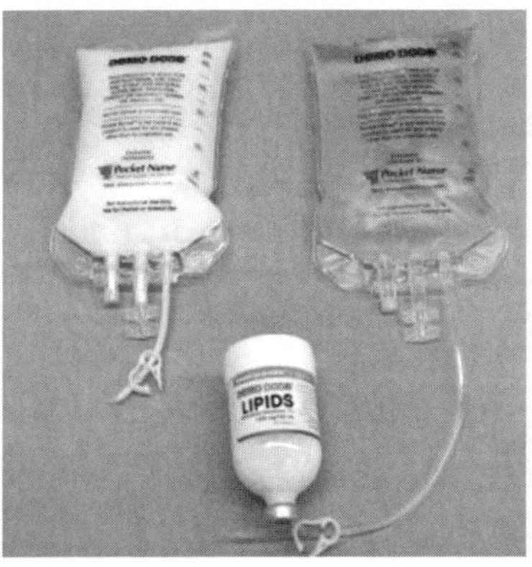
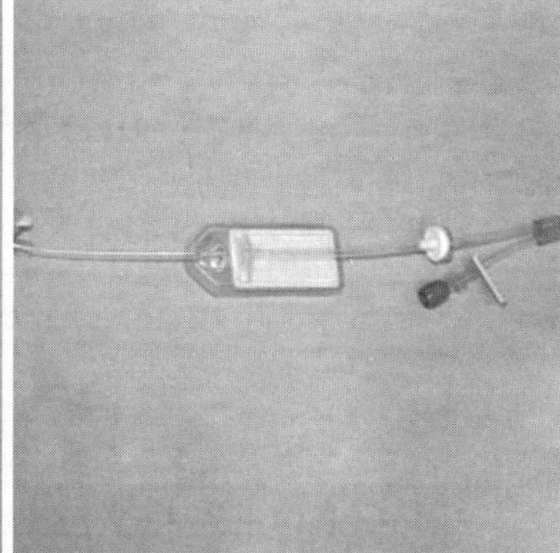

Fluids and Electrolytes in Parenteral Nutrition

Patients on PN require an appropriate amount of fluid and electrolytes. The volume will vary widely depending on oral intake, excess losses, and other medical conditions, such as cardiac or renal failure. Inpatients may also have other intravenous drugs prescribed, containing significant amounts of electrolytes in variable volumes of fluid. Although the basal requirement for water is quoted as 25–35 mL/kg/day, the above factors lead to wide variations in the total volume and electrolyte content of PN.

Macronutrients in Parenteral Nutrition

Carbohydrate

Carbohydrate in PN is provided by glucose, an energy source that is available in a range of concentrations (5–70%). It is generally provided in amounts up to 60% of total energy provided per day. While the inclusion of some carbohydrate is essential for central nervous system

(CNS) function, the maximum glucose oxidation rate (4–7 mg/kg/min/day) should not be exceeded as this may result in hyperglycemia, hepatic steatosis and impaired respiratory function with increased CO_2 production. Glucose tolerance may be impaired in patients with an inflammatory response and concurrent insulin treatment may be necessary to prevent hyperglycemia. It is recommended that insulin be given as a separate infusion and not added to the PN solution. Hyperglycemia in hospitalized patients is associated with a higher risk of complications and should be avoided (Krinsley, 2003).

Nitrogen

Nitrogen requirements are generally provided in a range of 0.17–0.3 g/kg/day depending on degree of metabolic stress and catabolism present. Amino acid solutions are available with a range of nitrogen content (e.g., 6–20 g). In addition, solutions enriched with certain amino acids have become available, e.g., glutamine. Glutamine, although not an essential amino acid, may become a conditionally essential amino acid during metabolic stress. There are problems providing glutamine in PN solutions due to its instability and low solubility in aqueous solutions.

Lipid

Lipid in PN solutions provides a concentrated form of energy reducing the need for infusion of large amounts of glucose, minimise respiratory and metabolic stress, preventing essential fatty acid deficiency and allows peripheral infusion of nutrients. It is available in 10%, 20% and 30% concentrations and generally used to provide 20–30% of daily energy requirements. Lipid can accumulate in the reticuloendothelial system, impairing its ability to remove bacteria and endotoxins and increasing susceptibility to infection. It is therefore recommended that lipid content of PN should not exceed 1–1.5 g/kg/day. Cholestatic complications have also been noted to be associated with higher lipid content. Soybean emulsions, e.g., Intralipid®, are the oldest lipid emulsions available. They provide essential fatty acids and fat soluble vitamins but contain a high proportion (>60%) of the polyunsaturated fatty acids (PUFA); linoleic acid (52–54%) and alpha linolenic acids (7–9%). These emulsions, rich in n-6 fatty acids, in conditions of stress may be pro-inflammatory and exert immunosuppressive effects. Novel or so called third generation lipids have been developed with the intention of modulating inflammatory responses and improving outcomes. These include emulsions containing medium chain triglycerides (MCT), olive oil and fish oil in various combinations as a partial replacement for soybean oil. Supplying n-3 fatty acids may have anti-inflammatory effects the opposite effect to fatty acids of the n-6 series. Lipid preparations based on olive oil can also be used to decrease the intake of PUFA and may be less susceptible to lipid peroxidation than n-6 and n-3 PUFA. Such novel lipids have been shown to be safe and may offer some advantages over the use of soybean oil alone but there is a lack of evidence on the differential effects of lipid emulsions on clinical endpoints. More work is needed to evaluate these emulsions before recommendations can be made.

Micronutrients in Parenteral Nutrition

An adequate supply of micronutrients is essential for patients on PN to prevent clinical and subclinical deficiency states. Commercially prepared mixtures are available that provide well-balanced amounts of all essential vitamins and trace elements. Requirements for parenteral vitamins, trace elements and minerals will vary among patients depending on clinical and metabolic status and the need to replace any losses or prevent toxicity, e.g., in renal patients.

Further supplements may be appropriate in certain circumstances. For example, starved patients may require additional thiamine as reserves would be expected to be low. Electrolytes are added according to anticipated patient requirements. Excessive electrolyte losses from wounds, surgical drains, vomiting and diarrhea need to be replaced in the PN formulation or other IV fluids.

Parenteral nutrition can be administered via peripheral or central veins:

1. *Choice of nutrient solution for peripheral administration:* Hyperosmotic solutions are poorly tolerated by peripheral veins, and could cause pain, thrombophlebitis and thrombosis. The inclusion of lipid and an increase in volume of solution may reduce osmolarity. Furthermore, lipid emulsion-based admixtures may also have a pH better tolerated by small vessels. Electrolyte content is an important consideration, as additions of electrolytes will increase the tonicity and affect the pH. Solutions <1200 mosm/L have been shown to be tolerated when infused into peripheral veins.

2. *Choice of nutrient solution for central administration:* The delivery of PN solutions into a large diameter high flow vein, such as the superior or inferior vena cava enables highly concentrated nutrient solutions to be infused. Consequently, central PN will be required for patients with special nutrient requirements, e.g., lipid free, high nutrient requirements or reduced fluid requirements or for patients who do not have suitable peripheral access.

ASSESSMENT OF A PATIENT WITH TPN

Assessment	Additional Information
CVC/peripheral IV line	Intravenous line should remain patent, free from infection. Dextrose in TPN increases risk of infection. Assess for signs and symptoms of infections at site (redness, tenderness, discharge) and systemically (fever, increased WBC, malaise). Dressing should be dry and intact.
Daily or biweekly weights	Monitor for evidence of edema or fluid overload. Over time, measurements will reflect weight loss/gain from caloric intake or fluid retention.
Capillary or serum blood glucose levels	QID (4 times a day) capillary blood glucose initially to monitor glycemic control, then reduce monitoring when blood sugars are stable or as per agency policy. May be done more frequently if glycemic control is difficult. Indicates metabolic tolerance to dextrose in TPN solution and patient's glycemic status.
Monitor intake and output	Monitor and record every eight hours or as per agency policy. Monitor for signs and symptoms of fluid overload (excessive weight gain) by completing a cardiovascular and respiratory assessment. Assess intakes, such as IV (intravenous fluids), PO (oral intake), NG (nasogastric tube feeds). Assess outputs: NG (removed gastric content through the nasogastric tube), fistula drainage, BM (liquid bowel movements), colostomy/ileostomy drainage, closed suction drainage devices (Penrose or Jackson-Pratt drainage) and chest tube drainage.
Daily to weekly blood work	Review lab values for increases and decreases out of normal range. Lab values include CBC, electrolytes, calcium, magnesium, phosphorus, potassium, glucose, albumin, BUN (blood urea nitrogen), creatinine, triglycerides, and transferrin.
Mouth care	Most patients will be NPO. Proper oral care is required as per agency policy. Some patients may have a diet order.
Vital signs	Vital signs are more frequently monitored initially in patients with TPN.

TPN may be administered in the hospital or in a home setting. Generally, patients receiving TPN are quite ill and may require a lengthy stay in the hospital. The administration of TPN must follow strict adherence to aseptic technique, and includes being alert for complications, as many of the patients will have altered defense mechanisms and complex conditions. To administer TPN, follow the steps in checklist:

CHECKLIST: TPN ADMINISTRATION

Disclaimer: Always review and follow your hospital policy regarding this specific skill.

Safety considerations:
- Compare the patient's baseline vital signs; electrolyte, glucose, and triglyceride levels; weight; and fluid intake and output with treatment values, and investigate any rapid change in such values.
- To identify signs of infection early, be aware of the patient's recent temperature range.
- Use strict aseptic technique when caring for central venous catheters and PICC lines.
- Do not use TPN solution if it has coalesced, as evidenced by formation of a thick, dense layer of fat droplets on its surface. If the solution appears abnormal in any way, request a replacement from the pharmacy.
- Never try to catch up with a delayed infusion.

Steps	*Additional Information*
1. Review physician's orders and compare to MAR and content label on TPN solution bag and for rate of infusion. Each component of the TPN solution must be verified with the physician's orders.	Check date and time of last TPN tubing change, lab values, and expiry date of TPN to prevent medication error. Assess CVC, WBC, and patient for malaise. Medications may be added to the TPN. Ensure the rate of infusion is verified in the doctor's order each time new TPN bag is initiated.
2. Collect supplies, prepare TPN solution, and prime IV tubing with filter as per agency protocol. TPN requires special IV tubing with a filter.	Generally, new TPN tubing is required every 24 hours to prevent catheter-related bacteremia. Follow agency policy. Ensure tubing is primed correctly to prevent air embolism. 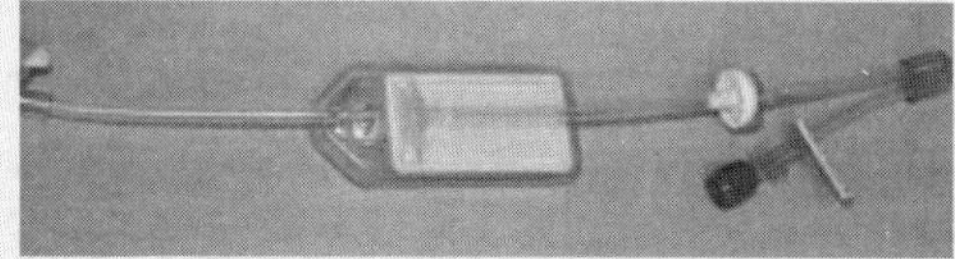 TPN tubing with special filter
3. Perform hand hygiene, identify yourself, and identify patient using two patient identifiers. Compare the MAR to the patient's wristband. Explain the procedure to the patient.	Hand hygiene prevents the spread of microorganisms. Proper identification prevents patient errors. 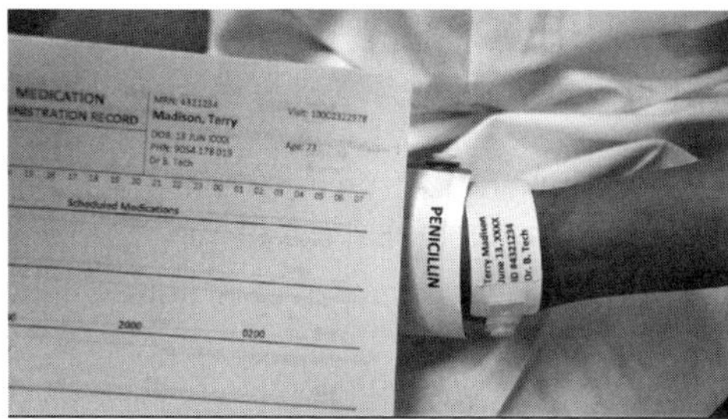 Compare MAR to patient wristband

Contd...

Contd...

Steps	Additional Information
4. Complete all safety checks for CVC as per agency policy.	This adheres to safety policies related to central line care.
5. If changing TPN solution, pause EID and remove old TPN administration set. Disinfect connections and change IV tubing as per agency policy. If starting TPN for the first time, flush and disinfect CVC lumens as per agency policy.	Change TPN IV tubing as per agency policy. Use strict aseptic technique with IV changes as patients with high dextrose solutions are at greater risk of developing infections.
6. Insert new TPN solution and IV tubing into EID.	EID must be used with all TPN administration.
7. Start TPN infusion rate as per physician orders.	Prevents medication errors.
8. Discard old supplies as per agency protocol, and perform hand hygiene.	These steps prevent the spread of microorganisms.
9. Monitor for signs and symptoms of complications related to TPN.	List of complications related to TPN.
10. Complete daily assessments and monitoring for patient on TPN as per agency policy.	Flow rate may be monitored hourly.
11. Document the procedure in the patient chart as per agency policy.	Note time when TPN bag is hung, number of bags, and rate of infusion, assessment of CVC site and verification of patency, status of dressing, vital signs and weight, client tolerance to TPN, client response to therapy, and understanding of instructions.

TPN COMPLICATIONS, RATIONALE, AND INTERVENTIONS

Complication	Rationale and Interventions
Catheter-related bloodstream infection (CR-BSI), also known as sepsis	CR-BSI, which starts at the hub connection, is the spread of bacteria through the bloodstream. There is an increased risk of CR-BSI with TPN, due to the high dextrose concentration of TPN. Symptoms include tachycardia, hypotension, elevated or decreased temperature, increased breathing, decreased urine output, and disorientation. **Interventions:** Strict adherence to aseptic technique with insertion, care, and maintenance; avoid hyperglycemia to prevent infection complications; closely monitor vital signs and temperature. IV antibiotic therapy is required. Monitor white blood cell count and patient for malaise. Replace IV tubing frequently as per agency policy (usually every 24 hours).
Localized infection at exit or entry site	Due to poor aseptic technique during insertion, care, or maintenance of central line or peripheral line **Interventions:** Apply strict aseptic technique during insertion, care, and maintenance. Frequently assess CVC site for redness, tenderness, or drainage. Notify health care provider of any signs and symptoms of infection.

Contd...

Contd...

Complication	Rationale and Interventions
Pneumothorax	A pneumothorax occurs when the tip of the catheter enters the pleural space during insertion, causing the lung to collapse. Symptoms include sudden chest pain, difficulty breathing, decreased breath sounds, cessation of normal chest movement on affected side, and tachycardia. **Interventions:** Apply oxygen, notify physician. Patient will require removal of central line and possible chest tube insertion.
Air embolism	An air embolism may occur if IV tubing disconnects and is open to air, or if part of catheter system is open or removed without being clamped. Symptoms include sudden respiratory distress, decreased oxygen saturation levels, shortness of breath, coughing, chest pain, and decreased blood pressure. **Interventions:** Make sure all connections are clamped and closed. Clamp catheter, position patient in left Trendelenburg position, call healthcare provider, and administer oxygen as needed.
Hyperglycemia	Related to sudden increase in glucose after recent malnourished state. After starvation, glucose intake suppresses gluconeogenesis by leading to the release of insulin and the suppression of glycogen. Excessive glucose may lead to hyperglycemia, with osmotic diuresis, dehydration, metabolic acidosis, and ketoacidosis. Excess glucose also leads to lipogenesis (again caused by insulin stimulation). This may cause fatty liver, increased CO_2 production, hypercapnea, and respiratory failure. **Interventions:** Monitor blood sugar frequently QID (four times per day), then less frequently when blood sugars are stable. Follow agency policy for glucose monitoring with TPN. Be alert to changes in dextrose levels in amino acids and the addition/removal of insulin to TPN solution.
Refeeding syndrome	**Refeeding syndrome** is caused by rapid refeeding after a period of malnutrition, which leads to metabolic and hormonal changes characterized by electrolyte shifts (decreased phosphate, magnesium, and potassium in serum levels) that may lead to widespread cellular dysfunction. Phosphorus, potassium, magnesium, glucose, vitamin, sodium, nitrogen, and fluid imbalances can be life-threatening. High-risk patients include the chronically undernourished and those with little intake for more than 10 days. Patients with dysphagia are at higher risk. The syndrome usually occurs 24 to 48 hours after refeeding has started. The shift of water, glucose, potassium, phosphate, and magnesium back into the cells may lead to muscle weakness, respiratory failure, paralysis, coma, cranial nerve palsies, and rebound hypoglycemia. **Interventions:** Rate of TPN should be based on the severity of undernourishment for moderate- to high-risk patients. TPN should be initiated slowly and titrated up for four to seven days. All patients require close monitoring of electrolytes (daily for one week, then usually three times/week). Always follow agency policy. Blood work may be more frequent depending on the severity of the malnourishment.
Fluid excess or pulmonary edema	Signs and symptoms include fine crackles in lower lung fields or throughout lung fields, hypoxia (decreased O_2 sats). **Interventions:** Notify primary healthcare provider regarding change in condition. Patient may require IV medication, such as Lasix to remove excess fluids. A decrease or discontinuation of IV fluids may also occur. Raise head of bed to enhance breathing and apply O_2 for oxygen saturation <92% or as per agency protocol. Monitor intake and output. Pulmonary edema may be more common in the elderly, young, and patients with renal or cardiac conditions.

Hygiene

UNIT OUTLINE

- Hygienic care
- Care of the skin
- Pressure ulcers
- Perineal care/meatal care
- Oral care
- Care of eyes, ears and nose including assistive devices

LEARNING OBJECTIVES

At the end of this unit, the reader will be able to:
- Introduce hygiene.
- Explain factors influencing hygiene.
- State effect of poor hygiene.
- Practice care of skin.
- Perform care of hair and nails, feet.
- Define pediculosis and treatment.
- Describe pressure points.
- List out causes of pressure ulcers.
- Identify preventive measures for pressure ulcers.
- Analyze assessment methods and scales for pressure ulcers.
- Explain treatment measure and nursing responsibilities.
- Impart health education for pressure sores.
- Categorize stages of pressure sores.
- Explain wound management.
- Practice perineal/meatal care.
- Define oral hygiene care of dentures.
- Perform care of eyes and drug instillation.
- Define eye irrigation.
- Perform care of ear and drug instillation.
- Visual aids.
- Hearing aids.

Physical hygiene is necessary for comfort, safety, and well-being. Ill patients require assistance with personal hygiene. Several factors influence a patient's hygiene practices, such as culture and age. Good hygiene techniques promote normal structure and function of tissues.

Personal hygiene involves care and cleanliness of our physical as well as mental being. The word 'hygiene' is derived from the Greek word 'Hygeia' the goddess of health who was supposed to look after the health of the people. Hygiene deals both with the individual and community—what the individual has to do to preserve and to improve the health of his body and mind comes under the scope of personal hygiene, and what the organized community needs to do to maintain, protect and improve the health of the people as a whole comes under the scope of public health. That aspect of public health which is concerned with keeping the external surroundings clean and healthy is termed sanitation. Environmental sanitation is concerned with all those things in a man's surroundings that affect his body and mind's development, his health and his life. It is concerned with safe drinking water, pollution-free air and surroundings, proper sewage disposal, sanitary conditions and food supply, regulation for house and building construction, pest control, etc.

Personal hygiene refers to maintaining cleanliness of one's body and clothing to preserve overall health and well-being. Personal hygiene involves a number of activities like bathing, washing hands, cleaning teeth, changing into clean clothes, etc.

The word contamination is sometimes used to denote the presence of germs outside—on surface of various articles, in the food, water and other eatables. Thus, when we consider ourselves healthy, it means that our body is functioning properly, we are emotionally stable, effectively face challenges and opportunities in our life and can live harmoniously with other members of society. In other words, being healthy means that we are not healthy just because we are not ill. We should not only be free from illness but should also lead a purposeful and productive life while maintaining good relationships with people.

The word hygiene is derived from Hygeia, the Greek goddess of health in Greek mythology. She is represented as beautiful women holding in her hand a bowl from which a serpent is drinking. In Greek mythology the serpent testifies the art of healing.

FACTORS INFLUENCING HYGIENE

Social patterns Ethnic, social, and family influences on hygiene patterns	**Personal preferences** Dictate hygiene practices
Body image A person's subjective concept of his or her body appearance	**Socioeconomic status** Influences the type and extent of hygiene practices used
Health beliefs and motivation Motivation is the key factor in hygiene	**Cultural variables** People from diverse cultures practice different hygiene rituals
Developmental stage Affects the patient's ability to perform hygiene care	**Physical condition** May lack physical energy and dexterity to perform self-care

❖ **Energy of the individual**: People in sickness may not have the health and energy to take care of hygiene (cleanliness). For example, people who are sick for long time, who have plasters, paralysis, may not have enough energy or strength to take care of themselves. So help the clients according to their abilities and energy to meet cleanliness needs.

❖ **Habits and culture:** Some people prefer to take bath twice a day and some once a day. They may have choices for some shampoos, soaps, toothpaste or when to bathe, shave. So these choices have to be kept in mind while giving care. In some cultures, personal hygiene is considered very important so people take bath everyday while some take bath during fast even though they have fever or other illness. So according to cultural practices hygienic care can be planned. During the long-term illness these habits are ignored by family members. So these choices have to be kept in mind while planning care of the patient.

❖ **Knowledge:** Knowledge about importance of hygienic practices influence hygiene of client. For example, when diabetic clients learn that proper foot care will help in prevention of developing foot ulcer, then they will do proper foot care.

Cultural Variables

People from diverse cultural backgrounds may follow different hygiene practices. Different groups of people regard cleanliness according to their own culture. Americans tend to bath daily. Individuals from others parts of the world may bath less frequently. Body odor is not always offensive in other cultures.

❖ Avoid forcing changes in hygiene practices unless the practice effects the patient's health.
❖ Use tact, provide information, and allow choice.
❖ Remember that religious practice can also influence hygiene practices.

The role that critical thinking plays in hygiene:

❖ Nurse must use past experiences and personal knowledge to make clinical judgements regarding patient hygiene practice.
❖ Remember the patient's condition is always changing, requiring continued critical thinking to apply other methods of care or instruction.
❖ Be aware of the impact of critical thinking attitudes on the patient. Be sensitive and non-judgmental in offering instruction on hygiene.
❖ Allow the patient to incorporate their own practices and routines when safe.
❖ Rely on professional standards of care when teaching a patient.

A patient with certain types of physical limitations or disabilities associated with disease and injury lack the physical energy and skill to perform hygiene self-care safely.

These patients may need assistance from a home health nurse or a family member to meet their hygiene needs.

This is the patient's subjective concept of their body and it affects the way the individual maintains their hygiene.

Some patients may need further education on the importance of hygiene.

Surgery, illness, and changes in emotional status can affect the patient's body image. Pain, discomfort and emotional stress may cause the patient to be less interested or motivated to maintain personal hygiene.

Developmental Stages

As we age, the body goes through many changes. It is expected that a person's developmental stage affects the ability of the patient to perform hygiene care and the type of care needed.

Physical Condition

Social Practices

❖ Parents perform hygiene for children.
❖ Family custom can determine hygiene habits, such as how often you should bath, and which hygiene practices should be performed.
❖ Involvement with friends and peer groups helps shape your hygiene practices.

Personal Preferences

❖ Patients have their own desires for personal hygiene, e.g., some prefer showers and other baths.
❖ Learn the patient's preferences. You may need to help the patient learn new hygiene practices if it is indicated for a condition or illness, e.g., proper foot care for diabetes.
❖ Always promote patient independence in decision making.
❖ Body image

Socioeconomic Status

❖ A person's resources will affect the type and extent of hygiene practices used.
❖ Some patients may not be able to afford hygiene items that others would consider basic or necessary. When this is the case, it may be difficult to take a role in assisting the patient in improving personal hygiene.

Health Beliefs and Motivation

❖ Knowledge about hygiene may not motivate a patient to make changes to their current practices.
❖ The nurse should provide hygiene teaching that is related to the patient's health-related issues.
❖ "Patient perception of the benefits of hygiene care and the susceptibility to and seriousness of developing a problem affect the motivation to change behavior".
❖ Patients are more willing to make necessary changes in hygiene practice if there is a need and reasonable effort can be made to accomplish the change.

Definition

Hygiene may define as the practice or activity that individual do to keep things healthy and clean.

For example, good oral hygiene includes brushing and cleaning your teeth, and working in a clean kitchen helps promote food hygiene.

The effects of poor hygiene are far-reaching beyond the obvious health concerns. Failing to frequently wash your hands, brush your teeth, and take showers does not just affect you. It affects everyone you interact with.

Poor personal hygiene arises from either intentional or unintentional neglect of your body's cleanliness and health requirements.

Effects of Poor Hygiene

The consequences of patient neglect are very serious. Neglect can result in malnutrition, bed sores, atrophy, unsanitary personal hygiene, and untreated medical conditions.

Body Odor

This is probably the most common evidence of poor personal hygiene. Not only does it lead to discomfort and an embarrassing situation for those around you, but there are also other consequences. Person could develop allergies, constant itching, and the result of being socially isolated due to these conditions.

When your sweat and the bacteria produced from your apocrine glands interact, it produces body odor. So the more there's unwashed sweat, the bacteria increases, and the odor gets even worse. But it all starts with poor personal hygiene and bad behaviors like:

* Infrequent showering.
* Wearing dirty, smelly socks
* Not airing shoes
* Not taking the time to wash feet
* Wearing smelly, stained, or dirty clothes each day
* Not changing your undergarments regularly.

Bad Breath

Bad breath (or halitosis) is another effects of poor hygiene that impacts your oral health. When you eat, the bacteria that are present on the food particles get stuck on your teeth. Unfortunately, as these bacteria digest, they produce a strong unpleasant odor that is associated with halitosis.

Poor oral hygiene leads to other problems like tooth decay and bleeding gums. The behaviors that lead to these oral diseases include:

* Irregular brushing of your teeth
* Not flossing every time you brush your teeth
* Neglecting to clean your tongue when brushing your teeth
* Drinking too many acidic drinks too often
* Excessive smoking

Lice Infestation

Body lice infestation is quite uncomfortable and hazardous to your health. These lice are small insects that live and lay eggs in clothing and bedding. They also feed on the residues found on your skin.

Lice tend to colonize in your armpits and groin, as these are the areas with a lot of humidity. So, it is important to take regular baths, and wear clean, fresh clothes each day to avoid any lice infestation.

Avoid doing the following to stave off any such infestation:

* Infrequent showering
* Not changing your bedding at least every week
* Not washing your clothes very well
* Wearing dirty and/or smelly clothes

HEALTH

"The first duty of mankind is preservation of self" (Rig-Veda) Sharir Madyam Khalu Dharm Sadhnam (the body is the vehicle of fulfilling all duties) has been the central thought in the Indian tradition. Also, it has been said that a healthy mind lives in a healthy body. Thus, it is of utmost importance to keep body and mind healthy to live a happy and nurturing life. Adolescence is the period where the seeds of habits are sown and if healthy habits are nurtured, they can prevent up to 70% of diseases.

World Health Organization (WHO) defines health "a state of complete physical, mental, and social well-being and not merely the absence of disease or infirmity." Let us understand what it means.

* Physical means concerned with the body.
* Mental means concerned with the functioning of mind and emotions.
* Social means concerned with other members of society.
* Disease or infirmity means sickness or ill health, i.e., one or more organs of our body are not able to function in the normal way.

Disease is caused by presence of harmful germs in and outside of our body or wear and tear in our body. The germs can be bacteria, viruses or certain fungi. The germs when enter our body and stay there, it is called infection. Our body has a defense mechanism to kill these germs but sometimes it is overpowered by germs and it results in disease.

CARE OF SKIN

Taking Bath Daily

Taking a bath has been recognized one of the healthy practices in all the cultures since antiquity. People used to take bath in community hammams as well as personal bathrooms.

Taking a bath daily not only removes sweat, dirt and accompanying germs from our body but it also gives a sense of freshness.

Following are the general guidelines for taking a bath:
* Take at least one bath a day.
* Change the undergarments after a bath as the sweat makes them smell badly and helps the germs to grow.
* Use your own towel only to wipe your body after taking the bath. Using other's towel can lead to skin infections.
* Use running water (preferably) and soap for taking the bath.
* If it is not possible to take bath (as in special medical conditions when you are bedridden) use warm and clean water and a towel to wipe your body at least once a day.
* Any bath soap is good for taking bath. The choice of a particular brand, color or shape and size is individual choice.
* Costly, fragrant and imported soaps are no better than ordinary bath soap.
* Baby soaps (e.g., Johnson baby soap) are recommended for children as their skin is delicate and requires mild soap.
* Special soaps (e.g., containing moisturizer, mild detergents) can be used on recommendation of the physician for any specific reason.
* Using oil over the body after taking bath is not essential except for dry skin.
* Avoid taking bath in ponds which usually have stagnant water and are also used by animals. It can lead to infections. After religious rituals involving taking a dip in a pond and/or river which is contaminated. It is advisable to take a bath with clean water and soap as soon as you get clean water.
* Be cautious in taking bath in rivers. It can be dangerous because of dirty water, striking with rocks, dangerous animals like crocodiles and accidental slippage and drowning.

CARE OF FEET

In our country, most of us wear some kind of an open footwear if not, none at all. The reason is partly the climate in a major part of the country being tropical, you feel more comfortable with open footwear most of the year round. It is also economical they are cheaper to buy. Anyway, the result of wearing open shoes in a large number of cases is development of calluses on the heels hard and thick skin with cracks in it. This not only looks dirty and ugly, but it can be a source of pain and infection. The simplest is not to allow calluses to develop. This can be ensured by scrubbing the soles of your feet, particularly the heels, with something which can have a scrubbing action, every time you have a bath. Pumice is a good stone for this. This also means you should have a low stool in your bathroom to sit upon and scrub your heels. Once you do this regularly it becomes a habit and you are likely to feel unclean if you do not do it. There are special creams ointments available to remove calluses.

CARE OF HAIR AND NAILS

Hair originates in tiny sacs or follicles deep in the dermis layer of skin tissue. Hair follicles are closely connected to the sebaceous glands, which secrete oil to the scalp and give hair its natural sheen. The texture of the hair differs among individuals and also among the different races. It also differs from one part of the body to another. In some areas it may be soft and downy; in others, tough and bristly. Hair texture also differs between the sexes. Properly cared hair looks clean, shiny and alive. Hair should be washed about once a week. Oily hair may need washing more often. No matter what kind of soap or detergent you use, a thorough rinsing of hair is essential to eliminate any deposits of soap left over. If the water you use is hard, a detergent shampoo is more easily rinsed off than one containing soap. Drying hair in sunlight or letting them dry on their own is more satisfactory than rubbing them dry with a towel, gentle brushing during drying reactivates the natural oils that give hair its shine. Brushing in general is excellent for the appearance of the hair. Both comb and brush however should be washed and kept clean regularly. Under normal combing, brushing and shampooing a person looses anywhere from 25 to 100 hairs a day but because new hair grow each day, the loss and replacement usually balance each other. When however, the loss rate is greater than the replacement rate, thinning and baldness result. Baldness is basically related to sex, age and heredity, but bacterial or fungal infections, allergic reactions to particular medicines, radiation, or continual friction may also cause baldness. Constant stress from hair curlers or tightly pulled hair styles can cause loss of hair. These forms of baldness, however, disappear when the cause is eliminated. Poor nutrition can result in hair that is dry, dull and brittle. Serious illness can lead to hair loss as well. Women ordinarily lose some of their hair at the end of pregnancy, after delivery and during menopause, but it often grows back. Dandruff is a condition in which the scalp begins to itch and flake a few days after the hair has been washed. There is no evidence that the problem is related to germ infection. There are medicines that control it but it cannot be cured totally. The average male removes (shaves) hair from at least part of his face once a day. Feminine shaving practices are however a recent phenomena. It is a part of body cleanliness and good grooming for women as well as men to remove hair from the arm pits as often as twice a week. Since wet hair is much easier to cut, the most effective time to shave the arm pits is during or immediately after a bath.

Sycosis or barber's itch is a bacterial infection of the hair follicles of the beard. It is accompanied by inflammation, itching, and the formation of pus-filled pimples. Doctors prescribe antibiotics to treat it. One should not share shaving equipment to avoid such infections.

Hair and nails are the parts of human body which played an important role in prehistoric times when our ancestors were living in jungles without clothes and killing animals for their food. Hair provided them warmth and nails were used like weapons. Nowadays, they have only aesthetic value and for this they need to be regularly trimmed and cleaned. Following points are worth considering for care of hair and nails:

Hair

- ❖ Wash your hair with soap and water at the time of taking bath to clean the dirt. In adolescents it is more required because the sweat glands are more active and thus, hair attract more dirt.
- ❖ There should be regular cutting/trimming of hair.
- ❖ The hair in the armpits and genital region should be removed regularly as they cause bad smell due to sweat and can have infections.
- ❖ Some medicated shampoos are helpful in medical conditions for which medical advice should be taken. Dandruff is one of such conditions which is caused by a fungus. It leads to itching, flakes and hairfall but is treatable.
- ❖ Hair fall and whitening is common in males after middle age but a skin specialist should be consulted for any untoward hair fall, itching and whitening of hair.
- ❖ Poor hygiene and sharing clothes and combs may lead to hair infections like dandruff and lice and hence, should be avoided.

TYPES OF HAIR CARE FOR PATIENT

General

A patient's hair should be combed daily. In addition to other care provided to patient it is necessary to:
- ❖ Enhance morale.
- ❖ Stimulate circulation of the scalp.
- ❖ Prevent tangled, matted hair.

Daily Care

Encourage the patient to rub his scalp with fingertips to stimulate circulation. This can be done by the relatives of patient also. Comb hair in a suitable style which patient wants. Assist a patient to comb matted and tangled hair, first comb the ends and progress toward the scalp. Hold the lock of hair being combed between the scalp and the comb to avoid pulling. Brush the hair as necessary.

Hair Cutting

Barber service is provided in most service hospitals. The barber makes regular rounds on the ward or comes by appointment. The patient receiving the service pays the fee directly to the barber. Ambulatory patients go to the barber shop or beauty parlor, if the medical officer approves. Hair is cut and shaved by barbers. Barbers can provide hair cutting services in the hospital as and when requested.

Shampoo

The patient confined to bed will require a cleansing shampoo at least every two weeks. With the approval of the medical officer, plan the shampoo for a time when the patient feels comfortable and has no conflicting treatments or appointments. If the patient can be moved to a stretcher, do so and take him to a convenient sink. If this is not possible, do the shampoo in bed.

PEDICULOSIS AND ITS TREATMENT

Due to lack of proper hygiene, parasites can infest hair. The most common infection is pediculosis or lice. They are tiny, greyish white parasite insects that infest mammals. They are of three types:

1. Pediculosis capitis (head lice)
2. Pediculosis corporis (body lice)
3. Pediculosis pubis (crab lice)

Symptoms of Pediculosis Capitis

The symptoms of lice infestation are not visible in the first 2–6 weeks, but some of the common signs and symptoms are:

* Continuous itching in the scalp, neck and ears.
* Visibility of lice on the scalp.
* Lice eggs on hair shafts. The lice can only be spotted around the ears or near the hairline of the neck. Medical care should be taken immediately if suspected of the above symptoms.

Treatments of Pediculosis Capitis

The doctors usually recommend an over-the-counter (OTC) treatment that is helpful in removing the lice from the scalp. OTC treatment is based on pyrethrin, which is toxic to lice. The doctors will recommend washing the hair with shampoo before taking these treatments. In some cases, if OTC treatments are not successful, the doctors may also recommend, one of the following:

* Benzyl alcohol treatment for children above 6 months of age.
* Malathion, a medicated shampoo for children above 6 years of age.
* Lindane shampoo treatment.

Articles Required for Pediculosis Treatment

* Anti lice agent (either liquid or powder form, e.g., Lysil, Medikr, Vinegar or DDT powder mixed with oil or powder 1:9)
* Vaseline
* A pair of gloves and a mask
* Cotton swabs in a container
* Face towel to protect the eyes
* Mackintosh with cover
* Kidney tray with carbolic solution
* Paper bag
* Apron
* Screen

Procedure Steps

* Explain the procedure to the patient.
* Wash hands.
* Assemble all the articles and take them to the bedside.
* Screen the patient.

- Put on the gown, and position the patient, preferably in a sitting up position.
- Place the Mackintosh with cover over the patient's shoulders if they are in a sitting up position, or under the head and over the pillow if they are lying down.
- Cover the patient's eyes with the face towel.
- Put on the gloves.
- Apply Vaseline on the skin around the hair line.
- Apply the anti-lice agent to the hair and scalp, following the prescribed instructions whenever necessary.
- Cover the hair with a towel or a triangular bandage and leave it on overnight, or for the amount of time prescribed by the anti-lice agent being used.
- Remove the articles.
- Clean and disinfect the articles.
- Wash hands.
- Record the time, treatment, type of agent used and condition of the patient.
- Shampoo hair or wash it with soap the next day.
- Repeat the procedure if required after one week.

Anti-lice agents which can be used are:
- DDT powder 1:9 ratio (mixed with oil or powder)
- Kerosene mixed with sweet oil (1:1)
- Warm vinegar
- Commercial anti-lice agents (e.g., Medikar, Lysil)

Special points to remember:
- Protect yourself and others from an infestation.
- Repeat the procedure as and when necessary.

NAIL CARE

Nails keeping big nails is a fashion in some ladies and men too. However, they may be harmful as:
- They can injure other persons, particularly small babies.
- The eggs of the worms are transferred to nails while washing toilet and it spreads worm infection to whole of the family through preparing and serving the food.
- Disease producing germs can be transferred through dirt collected in the nails. Thus, nails should be cut and brushed regularly.

Gather Equipment

Basin, warm water, soap, lotion, two washcloths, one towel, barrier, gloves, manicure stick, emery board, nail clipper, and linen bag or hamper

Routine Pre-procedure Steps

- Knock on the resident's door.
- Perform hand hygiene.
- Maintain respectful, courteous, and professional communication at all times.
- Introduce yourself and identify the resident.
- Provide for privacy.
- Explain the procedure to the resident.

Procedure Steps

- ❖ Put on gloves.
- ❖ Fill the basin with warm water and place it on a flat surface with a barrier underneath. Have the resident check the water temperature by placing their hand in the basin or putting a wet washcloth on the back of their hand.
- ❖ Have the resident perform hand hygiene with sanitizer.
- ❖ Immerse the client's hands in warm water for 5–20 minutes.
- ❖ Place their hand on a barrier.
- ❖ Using a manicure stick, clean underneath each nail, wiping any debris on the barrier after each nail.
- ❖ If necessary, trim nails using a clipper. Sanitize the clipper prior to and after use.
- ❖ Using an emery board, file each nail from the outside of the nail towards the middle of the nail.
- ❖ Check each nail for snags and file until smooth.
- ❖ Rinse the hand in water, return to the barrier, and dry.
- ❖ Repeat the procedure for the second hand.
- ❖ Offer lotion. If applying lotion, wear gloves.
- ❖ Rub the lotion gently into the skin if requested.
- ❖ Wipe off any excess lotion with a dry towel.
- ❖ While wearing gloves, empty the equipment.
- ❖ Rinse the equipment.
- ❖ Dry the basin.
- ❖ Return the equipment to storage.
- ❖ Dispose of soiled linen in a designated laundry hamper.
- ❖ Remove the gloves, turning them inside out.

Post-procedure Steps

- ❖ Perform hand hygiene.
- ❖ Check for resident comfort and ask if anything else is needed.
- ❖ Ensure the bed is low and locked. Check the brakes.
- ❖ Place the call light or signaling device within reach of the resident.
- ❖ Open the door and privacy curtain.
- ❖ Perform hand hygiene.
- ❖ Document and report any skin or nail issues or changes noted with the resident.

CARE OF PRESSURE POINTS

Pressure sores are wounds that develop when constant pressure or friction on one area of the body damages the skin. Constant pressure on an area of skin stops blood from flowing normally, so the cells die, and the skin breaks down.

Other names for pressure sores are bedsores, pressure ulcers and decubitus ulcers.

Definition: decubitus ulcer or bedsore or pressure sore is an ulcerated sloughed area of tissue resulting from pressure, slowing of circulation and causing death of cells (also called decubitus).

Common sites: This may happen more frequently over the bony prominences of the body where there is no rich supply of blood for nourishment and also where there is a thin layer of skin.

When the patient is in supine position the pressure point are:
* Nape of the neck
* Back of the head (occiput)
* Scapula
* Sacral region-most common area
* Elbows and heels

When patient is in side lying position, pressure points are:
* Ears
* Acromion process of the shoulder
* Ribs, iliac crest
* Greater trochanter of the hips
* Medial and lateral condyles of the knee
* Malleolus of the ankle joint

When patient is in prone position, pressure points are:
* Back of the ears and cheek
* Acromion process, knees and toes

Other area that should be watch carefully are between the folds of flesh such as breasts in females and genitalia in males. The skin of patients who are very thin or obsess may breakdown quickly.

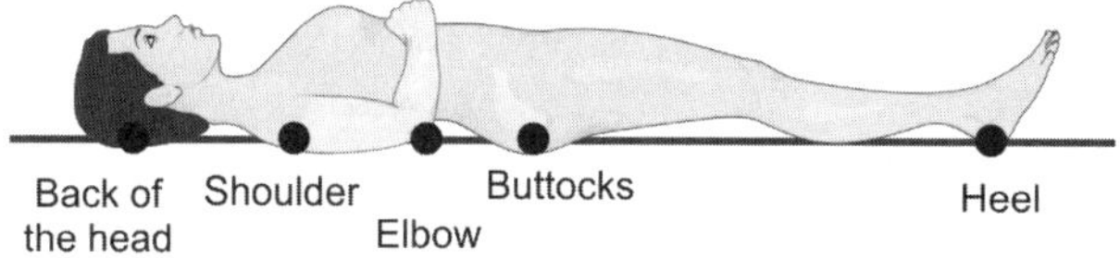

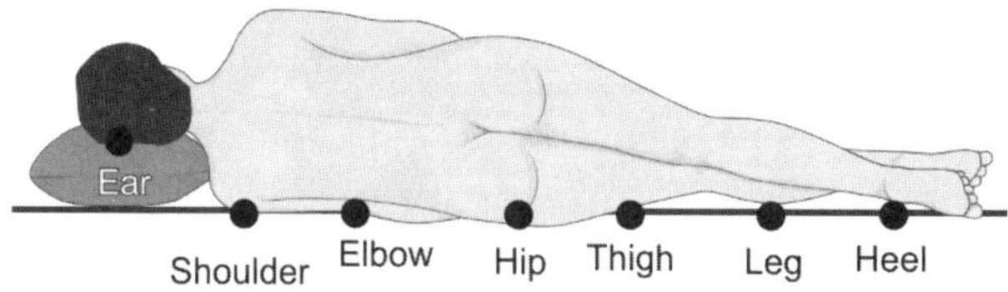

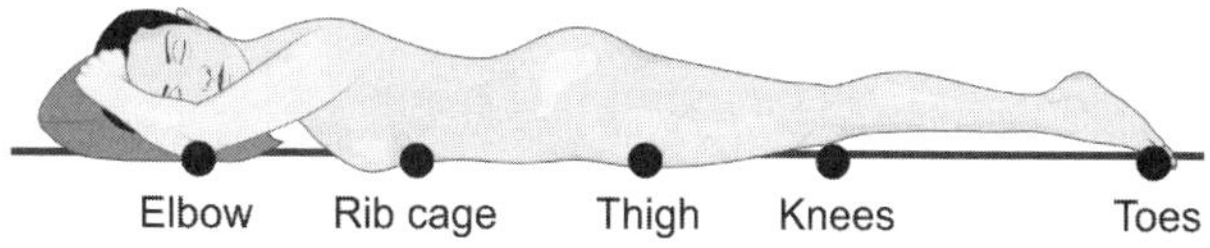

Causes of Bedsore

Predisposing causes which may lead to bedsore formation are as follows:
* Impaired circulation, which is the main cause due to interference in circulation, e.g., people with multiple fractures.
* Lowered vitality—due to disease, e.g., typhoid and due to old age and starvation.
* Emaciation (thinness).

❖ Edema.

❖ Deficient nerve supply.

Direct or immediate causes are as follows:

❖ **Pressure:** Form lying in one position for a long time causing pressure due to constant contact with bed.

❖ **Lack of cleanliness:** Directly act as an agent.

❖ **Friction:** Rough surfaces, patches, seams or wrinkles on the bed linen or garments or other foreign bodies like orange peels, breadcrumbs, rice and food particles, movement of the patients, rubbing of two skin surfaces together, etc., can cause friction on skin.

❖ **Moisture:** Resulting from perspiration, urine, feces and vaginal discharges irritate the skin.

❖ **Heat:** It is another cause for bedsore due to sameness of position or keeping the patient directly on rubber sheets.

❖ **Presence of pathogenic organism:** Lack of cleanliness accumulate pathogenic organisms and cause infection on the skin.

Pressure Ulcers: Pathogenesis and clinical findings

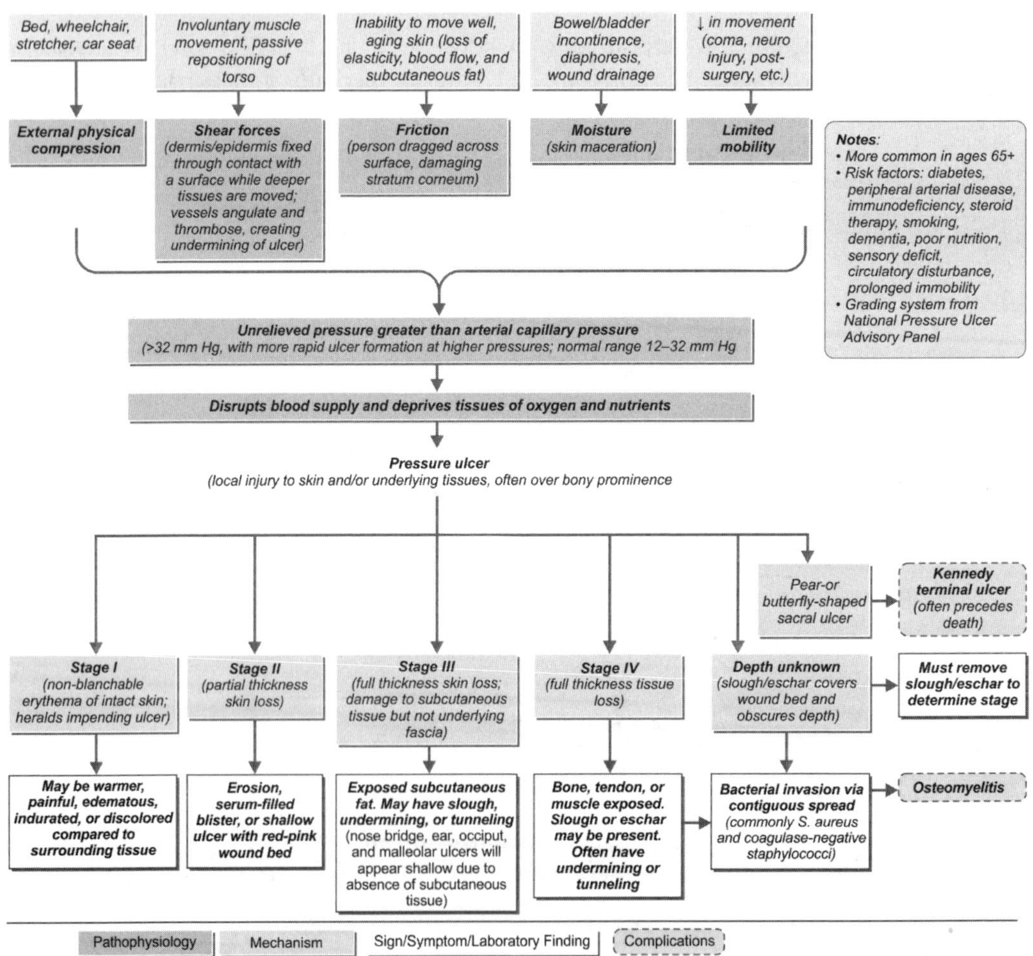

Source: www.thecalgaryguide.com

Type of Patients Most Susceptible to Bedsore

* Very tin, very fat and very old people.
* Persons for whom movement is difficult; as one with multiple fracture.
* Person with long wasting diseases such as typhoid (because body tissues became poorly nourished).
* Person with paralysis.
* Patients who have incontinence of urine and motion.
* Unconscious patients.
* Patients with anemia, cancer and diabetes and other whose circulation is poor because of age, heart disease, etc.
* Obese patients or edematous patients especially edema of the sacrum and buttocks.
* Acutely ill patients whose general condition is very poor and rapidly deteriorating.
* Elderly patients who move very little in the bed.
* Sedated patients who do not move in bed frequently.
* Neurologic patients with lack of sensation in bony prominences.
* Surgical patients with limited movements in bed.
* Patients with hyperpyrexia who sweat profusely.
* Patients with excessive discharge and drainage from wounds.
* Chronic conditions like diabetes who are in bed for a long time
* Any bed patients who are neglected and getting poor nursing care.
* Malnourished patients or patients with deficiency diseases.

Prevention of Bedsore

Absolute Cleanliness

* Keep patients clean by daily sponging. Careful back care twice a day or every four hours or often if necessary and daily observation of bed ridden patients.
* Keep the bed linen clean and dry and free from wrinkles and crumbs.
* Wash the back with warm water to stimulate circulation. Rub with methylated spirit for cooling, refreshing and to toughen the skin.
* Massage back thoroughly to stimulate circulation.
* If the skin is dry and in danger of cracking, use oil instead of spirit.
* Teach the patient and relatives the hygienic care of the skin.

Prevent Moisture

* Keep the patient dry always. If a patient perspires profusely or is incontinent, change the linen frequently and wash the patient well. Washing with a sodabicarb solution neutralizes the acid irritation of urine and feces. Keep skin dry by use of talcum powder.
* Protect the skin from urine and feces by rubbing on an oily ointment such as castor oil or zinc ointment.
* The use of retention catheter eliminates wetting with urine.

Relief of Pressure

* Change the patient's position frequently at least once in 2 hours or as often as necessary and encourages the patient to move in bed as far as possible.

- Careful use of bedpan and padding the edge of the bedpan to prevent undue pressure on susceptible areas. Never allow to patient to remain on the bedpan too long.
- Use air rings or cotton rings to remove pressure on susceptible sites.
- Use an air mattress or rubber sponge mattress for every susceptible patients to equalize the support to all parts of the body. Use extra – pillows. Water mattress is good for such patients.

Eliminate Friction

- Do not use chipped bedpan or drag bedpan from under the patient without lifting him. Pad the chipped edge of the bedpan if it has to be used.
- Splints when used should be well padded, prevent friction resulting from plaster casts by careful use of cotton or other suitable material.
- Prevent friction between two skin surface by careful drying of the part and application of the talcum powder. Pad and bandage the limbs that are being constantly rubbed back and forth or against each other.
- Bed cradles may be used to remove friction due to bed clothes.
- Keep the bed linen and mackintosh free from wrinkles.
- Build up the body resistance by good nutrition.
- Observe carefully for the presence of any reddened areas or skin abrasions and report promptly and see the appropriate measures are taken to prevent progress of formation of the ulcer.

Symptoms of Bedsore

If the patient is conscious he may experience and complain discomfort on pressure sore developing area. But before that the nurse should observe the following early symptoms. Remember that developing bedsore is a discredit to the healthcare workers and the hospital.

Early Symptoms

Heat, redness, tenderness, discomfort and smarting of the affected area. If pressure is not relieved, the tissues became congested. This congestion makes the part blue, or mottles, like a bruise. It is also cold and insensitive. If the pressure is not immediately relieved and normal circulation restored, gangrene may result. The formation of true bedsore is decubitus ulcer comes with the breaking of the skin, the death of tissues, formation of slough which later separates forming an ulcer.

Treatment of Bedsore

Curative Treatment of Pressure Sores

- Treatment may differ, but general principles remain the same. Report any symptom (if skin is broken or abraded or red) noted promptly to the sister in-change so that step may be taken to prevent further damage.
- Keep the patient off her back or off the area where the sore is, if it is possible to do so, keep the area dry and clean—protect the wound with surgical dressing. If the skin is broken, strict aseptic technique must be carried out in taking care of the part.
- The surrounding area should be given routine preventive treatment as often as necessary.
- The wound is usually cleansed with an antiseptic solution as ordered by doctor after cleaning the wound thoroughly (any reaction to penicillin should be ascertained before applying).

❖ When slough is present, clean the area thoroughly twice a day with hydrogen peroxide and sterile water. Then clean with sterile boric lotion or normal saline and apply hot wet dressing or as ordered by the doctor.

❖ If slough is removed by the doctor, stimulate healing by using some preparation as penicillin cream, powder, sulfanilamide powder, etc.

❖ Other treatments used are exposure to sunlight or ultraviolet light and vitamin therapy (administration of vitamins).

❖ Improve the general health of the patient by nourishing food in the possible method.

Tips to Prevent Pressure Sores

The following tips can help to prevent pressure sores:

Relieving direct pressure

❖ Change position and keep moving as much as possible.

❖ Ask for a painkiller if patient have pain and find moving position painful.

❖ Make patient stand up to relieve pressure if he/she can.

❖ Reposition patients regularly if they cannot move.

❖ Change position at least frequently, this may be from as often as every 15 minutes to every 6 hours depending on client's situation.

❖ Use special pressure relieving mattresses and cushions.

❖ Do not drag patient's heels or elbows when moving in bed or chair.

❖ Equipment are available to help the patients move in bed.

Skin Care

❖ Keep skin clean and dry.

❖ Avoid scented soaps as they can be more drying.

❖ Moisturize skin thoroughly after washing.

❖ Avoid using talcum powder as this dries the skins natural oils.

❖ Keep skin well moisturized.

❖ Do not massage or rub the skin to prevent pressure ulcers.

General Tips

❖ Make sure the bedsheets are smooth and not wrinkled when patents are lying in bed.

❖ Sheets should be cotton or silk like fabric.

❖ Give a well-balanced diet.

❖ Provide at least 2 L of fluid a day.

ASSESSMENT OF PRESSURE ULCERS

Pressure Injury

Pressure injury (PI) a localized area of tissue destruction that develops when soft tissue is compressed between a bony prominence, as a result of pressure, shearing forces and/or friction, or a combination of these.

Factors Associated with Increased Risk

Several factors may influence an individual's risk of developing pressure injuries. In the prevention of PIs, it is essential that patients at risk are identified so an individualized prevention plan can be implemented to mitigate the risks. A risk factor is any element that either diminishes the skins tolerance to pressure or contributes to increased exposure of the skin to excess pressure.

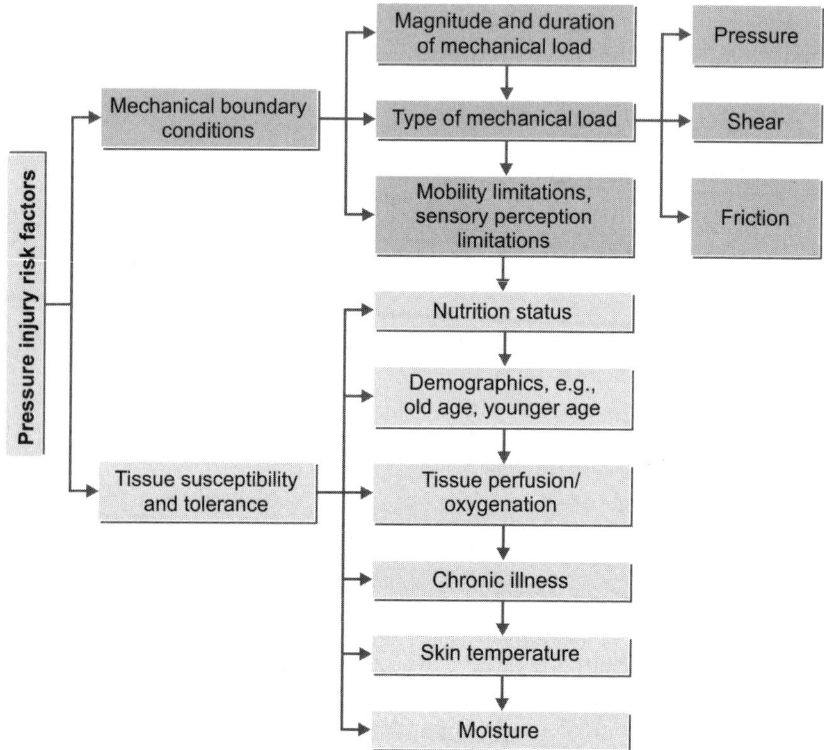

Methods of Risk Assessment

Pressure injury risk assessment tools are the key to determining if a patient is susceptible to PIs. Validated risk assessment tools for patients are effective for identifying those at risk and increasing awareness of potential pressure-related injuries, however they cannot embody every possible circumstance. Therefore, clinicians need to use their experience, clinical judgment and knowledge to prevent tissue damage and protect the skin in conjunction with the risk screening tool.

Braden Scale

The Braden pressure ulcer risk assessment tool and training; risk assessment using clinical judgement and training; and risk assessment using clinical judgement alone. The Braden pressure ulcer risk assessment tool comprises six sub-scales: sensory perception, moisture, activity, mobility, nutrition and friction/shear. Each sub-scale is ranked numerically from 1 to 4; a score of 4 indicates no problem with regard to the specific sub-scale, whereas a score of 1 indicates a significant problem. The friction and shear sub-scale is scored 1 to 3. The scores for each of the sub-scales are totalled to give a final score ranging from 6 to 23; as scores become lower, predicted risk becomes higher (Braden 1987).

Braden risk assessment scale (abridged version)				
Sensory perception	1. Completely limited	2. Very limited	3. Slightly limited	4. No impairment
Moisture	1. Constantly moist	2. Very moist	3. Occasionally moist	4. No impairment
Activity	1. Bedfast	2. Chairfast	3. Walks occasionally	4. Walks frequently
Mobility	1. Completely immobile	2. Very limited	3. Slightly limited	4. No limitation
Nutrition	1. Very poor	2. Probably inadequate	3. Adequate	4. Excellent
Friction and shear	1. Problem	2. Potential problem	3. No apparent problem	

Source: Barbara Braden and Nancy Bergstrom, 1988, reprinted with permission

Norton Scale

The Norton scale was developed in the 1960s and is widely used to assess the risk for pressure ulcer in adult patients. The five subscale scores of the Norton scale are added together for a total score that ranges from 5 to 20. A lower Norton score indicates higher levels of risk for pressure ulcer development. Generally, a score of 14 or less indicates at-risk status.

Norton scale						
		Physical condition	*Mental condition*	*Activity*	*Mobility*	*Incontinent*
		Good 4 Fair 3 Poor 2	Alert 4 Apathetic 3 Confused 2	Ambulant 4 Walk/help 3 Chair-bound 2	Full 4 Slightly limited 3 Very limited 2	Not 4 Occasionally 3 Usually/urine 2
Name	*Dale*	*Very bad 1*	*Stupor 1*	*Stupor 1*	*Immobile 1*	*Doubly 1*	*Total score*

Nursing Responsibilities

Every inpatient at RCH should have a Glamorgan Pressure Injury Risk Assessment Tool completed:

* On admission or as soon as practical after the admission (within 6 hours).
* At the commencement of every shift as required nursing documentation.
* When a patient's condition changes.
* When the patient is transferred from one ward/department to another.
* Once completed, the risk assessment should be documented on the primary assessment flowsheet within the EMR.
* Any patient deemed "At Risk" (risk score of +10) of pressure injury should have an individualized prevention plan developed and documented in the primary assessment flowsheet in the EMR. This plan should be reviewed for appropriateness following every pressure injury risk assessment completion. If a patient's pressure injury risk assessment score changes, a new pressure injury prevention plan needs to be completed and implemented to address the new level of risk.

Skin Assessment

Skin assessment is key to pressure injury prevention, classification/diagnosis, and treatment. All inpatients should have a skin assessment to determine its' general condition and identify factors that increase the risk for PI development. The status of the patient's skin is the most important early indicator of the skin's reaction to pressure exposure and the continuing risk of pressure injury.

Conducting the Assessment

Complete a general visual check of the skin including analysis of the entire skin surface to assess its integrity and identify any characteristics indicative of pressure damage.

Monitor and check the skin beneath dressings, prosthesis and devices when clinically appropriate.

Check for areas of localized heat, skin breakdown, edema, areas of redness that do not blanch and induration of the wound.

Particular attention should be paid to areas of bony prominence, which are at an increased risk for pressure injury due to pressure, friction and shearing forces. High-risk areas include; sacrum, heels, elbows, wrists, temporal region of skill, ears, shoulders, back of head (especially in children less than 36 months of age), knees, and toes.

Frequency of Assessment

As with the pressure injury risk assessment tool, a patient's skin should be assessed:
* ❖ On admission or as soon as practical after the admission (within 6 hours).
* ❖ At the commencement of every shift as required nursing documentation.
* ❖ When a patient's condition changes.
* ❖ When the patient is transferred from one ward/department to another.
* ❖ As well as, upon discharge (to ensure discharge planning is complete).
* ❖ Document skin assessment findings in the focused assessment flowsheet within the EMR.

Patient and Family Education

Parents and carers play a vital role in the care of their child; and therefore, their engagement is vital in helping to prevent the formation of pressure injuries. Carers and parents should be educated around the risk of their child developing pressure injuries whilst in hospital and be provided with effective and age-appropriate strategies to mitigate these risks.

The PI prevention factsheet should be provided to all carers and parents of patients that have been identified to be at risk of developing a pressure injury.

Nutrition and Hydration

Malnourished children are at increased risk of pressure injury development due to their compromised ability to maintain healthy skin and mucosa. Hydration and nutritional support should be aimed at preventing and correcting these deficits.

Maintenance of a positive nitrogen balance and serum albumin levels are vital in maintaining adequate skin integrity and hydration. Monitoring patient weight loss as well as protein and micronutrient intake have been identified as key factors in nutrition to support immunity and skin integrity.

Patients at risk should be offered frequent fluids and diet to maintain adequate nutrition and hydration.

Patients considered high risk or very high risk should follow the advice of the pediatric Nutritional Screening Tool and be referred to a dietician for assessment.

Moisture Control and Skin Care

Increased moisture on the skin or excessive dryness can exacerbate pressure injury development due to the risk of skin breakdown and altered skin integrity.

❖ Keep the skin clean and dry.

❖ Clean skin daily to remove unwanted substances and allow to dry.

❖ Do not vigorously rub or massage the patient's skin.

❖ Use a pH neutral or slightly acidic skin cleanser (pH 4–7) ~ Alkaline products (pH >7) should be avoided.

❖ Utilize a fragrance-free moisturizer to avoid dryness (e.g., SorboleneTM).

❖ Investigate and manage incontinence.

❖ Clean skin promptly after episodes of incontinence.

❖ Use appropriately sized incontinence products for maximum absorption.

❖ Consider referral to occupational therapy if the child was previously continent and support with return to toileting is required.

❖ Apply barrier creams. Barrier creams place a physical barrier between the skin and contaminants that may irritate skin and cause breakdown.

Area	*Treatment aim*	*Treatment/product*
Low-risk areas/normal skin hygiene	Support skin health and maintain hydration	Mild pH, fragrance-free moisturiser, e.g., Sorbolene™
High-risk areas (e.g., nappy region)	Create a protective physical barrier from moisture and irritants that promotes skin health and healing	Barrier wipes, e.g., 3MTM CavilonTM no sting barrier wipes. These wipes create a transparent barrier preventing incontinence associated skin irritation and nappy rash without impacting the absorbency of incontinence products. When used in nappy cares, barrier wipes have been shown to decrease redness and pain by preventing breakdown and can be used in a similar way to traditional barrier creams. Barrier wipes also allow for ongoing integumentary assessments and do not require removal. Zinc-oxide based creams, e.g., Sudocrem®
Broken down skin	Promote skin healing and prevent further breakdown in areas that are red or excoriated	Zinc-oxide based creams, e.g., Sudocrem® Consultation with medical team/Stomal Therapy Clinical Nurse Consultant if required.

Mobility and Positioning

Consider the patient's baseline level of mobility and their current level of mobility.

For patients who can move independently or assist in moving themselves, it is recommended that they be encouraged and/or assisted (as required) to change their position regularly, either in bed or out of bed (if able).

For patients who are unable to assist with moving themselves, it is recommended that they be repositioned every two hours. Employ appropriate manual handling techniques in line with Occupational Health and Safety guidelines when transferring and repositioning patients. Please refer to the Smart Move Smart Lift Training Program.

Positions will vary based on age, developmental stage, physical ability and medical stability; however, they may include lying in bed in a prone, supine, left side lying, or right side lying position, seated in bed, seated in a chair or on a parents' lap, or playing on a floor mat. Pillows or rolled towels can be used to help maintain a change in position.

For high-risk patients, limit time spent sitting in bed with head elevated > thirty degrees to no more than two hours due to the increased pressure on the sacrum.

Always check the positioning of the bony prominences (e.g., shoulders, elbows, ankles, ears) and heels when repositioning the patient into any position. Heels should be suspended off the bed using pillows or gel pads for patients spending prolonged periods in bed.

Consider smaller more frequent (e.g., 1-2 hourly) shifts in position of patients who cannot tolerate major changes in body position to redistribute pressure (e.g., patients with pulmonary hypertension, on ECMO support).

Patients in pain are at an increased risk of pressure injury. If pain is managed appropriately, they are more likely to move or be moved at frequent intervals. Monitor the patient's level of pain and ensure appropriate pain relief is provided to support and encourage mobility. Refer to Pain Management Clinical Practice Guidelines. Ensure the analgesia has adequate time to take effect prior to attending to pressure area care to reduce the patient's pain on moving—this will be dependent on the medication itself and the route of administration (i.e., IV vs oral).

For patients at higher risk of pressure injuries or with existing pressure injuries requiring additional support to manage their mobility and positioning, consider referral to:
❖ Physiotherapy referral for assistance/advice on positioning and repositioning, transferring and supporting mobility.
❖ Occupational therapy referral for assistance/advice on positioning and repositioning and selection of the most appropriate support surface.

Friction and Shear

For patients who are unable to assist in moving themselves, use appropriate transfer assistance devices (e.g., hoist, slide sheets) to reduce friction and shear forces. Always lower the bed head before repositioning patients.

Do not use incontinence bed pads to move/slide patient up the bed.

To reduce shear forces on the sacrum, the head of the bed should be raised in conjunction with the knee bend and/or pillows under the knee.

Medical Devices

Any object that comes into direct contact with the patient's skin has the potential to cause a pressure injury. This is exacerbated in the pediatric inpatient population with device related pressure injuries causing the majority of all pediatric pressure injuries due to the immature skin barrier and decreased tissue tolerance. With increasing complexity of care and advances in technology, incorporating more devices into patient care, nurses must correctly assess and protect a patient's skin from the formation of device related pressure injuries.

Key Points

❖ Regular repositioning and inspection of the patient to ensure that they are not unintentionally lying on devices.
❖ Conduct more frequent assessments at the skin—device interface in patients vulnerable to fluid shifts and exhibiting localized or generalized edema.

❖ Use the correct size equipment suitable to the patient's anatomical size.

❖ When equipment is secured to the patient using tapes, ensure that they are not applied too tightly and that where possible they have some elasticity and stretch (e.g., Hypafix®, Tegaderm™).

❖ Use the minimal amount of strapping or tape to safely secure the device to allow for maximal visualization of the patient's skin.

❖ Devices that are unable to be easily repositioned should be managed with appropriate dressing and skin care.

General Advice

Prior to the application of medical devices and associated preventative dressings, barrier products (e.g., 3M™ Cavilon™ no sting barrier wipes) should be used as a transparent barrier to protect the patient's skin. These products repel moisture and provide protection from fluids and friction, which can prevent skin breakdown in areas with frequent dressing changes or repositioning.

Dressings should be changed as appropriate or when soiled, however, removal within the first 24 hours of application should be avoided due to the increased risk of shearing force that can cause trauma to patient skin.

Where appropriate adhesive removal products (e.g., Convacare® removal wipes) should be used to promote comfort and reduce skin trauma when dressings are difficult to remove.

High-Risk Patient Populations

Patients in the Operating Room

Pressure injuries that originate in the operating room may not appear until 1–4 days postoperatively, highlighting the importance of thorough skin assessment and prevention interventions as the child continues their journey through the pre-operative, surgery and post-operative phase at the RCH.

Preoperative

Before going to theater, the perioperative nurse performs a preoperative assessment to assess for factors that may increase an individual child's risk for pressure injury during surgery. Assessment taken should be documented on the preoperative assessment through EMR. Factors that should be assessed include:

❖ Medical devices (catheter, tubes, drains)

❖ Jewellery or body piercings

❖ Braided hair, hair accessories, hair extensions

❖ Implants

❖ Prosthetics

❖ Comorbidities

❖ Skin condition

❖ Nutritional status

Intraoperative

Research suggests surgery that lasts longer than two hours has been associated with an increased risk of PIs. Anesthetized patients that are positioned on specialized frames in the prone position, may be at an even higher risk of developing PIs in uncommon areas such as the—chest, iliac crest, face (tip of the nose, chin and forehead) and heels.

There are many factors that contribute to the incidence of PI's in the operating theatre such as:
- Intense or prolonged pressure during lengthy surgical procedures.
- Increased pressure on bony prominences from positioning.
- Exposure to friction or shear during transfer to the operating table and positioning.

Risks for patients undergoing surgery should be determined by:
- Length of the operation
- Increased hypotensive episodes intraoperatively
- Low core temperature during surgery
- Reduced mobility on day one postoperatively
- Prolonged placement of equipment and medical devices, e.g., neurosurgical head frame, arm boards, monitoring equipment.
- The RCH operating tables are all fitted with high density pressure-redistributing foam to reduce the risk of pressure injury development.

Other methods of managing a patient to reduce the risk of pressure injuries include:
- The use of Gel Pads and Perspex boxes for complex theatre cases.
- Patients should be positioned to reduce the risk of pressure injury development during surgery.
- Heels should be completely elevated in such a way as to distribute the weight of the leg along the calf without putting all the pressure on the Achilles tendon. The knee should be in slight flexion.
- Hyperextension of the knee may cause obstruction of the popliteal vein, and this could predispose the individual to deep vein thrombosis.
- Pay attention to pressure redistribution prior to and after surgery. Position the individual in a different posture preoperatively and postoperatively than the posture adopted during surgery where possible.
- Patient supports and patient positioning aids, including the most appropriate support surface.

Actions/interventions taken should be documented on the EMR intraoperative nursing record including patient positioning and assessment of the integumentary system.

Postoperative

In the postoperative phase, a full integumentary assessment is required. Any altered skin integrity must be documented on the EMR flow sheet and communicated to the multidisciplinary team.

Neonatal Patients

Pressure injury prevention in this specialized population should be managed carefully, considering the effect of various dressing and barrier products on underdeveloped skin. Consultation with neonatal specialists is suggested before application of new products.

Pediatric Intensive Care Patients

Patients admitted to the pediatric intensive care unit (PICU) have a higher incidence of PI's and are usually more severe due to patient complexities and prolonged length of stay.

The ICU environment has several main contributing factors:
* Multiple invasive devices
* Low cardiac output state
* Inotrope, vasopressor and muscle relaxant use
* Impaired level of consciousness
* Immobility
* Poor peripheral and central blood flow
* Suboptimal nutrition

Patients should have existing PIs assessed every second hour and be repositioned based on their mobility status identified daily on medical ward from the 'Early Mobilization Traffic Light Guideline'. If the patient is identified as too clinically unstable to attend to major pressure area care and repositioning, an alternative pressure injury prevention plan needs to be discussed with the multidisciplinary team.

Orthopedic Patients

Orthopedic patients are considered to be at high risk of pressure injuries due to the prolonged presence of fixed devices such as external fixation, traction, plasters casts and braces. These devices can cause sheering force and friction, so should be regularly monitored and assessed. These patients are also at higher risk of immobilization due to painful procedures and extended periods of bed rest or reduced weight bearing capacity.

Elevation of limbs on pillows and towels where possible to reduce pressure, particularly on the heels.

Monitoring of neurovascular compromise or increased pain levels as this can decrease skin integrity and indicate the formation of pressure injuries.

Orthopedic patients with developmental delays are at increased risk of pressure injuries due to their compromised ability to communicate changes in sensation. Therefore, pain cues should be monitored closely in this population.

Patients with epidural analgesia should adhere to strict pressure area cares and frequent repositioning as they have extremely compromised movement and sensation.

Referral to Prosthetics + Orthotics for review of braces/splints/collars where required.

Support Surfaces

Support surfaces are devices (e.g., air mattresses, cushions) that are used to assist with pressure redistribution to manage the pressure load on the integumentary system. Support surfaces typically support pressure redistribution through either immersion to increase the body surface area in contact with the surface, or by alternating and offloading the area of the body in contact with the support surface.

Decisions about an appropriate support surface to use for pressure injury prevention should be based on an overall assessment of the patient, including their weight, and their Glamorgan screening tool score. Selection of an appropriate support surface should also take into consideration factors such as the individual's level of mobility within the bed, his/her comfort, and the need for microclimate control. The LINK Bariatric procedure should be referred to for guidance regarding suitable support surfaces for patients above 100 kg.

For support surfaces to be effective, there must be minimal layering in between the device and the person. The use of additional sheets, kylie pads, dry-flows and towels can alter the pressure relieving qualities of pressure redistribution equipment and should be avoided where possible. A single sheet that can be kept dry and crease free is optimal.

Please note: Support surfaces facilitate the redistribution of body weight but do not negate the need for regular repositioning of patients or pressure area care. For patients that are very high risk, these surfaces may allow a decrease in turning frequency overnight to 3–4 hourly to encourage rest patterns, however, this should be considered carefully on a case-by-case basis. If the patient is spending time sitting with the bed head raised, the mattress should be checked to ensure it is not 'bottoming out' underneath the patient.

Please consider the sudden infant death syndrome (SIDS) risk reduction recommendations when using support surfaces for infants. Monitoring is required for infants nursed outside of these recommendations.

Consider occupational therapy referral for assistance with assessment of causal factors and advice on pressure injury prevention or management plans, including selection of most appropriate support surfaces.

The following should NOT be used as a support surface:
- Sheepskins
- Doughnut shaped gels—this type of device may impair lymphatic drainage and circulation*.
- Water filled gloves under heels—these are not effective as the water filled glove is unable to redistribute pressure and it only supports a small surface of the heel.

***Note:** Doughnut shaped gel rings are still currently used in special circumstances in operating theaters only with careful consideration and application. Assessment of the occiput and surrounding tissue should take place before and after doughnut shaped gel ring use.

Characteristics of Support Surfaces

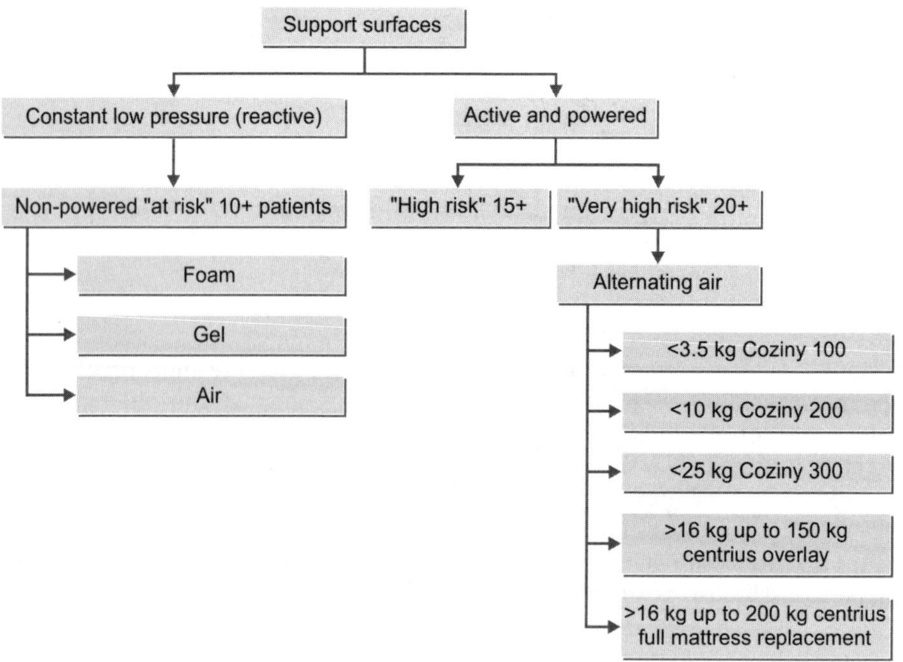

Alternating Air Mattresses

Pressure Injury Stages

Pressure injury staging or classification describes the extent of skin and tissue damage. Staging of a pressure injury is essential for the development and implementation of a management plan.

Stage	Description	Lightly pigmented skin	Darkly pigmented skin
Stage 1	Localized area of non-blanchable erythema of intact skin		
Stage 2	Partial-thickness skin loss with exposed dermis. Wound bed is viable, pink/red and can be moist, shiny or dry		
Stage 3	Full thickness skin loss. Adipose (fat) tissue is visible		
Stage 4	Full thickness skin and tissue loss. Exposed fascia, muscle, tendon, ligament, cartilage or bone		
Unstageable	Obscured full thickness skin and tissue loss. Extent of tissue damage cannot be determined as it is obscured by slough or eschar		
Deep tissue	Persistent non-blanchable deep red/purple discoloration. Skin can be intact or non-intact		

Pressure Injury/Wound Management

Basic Principles

❖ Avoid positioning patients directly on an existing pressure injury or body surface that remains damaged or erythematous, where possible.

❖ Ensure the patient is on the most suitable support surface. Consider referral to occupational therapy for further advice/support if required.

❖ Always consider patient nutrition and hygiene and refer for support if required.

Wound Management

❖ Utilize appropriate pain management.

❖ Clean the pressure injury with sterile water or 0.9% sodium chloride solution.

❖ If required, debride dead or devitalized tissue. This can be done using autolytic debridement through dressing selection or surgical debridement.

❖ Assess and document the size and appearance of the pressure injury in the LDA.

❖ Select a wound dressing that promotes a warm, moist environment for wound healing.

❖ If the wound appears infected antibiotics can be used. Topical antiseptics are not routinely used on pressure injuries, but topical antimicrobials should be considered if clinically indicated.

❖ Remove dressings with adhesive remover wipe or spray to gently remove tapes.

❖ Do not use gauze to treat pressure injuries.

❖ Wound management plan should be documented in the EMR progress notes.

Stage	Management goals	Dressing selection
Stage 1: Non-blanchable erythema	Protect skin to prevent further injury	Silicone adhesive, non-adherent foam or transparent hydrocolloid adhesive dressing Silicone, e.g., Mepilex® Border, Mepilex® Lite or Allevyn™ helps to reduce effects of friction and can be left in-situ for 7 days (must be changed if soiled) Hydrocolloid, e.g., Comfeel® has very little a sorbency so should only be used on wounds with no or low exudate. It should only be used if it can be left on for 7 days Apply 3M™ Cavilon™ No sting barrier wipe underneath to prevent adhesive trauma upon removing the Comfeel®
Stage 2: Partial thickness skin loss	Relieve pressure and protect wound from further trauma/ contamination	Silicone adhesive or non-adherent foam Silicone, e.g., Mepilex® Border, Mepilex® Lite or Allevyn™ has an absorption layer that draws moisture and exudate from the wound while protecting the surrounding healthy skin from maceration. It mounds well to the skin without sticking to the wound Silicone dressings can be left on for up to 7 days but should be changed PRN depending on exudate/as guided by stomal therapy Silicone properties prevent trauma upon removal
Stage 3: Full thickness skin loss	Relieve pressure and protect wound from further trauma/ contamination	Hydrogel, adhesive foam, hydrofiber or silicone dressing Hydrogel, e.g., intrasite™ gel absorbs slough/exudate while creating a moist healing environment Hydrofiber, e.g., Aquacel® is 100% sodium carboxylmethyl-cellulose which converts to a soft gel when in contact with wound exudate to absorb exudate and maintain a moist wound environment for healing

Contd...

Contd...

Stage	Management goals	Dressing selection
Stage 4: Full thickness tissue loss	Relieve pressure and protect wound from further trauma/ contamination	Alginate, hydrogel, adhesive foam, hydrofiber or silicone dressing Alginate dressings, e.g., Kaltostat® are used when there is active bleeding. It is made from brown seaweed and forms a gel when in contact with a wound surface to absorb the exudate and promote hemostasis
Unstageable depth unknown	Unable to determine prior to debridement	Surgical debridement required as determined by surgical team

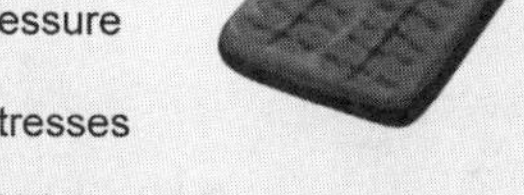

Preventive devices used to prevent pressure ulcers

- Bed cradle
- Heel and elbow protectors
- Flotation pads or cushions
- Pillows
- Water beds
- Alternating pressure mattresses
- Eggcrate mattresses

OPS Approved Canal14 14

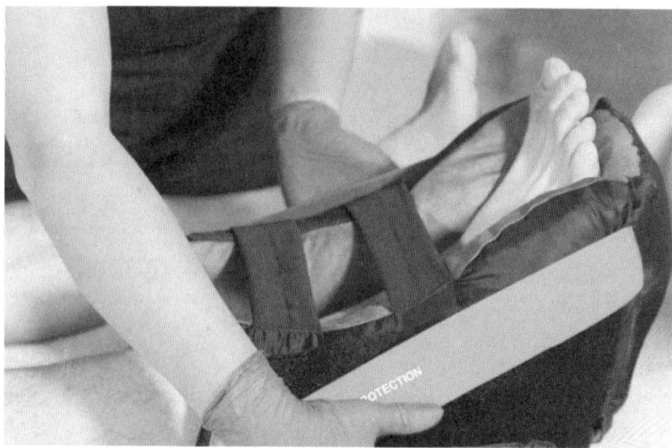

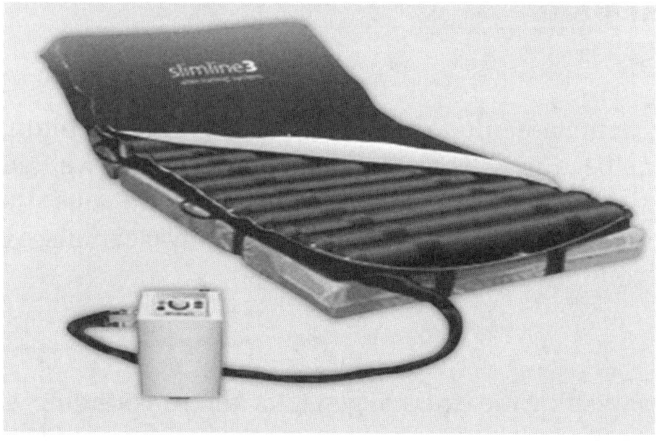

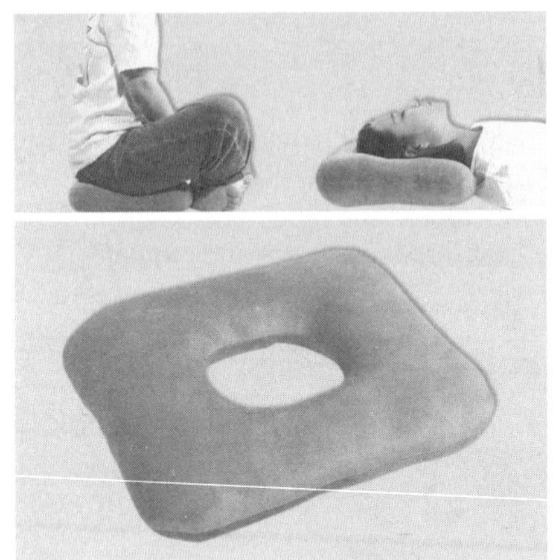

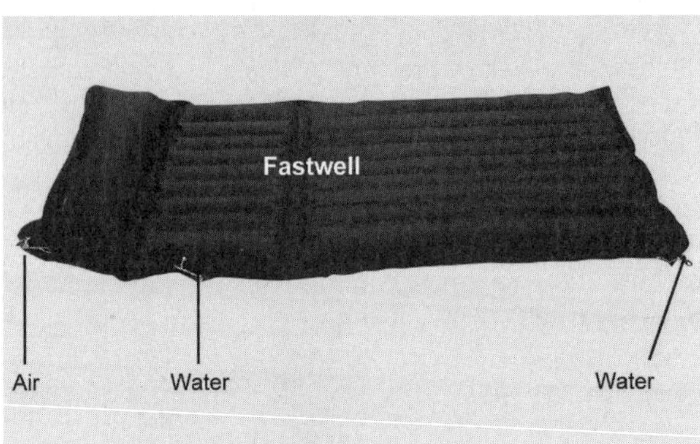

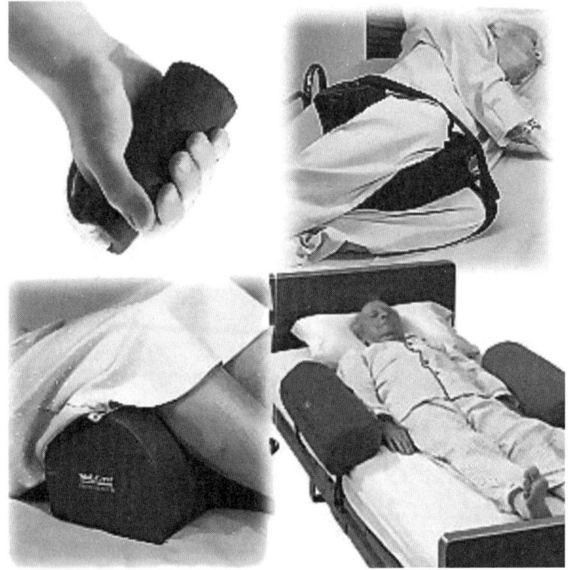

PERINEAL/MEATAL CARE

Introduction

It is also defined as perineal-genital care. The perineal area is conducive to the growth of pathogenic organisms because it is warm, moist and it is not well-ventilated. Since there are many orifices, e.g., urinary meatus, vaginal orifice and the anus situated in this area, the pathogenic organisms can enter into the body. Thoroughly cleanliness is essential to prevent bad odor to promote comfort.

Definition

Perineal care involves washing the external genitalia and surrounding with soap and water or with water alone or in combination with any commercially prepared peri-wash.

Principle

Clean the perineum from the cleanest to less clean area.
Patient who require special attention to perineal area.

- Patient who are unable to do self-care.
- Patient with genitourinary tract infection.
- Patient with incontinence of urine and stool.
- Patient with indwelling catheters.
- Postpartum patients.
- Patients after surgery on the genitourinary system.
- Patients with injury, ulcer or surgery on perineal area.

Preliminary Assessment (for Female Client)

- Assess the condition of perineal skin—any itching, irritation, ulcers, edema, drainage, etc.
- Assess the need and frequency of perineal care.
- Assess whether perineal care should be done under an aseptic technique or a clean technique.
- Check the physician's order for any specific instructions.
- Assess the patient ability for self-care.
- Assess the patient mental state to follow instructions.
- Check the articles available in patients unit.

Preparation of Articles

A Tray Containing

- Mackintosh
  Purpose: To protect the bed.
- Wet cotton ball or rag pieces in a bowl.
  Purpose: To clean perineum.
- A jug with warm water or antiseptic solution.
  Purpose: Gauze or rag pieces in a container.
- Long artery forceps in kidney tray.
  Purpose: To hold swabs for cleaning.
- Paper bag.
  Purpose: To receive wastes.
- Clean linen, pads, dressing, etc., as needed.
  Purpose: To keep patient clean.
- Bed pan.
  Purpose: If the patient is in need to passing urine or stool.

Preparation of Patient

- Explain procedure to the patient.
- Provide privacy by screens and drapes. Drape the patient as for vaginal examinations.
- Remove all articles that may interfere with the procedure, e.g., air cushion.
- Give extra pillows to raise the head.
- Roll the draw sheet to opposite side to prevent soiling when bedpan is placed under buttocks, over draw sheet.

- ❖ Offer bed pan. Keep the clean bed-pan on the bed on your working side.
- ❖ Untie the pads, if any and observe the discharges its color, odor, amount, etc.
- ❖ Leave the patient for sometime so that she may pass urine or stool if necessary.
- ❖ Get the toilet tray and arrange the articles conveniently on bed side table.

Procedure Steps

- ❖ Wash hands
  Reason: To prevent cross infection.
- ❖ Pour water over perineum.
  Reason: To wash off the discharge from the perineal area.
- ❖ Clean the perineum using the wet swabs.
  Reason: To prevent the entrance of bacteria from the colon into urinary tract.
- ❖ Hold the swabs with forceps and clean from above.
- ❖ Use one swab for one swabbing.
- ❖ Clean perineum from the midline outward in following order
  - ◆ The vulva
  - ◆ The labia
  - ◆ Inside of labia on both sides.
  - ◆ Outside of labia on both sides.
- ❖ Clean the perineal region and anus thoroughly.
- ❖ Remove the bed pan by supporting the hip as before. Turn the patient to one side and dry the buttocks with dry rag piece.

After Care

- ❖ Apply the medicine and pad if necessary.
- ❖ Remove the Mackintosh if extra one is used.
- ❖ Change linen if necessary straighten the bed clothes. Arrange the bed linen.
- ❖ Make patient comfortable.
- ❖ Take the bed pan to sanitary annex. Remove cotton swabs, and empty the contents into toilet.
- ❖ Clean all articles.
- ❖ Boil forceps.
- ❖ Replace articles.

ORAL HYGIENE AND CARE OF TEETH

Mouth is a general term covering the space containing tongue, teeth, etc. But the right term is oral cavity and the mouth is the outer area covered by lips. Our oral cavity is a place where multiple functions and the process of eating are performed namely—tasting, chewing and swallowing.

Various ways to maintain oral hygiene and care of teeth are:

- ❖ Do not take very cold and very hot food and liquids. It may damage the inner sensitive lining as well as teeth.
- ❖ It is a good habit to rinse you mouth with water every time you finish eating or drinking something other than water. This helps to clean the food particles which, otherwise, may ferment and lead to infection.
- ❖ Do not put your finger in the mouth unnecessarily. This may transfer germs from outside into the mouth.

❖ Cleaning the tongue while brushing the teeth is essential as it removes the bad breath generated by white/yellow coating of the tongue and associated germs.

❖ Chewing tobacco/gutka and smoking in long run leads to cancer of the mouth.

Contact your doctor when:

❖ Your mouth smells badly, there may be infection in the tonsils or teeth.

❖ There is pain in the throat.

❖ There is difficulty in swallowing.

❖ There is toothache (pain in the tooth).

❖ There is swelling inside the mouth or around the jaws.

❖ There is bleeding inside the mouth.

❖ There is an open wound in the mouth or on and around the area of lips and nose.

❖ Any tooth/teeth are heat/cold sensitive.

❖ Swollen/painful/white or bleeding tonsils.

Our teeth not only give us aesthetic beauty and maintain the shape of our mouth, but also helps in digestion of food by chewing it and mixing with saliva. Cleaning the teeth is essential for keeping them healthy. The following guidelines are recommended to keep your gums and teeth healthy:

❖ Brush your teeth twice a day after meals with a soft brush and tooth paste. Brushing in the night is particularly needed as it is proved to reduce dental decay and cavities.

❖ Brushing should be done at least for 3–4 minutes.

❖ Use a soft brush to avoid damage to gums.

❖ The teeth should be cleaned from all sides. You should learn correct technique of brushing from your dentist to avoid deposition of plaque/tartar on your teeth. The food decay and plaque irritates the gums, cause infection and the gums can start bleeding.

❖ Any tooth paste is good and to choose a particular color or brand is an individual choice.

❖ Some tooth pastes are good for heat and cold sensitive teeth. These can be advised by the dentist.

❖ Use a diamond-shaped brush as it is suitable to the space between cheek and gums. Small size brush is needed for children.

❖ When tooth brush/toothpaste is not available, Neem/Keeker/Babool datun can be used but proper use is important to avoid damage to the gums.

❖ Always use the tooth powder from a standard company and never use cheap, granular powder as it can harm your teeth and gums.

❖ Never use any tobacco based toothpaste/toothpowder.

❖ If you have a painful tooth, contact the dentist immediately. It may be due to infection which can be treated and you can save your tooth from extraction.

❖ Broken and damaged tooth can be replaced with artificial tooth. Take the advice of your dentist for it.

❖ Never use alpins/tooth picks to remove food particles from your teeth. It can damage the teeth. Instead, use tooth brush or dental floss.

❖ Never open bottles, hairpins and break walnuts/chestnuts using your teeth. The upper covering of your teeth can be damaged making it heat or cold sensitive. Even your teeth can break!!

❖ Dental flossing is recommended once a day. It is using a special thread (dental floss) to remove the food particles in between the teeth.

- Never apply any chemicals (e.g., baking soda and lemon, etc.) to your teeth to bring shining. The teeth can be damaged.
- Nail biting is a bad habit as it leads to infection in the oral cavity and damages the gums.
- Smoking, alcohol and chewing tobacco, supari and spices stain the teeth, pollute the environment, cause bad breath. They also causes cancer of the oral cavity in long run.
- Chewing gums help only in massaging the gums and not cleaning the teeth. The teeth need to be cleaned by toothbrush and paste only!
- You must have a dental check up at least 6 monthly. The dentist can clean the dirt/tartar on your teeth by the process of scaling and also find out any decay of the tooth.
- Mouthwash are medicated solutions which can be used for foul smell (bad breath) and improving oral hygiene but temporarily. The dentist should be consulted to find out the cause and treat the bad breath.
- Artificial teeth/teeth set (dentures) are an important and essential option for the people who have lost/damaged their teeth. However, dentists should be consulted for it. It should be well fitting as the loose denture can damage the inner lining of mouth. They need to be cleaned regularly by brushing.
- The alignment/shape of the teeth can be corrected by applying metal strings called braces. This is helpful aesthetically but the braces should be cleaned regularly after every meal to prevent tooth decay by food particles.

CARE OF DENTURES

Plaque can accumulate on dentures and can promote or pharyngeal colonization of pathogens. Diligent oral hygiene care can improve oral health and limit the growth of pathogens in the oropharyngeal secretions, decreasing the incidence of aspiration pneumonia and other systemic diseases. Dentures should be cleaned at least daily, to prevent irritation and infection. They may be cleaned more often, based on need and the patient's personal preference. Dentures are often removed at night. Handle dentures with care to prevent breakage.

Equipment

The equipment necessary to clean dentures follows:
- Soft toothbrush or denture brush
- Toothpaste
- Denture cleaner (optional)
- Denture adhesive (optional)
- Glass of cool water
- Emesis basin
- Denture cup (optional)
- Non sterile gloves
- Additional PPE, as indicated
- Towel
- Mouthwash (optional)
- Washcloth or paper towel
- Lip lubricant (optional)
- Gauze

Care action	Rationale
Perform hand hygiene and put on PPE, if indicated.	Hand hygiene and PPE prevent the spread of microorganisms. PPE is required based on transmission precautions.
Identify patient. Explain procedure to patient.	Identifying the patient ensures the right patient receives the intervention and helps prevent errors. Explanation facilitates cooperation.
Assemble equipment on over bed table within reach.	Organization facilitates performance of task
Provide privacy for patient.	Cleaning another person's mouth is invasive and may be embarrassing. Patient may be embarrassed by removal of dentures.
Lower side rail and assist patient to sitting position, if permitted, or turn patient onto side. Place towel across patient's chest. Raise bed to a comfortable working position, usually elbow height of the caregiver. Put on gloves.	Sitting or side-lying position prevents aspiration of fluids into the lungs. The towel protects the patient from dampness. Proper bed height helps reduce back strain while performing the procedure. Gloves prevent the spread of microorganisms.
Apply gentle pressure with 3 × 3 gauze to grasp upper denture plate and remove it. Place it immediately in denture cup. Lift lower dentures with gauze, using slight rocking motion. Remove, and place in denture cup.	Rocking motion breaks suction between denture and gum. Using 3 × 3 gauze prevents slippage and discourages spread of microorganisms.
Place paper towels or washcloth in sink while brushing. Using the toothbrush and paste, brush all surfaces gently but thoroughly. If patient prefers, add denture cleaner to cup with water and follow directions on preparation.	Putting paper towels or a washcloth in the sink protects against breakage. Dentures collect food and microorganisms and require daily cleaning.
Rinse thoroughly with water. Apply denture adhesive, if appropriate.	Water aids in removal of debris and acts as a cleaning agent. Cleaning removes food particles and plaque, permitting proper fit and preventing infection.
Use a toothbrush and paste to gently clean gums, mucous membranes, and tongue. Offer water and/or mouthwash so patient can rinse mouth before replacing dentures.	Mouthwash leaves a pleasant taste in the mouth.
Insert upper denture in mouth and press firmly. Insert lower denture. Check that the dentures are securely in place and comfortable. This ensures patient comfort.	This ensures patient comfort.
If the patient desires, dentures can be stored in the denture cup in cold water, instead of returning to the mouth. Label the cup and place in the patient's bedside table.	Storing in water prevents warping of dentures. Proper storage prevents loss and damage.
Remove equipment and return patient to a position of comfort. Remove your gloves. Raise side rail and lower bed.	Promotes patient comfort and safety. Removing gloves properly reduces the risk for infection transmission and contamination of other items
Perform hand hygiene.	

CARE OF EYES

The eye is a delicate organ, highly susceptible to infection and injury. For maximal safety for the patient, the equipment, solutions, and ointments introduced into the conjunctival sac should be sterile. The medicine should be given as per doctor's prescription.

Guidelines for preparing the equipment needed for eye care:

You may need to arrange following:
a. Clean trolley.
b. Sterile dressing packs inclusive of galipot, gauze swab and disposable towel or napkins as per instructions of nursing officer.
c. Sterile 0.9% sodium chloride.
d. Sterile gloves.
e. Eye drops (as prescribed by ophthalmologist).
f. Sufficient amount of light into the room.
g. Disposable garbage bag.

Guidelines for Preparation of Patient for Ear Care

The patient must sit or lie keeping his/her head tilted backwards and chin must point in upward direction. This facilitates easy accessibility to the eyes and makes up to be a good position for care givers in treating and for patient's comfort.

1. Explain the procedure to the patient.
2. The bed area must be clean to enable movement around the bed freely and ensure that you have all the equipment handy and there is no further need of leaving the patient in the middle of the treatment.
3. Patient should be in comfortable position.
4. Ensure sufficient amount of light in the room.
5. Patient's privacy should be ensured.
6. Hand hygiene should be taken care of, disposable towel should be placed around the neck of the patient.
7. Patient's eyelids have to be closed to prevent cornea damage.
8. Using a gauze swab (dampened in 0.9% solution), gently clean from the inwards (nasal corner) to outwards. New swab should be used every time until all crust and discharged is removed.
9. The procedure has to be repeated for other eye too.
10. Patient's eye has to be dried of excess fluid.
11. The disposable equipment are to be disposed and patient's comfort has to be taken care of;.
12. Hand hygiene is to be carried out.
13. If required, eye drops or eye ointments are to be given as prescribed and their expiry date has to be checked before giving to the patient.
14. Patient is to be given prior warning that he/she has to report if any irritation or itching is there after eye drop.
15. Always put the date on eye drop when its seal has been open. As we should not use eye ointment after one month of it opening.

Eye Drop Instillation

Articles Required

- ❖ Gloves
- ❖ Personal predictive equipment (if indicated)
- ❖ Medication as ordered by the doctor
- ❖ Tissues
- ❖ Normal saline
- ❖ Washcloth
- ❖ Cotton balls, or gauze piece.

Nursing action	Rationale
Gather equipment	Helps to avoid interruptions during procedure and prevents errors that may have occurred when orders were transcribed
Perform hand hygiene	Prevents the spread of microorganisms
Check expiration dates	Facilitates error-free administration
Transport medications to the patient's bedside carefully, and keep the medications in sight at all times	Careful handling and close observation prevent accidental or deliberate disarrangement of medications
Perform hand hygiene and put on PPE, if indicated	Prevent the spread of microorganisms
Identify the patient. Check the name and identification number on the patient's identification band	Ensures the right patient receives right medications and prevent errors
Ask the patient about allergies.	A prerequisite to administration of medications
Explain the purpose and action of each medication to the patient a prerequisite to administration of medications	A prerequisite to administration of medications
Put on gloves	Gloves protect from potential contact with mucous membranes and body fluids
Offer tissue to patient	Solution and tears may spill from the eye during the procedure
Cleanse the eyelids and eyelashes (any drainage) with a wash—cloth, cotton balls, or gauze piece moistened with normal saline solution. Use each area of the cleaning surface once, moving from the inner toward the outer canthus	Debris can be carried into the eye when the conjunctival sac is exposed. Using each area of the gauze once and moving from the inner canthus to the outer canthus prevents carrying debris to the lacrimal ducts thus prevent infection to lacrimal duct
Tilt the patient's head back slightly if sitting, or place the patient's head over a pillow if lying down. The head may be turned slightly to the affected side to prevent solution or tears from flowing toward the opposite eye	Tilting patient's head back slightly makes it easier to reach the conjunctival sac. Pillow should be avoided if the patient has a cervical spine injury. Turning the head to the affected side helps to prevent solution or tears from flowing toward the opposite eye
Remove the cap from the medication bottle, being careful not to touch the inner side of the cap	Touching the inner side of the cap may contaminate the bottle of medication

Contd...

Contd...

Nursing action	Rationale
Instruct patient to look up and focus on something on the ceiling. Place thumb or two fingers near margin of lower eyelid immediately below eyelashes, and exert pressure downward over bony prominence of cheek. Lower conjunctival sac is exposed as lower lid is pulled down	By having the patient look up and focus on something else, the procedure is less traumatic and keeps the eye still
Hold dropper close to eye, but avoid touching eyelids or lashes. Squeeze container and allow prescribed number of drops to fall in lower conjunctival sac	Touching the eye, eyelids, or lashes can contaminate the medication in the bottle. The eye drop should be placed in the conjunctival sac, not directly on the eyeball
Release lower lid after eye drops are instilled. Ask patient to close eyes gently. Apply gentle pressure over inner canthus to prevent eye drops from flowing into tear duct	This allows the medication to be distributed over the entire eye. This minimizes the risk of systemic effects from the medication
Instruct patient not to rub affected eye	
Remove gloves	
Assist patient to a comfortable position. Remove additional PPE, if used	
Perform hand hygiene	
Document the administration of the medication immediately after administration	Timely documentation helps to ensure patient safety
Observe the patient's response to medication within appropriate time frame	Observe the patient's response to medication within appropriate time frame

Note: Immediately after the procedure, including date, time, dose, route of administration, and site of administration, specially right, left, or both eyes, on the record. PRN medications require documentation of the reason for administration. Prompt recording avoids the possibility of accidentally repeating the administration of the drug. If the drug was refused or omitted, inform this also to notify the nursing officer. This verifies the reason medication was omitted and ensures that the nursing officer is aware of the patient's condition.

Eye Ointment Administration

❖ Follow medication order and the patient's chart for allergies under supervision of nursing officer. As nursing officer know the actions, special nursing considerations, safe dose ranges, purpose of administration, and adverse effects of the medications to be administered.
❖ Perform hand hygiene.
❖ Prepare medicine for administration in the medication area under supervision of nursing officer.
❖ Transport medications and equipment to the patient's bed-side carefully, and keep the medications in sight at all times.
❖ Perform hand hygiene and put on PPE, if indicated.
❖ The patient should be identified using proper method.
❖ Provide privacy.
❖ Nursing officer may complete necessary assessments before administering medications.
❖ Put on gloves. Offer the patient a tissue.

❖ Cleanse the eyelids and eyelashes of any drainage with cotton balls or gauze piece moistened with normal saline solution. Use each area of the gauze once, moving from the inner toward the outer canthus.

❖ Instruct patient to look up and focus on some-thing on the ceiling.

❖ Place thumb or two fingers near margin of lower eyelid immediately below eyelashes and exert pressure downward over bony prominence of cheek. Lower conjunctival sac is exposed as lower lid is pulled down.

❖ Hold the ointment tube close to eye, but avoid touching eyelids or lashes. Squeeze container and apply about 1 inch of ointment from the tube along the exposed sac. Apply the medication moving from the inner canthus to the outer canthus. Twist tube to break off ribbon of ointment. Do not touch the tip to the eye.

❖ Release lower lid after ointment is instilled. Ask patient to close eyes gently. The warmth helps to liquefy the ointment.

❖ Instruct the patient to move the eye, because this helps to spread the ointment under the lids and over the surface of the eyeball. Assist the patient to a comfortable position. Explain that the ointment may temporarily blur vision; encourage the patient not to rub the eye.

❖ Remove gloves and additional PPE, if used. Perform hand hygiene.

❖ Document medication administration immediately after the procedure. Evaluate the patient's response to medication within appropriate time frame.

Safety

❖ Care should be taken for avoiding cross infection.

❖ Hands should be washed properly and gloves should be worn.

❖ The eyes should be cleaned from inner corner nasal corner towards outward direction.

❖ The procedure should always begin with cleaner eye and new swab should be used for each eye.

Eye Irrigation

The main purpose of eye irrigation is to remove secretions or foreign bodies or to cleanse and soothe the eye. When irrigating one eye, care should be taken to prevent over flowing irrigation fluid does not contaminate the other eye.

Articles Required

❖ Sterile irrigation solution [warmed to 37°C (98.6°F)]

❖ Sterile irrigation set (sterile container and irrigating or bulb syringe)

❖ Emesis basin (kidney tray) or irrigation basin

❖ Washcloth

❖ Waterproof pad or Mackintosh

❖ Towel

❖ Disposable glove

Medication Administration Record

Nursing action	Rationale
Gather equipment	Helps to avoid interruptions during procedure and prevents errors that may have occurred when orders were transcribed

Contd...

Contd...

Nursing action	Rationale
Perform hand hygiene and put on PPE, if indicated	Hand hygiene and PPE prevent the spread of microorganisms. PPE is required based on transmission precautions
Identify the patient. Check the name and identification number on the patient's identification band. Ask the patient to state his or her name. If the patient cannot identify him or herself, verify the patient's identification with a staff member who knows the patient	Ensures the right patient receives right medications and prevent errors. This is the most reliable method. Do not use the name on the door or over the bed. Provides an additional check to ensure that the medication is given to the right patient
Explain procedure to patient	To facilitates cooperation and reassures patient
Assemble equipment at patient's bedside	For an organized approach to the task
Have patient sit or lie with head tilted toward side of affected eye. Protect patient and bed with a waterproof pad or Mackintosh	This help flow of irrigation solution away from unaffected eye and from the inner canthus of the affected eye toward the outer canthus
Put on gloves. Clean lids and lashes with washcloth moistened with normal saline or the solution ordered for the irrigation. Wipe from inner canthus to outer canthus. Use a different corner of washcloth with each wipe	Gloves protect from contact with mucous membranes, body fluids, and contaminants. Materials lodged on lids or in lashes may be washed into eye. This cleaning motion protects nasolacrimal duct and other eye
Place kidney tray at cheek on the side of the affected eye to receive irrigating solution. If patient is able, ask him or her to support the basin	Prevent soiling of linen
Expose lower conjunctival sac and hold upper lid open with your non-dominant hand	Solution is directed into lower conjunctival sac because the cornea is sensitive and easily injured. This also prevents reflex blinking
Fill the irrigation syringe with the prescribed fluid. Hold irrigation syringe about 2.5 cm (1 inch) from eye. Direct flow of solution from inner to outer canthus along conjunctival sac	This minimizes the risk for injury to the cornea. Directing solution toward the outer canthus helps to prevent the spread of contamination from the eye to the lacrimal sac, the lacrimal duct, and the nose
Irrigate until the solution is clear or all the solution has been used. Use only enough force to remove secretions gently from the conjunctiva. Avoid touching any part of the eye with the irrigating tip	Directing solutions with force may cause injury to the tissues of the eye as well as to the conjunctiva. Touching the eye is uncomfortable for the patient and may cause damage to the cornea
Pause irrigation and have patient close the eye periodically during procedure	Movement of the eye when the lids are closed helps to move secretions from the upper to the lower conjunctival sac
Dry periorbital area after irrigation with gauze sponge. Offer a towel to the patient if face and neck are wet	Leaving the skin moist after irrigation is uncomfortable for the patient
Remove gloves. Assist the patient to a comfortable position	This ensures patient comfort
Remove additional PPE, if used. Perform hand hygiene	Removing PPE properly reduces the risk for infection transmission and contamination of other items. Hand hygiene prevents the spread of microorganism
Evaluate the patient's response to medication within appropriate time frame	The patient needs to be evaluated for therapeutic and adverse effects from the medication

EAR CARE

Ear Drop Instillation

Drugs are instilled into the auditory canal for their local effect. They are used to soften wax, relieve pain, apply local anesthesia, and treat infections. The tympanic membrane separates the external ear from the middle ear. Normally, it is intact and closes the entrance to the middle ear completely. If it is ruptured or has been opened by surgical intervention, the middle ear and the inner ear have a direct passage to the external ear. When this occurs, perform instillations with the greatest of care to prevent forcing materials from the outer ear into the middle ear and the inner ear. Use sterile technique to prevent infection.

Articles Required

❖ Medication [warmed to 37°C (98.6°F)]
❖ Dropper
❖ Tissue
❖ Cotton ball (optional)
❖ Gloves
❖ Additional PPE, as indicated
❖ Washcloth (optional)
❖ Normal saline solution

Assess the affected ear for redness, erythema, edema, drainage, or tenderness. Assess the patient for allergies. Verify patient name, dose, route, and time of administration. Assess the patient's knowledge of medication and procedure. Assess the patient's ability to cooperate with the procedure.

Nursing action	Rationale
Gather equipment as per nursing officer advice	Helps to identify errors that may have occurred when orders were transcribed
Perform hand hygiene	prevents the spread of microorganisms
Assist nursing officer in preparing medicine for administration in the medication area. Prepare medications for one patient at a time	Facilitates error-free administration and saves time
Assist in selection the proper medication from the patient's medication drawer or unit stock. Read and compare the label with the order	This prevents errors in medication
Transport medications to the patient's bedside carefully, and keep the medications in sight at all times	Careful handling and close observation prevent accidental or deliberate disarrangement of medications
Ensure that the patient receives the medications at the correct time	
Perform hand hygiene and put on PPE, if indicated	Hand hygiene and PPE prevent the spread of microorganisms. PPE is required based on transmission precautions
Identify the patient. Check the name and identification number on the patient's identification band. Ask the patient to state his or her name. If the	Ensures the right patient receives right medications and prevent errors. This is the most reliable method. Do not use the name on the door or over

Contd...

Contd...

Nursing action	Rationale
patient cannot identify him- or herself, verify the patient's identification with a staff member who knows the patient. Ask the patient about allergies. Explain the purpose and action of each medication to the patient.	the bed. Provides an additional check to ensure that the medication is given to the right patient.
Put on gloves	Gloves protect from potential contact with contaminants and body fluids.
Cleanse external ear of any drainage with cotton ball or wash—cloth moistened with normal saline.	Debris and drainage may prevent some of the medication from entering the ear canal.
Place patient on his or her unaffected side in bed, or, if ambulatory, have patient sit with head well tilted to the side so that affected ear is uppermost.	Maximum benefit of the drug. Prevents the drops from escaping from the ear.
Draw up the amount of solution needed in the dropper. Do not return excess medication to stock bottle.	Risk for contamination is increased when medication is returned to the stock bottle.
Straighten auditory canal by pulling cartilaginous portion of pinna up and back for an adult.	Helps to straighten the canal properly for ear drop instillation.
Hold dropper in the ear with its tip above the auditory canal. Do not touch the dropper to the ear. Allow drops to fall on the side of the canal.	Most of the medication will enter the ear canal. Touching the dropper to the ear contaminates the dropper and medication it is uncomfortable for the patient if the drops fall directly onto the tympanic membrane.
Release pinna after instilling drops, and have patient maintain the position to prevent escape of medication.	Medication should remain in ear canal for at least 5 minutes.
Gently press on the tragus a few times.	Allows medication from the canal to move toward the tympanic membrane.
Loosely insert a cotton ball into the ear canal, If ordered.	A cotton ball can help prevent medication from leaking out of ear canal.

Maintenance of Visual Aids

- ❖ Always keep glasses clean and smudge free to prevent scratches.
- ❖ Store them in a hard box when not in use.
- ❖ Use microfiber cloth to clean glasses as it clear grease and dirt.
- ❖ Do not wipe glasses with tissue, clothes and paper towel to avoid scratches.

Contact Lenses

Contact lenses are a convenient way to correct vision without wearing glasses. It is important to keep them always clean to prevent infection to eyes:

- ❖ Always clean hands with mild soap and water before handling contact lenses (avoid using sanitizers and other lotions which may irritate eyes).
- ❖ Use lint free towel to dry hands.
- ❖ Open one side of the contact lens case at a time to avoid mixing up (both eyes may not have same power) and place the lens in the appropriate side of contact lens case.

- Make a habit of taking out the lens in the same order each night.
- Use suction cup to remove rigid contact lens, rinse suction cup with contact lens solution after each use.
- Check lens for any damage before use because lenses are soft it may get torn easily, especially around the edges, which cause irritation and also allow microorganism to collect in the damaged spot.
- Always clean contact lenses using the solution provided for them, not with water and other solution.
- Soak lens overnight (at least 6 hours) with the solution provided for them to disinfect (rigid lens need more soaking time).
- Change lens according to doctor's order.
- Refill contact lens case with fresh solution each time (never top off the lens case).
- Sterilize case daily using contact solution and allow to air dry—follow manufactures instruction.
- Switch to a new case every 3 months, or as recommended (sterilize case by boiling it at least once every 3 months as an alternative method).
- Avoid wearing contact lenses while swimming, showering, or bathing.
- Avoid placing contact lenses on hard surface.
- Always keep them in a hard shell case, which is fit for the lens to prevent damage.

Eye Glasses

Eye glasses can be cleaned with soap and water as well as with eyeglass cleaner soap and water:
- Run a gentle stream of tap water over glasses. Rotate them to wet both sides of each lens, the frame, and earpieces. Hot water is bad for lenses, protective coatings, and the frame, so be sure to use warm water.
- Add a small drop of mild soap to each lens. Make gentle circular motions with fingertips to lather the soap over both sides of the lenses, around the frame, and down each earpiece. Clean the nose pads with a cotton swab or soft toothbrush. Use gentle pressure to scrub the nose pads and the crevices between them and the frame. Use only soft-bristled toothbrush, avoid grazing the lenses with the toothbrush, even if it is soft-bristled.
- Use cotton swab to clean between the lenses and the frame.
- Hold the glasses under running water again to rinse away soap.
- Shake off excess water and make sure your lenses are clean.
- Dry glasses with a microfiber cloth use soft circular motions with your fingertips to dry it, repeat on the other lens.

Eyeglass Cleaner

- Spray your glasses liberally with eyeglass cleaner.
- Wipe away the cleaner with a microfiber cloth. Eyeglasses also can be cleaned with wet wipes, gently rub them with a wet wipe using soft, circular motions. After cleaning them, dry them with a microfiber cloth.

Prosthetic (False) Eyes

A person who has had an eye removed due to illness or disease may wear prosthetic (false) eyes. Prosthetic eyes are custom-made for the person and can be very expensive to replace. If a person in your care has a prosthetic eye and needs help caring for it, the nurse will show you how to assist the person with removing, cleaning and re-inserting the prosthesis. It is important to care for the prosthetic eye properly to prevent injury to the eye socket and eyelid. Always handle a prosthetic eye carefully, and with clean hands.

Hearing Aids

Hearing aid is an electronic device which is designed to make some sounds louder so that people with hearing impairment are able to listen, communicate and indulge in daily life activities to the fullest. Hearing aid is helpful in both quiet and noisy situations. Hearing aids are delicate instruments that need attention to ensure good operation. Before you put the hearing aid on your patient, you should give it a quick visual inspection and listening check. Here is a checklist you should follow every day:

Hearing aid consists of the following:
* Microphone—it receives sound.
* Amplifier—for increasing the loudness of sound.
* Receiver—for reproducing the sound and then transmitting it into the ear.
* Battery—to supply power to the unit. Hearing aids may differentiate with each other in order to assist different types of hearing loss respectively.

Styles of Hearing Aid

There are three styles of hearing aids:
1. Behind the ear
2. In the ear
3. Canal

Behind the ear: It fits behind the ear and is enclosed in a small curved case and consists of a custom ear piece which designed in the shape of outer ear. It is best suited for children, since the only change required with respect to the age and size of child, is the design of ear mould, which is required to be replaced accordingly. These are the most powerful hearing aid available as these serve to be the best option for people with intense to profound hearing impairment. For some people, there are ear wax issues, open fit hearing aid act as a better choice.

In the ear: This style of hearing aid fits completely into the external ear and is used for mild to intense hearing loss. The electronic components are encased into a hard plastic case. Some aids have telecoils installed in them. The telecoil refers to a small magnetic coil which allows the aid user to receive sound with the help of the circuitry of hearing aid instead of the microphone. This enables easy telephonic conversation. It helps people hear in public ceremonies wherein there are special sound devices, known as Induction Loop System installed. Young children are not allowed to wear these hearing aids as these are required to be replaced as the ear grows in size.

Canal aids: These fit into the ear canal and are available in two styles. This type of hearing aid is designed to fit in the size and shape of the user's ear canal. It is almost hidden in the ear canal and is not easily visible to the other person. Both the styles of canal aid are used for mild to intense hearing loss. These are a little difficult for the user to adjust or remove due to their small size. These aids do not have enough space for battery and telecoils and as result these are not advisable to children and people with severe to profound hear loss since their reduced size generally limits the power and volume.

Elimination Needs

UNIT OUTLINE

- Urinary elimination
- Factors influencing urination
- Alteration in urinary elimination
- Facilitating urine elimination
- Providing urinal/bed pan
- Condom drainage
- Intermittent catheterization
- Indwelling urinary catheter and urinary drainage
- Urinary diversions
- Bladder irrigation
- Bowel elimination
- Physiology of bowel elimination, composition and characteristics of feces
- Enemas
- Bowel wash
- Digital evacuation of impacted feces
- Care of patients with ostomies

LEARNING OBJECTIVES

At the end of this unit, the reader will be able to:
- Analyze composition of urine.
- List down characteristics of urine.
- Describe physiology of urine elimination.
- Enumerate factors affecting urine elimination.
- Identify factors affecting urination.
- Describe measures to facilitate urination.
- Define nursing measures to induce micturition.
- Explain incontinence of urine.
- Classify urine incontinence.
- Practice to providing urinal/bed pan.
- Perform care for patient with indwelling catheter.
- Define urinary diversion.
- Classify types of urinary diversion.
- Practice care for stoma.
- Define bladder irrigation and its types.
- Introduce bowel elimination.
- Explain characteristics of feces.
- Categorize the types of stool.
- Analyze composition of feces.
- Define enema.
- Enumerate purposes and indications of enema.
- Classify the types of enema
- Explain colon hydrotherapy
- Define digital evacuation of feces—definition, purposes, procedure

INTRODUCTION

In the kidney, a fluid that resembles plasma is filtered through the glomerular capillaries into the renal tubules (glomerular filtration). As this glomerular filtrate passes down the tubules, its volume is reduced and its composition altered by the process of tubular reabsorption (removal of water and solutes from the tubular fluid) and tubular secretion (secretion of solutes into the tubular fluid) to form the urine that enters the same pelvis. From here, the urine passes into the bladder and is expelled out by the process of urination or micturition.

COMPOSITION OF URINE

Human urine is composed primarily of water (95%). The rest is urea (2%), creatinine (0.1%), uric acid (0.03%), chloride, sodium, potassium, sulfate, ammonium, phosphate and other ions and molecules in lesser amounts.

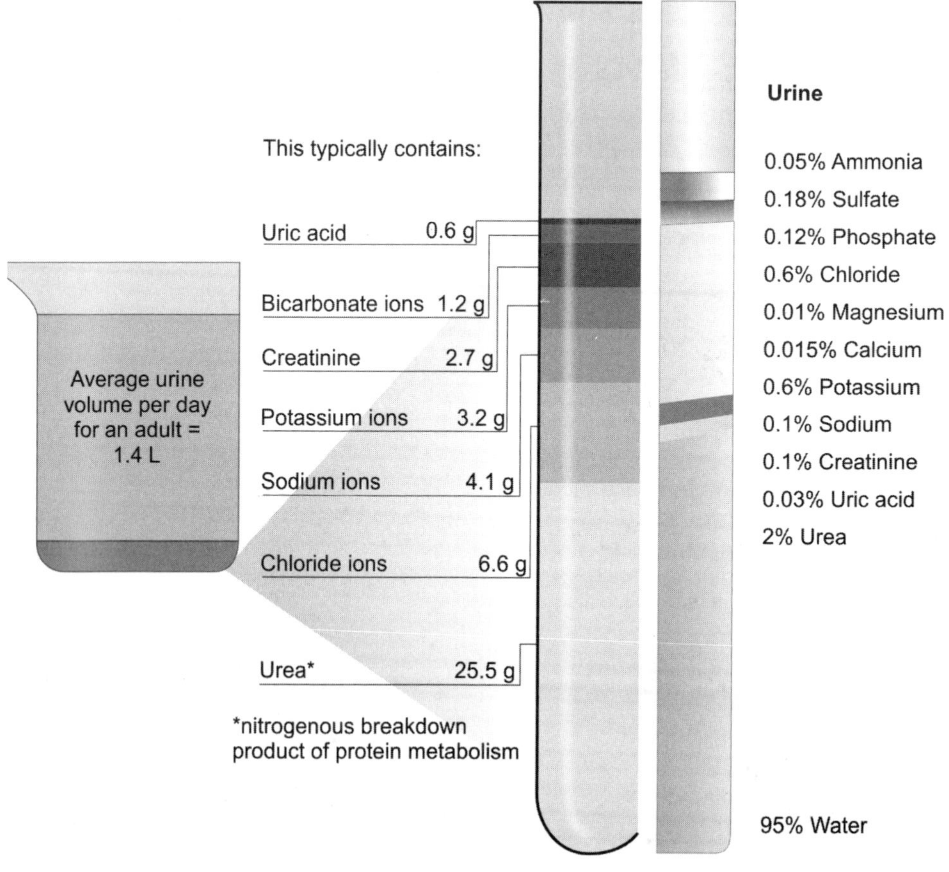

Composition of urine.

Physiological ranges of selected compounds in healthy human urine

Property and composition	Molar mass (g/mol)	Normal Range in humans (reference age in years)	Molarity (mmol/1.5 L)
Volume		0.8–2 L	
pH		4.5–8.0	
Specific gravity (SG)		1.002–1.030 g/mL (all)	
Osmolality		150–1150 mOsm/kg (>1)	
Urea (CH_4N_2O)	60.06	10–35 g/d (all)	249.750
Uric Acid ($C_5H_4N_4O_3$)	168.11	<750 mg/d (>16)	1.487
Creatinine ($C_4H_7N_3O$)	113.12	Males: 955–2936 mg/d	7.791
		Females: 601–1689 mg/d (18–83)	
Citrate ($C_6H_5O_7^{-3}$)	192.12	221–1191 mg/d (20–40)	2.450
Sodium (Na^+)	22.99	41–227 mmol/d (all)	92.625
Potassium (K^+)	39.10	17–77 mmol/d (all)	31.333
Ammonium (NH_4^+)	18.05	15–56 mmol/d (18–77)	23.667
Calcium (Ca^{2+})	40.08	Males: <250 mg/d	1.663

PHYSICAL CHARACTERISTICS OF URINE

Urine specimen is in itself, very informative. It can give us some idea regarding the status of the sample whether it is a normal one or from a patient with a certain abnormality. The following features are important in the analysis of urine:

1. **Color:** Normally, the urine is colorless or straw colored (due to the presence of urochrome). A deep yellow color is indicative of mild to severe dehydration, jaundice, vitamin B complex therapy.
   A color of red to brown suggests hematuria, hemoglobinuria, myoglobinuria, porphyria, etc. Brown to black color is due to alkaptonuria, methemoglobinuria, etc.
2. **Appearance:** Normal urine is perfectly clear and transparent, when freshly voided. It may become turbid, if exposed for a long time, due to the urea getting converted into ammonium carbonate by bacteria.
3. **Turbidity:** It may be due to:
   - Phosphate excretion in alkaline urine
   - Pus cells
4. **Specific gravity:** This is measure of the capacity of kidney to concentrate the urine. Normal value: 1.002–1.028. This depends upon the state of hydration and solute load. Values more than 1.028 imply:
   - Severe dehydration
   - Diabetes mellitus
   - Adrenal insufficiency
   Values less than 1.002 indicates:
   - Increased water intake
   - Diabetes insipidus
   - Chronic nephritis: It is important to note that, a fixed specific gravity, even on fluid restriction, denotes loss of concentrating power by the kidney and is usually seen in chronic renal failure.

5. **Volume normal value:** 700–2000 mL/day. It depends on fluid intake, solute load and loss of fluid by skin or otherwise.
   a. **Polyuria:** More than 3 L/day. This may be due to:
      ◊ Diabetes mellitus
      ◊ Diabetes insipidus
      ◊ Recovery from acute renal failure
      ◊ Diuretic therapy
   b. **Oliguria:** Less than 400 mL/day. This could be due to:
      ◊ Vomiting, fever, burns
      ◊ Edema
      ◊ Acute renal failure
   c. **Anuria:** Less than 50 mL/12 hours.
6. **pH**
   a. **Normal range:** 4.5–8.5. Average value is 6.0 in 24 hours sample.
   b. **pH >8.5:** After heavy meals, proteus infection.
   c. **pH <4.5:** After heavy exercise, metabolic acidosis, chronic respiratory acidosis.

PHYSIOLOGY OF URINE ELIMINATION

Urination or micturition primarily functions in the excretion of metabolic products and toxic wastes. The urinary tract also serves as a storage vessel of the waste filtered from the kidneys. Urine stored in the bladder is released from the bladder through the urethra upon a complex network of neurological function.

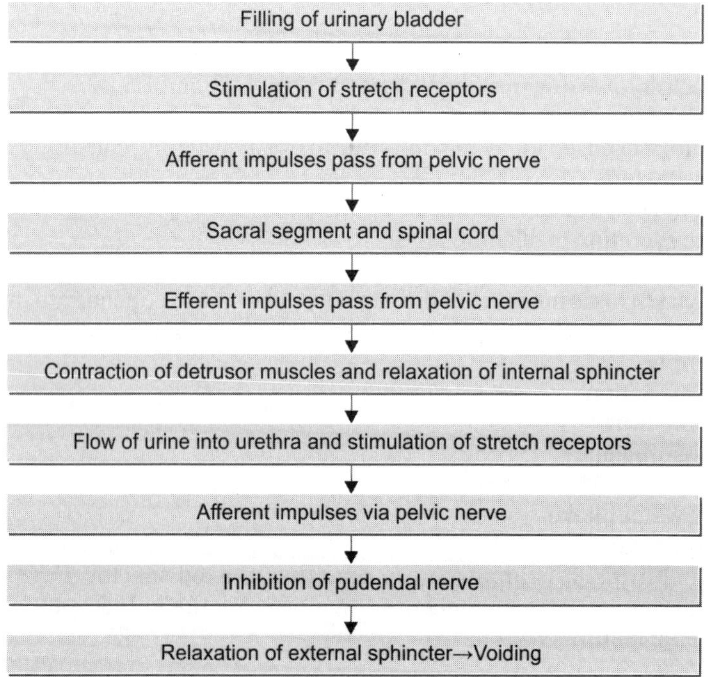

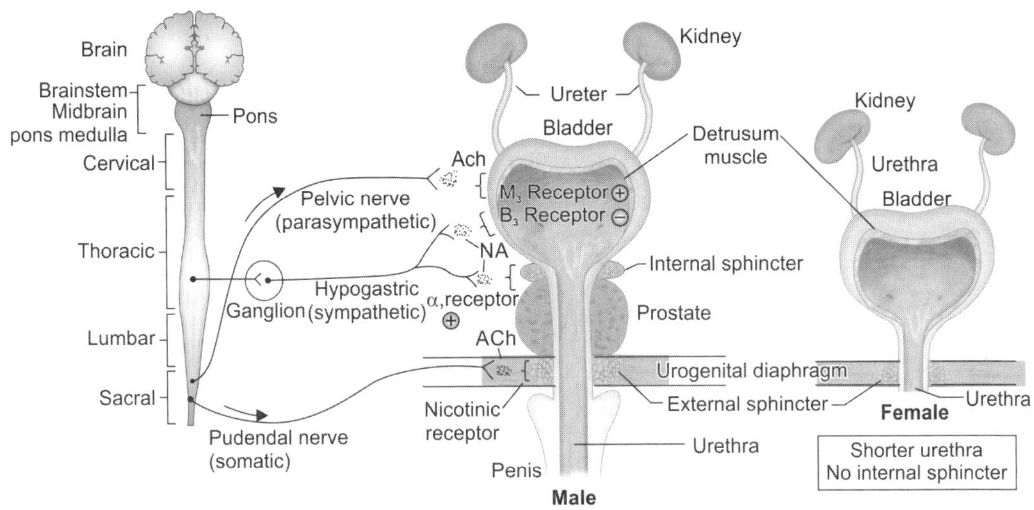

Physiology of micturition.

Mechanism

The brain, spinal cord, and peripheral ganglia all affect the micturition reflex. Afferent pathways from the bladder to the brain include the dorsal system and the spinothalamic tract. Efferent pathways from the brain to the bladder exist for micturition and storage, requiring the bladder and an outlet (bladder neck, urethra, and urethral sphincter). Sympathetic fibers originating from the T11–L2 spinal segments travel in the hypogastric nerve and link to the base of the bladder and urethra through the β3 adrenergic and α1 adrenergic receptor, respectively.

Parasympathetic preganglionic fibers from the S2–S4 spinal segments travel in the pelvic nerves and link to the bladder wall through the M3 muscarinic receptor. Somatic motor nerves from the S2–S4 motor neurons travel in the pudendal nerves and link to the striated muscles of the external urethral sphincter through the nicotinic cholinergic receptor.

When sympathetic postganglionic neurons release noradrenaline (NA), the β3 receptors are stimulated to relax the bladder smooth muscle while the α1 receptors become stimulated to contract the urethral smooth muscle to store urine. When the parasympathetic postganglionic axons release acetylcholine (ACh), the M3 receptors are stimulated to contract the bladder smooth muscle (detrusor). When the somatic axons release ACh, the nicotinic receptors become stimulated to contract the external urethral sphincter. These pathways conjunctively lead to urination.

Urinary Bladder

When smooth muscle in the wall of the bladder stretches, the micturition reflex (urination) is triggered. Urine produced in the kidneys travels down the ureters into the urinary bladder. The bladder expands like an elastic sac to hold more urine. As it reaches capacity, the process of micturition, or urination, begins. Involuntary muscle movements send signals to the nervous system, putting the decision to urinate under conscious control.

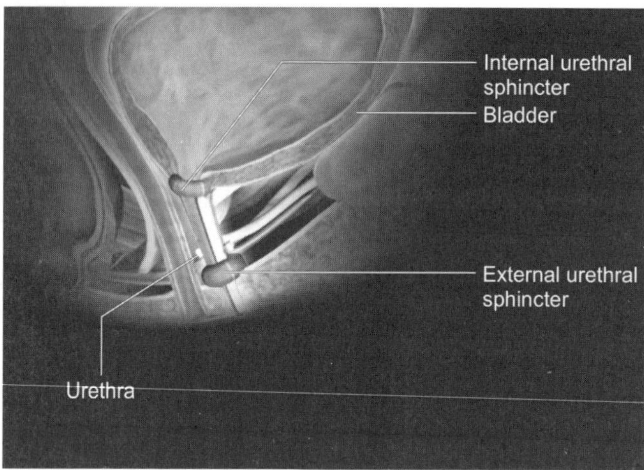

Internal and external sphincters.

The internal urethral sphincter and the external urethral sphincter both provide muscle control for the flow of urine. The internal sphincter is involuntary. It surrounds the opening of the bladder to the urethra and relaxes to allow urine to pass. The external sphincter is voluntary. It surrounds the urethra outside the bladder and must be relaxed for urination to occur.

The Bladder Expands as it Fills with Urine

The bladder is shaped like a pyramid when empty. It becomes more oval as it fills with urine and expands. A smooth muscle called the detrusor surrounds the bladder, and folds called rugae line the interior wall. These structures give the bladder elasticity and allow it to expand. The floor of the bladder includes a funnel-like region called the trigone, formed by the two ureteral orifices and the internal urethral sphincter. Urine flows into the bladder via the ureteral orifices and out through the internal sphincter.

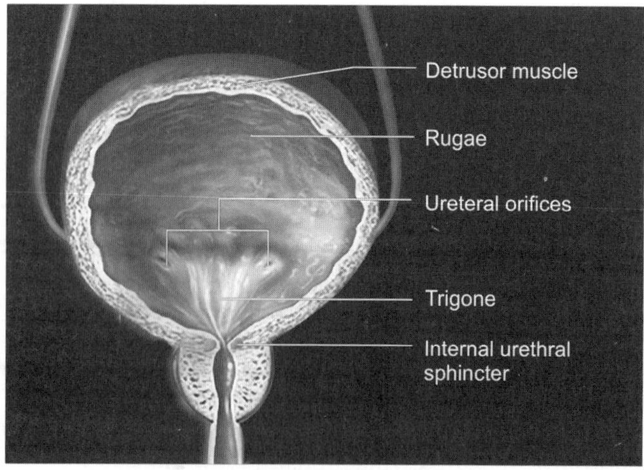

Bladder anatomy.

Muscles of micturition: The detrusor and urethral sphincters

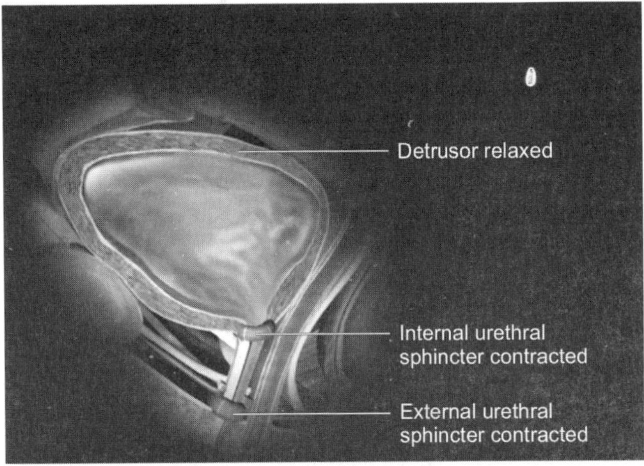

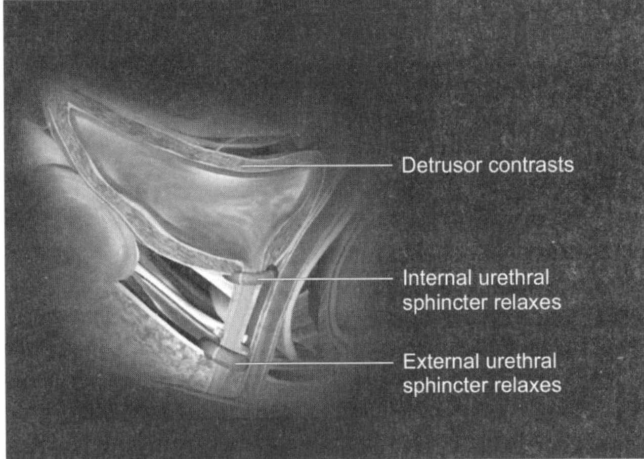

Micturition.

Micturition, or urination, is the act of emptying the bladder. When the bladder is full of urine, stretch receptors in the bladder wall trigger the micturition reflex. The detrusor muscle that surrounds the bladder contracts. The internal urethral sphincter relaxes, allowing for urine to pass out of the bladder into the urethra. Both of these reactions are involuntary. The external urethral sphincter is voluntary. It must be relaxed for urine to flow through the urethra and outside the body.

The bladder expands as urine flows in from the ureters, but there is a limit to the volume it can contain. At about 200 mL of urine, the detrusor muscle begins to contract and the internal urethral sphincter muscle begins to relax. This sends signals through the nervous system and creates the "urge" to urinate. If this urge is ignored, continence may be threatened. At about 500 mL, detrusor muscle contractions begin to force open the internal urethral sphincter. Unless the external urethral sphincter is powerful enough to prevent it, micturition (urination) will occur involuntarily.

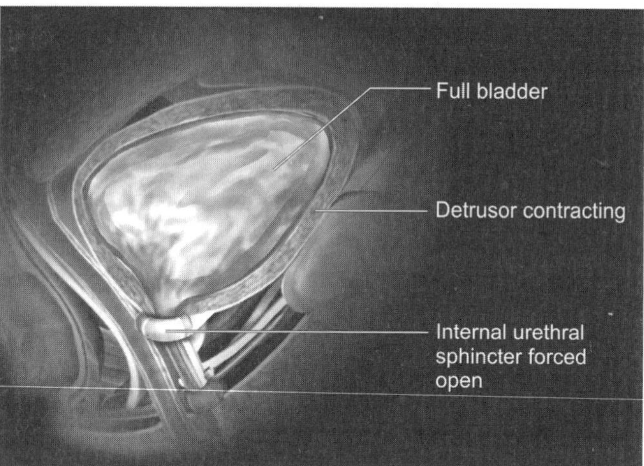

Emptying the bladder.

Bladder Stretch Triggers the Nervous System to Initiate and Control Micturition

Smooth muscle stretch initiates the micturition reflex by activating stretch receptors in the bladder wall. This autonomic reflex causes the detrusor muscle to contract and the internal urethral sphincter muscle to relax, allowing urine to flow into the urethra. The stretch receptors also send a message to the thalamus and the cerebral cortex, giving voluntary control over the external urethral sphincter. We usually gain this control of urination between the ages of 2 and 3, as our brains develop.

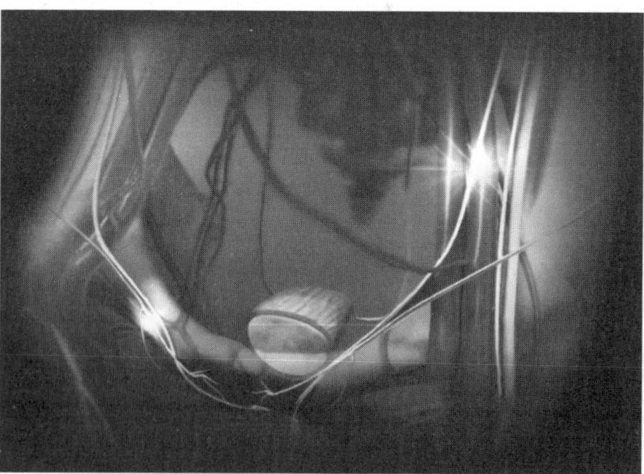

Control of urination.

FACTORS INFLUENCING URINARY ELIMINATION

Many factors influence the volume and quality of urine and the patient's ability to urinate. Some pathophysiological conditions are acute and reversible [urinary tract infection (UTI)], whereas others are chronic and irreversible (slow, progressive development of renal dysfunction).

Sociocultural factors, psychological factors, fluid balance, and surgical and diagnostic procedures affect urine and urination in several ways. In addition, medications, including anesthesia, interfere with both the production and characteristics of urine, affect the act of urination, and affect the ability to completely empty or control voiding.

Disease Conditions

Disease processes that affect urine elimination affect renal function (changes in urine volume or quality), the act of urine elimination, or both. Conditions that affect urine volume and quality are generally categorized as prerenal, renal, or postrenal in origin.

Decreased blood flow to and through the kidney (prerenal), disease conditions of the renal tissue (renal) and obstruction in the lower urinary tract that prevents urine flow from the kidneys (postrenal) sometimes alter renal function. Conditions of the lower urinary tract, including narrowing of the urethra, altered innervation of the bladder, or weakened pelvic and/ or perineal muscles, affect urinary elimination.

Diabetes mellitus and neuromuscular diseases such as multiple sclerosis cause changes in nerve functions that can lead to possible loss of bladder tone, reduced sensation of bladder fullness, or inability to inhibit bladder contractions. Older men often suffer from benign prostatic hyperplasia (BPH), which makes them prone to urinary retention and incontinence. Some patients with cognitive impairments, such as Alzheimer's disease, lose the ability to sense a full bladder or are unable to recall the procedure for voiding. Diseases that slow or hinder physical activity interfere with the ability to void. Degenerative joint disease and Parkinsonism are examples of conditions that make it difficult to reach and use toilet facilities.

Diseases that cause irreversible damage to kidney tissue result in end-stage renal disease (ESRD). Eventually the patient has symptoms resulting from uremic syndrome. An increase in nitrogenous wastes in the blood, marked fluid and electrolyte abnormalities, nausea, vomiting, headache, coma, and convulsions characterize this syndrome. As the uremic symptoms worsen, aggressive treatment is indicated for survival. These treatments are renal replacement therapies.

Sociocultural Factors

The degree of privacy needed for urination varies with cultural norms. North Americans expect toilet facilities to be private, whereas some European cultures accept communal toilet facilities. Social expectations (e.g., school recesses) influence the time of urination.

Psychological Factors

Anxiety and emotional stress cause a sense of urgency and increased frequency of urination. Anxiety often prevents a person from being able to urinate completely; as a result, the urge to void returns shortly after voiding. Emotional tension makes it difficult to relax abdominal and perineal muscles. Attempting to void in a public restroom sometimes results in a temporary inability to void. Privacy and adequate time to urinate are usually important to most people.

Fluid Balance

The kidneys primarily maintain the balance between retention and excretion of fluids. If fluids and the concentration of electrolytes and solutes are in equilibrium, an increase in fluid intake causes an increase in urine production. This amount varies with food and fluid intake. The volume of urine formed at night is about half of the volume formed during the day because both intake and metabolism decline. Nocturia (awakening to void one or more times at night) is often a sign of renal alteration. In a healthy person the intake of water in food and fluids balances the output of water in urine, feces, and insensible losses in perspiration and respiration. An excessive output of urine is polyuria. A urine output that is decreased despite normal intake is called oliguria. Oliguria often occurs when fluid loss through other means (e.g., perspiration, diarrhea, or vomiting) increases. It also occurs in early kidney disease. Often in severe kidney disease no urine is produced (anuria).

Ingestion of certain fluids directly affects urine production and excretion. Coffee, tea, cocoa, and cola drinks that contain caffeine promote increased urine formation (diuresis). Alcohol inhibits the release of antidiuretic hormone (ADH), also resulting in increased water loss in urine.

Febrile conditions affect urine production. A patient with excessive perspiration loses a large amount of fluids through insensible water loss, which decreases urine production. Fever causes an increase in body metabolism and accumulation of body wastes. Although urine volume is reduced, it is highly concentrated.

Surgical Procedures

The stress of surgery initially triggers the general adaptation syndrome. Preoperative orders of nothing-by-mouth or an underlying disease condition affect fluid balance before surgery, which reduces urine output. In addition, the stress response releases an increased amount of ADH, which increases water resorption. Stress also elevates the level of aldosterone, causing retention of sodium and water. Both of these substances reduce urine output in an effort to maintain circulatory fluid volume.

Anesthetics and narcotic analgesics slow the glomerular filtration rate, reducing urine output. These pharmacological agents also impair sensory and motor impulses traveling among the bladder, spinal cord, and brain. Patients are often unable to sense bladder fullness and initiate or inhibit micturition. Spinal anesthetics, in particular, create the risk of urinary retention because of an inability to sense the need to void and a possible inability of the bladder muscles and urethral sphincters to respond.

Surgery of lower abdominal and pelvic structures sometimes impairs urination because of local trauma to surrounding tissues. After returning from surgery involving the ureters, bladder, and urethra, patients routinely have urinary catheters.

Medications

Many medications directly or indirectly contribute to urinary dysfunction. Antipsychotics, antidepressants, alpha-adrenergic agonists, and calcium channel blockers can cause urinary retention and overflow incontinence. Alpha-antagonists, diuretics, sedative hypnotics, opioid analgesics, angiotensin-converting enzyme (ACE) inhibitors, and antihistamines can cause urinary incontinence. Antiparkinson medications may cause urinary urgency and subsequent incontinence. Always consider these medications as the cause of new-onset urinary incontinence, especially in older adults.

Some medications change the color of urine. For example, phenazopyridine (Pyridium) colors the urine a bright orange to rust; amitriptyline causes a green or blue discoloration, whereas levodopa discolors the urine to brown or black. Cancer chemotherapy drugs also color the urine and are often toxic to the bladder and/or kidneys. Patients with impaired kidney function require dosage adjustments in medications excreted by the kidneys.

Diagnostic Examination

Examination of the urinary system influences micturition. Some procedures such as an intravenous pyelogram (IVP) require patients to limit fluids before the test. A restriction in fluid intake commonly lowers urine output. Diagnostic examinations (e.g., cystoscopy) involving direct visualization of urinary structures cause localized edema of the urethral passageway and spasm of the bladder sphincter. After the procedure, a patient may have difficulty voiding or have red or pink urine because of trauma to the urethral or bladder mucosa.

ALTERATIONS IN URINARY ELIMINATION

Elimination refers to the bodily process of expelling waste products from the body by emptying either the bowels or the bladder. When patients experience an alteration in bowel or bladder habits, they often feel embarrassment and are reluctant to seek help.

Most patients with urinary problems are unable to store urine or fully empty the bladder. These disturbances result from impaired bladder function, obstruction to urine outflow, or inability to voluntarily control micturition.

Some patients may have permanent or temporary changes in the normal pathway of urinary excretion. The surgical formation of a urinary diversion temporarily or permanently bypasses the bladder and urethra as the exit routes for urine. Permanent urinary diversions are often necessary in the patient with cancer of the bladder. The patient with a urinary diversion has a stoma (artificial opening) on the abdomen to drain urine. He or she has many special needs because urine drains to the outside through a stoma.

Urinary Retention

Urinary retention is an accumulation of urine resulting from an inability of the bladder to empty properly. Normally urine production slowly fills the bladder and prevents activation of stretch receptors until it distends to a certain level of stretch. The micturition reflex occurs, and the bladder empties. In urinary retention the bladder is unable to respond to the micturition reflex and thus is unable to empty. Urine continues to collect in the bladder, stretching its walls and causing feelings of pressure, discomfort, tenderness over the symphysis pubis, restlessness, and diaphoresis (sweating).

As retention progresses, retention with overflow develops. Pressure in the bladder builds to a point at which the external urethral sphincter is unable to hold back urine. The sphincter temporarily opens to allow a small volume of urine (25–60 mL) to escape. As urine exits, the bladder pressure falls enough to allow the sphincter to regain control and close. With retention a patient may void small amounts of urine 2 or 3 times an hour with no real relief of discomfort or may continually dribble urine. Be aware of the volume and frequency of voiding to assess for urinary retention. Assess the abdomen for evidence of bladder distention and tenderness.

In acute retention key signs are bladder distention and absence of urine output over several hours. A patient under the influence of anesthetics or analgesics often feels only pressure, but the alert patient has severe pain as the bladder distends beyond its normal capacity. In severe urinary retention the bladder holds as much as 2,000 to 3,000 mL of urine. Retention occurs as a result of urethral obstruction, surgical or childbirth trauma, and alterations in motor and sensory innervation of the bladder such as occurs with neuropathy secondary to diabetes. It may occur after removal of an indwelling catheter. Medication side effects or anxiety may also result in urinary retention. If a patient cannot void or completely empty the bladder, he or she must be catheterized because a UTI, kidney stones, and hyperreflexia can occur.

Retained or residual urine, also referred to as postvoid residual (PVR), occurs if a patient has urinary retention or cannot empty the bladder completely. You can use a portable noninvasive bladder ultrasound device (bladder scanner) or the technique of straight/intermittent catheterization to assess for PVR. Bladder scanners are often not readily available for nurses to use in all clinical settings, and straight/intermittent catheterization may be the only means to determine bladder urine volume. Regardless of the method used to determine PVR, assess the amount of urine left in the bladder within 10–15 minutes after a patient voids. Instruct the patient not to void again before measurement. At least two residuals should be obtained since a patient may empty well one time and not the next.

Spastic bladders and some medications and problems such as using a bedpan or not sitting upright to void cause inconsistent emptying. In normal micturition or in a normal void the bladder should empty completely.

Urinary Tract Infections

Urinary tract infection (UTI) is the most common health care-acquired infection; 80% of these infections result from the use of an indwelling urethral catheter. Catheterization results in over 1 million UTIs each year in the United States. Infection frequently occurs after placement of urinary catheters, and each day a catheter is in place there is a 5% increase in bacteria in the urine. Catheter-associated UTIs (CAUTIs) are associated with increased hospitalizations, increased morbidity and mortality, longer hospital stay, and increased hospital costs. Consequently, there has been a shift in reimbursement practices from its traditional focus on early recognition and prompt treatment to one of prevention.

Although several different microorganisms cause CAUTIs, the patient's own colonic flora, including *Escherichia coli*, remains the most common causative pathogen. Bacteriuria (bacteria in the urine) leads to the spread of organisms into the kidneys and possibly to bacteremia or urosepsis (bacteria in the bloodstream). Microorganisms commonly enter the urinary tract through the ascending urethral route. Bacteria inhabit the distal urethra and external genitalia in men and women and the vagina in women. Organisms enter the urethral meatus easily and travel up the inner mucosal lining to the bladder. Women are more susceptible to infection because of a short urethra and the proximity of the anus to the urethral meatus. In men prostatic secretions containing an antibacterial substance and the length of the urethra reduce the susceptibility to UTIs. However, men are at increased risk for infection-related renal disease. Older adults and patients with progressive underlying disease or decreased immunity are also at increased risk.

In a healthy person with good bladder function, organisms are flushed out during voiding. Residual (retained) urine in the bladder becomes more alkaline and is an ideal site for microorganism growth. Any condition resulting in urinary retention such as a kinked, obstructed, or clamped catheter increases the risk of a UTI.

Poor perineal hygiene is another cause of UTIs in women. Inadequate hand washing, failure to wipe from front to back after voiding or defecating, and frequent sexual intercourse predispose women to infection.

Patients with lower UTIs have pain or burning during urination (dysuria) as urine flows over inflamed tissues. Fever, chills, nausea, vomiting, and malaise develop as an infection worsens. An irritated bladder (cystitis) causes a frequent and urgent sensation of the need to void. Irritation to bladder and urethral mucosa results in blood-tinged urine (hematuria). The urine appears concentrated and cloudy because of the presence of white blood cells (WBCs) or bacteria. If infection spreads to the upper urinary tract (kidneys—pyelonephritis), flank pain, tenderness, fever, and chills are common.

Another common cause of infection is the introduction of instruments into the urinary tract. For example, the introduction of a catheter through the urethra provides a direct route for microorganisms. With an indwelling catheter bacteria ascend along the outside of the catheter on the urethral wall or travel up its lumen. Local irritation to the urethra or bladder predisposes tissues to bacterial invasion.

Urinary Incontinence

Urinary incontinence is the involuntary leakage of urine that is sufficient to be a problem. It can be either temporary or permanent, continuous or intermittent. Urinary incontinence related to urinary causes is called either stress or urge urinary incontinence. Urge incontinence is more common in younger women and may be caused by local irritating factors such as UTIs. Individuals sense the urge to urinate but cannot keep from urinating long enough to reach a toilet. Stress incontinence occurs more often in older women when intra-abdominal pressure exceeds urethral resistance. Muscles around the urethra become weak; thus even a small amount of urine may leak spontaneously. Some patients may have a mixed form of incontinence that has features of both stress and urge urinary incontinence. Describes the types of urinary incontinence, their symptoms, and treatment interventions. Hyperactive or overactive bladder (OAB) is associated with individuals of all ages, but older adults are more likely to have incontinence associated with it following physical and cognitive decline associated with aging and effects of medications. OAB results from sudden, involuntary contraction of the muscles of the urinary bladder, resulting in an urge to urinate (urge incontinence). Common abnormalities of the nervous system that cause OAB include cerebrovascular accident (CVA) and other head injuries, spinal cord injury, and diabetic neuropathy. Other causes include UTI and anxiety.

Approximately 15–30% of adult women experience urinary incontinence. It is present in as many as 30–70% of nursing home residents and in 30% of adults living at home. Incontinence can impair body image and often leads to a loss of independence. Clothing becomes wet with urine, and the accompanying odor adds to the embarrassment. As a result, patients with this problem often avoid social activities. They often fail to discuss this condition with healthcare providers or nurses, and as a result urinary incontinence is underreported and undertreated. Physical limitations and environmental barriers are risks for incontinence. People with restricted mobility have greater chances of being incontinent because of their inability to reach toilet facilities in time. Low-set chairs and beds raised well above the floor are obstacles for people who must get up to reach a toilet. Some patients often lack the energy to walk very far at one time. The toilet is sometimes too far away for patients with urge incontinence. Patients who have difficulty undoing buttons or manipulating zippers face another obstacle.

Continued episodes of incontinence is a risk for impaired skin integrity. The character of urine changes when it remains in contact with skin, causing skin breakdown. The immobilized patient with frequent incontinence is especially at risk for pressure ulcers.

FACILITATING URINE ELIMINATION

Common nursing interventions related to facilitating elimination include inserting and managing urinary catheters, obtaining urine specimens, caring for ostomies, providing patient education to promote healthy elimination, and preventing complications.

Urinary Elimination Devices

This section will focus on the devices used to facilitate urinary elimination.

Urinary Catheterization

This is the insertion of a catheter tube into the urethral opening and placing it in the neck of the urinary bladder to drain urine. There are several types of urinary elimination devices, such as indwelling catheters, intermittent catheters, suprapubic catheters, and external devices. Each of these types of devices is described in the following subsections:

1. **Indwelling catheter:** An indwelling catheter, often referred to as a "Foley catheter," refers to a urinary catheter that remains in place after insertion into the bladder for the continual collection of urine. It has a balloon on the insertion tip to maintain placement in the neck of the bladder. The other end of the catheter is attached to a drainage bag for the collection of urine.

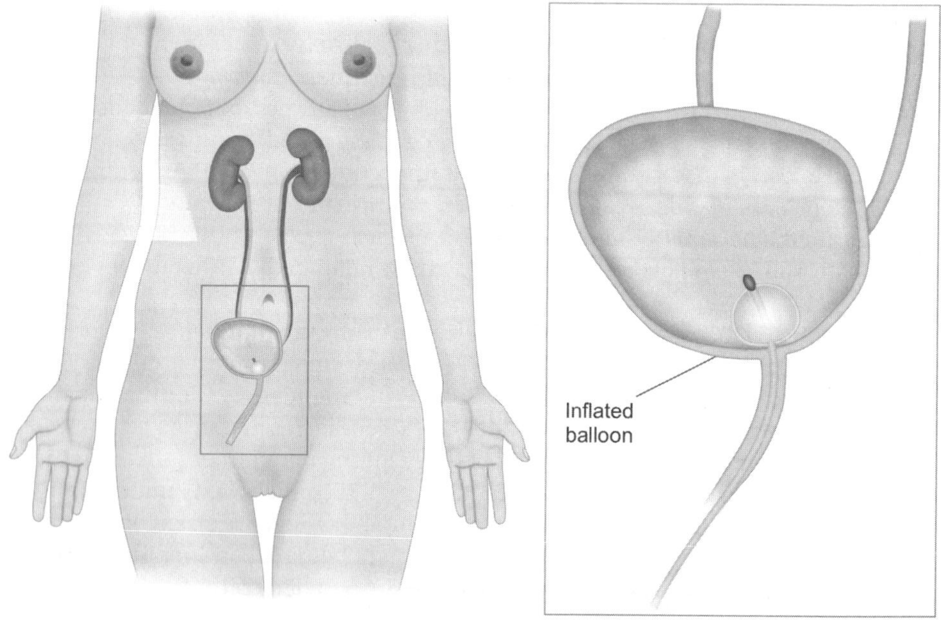

Anatomical placement of an indwelling catheter.

The distal end of an indwelling catheter has a urine drainage port that is connected to a drainage bag. The size of the catheter is marked at this end using the French catheter scale. A balloon port is also located at this end, where a syringe is inserted to inflate the balloon after it is inserted into the bladder. The balloon port is marked with the amount of fluid required to fill the balloon.

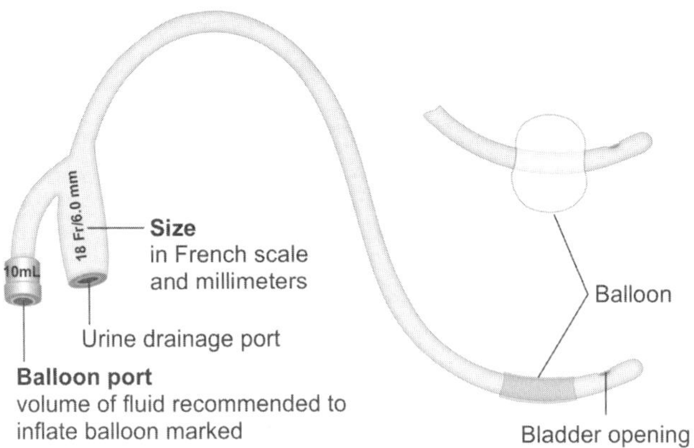

Parts of an indwelling catheter.

Catheters have different sizes, with the larger the number indicating a larger diameter of the catheter.

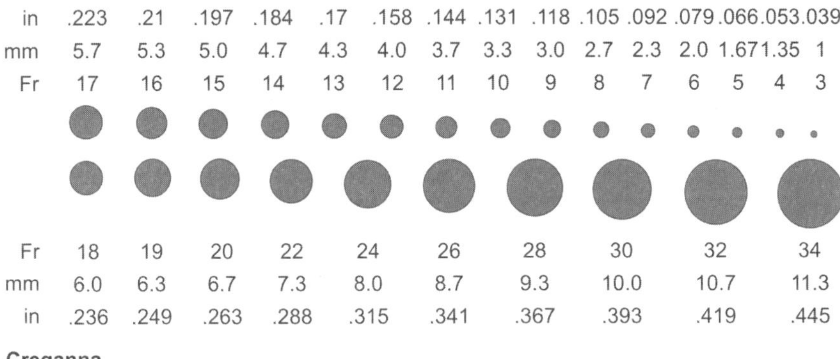

An image of the French catheter scale.

There are two common types of bags that may be attached to an indwelling catheter. During inpatient or long-term care, larger collection bags that can hold up to 2 liters of fluid are used. An image of a typical collection bag attached to an indwelling catheter. These bags should be emptied when they are half to two-thirds full to prevent traction on the urethra from the bag. Additionally, the collection bag should always be placed below the level of the patient's bladder so that urine flows out of the bladder and urine does not inadvertently flow back into the bladder. Ensure the tubing is not coiled, kinked, or compressed so that urine can flow unobstructed into the bag. Slack should be maintained in the tubing to prevent injury to the patient's urethra. To prevent the development of a urinary tract infection, the bag should not be permitted to touch the floor.

An illustration of the placement of the urine collection bag when the patient is lying in bed.

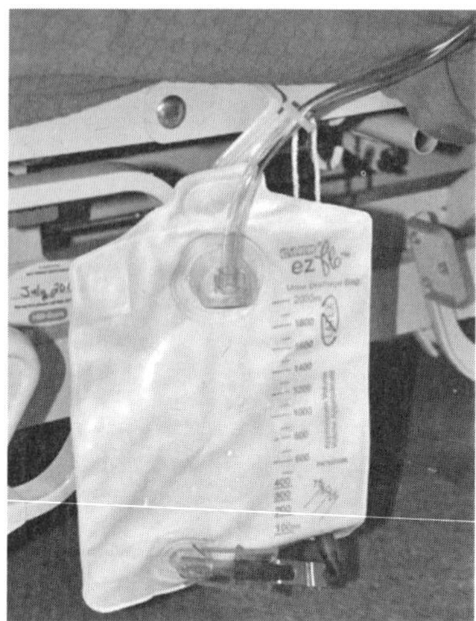

Urine collection bag.

Closed urinary drainage

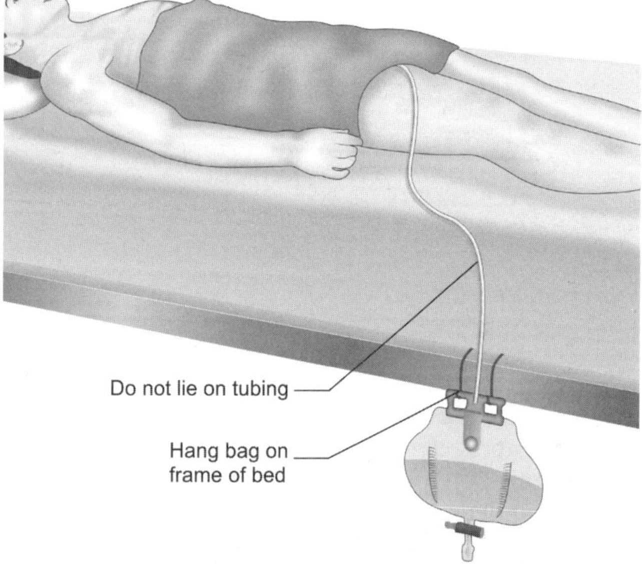

Placement of urine collection bag.

Leg bag: A second type of urine collection bag is a leg bag. Leg bags provide discretion when the patient is in public because they can be worn under clothing. However, leg bags are small and must be emptied more frequently than those used during inpatient care.

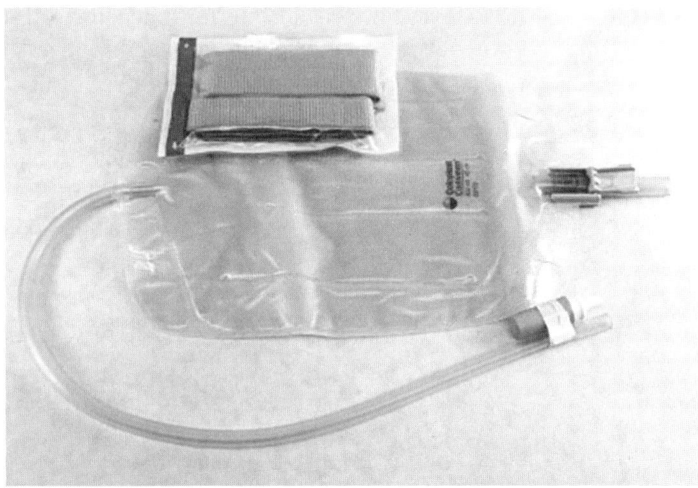

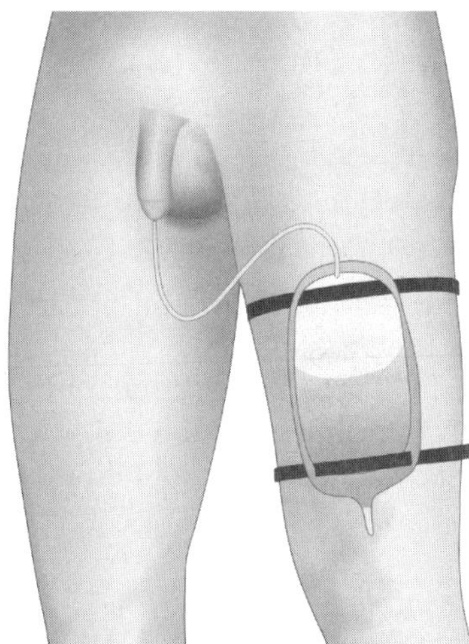

Indwelling catheter attached to leg bag.

2. **Straight catheter:** A straight catheter is used for intermittent urinary catheterization. The catheter is inserted to allow for the flow of urine and then immediately removed, so a balloon is not required at the insertion tip.

Intermittent Catheterization

This is used for the relief of urinary retention. It may be performed once, such as after surgery when a patient is experiencing urinary retention due to the effects of anesthesia, or performed several times a day to manage chronic urinary retention. Some patients may also independently perform self-catheterization at home to manage chronic urinary retention caused by various medical conditions. In some situations, a straight catheter is also used to obtain a sterile urine specimen for culture when a patient is unable to void into a sterile specimen cup. According to the Centers for Disease Control and Prevention (CDC), intermittent catheterization is preferred to indwelling urethral catheters whenever feasible because of decreased risk of developing a urinary tract infection.

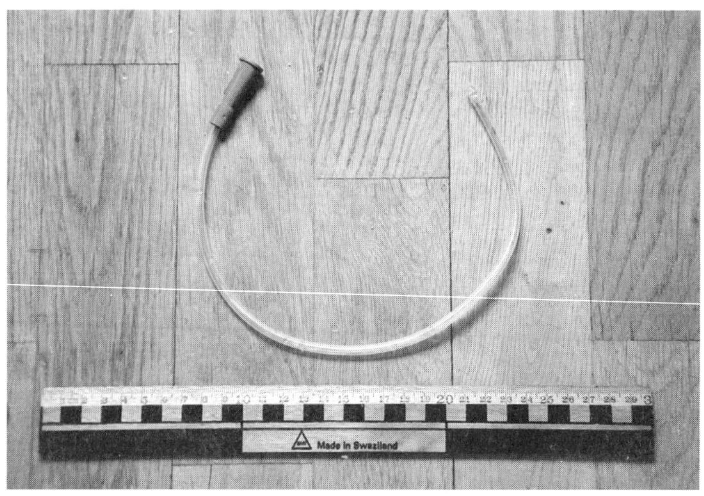

Straight catheter.

Other Types of Urinary Catheters

a. **Coude catheter:** Tips are curved to follow the natural curve of the urethra during catheterization. They are often used when catheterizing male patients with enlarged prostate glands. During insertion, the tip of the Coude catheter must be pointed anteriorly or it can cause damage the urethra. A thin line embedded in the catheter provides information regarding orientation during the procedure; maintain the line upwards to keep it pointed anteriorly.

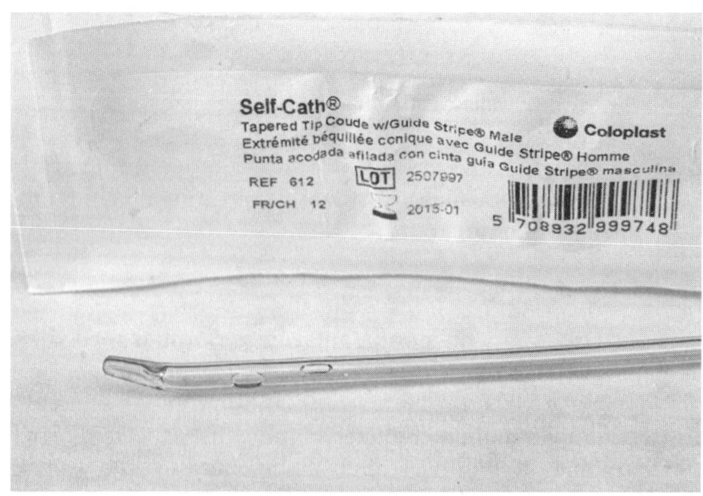

Coude tipped catheter.

b. **Irrigation catheter:** Irrigation catheters are typically used after prostate surgery to flush the surgical area. These catheters are larger in size to allow for larger amounts of fluid to flush. An image comparing a larger 20 French catheter (typically used for irrigation) to a 14 French catheter (typically used for indwelling catheters).

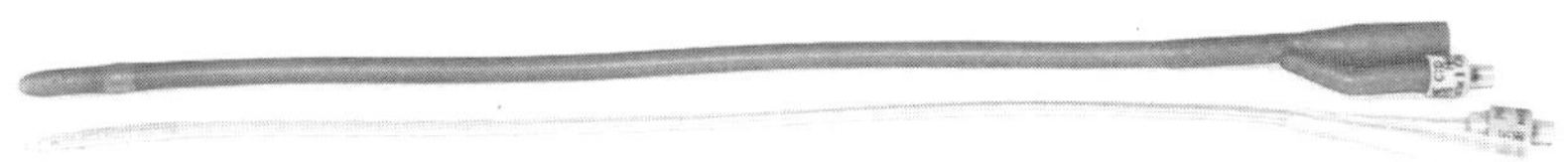

Comparison of a 20 French and a 14 French catheter.

c. **Suprapubic catheters:** Suprapubic catheters are surgically inserted through the abdominal wall into the bladder. This type of catheter is typically inserted when there is a blockage within the urethra that does not allow the use of a straight or indwelling catheter. Suprapubic catheters may be used for a short period of time for acute medical conditions or may be used permanently for chronic conditions. The insertion site of a suprapubic catheter must be cleaned regularly according to agency policy with appropriate steps to prevent skin breakdown.

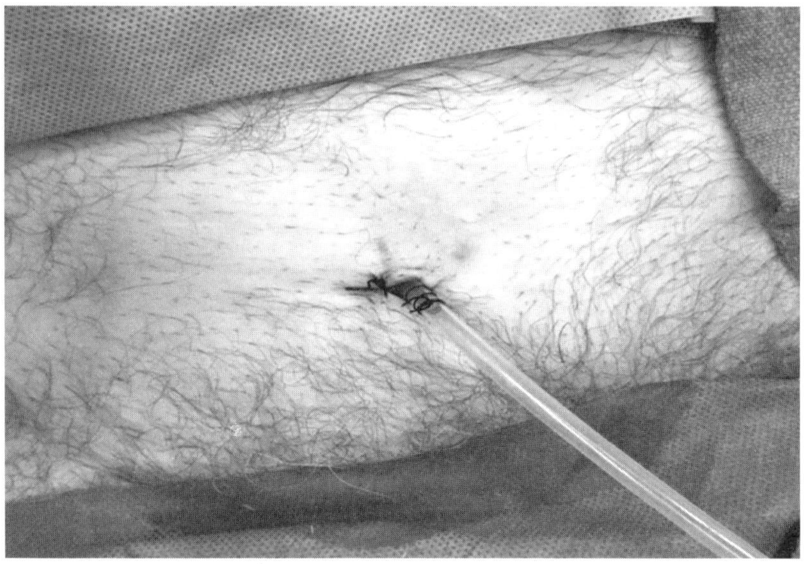

Suprapubic catheter.

d. **Male condom catheter:** A condom catheter is a noninvasive device used for males with incontinence. It is placed over the penis and connected to a drainage bag. This device protects and promotes healing of the skin around the perineal area and inner legs and is used as an alternative to an indwelling urinary catheter.

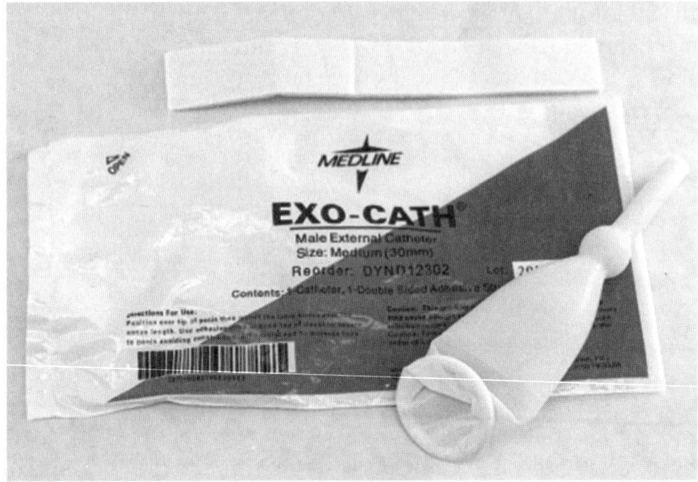

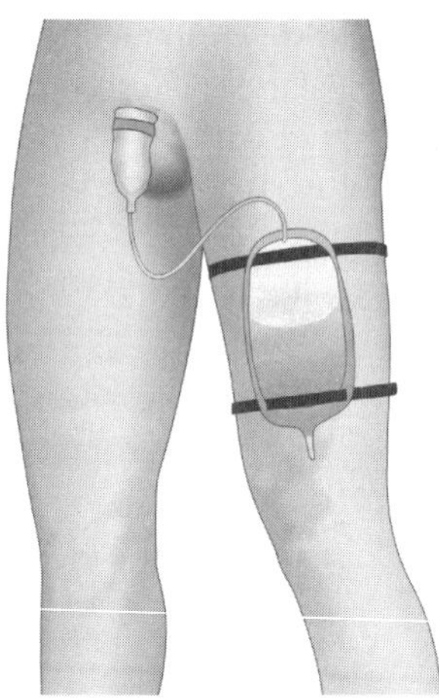

Strap the drainage bag to the thigh

Male condom catheter.

e. **Female external urinary catheter (FEUC):** It have been recently introduced into practice to reduce the incidence of catheter-associated urinary tract infection (CAUTI) in women. The external female catheter device is made of a purewick material that is placed externally over the female's urinary meatus. The wicking material is attached to a tube that is hooked to a low-suction device. When the wick becomes saturated with urine, it is suctioned into a drainage canister. Preliminary studies have found that utilizing the FEUC device reduced the risk for CAUTI.

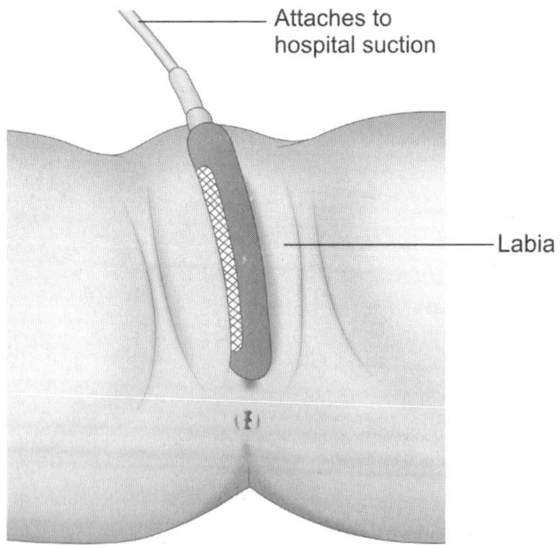

Female external urinary catheter.

Measures to Induce Micturition

When a client is experiencing difficulty in passing urine, the cause must be identified and treated. Difficulty in passing urine may result from an obstruction to the outflow of urine but may also be caused by other factors such as:

❖ Anxiety, stress, nervousness or embarrassment associated with the need to use toilet aids.
❖ The need to remain in a supine position when using toilet aids.
❖ The effects of medications, anesthesia or the acute stress of surgery.
❖ Pain, which can lead to tension in the muscles controlling the urethral opening.

Nursing actions that may be implemented to induce micturition include:
1. **Relieving pain:** If a client is experiencing pain, the cause should be identified and treated. Nursing actions to relieve pain include ensuring that the client is positioned comfortably, checking any splints or dressings to detect whether they are causing the pain, and reporting to the RN for the administration of any prescribed analgesia.
2. **Ensuring adequate privacy and sufficient time for the client to void:** If possible, the client should be left alone to use the toilet aids (e.g., bedpan or urinal) as they are generally self-conscious about the need to eliminate in the presence of others. Ensure the client's safety and that the call bell is accessible.
3. **Assisting the client to assume a natural voiding position:** Whenever possible the client should be permitted to use the toilet but, if this is contraindicated, an upright position may assist. Males may find it easier to pass urine if allowed to stand.
4. **Helping the client to relax:** Unless contraindicated, a warm shower or bath may be beneficial. The RN should be consulted as to the advisability of pouring warm water over the genitalia of a female, as this action sometimes helps to stimulate micturition.
5. **Stimulating the micturition response:** This can often be achieved by providing the sound of running water (e.g., turning on a nearby tap).
6. Encouraging the client to drink adequate amounts of fluids, unless this is contraindicated.
   If these actions fail to induce micturition and the client is uncomfortable because of a distended bladder, it may be necessary to implement further actions, such as inserting a urinary catheter. This is ordered by a medical officer and performed by an RN.

INCONTINENCE OF URINE

Incontinence is the inability to control the excretion of urine and may result from a variety of local or generalized conditions that include:
❖ Sphincter incompetence; for example, as a result of urethral trauma, surgery to the bladder, or after childbirth
❖ Urinary tract infections (UTIs)
❖ Neurological lesions
❖ Bladder tumors or stones
❖ Impaired consciousness or awareness
❖ Medications that increase urinary output; for example, diuretics, or those that affect awareness
❖ Environmental causes such as difficult access to toilet facilities.

Incontinence of urine may be classified into six types:
1. Total incontinence, when the person experiences a constant involuntary loss of urine that is unpredictable and the client is unaware that it has occurred.
2. Functional incontinence, when the person experiences an involuntary loss of urine that is unpredictable.
3. Stress incontinence, when the person loses less than 50 mL of urine while sneezing, coughing, laughing, during exercise or other activities that result in increased intra-abdominal pressure.

4. Urge incontinence, when the client experiences a strong sense of urgency to void, followed immediately by involuntary urination.
5. Overflow incontinence, which is characterized by constant dribbling while the bladder remains full.
6. Reflex incontinence — an involuntary loss of urine occurring when a specific bladder volume is reached. It may be predictable.

Urinary Elimination Assessment

Assessment of the urinary system includes asking questions about voiding habits, frequency, and if there is difficult or painful urination. The bladder may be palpated above the symphysis pubis for distention.

If the patient has incontinence, the perineal area should be inspected for skin breakdown. If urinary retention is suspected, a post-void residual amount may be measured by using a bladder scanner or by straight urinary catheterization.

PROVIDING URINAL OR BEDPAN

If the patient is not able to get out of the bed or not able to stand and walk the assistive equipment like urinal can and bedpan can be provided.

The following are the steps in providing bed pan to the patient.

Preparation

Articles needed: Bedpan/urinal, clean gloves, towel/toilet wipes, waterproof disposable pad or rubber sheet.

Steps of the procedure to help the patient to use bed pan:
1. Explain the procedure to the patient and tell him/her clearly that you are going to assist him in using the bedpan/urinal to ease the fear and discomfort. Call for help if you are not be able to support the patient by yourself to avoid injury to you as well as to the patient.
2. Close the door and put curtains to provide privacy to the patient.
3. Make the bed flat by lowering the head end of the bed to help the patient to roll. Ensure with the assigned staff nurse that making the patient in flat supine position is permitted by the doctor. Check with the patient that they are comfortable.
4. Put on the disposable gloves.
5. Put the side rails on the other side of the bed and assist the patient to gently roll to the other side of the bed holding the side rails. If the patient is not able to roll tell the other person to hold the patient from the other side.
6. Place the rubber sheet or waterproof disposable pad under the patient and ensure proper position.
7. Bring warm bedpan to patient rinsed it with warm water because if the bed pan is chill it will cause discomfort. Place the curved end of the bedpan correctly under patient's buttocks. To make sure that the bedpan has been rightly placed, ask the patient to spread the legs.
8. After positioning patient on bedpan, raise head of the bed to bring patients to normal toileting position.

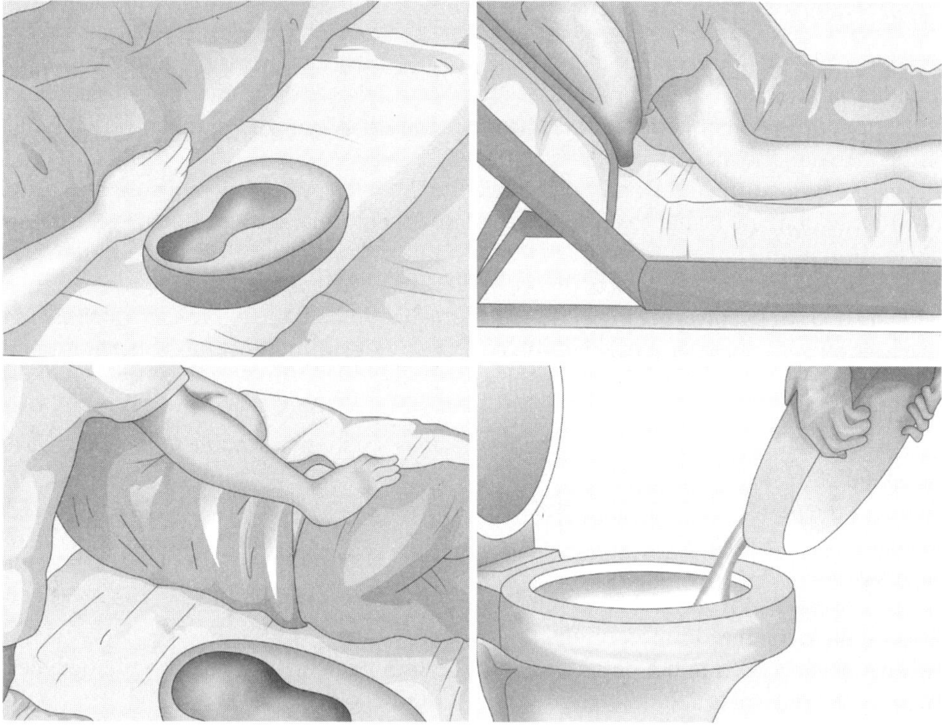

Steps of the procedure to help the patient to use bed pan.

9. Tell the patient you will be standing nearby with in the call By no means leave the bedpan in place for longer periods of time, bedsores and severe skin irritation can result.
10. When the patient is done, lower the head of the bed, help the patient to turn his/her side by holding the side rails. Remember to support the bedpan while the patient is turning.
11. Gently remove the bedpan and cover it with the lid and place it under the bed.
12. Keeping the patient stay inside lying position clean the buttock and genital of the patients with wet towel or wipes and dry with tissue paper or towel. Clean in between the legs also. In female patients ensure that you clean from front to back to prevent ascending infection. If the patients is able to clean by themselves then provide the cloth to the patient hand and encourage them to clean properly.
13. Remove the rubber sheet or waterproof disposable pad.
14. Allow the patient to return to a comfortable position as before. Provide him with a wet towel or cloth to clean the hands, if he or she wishes to do so.
15. Ensure that the patient is comfortable and ask them whether they want anything else before you leave.
16. In case of urine measure it with measuring jar and report to the staff.
17. Empty the contents in to the toilet and flush them away.
18. Clean the bedpan with soap and water and replace in the utility room.
19. Remove gloves and wash hands.

HELPING PATIENT TO USE URINAL

In case the patient who is unable to get out of the bed wants to pass urine then urinals can be provided in the bed itself. Remember separate urinals are available for the male and the female patients' nurses can differentiate it from its mouth shape. The following are the steps in providing urinal to the patient.

1. Explain the procedure to the patient and tell him/her clearly that you are going to assist him in using the bedpan/urinal to ease the fear and discomfort. Call for help if you are not be able to support the patient by yourself to avoid injury to you as well as to the patient.
2. Close the door and put curtains to provide privacy to the patient.
3. Make the bed flat by lowering the head end of the bed to help the patient to roll. Ensure with the assigned staff nurse that making the patient in flat supine position is permitted by the doctor. Check with the patient that they are comfortable.
4. Put on the disposable gloves.
   - Ask the patient to put the urinal between his legs if patient is unable to do then you assist in placing the urinal.
   - Spread the patient's legs if he cannot do it himself.
   - If the patient is male and needs extra help, place his penis into the opening at the top of the urinal.
   - Position the urinal and hold it gently while the person urinates.
   - When the person is done, carefully remove the urinal.
   - Provide wash cloth to the patient and advise him to clean and gently wipe between the legs. If the patient is a female, clean from front to back.
   - Dry the area between the person's legs.
   - Provide him with a wet towel or cloth to clean the hands, if he or she wishes to do so.
   - Ensure that the patient is comfortable and ask them whether they want anything else before you leave.
   - Measure the urine and inform to the assigned the nurse.
   - Wash the urinal with soap and water, dry it and keep in the utility room.
   - Remove gloves and wash hands thoroughly.

CARE OF PATIENTS WITH INDWELLING URINARY CATHETER

Catheter care is given for patients with retention, i.e., not able to pass urine normally and who are bed ridden. The areas around catheter such as urethral meatus (opening), skin surrounding the catheter insertion site and perineum need to be cleaned to prevent infection.

Purpose

The purposes of this procedure are to:
- Prevent or reduce chances of developing urinary tract infection.
- Provide emotional and physical comfort.
- Secure the catheter well, to enable the patient to move freely on the bed.

Articles Required

A clean tray containing:
- Clean towels -2 in number.
- Warm water and soap.

* Antiseptic lotion.
* Mackintosh and bed sheet.
* Antiseptic ointment.
* Disposable gloves.

Procedure

* Arrange the articles at the bedside.
* Explain the procedure to the patient.
* Position the patient with the knees flexed.
* Avoid unnecessary exposure.
* Clean the perineal area by using clean cotton, soap and water. Make sure to clean each side and dry well again. Make sure that soap is fully removed.
* Reassess urethral meatus for any discharge.
* Change the gloves and clean the perineal area by using sterile cotton swabs dipped in antiseptic solution. From center to periphery in straight strokes from front to back, using one cotton ball for each stroke.
* Use each swab only once.
* Repeat the same using cotton swabs soaked in sterile (boiled and cooled) water.
* Apply antiseptic ointment at urethral meatus and 2.5 cm of catheter. Fix catheter tubing to the inner thigh with a strip of plaster properly to allow free movement in the bed.
* Place the patient in a comfortable position.
* Remove gloves, dispose the contaminated items, wash hands.

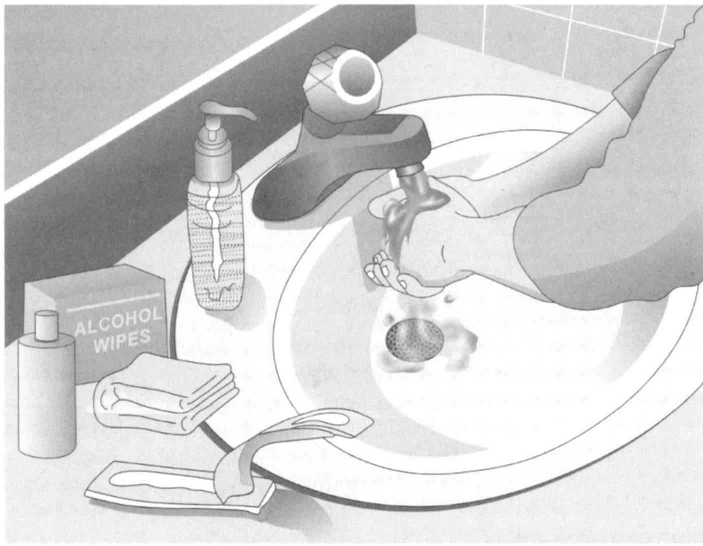

Hand wash.

URINARY DIVERSION

A urinary diversion is surgery that makes a new way for urine (pee) to leave the body. Urine is your body's liquid waste. A urinary diversion is done when the normal flow of urine is blocked or the bladder can't store urine. The most common reason to have a urinary diversion is after the whole bladder is removed for bladder cancer.

Normal Condition

The urinary tract is like a plumbing system, with special 'pipes' that allow water and salts to flow through them. The urinary tract is made up of 2 kidneys, 2 ureters, the bladder, and the urethra.

The kidneys act as a filter for the blood. They remove toxins and keep the useful sugar, salts, and minerals. Urine, the waste product, is made in the kidneys and flows down 2, 10 to 12-inch-long tubes called ureters into the bladder. The ureters are about a quarter inch wide and have muscled walls which push the urine into the bladder. The bladder can swell to store the urine until you are ready to drain it by peeing. It also closes the pathways into the ureters so urine can't flow back into the kidneys. The tube that carries the urine from the bladder out of the body is called the urethra.

Indication of Urinary Diversion

Urinary diversion is when the normal structures are bypassed and an opening is made in the urinary system to bring the urine out another way. This might need to be done if your bladder stops working the right way or needs to be removed because of cancer or an injury. The flow of urine is diverted to a replacement bladder ("neobladder") or through an opening in the abdominal wall (called a "stoma").

A urinary diversion may also be called a urinary tract diversion or bladder diversion.

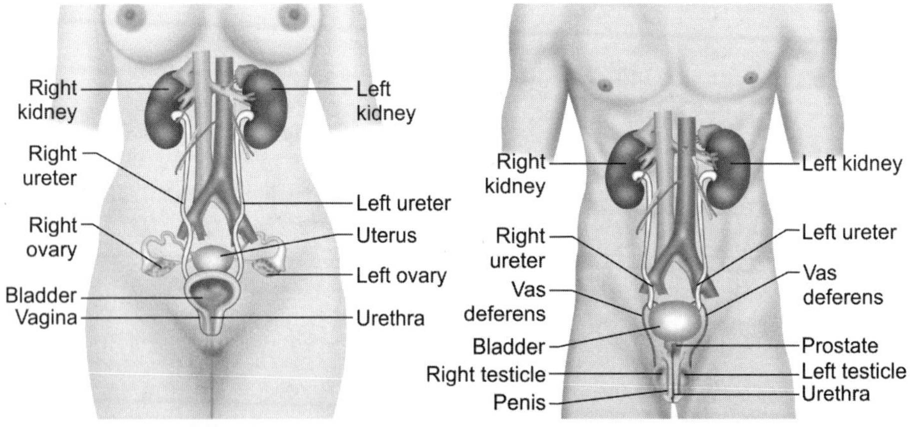

Male and female urinary tracts.

A urinary diversion can be done:
- ❖ For bladder cancer when the whole bladder is removed (called a radical cystectomy)
- ❖ After pelvic exenteration surgery for some advanced cancers.
- ❖ To go around a blockage (obstruction) and relieve blocked urine flow.
- ❖ When there is damage to the bladder from radiation therapy or other cancer treatments.

❖ For noncancerous (benign) reasons such as urinary tract stones, an enlarged prostate, birth defects, nerve problems and tumors.

The main types of urinary diversion include:
❖ Bladder catheterization
❖ Cystostomy
❖ Nephrostomy
❖ Ureteral stent
❖ Urostomy
❖ Continent urinary diversion
❖ Noncontinent urinary diversion

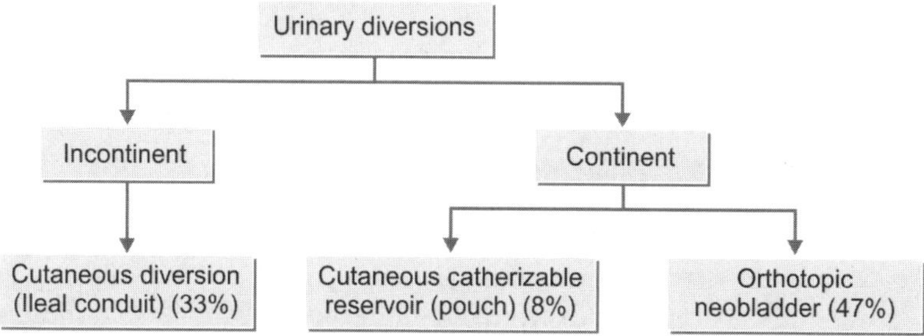

Noncontinent urinary diversions: Noncontinent urinary diversions often involve linking the ureters to a piece of intestine that is brought out of the belly. The urine then drains continuously into an ostomy bag wear under the clothes. Patient still be able to take part in strenuous physical activity, as well as daily routines.

Continent urinary diversion: For continent urinary diversion, the surgeon will make a pouch inside body from part of intestines to hold urine.

There are two basic types:
❖ Those that have a stoma brought out of the belly.
❖ Those in which a neobladder is made. With a neobladder, patients are able to pee in a normal way.
   With a surgical stoma, patient will need to insert a tube into the stoma to drain the urine 4 or 5 times a day.

CYSTOSTOMY

A cystostomy is a surgical procedure where a doctor inserts a small tube into the bladder through the skin of the lower abdomen. The tube allows urine to drain from the bladder into a bag outside your body.

NEPHROSTOMY

Similar to a cystostomy, during a nephrostomy a surgeon or radiologist makes a tiny incision and inserts a small tube, called a nephrostomy tube, through the skin of back into client's kidney. The nephrostomy tube allows urine to drain from kidney into a bag outside client's body.

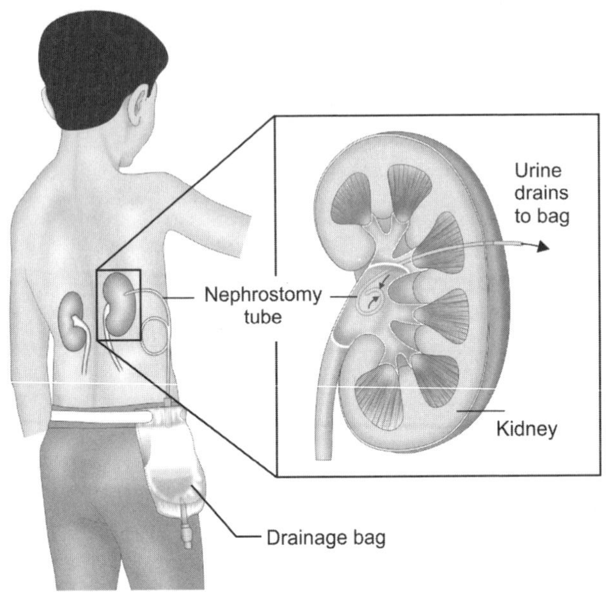

Nephrostomy.

Patient may need a nephrostomy when being treated for a kidney stone or when their ureters are narrowed, blocked, or inflamed. Depending on the reason for the nephrostomy and how quickly body heals, the nephrostomy tube may be used for different lengths of time.

URETERAL STENT

A ureteral stent is a thin flexible tube that is inserted into the ureter to help urine flow from the kidney to the bladder. The ureteral stent is guided with a cystoscope into ureter, then one end of the stent is placed in the kidney and the other end is placed in the bladder.

Patients may need a ureteral stent if one of their ureters is blocked as a result of surgery, a kidney stone, a tumor, or infection. A ureteral stent is usually temporary but, in some cases, can be used to permanently manage a blockage of the ureter. Ureteral stents that are in place for longer periods of time need to be replaced periodically.

UROSTOMY

A urostomy is used to continuously drain urine from the body through a stoma. The

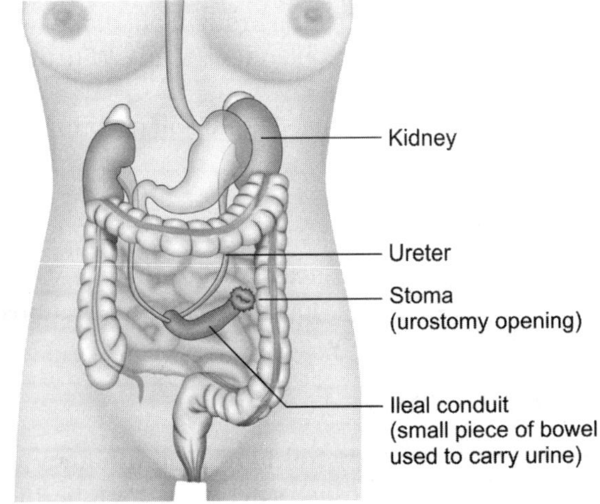

Urostomy.

urine is collected in a small bag worn outside of the body (called a urostomy bag, appliance or pouching system). This type of diversion is used more often for people who are older or in poor health.

A urostomy is a stoma, or opening, in abdomen that connects to urinary tract to allow urine to drain freely from body. Urine is collected and stored in a small bag, called a urostomy pouch, which can empty at patient's convenience. The pouch is attached to the skin around stoma and worn outside the body.

The two main types of urostomy include:

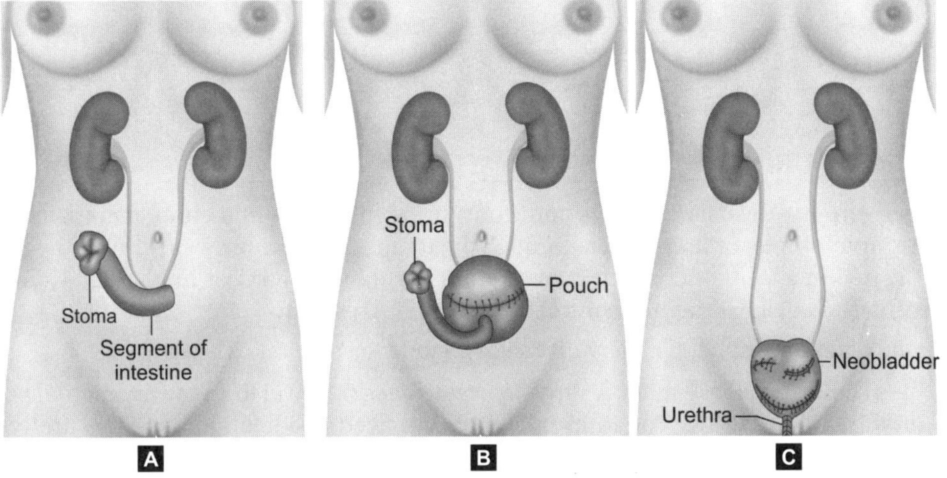

(A) Ileal conduit (incontinent diversion to skin); (B) Continent cutaneous reservoir (continent diversion to skin); (C) Orthotopic neobladder (continent diversion to urethra).

1. **Ileal conduit:** A surgeon removes a piece of intestine to create a passageway for urine. The ureters are attached to the piece of intestine, then the intestine is attached to an opening in abdomen, creating a stoma. The urine flows from the ureters, through the piece of intestine, and out the stoma.
   An ileal conduit (also called a loop diversion) is the most common type of urinary diversion done. The surgeon removes a piece of the small intestine (ileum) and uses it as a passageway (conduit) for urine. Sometimes a piece of the colon is used instead (called a colon conduit), but this isn't as common. The ureters are placed into the piece of intestine and then each ureter is surgically attached to it. An open end of the intestine is attached to an opening (called a stoma) made in the wall of the abdomen and skin. Urine travels from the kidneys, through the ureters, into the piece of intestine and then out through the stoma. Every 3–4 hours, patient empty the bag that collects the urine.
2. **Cutaneous ureterostomy:** A surgeon attaches one or both ureters directly to a stoma in abdomen.
   A cutaneous ureterostomy is when the surgeon attaches one or both of the ureters directly to the wall of the abdomen. The urine drains out of 1 or 2 stomas. This surgery is not done very often because of the increased risk of serious problems, such as kidney failure.

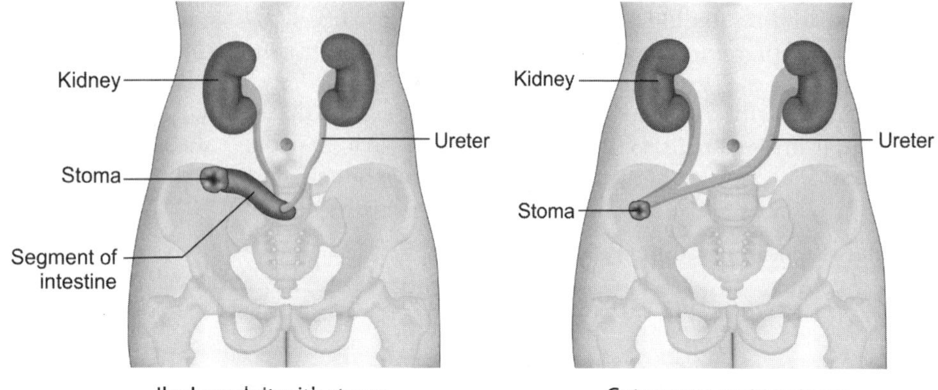

Ileal conduit with stoma.   Cutaneous ureterostomy.

CONTINENT URINARY DIVERSION

Continent urinary diversion collects and stores urine inside the body until patient drain the urine using a catheter or they urinate through the urethra. The urine flows through the ureters and is stored in an internal pouch created from part of the bowel or in bladder. Continent urinary diversion allows them to control when urine leaves body.

The main types of continent urinary diversion include:

Continent cutaneous reservoir: A surgeon uses a piece of bowel to create an internal pouch, or reservoir, to hold urine. The internal pouch is placed inside abdomen. The ureters are attached to the internal pouch, and the internal pouch is attached to a stoma in abdomen. Urine flows through the ureters and into the internal pouch, where it is stored until patient drain the urine by inserting a catheter into the stoma. The stoma is the end of a channel that connects to the reservoir. The channel has a valve that prevents urine from exiting the body until a catheter is inserted. The channel can be created from a piece of intestine or by using the appendix.

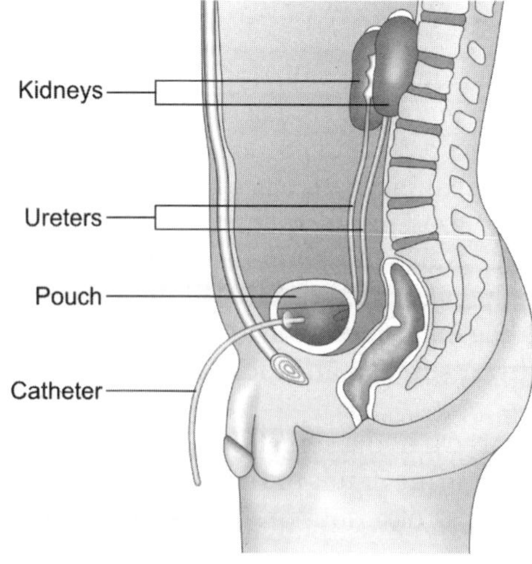

Continent urinary diversion.

Bladder substitute or neobladder: A surgeon uses a piece of bowel to create an internal reservoir, called a bladder substitute or neobladder, to hold urine. The bladder substitute is placed in the pelvis. The ureters are attached to the bladder substitute, and the bladder substitute is attached to the urethra. Urine flows through the ureters, into the bladder substitute, and patient may urinate through the urethra.

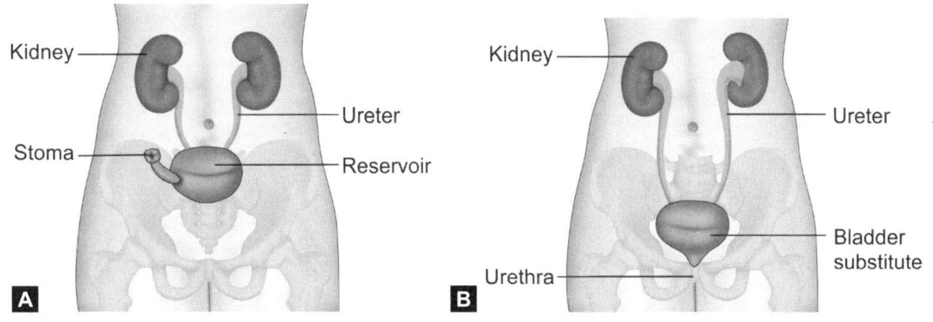

(A) Continent cutaneous reservoir; (B) Bladder substitute.

CARING FOR A STOMA

Care for the stoma every day to keep the stoma and skin around the stoma clean and healthy.

* Gently wipe away mucus.
* Wash the stoma and surrounding skin with warm water.
* If using soap, choose mild soap only.
* Rinse the stoma and surrounding skin thoroughly.
* Avoid products that contain oils, fragrance, deodorants, alcohol, or harsh chemicals.
* Gently pat the stoma and surrounding skin dry completely.
* Inspect the stoma and surrounding skin and contact your healthcare professional if you notice any skin changes or irritation.

Urostomy pouch: If patient have an ileal conduit or cutaneous ureterostomy, you need to care for your urostomy pouch, also called a pouching system. You either have a two-piece pouching system with a barrier that sticks to the skin and a pouch that attaches to the barrier, or a one-piece system with a skin barrier and pouch combined as a single unit. The skin barrier, also called a wafer, fits over your stoma and is designed to protect your skin. You empty the urine by opening a valve on the pouch and drain the urine into a toilet.

Steps to care for pouch include:

a. **Emptying the pouch:** Often empty the pouch when it is one-third to one-half full to avoid leaks, skin irritation, and odor.

b. **Changing the pouch regularly:** Most pouches need to be changed 1 to 2 times per week, but how often you need to change your pouch depends on

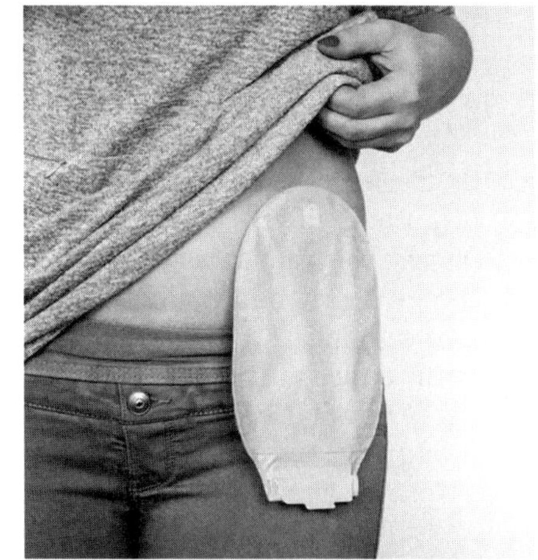

Urostomy pouch.

the type of pouch you wear, how well the skin barrier fits, the condition of the skin around your stoma, your activity level, your body shape, and your level of perspiration.

c. **Keeping the skin around the stoma clean:** Each time you change the pouch, gently clean the skin around the stoma and dry the skin completely before putting on a new pouch.

BLADDER IRRIGATION

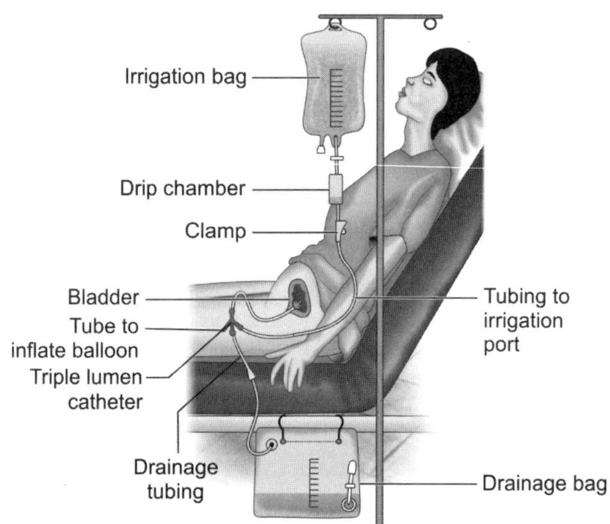

Bladder irrigation.

Definition

It is defined as flushing out/washing out the urinary bladder with specified solution.

Purposes

1. To flush clots and debris out of the catheter and bladder.
2. To instill medication to bladder lining.
3. To restore patency of the catheter.

Articles

1. Disposable gloves.
2. Disposable, water resistant, sterile towel/mackintosh.
3. Three-way retention catheter in situ.
4. Sterile drainage tubing and bag in place.
5. Sterile antiseptic swab.
6. Sterile receptacle.
7. Sterile irrigating solution warmed or at room temperature
   a. Normal saline.
   b. Distilled water.
   c. Solution as prescribed by physician.

8. Infusion tubing.
9. IV pole.
10. Kidney basin.

Procedures

Nursing action	Rationale
1. Check physician's order and nursing care plan for type, amount and strength of irrigating fluid and reason for irrigation	
2. Prepare the patient. A. Explain the procedure and its purpose to the patient. B. Provide for privacy and drape the patient. C. Empty, measure and record the amount and appearance of urine present in the urine bag.	A. Clear explanation reduces anxiety C. Emptying the bag allows for more accurate measurement of urinary output after irrigation. Assessment of character of urine helps in obtaining a baseline assessment data for later comparison.
3. Prepare the equipment. A. Wash hands. B. Connect the irrigation infusion tubing to the irrigating solution and flush the tubing with solution. C. Connect the irrigation tube to the input of 3-way catheter. Connect the drainage bag and tubing to the urinary drainage part if not already in place.	A. Reduces transmission of micro-organisms. B. Flushing the tubing removes air and prevents it from being instilled into the bladder.

4. Irrigate bladder.
A. Intermittent irrigation:
  a. Instill the prescribed amount of irrigant. If specific amount is not ordered, fill up to 150 mL of irrigant.
  b. Clamp the irrigant tubing.
  c. If the physician has ordered the irrigant remain in the bladder, for a measured length of time, clamp the drainage tube and wait for the prescribed length of time.
  d. Open the drainage tube (the clump) and monitor the drainage as it flows into the drainage bag.
B. Continuous bladder irrigation:
  a. Adjust the clump on the irrigation tube to allow the prescribed rate of irrigant to flow into the catheter and bladder.
  b. Monitor to color, clarity, debris and volume as it flows back into the drainage bag.
	a. The bladder normally feels full when it contains 300 mL of urine.
	b. Prevents further instillation of irrigant.
	c. Some irrigation solution contain medication and are meant to remain in contact with the bladder wall for a prescribed length of time.
	d. Assess the drainage for volume, color, clarity and the presence of any clots or debris.
	
	a. Regulates the amount of irrigant flowing in and out of the bladder to prevent distention or damage to any surgical site.
	b. Assess for bleeding, clotting and blockage of urine drainage or other complications.

5. Tape the catheter securely to the thigh.	Prevents the catheter from dislodging.
6. Assess the patient's condition and tolerance of procedure.	
7. Discard all used disposable articles, clean and replace reusable articles.	
8. Wash hands.	Prevents spread of microorganisms.
9. Record procedure in Nurse's Record.	

BOWEL ELIMINATION

Introduction

Defecation is the term given for the act of expelling feces from the digestive tract via the anus. It is a complex function that requires coordinated involvement from the gastrointestinal system, the nervous system, as well as the musculoskeletal system. The frequency of defecation within a 24-hour period varies depending on age and diet, but most people tend to have a bowel movement 1 to 3 times daily.

Cellular Level

The lining of the anus and rectum primarily columnar epithelium. This shifts to squamous epithelium in an area known as the transitional zone, located just superior to the dentate line. Two sphincters control the act of defecation. The internal anal sphincter consists of smooth muscle cells under involuntary control, whereas the external anal sphincter consists of voluntarily-controlled striated muscle cells.

Development

Defecation begins as an involuntary process early in life. Through the process of toilet training, children learn to control the urge to defecate and only perform the action when it is socially acceptable to do so. The age for acquiring this skill depends on the age that toilet training began for the child, as well as the method of training used.

Organ Systems Involved

The colon is responsible for propelling feces toward the rectum and beginning the urge to defecate. The external anal sphincter and the puborectalis muscle relax to allow the passage of feces out of the rectum. Valsalva maneuver and abdominal muscle contraction are performed to increase intra-abdominal pressure and expel feces more rapidly. Rectal afferent nerves are responsible for the sensation of rectal fullness and the urge to defecate. Sacral nerves S2-S4 supply innervation to the muscles most involved in the act of defecation via the pudendal nerve.

Function

Defecation is necessary to expel undigested portions of food in addition to metabolic waste products like stercobilin from the body in the form of stool. Stool also contains bacteria and cellular debris from the gastrointestinal tract.

Mechanism

Colonic mass movements and peristalsis move intestinal contents distally into the rectum. Rectal filling activates mechanoreceptors in the rectal wall causing awareness of the need to defecate. As stool reaches the rectum, a small amount is allowed to pass through to the anal canal by an involuntary relaxation of the internal anal sphincter. This action, known as the rectoanal inhibitory reflex, is necessary for anal sampling, which is the process of determining if the rectal contents are of the gaseous, solid, or liquid form. At this time, if defecation is not socially acceptable or convenient, the rectal wall relaxes, and the need to defecate subsides temporarily. If it is a proper time to defecate, the person generally either sits or squats depending on their environment. Next, contraction of the abdominal muscles and performing the Valsalva maneuver while simultaneously relaxing the external anal sphincter and puborectalis muscle will expel feces from the body due to the pressure gradient generated between the rectum and anal canal. After fecal expulsion, the closing reflex occurs, which involves the external anal sphincter regaining its tone to maintain continence at rest.

Characteristics of Feces

Human feces is the solid or semisolid remains of food that could not be digested or absorbed in the small intestine of humans, but has been further broken down by bacteria in the large intestine. It also contains bacteria and a relatively small amount of metabolic waste products such as bacterially altered bilirubin, and the dead epithelial cells from the lining of the gut. It is discharged through the anus during a process called defecation.

Normally human feces are semisolid, with a mucus coating. Small pieces of harder, less moist feces can sometimes be seen impacted in the distal (final or lower) end. This is a normal occurrence when a prior bowel movement is incomplete, and feces are returned from the rectum to the large intestine, where water is further absorbed.

In the medical literature, the term "stool" is more commonly used than "feces".

Human feces together with human urine are collectively referred to as human waste or human excreta.

Soft, formed, light yellowish brown to dark brown, slightly odiferous, slightly curved shape.

a. Sometimes may be a different color such as red or green because of variance in diet—spinach may result in greenish black streak, Iron supplements causes stools to be very dark brown or black.
b. Like frequency, expected color and consistency are different across lifespan.
   1. Newborns: Black, shiny, sticky stools called meconium.
   2. Infants who breast-feed: Bright yellow, seedy appearing stool
   3. Infants who receive formula or cows milk: Darker yellowish-brown or tan colored stool much more firm and formed.

Abnormal characteristics:
a. **If patient has in adequate fluid intake or if transit time is prolong:** Stool harder consistency and maybe passed in smaller balls or clumps rather than softer, longer, curved shape.
b. **If transit time is short:** Stool will be liquid or semiliquid, rapid transit time does not allow bio to go through it's typical chemical changes giving feces a green color.
c. **Diarrhea:** Several liquid or watery stools per day.
d. Consistency and shape may change due to variation in amount of fiber intake, increase amount of ingested fat, or change of structure of the intestine. Fiber intake affects bulk of stool.
e. **Frank blood:** Visible to the naked eye.
f. **Occult blood:** Hidden or not visible-guaiac test must be performed to determine. Indicates bleeding in digestive tract soft, formed, light yellowish-brown to dark brown, slightly odiferous, slightly curved shape.

Classification

The Bristol stool scale is a medical aid designed to classify the form of human feces into seven categories. It was developed by K.W. Heaton at the University of Bristol and was first published in the Scandinavian Journal of Gastroenterology in 1997. The form of the stool depends on the time it spends in the colon.

The seven types of stool are:
1. Separate hard lumps, like nuts (hard to pass)
2. Sausage-shaped but lumpy
3. Like a sausage but with cracks on the surface
4. Like a sausage or snake, smooth and soft
5. Soft blobs with clear-cut edges
6. Fluffy pieces with ragged edges, a mushy stool
7. Watery, no solid pieces. Entirely liquid.
   - Types 1 and 2 indicate constipation.
   - Types 3 and 4 are optimal, especially the latter, as these are the easiest to pass.
   - Types 5–7 are associated with increasing tendency to diarrhea or urgency.
   - Meconium is a newborn baby's first feces.

Color

Human fecal matter varies significantly in appearance, depending on diet and health.

Brown

Human feces ordinarily has a light to dark brown coloration, which results from a combination of bile, and bilirubin derivatives of stercobilin and urobilin, from dead red blood cells. Normally it is semisolid, with a mucus coating.

Yellow

Yellowing of feces can be caused by an infection known as giardiasis, which derives its name from Giardia, an anaerobic flagellated protozoan parasite that can cause severe and communicable yellow diarrhea. Another cause of yellowing is a condition known as Gilbert's syndrome. Yellow stool can also indicate that food is passing through the digestive tract relatively quickly. Yellow stool can be found in people with gastroesophageal reflux disease (GERD).

Pale or Gray

Stool that is pale or gray may be caused by insufficient bile output due to conditions such as cholecystitis, gallstones, giardia parasitic infection, hepatitis, chronic pancreatitis, or cirrhosis. Bile pigments from the liver give stool its brownish color. If there is decreased bile output, stool is much lighter in color.

Black or Red

Feces can be black due to the presence of red blood cells that have been in the intestines long enough to be broken down by digestive enzymes. This is known as melena, and is typically due to bleeding in the upper digestive tract, such as from a bleeding peptic ulcer. Conditions that can also cause blood in the stool include hemorrhoids, anal fissures, diverticulitis, colon cancer, and ulcerative colitis. The same color change can be observed after consuming foods that contain a substantial proportion of animal blood, such as black pudding or tiết canh. Black feces can also be caused by a number of medications, such as bismuth subsalicylate (the active ingredient in Pepto-Bismol), and dietary iron supplements, or foods such as beetroot, black liquorice, or blueberries.

Hematochezia is similarly the passage of feces that is bright red due to the presence of undigested blood, either from lower in the digestive tract or from a more active source in the upper digestive tract. Alcoholism can also provoke abnormalities in the path of blood throughout the body, including the passing of red-black stool. Hemorrhoids can also cause surface staining of red on stools, because as they leave the body the process can compress and burst hemorrhoids near the anus.

Blue

Prussian blue, or blue, a coloring used in the treatment of radiation, cesium, and thallium poisoning, can turn the feces blue. Substantial consumption of products containing blue food dye, such as blue curacao or grape soda, can have the same effect.

Silver

A tarnished-silver or aluminum paint-like feces color characteristically results when biliary obstruction of any type (white stool) combines with gastrointestinal bleeding from any source (black stool). It can also suggest a carcinoma of the ampulla of Vater, which will result in gastrointestinal bleeding and biliary obstruction, resulting in silver stool.

Green

Feces can be green due to having large amounts of unprocessed bile in the digestive tract and strong-smelling diarrhea. This can occasionally be the result from eating liquorice candy, as it is typically made with anise oil rather than liquorice herb and is predominantly sugar. Excessive sugar consumption or a sensitivity to anise oil may cause loose, green stools. It can also result from consuming excessive amounts of blue or green dye.

Violet or Purple

Violet or purple feces is a symptom of porphyria or more likely the consumption of beetroot.

Odor

Feces possesses physiological odor, which can vary according to diet and health status. For example, meat protein is rich in the amino acid methionine, which is a precursor of the sulfur-containing odorous compounds listed below. The odor of human feces is suggested to be made up from the following odorant volatiles:

- Methyl sulfides
- Methylmercaptan/methanethiol (MM)
- Dimethyl sulfide (DMS)
- Dimethyl disulfide (DMDS)
- Dimethyl trisulfide (DMTS)
- Benzopyrrole volatiles
- Indole
- Skatole
- Hydrogen sulfide (H_2S)

(H_2S) is the most common volatile sulfur compound in feces. The odor of feces may be increased when various pathologies are present, including:

- Celiac disease
- Crohn's disease
- Ulcerative colitis
- Chronic pancreatitis
- Cystic fibrosis
- Intestinal infection, e.g., *Clostridium difficile* infection.
- Malabsorption
- Short bowel syndrome

Attempts to reduce the odor of feces (and flatus) are largely based on animal research carried out with industrial applications, such as reduced environmental impact of pig farming. Many dietary modifications/supplements have been researched, including:

- Activated charcoal (it was found that activated charcoal at a dose of 0.52g four times a day did not appreciably influence the liberation of fecal gases)
- Bismuth subsalicylate
- Chlorophyllin
- Herbs such as rosemary
- Yucca schidigera
- Zinc acetate

Average Chemical Characteristics of Feces

On average humans eliminate 128 g of fresh feces per person per day with a pH value of around 6.6. Fresh feces contain around 75% water and the remaining solid fraction is 84–93% organic solids.

These organic solids consist of: 25–54% bacterial biomass, 2–25% protein or nitrogenous matter, 25% carbohydrate or undigested plant matter and 2–15% fat. Protein and fat come from the colon due to secretion, epithelial shedding and gut bacterial action. These proportions vary considerably depending on many factors such as mainly diet and body weight.

The remaining solids are composed of calcium and iron phosphates, intestinal secretions, small amounts of dried epithelial cells, and mucus.

The fecal pH test for healthy humans is a pH of 6.6.

Composition of Feces

Normally, feces are made up of 75% water and 25% solid matter. About 30% of the solid matter consists of dead bacteria; about 30% consists of indigestible food matter such as cellulose; 10–20% is cholesterol and other fats; 10–20% is inorganic substances such as calcium phosphate and iron phosphate; and 2–3% is protein. Cell debris shed from the mucous membrane of the intestinal tract also passes in the waste material, as do bile pigments (bilirubin) and dead leukocytes (white blood cells). The brown color of feces is due to the action of bacteria on bilirubin, which is the end product of the breakdown of hemoglobin (red blood cells). The odor of feces is caused by the chemicals indole, skatole, hydrogen sulfide, and mercaptans, which are produced by bacterial action.

	Feces	*Urine*
Amount	150–300 g/person/day	1–1,3 1/person/day
Moisture content	66–80%	93–96%
Dry matter	40–81 g/person/day	50–70 g/person/day
In the dry matter:		
Organic compounds	88–97%	65–85%
N	5–7%	15–19%
P (as P_2O_5)	3–5,4%	2,5–5%
K (as K_2O)	1–2,5%	3,0–4,5%
C	40–55%	11–17%
Ca (as CaO)	4–5%	4,5–6%

Factors that Influence Bowel Elimination

1. Age
2. Diet
3. Position
4. Pregnancy
5. Fluid intake
6. Activity
7. Psychological
8. Personal habits
9. Pain
10. Medications
11. Surgery/anesthesia

Age: Age affects both elimination and ability to control it. Children lack elimination control, while we lose the same as we age. Elderly people experience reduced muscle torus, causing difficulty in elimination leading to constipation.

Diet: It is the main factor that affects this process. High fiber diets and fruits enhance elimination while malnutrition causes abnormalities of GI system. Low fiber foods cause constipation.

Fluid: Equally important as diet; more fluid means less constipation and proper bowel movements and vice versa.

Physical and psychological factors: Physical activity aids in maintaining proper muscle tone whereas psychological stress exerts adverse effects.

Temperature: Elevated temperature results in dehydration and consequently constipation.

Other factors that influence bowel movements are personal habits, pain, position, pregnancy, surgery and anesthesia, and medications.

Interventions that aid to restore altered bowel elimination are laxatives and cathartics, enemas, suppositories, and digital removal.

Suppository

Suppository is a solid medical preparation in a conical/cylindrical shape designed to dissolve after insertion into the rectum.

Purpose

The purposes of this procedure are to:
- Stimulate peristalsis (movement of intestine)
- Promote defecation (passing of stool)
- Relieve abdominal distension
- Act as pain reliever

Articles Required at Home

- Rectal suppository.
- A mackintosh and a towel.
- Lubricating jelly.
- Disposable gloves.
- Tissue paper (or) clean cloth.
- Kidney tray (or) paper bag.

Procedure

Talk to the patient in general to enquire about the bowel pattern.
- Check the general condition of the patient.
- Keep the required articles near bedside.
- Provide privacy by closing the door at the room (or) pulling the curtain
- Avoid unnecessary exposure.
- Place a mackintosh with a towel under the patient's buttocks to protect the bed.
- Wash your hands thoroughly before and after the procedure.
- Assist patient in assuming left side lying position with upper leg flexed.
- Wear gloves.
- Remove suppository from its package and lubricate the rounded end with jelly. Lubricate your gloved index finger also with jelly.
- Ask patient to take slow deep breath through mouth and to relax anal sphincter.
- Separate the buttocks with the left hand and insert the suppository into the anus.
- Once it has gone inside the anus, push it further (at least 10 cm in adults and 5 cm in children) with the lubricant gloved index finger.
- Withdraw finger and wipe patient's anal area with tissue paper (or) clean cloth.
- Discard gloves turning them inside out.
- Ask patient to remain flat or on the side for 5 minutes.
- Make sure that the suppository is in place.
- Instruct the patient to retain the suppository as long as it is possible and comfortable (at least for 20–30 minutes)
- Help the patient to go to the toilet if s/he ewants to pass stool or ask about relieve in pain.
- Replace the articles after cleaning them.
- Keep the bed pan close by if the patient is not able to move out of the bed.
- Ensure comfort and safety of the patient.

Points to Keep in Mind

❖ Suppository must be kept in the refrigerator as they melt at room temperature and insertion becomes difficult.

❖ Suppository to be inserted shortly before the patient's usual time of defection or immediately after a meal.

Observation, Recording and Reporting

Observe and record the result of the suppository insertion. Record the time of insertion, duration of its retention, i.e., for how long patient kept it inside the body, result and any other observation.

Giving Enema

It is an introduction of solution into the large intestine for removing feces and cleansing the bowel.

An enema is the introduction of a liquid through the anus and into the large intestine. An enema may be given to treat constipation or to administer medication. It also may be used as part of the procedure to empty the contents of the bowel before a test, as with a colonoscopy preparation.

An enema is a liquid administered via the rectal route either to aid bowel evacuation or to administer medication.

Indications

❖ Evacuate the bowel before surgery, X-ray or for bowel examinations such as an endoscopy.

❖ Treat severe constipation when less invasive methods have failed.

❖ Administer prednisolone for patients with rectal and rectosigmoidal ulcerative colitis or rectal and rectosigmoidal Crohn's disease.

Classification/Types

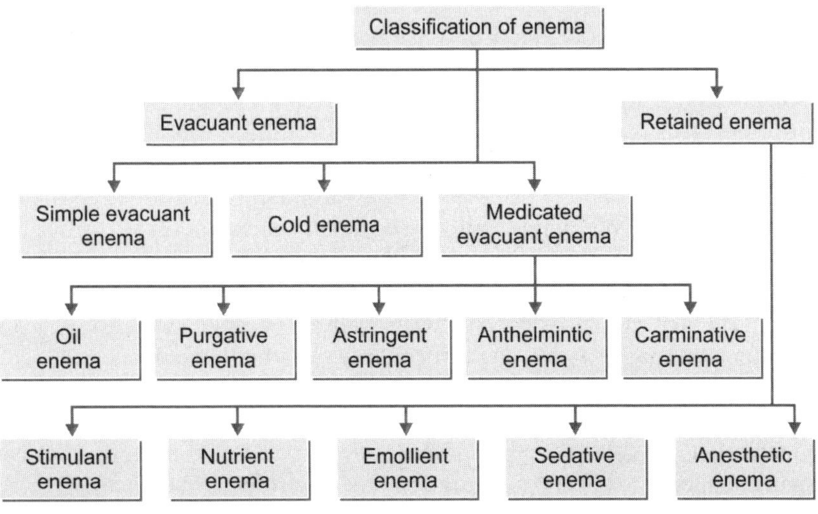

Some commonly used enema solutions include:
1. **Normal saline solution:** It is a combination of salt and water. The salt of the mixture sends the body's water into the bowels to make the feces soft.
2. **Glycerin:** It stimulates the lining of the colon to cause bowel movements.
3. **Castile soap:** It is a mild soap made of many oils, like olive oil. This mild soap is added to saline solution, which is then inserted through an enema. This solution stimulates the bowel to create movements.
4. **Coffee:** It is a mixture of brewed coffee and water, used to remove bile from the colon.
5. **Phosphate solution:** A phosphate solution enema attracts water into the bowel to soften the hardened feces.

Purpose

The purposes of this procedure are to:
- ❖ Stimulate defecation.
- ❖ Treat constipation or fecal impaction.
- ❖ Help to establish regular bowel function.
- ❖ Relieve gaseous distension by stimulating the peristalsis.
- ❖ Cleanse the bowel before surgery.
- ❖ Stimulate uterine contractions and to speed up the child birth.

Types

1. **Cleansing enema:** A cleansing enema is used to cleanse the bowels and digestive organs. The 3 main types of cleansing enemas include:
   A. **Large volume cleansing enema** (500–1000 mL): Enema solution (differs depending on the purpose of enema) cleanses the colon and most of the large intestine. This type of enema may cause damage to the external tissue of bowels.
   B. **Small volume cleansing enema (50–200 mL):** For younger users or elderly patients who may have more sensitive external tissue in their bowels. This rarely causes complications in children.
   C. **Packaged predisposable enema:** These are enemas designed for use at home for users who can do it themselves. These single-use packages come with sodium phosphate solutions. The largest side effects of these are water and electrolyte imbalances, which can be dangerous for the elderly.
2. **Retention enema:** A retention enema is, when a specific solution is released into the bowel to be absorbed. This is held in for varying periods of time without expulsion of any of the solution. Even though it may be quite uncomfortable, holding it in allows time for the colon to absorb most of the solution (e.g., medication administration).
3. **Barium enema:** Barium enema is an X-ray imaging preparation that physicians use to examine and evaluate the lower intestinal tract. The barium solution used helps provide more clear and accurate imaging results. If proper equipment and careful techniques are used by your medical caregiver during this procedure, complications are very rare.
4. **Salt water fleet enema:** Fleet enemas are primarily used for the preparation of a colonoscopy and for constipation. The bowel-cleansing solution of sodium phosphate or sodium chloride mixed with water stimulates bowel movements within minutes of the enema. It is more effective in bowel cleansing for colonoscopy preparation than its oral equivalent, with both having similar side effects (dehydration and electrolyte imbalance).

5. **Mineral oil enema:** Mineral oil enemas are used to treat constipation and to clean out the intestines and digestive organs.

6. **Evacuant enema**
   - **Simple evacuant enema:**
     ◊ Purpose: To treat constipation
     ◊ To stimulate defecation
   Solution:
     ◊ Soap jelly solution: 50 mL + 1 L water
     ◊ NS enema: 1 teaspoon to 500 mL water

7. **Oil enema:**
   - *Purpose:* To soften the hard fecal matter.
   - Severe constipation, to avoid staining of suture after surgery
   Solution:
   - Olive oil
   - Caster oil + olive oil (1 : 2)
   Amount: 115–175 mL
   Temperature of oil: 100°F

8. **Purgative enema:**
   - **Purpose:**To induce peristalsis movement
   Solution:
   - Pure glycerin (15–30 mL)
   - Glycerin + Water = 1 : 2
     ◊ $MgSO_4$ (60–120 mL with water)
     ◊ Glycerin and castor oil (1 : 1)

9. **Anthelmintic enema:**
   - **Purpose:** To kill and destroy intestinal parasite.
   Solution:
   - Infusion of Quassia:15 g in 600 mL water.
   - Hypertonic saline solution: 60 mL NS in 600 mL water.

10. **Carminative enema**

11. **Antispasmodic enema**
   - **Purpose:** To relieve gaseous distension.
   - To pass flatus (abdominal gas)
   Solution:
   - Turpentine: 8–16 mL + 600–1200 mL soap solution
   - Tr. Asafoetida: 8–18 mL + 600–1200 mL soap solution.
   - Milk: 90–230 mL + Molasses: 90–230 mL

12. **Astringent enema:**
   - **Purpose:** To relieve inflammation and prevent bleeding
   Solution:
   - Tanic acid 2 g + 600 mL water
   - Silver nitrate –2% with water
   - Alum: 30 g + 600 mL water

13. **Cold enema/ice enema:**
   - **Purpose:** To treat hyperpyrexia and heat stroke (water temperature 80–90°F)

14. **Retained enema:**
    - **Stimulant enema**
      Purpose:
      ◊ In case of shock, collapse and opium poisoning.
      Solution:
      ◊ Black coffee 1 table spoon + 300 mL water
      ◊ Brandy 15 mL + 120–180 mL glucose saline.
    - **Emollient enema:**
      Purpose:
      ◊ To protect and soothe mucus membrane of intestine and to check diarrhea.
      Solution:
      ◊ Starch and opium 1–2 mL opium.
    - **Nutrient enema:**
      Purpose:
      ◊ To give nutrient and fluid.
      Solution:
      ◊ Normal saline
      ◊ Glucose saline
      ◊ Peptonised milk
      Amount: 180–270 mL 4 hourly and Temp. 100°F
    - **Anesthetic enema:**
      Purpose:
      ◊ To induce anesthesia
      Solution:
      ◊ Avertin 150–300 mg/kg
    - **Sedative enema:**
      Purpose:
      ◊ To administer sedative medication
      Solution:
      ◊ Potassium bromide
      ◊ Choral hydrate
      ◊ Paraldehyde
    - **Barium enema:**
      Purpose:
      ◊ To make diagnosis
      Solution:
      ◊ Barium sulfate (dose 2–3 pint)

Important Points

1. **Size of rectal tube/catheter:**
   - Adult: 22 French
   - School age children:14–18 French
   - Infant: 12 French
2. **Tube insertion:**
   - Adult: 3–4 inch
   - Child: 2–3 inch
   - Infant: 1–1.5 inch

3. **Position for enema:**
   Left lateral or Sims position
4. **Height:**
   - Cleaning enema: 18 inch (45 cm)
   - Retained enema: 8 inch (20 cm)
5. **Lubricants:**
   Use of water-soluble jelly to lubricate 2–4 inch.

Articles Required for Giving an Enema

- Disposable gloves.
- Packet of enema.
- Toilet tissues (or)
- Soap and water.
- Kidney tray.
- Mackintosh.
- Bath sheet (or) bed sheet.
- Lubricant jelly.
- Bed pan with cover in case of bed ridden patient.

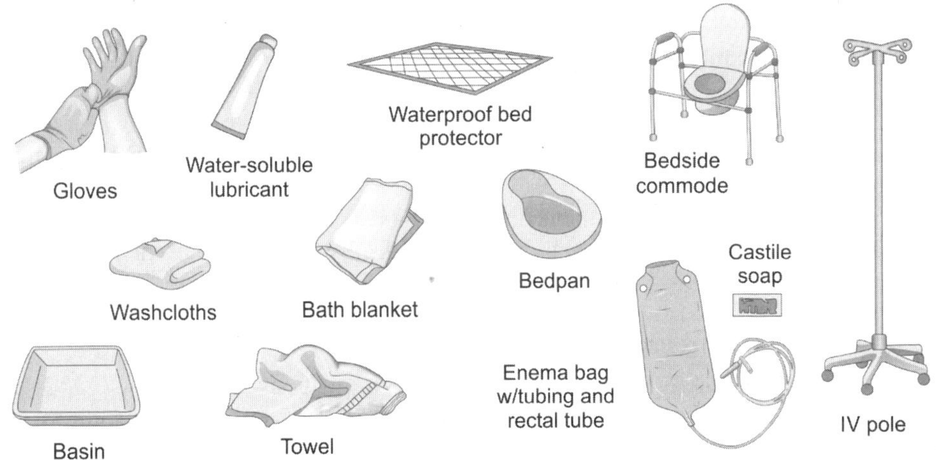

Articles required for giving an enema.

Procedure

- Assess the status of patient (last bowel movement, normal bowel pattern, abdominal pain and piles, etc.)
- Explain the procedure to the patient to get his cooperation.
- Provide privacy by closing the door (or) pulling the curtain.
- Keep all articles near the bedside.
- Wash hands and wear gloves to prevent (or) reduce infection.
- Place the mackintosh under the patients hip.
- Position the patient in left side -lying with right knee flexed.
- Cover the patient with a bath sheet (or) bed sheet exposing only anal area.

- ❖ Keep the bed pan in an easily accessible position.
- ❖ Remove plastic cap from the tip of an enema pocket.
- ❖ Lubricate the tip with jelly if needed. The tipis already lubricated.
- ❖ Gently separate the buttocks and locate anus as done while inserting rectal thermometer also.
- ❖ Ask patient to relax by breathing through mouth.
- ❖ Insert tip of an enema pocket gently in to the rectum. Approximately 7.5–10 cm to be inserted if the patient is adult, in case of child 5–7.5 cm to be inserted.
- ❖ Squeeze the pocket until all the solution has entered into the rectum and colon.
- ❖ Explain that the feeling of distension is normal.
- ❖ Instruct the patient to retain solution until an urge to defecate occurs. It occurs usually in 5–10 minutes.
- ❖ Place toilet tissue (or) cloth piece around the tube at anus and withdraw the tube.
- ❖ Discard the disposable items in proper container.
- ❖ Assist patient to go to the toilet (or) help to position on bed pan.
- ❖ Observe the fecal matter and expelled solution.
- ❖ Remove gloves and discard. Wash hands.
- ❖ Assess the condition of patient.

Points to Keep in Mind

- ❖ Listen to the complaint of the patient. You should not ignore any discomfort, however small it may be.
- ❖ Patients with hemorrhoids (piles) may experience discomfort/bleeding when enema is administered. Extra care should be taken to use lubricating jelly and while inserting the catheter.
- ❖ Warm sitz bath can be given to relieve discomfort after the procedure.
- ❖ Look for rectal bleeding and keep the dressing materially ready to clean the patient.
- ❖ Pad may need to be applied in case of bleeding.

Observation, Recording and Reporting

Observe and record the characteristics (color, amount and consistency) of fecal return (stool and the gas passed by the patient) and also whether the procedure has provided comfort to the patient.

CARE OF PATIENTS WITH OSTOMIES

Colostomy care is given by regular emptying of colostomy bag, cleaning colostomy site and applying the dressings and observation of the surrounding of the colostomy area.

Purposes

The purposes of this procedure are to:
- ❖ Prevent leakage
- ❖ Prevent excoriation of skin and stoma.
- ❖ Observe stoma and surrounding tissue.
- ❖ Teach patient and relatives about care of colostomy.

Articles Required

- Rubber sheet
- Long sheet
- Towel
- Clean gloves
- Wash clothes, cotton swabs and gauze pieces
- Water in basin and soap
- Disposable colostomy bag.
- Zinc oxide ointment.
- Bed pan with cover.

Steps of Procedure

- Explain the procedure to the patient.
- Keep the articles nearby.
- Provide privacy by closing the door of the room.
- Place the rubber sheet under the patient to protect the bed.
- Wash hands and wear gloves.
- Remove the appliance (colostomy bag) slowly beginning at the top by keeping the abdominal skin intact. If needed, use warm water for easy removal.
- Use tissue paper (or) gauze pieces to remove excess stool from the stoma (opening).
- Cover stoma with a gauze pad. It will absorb any drainage from the stoma while cleaning the skin.
- Gently clean the area around the stoma with mild soap and water.
- Check the area around the stoma. A moist reddish-pink stoma is considered normal.
- Apply Zinc-Oxide paste. It provides a smooth surface for applying skin barrier and pouch.
- Allow it to dry for 1–2 minutes.
- Select the size of stoma opening cut an opening at the center of the skin barrier (at the back side) by using scissors.
- The opening should be 1 inch larger than the stoma.
- Remove the backing to expose the sticky side.
- Remove gauze pad covering stoma.
- Apply barrier and pouch over the stoma gently.
- Hold the pouch in place for 2–3 minutes.
- Instill deodorant in bag.
- Close the pouch.
- Dispose the used items, discard gloves
- Wash hands thoroughly.

Points to Keep in Mind

- Flatus may cause a pouch to balloon out. It needs to be released immediately otherwise pouch may separate from the skin barrier and cause leaking of fecal contents and odor. So the clamp needs to be opened and the flatus to be released.
- Advise patient to avoid taking gas forming foods, e.g., pulses, cabbage, onion, turnip, radish, carrot, ladies finger, bitter gourd, potato, spinach, pumpkin, banana, fried food, fish, meat, egg, bread, etc.
- Stoma site should always be dry. Moisture will cause infection.

Observation, Recording and Report

- ❖ Observe the stoma site and record the appearance of stoma, skin area around the stoma and patient's condition.
- ❖ Check the appliance for quality and quantity of discharge and record it.

BOWEL WASH/COLON HYDROTHERAPY

It is the process of cleansing and flushing out colon or large intestine. The treatment is similar to an enema but is more extensive. It uses clean filtered water under gentle pressure (without pain) to wash out or detoxify colon of stagnated fecal materials. The number of sessions will depend on individual. Most people require a series of 3–6 treatments to receive a thorough cleansing of the colon.

Indications

- ❖ Rectal washouts are performed to decompress the lower intestine and deflate the abdomen by removing gas and stool using small amounts of sodium chloride 0.9% (normal saline).
- ❖ They are performed in babies and children to relieve low bowel obstruction, e.g., suspected Hirschsprung disease (HD), meconium plug disease, meconium ileus or intestinal dysmotility.
- ❖ This is used as a mode of temporary management in proven cases of Hirschsprung disease until definitive surgery is performed.
- ❖ This is used in the management of patients admitted with Hirschsprung-associated enterocolitis (HAEC).
- ❖ Used preoperatively in patients undergoing closure of stoma procedures.
- ❖ May be used in the management of constipation in children.

Physical Assessment

Assess and record any signs of bowel obstruction in the EMR flowsheets. These include:
- ❖ Vomiting
- ❖ Frequency
- ❖ Color (containing bile, blood)
- ❖ Amount
- ❖ Increasing nasogastric aspirate
  Note: Green vomitus/nasogastric aspirate indicates the presence of bile, making bowel obstruction more likely. If present, notify surgical team immediately.

Abdominal Distension

- ❖ Describe, e.g., tight, shiny, soft, firm, visible bowel loops, visible veins.
- ❖ Describe degree of distension of the abdomen prior to performing rectal washout.

Bowel Action

- ❖ Time of each bowel action
- ❖ Note—frequency, amount, consistency, color, +/- blood
- ❖ Odor—malodorous stools are more common in HAEC

Note: Routine measurement of abdominal girth is not used as an accurate method of determining abdominal distension.

Investigations that may be required prior to a washout:

❖ Abdominal X-ray
❖ Lower gastrointestinal contrast study
❖ Upper gastrointestinal contrast study
❖ Rectal biopsy

Medical Orders

❖ Medical orders by the treating surgeons/senior medical staff must be active in the EMR.
❖ Washouts need to be ordered on the MAR and should include:
  ◆ Frequency
  ◆ Size of catheter (in French)
  ◆ Amount (mL) of 0.9% Sodium Chloride solution to be instilled (Maximum 20 mL/kg per procedure)

Note: Use only Sodium Chloride 0.9% solution

Procedure

Perform the rectal washout as prescribed. The frequency of washouts is determined according to the effectiveness of decompression of the bowel and treatment protocols should be individualized based on the underlying condition. Notify the surgical team if the washout fails to achieve abdominal decompression.

Equipment

1. Nelaton catheter with a round tip end and side holes
2. Water-based lubricant
3. 60 mL catheter tip syringe
4. 0.9% sodium chloride. This can be the 500 mL bottles or 30 mL sachets, depending on volume required.

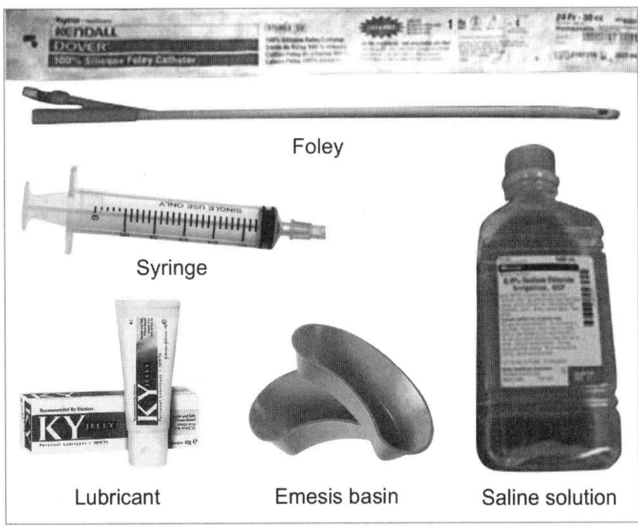

Equipment for rectal washout.

5. Blueys/incontinence sheets
6. Gloves

Nelaton Catheters Sizing

Confirm orders with treating surgeon/doctor if they vary from the below guide. Nelaton catheters can be found in the store room of most wards and in the operating theater.

Weight (kg)	Size (French)	Length to be inserted (cm)
<2 kg	8	2–3 cm
2–4 kg	8–10	2–5 cm
4–6 kg	10–14	5 cm
>6 kg	14–16	5 cm

Considerations Prior to the Washout

* Ensure procedural consent obtained by treating surgical team before commencement.
* Performing the washout in a treatment room, away from the client's bedside.
* The use of sedation.
* Nonpharmacological pain management strategies, should follow.
* A second staff member or attender to assist
* Ensure the 0.9% sodium chloride is warmed prior to use (do not use the microwave). Children may cool quite rapidly if the solution is cold.
* Ensure that the client remains warm throughout the procedure. Consider using a blanket or towel to cover their top half.

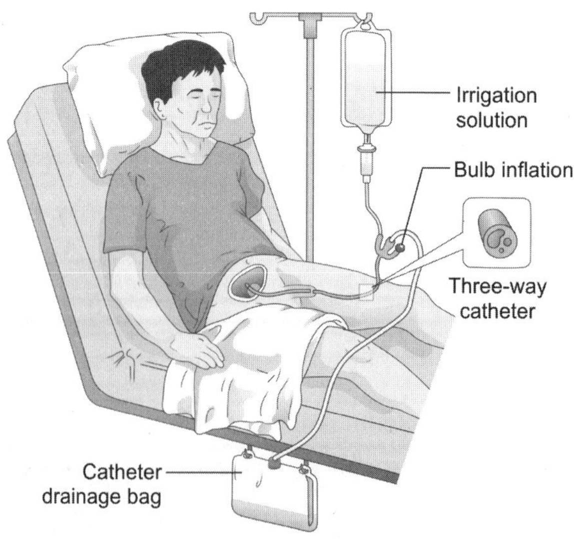

Continuous bladder irrigation.

Step by Step Guide

❖ Perform hand hygiene
❖ Prepare equipment prior to starting the washout
❖ Warm 0.9% Sodium Chloride sachets (in a jug of warm tap water)
❖ Position the client on his/her back with legs in the frog position
❖ You may position an older child on their left side.
❖ Perform hand hygiene and don gloves.
❖ Select appropriately sized catheter for use.
❖ Lubricate tip of catheter and gently insert into the rectum
❖ Initially place an empty catheter into the rectum to dispel any gas
❖ Remove catheter and then prime with warmed 0.9% Sodium Chloride
❖ Leave syringe attached to ensure no air enters the catheter
❖ Lubricate tip of catheter again and gently insert into the rectum
❖ Length to be determined by the table above
❖ Instill 0.9% Sodium Chloride solution in 10–30 mL aliquots (by pushing in with syringe plunger) over 1–2 minutes (there should be no resistance when injecting the normal saline)
❖ Remove syringe and let fluid run into nappy/kidney dish/emesis bag.
❖ Continue to repeat until the prescribed amount of 0.9% Sodium Chloride solution has been used
❖ Remove catheter from the rectum and leave the patient clean and dry
❖ Remove gloves and perform hand hygiene
❖ Clean area, dispose of waste and perform hand hygiene
❖ Note and record results of rectal washout accurately on the MAR and the fluid balance section of the EMR flow sheets.
❖ Do not use excessive force if resistance is felt. Contact medical staff if unsure.
❖ Do not pull back on syringe to aspirate. Allow the 0.9% Sodium Chloride to run out naturally. Sometimes manipulating the catheter in and out a few centimeters gently and massaging the abdomen may encourage fluid returns to be expelled.
❖ Do not exceed maximum of 20 mL/kg
❖ If there is 0.9% sodium chloride retention or return volume cannot be determined, contact surgeon

Monitor for Signs of Hirschsprung's Associated Enterocolitis (HAEC) including:

❖ Offensive smelling stools
❖ Unusual color of stools
❖ Looser consistency, explosive stools
❖ Blood in stool
❖ Documentation
❖ Note any reduction in abdominal distension and/or abdominal decompression in the progress notes.
❖ Document the washout result including, Signing the MAR.
❖ Updating the fluid balance chart via flow sheets.
❖ Color, consistency and type of substance expelled, e.g., stool/meconium/instilled fluid
❖ Complications
  ◆ Reabsorption of 0.9% sodium chloride, especially if most of the solution is not expelled.

- ❖ In the case of retention of instilled solution:
- ❖ Contact the surgical/neonatal team
- ❖ Record volume of fluid retained.
- ❖ Bowel perforation
- ❖ Nausea and vomiting
- ❖ Abdominal discomfort

DIGITAL EVACUATION OF FECES

A fecal impaction or an impacted bowel is a solid, immobile bulk of feces that can develop in the rectum as a result of chronic constipation (a related term is fecal loading which refers to a large volume of stool in the rectum of any consistency). Fecal impaction is a common result of neurogenic bowel dysfunction and causes immense discomfort and pain. It treatment includes laxatives, enemas, and pulsed irrigation evacuation (PIE) as well as digital removal.

Digital disimpaction is the use of fingers to manually remove stool from the rectum. This may be done by a person with constipation or by a medical professional assisting someone with fecal impaction or conditions (like a spinal cord injury) that prevent defection.

For this procedure, a single finger of a gloved hand is lubricated and inserted into the rectum. The stool is gently broken up and removed in pieces until the rectum is cleared. Digital

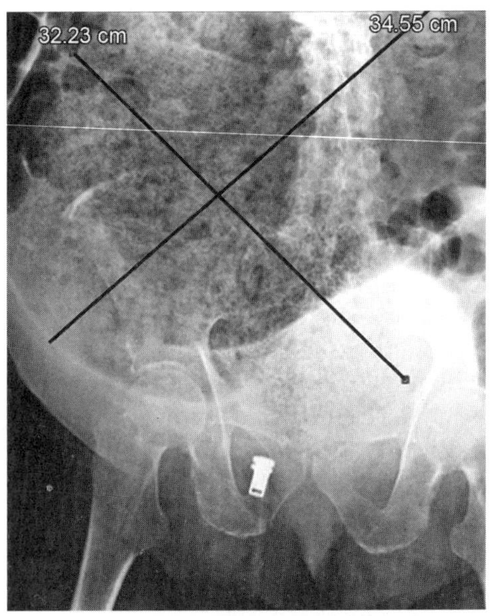

Digital evacuation of feces.

disimpaction can be performed on its own or in tandem with rectal irrigation (douching).

Digital removal of feces is often carried out for patients with spinal injuries, spina bifida and multiple sclerosis as part of their routine bowel management in conjunction with a fiber-rich diet, digital stimulation, suppositories, enemas, abdominal massage and stool softeners. Digital stimulation is a method of initiating the defecation reflex by dilating the anus either using a finger or an anal dilator. It is important to note that this procedure is useful only if the rectum is full advances in oral medications and rectal and surgical treatments have reduced the need for the digital removal of feces in patients.

Digital removal of feces should be performed only by a nurse deemed competent, with the correct knowledge, skills and ability required for safe practice Competent nurses should have successfully completed bowel-dysfunction training, which includes the practical and theoretical aspects of digital removal of feces, and follow local protocols and policies.

Autonomic Dysreflexia

Autonomic dysreflexia is an abnormal response from the autonomic nervous system to a painful stimulus unique to patients with a spinal cord injury at the sixth thoracic vertebrae or above. A distended bowel caused by constipation can lead to autonomic dysreflexia.

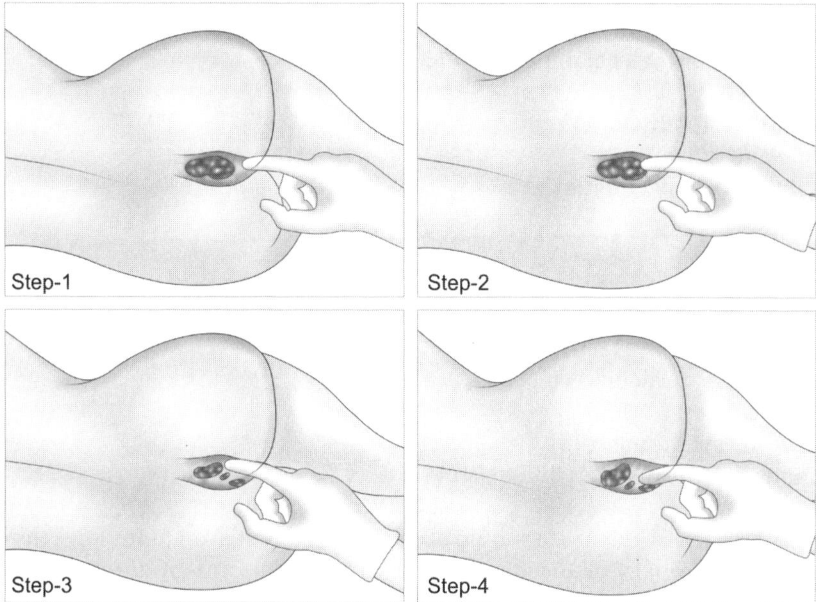

Digital removal of fecal impaction.

Nurses should be aware that acute autonomic dysreflexia can be a response to digital interventions and must assess for the signs and symptoms throughout the procedure. These include headache, hypertension, brachycardia, sweating, flushes, nasal obstruction, pallor below the level of spinal injury and hypertension. Severe hypertension may lead to life-threatening complications such as intracranial bleeding, seizure or retinal detachment. Note that the most significant symptom is the rapid onset of a severe headache. If this occurs the invention should be stopped immediately and the patient monitored until symptoms desist.

Definition

The digital (manual) removal of feces is defined as an invasive procedure that involves the manual removal of feces from the rectum using a gloved finger. This should only be performed following a complete bowel assessment to understand the patient's normal bowel habits bowel history including constipation, complications, current medication and medical history.

Indications

Digital removal of feces should only be performed following a complete bowel assessment and for the following indications:
* Fecal impaction/loading
* Incomplete defecation
* An inability to defecate
* When other methods of bowel emptying have failed, or are deemed inappropriate
* If a patient has a neurogenic bowel dysfunction
* For patients with a spinal cord injury.

Causes and Risk Factors

Causes and risk factors of fecal impaction include:

* Physical inactivity
* Chronic or severe dehydration
* Not eating enough fiber
* Holding in bowel movements
* Opioid drug use
* Barium enemas
* Foreign object obstruction
* Enlarged prostate
* Pregnancy
* Being in traction (particularly if obese)
* Celiac disease
* Irritable bowel syndrome (IBS)
* Inflammatory bowel disease (IBD)
* Hypothyroidism

During the procedure, the nurse should observe the patient at all times for signs of distress, which could include pain or discomfort, bleeding, symptoms of autonomic dysreflexia or collapse. Nurses should not perform digital removal of feces if the patient has recently undergone rectal surgery or if there is any indication of trauma to the anal or rectal area.

The digital removal of feces can be a distressing, painful and dangerous procedure. Nurses must ensure that they follow best practice guidelines and local policies when performing this role. Caution should be taken to avoid damage to the vagus nerve in the rectal wall as this can slow the patient's heart rate. Take care to minimize the risk of bowel perforation, bleeding or rectal trauma. The equipment required to perform digital removal of feces is listed below:

Equipment

* Disposable apron and two pairs of gloves
* Lubricating gel
* Swabs
* Commode or bedpan
* Specimen pot (if required)
* Local anesthetic gel (if prescribed)
* Disposable incontinence pad
* Clinical waste bag

Procedure

* Confirm the patient's identity, and explain and discuss the full procedure.
* Obtain consent verbal, written or implied. Ask the patient if they would like to have a chaperone present. The procedure must be stopped at any time if the patient requests this. If the patient lacks capacity, practitioners must act in accordance with the Mental Capacity Act.
* Assess the patient's specific requirements and the reason for intervention. If the patient is constipated a full physical, psychological and social assessment should be completed.
* Check for any allergies such as latex.

❖ Wash hands and put on an apron and one pair of non-latex gloves. This is to ensure that hygiene and infection control measures are maintained.

❖ Close the door or draw the curtains to maintain privacy and dignity.

❖ Record the patient's pulse rate before and during the procedure.

❖ Record the patients' blood pressure before and during the procedure.

❖ Encourage the patient to empty their bladder first. A full bladder can create discomfort during the procedure.

❖ Place the waterproof pad underneath the patient.

❖ Remove the patient's clothing from the waist down if they are unable to do this themselves.

❖ The patient should lie on their left side, knees flexed, with the upper knee higher than the lower knee and buttocks near the edge of the bed. This supports the easy passage of the finger into the rectum. Note that patients with musculoskeletal conditions may not be able to lie in this position. Ensure you have adequate lighting and that the patient is not at risk of falling from the bed.

❖ Observe the anal area for evidence of skin soreness, swelling, excoriation, hemorrhoids, anal skin tags, infestation, foreign bodies or a rectal prolapse. Swelling may be indicative of a mass or abscess. Report any abnormalities such as bleeding, discharge or prolapse and do not continue the procedure but seek additional advice.

❖ If the patient has a spinal injury, observe for signs of autonomic dysreflexia throughout the procedure

❖ Put on an additional pair of gloves.

❖ Place lubricating gel on a gloved finger.

❖ Inform the patient that the procedure is about to begin.

❖ Proceed with caution. Gently insert the lubricated finger into the anus and slowly advance into the rectum.

❖ For digital rectal stimulation insert the lubricated gloved finger into the anus and slowly rotate the finger in circular movements. Contact should be maintained with the rectal mucosa. Gently stretch the anal canal, this helps the sphincter to relax and the rectum contract.

❖ Check the stool type. If it is type 1 on the Bristol Stool Form Scale, remove one lump at a time until no more fecal matter can be felt. This will relieve patient discomfort. If the stool is soft gently circle the finger continuously to remove feces.

❖ If the matter is solid, use the index finger to split it and remove individual pieces at a time, taking care not to cause rectal trauma. Avoid using a hooked finger to remove feces, this may cause damage to the rectal mucosa and anal sphincter. Using a hooked finger can cause scratching or scoring of the mucosa.

❖ During the procedure carry out abdominal massage.

❖ If the fecal matter is more than 4 cm across and is too hard and solid to break up, discontinue the procedure to avoid any pain or damage to the anal sphincter and discuss other approaches with the multidisciplinary team. It may be necessary for the procedure to be carried out under anesthetic.

❖ Place the feces in an appropriate receiver for disposal as it is removed to reduce the likelihood of contamination and cross-infection.

❖ Allow the patient to rest if needed. If appropriate, ask the patient to breathe in and force air out of the mouth with the nose closed. This is the Valsalva maneuver and can assist with the passage of feces into the rectum.

❖ Observe the patient throughout for any signs of distress and stop if the patient complains of pain or asks you to stop. If there are any signs of autonomic dysreflexia discontinue immediately. It may be necessary to refer spinal injury patients to the local spinal unit.

❖ Once the rectum is empty, carry out a final digital check after 5 minutes to ensure evacuation is complete.

❖ Remove top layer of gloves. Wash and dry the buttocks and anal area.

❖ Remove gloves and apron and dispose of appropriately in clinical waste. Wash hands.

❖ Assist the patient to a comfortable position.

❖ For spinal injury patients, record blood pressure.

❖ Document color, consistency and amount using the Bristol scale.

❖ Document any abnormalities and report any findings to the multidisciplinary team if necessary.

Diagnostic Testing

UNIT

6

UNIT OUTLINE

- Complete blood count
- Serum electrolytes
- LFT
- Lipid/lipoprotein profile
- Serum glucose—AC, PC, HbA1c of monitoring capillary blood glucose (glucometer random blood sugar—GRBS)
- Stool routine examination
- Urine testing—albumin, acetone, pH, specific gravity of urine culture, routine, timed urine specimen
- Sputum culture
- Radiologic and endoscopic procedures

LEARNING OBJECTIVES

At the end of this unit, the reader will be able to:

- Define laboratory testing.
- Categories phases of laboratory testing.
- Interpret complete blood count.
- Enumerate purposes of CBC.
- Define serum electrolyte critical findings.
- Perform liver function test.
- Interpret lipid profile.
- Analyze blood glucose test.
- Perform glucose tolerance test.
- Define stool routine examination.
- Categories types of stool tests.
- Define urine testing.
- Analyze urine culture, routine urine test.
- Practice sputum culture.
- Define radiodiagnosis.
- Explain endoscopic procedures.

Diagnostic testing may occur in successive rounds of information gathering, integration, and interpretation, as each round of information refines the working diagnosis. In many cases, diagnostic testing can identify a condition before it is clinically apparent; for example, coronary artery disease can be identified by an imaging study indicating the presence of coronary artery blockage even in the absence of symptoms.

Getting the right diagnosis is a key aspect of healthcare—it provides an explanation of a patient's health problem and informs subsequent healthcare decisions. The diagnostic process is a complex, collaborative activity that involves clinical reasoning and information gathering to determine a patient's health problem. According to improving diagnosis in healthcare, diagnostic errors-inaccurate or delayed diagnoses-persist throughout all settings of care and continue to harm an unacceptable number of patients. It is likely that most people will experience at least one diagnostic error in their lifetime, sometimes with devastating consequences. Diagnostic errors may cause harm to patients by preventing or delaying appropriate treatment, providing unnecessary or harmful treatment, or resulting in psychological or financial repercussions. The committee concluded that improving the diagnostic process is not only possible, but also represents a moral, professional, and public health imperative.

Three Phases of Laboratory Testing

1. **Pre-analytical phase:** Selecting the appropriate test, obtaining the specimen, labeling it with the patient's name, providing timely transport to the laboratory, registering receipt in the laboratory, and processing before testing.
2. **Analytical phase:** Performing the test and interpreting the result.
3. **Post-analytical phase:** Preparing a report detailing the result and its interpretation, authorizing the report, and transmitting the report to the clinician so that the clinician can institute appropriate action.

COMPLETE BLOOD COUNT (CBC)

A CBC test is a medical blood test. It counts blood cells or blood components that include:
1. Red blood cells (RBC)
2. White blood cells (WBC)
3. Platelets
4. Total leukocyte count (TLC)
5. Differential leukocyte count (DLC)

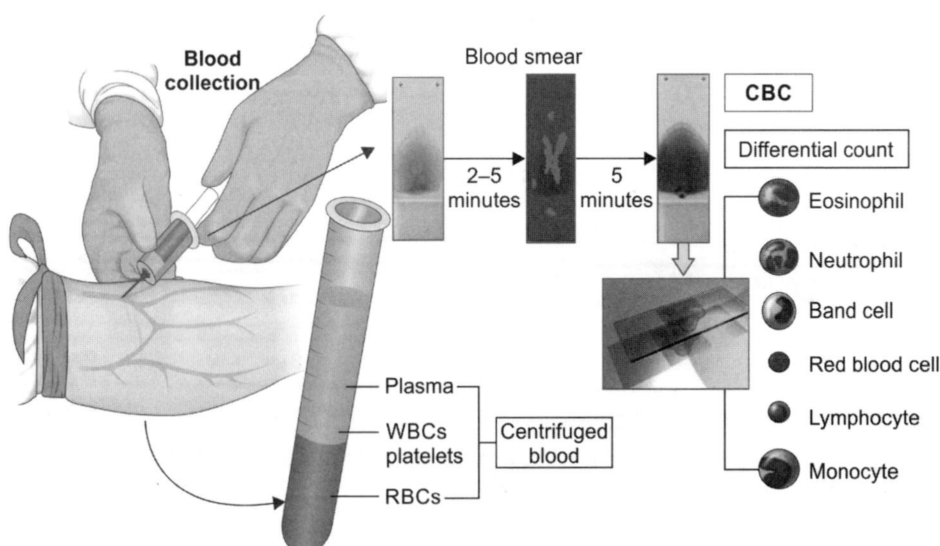

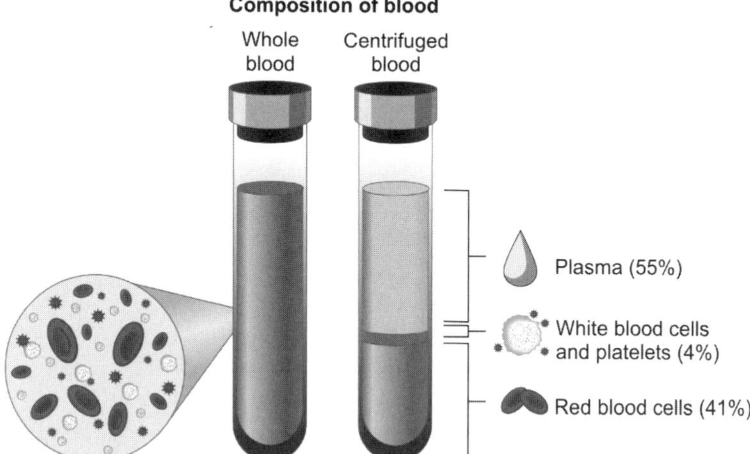

A CBC is a series of tests used to evaluate the composition and concentration of the cellular components of blood.

It measures the following:
1. The number of red blood cells (RBCs)
2. The number of white blood cells (WBCs)
3. The total amount of hemoglobin in the blood
4. The fraction of the blood composed of red blood cells (hematocrit)
5. The mean corpuscular volume (MCV)—the size of the red blood cells
6. CBC also includes information about the red blood cells that is calculated from the other measurements.
7. MCH (mean corpuscular hemoglobin)
8. MCHC (mean corpuscular hemoglobin concentration)
9. The platelet count is also usually included in the CBC.

Purpose of CBC Test

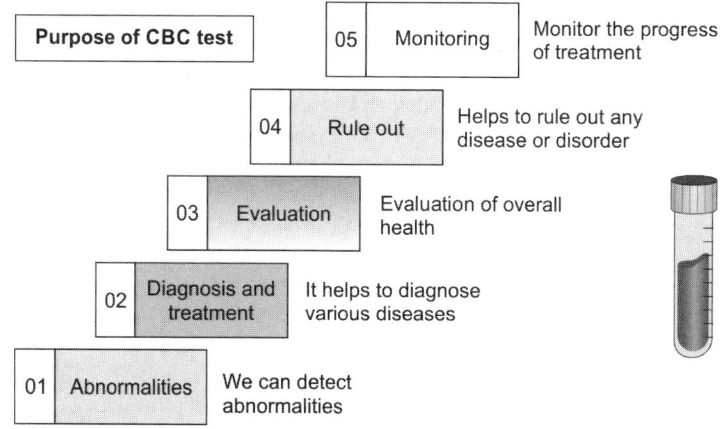

Counts of different components of blood indicate our overall wellness. In particular, a complete blood count test detects anemia, infections, inflammation and cancer. The test helps the healthcare provider to evaluate all the aspects of blood for better diagnosis and treatment. The CBC provides valuable information about the blood and to some extent the bone marrow, which is the blood-forming tissue. The CBC is used for the following purposes:

- ❖ Abnormalities in the blood
- ❖ Evaluation of overall health
- ❖ Rule out any disease or disorder
- ❖ Monitoring the treatment
- ❖ Diagnosis and treatment of various diseases
- ❖ As a preoperative test to ensure both adequate oxygen carrying capacity and hemostasis.
- ❖ To identify persons who may have an infection
- ❖ To diagnose anemia—those who suffer from anemia might take medication similar to methylfolate 15 mg to help with creating healthy red blood cells
- ❖ To identify acute and chronic illness, bleeding tendencies, and white blood cell disorders such as leukemia.
- ❖ To monitor treatment for anemia and other blood diseases detected in human plasma and blood cells.
- ❖ To determine the effects of chemotherapy and radiation therapy on blood cell production.

Procedure to Take CBC Sample

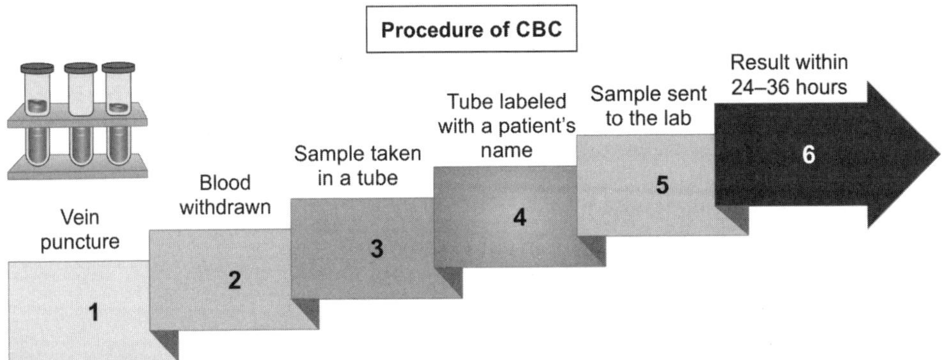

Blood is drawn from a vein, usually from the inside of the elbow or the back of the hand. The puncture site is cleaned with antiseptic. An elastic band is placed around the upper arm to apply pressure and cause the vein to swell with blood.

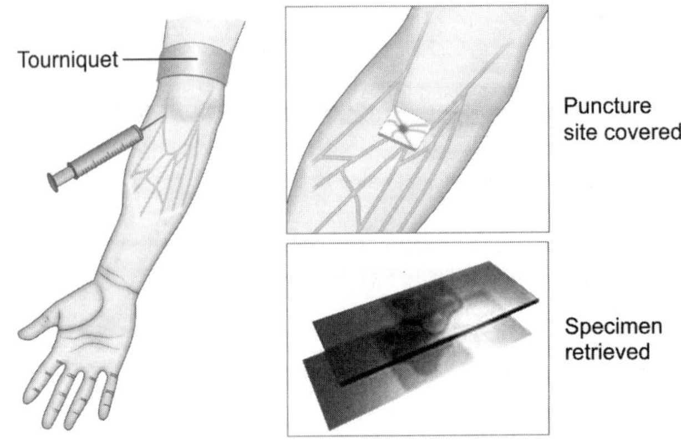

A needle is inserted into the vein, and the blood is collected in an air-tight vial or a syringe. During the procedure, the band is removed to restore circulation. Once the blood has been collected, the needle is removed, and the puncture site is covered to stop any bleeding.

In infants or client, the area is cleansed with antiseptic and punctured with a sharp needle or a lancet. The blood may be collected in a pipette (small glass tube), on a slide, onto a test strip, or into a small container. A bandage may be applied to the puncture site if there is any bleeding.

Tests

- ❖ **White blood cell count (WBC):** Presence of infection
- ❖ **Differential white blood cell count:** Specific patterns of WBC
- ❖ **Red blood cell count (RBC):** Carries oxygen and carbon dioxide from lungs to tissue and vice versa
- ❖ **Hematocrit (Hct):** Measures RBC mass
- ❖ **Hemoglobin (Hgb):** Main component of RBC
- ❖ **Red blood cell indices:** Calculated values of size and Hgb content of RBCs, important in anemia evaluation
- ❖ **Platelet count:** Necessary for clotting and control of bleeding
- ❖ **Red blood cell distribution width (RDW):** Indicates degree variability and abnormal cell size
- ❖ **Mean platelet volume (MPV):** Index of platelet production

Normal Values

Test	Normal Values
Leukocyte (white blood cell)	X1000 cells/mm^3 (µL)
Birth	9.0–30.0
24 hours	9.4–34.0
1 month	5.0–19.5
1–3 years	6.0–17.5
4–7 years	5.5–15.5
8–13 years	4.5–13.5
Adult	4.5–11.0
Neutrophils bands	3–5% (total WBC count)
Segs	54–62%
Lymphocytes	25–33%
Monocytes	3–7%
Eosinophils	1–3%
Basophils	0–0.75%
Erythrocytes (red blood cells)	
Cord	3.9–5.5 million/mm^3
1–3 days	4.0–6.6 million/mm^3
1 week	3.9–6.3 million/mm^3

Contd...

Contd...

Test	Normal Values
2 weeks	3.6–6.2 million/mm^3
1 month	3.0–5.4 million/mm^3
2 months	2.7–4.9 million/mm^3
3–6 months	3.1–4.5 million/mm^3
0.5–2 years	3.7–5.3 million/mm^3
2–6 years	3.9–5.3 million/mm^3
6–12 years	4.0–5.2 million/mm^3
12–18 years (male)	4.5–5.3 million/mm^3
12–18 years (female)	4.1–5.1 million/mm^3
Hemoglobin	
1–3 days	14.5–22.5 g/dL
2 months	9.0–14.0 g/dL
6–12 years	11.5–15.5 g/dL
12–18 years (male)	13.0–16.0 g/dL
12–18 (female)	12.0–16.0g/dL
Hematocrit	
1 day	48–69%
2 days	48–75%
3 days	44–72%
2 months	28–42%
6–12 years	35–45%
12–18 years (male)	37–49%
12–18 years (female)	36–46%
Mean corpuscular volume (MCV)	
1–3 days	95–121 µm^3
0.5–2 years	70–86 µm^3
6–12 years	77–95 µm^3
12–18 years (male)	78–98 µm^3
12–18 years (female)	78–102 µm^3
Mean corpuscular hemoglobin (MCH)	
Birth	31–37 pg/cell
1–3 days	31–37 pg/cell
1 week–1 month	28–40 pg/cell
2 months	26–34 pg/cell
3–6 months	25–35 pg/cell
0.5–2 years	23–31 pg/cell

Contd...

Contd...

Test	Normal Values
2–6 years	24–30 pg/cell
6–12 years	25–33 pg/cell
12–18 years	25–35 pg/cell
Mean corpuscular hemoglobin concentration (MCHC)	
Birth	30–36 g Hg/dL RBC
1–3 days	29–37 g Hg/dL RBC
1–2 weeks	28–38 g Hg/dL RBC
1–2 months	29–37 g Hg/dL RBC
3 months–2 years	30–36 g Hg/dL RBC
2–18 years	31–37 g Hg/dL RBC
Reticulocyte count	
Infants	2–5% of RBCs
Children	0.5–4% of RBCs
12–18 years (male)	0.5–1% of RBCs
12–18 years (female)	0.5–2.5% of RBCs
Platelet count	
Birth–1 week	84,000–478,000/mm^3
Thereafter	150,000–400,000/mm^3
Erythrocyte sedimentation rate (ESR)	
Test	Normal value
Westergren	
Child	0–10 mm/hour
Adult (male)	0–15 mm/hour
Adult (female)	0–20 mm/hour
Wintrobe	
Child	0–13 mm/hour
Adult (male)	0–9 mm/hour
Adult (female)	0–20 mm/hour

What Abnormal Results Mean

a. High numbers of RBCs may indicate:
- Low oxygen tension in the blood
- Congenital heart disease
- Cor pulmonale
- Pulmonary fibrosis
- Polycythemia vera
- Dehydration (such as from severe diarrhea)
- Renal (kidney) disease with high erythropoietin production

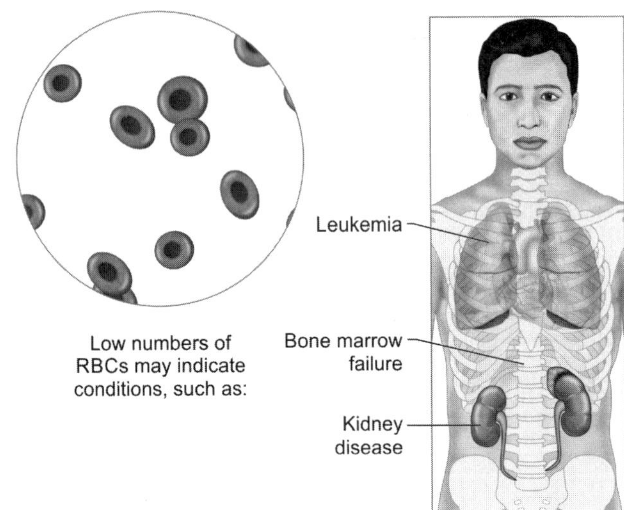

b. Low numbers of RBCs may indicate:

- Blood loss
- Anemia (various types)
- Hemorrhage
- Bone marrow failure (for example, from radiation, toxin, fibrosis, tumor)
- Erythropoietin deficiency (secondary to renal disease)
- Hemolysis (RBC destruction)
- Leukemia
- Multiple myeloma
- Malnutrition (nutritional deficiencies of iron, folate, vitamin B12, or vitamin B6)

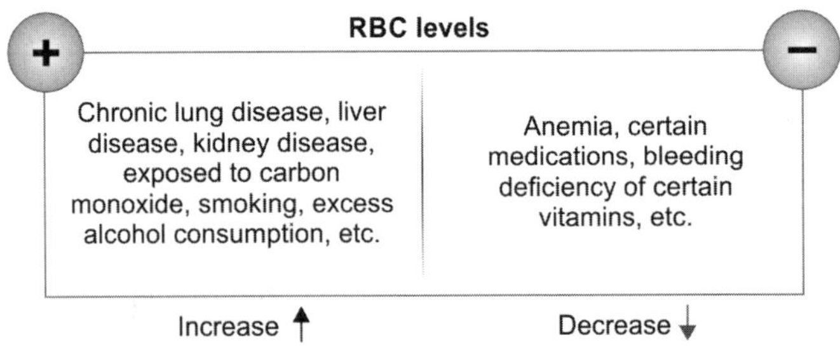

c. Low numbers of WBCs (leukopenia) may indicate:

- Bone marrow failure (for example, due to infection, tumor or fibrosis)
- Presence of cytotoxic substance
- Autoimmune/collagen-vascular diseases (such as lupus erythematosus)
- Disease of the liver or spleen
- Radiation exposure
- High numbers of WBCs (leukocytosis) may indicate:
  ◊ Infectious diseases
  ◊ Inflammatory disease (such as rheumatoid arthritis or allergy)

◊ Leukemia
◊ Severe emotional or physical stress
◊ Tissue damage (such as burns)

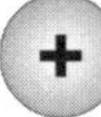

d. Low hematocrit may indicate:
- Anemia (various types)
- Blood loss (hemorrhage)
- Bone marrow failure (for example, due to radiation, toxin, fibrosis, tumor)
- Hemolysis (RBC destruction) related to transfusion reaction
- Leukemia
- Malnutrition or specific nutritional deficiency
- Multiple myeloma
- Rheumatoid arthritis
- High hematocrit may indicate:
  ◊ Dehydration
  ◊ Burns
  ◊ Diarrhea
  ◊ Polycythemia vera
  ◊ Low oxygen tension (smoking, congenital heart disease, living at high altitudes)
- Low hemoglobin values may indicate:
  ◊ Anemia (various types)
  ◊ Blood loss

The test may be performed under many different conditions and in the assessment of many different diseases.

Nursing Considerations

1. Explain test procedure. Explain that slight discomfort may be felt when the skin is punctured.
2. Encourage to avoid stress if possible because altered physiologic status influences and changes normal hematologic values.
3. Explain that fasting is not necessary. However, fatty meals may alter some test results as a result of lipidemia.
4. Apply manual pressure and dressings over puncture site on removal of dinner.
5. Monitor the puncture site for oozing or hematoma formation.
6. Instruct to resume normal activities and diet.

SERUM ELECTROLYTES

Electrolytes are essential for basic life functioning, such as maintaining electrical neutrality in cells and generating and conducting action potentials in the nerves and muscles.

Significant electrolytes include sodium, potassium, chloride, magnesium, calcium, phosphate, and bicarbonates. Electrolytes come from our food and fluids.

These electrolytes can be imbalanced, leading to high or low levels. High or low levels of electrolytes disrupt normal bodily functions and can lead to life-threatening complications.

An electrolyte panel is a blood test to measure electrolytes (minerals) in blood. An electrolyte imbalance may be a sign of a heart, lung or kidney problem. Dehydration also causes electrolyte imbalances. Client provider may order an anion gap test along with the electrolyte panel to determine why certain electrolyte levels are too high or low.

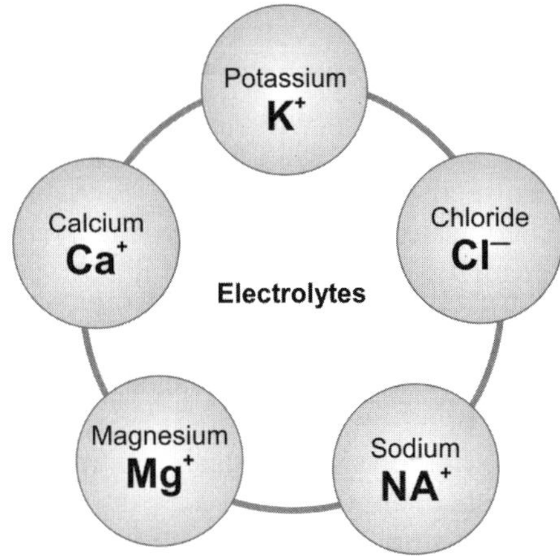

Electrolytes are electrically charged minerals that help control the amount of fluids and the balance of acids and bases in client's body. They also help control muscle and nerve activity, heart rhythm, and other important functions. An electrolyte panel, also known as a serum electrolyte test, is a blood test that measures levels of the body's main electrolytes:

- ❖ Sodium, which helps control the amount of fluid in the body. It also helps client's nerves and muscles work properly.
- ❖ Chloride, which also helps control the amount of fluid in the body. In addition, it helps maintain healthy blood volume and blood pressure.
- ❖ Potassium, which helps client's heart and muscles work properly.
- ❖ Bicarbonate, which helps maintain the body's acid and base balance. It also plays an important role in moving carbon dioxide through the bloodstream.

Sodium

Sodium, an osmotically active cation, is one of the essential electrolytes in the extracellular fluid. It is responsible for maintaining the extracellular fluid volume and regulating the membrane potential of cells. Sodium is exchanged along with potassium across cell membranes as part of active transport.

Sodium regulation occurs in the kidneys. The proximal tubule is where the majority of sodium reabsorption takes place. In the distal convoluted tubule, sodium undergoes reabsorption. Sodium transport occurs via sodium-chloride symporters, controlled by the hormone aldosterone.

Among the electrolyte disorders, hyponatremia is the most frequent. Hyponatremia is diagnosed when the serum sodium level is <135 mmol/L. Hyponatremia has neurological manifestations. Patients may present with headaches, confusion, nausea, and delirium. Hypernatremia occurs when serum sodium levels are >145 mmol/L. Symptoms of hypernatremia include tachypnea, sleeping difficulty, and restlessness. Rapid sodium corrections can have severe consequences, such as cerebral edema and osmotic demyelination syndrome (ODS). Other factors, such as chronic alcohol misuse disorder and malnutrition also play a role in the development of ODS.

Potassium

Potassium is mainly an intracellular ion. The sodium-potassium adenosine triphosphatase pump is primarily responsible for regulating the homeostasis between sodium and potassium, which pumps out sodium in exchange for potassium, which moves into the cells. In the kidneys, the filtration of potassium takes place at the glomerulus. Potassium reabsorption occurs at the proximal convoluted tubule and thick ascending loop of Henle. Potassium secretion occurs at the distal convoluted tubule. Aldosterone increases potassium secretion. Potassium channels and potassium-chloride co-transporters at the apical tubular membrane also secrete potassium.

Potassium derangements may result in cardiac arrhythmias. Hypokalemia occurs when serum potassium levels are under 3.6 mmol/L. The features of hypokalemia include weakness, fatigue, and muscle twitching. Hypokalemia paralysis is generalized body weakness that can be either familial or sporadic. Hypokalemia occurs when the serum potassium levels are above 5.5 mmol/L, which can result in arrhythmias. Muscle cramps, muscle weakness, rhabdomyolysis, and myoglobinuria may be presenting signs and symptoms of hyperkalemia.

Calcium

Calcium has a significant physiological role in the body. It is involved in skeletal mineralization, contraction of muscles, and the transmission of nerve impulses, blood clotting, and secretion of hormones. The diet is the predominant source of calcium. Calcium is a predominately extracellular cation. Calcium absorption in the intestine is primarily controlled by the hormonally active form of vitamin D, which is 1,25-dihydroxy vitamin D3. Parathyroid hormone also regulates calcium secretion in the distal tubule of the kidneys. Calcitonin acts on bone cells to increase the calcium levels in the blood.

Hypocalcemia diagnosis requires checking the serum albumin level to correct for total calcium. Hypocalcemia is diagnosed when the corrected serum total calcium levels are less than 8.8 mg/dL, as in vitamin D deficiency or hypoparathyroidism. Checking serum calcium levels is a recommended test in post-thyroidectomy patients. Hypercalcemia is when corrected serum total calcium levels exceed 10.7 mg/dL, as seen with primary hyperparathyroidism. Humoral hypercalcemia presents in malignancy, primarily due to PTHrP secretion.

Bicarbonate

The acid-base status of the blood drives bicarbonate levels. The kidneys predominantly regulate bicarbonate concentration and maintain the acid-base balance. Kidneys reabsorb the filtered bicarbonate and generate new bicarbonate by net acid excretion, which occurs by the excretion of titrable acid and ammonia. Diarrhea usually results in bicarbonate loss, causing an imbalance in acid-base regulation. Many kidney-related disorders can result in imbalanced bicarbonate metabolism leading to excess bicarbonate in the body.

Magnesium

Magnesium is an intracellular cation. Magnesium is mainly involved in adenosine triphosphate (ATP) metabolism, proper functioning of muscles, neurological functioning, and neurotransmitter release. When muscles contract, calcium re-uptake by the calcium-activated ATPase of the sarcoplasmic reticulum is brought about by magnesium. Hypomagnesemia occurs when the serum magnesium levels are <1.46 mg/dL. Alcohol use disorder, gastrointestinal conditions, and excessive renal losses may result in hypomagnesemia. It commonly presents with ventricular arrhythmias, which include torsades de pointes. Hypomagnesemia may also result from the use of certain medications, such as omeprazole.

Chloride

Chloride is an anion found predominantly in the extracellular fluid. The kidneys predominantly regulate serum chloride levels. Most chloride, filtered by the glomerulus, is reabsorbed by both proximal and distal tubules (majorly by proximal tubule) by both active and passive transport.

Hyperchloremia can occur due to gastrointestinal bicarbonate loss. Hypochloremia presents in gastrointestinal losses, such as vomiting or excess water gain, such as congestive heart failure.

Phosphorus

Phosphorus is an extracellular fluid cation. Eighty-five percent of the total body phosphorus is in the bones and teeth in the form of hydroxyapatite; the soft tissues contain the remaining 15%. Phosphate plays a crucial role in metabolic pathways. It is a component of many metabolic intermediates and, most importantly, of ATP and nucleotides. Vitamin D3, PTH, and calcitonin regulate phosphate simultaneously with calcium. The kidneys are the primary avenue of phosphorus excretion.

Phosphate imbalance is most commonly due to one of three processes—impaired dietary intake, gastrointestinal disorders, and deranged renal excretion.

Electrolytes play a critical role in:
- Balancing fluids in client's body.
- Controlling client's heart rate and rhythm.
- Promoting bone and dental health.
- Supporting nerve and muscle function.
- Stabilizing blood pressure.
- Transport nutrients into cells.
- Send the waste products out.
- Keep normal water levels and pH levels in client's body.
- Balance the acidity and alkalinity of client's blood.

Indications

Indications to order serum electrolyte panels are numerous. Some indications are:
- Routine blood investigations
- Routine monitoring of hospitalized patients on medications, receiving fluid therapy, undergoing dietary changes, or being treated for ongoing illnesses.
- Any illness that can cause electrolyte derangements, such as malnutrition, gastrointestinal disorders, cardiac disorders, kidney dysfunction, endocrine disorders, circulatory disorders, lung disorders, and acid-base imbalance.
- Arrhythmias
- Use of diuretics or any medications that can interfere with fluid and electrolyte homeostasis

❖ Burns
❖ Cancer
❖ Dehydration due to not drinking enough liquids or from excessive vomiting, diarrhea, sweating (hyperhidrosis) or fever.
❖ Diabetes
❖ Cardiovascular disease, heart failure or high blood pressure
❖ Liver disease, such as cirrhosis.

Normal and Critical Findings

Laboratory Values

a. Serum sodium
  - *Normal range:* 135 to 145 mmol/L
  - *Mild to moderate hyponatremia:* 125 to 135 mmol/L
  - *Severe hyponatremia:* <125 mmol/L
  - *Mild to moderate hypernatremia:* 145 to 160 mmol/L
  - *Severe hypernatremia:* >160 mmol/L

b. Serum potassium
  - *Normal range:* 3.6 to 5.5 mmol/L
  - *Mild hypokalemia:* <3.6 mmol/L
  - *Moderate hypokalemia:* <2.5 mmol/L
  - *Severe hypokalemia:* <2.5 mmol/L
  - *Mild hyperkalemia:* 5 to 5.5 mmol/L
  - *Moderate hyperkalemia:* 5.5 to 6.5 mmol/L
  - *Severe hyperkalemia:* 6.5 to 7 mmol/L

c. Serum calcium
  - *Normal range:* 8.8 to 10.7 mg/dL
  - *Hypocalcemia:* <8.8 mg/dL
  - *Mild to moderate hypercalcemia:* >10.7 to 11.5 mg/dL
  - *Severe hypercalcemia:* >11.5 mg/dL

d. Serum magnesium
  - *Normal range:* 1.46 to 2.68 mg/dL
  - *Hypomagnesemia:* <1.46 mg/dL
  - *Hypermagnesemia:* >2.68 mg/dL

e. Bicarbonate
  - *Normal range:* 23 to 30 mmol/L
  - It increases or decreases depending on the acid-base status.

f. Phosphorus
  - *Normal range:* 3.4 to 4.5 mg/dL
  - *Hypophosphatemia:* <2.5 mg/dL
  - *Hyperphosphatemia:* >4.5 mg/dL

Procedure

The procedure is similar to regular blood tests. The skin is cleaned by swabbing with 70% isopropyl alcohol to prevent any contamination. The lab technician then usually wraps an elastic band around (tourniquet) client's arm close to the venipuncture site to allow client's veins to fill with blood. A needle is then used to draw the required number of samples of blood from the vein. After the drawing of the blood, the venipuncture site is covered with a Band-Aid. The blood sample is then submitted to a laboratory where the serum is tested, the test results are usually available within 24 hours.

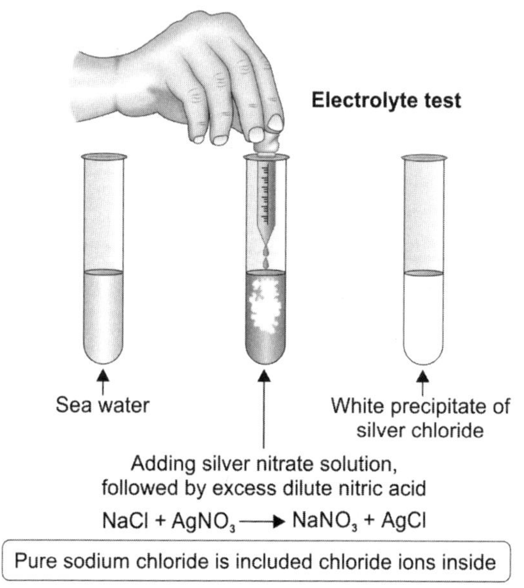

Requirements

Specimen: Serum (preferred) or plasma

Volume: 2 mL

Container: Gel-barrier tube (send entire tube) preferred. Red-top tube or green-top (heparin) tube is acceptable if centrifuged within 45 minutes and the serum or plasma is removed and placed in a tightly-stoppered secondary tube.

LIVER FUNCTION TEST (LFT)

Liver

The liver is the largest internal organ. It sits in the tummy (abdomen), under diaphragm on the right-hand side. It is usually tucked under the ribs, which protect it, although in some people the edge of the liver protrudes slightly. If the liver is swollen, through inflammation or disease, it can swell out from under the ribs and make client's tummy swollen.

Liver Function

The liver is a factory for the production and breakdown of carbohydrates, fats, proteins, hormones and other essential body chemicals, and helps dispose of waste products. This work is mainly carried out by liver cells (hepatocytes). Some of the most important functions include:

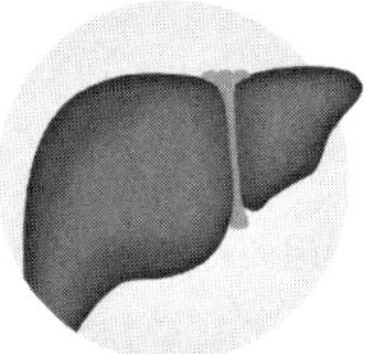

To check for damage
from liver infections or
diseases

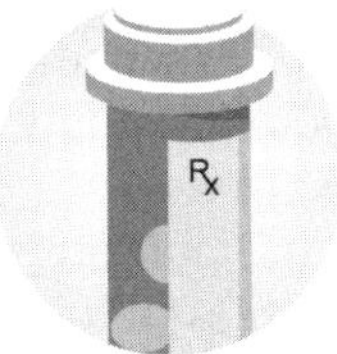

To monitor side effects
of medications

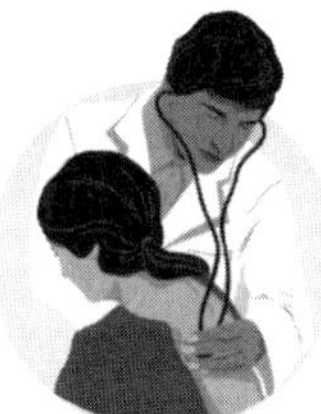

To assess treatment
for a disease

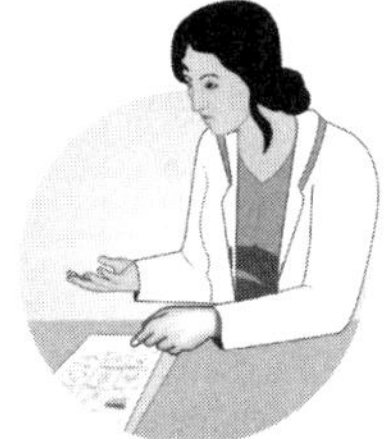

To diagnose symptoms
of a liver disorder

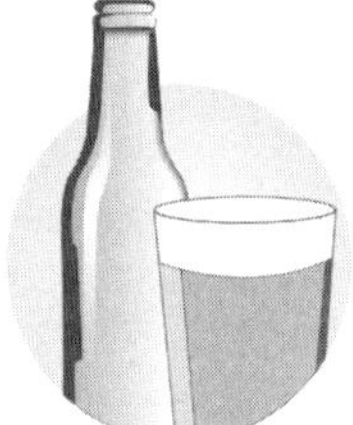

To check for liver damage
from heavy alcohol use

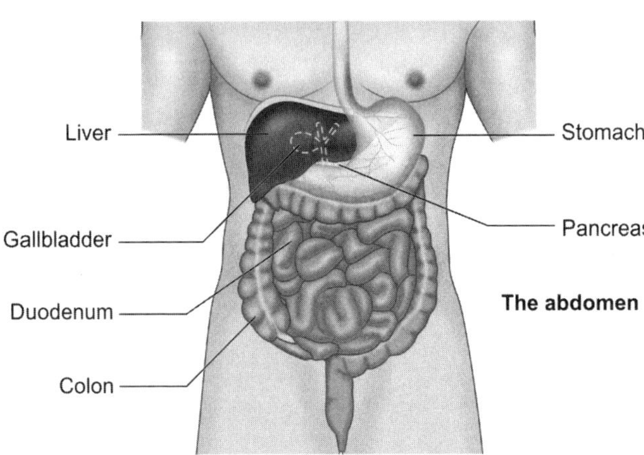

Production of these Substances

* ❖ Glycogen (a carbohydrate energy store), which it makes from glucose.
* ❖ Glucose, made and released into the blood from glycogen, proteins and fats.

- Many essential proteins and amino acids (building blocks of proteins).
- Many of the clotting factors that help client's blood to clot normally.
- Plays a part in red blood cell production.
- Albumin, one of the main proteins in client's blood, which bulks out client's serum and enables it to carry essential substances around the body.
- Angiotensinogen, which plays a role in blood pressure control.
- Thrombopoietin, which regulates some of the work of client's bone marrow.
- Cholesterol, triglycerides, lipoproteins and fats—as part of the management of fat stores in client's body.
- Bile, excreted into the intestine for absorbing fats and vitamin K.
- Hormones that help children grow and that build muscle in adults.
- Breakdown of these substances
- Excess hormones, including insulin.
- Bilirubin, which is a waste product from worn-out blood cells.
- Many waste products.
- A wide range of toxic substances and medicines, including alcohol.
- Foreign proteins that reach it from the digestive system (trapped and destroyed by specialized immune cells in the liver).

Storage of these (and other) Substances

- Glucose (as glycogen).
- Vitamin A (1–2 years' supply).
- Vitamin D (1–4 months' supply).
- Vitamin B12 (3–5 years' supply).
- Vitamin K.
- Iron and copper.

Liver function tests measure a series of chemicals which relate to the way the liver works. They include substances that are made in the liver or affected by the health of the liver cells, chemicals which are processed or excreted by the liver, and hormones that the liver makes in order to do its work.

Purpose

Liver function tests are aimed at giving a picture of the 'state' of liver. They are a sensitive way of looking for liver strain or liver damage, as they often show this well before client get any symptoms or problems with liver. This means that the cause of liver strain or damage can be diagnosed and, often, reversed.

Liver function tests are also used for monitoring in cases of known liver inflammation, injury or disease.

The usual liver function tests typically include the following:
- Bilirubin.
- Albumin.
- Total protein.
- Transferases (AST or SGOT and ALT or SGPT).
- Gamma GT.
- Creatine kinase.

❖ Calcium and corrected calcium.

❖ Prothrombin time or International normalized ratio (INR).

Each of these is discussed below. The liver performs hundreds of different functions, so there are many other possible tests that look at its health. These would normally be done if an abnormality is found with the basic liver function tests described here, or if a specific problem is suspected. They might include:

❖ Virus tests, for example, hepatitis A, B or C—to look for the cause of disease.

❖ Autoantibody tests (to detect and monitor immune diseases).

❖ Immunoglobulins (antibodies made in response to various challenges including allergies, infections, some blood disorders and some cancers).

❖ Serum ferritin and transferrin saturation (measures of iron storage and management by client's body).

❖ Alpha-fetoprotein (maternal levels help look at the health of the baby during pregnancy, and levels are also raised in some cancers).

❖ Copper/caeruloplasmin (measures of copper management by the body).

❖ Alpha-1 antitrypsin (a hormone involved in protecting liver and lung cells from injury).

❖ Clotting factors (particularly if there is a suspicion that client's blood is not clotting well or client have severe liver disease).

Causes of Liver Function Tests to be Abnormal

Client's liver function tests can be abnormal because: There is a build up of fat in the liver, due to being overweight or obese (called non-alcoholic fatty liver disease, or NAFLD). However this does not always cause abnormal liver function tests, and can also be picked up on an ultrasound scan of the liver. If NAFLD is diagnosed, further blood tests including NAFLD score, and ELF (enhanced liver fibrosis) test, and a fibroscan (a special type of ultrasound to look for more advanced signs, such as fibrosis/cirrhosis) may be done to assess the severity of the condition.

❖ Liver is inflamed (for example, by infection, toxic substances like alcohol and some medicines, or by an immune condition).

❖ Liver cells have been damaged (for example, by toxic substances, such as alcohol, paracetamol, poisons).

❖ Liver is having to work harder to process medicines or toxic substances (for example, alcohol, paracetamol, poisons).

❖ The bile drainage from liver is blocked, for example, by a gallstone.

❖ There is a swelling inside liver (for example, an abscess or a tumour), have an underlying condition that affects the liver's production and storage abilities (for example, Wilson's disease, hemochromatosis, Gilbert's syndrome).

❖ Liver is physically injured (for example, trauma).

An Abnormal Bilirubin Level

Bilirubin comes from the breakdown of red blood cells in the body. The liver processes (conjugates) bilirubin so that it can be excreted via the kidneys. A high bilirubin level can make client appear jaundiced (with a yellow tinge to the skin and to the whites of the eyes).

The most likely cause of raised bilirubin depends on whether the rise is in bilirubin that the liver has already processed (conjugated bilirubin), in the bilirubin that the liver has not yet processed (unconjugated bilirubin), or in both.

A Rise in Both Types of Bilirubin

Conjugated bilirubin tends to rise if the flow of bile in the tiny tubes within the liver is blocked, and unconjugated bilirubin tends to rise if the liver calls cannot do their work (or there is too much work for them to do). If the liver is both damaged (not working properly) and swollen or scarred (blocking the drainage system) then both types of bilirubin will tend to rise.

An Isolated Rise in Unconjugated Bilirubin

Unconjugated bilirubin may increase because the liver cannot process the bilirubin, or because the body is making an excess of bilirubin by breaking down too many blood cells, and the liver is normal but cannot keep up.

In adults, the most common causes are breakdown of blood cells (hemolysis) and Gilbert's syndrome.

Hemolysis is a condition of the blood. Further tests will be needed to identify the cause and client may need to see a hematologist. Causes can include reactions to medicines, lifelong (congenital) blood cell abnormalities, such as hereditary spherocytosis and, in babies, breast milk jaundice, severe infection (sepsis) and hemolytic disease of the newborn.

An Isolated Rise in Conjugated Bilirubin

Increased conjugated bilirubin suggests that the liver is conjugating the bilirubin properly (the job of liver cells) but not excreting it properly via the bile ducts. Causes include:

Reactions to some medicines, including common ones, such as blood pressure tablets, hormones (for example, estrogen), antibiotics (particularly erythromycin and flucloxacillin), tricyclic antidepressants and anabolic steroids.

* Some autoimmune diseases that affect bile excretion.
* Blockage of the bile ducts, for example, by a gallstone.
* Dubin-Johnson syndrome and Rotor's syndrome.

In babies a rise in conjugated bilirubin can signify rare but serious problems with the development of the bile drainage system in the liver, such as biliary atresia.

An Abnormal Albumin Level

Albumin is the main protein in client's serum, and its level is a good guide to long-term liver health. Albumin levels that are abnormally low have the greatest significance for the liver.

Low Levels of Albumin

This can be due to:

* Severe liver disease.
* Poor nutrition.
* Malabsorption of protein (for example, in Crohn's disease or in coeliac disease).
* Bowel conditions which result in leakage of protein (for example, severe bowel inflammation or infection, such as cholera).
* Protein loss through kidney problems (for example, nephrotic syndrome).
* Failure of protein manufacture through severe liver inflammation.
* Albumin levels also fall if client lose protein through client's skin (for example, in extensive skin inflammation and widespread burns).
* Albumin levels decrease during pregnancy, when client's blood is more dilute.

High Levels of Albumin

This is usually due to having the tourniquet on for too long before client's blood sample is taken. Sometimes, it can be due to a very high-protein diet, as in bodybuilders, or to lack of fluid in the body (dehydration), when the blood is more concentrated.

An Abnormal Total Protein Level

Total protein measures the total of albumin and globulins. It is usually normal in liver disease even if albumin levels are low, as globulin levels tend to increase as albumin levels fall.

High values of total protein are seen in chronic active hepatitis and alcoholic hepatitis.

High values of total protein are also seen in conditions outside the liver which increase globulins (such as myeloma) and conditions involving overactivity of the immune system (such as severe infection and chronic inflammatory disease).

Low levels of total protein can sometimes be seen in severe liver disease, in conditions of severe protein loss (such as widespread burns) and in severe malnutrition.

Abnormal ALT (SGPT), AST (SGOT) or Creatine Kinase Level

These substances are also called transferases. They are liver hormones (proteins which help do the work of the liver) which are normally found inside liver cells rather than in the blood.

ALT stands for alanine transaminase and is also called SGPT (serum glutamic-pyruvic transaminase).

AST stands for aspartate transaminase and is also called SGOT (serum glutamic oxaloacetic transaminase).

Creatine kinase is sometimes checked along with AST and ALT.

If blood levels of transaminases go up this suggests leakage from damaged liver cells due to inflammation or cell death. AST and ALT tend to be high in liver disease and very high in liver inflammation.

ALT is mainly found in the liver. AST is also found in muscle and red blood cells.

ALT rises more than AST in acute liver damage, e.g., viral hepatitis.

In chronic liver disease (for example, alcoholic cirrhosis), AST is higher than ALT.

Lower-than-normal levels of transaminases do not signify disease.

Creatine kinase comes mainly from muscle, so if it is raised alongside AST and ALT it suggests that the liver may not be the main source of the problem. Creatine kinase can be very raised if client have a heart attack. However, a different blood test called troponin is now used if client have a suspected heart attack.

Causes of Mild Rises in Transferases

These include:

* ❖ Non-alcoholic fatty liver disease (the most common cause).
* ❖ Chronic hepatitis C infection.
* ❖ Coeliac disease.
* ❖ Hemochromatosis (a genetic condition that tends to come on in client's 40s or 50s).
* ❖ Autoimmune hepatitis.

Causes of Marked Increases in Transferases

Marked increases are usually caused by acute injury to the liver by viruses, shortage of oxygen (ischemia) or toxic substances. Causes include:

- Acute alcoholic hepatitis.
- Viral (hepatitis A, hepatitis B, hepatitis C, hepatitis D or hepatitis E). Hepatitis A and B tend to have the greatest increases.
- Autoimmune hepatitis.
- Chronic hepatitis and liver cirrhosis.
- Very high levels (>75 times upper reference limit) suggest ischemic or toxic (poison or medicine-related) injury to the liver.

Ischemic liver damage is mostly seen in patients with other serious illnesses, such as septicemia or collapse.

An Abnormal Gamma-Glutamyl Transferase Level

Gamma-glutamyl transferase (GGT) levels increase in most liver diseases. This liver function test is very sensitive, although it also goes up in some heart, lung and kidney conditions.

The most common reason for GGT increasing as a single abnormality is drinking more alcohol than liver can easily cope with. GGT levels can be 10 times normal. The rise is a sign client's liver is under strain and is at risk of being damaged by alcohol.

GGT rises to 2–3 times the upper limit of normal in non-alcoholic fatty liver disease (NAFLD). This condition is increasingly common and can progress to scarring or inflammation of the liver. Transaminase levels also tend to rise in NAFLD.

Some prescribed and over-the-counter medicines can increase GGT levels.

GGT rises in some patients with chronic hepatitis C infection.

In chronic liver disease, a rise in GGT suggests bile duct damage and scarring.

An Abnormal Alkaline Phosphatase Level

Alkaline phosphatase (ALP) comes mainly from the cells lining bile ducts and from bones—particularly growing bones. Therefore, it is commonly raised during childhood and puberty. It rises if there is slow or blocked flow in the bile ducts, if the bile ducts are damaged and in bone disorders. If the cause is in the liver, the GGT is also abnormal, whereas if it is the bone, the GGT is usually normal. ALP is also raised during the third trimester of pregnancy.

Common causes of raised ALP with other abnormalities on liver function tests include:

- Gallstones.
- Hepatitis of any cause.
- Cirrhosis.
- Bile duct blockage of any cause.
- Isolated raised ALP can occur in:
- Sarcoidosis.
- Bone fractures.
- Paget's disease of bone.
- Osteomalacia.
- Primary sclerosing cholangitis.

❖ Primary biliary cholangitis.
❖ Cancer in bones or in the liver.

Abnormal Calcium and Corrected Calcium Levels

About 99% of the body's calcium is stored in the bones, with the remaining 1% stored in other tissues, including the blood plasma. The calcium test measures the total calcium in the blood plasma. About half of this is tightly attached to the protein, albumin, which forms the bulk of the protein in client's plasma. The calcium level that really counts is the 'free', or unbound, calcium that floats unattached in the plasma.

If client have low albumin levels, the total calcium in client's blood will be lower. However, because the amount attached to the albumin is reduced (because there is less albumin), the actual free levels of calcium may be normal (or even raised). Corrected calcium corrects the figure to give the actual, free amount of calcium.

Causes of Low (Corrected) Calcium Levels

Calcium levels are regulated by the kidney, thyroid and parathyroid glands, using the hormones parathyroid hormone, calcitonin and vitamin D. Low levels are uncommon. Causes include:
❖ Hypoparathyroidism (client's parathyroid glands do not make enough of their hormone).
❖ Just after parathyroid surgery.
❖ Severe chronic kidney disease.
❖ Severe liver disease.
❖ Pancreatitis.
❖ Severe vitamin D deficiency.
❖ High phosphate ingestion (we can take in phosphate from enemas, from baby milks and from some flours, for example, chapati flour).
❖ Magnesium deficiency (often due to dietary deficiency and to prescribed medicines, including some antibiotics, diuretics and painkillers).

Causes of Raised (Corrected) Calcium Levels

❖ Primary hyperparathyroidism (overactive parathyroid glands) cause 8 out of 10 cases.
❖ Cancer of many different kinds can increase calcium levels, and accounts for about 2 out of 10 cases.
❖ Overconsumption of antacids.
❖ Sarcoidosis.
❖ Pulmonary tuberculosis.
❖ Addison's disease.
❖ Prolonged bed rest—especially in teenagers whose bones are growing fast.
❖ Vitamin A and/or D overdose.
❖ A number of medicines, including lithium, tamoxifen and diuretics.
❖ Kidney dialysis.

Abnormal Prothrombin Time and INR

Prothrombin time (PT) or international normalized ratio (INR) are sometimes measured as a part of standard liver function tests.

PT and INR are ways of measuring the ability of client's blood to clot. Conditions which impair this clotting (prolonging the PT and increasing the INR) include:

❖ Acute and severe liver disease (including liver failure and severe paracetamol overdose).

❖ Use of anticoagulant medicines (in this case, lengthening the prothrombin time and increasing the INR is the intention).

Measures for Healthy Liver Function

There is a difference between what client need to do to keep client's liver healthy most of the time and what client need to do if client's liver is inflamed or damaged.

The liver does not need a detox diet, which will not help it and will often (if it is very low-calorie, for instance) make it work harder. The liver is a digesting, storage and detoxing organ. If client are well, the way to look after client's liver is by:

❖ A balanced diet with a good fiber content.

❖ Regular exercise.

❖ Keeping client's weight within healthy limits.

❖ Avoiding 'fad' diets (which can challenge the kidneys and liver hard).

❖ Avoiding unnecessary medicines and supplements including paracetamol

❖ Stopping smoking.

❖ Saying within the recommended limits for alcohol (both daily and weekly).

If liver is inflamed and injured (for example, client have hepatitis and are jaundiced) or have advanced liver disease (for example, cirrhosis) then, depending on the severity, client may be advised to have a special diet. This involves using carbohydrates as major source of calories, eating fat moderately and cutting down on protein. Also may be advised to take vitamin supplements, and if client are retaining fluid client should reduce client's salt consumption to less than 1500 milligrams per day.

A few things to remember about abnormal liver function tests

Liver function tests are not a diagnosis; they are a set of clues which help doctors make a diagnosis.

Liver function tests are a sensitive early warning system for problems in the liver and, in some cases, elsewhere.

Because 'normal ranges' used by laboratories are the levels between which about 19 out of 20 of people's tests will fall, about 1 person in 20 will have an abnormal test without cause. About half of these people will have slightly high tests and about half will have slightly low tests, but their levels either way should not be extreme.

The most likely cause of any particular pattern of abnormal liver function tests varies between patients (because of difference in age and sex) and between populations (because of variations in genetics and because different things are more common in different parts of the world).

Almost any pattern of liver function test abnormality can be caused by medicines (including over-the-counter medications), by herbal remedies and traditional medicines from other cultures, and by poisonous substances.

Many liver conditions cause no symptoms, at least at first; so, if client have several abnormal tests (or one test is markedly abnormal), it is very important to follow this up.

Although single, mildly abnormal tests are not usually significant, any unexplained abnormality generally needs a check that client are well and may need a repeat test.

Abnormal liver function tests in a person who is also sick are more worrying than those in a person who is well.

On average, normal ranges are:
1. *Alanine transaminase (ALT):* 0 to 45 IU/L.
2. *Aspartate transaminase (AST):* 0 to 35 IU/L.
3. *Alkaline phosphatase (ALP):* 30 to 120 IU/L.
4. *Gamma-glutamyl transferase (GGT):* 0 to 30 IU/L.
5. *Bilirubin:* 2 to 17 micromoles/L.
6. *Prothrombin time (PT):* 10.9 to 12.5 seconds.
7. *Albumin:* 40 to 60 g/L.
8. *Total proteins:* 3 to 8.0 g/dL.

LIPID PROFILE

A lipid profile test is usually done to measure the lipids (cholesterol + triglycerides) in an individual's blood. Lipids include all the fatty substances that get circulated in the blood and stored in the tissues. Lipids are generally used by the body as a source of energy. Lipids can become abnormal due to various factors, such as age, use of certain medications, eating disorders, unhealthy lifestyle habits, etc. A lipid profile test helps to identify and detect any abnormality in lipids levels.

The lipid profile test is performed to determine the level of cholesterol in the blood. The different types of cholesterol (good and bad) and other fats in the body are together known as lipids. A lipid profile test measures the levels of lipids, which are crucial for bodily functions up to a certain level, above which, they can lead to several health conditions, such as blood clots, blockage in the arteries, heart problems, and much more. The lipid profile indicates the levels of high-density lipoprotein (HDL or good cholesterol), low-density lipoprotein (LDL or bad cholesterol), very low-density lipoprotein (VLDL), total cholesterol, etc.

A lipid profile, also known as a lipid test, cholesterol panel, coronary risk panel, or lipid panel, determines the levels of good and bad cholesterol as well as triglycerides in the blood. The lipid profile includes tests for measuring:
* Total cholesterol/HDL Ratio
* Triglyceride
* HDL cholesterol
* LDL cholesterol
* VLDL cholesterol
* Cholesterol
* Non-HDL cholesterol
* HDL/LDL

Procedure

Standard practice requires overnight fasting before a lipid profile test as the food ingested by a person can affect the levels of cholesterol molecules in the blood. So, fasting before the lipid profile test is a very common precaution people are asked to take before sample collection.

To take the blood sample, a tourniquet (elastic) band is placed tightly on the upper arm. The patient is asked to make a fist. This helps in the build up of blood filling the veins and it becomes easy to collect the blood. The skin is cleaned before inserting the needle in the vein in order to prevent bacteria from entering. The needle is then inserted into the vein in the arm and the blood sample is collected in the vacutainer.

Lipid Profile Normal Ranges

	Adult		Children: 1–12 years	
Total cholesterol	Desirable	<200 mg/dL	Acceptable	<170 mg/dL
	Borderline high	200–239 mg/dL	Border Line	170–199 mg/dL
	High	≥240 mg/dL	High	≥200 mg/dL
HDL	Low HDL	<40 mg/dL		
	High HDL	≥60 mg/dL		
LDL	Optimal	<100 mg/dL		
	Near optimal/above optimal	100–129 mg/dL		
	Borderline high	130–159 mg/dL		
	High	160–189 mg/dL		
	Very high	≥190 mg/dL		
Triglyceride	Normal	<150 mg/dL		
	Borderline high	150–199 mg/dL		
	High	200–499 mg/dL		
	Very high	≥500 mg/dL		
VLDL	Normal	<30 mg/dL		
Total cholesterol/ HDL ratio	Normal	0–4.9		

Causes of High Serum Lipids

High serum lipids refer to a high lipid profile (serum) or high levels of LDL and/or triglycerides in the blood. There are several lifestyle habits that can cause a high lipid profile (serum). These include:

❖ Smoking
❖ Excessive alcohol consumption
❖ Having a diet with too many saturated or trans fats
❖ Sedentary lifestyle
❖ Stress
❖ Genetics
❖ Obesity
❖ Certain conditions, such as hypothyroidism, diabetes, kidney disease or liver diseases, etc., and certain medications, such as steroids, blood pressure medicines, birth control pills, etc., can also lead to a spike in the lipid profile test results.

Findings of Report

A lipid test report provides an overview of the levels of various fat molecules and lipids in the blood. The report clearly lists the parameters that are being measured, against which the result as well as what the normal range should be are mentioned. In general, a lipid test report will display the following, along with their generally expected normal ranges:

1. **Total cholesterol:** This is the estimated total level of all types of cholesterol in the blood, which should generally be below 200 mg/dL. If the levels are higher than normal, the ratio of LDL and HDL must be taken into consideration to determine one's risk of developing cardiovascular issues.

2. **Triglycerides:** This is a form of fat that is generally associated with diabetes and heart diseases. Normal triglyceride levels should be less than 150 mg/dL, whereas 150–199 mg/dL is considered to be borderline; high up to 499 mg/dL; and very high if they are above 500 mg/dL.

3. **High-density lipoprotein (HDL):** The good cholesterol, HDL helps carry the bad cholesterol out of the bloodstream. Generally, HDL levels over 60 mg/dL are considered to be good and 'at risk' if they are below 40 mg/dL.

4. **Low-density lipoprotein (LDL):** The bad cholesterol, LDL increases the risk of heart diseases. Barring any mitigating health conditions, <100 mg/dL is the optimal level for LDL, which is also considered as near-optimal up to 129 mg/dL. On the other hand, 130–159 mg/dL is borderline high, with 160–189 mg/dL being considered as high.

A person's normal cholesterol levels or the levels they should aim to reach will vary depending on the medication they are taking (if any), their overall health, underlying health conditions, age, etc., so it is best to consult a doctor with the lipid test report for a proper diagnosis.

Deep-fried foods, sugary items, cakes and pastries, processed foods and food cooked using unhealthy oils can increase cholesterol levels.

6 ways to maintain healthy cholesterol levels

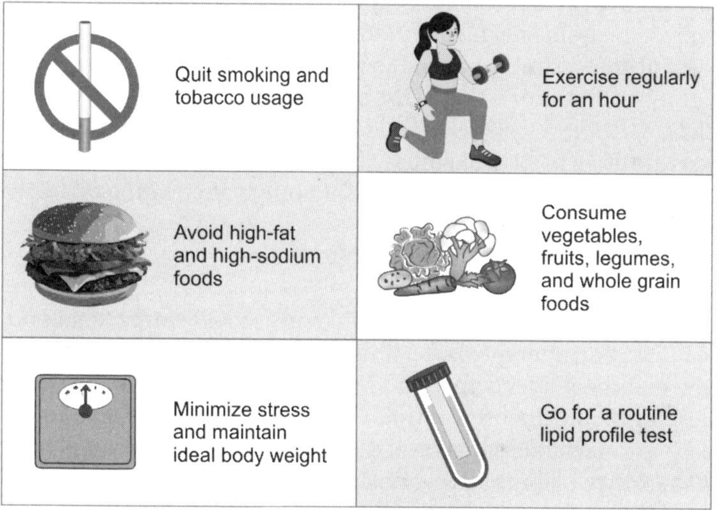

Lipid profile

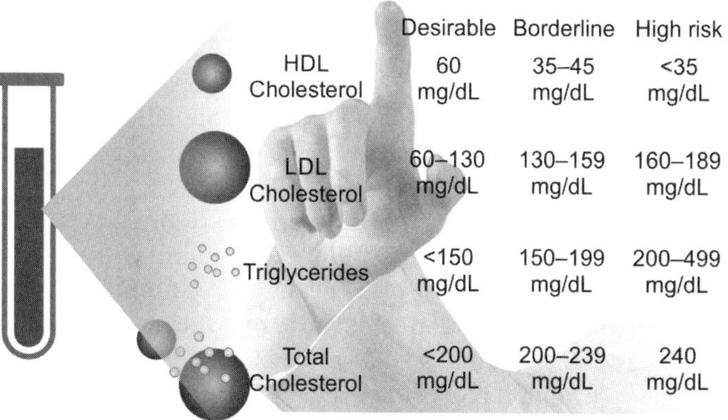

	Desirable	Borderline	High risk
HDL Cholesterol	60 mg/dL	35–45 mg/dL	<35 mg/dL
LDL Cholesterol	60–130 mg/dL	130–159 mg/dL	160–189 mg/dL
Triglycerides	<150 mg/dL	150–199 mg/dL	200–499 mg/dL
Total Cholesterol	<200 mg/dL	200–239 mg/dL	240 mg/dL

Blood Glucose Test

Many types of glucose tests exist and they can be used to estimate blood sugar levels at a given time or, over a longer period of time, to obtain average levels or to see how fast body is able to normalize changed glucose levels. Eating food for example leads to elevated blood sugar levels. In healthy people, these levels quickly return to normal via increased cellular glucose uptake which is primarily mediated by increase in blood insulin levels.

Glucose tests can reveal temporary/long-term hyperglycemia or hypoglycemia. These conditions may not have obvious symptoms and can damage organs in the long-term. Abnormally high/low levels, slow return to normal levels from either of these conditions and/ or inability to normalize blood sugar levels means that the person being tested probably has some kind of medical condition, such as type 2 diabetes which is caused by cellular insensitivity to insulin. Glucose tests are thus often used to diagnose such conditions.

Testing Methods

Tests that can be performed at home are used in blood glucose monitoring for illnesses that have already been diagnosed medically so that these illnesses can be maintained via medication and meal timing. Some of the home testing methods include:

1. Fingerprick type of glucose meter—need to prick self finger 8–12 times a day.
2. Continuous glucose monitor—the CGM monitors the glucose levels every 5 minutes approximately.
3. Laboratory tests are often used to diagnose illnesses and such methods include fasting blood sugar (FBS), fasting plasma glucose (FPG): 10–16 hours after eating
4. **Glucose tolerance test:** Continuous testing
5. **Postprandial glucose test (PC):** Two hours after eating
6. Random glucose test

AC (Ante Cibum) and PC (Post Cibum) meal markers provide more details on the test results of blood glucose before and after meals. Testing the blood glucose both before and after meals, allows to see how that meal affects the blood glucose levels and helps to understand which meals may be best for blood glucose control. During the day, levels tend to be at their lowest just before meals. A normal blood sugar level is <100 mg/dL after not eating (fasting) for at least 8 hours and <140 mg/dL two hours after eating. The most powerful influence on blood glucose levels comes from food. Whether client have type 1 or type 2 diabetes, the peak blood glucose levels are often likely to occur around two hours after a meal.

HbA1c Test

The A1C test is sometimes called the hemoglobin A1C, HbA1c, glycated hemoglobin, or glycohemoglobin test. Hemoglobin is the part of a red blood cell that carries oxygen to the cells. Glucose attaches to or binds with hemoglobin in client's blood cells, and the A1C test is based on this attachment of glucose to hemoglobin.

The higher the glucose level in client's bloodstream, the more glucose will attach to the hemoglobin. The A1C test measures the amount of hemoglobin with attached glucose and reflects client's average blood glucose levels over the past three months.

The A1C test result is reported as a percentage. The higher the percentage, the higher client's blood glucose levels have been. A normal A1C level is below 5.7%.

Hemoglobin A1c test to evaluate glucose levels in the blood over the last 2 to 3 months. This test is essential in managing one's diabetes. Researchers believe that keeping the blood sugar in the body within a normal range can help people with diabetes avoid many of the risks and side effects of diabetes. For many people with diabetes, the goal is to keep the level below 7%. Additionally, a significant benefit of the hemoglobin A1c blood test is that it provides information on overall glycemic health over several months. Other blood tests that evaluate glucose levels are highly sensitive to determining glucose levels at the time of collection, but they do not give information on average glucose blood levels.

Common risks and side effects associated with unmanaged higher A1C levels include:

- Eye disease
- Heart disease
- Kidney disease
- Nerve damage
- Stroke

Hemoglobin is stored in the red blood cells. When glucose levels are high, the sugar starts to combine with the hemoglobin. It takes the body 8 to 12 weeks to bring hemoglobin A1c levels back to normal. Therefore, if hemoglobin A1c levels are high, there has been a high glucose level in the blood over the last 2 to 3 months.

The hemoglobin (Hb) A1c blood test results are interpreted by looking at the hemoglobin A1c levels in the blood. Hemoglobin A1c results are represented as a percentage of glucose in the blood. Glucose is measured in milligrams per deciliter (mg/dL). Normal results vary based on what test is being used. The following results represent numbers found on the hemoglobin blood test A1c.

- Normal: < 5.7%
- Pre-diabetes/increased risk of diabetes 5.7–6.4%
- Diabetes: >6.5%

It is important to note that other underlying health factors or conditions unrelated to diabetes may cause a higher or lower hemoglobin A1c result. Other factors that may affect hemoglobin A1c levels include:

I. Anemia
II. High-dose aspirin
III. Iron, vitamin B12, or folate deficiency
IV. Pregnancy
V. Chronic kidney disease and its treatment
VI. Blood transfusion recipients
VII. Hereditary disorders (sickle cell disease)
VIII. High alcohol consumption

Collection container:

Adults: 3.4 mL whole blood K-EDTA

Pediatrics: 1.2 mL whole blood K-EDTA

Type and volume of sample: Whole blood, minimum 1.0 mL

Specimen transport/special precautions: None

Blood Glucose PC Test

Measuring blood glucose (glycemia) 2 hours PC (after a meal) is one of several tests used to monitor diabetes. This test is different from hyperglycemia 2 hours post 75 grams of glucose, which is used to diagnose diabetes. The blood glucose 2 hours PC better reflects fluctuations in glucose levels in the patient's environment (eating habits, medication-related, etc.) and complements diabetes self-monitoring performed at home with a blood glucose monitor or monitoring in the lab with a measure of glycosylated hemoglobin (HbA1c).

Glycemia, exactly 2 hours after the end of a balanced meal containing sufficient carbohydrates (sugars) but also other elements from each of the major food groups, must be lower than 7.8 millimoles of glucose per liter of blood (mmol/L).

Glucose levels over 7.8 mmol/L (or more rarely below 3.9 mmol/L) may indicate that the diabetes is not being controlled optimally, but these levels must be interpreted along with all elements of the case (diabetes type, treatment type and targets, in-home self-monitoring results, HbA1c level, risk of hypoglycemia, etc.).

Testing Methods

Tests that can be performed at home are used in blood glucose monitoring for illnesses that have already been diagnosed medically so that these illnesses can be maintained via medication and meal timing. Some of the home testing methods include:

1. **Fingerprick** type of **glucose meter**—need to prick self finger 8–12 times a day.
2. **Continuous glucose monitor**—the cgm monitors the glucose levels every 5 minutes approximately.

Laboratory tests are often used to diagnose illnesses and such methods include:

1. **Fasting blood sugar (FBS), fasting plasma glucose (FPG):** 10–16 hours after eating
2. **Glucose tolerance test:** Continuous testing
3. **Postprandial glucose test (PC):** 2 hours after eating
4. **Random glucose test**

Some laboratory tests do not measure glucose levels directly from body fluids or tissues but still indicate elevated blood sugar levels. Such tests measure the levels of glycated hemoglobin, other glycated proteins, 1,5-anhydroglucitol, etc., from blood.

- ❖ Use in medical diagnosis
- ❖ Glucose testing can be used to diagnose or indicate certain medical conditions
- ❖ High blood sugar may indicate
- ❖ Gestational diabetes. This temporary form of diabetes appears during pregnancy, and with glucose-controlling medication or insulin symptoms can be improved.
- ❖ Type 1 and type 2 diabetes or prediabetes. If diagnosed with diabetes, regular glucose tests can help manage or maintain conditions. Type 1, is commonly seen in children or teenagers whose bodies are not producing enough insulin. Type 2 diabetes, is typically seen in adults who are overweight. The insulin in their bodies are either not working normally, or there is not being enough produced.
- ❖ Pancreatic cancer
- ❖ Pancreatitis
- ❖ Underactive thyroid

Low blood sugar may indicate:

- ❖ Insulin overuse
- ❖ Starvation
- ❖ Underactive thyroid
- ❖ Addison's disease
- ❖ Insulinoma
- ❖ Kidney disease

Preparing for Testing

Fasting prior to glucose testing may be required with some test types. Fasting blood sugar test, for example, requires 10–16 hour long period of not eating before the test.

Blood sugar levels can be affected by some drugs and prior to some glucose tests these medications should be temporarily given up or their dosages should be decreased. Such drugs may include salicylates (Aspirin), birth control pills, corticosteroids, tricyclic antidepressants, lithium, diuretics and phenytoin.

Some foods contain caffeine (coffee, tea, colas, energy drinks, etc.). Blood sugar levels of healthy people are generally not significantly changed by caffeine, but in diabetics caffeine intake may elevate these levels via its ability to stimulate the adrenergic nervous system.

Fasting Blood Sugar

A level below 5.6 mmol/L (100 mg/dL) 10–16 hours without eating is normal. 5.6–6 mmol/L (100–109 mg/dL) may indicate prediabetes and oral glucose tolerance test (OGTT) should be done for high-risk individuals (old people, those with high blood pressure, etc.). 6.1–6.9 mmol/L (110–125 mg/dL) means OGTT should be done even if other indicators of diabetes are not present. 7 mmol/L (126 mg/dL) and above indicates diabetes and the fasting test should be repeated.

Glucose Tolerance Test

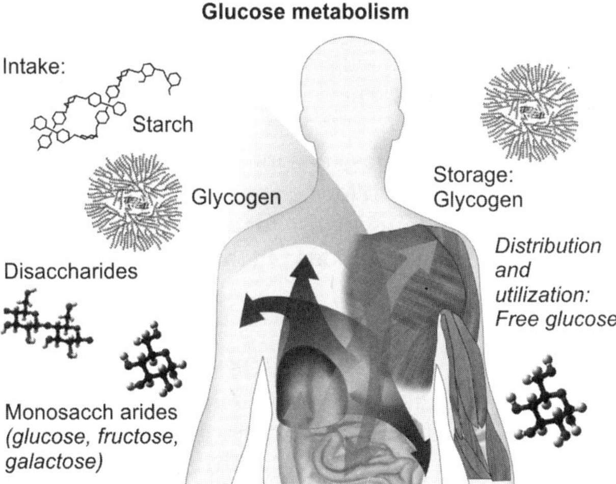

The glucose tolerance test (GTT) is a medical test in which glucose is given and blood samples taken afterward to determine how quickly it is cleared from the blood. The test is usually used to test for diabetes, insulin resistance, impaired beta cell function, and sometimes reactive hypoglycemia and acromegaly, or rarer disorders of carbohydrate metabolism.

In the most commonly performed version of the test, an oral glucose tolerance test (OGTT), a standard dose of glucose is ingested by mouth and blood levels are checked two hours later. Many variations of the GTT have been devised over the years for various purposes, with different standard doses of glucose, different routes of administration, different intervals and durations of sampling, and various substances measured in addition to blood glucose.

Preparation

The patient is instructed not to restrict carbohydrate intake in the days or weeks before the test. The test should not be done during an illness, as results may not reflect the patient's glucose metabolism when healthy. A full adult dose should not be given to a person weighing less than 42.6 kg (94 lb), or the excessive glucose may produce a false positive result. Usually, the OGTT is performed in the morning as glucose tolerance can exhibit a diurnal rhythm with a significant decrease in the afternoon. The patient is instructed to fast (water is allowed) for 8–12 hours prior to the tests. Medication such as large doses of salicylates, diuretics, anticonvulsants, and oral contraceptives affect the glucose tolerance test.

Procedure

A zero time (baseline) blood sample is drawn.

The patient is then given a measured dose (below) of glucose solution to drink within a 5 minute timeframe.

Blood is drawn at intervals for measurement of glucose (blood sugar), and sometimes insulin levels. The intervals and number of samples vary according to the purpose of the test. For simple diabetes screening, the most important sample is the 2 hour sample and the 0 and 2 hour samples may be the only ones collected. A laboratory may continue to collect blood for up to 6 hours depending on the protocol requested by the physician.

Dose of Glucose and Variations

About 75 g of oral dose is the recommendation of the WHO to be used in all adults, and is the main dosage used in the United States. The dose is adjusted for weight only in children. The dose should be drunk within 5 minutes.

A variant is often used in pregnancy to screen for gestational diabetes, with a screening test of 50 g over one hour. If elevated, this is followed with a test of 100 g over three hours.

In UK general practice, the standard glucose load was provided by 394 mL of the energy drink Lucozade with original carbonated flavour, but this is being superseded by purpose-made drinks.

Substances Measured and Variations

If renal glycosuria (sugar excreted in the urine despite normal levels in the blood) is suspected, urine samples may also be collected for testing along with the fasting and 2 hour blood tests.

Results

Fasting plasma glucose (measured before the OGTT begins) should be below 5.6 mmol/L (100 mg/dL). Fasting levels between 5.6 and 6.9 mmol/L (100 and 125 mg/dL) indicate prediabetes ("impaired fasting glucose"), and fasting levels repeatedly at or above 7.0 mmol/L (>126 mg/dL) are diagnostic of diabetes.

For a 2 hour GTT with 75 g intake, a glucose level below 7.8 mmol/L (140 mg/dL) is normal, whereas higher levels indicate hyperglycemia. Blood plasma glucose between 7.8 mmol/L (140 mg/dL) and 11.1 mmol/L (200 mg/dL) indicate "impaired glucose tolerance", and levels at or above 11.1 mmol/L at 2 hours confirm a diagnosis of diabetes.

For gestational diabetes, the American College of Obstetricians and Gynecologists (ACOG) recommends a two-step procedure, wherein the first step is a 50 g glucose dose. If after 1 hour the blood glucose level is more than 7.8 mmol/L (140 mg/dL), it is followed by a 100 g glucose dose. The diagnosis of gestational diabetes is then defined by a blood glucose level meeting or exceeding the cutoff values on at least two intervals, with cutoffs as follows:

Before glucose intake (fasting): 5.3 mmol/L (95 mg/dL)
1 hour after drinking the glucose solution: 10.0 mmol/L (180 mg/dL)
2 hours: 8.6 mmol/L (155 mg/dL)
3 hours: 7.8 mmol/L (140 mg/dL)

Sample Method

The diagnosis criteria stated above by the World Health Organization (WHO) are for venous samples only (a blood sample taken from a vein in the arm). An increasingly popular method for measuring blood glucose is to sample capillary or finger-prick blood, which is less invasive, more convenient for the patient and requires minimal training to conduct. Though fasting blood glucose levels have been shown to be similar in both capillary and venous samples, postprandial blood glucose levels (those measured after a meal) can vary. The diagnosis criteria issued by the WHO are only suitable for venous blood samples. Given the increasing popularity of capillary testing, the WHO has recommended that a conversion factor between the two sample types be calculated, but as of 2017 no conversion factor had been issued by the WHO, despite some medical professionals adopting their own.

Variations

A standard two-hour GTT (glucose tolerance test) is sufficient to diagnose or exclude all forms of diabetes mellitus at all but the earliest stages of development.

Longer tests have been used for a variety of other purposes, such as detecting reactive hypoglycemia or defining subsets of hypothalamic obesity. Insulin levels are sometimes measured to detect insulin resistance or deficiency.

The GTT (glucose tolerance test) is of limited value in the diagnosis of reactive hypoglycemia, since normal levels do not preclude the diagnosis, abnormal levels do not prove that the patient's other symptoms are related to a demonstrated atypical OGTT, and many people without symptoms of reactive hypoglycemia may have the late low glucose.

Oral Glucose Challenge Test

The oral glucose challenge test (OGCT) is a short version of the OGTT, used to check pregnant women for signs of gestational diabetes. It can be done at any time of day, not on an empty stomach. The test involves 50 g of glucose, with a reading after one hour.

Limitations of OGTT

The OGTT does not distinguish between insulin resistance in peripheral tissues and reduced capacity of the pancreas beta-cells to produce insulin. The OGTT is less accurate than the hyperinsulinemic-euglycemic clamp technique (the "gold standard" for measuring insulin resistance), or the insulin tolerance test, but is technically less difficult. Neither of the two technically demanding tests can be easily applied in a clinical setting or used in epidemiological studies. HOMA-IR (homeostatic model assessment) is a convenient way of measuring insulin resistance in normal subjects, which can be used in epidemiological studies, but can give erroneous results for diabetic patients.

A postprandial glucose (PPG) test is a blood glucose test that determines the amount of glucose, in the plasma after a meal. The diagnosis is typically restricted to postprandial hyperglycemia due to lack of strong evidence of co-relation with a diagnosis of diabetes.

American Diabetes Association do not recommend a PPG test for determining diabetes; it though notes that postprandial hyperglycemia does contribute to elevated glycated hemoglobin levels (a primary factor behind diabetes) and recommends testing and management of PPG levels for those patients who maintain optimum pre-prandial blood glucose levels but have high A1C values.

Carbohydrate in the form of glucose is one of the main constituents of foods and assimilation starts within about 10 minutes. The subsequent rate of absorption of carbohydrates in conjunction with the resultant rates of secretion of insulin and glucagon secretion affects the time-weighed PPG profile.

In non-diabetic individuals, levels peak at about an hour after the start of a meal, rarely exceed 140 mg/dL, and return to preprandial levels within 2–3 hours. These time-profiles are heavily altered in diabetic patients.

Typically, PPG levels are measured after about 2 hours from the start of the meal which corresponds to the time-span in which peak values are typically located, in case of diabetic patients.

A random glucose test, also known as a random blood glucose test (RBG test) or a casual blood glucose test (CBG test) is a glucose test (test of blood sugar level) on the blood of a non-fasting person. This test assumes a recent meal and therefore has higher reference values than the fasting blood glucose (FBG) test.

Most mentions of capillary blood glucose (CBG) tests refer to random, nonfasting instances thereof, but the real distinction in that term is capillary blood glucose versus venous blood glucose, arterial blood glucose, or interstitial fluid glucose; any fingerstick or optical transdermal glucose test, fasting or non-fasting, measures capillary blood glucose level.

STOOL ROUTINE EXAMINATION

A stool routine test is a non-invasive and painless test done to detect the presence of blood in the stool and any fungi, bacteria, or viruses. Simply collect the stool in a container and send it to the lab for analysis. Most useful to detect any gastrointestinal problems.

A stool test is also known as stool culture, fecal sample test or stool sample test. The test helps in diagnosing medical conditions, such as inflammatory bowel disease, gastric or colon cancer, anal fissures, hemorrhoids, as well as to detect the presence of blood in client's stool sample.

Stool tests helps to determine whether a bacteria or any other microorganism has infected the intestines or not. But not all microorganisms in the gut are harmful some are necessary for normal digestion. If harmful bacteria or parasites infect client's intestines, they cause bloody diarrhoea and testing the stool may help find the cause of this condition.

Types of Stool Test

1. Rotavirus Test
2. Yersinia Test

3. Giardia Antigen Test
4. Salmonella Culture Test
5. White Blood Cell Test
6. Calprotectin Test
7. Fecal Occult Blood Test
8. Trypsin/Chymotrypsin Test
9. Clostridium Difficile Toxin Test
10. Ova and Parasites Test
11. Fecal Fat Test
12. Campylobacter Culture Test

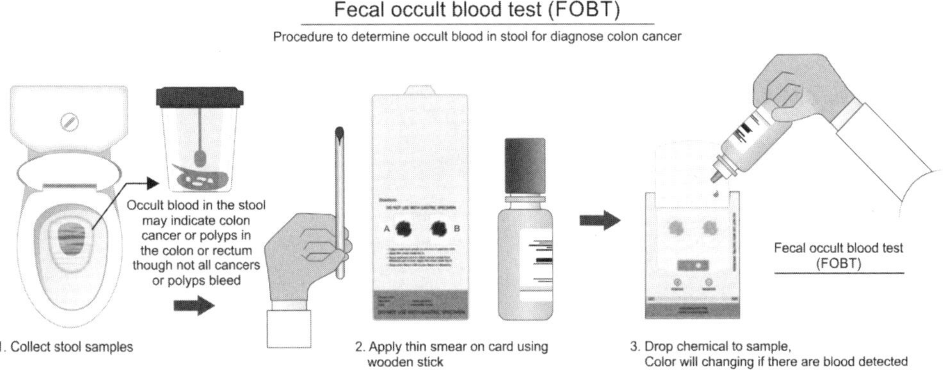

Ova and Parasites Test

The test is usually ordered if client are experiencing symptoms associated with an intestinal infection, such as:

- ❖ Presence of blood or mucus in client's stool
- ❖ Frequent diarrhea
- ❖ Fever
- ❖ Acute abdominal pain
- ❖ Headache
- ❖ Vomiting or nausea

Sample Required

- ❖ The fresh stools can be examined directly to detect moving organisms.
- ❖ Stools in 10% formalin can be used for helminths and protozoa.
- ❖ The stools in formalin-ethyl acetate can be used.
- ❖ The sample amount of stool test is 2–5 grams.

Safeguards for Sample

Patients are advised the following things for at least 48 hours before stool collection:
a. Avoid mineral oils.
b. Do not take bismuth.

c. Antibiotics such as tetracyclines are contraindicated.

d. Antidiarrheal medications are not advised.

e. If there is blood, that should be included in the stool. Because most pathogens are found in this substance.

f. Semiformed feces should be examined within an hour after collection.

g. Liquid wastes should be discussed within the first 30 minutes.

h. Solid stool should be addressed within the group examinations.

Physical Examination

* ❖ Quantity
* ❖ Gross Appearance
* ❖ Color
* ❖ Consistency

Chemical Examination

* ❖ pH
* ❖ Specific gravity
* ❖ Water contents
* ❖ Occult blood
* ❖ Reducing substances
* ❖ Porphyrins
* ❖ Urobilinogen
* ❖ Sodium
* ❖ Potassium
* ❖ Chloride
* ❖ Nitrogen
* ❖ Trypsin
* ❖ Lipids
* ❖ Osmolality

Microscopic Examination

* ❖ WBCs
* ❖ RBCs
* ❖ Parasites
* ❖ Yeast
* ❖ Bacteria
* ❖ Viruses

Sample Collection

A dry and clean container should be taken for stool sample collection. Client are not supposed to urinate while collecting the stool. To fault doing this, urinate first, and, once done, pass stool into the container. Close the lid and then wash client's hands. It is also advisable to wear gloves while collecting the stool sample.

Client need to collect stool samples at home, using latex gloves and plastic wrap. The plastic wrap should be covered in the toilet before using it. The sample should not contain urine or toilet water. After collecting the sample in a container, it should be returned to the lab right away, for getting accurate results.

Positive results may indicate that there is a presence of parasites and ova in client's stool sample. Bacteria in the stool that may cause an infection are:

* *Entamoeba histolytica*
* *Giardia*
* *Cryptosporidium*

The test may also detect:

* *Dientamoeba fragilis*
* *Balantidium coli*
* *Cyclospora cayetanensis*
* Roundworms
* Flatworms
* Hookworms
* Tapeworms

White Blood Cell Test

This test is often used to detect leukocytes or white blood cells in client's stool sample. WBC help client's body fight off infections, and it is usually a part of our immune system. Leukocytes in the stool may indicate a bacterial infection or an Inflammatory bowel disease a condition characterised by inflammation in the digestive system. Client's doctor may order this test if client experience any of the symptoms, such as: 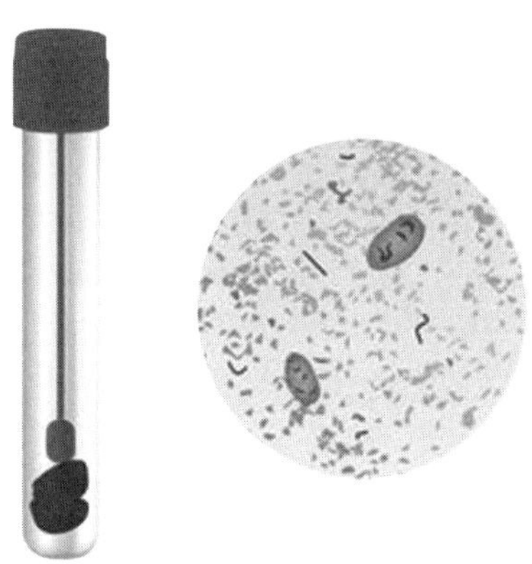

* Mucus or blood in the stool
* Watery diarrhoea that lasts for more than four days
* Fever
* Abdominal pain
* Fatigue

The healthcare provider will provide client with a special container to collect client's stool sample. Make sure that there is no urine, toilet paper or water in client's stool sample. After collecting the sample, seal it, and return it to the healthcare provider.

If white blood cell test results are negative, then it indicates that there are no leukocytes present in client's stool sample. The symptoms that client have experienced may not be caused by an infection.

If results are positive, then it indicates the presence of leukocytes in client's stool sample. There may be some kind of inflammation inside client's digestive tract. If there are more leukocytes in the sample, it means client have a higher chance for a bacterial infection.

H. Pylori Antigen Test

H. pylori or *Helicobacter pylori* is a bacteria that infects client's digestive system. Some people may never have any symptoms of infection, even though these bacteria infect them. But for others, *H. pylori* may cause gastrointestinal disorders, such as:

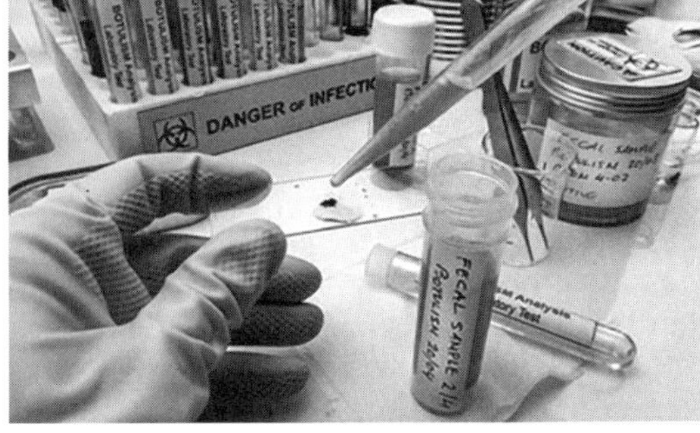

❖ Peptic ulcers (a condition characterized by sores in the esophagus, small intestine or stomach)

❖ Gastritis (inflammation of the stomach) or certain types of stomach cancer

The test is often used to:

❖ Detect *H. pylori* inside client's digestive tract.

❖ Check whether the digestive symptoms are caused by an infection.

❖ Determine whether the treatment for *H. pylori* infection is working or not.

❖ If client are experiencing symptoms that indicate a peptic ulcer, such as:

a. Abdominal pain
b. Nausea
c. Indigestion
d. Frequent vomiting
e. Bloated feeling

Collect the stool in the special container provided to client by the healthcare provider and return it, making sure that there is no presence of urine, toilet water or toilet paper in the sample. A small amount of stool sample is placed in vials and color developer, and chemicals are added to it. If the sample turns blue in color, then it is a sign of *H. pylori* in client's stool.

Fecal Occult Blood Test

This test helps in checking hidden or occult blood in a sample of client's stool. If there is small amount of blood in client's stool, it may indicate bleeding in client's digestive tract, due to conditions, such as:

a. Ulcers
b. Polyps (non-cancerous tissue growth on client's mucous membrane)
c. Diverticulosis (a medical condition in which small pouches develop in the digestive tract)
d. Colitis (inflammation or swelling of the colon)
e. Hemorrhoids (a condition characterized by swollen blood vessels around client's anus or rectum)
f. Colorectal cancer

If client are tested positive for any of the types of a faecal occult blood test, it can be a sign that client have bleeding in client's digestive tract. But this does not necessarily indicate that client have cancer. A positive fecal occult blood test also shows polyps, hemorrhoids, ulcers, or benign tumors.

Stool DNA Test

This type of stool test detects abnormal DNA, that occur normally because of colon polyps or colon cancer as well as traces of occult blood, in client's stool sample. A stool DNA test is a screening test for colon cancer and precancerous polyps for people who are not experiencing any signs and symptoms associated with it. If there are polyps or cancer in client's colon, they may shed cells having abnormal DNA into client's stool.

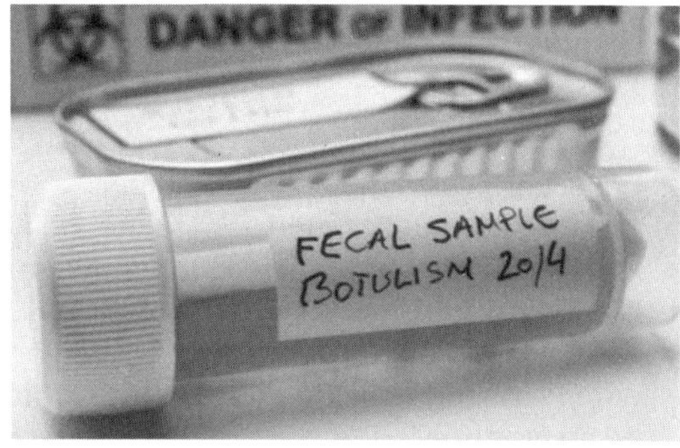

Client's test is considered positive if there are abnormal DNA changes associated with polyps or colon cancer or traces of occult blood in client's sample. client's test is considered negative if there are no abnormal DNA changes associated with polyps or colon cancer or traces of occult blood in client's sample.

Client need to take an additional test, such as colonoscopy to diagnose polyps or cancer inside client's colon. For those who take a stool DNA test, only a few get positive results, but no polyps or cancer are detected during colonoscopy. In such cases, further testing is normally not recommended.

URINE TESTING

pH

Kidney is an excretory organ that removes waste materials from the blood and excretes them from the body in the form of urine. It also maintains acid–base balance and the body's homeostasis. It plays an important role in maintaining pH 7.4 of the blood. The average pH of urine is, however, about 6.0 though it can range from acidic (pH 4.6) to alkaline (pH 8.0). The urine with pH <5 is considered acidic and urine with pH >8 is considered alkaline urine. The pH of human urine varies and depends on the diet. The acidic or alkaline pH of given sample (urine) can be determined by using pH strip, which is a special paper composed of different chemical compounds (dye) such as methyl red and bromothymol blue, etc. The color of the pH strip can be compared with a color disc which shows the relevant pH value for the varying shades of color.

Principle

To determine pH of the urine sample, a pH strip is dipped into given sample and the color change is recorded. The change in color is compared to the pH chart to determine approximate acidic or alkaline pH of the sample.

Materials Required

❖ Urine sample
❖ pH strip (commercial available)
❖ Color chart

A pH strip or dipstick is common diagnostic tool used to determine pH of urine sample. A pH strip is already colored and has about 10 different chemical pads or reagents which react to the sample when immersed in it.

Procedure

❖ Collect urine in a clean, dry container.
❖ Test the specimen as soon as possible. Do not add any preservatives.
❖ A pH strip into the container containing urine for few seconds more than 5 seconds).
❖ Dry the pH strip.
❖ Compare the color of the strip with the color chart on the vial label under well-lit conditions. While comparing, keep the strip horizontally to prevent possible mixing of chemicals if excessive urine is absorbed. Discard the used pH strips.

Result Observations

The change of the color of pH strip to red color indicates acidic pH of the urine while the appearance of blue indicates alkaline pH. The pH value of Urine ranges from pH 4.6 (acidic) to pH 8.0 (alkaline).

Precautions

❖ Store pH strips in a cool, dry place at temperatures between 2°–30°.
❖ Do not store the strips in a refrigerator or freezer. Store them away from moisture and light.
❖ Discoloration or darkening of the test strips may indicate deterioration.
❖ Draw the edge of the strip along the brim of the vessel to remove excess urine; don't let the test areas touch to the brim of the vessel.

Articles Required

❖ Clean or sterile dry containers for collection of urine. Wide mouthed preferable
❖ In acutely ill patient or in post-operative case
❖ Test tubes
❖ Test tube rack or stand
❖ Test tube holder
❖ Glass pipette (plain or graduated)
❖ Burner: Gas or spirit
❖ Chemical reagent
❖ Collection of urine

Procedure

Explain the procedure to the patient to collect urine in a bottle.

Ask the patient to void urine. First part of the urine is to be discarded. Collect the required amount from later part of urine in a clean dry wide mouthed container, i.e., mid stream urine. Amount of urine collected depends on tests to be performed. Mouth of the container is closed with a stopper. The container must be properly labelled with name of the patient, registration number date and time of collection.

Examination of urine helps in diagnosis, monitoring and management of diabetes mellitus. Chemical examination is useful to detect glycosuria proteinuria, ketonuria, i.e., glucose, protein, Ketone in urine respectively. Besides diabetes urine examination help in diagnosing some other metabolic and systemic diseases, diseases of kidney and urinary tract infection.

Benedict's Test

Glucose in urine is detected by Benedict's method and the test is known as Benedict's test. This test is used to detect glucose in urine (Glycosuria). Benedict's test is preferred by many and is economical.

Procedure

❖ Take 5 mL of Benedict's reagent in a test tube (150 × 18 mm) and boil for a minute by holding the tube over a burner flame with the help of a test tube holder.

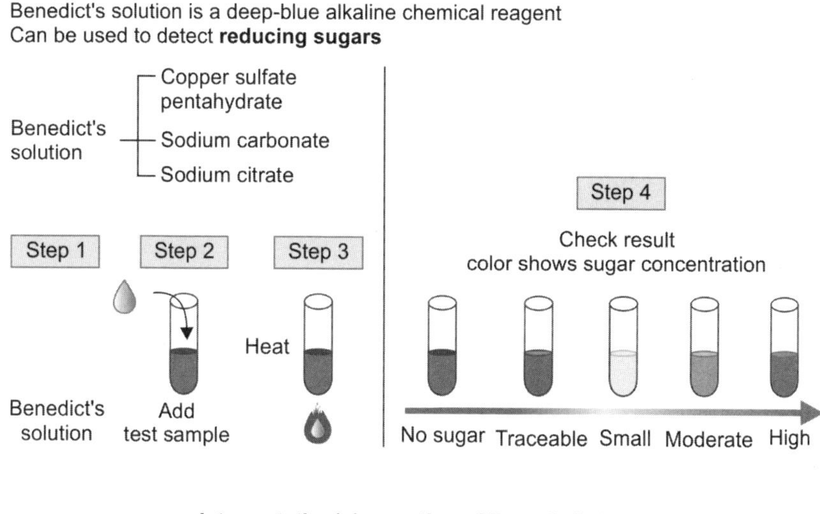

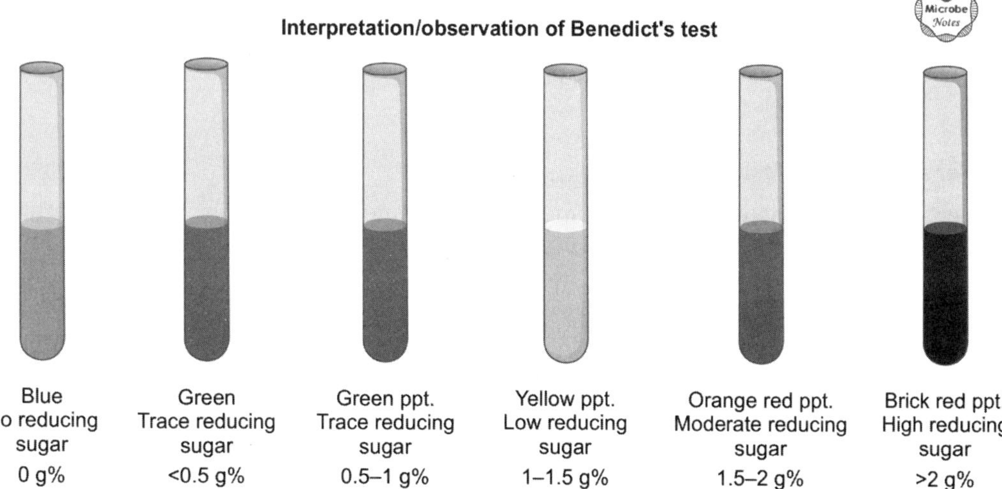

* Add 8 drops of urine from the collected sample by a pipette.
* Boil it further over the flame for another 2–3 minutes and cool.
* Observe the change in the color of the urine.

URINE TESTING FOR ALBUMIN AND KETONES

Testing for Albumin in Urine

A. Acetic Acid Test

About 2–8 mg/dL of protein is excreted in urine which is not usually detected by routine test. The testing of urine for protein of which albumin is the main organic constituents is widely used laboratory procedure. Detection of an abnormal amount of protein in urine is a reliable indicator of renal disorder including complications associated with diabetes mellitus.

Take urine in a clean test tube filling 2/3rd portion and boil upper portion of urine for 2 minutes by holding with a test tube holder over a burner flame. A white cloud appears in the heated portion if proteins (including albumin) and phosphates are present. Now client add 2–3 drops of 5–10% glacial acetic acid. If the cloudiness disappears it is due to phosphate, if it persists, then it implies proteinuria (Albuminuria).

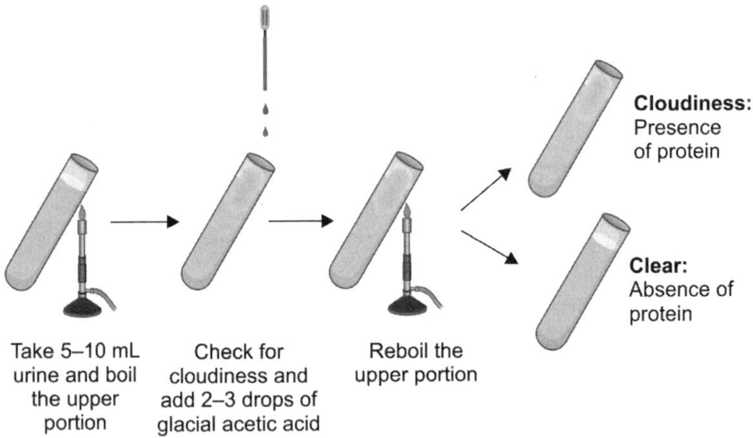

Heller's Nitric Acid Test

Heller's test is a biochemical test performed to detect proteins in a sample by the denaturation of those proteins by the addition of strong acids. Heller's test usually uses concentrated nitric acid for the denaturation of proteins. The test is performed for clinical purposes to detect abnormal proteins in biological fluids, including urine. Heller's test is a type of precipitation test where the precipitation is brought about by denaturation. Take 1 mL concentrated (fuming) nitric acid in a test tube and add 2 mL of urine by means of a pipette by the side of the test tube and layer on the top of the acid. A whitish ring of precipitate form at the junction of the two fluids due to formation of metaprotein due to albumin in urine.

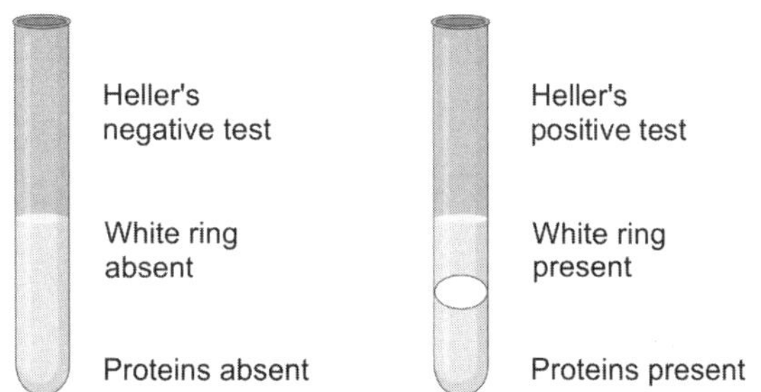

Procedure of Heller's Test

In a clean and dry test tube, 2 mL of concentrated nitric acid is taken.

To this, 2 mL of urine or other sample is added. The sample should be poured from the sidewall of the test tube in an inclined position in order to form a layer of the sample above the nitric acid.

The test tube is then observed for the formation of a white ring at the junction of the two layers.

Positive result: A positive result is represented by the formation of a white ring (precipitated protein) at the junction of the two distinct layers. This indicates the presence of proteins in the given sample.

Negative result: A negative result is represented by the absence of a white ring. This indicates the absence of protein in the sample.

B. Testing of Ketones in Urine

Ketones are also known as ketone bodies. Ketone bodies are catabolic products of free fatty acids and three ketone bodies that can be detected in urine are:
1. Acetone—2%
2. Acetoacetic acid (Ac Ac)—20%
3. B-Hydroxybutyric acid (BHBA)—78%

Determination of Ketone bodies in urine and blood are widely used in the management of patient, with diabetes mellitus specially monitoring of Diabetic Ketoacidosis (DKA). All patients with diabetes mellitus should test their urine for ketone bodies during acute illness, stress, persistent hyperglycemia, pregnancy or symptoms of DKA like nausea, vomiting or pain abdomen.

Rothera's Test

It is highly sensitive for both acetoacetic and acetone. Although it is one of the oldest methods still it is widely used.

Procedure

Take about 5 mL of urine in a test tube and saturate with ammonium sulphate and add few crystals (or about 0.5 mL of 20% aqueous solution) of sodium nitroprusside. If solid crystals are taken, shake well the tube to dissolve the crystals and wait for about 10 minutes.

Now carefully pour down the side of the test tube about 2–3 mL of concentrated ammonia (Liquor ammonia) so that it forms a layer on the top of saturated urine. Formation of a purple ring at the junction indicates positive test.

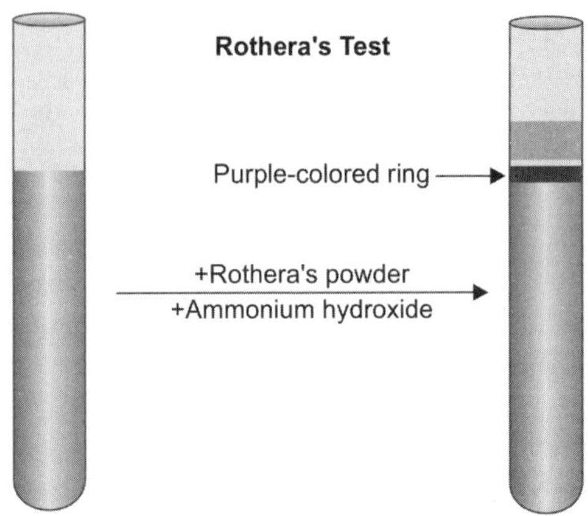

Dipstick Test

Plastic strips impregnated with a buffered mixture of sodium nitroprusside and glycine is now widely used. Usually it is available as single reagent strip for ketone detection or as Multi strip Reagent Strip for detection of Sugar, protein, ketone bodies and other substances in urine. The strips are available commercially produced by several manufacturers like Siemens, Boehringer, Miles, Ames, etc.

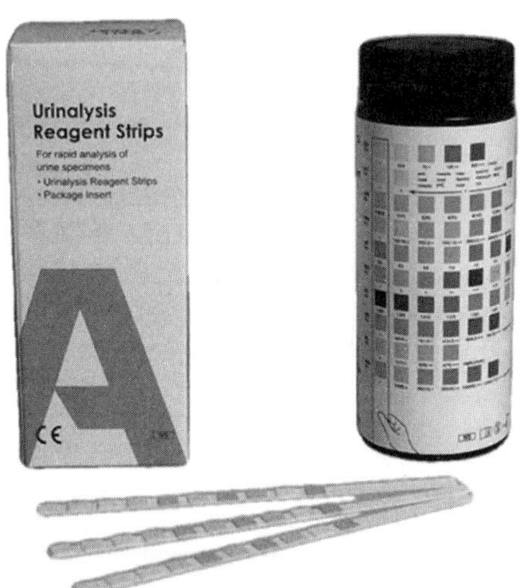

ANALYSIS OF URINE

Having learnt about the normal and abnormal constituents of urine let us learn about the analysis of urine samples. Let us begin with physical examination of urine and see how we perform physical examination and what do the results of such an examination indicate.

Physical Examination of Urine

The first step of urine analysis is its physical examination in terms of its color, appearance, odor (smell), amount, specific gravity (thickness) and reaction to litmus. The physical examination can also provide important lead into the diagnosis. Let us take up different physical examinations one by one.

Appearance: A normal fresh sample of urine is clear. A turbidity or cloudiness in the sample may be due to the,

❖ Presence of cellular material, like RBC, WBC or bacteria
❖ Presence of protein
❖ Precipitation of salts upon standing at room temperature or in the refrigerator
❖ Presence of fat globules

The presence of cellular material, like RBC, WBC or bacteria is established by microscopic examination while heat test (given later) is used to confirm the presence of protein. If, however, the turbidity disappears on adding a few drops of acid then turbidity is likely to be due to the precipitation of salts.

Color: Normal, fresh urine is pale yellow or amber in color due to the presence of the pigment *urochrome*. The color may be pale or dark depending on the volume of the urine excreted. However, an abnormal sample may have distinctly different colors.

A greenish yellow sample may indicate the presence of excessive amount of bile pigments, possibly due to jaundice.

A **red or red-brown** color could be from a food dye, eating fresh beets, a drug, or the presence of either hemoglobin or myoglobin, suggesting hemoglobinuria or myoglobinuria. If the sample contains many red blood cells, it would be cloudy as well as red.

A brownish black color is due to alkaptonuria, methemoglobinuria or may be due poisoning with lead, mercury or phenol, etc.

The presences of pus of fat globules impart a **milky** appearance to urine.

Specific gravity: Specific gravity (sp. gr.) is a measure of urine density, which is directly proportional the concentration of dissolved solutes. It is normally measured for a 24-hour sample and its value reflects the ability of the kidney to concentrate or dilute the urine over that of plasma. A value of specific gravity between 1.015 and 1.025 is considered normal. A value below this range indicates hydration while above it indicates relative dehydration.

The sp. gr. of urine may go down to 1.002 on ingesting a large amount of water while could increase on fluid restriction. If, however, sp. gr. is not >1.022 after a 12-hour period without food or water, renal concentrating ability is impaired and the patient either has generalized renal impairment or nephrogenic diabetes insipidus. Any urine sample having a specific gravity over 1.035 is either contaminated or contains very high levels of glucose. The specific gravity is measured with the help of a floating urinometer.

Odor: A fresh sample of urine has an aromatic odor; however, in the case of a disease urine may have abnormal smells. An ammoniacal smell is indicative of a urinary tract infection while a fruity smell of acetone is observed in ketosis. The presence of pus or decomposing tissues in the urine makes it smell putrid.

Volume: An adult normally excretes between 800–2000 cm³ of urine per day depending on the fluid intake and loss of fluid through skin or otherwise. The volume of urine may increase or decrease under pathological conditions.

A urine volume of more than 3,000 cm³ per day is referred to as **polyuria** and is indicative of diabetes, recovery from acute renal failure or a high protein diet. While **oliguria,** a condition wherein the urine volume goes below 400 cm³ per day could be due to acute renal failure, vomiting, fever, bums or edema. A condition when the urine output decreases to below 100 cm³ per day is called **anuria** and may be indicative of poisoning with heavy metal salts or acute nephritis.

Reaction to litmus: A normal sample of urine has a pH of about 6 and gives a **slightly acidic** response to litmus. A strongly acidic urine points to metabolic or respiratory acidosis, methanol poisoning, or metabolic disorders like phenylketonuria, while a strongly alkaline urine is indicative metabolic and respiratory alkalosis and urinary tract infection which should be confirmed by chemical and other means. In severe acidosis the pH of urine may go as low as 4 while in alkalosis the pH may go beyond 8.

URINE CULTURE

A laboratory test to check for bacteria, yeast, or other microorganisms in the urine. Urine cultures can help identify the type of microorganism that is causing an infection. This helps determine the best treatment. They may be used to help diagnose urinary tract infections, such as bladder infections. They may also be done after treatment for a urinary tract infection to make sure the microorganism that caused the infection is gone.

A urine culture test can be used to detect and identify urinary tract infection (UTI)-causing bacteria. In general, bacteria that cause UTIs enter the urinary tract via the urethra. These bacteria can flourish in the urinary tract's warm, moist environment and cause an infection.

Women tend to experience UTIs more than men because their urethra is shorter, and the proximity of the urethra to the anus is much closer than in men. Hence, the bacteria in the digestive tract gain easy access to the urinary system. The urethra is the entry point for bacteria that can cause an infection to spread to the bladder, ureters, and kidneys.

Indications

- ❖ Painful urination
- ❖ Clients has a frequent urge to urinate but are unable to empty the bladder efficiently.
- ❖ Client get sick or experience stomach pain for no apparent reason.
- ❖ Client urinalysis results show an abnormally high count of white blood cells.
- ❖ Client has just recovered from a UTI, and the doctor needs to check whether there is a chance of recurrence.

Procedure

The following are the steps that need to be followed for the collection of urine samples during a urine culture test:
- ❖ Thoroughly wash genital area and the surrounding skin area to eradicate any chances of contamination. Do this before taking a sample.

- ❖ Wash your hands thoroughly.
- ❖ Ask patient to start urinating till bladder is empty, and when you're about to finish, urinate a few drops into the sterile container given by doctor. Make sure your skin doesn't touch the inside of the container while doing it.

Specimen

Specimen type: Urine

Container: Sterile container. If anaerobes are suspected, use an anaerobic transport system (available in Microbiology).

Volume: 1–10 mL of urine from a first morning specimen

Collection: Catheterized specimen:

Straight Catheter, Female

- ❖ Place the client supine, with the thighs in a frog-leg position.
- ❖ Separate the labia and cleanse the area around the meatus with povidone-iodine swabs. Use anterior-to-posterior strokes to prevent fecal contamination. Rinse area with sterile water using cotton balls or sponges.
- ❖ Aseptically insert catheter into the bladder.
- ❖ Allow about 10 mL to pass, then collect 1–10 mL into sterile tube, or sterile container.
- ❖ After urine is collected, pull catheter out of the cap of the centrifuge tube, tighten cap (and depress spout, if using the kit).

Straight Catheter, Male

- ❖ Place the infant supine, legs extended.
- ❖ Cleanse the penis with povidone iodine swabs in a spiral motion from meatus outward, one sponge per stroke. Rinse area with sterile water.
- ❖ Aseptically insert catheter, holding the penis perpendicular to the body to straighten the urethra.
- ❖ Allow about 10 mL to pass, then collect 1–10 mL into sterile tube, or specimen container.
- ❖ After urine is collected, pull catheter out of the cap of the centrifuge tube, tighten cap (and depress spout, if using the container).

Vesicostomy

- ❖ Gather supplies (lubricant, sterile gloves, sterile specimen container, and appropriate catheter).
- ❖ Don sterile gloves.
- ❖ Swab stoma site with povidone iodine.
- ❖ Open catheter. Any catheter is appropriate to use, including a sterile self cath, or a Foley cath. The catheter should be larger than what would be placed in the urethra (10–16Fr.) Lubricate tip.
- ❖ Insert only 1–2 inches, until you see urine. Collect/transfer into sterile specimen container. You may need to leave catheter in place for a few minutes, as urine normally dribbles out slowly.

Indwelling Catheter

* Do not collect urine from drainage bag.
* Disinfect catheter collection port with 70% alcohol.
* Use a syringe to aseptically collect 1–10 mL of urine and transfer into a sterile container.

Clean Catch, Mid-stream Specimen

Males

* Clean glans with soap and water.
* Rinse area with wet gauze pads.
* While holding foreskin retracted, begin voiding.
* After several mL have passed, collect midstream portion without stopping flow of urine.
* Transfer specimen to a leak proof sterile container.

Females

* Thoroughly clean urethral area with soap and water.
* Rinse area with wet gauze pads.
* While holding labia apart, begin voiding.
* After several mL have passed, collect midstream portion without stopping flow of urine.
* Transfer specimen to a sterile leak proof container.

Bagged Specimen

(Caution: contamination rates may run as high as 70%):
* Clean glans or urethral area with soap and water.
* Rinse area with wet sponges.
* Place sterile urine bag over labia or penis.
* After 30 minutes, observe for presence of urine. If no urine is present, re-clean patient and attach a new bag.
* If impossible to obtain urine or if culture results yield a mixture of organisms, collect a catheterized specimen or collect urine by suprapubic aspiration.

Suprapubic Aspiration

* Expose area above pubis.
* Scrub area with povidone iodine. Allow to dry.
* Using a sterile needle and syringe, aspirate 1 mL of urine from bladder.
* Transfer into a sterile container. If anaerobic culture is desired, expel air bubbles and inject urine into an anaerobic transport device.

Transport/storage: Onsite collections: Transport to the laboratory immediately.

If unpreserved specimens cannot be processed within one hour of collection, specimens can be refrigerated up to 24 hours.

Offsite collections: Refrigerate specimen if Gray Boric acid tube cannot be immediately filled or if culture cannot be inoculated immediately. Transport to laboratory within 24 hours, refrigerated.

Gray Boric acid tube: Fill with urine, shake vigorously.

Note: Gray top minimum fill is 3.5 mL. Store and transport at refrigerated or room temperature for up to 48 hours.

Unpreserved specimens must be promptly transported to the laboratory refrigerated, with the next available courier, not to exceed 24 hours from the time of collection. Preserved specimens should be transported to the laboratory, not to exceed 48 hours from the time of collection. However, delayed transport causes a delay of test results.

Sample rejection: Unrefrigerated/unpreserved specimen with a transit time exceeding 1 hour after collection:

* Improperly labeled specimen;
* Specimens with prolonged transit time (see transport/storage for requirements);
* Specimen not submitted in appropriate transport container;
* Insufficient volume;
* External contamination;
* Preserved specimens exceeding 48 hours.

If an unacceptable specimen is received, the physician or nursing station will be notified and another specimen will be requested before the specimen is discarded.

Interpretive

Reference range: No growth

Alert value:

* Gram-negative rods identified as ESBL or carbapenemase producers will be called to the physician or patient's nurse. Infection prevention will be notified.
* If MRSA is isolated for the first time, and the patient location is not emergency department, the result will be called to the physician or patient's nurse.

ROUTINE URINE TEST

The urine routine test is analyzed to diagnose various liver, kidney, and urinary tract diseases, etc. It is also used to monitor the progress of certain conditions. The urine test is performed to examine its odor, color, and components. Your urine contains toxic components of food and medicine, which can tell a lot about your urinary and metabolic system.

The urine analysis is done as a part of a routine check-up or to analyze certain diseases like urinary tract infection (UTI), diabetes, and kidney or liver diseases in their early stages. It is also a part of pregnancy check-ups.

The urine routine test is analyzed in three ways, and your laboratory assistant may perform either or all of them.

1. **Visual test:** When your laboratory assistant examines the odor, color, and clarity of the urine with the naked eye, it is called a visual test. The color of the urine depends on its concentration and ranges from pale yellow to amber. Your urine might turn reddish or brown if it has traces of blood in it. It is also associated with kidney diseases. Likewise, cloudy urine indicates a urinary tract infection.
2. **Microscopic test:** Lab experts perform urine routine microscopy to examine substances in your urine. These substances are not visible to the naked eye; therefore, they must be analyzed under a microscope. Some common substances found in urine are RBC, WBC, cells, mucus, bacteria, crystals, urinary casts, etc.
3. **Rapid urine test:** A rapid urine test is performed to find the chemical components present in the urine. For the test, a dipstick strip is dipped in the urine for some time. After a while, the strip changes its color depending on the urine concentration. Then the lab technician

compares the strip color to the color table to analyze the chemical values in the urine. The rapid urine test is used to analyze urine pH levels, protein, sugar, RBC, WBC, nitrites, blood, etc.

A routine urine test is used to check and manage a wide range of disorders such as to diagnose of:

- Infection
- Diabetes
- Kidney stone
- Presence of bilirubin
- pH, or relative acidity or alkalinity
- Physical color and appearance
- Presence of blood and its components like RBC, hemoglobin and WBC
- Specific gravity
- Burning on urination
- Frequency to urinate
- Bloody or cloudy urine
- Symptoms of a urinary tract infection or bladder infection
- Symptoms of kidney failure
- Chills
- Fever
- Back pain
- High blood pressure
- Edema or swelling
- Loss of appetite
- Nausea, vomiting
- Fatigue, sleepiness
- Itching, twitching
- Metallic taste in the mouth

The Components of Urine Routine Tests

Urine routine test has three parts:

1. Physical examination—to evaluate the urine for color and appearance.
2. Chemical examination—to evaluate pH of urine. An abnormal pH signifies kidney stones, urinary infections, chronic kidney disease, or certain kidney disorders.
   - Protein signifies damage of kidney's filtering unit by kidney disease.
   - Sugar signifies diabetes.
   - Pus cells are signs of infection.
   - Bilirubin signifies liver disease.
   - Blood indicates renal stones and requires further evaluation.
   - Creatinine gives an estimate of the concentration of the urine.
   - Nitrites or leukocyte esterase signifies urinary tract infection.

Microscopic examination: This includes examining a small amount of urine under a microscope, which evaluates and look for the following:

- Red blood cells indicate kidney diseases that damage the kidneys, kidney stones, infections, bladder cancer, or a blood disorder like sickle cell disease.

* White blood cells indicate an infection or inflammation in the kidneys, bladder, or other areas.
* Bacteria indicates an infection in the body.
* Crystals may signify kidney stones.
* Casts may form as a result of kidney disorders.

Procedure and Prerequisites

Mid-stream urine should be collected, neither at the beginning nor at the end.
Collecting a clean catch urine sample.

For female client, use the following steps to get a clean catch urine sample:
* Start by sitting on the toilet with her legs spread apart.
* Instruct her using two fingers, spread labia open. Then, use one sterile wipe to clean the inner folds of labia, wiping from front to back.
* Use another sterile wipe to clean over urethra, the opening where urine flows out of body.
* Urinate a small amount into the toilet.
* Stop the flow of urine, and hold the specimen cup a few inches away from urethra.
* Urinate into the cup, filling it about half full or however full as instructed.
* Finish urinating into the toilet.

For male client, collecting a clean catch urine sample:
* Instruct the client use a sterile wipe to clean the head of penis. If penis is uncircumcised, first pull back foreskin to ensure a thorough cleaning.
* Instruct to urinate a small amount into the toilet.
* Stop the flow of urine, and hold the specimen cup a few inches from urethra, the opening where urine flows out of penis.
* Fill specimen cup about half full or however full your provider instructed you to.
* Finish urinating into the toilet.

Collecting a urine sample with a catheter:
A healthcare provider can also collect a urine sample with a catheter using the following steps:
* A healthcare provider will thoroughly clean the area around the opening of urethra with a germ-killing (antiseptic) solution.
* A provider will insert a thin rubber tube called a catheter through urethra.
* Urine will then drain into a sterile container.
* Will remove the catheter.

Reference Range

Color	Straw
Turbidity	Clear
pH	4.5–8
Specific gravity	1.001–1.030
Protein	Negative
Glucose	Negative
Ketone	Negative
Bile	Trace to 1 mg/dL

Contd...

Contd...

Urobilinogen blood	Negative
Leukocyte	Negative
Esterase	Negative
Nitrite	Negative

Microscopic

WBC	Male 0–2/ hpf Female 0–5/ hpf
RBC	Male 0–3/hpf Female 0–4/hpf
Casts	0–1 hyaline/lpf
Epithelial squamous	Varies with collection
Epithelial transitional	0–2
Bacteria clean catch	Occasional
Bacteria catheterized	Not seen

TIMED URINE SPECIMEN

Introduction

A 24-hour urinalysis is a timed urine collection used in the metabolic evaluation of urinary stone disease, proteinuria evaluation, and estimation of renal function via creatinine clearance, estimating residual renal function in end stage renal disease with urea and creatinine clearance. The testing is usually performed in an outpatient setting while the patient consumes their usual diet. Results are combined with detailed medical and dietary history, serum chemistry, and stone composition to guide prophylactic stone-reducing treatment.

This is a test of all the urine the body produces over a specific time period to find out how well the body is working. A 24-hour urine collection helps diagnose kidney problems. It is often done to see how much creatinine clears through the kidneys. It's also done to measure protein, hormones, minerals, and other chemical compounds.

Specimen Requirements and Procedure

Instructions for collecting a 24-hour urine sample vary by the laboratory. Typically, the patient's first voided morning urine is discarded. Subsequent urine produced for next 24 hours including the next morning's first voided specimen, is collected in containers that are provided by the laboratory. A preservative solution is added to the urine collection to stabilize the sample for later analysis. Once a full 24 hours of urine is collected, the total volume is recorded. A representative sample from the total collection is then submitted to the laboratory for analysis. Serum samples, usually calcium, potassium, uric acid, and phosphorus, are sometimes also included in the study. It is important for patients to adhere to their normal diet and activities during the collection.

Once the analysis is complete, a detailed report of the results is provided to the ordering clinician. These results are used to direct prophylactic medical management. Collecting a sample for a full 24 hours can be difficult for some patients and is certainly inconvenient.

However, it is necessary to accurately and reliably identify urinary chemistry risk factors for calculus formation as spot urine chemistry is inadequate.

A chemical composition analysis of any stone material is very helpful if available.

Diagnostic Tests

Various labs offer 24-hour urine testing which provides clinicians a detailed laboratory report stratifying stone risk based on the laboratory data points. Typically, 24-hour urine tests for nephrolithiasis prophylaxis will include urinary volume, pH, calcium, citrate, magnesium, phosphate, sulfate, oxalate, and uric acid. Supersaturation ratios for various stone types can then be calculated. In patients with a history of cystine stones or a positive cystine cyanide test, 24-hour cystine levels can also be measured.

Results, Reporting, and Critical Findings

Components of 24-hour urine exams vary by the laboratory. Components included in most standard 24-hour analyzes include urine volume, the concentration of urine calcium, oxalate, citrate and uric acid, urine pH level, and supersaturation values. Supersaturation of calcium oxalate, calcium phosphate, and uric acid are commonly reported. Other analytes include urine potassium, magnesium, phosphorus, ammonium, chloride, sulfate, and nitrogen in the form of urea. Reports typically include reference range values that help stratify the risk of stone formation. Specialized testing is also available for pediatric patients and patients with cystinuria. These tests include cysteine excretion, supersaturation, and urine pH. The interpretation of urine chemistry requires reference ranges. Urine chemistry is a continuous variable making the strict cut-off points and abnormal values somewhat arbitrary. As urinary constituents reach outside of normal or optimal ranges, the lithogenic risk increases.

Below is a summary of the key components of the 24-hour urinalysis and their importance.

Urine Volume and Creatinine

Decreased urine volume is a major risk factor for stone disease as concentrated urine raises the supersaturation of all stone-forming salts. A prospective trial by Borghi et al. in 1999 helped define a goal urinary volume level of 2,500 mL per day to reduce stone risk. Furthermore, urine volumes over this amount can decrease stone risk even further.

Urine creatinine excretion is used to determine the accuracy of a timed urine collection. As a byproduct of muscle metabolism, the excretion of creatinine is relatively stable based on muscle mass. The average daily excretion of creatinine for males is 18 to 24 mg/kg and 15 to 20 mg/kg for females. Thus, a lower than expected creatinine excretion suggests an incomplete collection.

pH

Human urine has a pH typically between 4.5 and 8.0. Urine pH is a critical data point as changes in urine pH can drive the crystallization of certain salts. Crystallization of calcium phosphate, calcium oxalate, uric acid, cystine, and struvite are all pH-dependent. Calcium oxalate precipitation is typically not as pH-dependent as the others. Uric acid stone risk is greatest in the acidic range below 5.5. Calcium phosphate crystals form in an alkaline environment of 6.5 and above. Average urine pH over a 24-hour period should fall between 5.7 to 6.3, which limits pH-dependent stone formation.

Sodium and Potassium

Urinary sodium excretion roughly equates to dietary sodium intake. As urinary sodium increases, urinary calcium excretion increases. Because of this relationship, control of dietary sodium is key to controlling hypercalciuria. Lower sodium diets typically allow for up to 1,500 mg of dietary sodium per day. Urinary potassium concentration is most useful in monitoring compliance of treatments such as potassium citrate. Potassium citrate supplements should result in marked increases in urinary potassium secretion.

Magnesium

Magnesium is an inhibitor of urinary crystallization thus decreasing stone risk. Roughly half of the dietary magnesium is excreted in the urine. Low urine magnesium is typically dietary in origin.

Calcium

Elevated urinary calcium concentration can be found in nearly half of patients forming calcium stones. Urine calcium concentration is dependent on dietary calcium, sodium intake, and protein intake. Moderate calcium intake is typically recommended to limit urinary excretion while maintaining bone health. Diets low in calcium can be lithogenic, due to increased oxalate absorption in a low calcium diet. Modulation of urine calcium is often accomplished with diet changes or medications depending on etiology.

Citrate

Citrate is a potent inhibitor of calcium salt crystallization. Hypocitraturia is a common risk factor for stone disease and can be found in up to a third of calcium stone formers. Low urinary citrate can be from a variety of factors including diet, metabolic acidosis, or hypokalemia. Hypocitraturia can also be idiopathic. Citrate can be found in foods such as citrus juice. Most patients with low urinary citrate require supplementation as dietary means alone is insufficient.

Concentrated citrate supplements such as potassium citrate are commonly available. Optimal urinary citrate levels are roughly 300 mg per 1,000 mL of urine. Low urinary citrate levels in the setting of thiazide therapy may correlate with hypokalemia. A 24-hour urine study is used to monitor urinary citrate concentration and resultant urinary pH level. Over alkalinizing, the urine can predispose to calcium phosphate stones if the pH consistently exceeds 7.0.

Oxalate

High urine oxalate is another common abnormality in the urine of calcium stone formers. Roughly a third of calcium stone formers will have elevated urine oxalate. Oxalate is both endogenous and dietary. Dietary oxalate is absorbed in the colon and distal portions of the ileum. Normal oxalate excretion ranges from around 40 to 50 mg per day. Reductions in excretion can have goals as low as 25 mg per day. Dietary sources of oxalate include black tea, nuts, chocolate and green leafy vegetables like spinach. Excessive vitamin C supplements are also metabolized to oxalate in the urine. For this reason, vitamin C supplements should be limited to 1000 mg or less daily. Enteric hyperoxaluria can be a significant risk factor for patients with inflammatory bowel disease, cystic fibrosis, pancreatic insufficiency, or previous bariatric bowel surgery.

SPUTUM CULTURE

A sputum culture is a test that checks for bacteria or another type of organism that may be causing an infection in lungs or the airways leading to the lungs. Sputum, also known as phlegm, is a thick type of mucus made in your lungs. If you have an infection or chronic illness affecting the lungs or airways, it can make you cough up sputum.

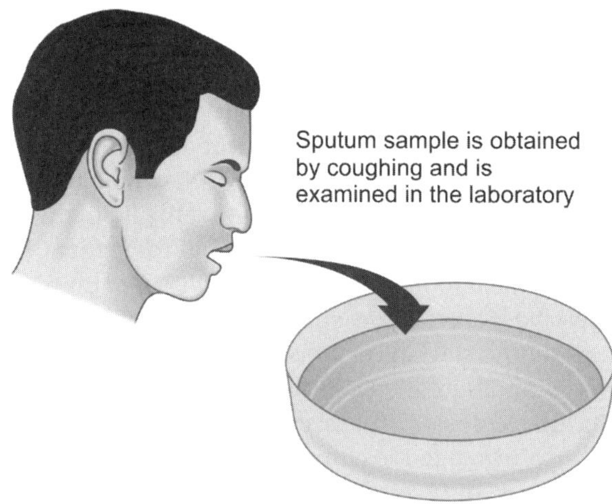

Mucus is the fluid secreted by the airways (also known as bronchial and windpipes) and lungs. In the setting of an infection or a longstanding health condition, the term phlegm is also used.

Sputum can be one of several different colors. The colors can help identify the type of infection. Patient may have or if a chronic illness has become worse:

❖ **Clear:** This usually means no disease is present, but large amounts of clear sputum may be a sign of lung disease.

❖ **White or gray:** This may also be normal, but increased amounts may mean lung disease.

❖ **Dark yellow or green:** This often means a bacterial infection, such as pneumonia. Yellowish-green sputum is also common in people with cystic fibrosis. Cystic fibrosis is an inherited disease that causes mucus to build up in the lungs and other organs.

❖ **Brown:** This often shows up in people who smoke. It is also a common sign of black lung disease. Black lung disease is a serious condition that can happen if you have long-term exposure to coal dust.

❖ **Pink:** This may be a sign of pulmonary edema, a condition in which excess fluid builds up in the lungs. Pulmonary edema is common in people with congestive heart failure.

❖ **Red:** This may be an early sign of lung cancer. It may also be a sign of a pulmonary embolism, a life-threatening condition in which a blood clot from a leg or other part of the body breaks loose and travels to the lungs.

❖ **Other names:** Respiratory culture, bacterial sputum culture, routine sputum culture.

Specimen Requirements and Procedure

The procedure of sputum specimen collection is usually non-invasive. In medicine, it is comparatively simple. However, in some clinical settings, the approach may be more vigorous due to the inability of the patient to expel such fluid from the upper respiratory tract. Thus, some maneuvers of physiotherapy may be considered adjuvant for getting some material for the analysis. Commonly, the "deep cough" sample of the early morning is collected before eating or drinking anything to avoid bias in interpreting the results. At first, the patients need to rinse out the mouth with clear water for 10–15 seconds to eliminate any contaminants in the oral cavity. After expelling saliva, the patients then breathe in deeply three times to cough at 2-minutes intervals until bringing up some sputum. The sputum is then released in a sterile well-closed container provided by the medical professionals to the patient.

The medical professionals will check the amount and gross qualities of the sputum, which should be thick to allow a proper investigation by the laboratory medical staff. In several institutions, clear and runny samples are not acceptable for further microscopic or microbiological studies. In some settings, the procedure can be repeated until 10 to 20 mL of sputum sample has been collected. It is paramount that the lid of the container where the first fluid is collected is changed to avoid contaminations. If the patient has difficulties coughing up enough sputum, the medical professionals may apply some physiotherapeutic maneuvers, which allow the progressive release of the sputum. Routine sputum culture requires that one sample is collected and sent to the lab on the same day of collection. If the patient leaves the specimen in the refrigerator after collection, there is often a tolerance range, which may run well over 24 hours. In tuberculosis (TB), three sputum samples must be collected on three consecutive days and be returned to the clinical lab each day.

Sputum induction is a procedure used to collect adequate lower respiratory secretions from patients who have trouble producing sputum to aid the diagnosis of TB. In particular, patients with suspicion of miliary tuberculosis and/or tuberculous pleural effusion are often targeted using this adjuvant procedure. In such settings, the patient inhales nebulized hypertonic saline solution to liquefy airway secretions. This solution stimulates the patient's coughing and promotes the expectoration of airway secretions. The medical professionals prepare a 20 mL 3% hypertonic saline solution and inject it into the nebulizer cup filled with water. Similar to the non-adjuvant procedure, the patients are always required to wash their mouths thoroughly.

Moreover, the patients wear the nebulizer cup to cover the face and nose after sitting in an upright position. The patients inhale and exhale through the mouthpiece. An expectorate saliva into an emesis bowl and expectorate sputum coughed up are collected into a sterile well-closed container. The medical staff turns on the nebulizer device to allow the patient to inhale the hypertonic mist for approximately five minutes. Then the patients take several deep breaths before attempting to cough. If there are difficulties for the patients to cough up the sputum, the medical staff may use gentle chest physiotherapy to aid the patients to produce sputum. During the procedure, the patients should be observed closely by the medical staff to identify any potential rupture of pleural bullae, triggering a life-threatening pneumothorax. The patients should stop when 1 to 2 mL sputum specimen is collected for each sample or reach 15 minutes of nebulization, or the patient complains of chest tightness, dyspnea, or wheeze. Imaging is advised if there is the persistence of these symptoms at the end of the sputum collection.

Bronchoscopy is a procedure used to investigate the throat and airway through a thin viewing camera. It is also used to collect the sputum samples in some special situations such as a persistent infection, cough, or something unusual seen on clinical laboratory tests or chest X-rays. The sputum specimen will be examined under a microscope to detect whether abnormal cells are present. Flexible bronchoscopy is used more often than rigid bronchoscopy to collect the sputum samples. Before having a flexible bronchoscopy, the doctor may give the patient anesthetic to relax the throat muscles and numb the mouth, nasal passages, or throat. The procedure is performed using a thin and lighted bronchoscope inserted through the mouth or nose, down to the throat into the windpipe (trachea), and then to the major bronchi leading to the lungs. Sputum samples may be taken using the devices passed through the bronchoscope by the doctor.

Diagnostic Tests

Clinical diagnostic sputum tests aim to detect the causes of lower respiratory tract infections and some other diseases. It also provides an efficacious tool for monitoring the effectiveness of clinical treatment. Sputum culture is the most common test needed to be performed when the patient has pneumonia. It is used to identify the bacteria or fungi causing the airways or lung infection.

Sputum smear microscopy is the initial step taken in laboratory sputum analysis. It is a fast and inexpensive technique, precisely, in resource-limited settings. Gram stain is used to differentiate bacteria into two broad groups (gram-positive and gram-negative microorganisms). The Gram stain is the first staining technique performed in preliminary bacterial identification, which helps determine if there is an adequate amount of pathogens in the culture and make a definitive diagnosis. It is also crucial because it can address antibiotic therapy more specifically. With the Gram stain, the bacterial species are distinguished into gram-positive and gram-negative groups by the differences in cell walls' physical and chemical properties. Some bacteria have a thick peptidoglycan layer cell wall stained with crystal violet (gram-positive).

In contrast, some other bacteria have a thinner peptidoglycan layer stained red or pink by counterstain (gram-negative). When the physician suspects that the patient may have TB, acid-fast bacilli (AFB), stain testing must be performed. TB is a lung infection disease caused by *Mycobacterium tuberculosis*. Mycobacteria are a group of rod-shaped acid-fast bacilli. They can be distinguished under the microscope after an AFB staining procedure where the bacilli retain the stain color after an acid-fast wash. The Grocott-Gomori's methenamine silver stain (GMS) is a standard staining method used to detect fungal microorganisms. GMS staining is critical in identifying Pneumocystis jirovecii. This microorganism first appeared in patients with human immunodeficiency virus (HIV) infection in the 1980s, and it was used to be classified as a protozoan. This microorganism, which is now classified as a fungus, was initially called Pneumocystis carinii. Colony morphology is a method that describes the characteristics of an individual colony of bacteria growing on agar in a Petri dish. It can help the lab technologist to identify some specific bacteria.

However, only relying on microscopic observation and colony morphology maybe not be enough to get the relevant information of the species and genus of etiologic microorganisms. Biochemical tests of bacterial growth are the next step to perform to recognize the bacteria.

The common biochemical tests used to identify bacterial growth include motility, McFarland standard, fluid thioglycollate medium (FTM), catalase, and oxidase tests.

Respiratory viruses have been tested in sputum specimens from patients with cystic fibrosis, asthma, and chronic obstructive pulmonary disease (COPD). Typically, viral testing is also performed on upper airway samples such as nasopharyngeal swabs or nasal washes. However, some viral pathogens such as severe acute respiratory syndrome (SARS) coronavirus, H1N1 influenza, Middle Eastern respiratory syndrome coronavirus (MERS-CoV), and SARS coronavirus 2 (SARS-CoV-2), the causative agent of Coronavirus Virus Disease 2019 (COVID-19), may be absent in upper airway secretions. So the sputum samples are also frequently used for viral diagnosis testing by using the clinical real-time polymerase chain reaction (RT-PCR) method or the newly developed next-generation sequencing (NGS) method. Potentially, face masks, which reduce the aerosol-related risk of transmission in the current era of the COVID-19 pandemic, may also represent a useful source for NGS investigations.

Sputum cytology examination is using a microscope to determine whether abnormal cells are present in sputum samples. The thin layer of sputum placed on a slide before specific staining and diagnosed directly under the microscope helps find out some abnormal cells. Sputum cytology helps detect both lung cancer cells and non-cancer cellular and acellular material useful for the diagnosis of conditions such as pneumonia, tuberculosis, interstitial lung diseases, or pneumoconiosis (e.g., asbestosis). Hematoxylin and eosin stain is the worldwide most performed tissue stain in medical laboratory diagnosis. It is often considered the gold standard. It is mostly used for suspected lung cancer samples. Periodic acid–Schiff (PAS) stain is used to detect polysaccharides and mucosubstances in tissue specimens. It is mainly helpful for the detection of living fungi in sputum specimens.

Further, Wright stain, Giemsa stain, and Wright-Giemsa mixture stain are used for staining the sputum smears. These stain methods facilitate the differentiation of blood cell types by using specific solutions. These staining methods help detect abnormal white blood cells of sputum, which are vital signs of lung infection.

Sputum molecular analysis is a new insight and advanced technique used to detect lung cancer-related biomarkers to assist in the early stage of a lung cancer diagnosis. Many DNA mutations, such as p53, KRAS, EML4-ALK, and GFR mutations, have been investigated on sputum specimens. DNA hypermethylation has also been reported in lung cancer sputum samples. Loss of heterozygosity (LOH) and microsatellite instability (MSI) have been found in lung cancer patients' sputum specimens by using DNA markers. MicroRNAs (miRNAs) such as miR-21 and miR-155, proteins such as proliferation-inducing ligand (APRIL) and complement factor H were significantly overexpressed, and some messenger RNAs (mRNAs) such as APRIL, MAGE, Telomerase, CEA, et al., have been found rapidly degraded in sputum specimens of lung cancer patients by RT-PCR and immunocytochemistry. Still, other molecular biomarkers such as free DNA and mitochondrial DNA (mtDNA) variants seem to exhibit some promise.

Finally, sputum antimicrobial susceptibility testing is performed on the bacteria or fungi, leading to lung infection after being identified in a sputum culture sample. The most common approaches consist of the disk diffusion and minimum inhibitory concentration (MIC) methods. These tests are used to detect the effectiveness of the specific antibiotics on the bacteria or to detect whether the bacteria have already developed resistance to certain antibiotics or not. The results of antimicrobial susceptibility testing help to select the most likely effective antibiotics in treating lung infection.

Testing Procedures

Sputum Culture Procedure

The sputum sample is added to a culture plate with a specific substance that promotes the growth of bacteria or fungi. Then cover the lid of the dish and place it in a 37°C incubator for bacteria and 30°C for fungus. The lab specialist should check the bacteria or fungi growth in the sputum plate every day. Once the sputum culture is positive, microscopy, colony morphology, or biochemical tests of bacterial growth will be performed to identify the specific type of bacterium or fungus.

Sputum Staining Tests Procedure

The sputum specimen is a smear on a microscope slide. Different staining dyes are added to the cells, bacteria, or fungi of the sample on the slides and then washed with water, alcohol, or acid solutions. The slides are then diagnosed under a microscope. If the bacteria, fungi, or specific cells are identified in the specimens, the results are positive.

Sputum Biochemical Tests Procedure

To identify a suspected organism, at first, the bacteria will be inoculated in a series of differential media. Then use different indicators to observe the specific end products of metabolism inside of the medium.

Sputum Cytology Examination Procedure

The smear sputum slide is stained with different dyes according to the instructions. Then the pathology specialist examines the stained slide under the microscope to find the abnormal cells from the sputum specimen.

Sputum Nucleic Acid Amplification Test Procedure

The RNA or DNA is extracted from the sputum specimen according to the instruction of different commercial kits. The DNA or RNA is added to a PCR reaction tube with designed primers, Taq polymerase, deoxynucleoside triphosphates [dNTPs], and a fluorescent-labeled probe. Then the tube with RT-PCR reaction mixture is placed in a real-time PCR device for amplifying the molecules at specific temperatures.

Sputum Antimicrobial Susceptibility Tests Procedure

For the MIC method, the bacteria or fungi isolated from sputum specimens were diluted in saline and swabbed onto the MIC panels. For the dish diffusion method, selected different concentrations of antibiotics are placed directly onto the bacteria swabbed agar plates. Panels or plates are incubated at 35°C for about 16 to 18 hours or longer. The minimal concentration of the antibiotic that inhibits the growth of organisms or MIC panel is read according to the guidelines of different manufacturers. Then the result is reported.

Interfering Factors

Many interfering factors affect the results of every step of the sputum diagnosis. Any deviation from the standard procedure of sample collection, culture, staining, biochemical, molecular, and antimicrobial susceptibility tests can significantly impact the diagnostic result, directly affecting the patient's clinical management. Therefore, strict laboratory workflow procedures and well-trained laboratory technologists are required to perform the sputum analysis.

Collecting a good quality sputum sample is the first step for getting and, the pathogens identified from sputum culture do not always originate from lower respiratory tract infections because they may be part of contaminant sites or preexisting in the oral flora. Thus, standard microbiological procedures for organisms' isolation and identification are critical for the sputum quality assessment (QA).

QA remains an essential tool in the lab for distinguishing the real respiratory pathogens from the possible colonizing flora. Finally, it is vital to check the quality of commercial products that need to be approved by the United States Food and Drug Administration, the Public Health Agency of Canada, and European and Australian similar agencies. Inferior quality culture plates, expired staining kits, or ineffective molecular biology kits are directly related to poor performance. Several agencies determine the quality performed in a laboratory, and the College of the American Pathologists plays a major in dictating laboratory standards and quality control procedures, which are essential to avoid different interfering factors.

Results, Reporting, and Critical Findings

Sputum Culture

If the pathogenicity organisms grow after 24 hours of incubation in the culture dish, the result is positive. Some sample dishes will keep incubating longer, depending on microbial flora present and the need to identify and semiquantitative isolates and perform antimicrobial susceptibility tests. Conversely, if no bacteria or fungi grow in 6 to 8 weeks for solid culture media or six weeks for liquid culture media, the result is negative.

Sputum Staining Tests

Gram stain test: The bacteria detected by the test will be gram-positive or gram-negative.

Common gram-positive bacteria include *Staphylococcus, Streptococcus, Bacillus, Listeria, Enterococcus,* and *Clostridium.*

Common gram-negative bacteria include *E. coli, Klebsiella, Proteus* and *Pseudomonas aeruginosa.*

AFB stain test: The bacteria detected by the test will be positive or negative.

- ❖ **AFB stain test positive result:** The acid-fast bacilli, such as *Mycobacterium tuberculosis,* retain the red or pink color.
- ❖ **AFB stain test negative result:** No red or pink bacteria are found in the stained slide.
- ❖ **GMS stain test:** The fungal organisms detected by the test will be positive or negative.
- ❖ **GMS test positive result:** Black or brown wall from fungal organisms or worms such as Pneumocystis jirovecii are found.
- ❖ **GMS test negative result:** No black or brown stained fungal organisms or worms are found.

Sputum biochemical tests: The motility, McFarland standard, catalase, and oxidase tests are positive or negative.

Organisms motility test: The test is performed in gram-negative enteric bacilli, and the result will be either motile or nonmotile.

Motile (positive): Organisms will spread out from the stab line and produce cloudiness or turbidity throughout the medium.

Nonmotile (negative): Organisms will remain along the stab line of inoculation.

McFarland standard test: The test is used to standardize the number of bacteria in liquid suspensions by the turbidity of bacteria in the McFarland standard vial or tube. The test result arises by comparing the turbidity of a bacterial suspension to different concentrations of McFarland standard solutions.

FTM test: The test is used to detect the aerotolerance of bacteria.

Obligate aerobes, such as *Pseudomonas spp.*, requiring oxygen for growth, will only grow toward the oxygen-rich surface layer.

Obligate anaerobes, which cannot grow with oxygen, will only grow on the bottom of the tube.

Microaerophiles frequently grow below the oxygen-rich layer.

Gram-negative, facultative or aerotolerant anaerobes generally can grow throughout the broth but will mostly grow between the oxygen-rich and oxygen-free area.

Catalase test: The test is used to differentiate staphylococci from streptococci by detecting the presence of catalase.

Catalase-positive: The organisms can produce catalase, which will generate oxygen bubbles after adding 3% hydrogen peroxide.

Catalase-negative: The organisms cannot produce catalase, and there is no reaction after adding 3% hydrogen peroxide.

Oxidase test: The test is used to detect the presence of cytochrome coxidases.

Oxidase-positive: There is a deep purple-blue or blue color change within 10 to 30 seconds.

Oxidase-negative: No purple-blue color or no color change.

Sputum Nucleic Acid Amplification Test

If the RT-PCR amplification is successful, the result is positive. However, if it is not successful, the result is negative.

Sputum Cytology Examination

If a few white blood cells and no abnormal cells have been found in the sputum sample, that means the sputum cytology examination is regular, and other reasons may cause the patient's symptoms.

Sputum Antimicrobial Susceptibility Test

If antibiotics inhibit the growth of an organism, that means the antibiotics are working to treat the patient infected by the organism, and the antibiotics are susceptible. Conversely, if the antibiotic does not inhibit the organism's growth, it means the antibiotics are not adequate for the patient's treatment, and the antibiotics are resistant.

RADIO DIAGNOSIS

Computed Tomography (CT)

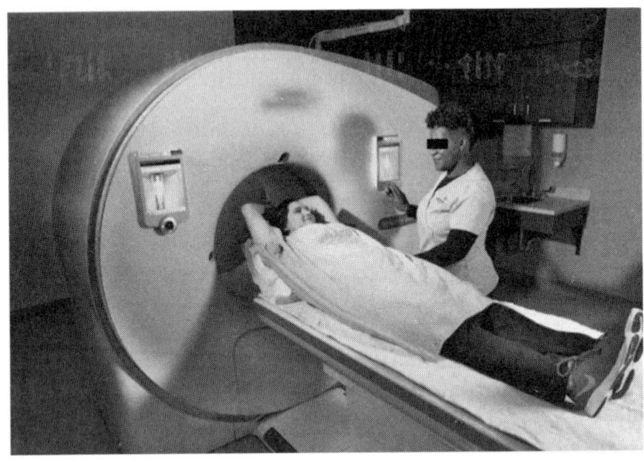

Breast Imaging

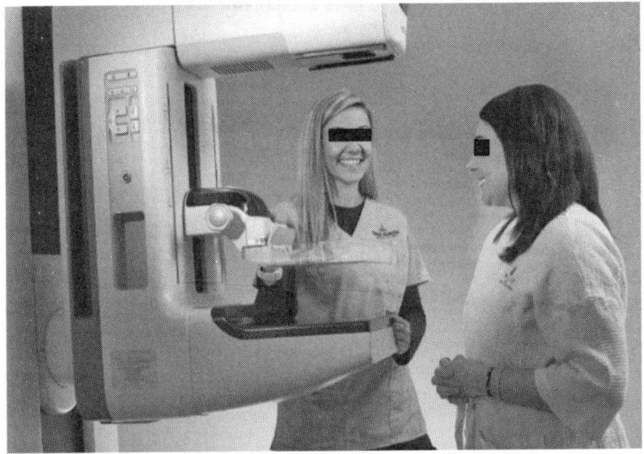

Ultrasound

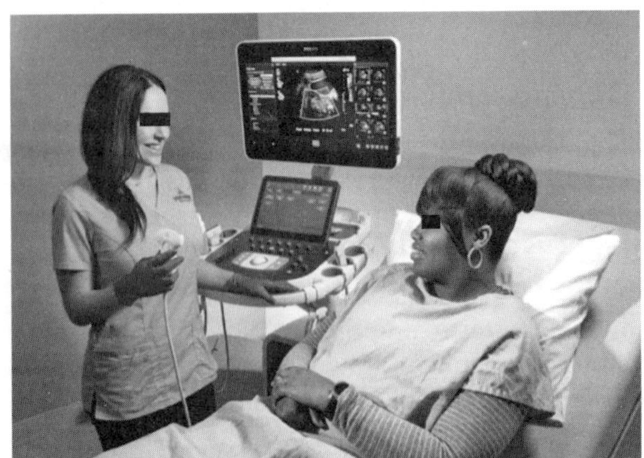

X-ray

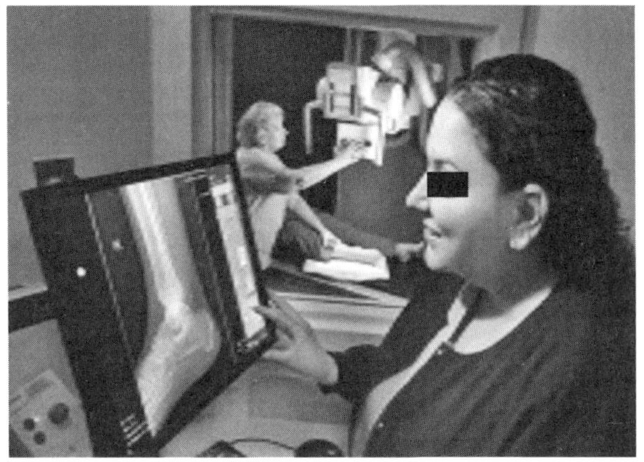

PET/CT

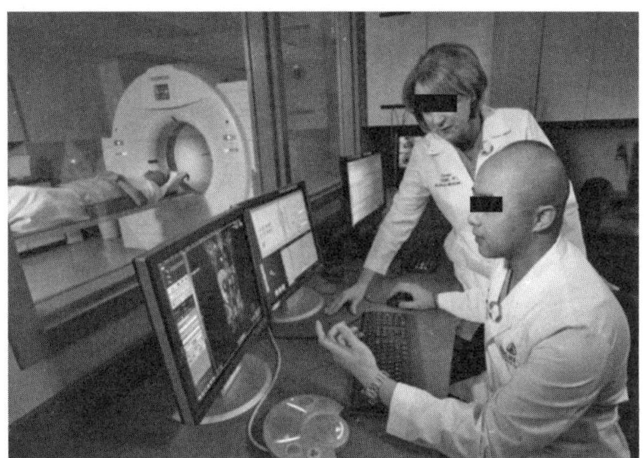

Central Venous Access Ports

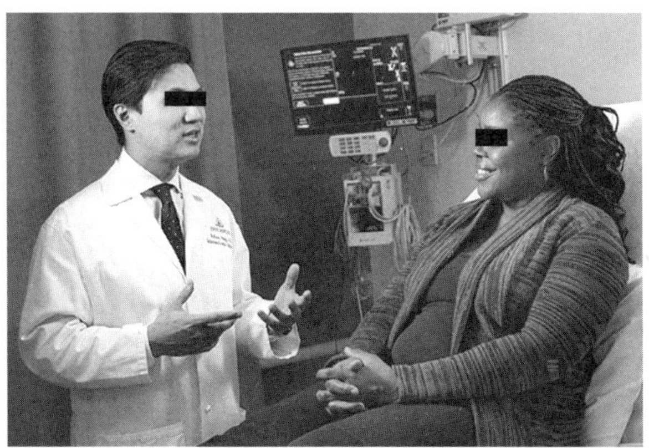

Pediatrics Imaging

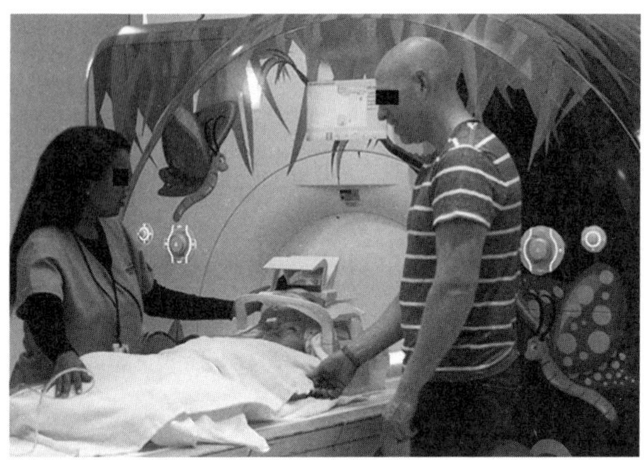

DEXA (Dual X-Ray Absorptiometry) Scan

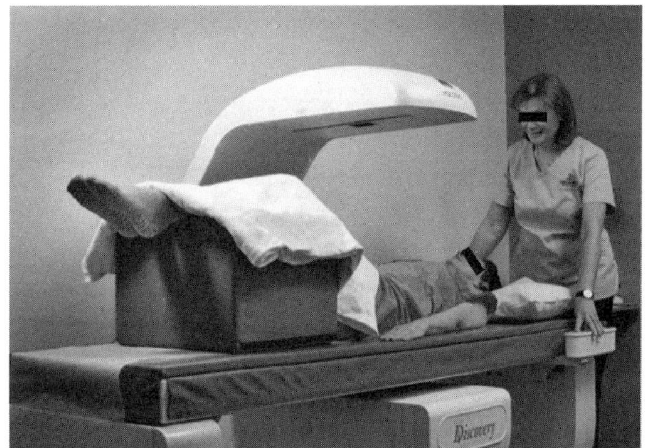

Prostate Artery Embolization

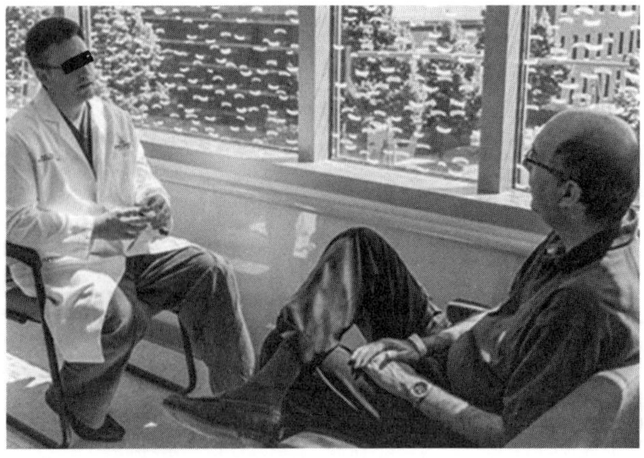

The Radio Diagnosis and Imaging Services as you know are one of the most important diagnostic armaments with any medical practitioner. With increasing complexities of disease profile, there is increasing need to improve diagnostic approach (early and precise) and therapeutic modalities to achieve best patient care. The metamorphoses in medical technology, with application of bio-physics and computer sciences, have made available the newer modalities in the field of Radiology and Imaging Services. However, with advancement, the service has also become more expensive and at times unaffordable and hence it is very essential to manage these activities very effectively and efficiently.

Radiology is the field of medicine that uses imaging techniques (such as X-rays) to diagnose and treat disease. It may be used diagnostically in order to determine if a medical condition is present or not (such as finding a lung cancer), interventionally as a procedure (such as removing a blood clot in an artery), or as a treatment. such as giving radiation therapy to treat cancer.

TYPES OF SERVICES

Conventionally radiology services are linked with X-rays. However, ever-changing need for more and more information and introduction of newer technology has definitely revolutionized these services to a great extent.

The radiology is linked to images of human body, and these images can be achieved either by transmission or by emission from a source. Transmission is a technique where there is a source which emits rays and which are picked up after reflection from body part and taken on plate or on screen (films) and studied by competent professional. The modalities under this group are X-rays, CT scan, ultrasound.

Emission is a technique which involves giving a dose of radioisotopes or radionuclides to the patient, which are picked up by target organs or cells and emitted gamma rays are recorded by gamma or scintillation camera.

X-rays

X-ray is oldest radio diagnostic tool. The principle is transmission of rays from a source to the specified part of body and images will be formed. It still remains effective modality and number of X-rays performed has been on increase, but total percentage has been declining with the advent of newer modalities.

Computed Tomography (CT)

Computed axial tomography (CAT scans or CT scans) use a series of X-rays plus a computer to produce a cross-sectional image of the inside of the body. CT provides more detail than an X-ray, and can better define areas where tissues overlap. CT scans can detect smaller abnormalities than can be found with a conventional X-ray.

The use of contrast dyes for CT scan can further improve visualization in some areas, such as the digestive tract. In some situations, CT procedures such as CT angiography may provide information that would otherwise require a more invasive procedure.

Magnetic Resonance Imaging (MRI)

Magnetic resonance imaging uses strong magnetic fields and radio waves to produce images of the inside of the body. While CT is often a better method for evaluating bones and blood vessels,

MRI is frequently a better test for evaluating soft tissue, such as the brain, spinal cord, nerves, muscles, tendons, and breast tissue.

With brain, spinal cord, and peripheral nerve disorders, MRI has allowed healthcare providers to diagnose conditions that could only be assumed clinically in the past. For example, practitioners can now diagnose multiple sclerosis with an MRI, a diagnosis that was limited to an assessment of symptoms alone before MRI was available (and could only be confirmed on an autopsy).

For breast cancer screening, MRI is more accurate than mammography, but the higher price makes it impractical for people who do not have underlying risk factors for breast cancer (such as a strong family history, BRCA mutation, or a history of childhood cancer). A newer technique called fast MRI is a rapid, much less expensive test that may be more accurate in detecting early breast cancer in the future.

Other than PET/CT (see below), most imaging techniques are structural but not functional. This means that they reveal the structure of an area of the body but do provide information as to function. One form MRI called functional MRI, can, however, give an estimate of brain activity.

As with CT, contrast is often used to better define regions that are being scanned, with a common agent being gadolinium. Magnetic resonance technology may also be used as an alternative to more invasive procedures at times, such as with magnetic resonance angiography (MRA).

An advantage of MRI is that it does not use ionizing radiation, which has been linked to an increased risk of cancer, especially in children. Three limitations include the cost, body mass index (MRI is difficult in very overweight people), and that it may not be used in people who have metal in their body.

Ultrasound

Ultrasound uses sound waves (acoustic energy) to produce moving images of a part of the body. Best known as a method for examining a fetus during pregnancy, ultrasound is particularly helpful with some medical conditions:

- ❖ Breast ultrasound can often distinguish breast cysts from masses. Cysts may be aspirated under ultrasound guidance and their disappearance can be reassuring as well (no further evaluation may be needed).
- ❖ Heart ultrasound (echocardiogram) can be used to evaluate the heart valves, heart motion, the pericardium (lining of the heart), and more. This procedure may be done by placing a transducer on the skin overlying the heart, or instead via a transducer that is threaded into the esophagus (transesophageal echocardiogram).
- ❖ Thyroid ultrasound can be used to evaluate thyroid nodules.
- ❖ Abdominal ultrasound is often used to look for gallstones as well as other medical conditions.
- ❖ Pelvic ultrasound is often used to look for ovarian cysts.

Ultrasound does not involve radiation, and is therefore safe in pregnancy. Since it is dependent on finding contrast (such as between a solid mass and a fluid-filled mass), it is less helpful in distinguishing conditions where such a contrast in tissue density is not present.

Fluoroscopy

Fluoroscopy uses X-rays, but in real time, to create moving images of the body. In some settings, these real-time images are particularly important.

For example, fluoroscopy may be used to note the change in flow of contrast in joints associated with different movements, in the digestive tract with an upper gastrointestinal or barium enema study, or to monitor progress during the insertion of a pacemaker.

Due to continuous monitoring (multiple images taken over time), the radiation exposure with fluoroscopy is significantly higher than that of conventional X-rays.

Nuclear Medicine Scans

Nuclear medicine imaging includes techniques that use radioactive material ("radioactive tracers") that are then detected by a camera in order to produce images of the inside of the body. While most imaging methods are considered structural, that is, they describe structures on the inside of the body, these scans are used to evaluate how regions of the body function.

In some cases, the radioactive substance may also be used to treat a cancer (such as the use of radioactive iodine to treat thyroid cancer).

Examples of nuclear medicine scans include:

Positron emission tomography (PET scan): With a PET scan, radioactive glucose (sugar) is injected into a vein, and then a positron emission scanner is used to record the radiation emitted. The radioactive glucose concentrates in areas of the body with a high metabolic rate (i.e., are actively growing). PET scans are commonly used to evaluate for the presence of cancer metastases anywhere in the body. They can be particularly helpful in some situations in which a diagnosis is uncertain. For example, in someone who has had cancer, it may be difficult to determine if an abnormal region in the lungs (or elsewhere) is due to a new and actively growing tumor, or instead is old scar tissue related to previous treatment.

Single Photon Emission Computed Tomography (SPECT)

Bone scan: With a bone scan, a radioactive tracer is injected which is taken up by bones. These scans may identify cancer in the bones, a bone infection (osteomyelitis), fractures (such as stress fractures that may be missed on a plain X-ray), and more.

Thyroid scan (radioactive iodine uptake test): In a thyroid scan, radioactive iodine is injected into a vein, and a camera determines the pattern of its uptake in the thyroid gland. It is used most commonly to look for causes of hyperthyroidism.

Thallium and Cardiolite stress tests: During a stress test, a radioactive tracer (thallium-201 or cardiolite) is injected. The tracer can help determine how different parts of the heart are functioning, and hence, the presence of coronary artery disease.

Arthrogram

Sentinel lymph node mapping/biopsy: With cancers such as breast cancer or melanoma, the cancer usually spreads first to specific lymph nodes referred to as the sentinel nodes. Evaluating these nodes for the presence of cancer can help stage the cancer. A tracer is injected directly into a tumor and allowed to follow the lymphatic pathway that would be followed by cancer cells as they spread. These nodes can subsequently be biopsied (by using a camera in order to locate them).

Virtual Colonoscopy

Molecular Imaging

Additional specialized techniques referred to as molecular imaging may also be used. This includes procedures such as CT perfusion, dual-energy CT, and optical imaging.

Interventional Radiology Procedures

There are now a multitude of interventional radiology procedures available. In many cases, these "minimally invasive" procedures can replace more invasive measures (such as surgery) that were used in the past.

In turn, these techniques may have fewer complications, involve smaller incisions, cause less discomfort, and help people recuperate more rapidly than had been possible in the past. They are often less expensive. Some of the conditions that may be treated in this way are listed below.

To Detect and Open a Blocked Blood Vessel

Blood vessels (either arteries or veins) that are blocked in the heart, legs, and lungs may be treated with interventional procedures.

Coronary artery blockages: Narrowing or blockages in the coronary arteries may be treated with angiography, angioplasty, and stent placement. In these procedures, a wire is inserted into the artery and a balloon used to open the narrowing in the artery. As an alternative, a clot busting medication may be injected to open the artery instead.

A stent may then be placed to keep the artery open and allow blood to flow to a portion of the heart that would otherwise be damaged. If an artery is blocked acutely in the heart (heart attack) or extremities, clot-blasting medicine may be injected to first open the artery followed by stent placement if needed.

Deep venous thrombosis (blood clots in the veins of the legs or pelvis): When detected, clot blasting medication (thrombolytics) may be injected via a catheter placed in a vein with the help of imaging. A balloon or stent placement may then be used.

Stents may also be placed in blood vessels that are compressed by a tumor and leading to complications.

Pulmonary emboli: When blood clots (deep vein thromboses) occur in the legs or pelvis, they may break off and travel to the lungs (pulmonary emboli). When there is a large clot in the lungs, a radiologist may sometimes insert a catheter into the artery to break up the clot.

For people who have recurrent clots in their legs, a radiologist may also insert a filter into the large blood vessel returning blood to the heart (the inferior vena cava). In this case, the filter may prevent pulmonary emboli from occurring.

To Block a Blood Vessel

Alternatively, interventional radiology may be used to block a vessel. Vein embolization may be done for varicose veins, whereas artery embolization (uterine artery embolization) may be done to treat fibroids.

Treatment of Aneurysms

Aneurysms are sections of an artery that are dilated and weak and hence, are subject to rupture or bleed. Via interventional radiology, a radiologist may place a stent graft in the region of an aneurysm thus essentially relining the blood vessel.

To Control Bleeding

As an alternative to surgery, interventional radiology may be used to control bleeding (hemorrhage) in conditions ranging from gastrointestinal bleeding, to postpartum bleeding, to trauma. Bleeding may be controlled by blocking a blood vessel (as noted above), placing a stent, using a balloon to apply pressure, and more.

Central Line Placement

When a person is seriously ill, or will be receiving caustic medications such as chemotherapy, rapid access to larger blood vessels for infusion is needed. (Peripheral veins, such as a vein in the hand or forearm, are often insufficient.) Examples of central lines include ports and PICC lines.

Feeding Tube Placement

The placement of feeding tubes (gastrostomy, jejunostomy) are a relatively common interventional radiology procedure. These are frequently used when a person is unable to eat food for any reason.

Tissue Biopsies

A number of different types of biopsy procedures may be performed by a radiologist, and are often guided by ultrasound or CT. Examples include needle biopsies and stereotactic biopsies.

Cancer Treatment

In addition to radiation therapy (discussed below), a number of interventional radiology procedures may be used to treat either a primary tumor or metastases (cancer that has spread).

Tumors may be addressed by ablative treatment (treatments that destroy tumors) such as radio frequency ablation or microwave ablation, or instead by tumor embolization (blocking a blood vessel that feeds a tumor so that the tumor dies).

Alternatively, either chemotherapy or radiation can be directly delivered to an area of tumor or metastasis (chemoembolization/radioembolization).

For Fractured Vertebrae

Procedures known as vertebroplasty or kyphoplasty can be used to treat collapsed vertebrae. In these procedures, a cement type substance is injected by the radiologist to effectively repair a fracture.

To Treat Blockages

When blockages occur in different regions of the body, an interventional radiologist may apply a stent. This may be done to open up a blocked esophagus, blocked bile ducts, a blockage of the ureter draining from the kidney, or a blockage in the bowel.

Drainage

When fluid collects in a region of the body, an interventional radiologist may insert a drain to remove fluid or pus. This might be done to drain recurrent pleural effusions (fluid buildup in the area around the lungs), in the brain (shunting), and much more.

Procedures to Treat Back Pain

Radiologists now use a wide array of procedures to treat chronic back pain:

* **Radiation therapy:** There are a number of ways in which radiation therapy or proton therapy may be given, and the particular use often depends on the goal of treatment. It's thought that roughly 50% of people with cancer will undergo some form of radiation therapy.
* **External beam radiotherapy:** In external beam radiotherapy, radiation is applied from outside of the body on a table resembling a CT machine. It may be used:
  * Before surgery (neoadjuvant radiation therapy) to reduce the size of a tumor
  * After surgery (adjuvant radiation therapy) to "clean up" any leftover cancer cells and reduce the risk of recurrence
  * As a palliative therapy to reduce pain (such as with bone metastases) or an obstruction due to a tumor
* **Brachytherapy:** Brachytherapy is similar to external beam therapy except that the radiation is delivered internally, often through beads that are inserted into an area during surgery or after.
* **Stereotactic body radiotherapy (SBRT):** Stereotactic body radiotherapy (SBRT) or Cyberknife refers to a procedure in which a high dose of radiation is directed to a localized area of tissue. Unlike traditional radiation therapy, SBRT is often used with a "curative" intent, or a hope to cure a cancer rather than simply extend life or reduce symptoms.
SBRT is sometimes used to treat small tumors as an alternative to surgery, especially in people who would not be expected to tolerate surgery as well. It is also often used to treat areas of metastases, such as brain metastases due to lung cancer or breast cancer.
* **Proton beam therapy:** Proton beam therapy is similar to conventional radiation therapy but uses high energy protons instead of photons or X-rays to damage tumors. It was first used in 1990, and offers similar effectiveness to radiation therapy.
Due to the way the radiation is delivered, it may be less likely to damage nearby healthy tissue. For this reason, proton beam therapy can sometimes be used in an area that was previously treated with radiation (and thus, cannot be treated again with conventional radiation).

Endoscopic Procedures

Risks of endoscopy may include:

* Over-sedation, although sedation is not always necessary
* Feeling bloated for a short time after the procedure

- ❖ Mild cramping
- ❖ A numb throat for a few hours due to the use of local anesthetic
- ❖ Infection of the area of investigation, which most commonly occurs when additional procedures are carried out at the same time (the infections are normally minor and treatable with a course of antibiotics)
- ❖ Persistent pain in the area of the endoscopy
- ❖ Perforation or tear of the lining of the stomach or esophagus, a rare but serious complication
- ❖ Internal bleeding, usually minor and sometimes treatable by endoscopic cauterization
- ❖ Complications related to preexisting conditions

Any of the following symptoms should be reported to a doctor:
- ❖ Dark-colored stool
- ❖ Shortness of breath
- ❖ Severe and persistent abdominal pain
- ❖ Chest pain
- ❖ Vomiting blood

Types of tools include:
- ❖ **Flexible forceps:** These tong-like tools take a tissue sample.
- ❖ **Biopsy forceps:** These remove a tissue sample or a suspicious growth.
- ❖ **Cytology brushes:** These take cell samples.
- ❖ **Suture removal forceps:** These remove stitches inside the body.

Indications

To screen for and prevent cancer: For example, doctors use a type of endoscopy called a colonoscopy to screen for colorectal cancer. During a colonoscopy, doctor may remove growths called polyps.

To diagnose a disease or find out the cause of symptoms: The type of endoscopy your doctor will recommend depends on the part of the body under examination.

To give treatment: Treatments that may involve an endoscope include:
- ❖ Laparoscopic surgery, which is done through small incisions in the skin
- ❖ Laser therapy, which uses a powerful beam of light to destroy cancer cells
- ❖ Microwave ablation, which uses heat to destroy cancerous tissue
- ❖ Endoscopic mucosal resection or endoscopic submucosal dissection, which is surgery using an endoscope inserted into the gastrointestinal tract
- ❖ Photodynamic therapy, which destroys a tumor with a laser after injecting it with a light-sensitive substance
- ❖ Medication delivery, also called medication administration
- ❖ Inflammatory bowel diseases (IBD), such as ulcerative colitis (UC) and Crohn's disease
- ❖ Stomach ulcer
- ❖ Chronic constipation
- ❖ Pancreatitis
- ❖ Gallstones
- ❖ Unexplained bleeding in the digestive tract
- ❖ Tumors

❖ Infections
❖ Blockage of the esophagus
❖ Gastroesophageal reflux disease (GERD)
❖ Hiatal hernia
❖ Unusual vaginal bleeding
❖ Blood in your urine
❖ Other digestive tract issues

Types of Endoscopy

The most common types of endoscopy are listed below:

Name of procedure	Name of tool	Area or organ viewed	How endoscope reaches target area
Anoscopy	Anoscope	Anus and/or rectum	Inserted through the anus
Arthroscopy	Arthroscope	Joints	Inserted through a small incision over the joint
Bronchoscopy	Bronchoscope	Trachea, or windpipe, and the lungs	Inserted through the mouth
Colonoscopy	Colonoscope	Entire length of the colon and large intestine	Inserted through the anus
Colposcopy	Colposcope	Vagina and cervix	Placed at the vagina's opening after a tool called a speculum dilates the vagina. It is not inserted in the body
Cystoscopy	Cystoscope	Inside of the bladder	Inserted through the urethra
Esophagoscopy	Esophagoscope	Esophagus	Inserted through the mouth
Gastroscopy	Gastroscope	Stomach and duodenum, which is the beginning of the small intestine	Inserted through the mouth
Laparoscopy	Laparoscope	Stomach, liver, or other abdominal organs, including female reproductive organs, including the uterus, ovaries, and fallopian tubes	Inserted through a small, surgical opening in the abdomen
Laryngoscopy	Laryngoscope	Larynx, or voice box	Inserted through the mouth
Neuroendoscopy	Neuroendoscope	Areas of the brain	Inserted through a small incision in the skull
Proctoscopy	Proctoscope	Rectum and sigmoid colon, which is the bottom part of the colon	Inserted through the anus
Sigmoidoscopy	Sigmoidoscope	Sigmoid colon	Inserted through the anus
Thoracoscopy	Thoracoscope	Pleura, which are the two membranes covering the lungs and lining the chest cavity, and structures covering the heart	Inserted through a small surgical opening in chest

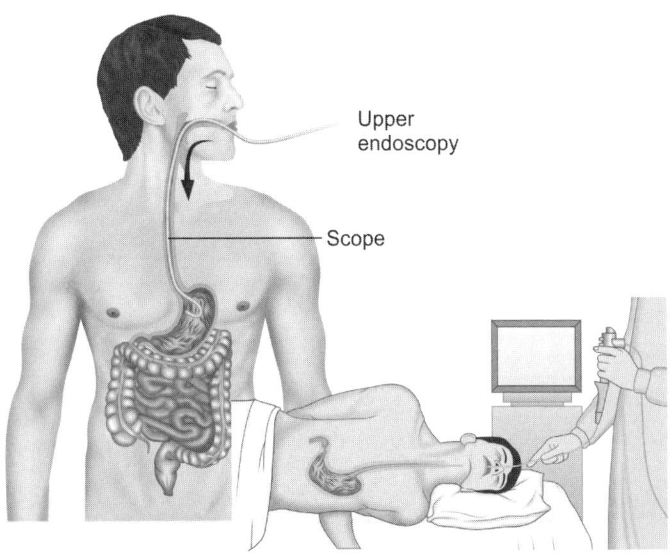

The Latest Techniques in Endoscopy Technology

Like most technologies, endoscopy is constantly advancing. Newer generations of endoscopes use high-definition imaging to create images in incredible detail. Innovative techniques also combine endoscopy with imaging technology or surgical procedures.

Here are some examples of the latest endoscopy technologies.

Capsule Endoscopy

A revolutionary procedure known as a capsule endoscopy may be used when other tests aren't conclusive. During a capsule endoscopy, you swallow a small pill with a tiny camera inside. The capsule passes through your digestive tract, without any discomfort to you, and creates thousands of images of the intestines as it moves through.

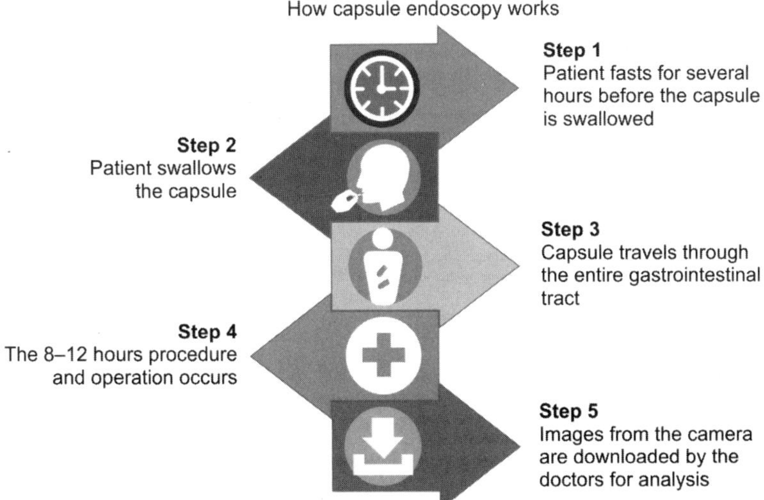

Endoscopic Retrograde Cholangiopancreatography (ERCP)

ERCP combines X-rays with upper GI endoscopy to diagnose or treat problems with the bile and pancreatic ducts.

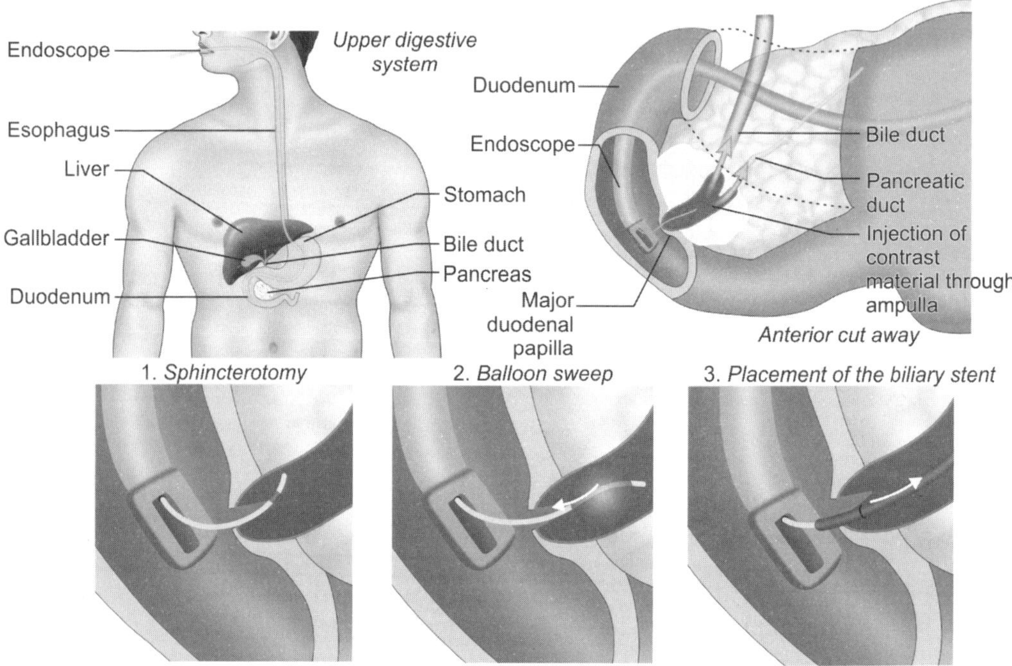

Chromoendoscopy

Chromoendoscopy is a technique that uses a specialized stain or dye on the lining of the intestine during an endoscopy procedure. The dye helps the doctor better visualize if there's anything abnormal on the intestinal lining.

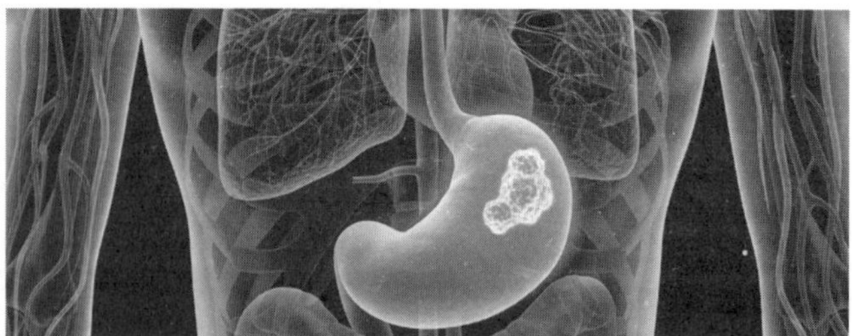

Endoscopic Ultrasound (EUS)

EUS uses an ultrasound in conjunction with an endoscopy. This allows doctors to see organs and other structures that aren't usually visible during a regular endoscopy. A thin needle can then be inserted into the organ or structure to retrieve some tissue for viewing under a microscope. This procedure is called fine needle aspiration.

Endoscopic Mucosal Resection (EMR)

EMR is a technique used to help doctors remove cancerous tissue in the digestive tract. In EMR, a needle is passed through the endoscope to inject a liquid underneath the abnormal tissue. This helps separate the cancerous tissue from the other layers so it can be more easily removed.

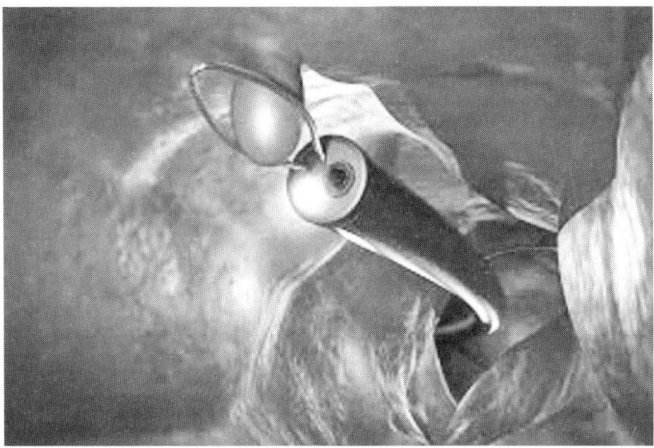

Narrow Band Imaging (NBI)

NBI uses a special filter to help create more contrast between vessels and the mucosa. The mucosa is the inner lining of the digestive tract.

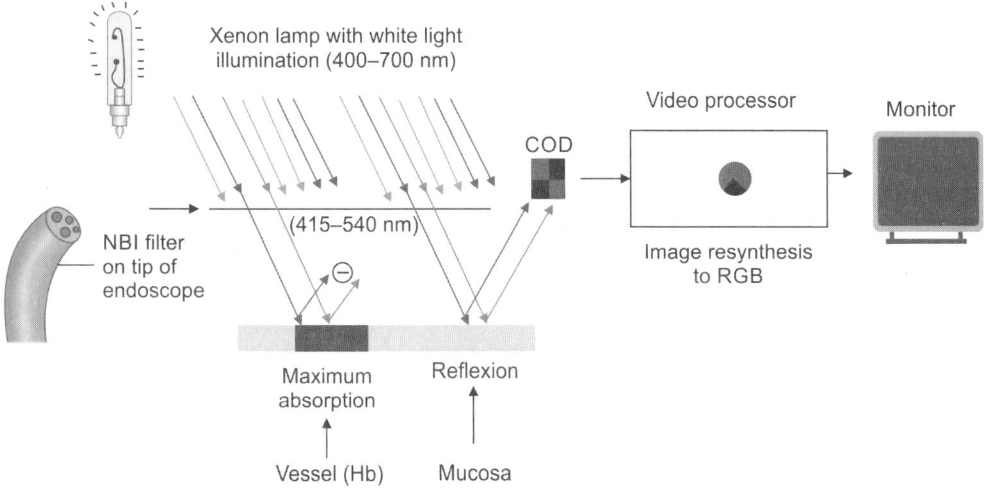

Enteroscopy

Enteroscopy allows for the examination of a large portion of the upper small bowel via the use of an extended length endoscope. It is about two and a half times as long as a standard upper endoscope. It is typically used to identify and treat potential sources of bleeding in patients whose previous endoscopy and colonoscopy results have been normal. In addition, enteroscopy may be performed in patients with suspected mucosal disease of the small bowel, whose tissues biopsies are obtained during the time of the procedure.

Esophageal Stenting

Esophageal stenting, also called enteral stenting, is performed for patients with obstruction of the digestive tract. Typically, these stents are placed in the esophagus, colon or the upper small bowel to relieve the obstruction caused by esophageal, colon and pancreaticoduodenal cancers. Stents usually are placed in patients with advanced, incurable cancer in order to help them to continue to eat. In addition, in patients with colon cancer who are candidates for surgery, it may allow for improved preoperative cleansing of the colon. This has the potential to allow for performing the excision of the cancer and reattachment of the colon with a single operation, rather than with two procedures.

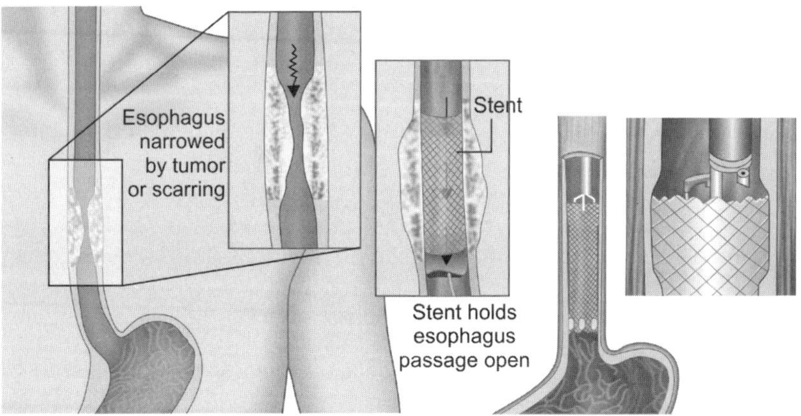

Endoscopic Therapies

We offer a variety of endoscopic therapies for the treatment of gastrointestinal bleeding. These include:

❖ Esophageal banding and sclerotherapy for variceal bleeding
❖ Bicap cautery, "endo-clipping" or injection therapy with epinephrine for ulcer bleeding
❖ Bicep-cautery or for the treatment of vascular ectasia of the stomach, colon or rectum
❖ Hemorrhoidal sclerotherapy for patients with hemorrhoidal bleeding

Many large polyps or early cancers that previously required a surgical approach may now be treated endoscopically. These improved techniques provide an alternative to surgery when noninvasive lesions are identified.

Endoscopic Ultrasound

Endoscopic ultrasound (EUS) is a method of combining endoscopy and ultrasound imaging technologies to obtain high-quality images of the digestive tract and its adjacent structures. An endoscope is a thin, flexible tube with a tiny video camera and light on the end, which offers a clear, detailed view of your digestive tract. Ultrasound is an imaging technique that uses sound waves to produce pictures.

In an endoscopic ultrasound, a special endoscope is used that has an ultrasound processor on its tip, which is called an EUS scope, or echoendoscope. These instruments allow examination of both the lining of your digestive tract with the endoscope, but also of the wall of the tract and its surrounding structures such as the liver, pancreas, bile ducts and lymph nodes. Many other structures can also be seen. Because of these unique capabilities, EUS can sometimes detect abnormalities or obtain information other imaging tests cannot. EUS procedures can be done via the mouth, called an upper EUS, or via the rectum, called a rectal or lower EUS.

EUS is primarily used to detect suspected cancers and evaluate how far a previously diagnosed cancer has spread in order to determine a patient's appropriate treatment plan. The process of determining the extent to which a cancer has spread is called staging. EUS is used to stage cancers of the esophagus, stomach, pancreas and rectum. If cancer has spread to adjacent lymph nodes and blood vessels, it can be determined by the imaging and fine-needle aspiration capabilities of EUS. EUS gives partial, but incomplete, information regarding the spread of these tumors to adjacent organs due to its limited depth of penetration. However, recent imaging enhancements allow for greater evaluation of adjacent organs than previously possible.

Other uses of EUS include:
- Identifying the nature of "lumps" and "bumps" seen on a previous endoscopic exam. These bumps may represent an adjacent structure compressing the digestive tract or represent a mass or fluid collection within the wall of the digestive tract.
- Evaluating disorders of the pancreas and bile ducts, the tubes that drain bile from your liver and gall bladder. The bile ducts are easy to see with EUS, and the pancreas can be evaluated for masses, cysts or changes that suggest chronic inflammation.
- Evaluating patients with fecal incontinence and stage lung cancers as well as evaluating for clots in the vessels of the abdomen with the use of a process known as Doppler ultrasound imagining.

Oxygenation Needs

UNIT OUTLINE

- Cardiovascular and respiratory physiology
- Factors affecting respiratory functioning
- Alterations in respiratory functioning
- Alterations in oxygenation
- Nursing interventions to promote oxygenation
- Chest physiotherapy
- Care of chest drainage
- Pulse oximetry
- Restorative and continuing care

LEARNING OBJECTIVES

At the end of this unit, the reader will be able to:
- Define respiration.
- Explain alterations in respiration.
- Identify factors affecting respiration.
- Describe indications of oxygenation.
- List down equipments for oxygenation.
- Implement nursing interventions to promote oxygenation.
- Define chest physiotherapy.
- Explain restorative and continuing care.

INTRODUCTION

Every living cell in a living organism consumes oxygen. Oxidation of substances within the cells results in the liberation of heat and energy and in the production of carbon dioxide. The end product of respiratory metabolism is continuously removed from the body. The exchange of oxygen and carbon dioxide between an organism and its environment is known as respiration. In vertebrates blood serves to transport oxygen and carbon dioxide.

RESPIRATION

Definition

"Human respiratory system is a network of organs and tissues that help us breathe. The primary function of this system is to introduce oxygen into the body and expel carbon dioxide from the body."

External respiration: The gas exchange between the environment and blood via the respiratory surface is referred to as external respiration.

Internal respiration: The utilization of oxygen for oxidation of nutrients within the cells and tissues may be termed as internal respiration.

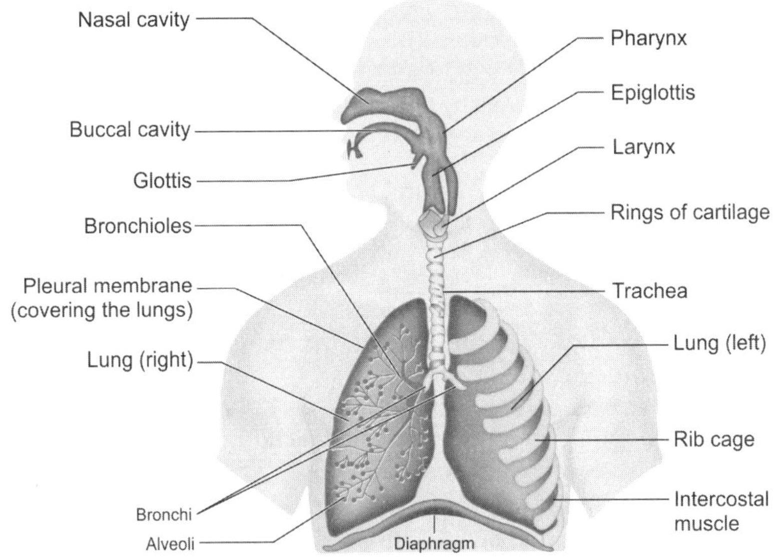

Respiratory system.

The importance of respiration in the body is given below, that it:
- Is required for the exchange of gases oxygen (O_2) and carbon dioxide (CO_2)
- Provides oxygen which causes oxidation of food materials for energy requirements of the body.
- Aids in maintaining the pH of the blood by eliminating CO_2.
- Helps in the excretion of volatile substances like ammonia, water vapor, etc.
- Also helps in maintaining the temperature of the body.
- Filters inspired air.

Organization and Structure

The respiratory system is structurally divisible into two parts:
1. The upper respiratory system which comprises of the nose, or nasal cavity, pharynx, and associated structures.
2. The lower respiratory system which includes the larynx, trachea, bronchi and lungs.

The respiratory system in humans is thus, composed of the following structures:
- Nasal canal or nasal cavity
- Pharynx
- Nasopharynx
- Larynx
- Trachea

- ❖ Bronchi and bronchioles
- ❖ Lungs and alveoli

On the basis of functions also the respiratory system can be divided into two parts:

i. **Conducting part:** Which consists of a series of interconnecting cavities and tubes both outside and within the lungs which is formed of the nose, pharynx, larynx, trachea, bronchi, bronchioles and terminal bronchioles. All these together form a passage for air to be filtered, warmed and moistened and conducted into the lungs.

ii. **Respiratory part:** Which consists of tissues within the lungs where gas exchange takes place. This respiratory part is formed by the respiratory bronchioles, alveolar ducts, alveolar sacs and alveoli (the main sites of gas exchange between air and blood).

Respiratory System Parts and Functions

Let us have a detailed look at the different parts of the respiratory system and their functions.

Nose

Humans have exterior nostrils, which are divided by a framework of cartilaginous structure called the septum. This is the structure that separates the right nostril from the left nostril. Tiny hair follicles that cover the interior lining of nostrils act as the body's first line of defense against foreign pathogens. Furthermore, they provide additional humidity for inhaled air.

Larynx

Two cartilaginous chords lay the framework for the larynx. It is found in front of the neck and is responsible for vocals as well as aiding respiration. Hence, it is also informally called the voice box. When food is swallowed, a flap called the epiglottis folds over the top of the windpipe and prevents food from entering into the larynx.

Pharynx

The nasal chambers open up into a wide hollow space called the pharynx. It is a common passage for air as well as food. It functions by preventing the entry of food particles into the windpipe. The epiglottis is an elastic cartilage, which serves as a switch between the larynx and the esophagus by allowing the passage of air into the lungs, and food in the gastrointestinal tract.

Have you ever wondered why we cough when we eat or swallow?

Talking while we eat or swallow may sometimes result in incessant coughing. The reason behind this reaction is the epiglottis. It is forced to open for the air to exit outwards and the food to enter into the windpipe, triggering a cough.

Trachea

The trachea or the windpipe rises below the larynx and moves down to the neck. The walls of the trachea comprise C-shaped cartilaginous rings which give hardness to the trachea and maintain it by completely expanding. The trachea extends further down into the breastbone and splits into two bronchi, one for each lung.

Bronchi

The trachea splits into two tubes called the bronchi, which enter each lung individually. The bronchi divide into secondary and tertiary bronchioles, and it further branches out into small air-sacs called the alveoli. The alveoli are single-celled sacs of air with thin walls. It facilitates the exchange of oxygen and carbon dioxide molecules into or away from the bloodstream.

Lungs

Lungs are the primary organs of respiration in humans and other vertebrates. They are located on either side of the heart, in the thoracic cavity of the chest. Anatomically, the lungs are spongy organs with an estimates total surface area between 50 to 75 m^2. The primary function of the lungs is to facilitate the exchange of gases between the blood and the air. Interestingly, the right lung is quite bigger and heavier than the left lung.

Respiratory Tract

The respiratory tract in humans is made up of the following parts:
- **External nostrils:** For the intake of air.
- **Nasal chamber:** Which is lined with hair and mucus to filter the air from dust and dirt.
- **Pharynx:** It is a passage behind the nasal chamber and serves as the common passageway for both air and food.
- **Larynx:** Known as the soundbox as it houses the vocal chords, which are paramount in the generation of sound.
- **Epiglottis:** It is a flap-like structure that covers the glottis and prevents the entry of food into the windpipe.
- **Trachea:** It is a long tube passing through the mid-thoracic cavity.
- **Bronchi:** The trachea divides into left and right bronchi.
- **Bronchioles:** Each bronchus is further divided into finer channels known as bronchioles.
- **Alveoli:** The bronchioles terminate in balloon-like structures known as the alveoli.
- **Lungs:** Humans have a pair of lungs, which are sac-like structures and covered by a double-layered membrane known as pleura.

Respiration is the movement of oxygen from the outside environment to the cells within tissues, and the removal of carbon dioxide in the opposite direction that's to the environment.

PHYSIOLOGY OF RESPIRATION

Lung Volumes

- Tidal volume (VT)—air that enters into lungs with each inspirium.
- Inspiratory reserve volume (IRV)—the air inspired with a maximal inspiratory effort to normal inspiratory volume (in excess of the quiet VT).
- Expiratory reserve volume (ERV)—the volume expired by an active expiratory effort after quiet passive expiration.
- Residual volume—air left in the lungs after a maximal exhalation—collapse air + minimal air-total lung capacity–air in the lungs after maximal inspiration.
- Vital capacity—the largest volume of the air that can be expired after a maximal inspiratory effort VC = ERV + VT + IRV.
- Forced vital capacity (FVC)—information about the strength of the resp. mm FVC in · 1 second—the fraction of the FVC expired in 1 second (reduced in Bronchoconstrictory disease—asthma).

Multinodular Goiter

This is an enlargement of the thyroid gland near the base of the neck. It's close to your windpipe, so if it grows, it can push the trachea to one side.

Mediastinal Lymphoma

Mediastinal lymphoma is a type of cancer that affects the mediastinal lymph nodes. These are located near your trachea.

Pleural Effusion

Pleural effusion is a condition in which extra fluid builds up around the lungs in the pleural cavity.

Pneumonectomy

Pneumonectomy is a type of lung removal surgery. It can cause pressure to be unevenly distributed throughout your chest cavity.

Atelectasis

This is a condition where only part of a lung has collapsed. It's usually caused when sacs of air in the lungs, called alveoli, can't hold air. This creates uneven pressure in the chest cavity, which can cause the trachea to move.

Pleural Fibrosis

This condition happens when the membrane that surrounds the lungs, known as the pleura, becomes inflamed.

Pulmonary Fibrosis

Pulmonary fibrosis happens when your lung tissue is scarred. The lungs can become stiff and create abnormal pressure in your chest cavity.

Factors Affecting Respiratory Function

- **Sleep**
    - **CO_2 is higher**
    - **O_2 is lower**
    - **Ventilation is lower**
    - **Inspiratory** decreases
    - Rib cage contribution to ventilation increases
    - Airway resistance
- **Obesity**
    - Adipose tissue around the rib cage and abdomen loads the chest wall, therefore reducing functional capacity
    - Decreased lung compliance
    - More weight to carry = More energy/O_2 used
    - Risks from surgery = Heart attacks, wound infection, nerve injury, urinary tract infection.

- ❖ **Smoking**
  - ◆ Leads to overproduction of mucus
  - ◆ Paralyses the cilia, meaning they do not work (cannot propel mucus upwards/cannot trap bacteria)
  - ◆ Tobacco can destroy lung elastic walls, decreasing expandability capacity
  - ◆ Cause lung cancer, many lung diseases, etc.
- ❖ **Stress**
  - ◆ Makes you breathe harder (leading to hyperventilation/panic attack)—leads you to exercise—leading to an increased metabolism of working muscles—increasing O_2 demands
  - ◆ Tidal volume increase
- ❖ **Immobility**
  - ◆ Lung volume changes = Tidal volume decreases/residual volume decreases/amount of air that can get into lungs is reduced
  - ◆ Mucus gets stuck in the airways easier- Diameter of airways decreases causing fewer but deeper breaths—decrease O_2 consumption as less energy is needed
- ❖ **Exercise**
  - ◆ Increases O_2 consumption, delivery and extraction
  - ◆ Benefits = Decrease in weight, increase muscle strength, get rid of fatty acids (cholesterol), Improves general health.

Factors Influencing Oxygenation

In addition to physiological factors, multiple developmental, lifestyle and environmental factors affect patients' oxygenation status. It is important to recognize these as possible risks or factors that impact their health care goals.

Developmental Factors

The developmental stage of a patient and the normal aging process affect tissue oxygenation.

Infants and Toddlers

Infants and toddlers are at risk for upper respiratory tract infections as a result of frequent exposure to other children, an immature immune system, and exposure to second-hand smoke. In addition, during the teething process some infants develop nasal congestion, which encourages bacterial growth and increases the potential for respiratory tract infection. Upper respiratory tract infections are usually not dangerous, and infants or toddlers recover with little difficulty.

School-age Children and Adolescents

School-age children and adolescents are exposed to respiratory infections and respiratory risk factors such as cigarette smoking or second-hand smoke. A healthy child usually does not have adverse pulmonary effects from respiratory infections. The American Lung Association (2008) reported a study showing that cigarette smoking in college students (19.2%) had declined in 2006 compared to those smoking in 1999 (30.6%). Although this is still higher than the national goal set by the US Department of Health and Human Services (12%), there is hope that the decline will continue. The biggest risk factor for those still smoking in college was if they started smoking in high school (American Lung Association, 2008). A person who starts smoking in adolescence and continues to smoke into middle age has an increased risk for cardiopulmonary disease and lung cancer.

Young and Middle-age Adults

Young and middle-age adults are exposed to multiple cardiopulmonary risk factors: an unhealthy diet, lack of exercise, stress, over-the-counter and prescription drugs not used as intended, illegal substances and smoking. Reducing these modifiable factors decreases a patient's risk for cardiac or pulmonary diseases. This is also the time when individuals establish lifelong habits and lifestyles. In 2007, 20.6% of adults were smokers (Lung USA, 2010). It is important to help your patients make good choices and informed decisions about their health care practices. The increased cost of cigarettes plus the state smoke-free air policies and laws that reduce smoking in public places have proven to be helpful in smoking cessation (American Lung Association, 2008).

Older Adults

The cardiac and respiratory systems undergo changes throughout the aging process. The changes are associated with calcification of the heart valves, SA node and costal cartilages. The arterial system develops atherosclerotic plaques.

FOCUS ON OLDER ADULTS

Oxygenation Changes in Older Adults

- The tuberculin skin test is an unreliable indicator of tuberculosis in older patients. They frequently display false-positive or false-negative skin test reactions.
- Older patients are at an increased risk for reactivation of dormant organisms that were present for decades as a result of age-related changes in the immune system.
- The standard 5-TU Mantoux test is given and repeated or repeated with the 250-TU strength to create a booster effect.
- If the older patient has a positive reaction, a complete history is necessary to determine any risk factors.
- Older adults have more atypical signs and symptoms of coronary artery disease (Meiner, 2011).
- The incidence of atrial fibrillation increases with age and is the leading contributing factor for stroke in the older adult (Meiner, 2011).
- Mental status changes are often the first signs of respiratory problems and often include forgetfulness and irritability.
- Older adults do not always complain of dyspnea until it affects the activities of daily living that are important to them.
- Changes in the older adult's cough mechanism lead to retention of pulmonary secretions, airway plugging, and atelectasis if patients do not use cough suppressants with caution.
- Age-related changes in the immune system lead to a decline of both cell-mediated and humoral immunity, resulting in an increased risk of respiratory infections (McCance and Huether, 2010).
- Changes in the thorax that occur from ossification of costal cartilage, decreased space between vertebrae, and diminished respiratory muscle strength lead to problems with chest expansion and oxygenation (Linton and Lach, 2007).

Osteoporosis leads to changes in the size and shape of the thorax. The trachea and large bronchi become enlarged from calcification of the airways. The alveoli enlarge, decreasing the surface area available for gas exchange. The number of functional cilia is reduced, causing a decrease in the effectiveness of the cough mechanism, putting the older adult at increased risk for respiratory infections (Meiner, 2011).

Lifestyle Factors

Lifestyle modifications are difficult for patients because they often have to change an enjoyable habit such as cigarette smoking or eating certain foods. Risk-factor modification is important and includes smoking cessation, weight reduction, a low-cholesterol and low-sodium diet, management of hypertension, and moderate exercise. Although it is difficult to change long-term behavior, helping patients acquire healthy behaviors reduces the risk for or slows or halts the progression of cardiopulmonary diseases (Meiner, 2011).

Nutrition

Nutrition affects cardiopulmonary function in several ways. Severe obesity decreases lung expansion, and increased body weight increases tissue oxygen demands. The malnourished patient experiences respiratory muscle wasting, resulting in decreased muscle strength and respiratory excursion. Cough efficiency is reduced secondary to respiratory muscle weakness, putting the patient at risk for retention of pulmonary secretions.

Patients who are morbidly obese and/or malnourished are at risk for anemia. Diets high in carbohydrates play a role in increasing the carbon dioxide load for patients with carbon dioxide retention. As carbohydrates are metabolized, an increased load of carbon dioxide is created and excreted via the lungs.

Dietary practices also influence the prevalence of cardiovascular diseases. Cardioprotective nutrition includes diets rich in fiber; whole grains; fresh fruits and vegetables; nuts; antioxidants; lean meats, fish, and chicken; and omega-3 fatty acids. The latest update by the Joint National Committee (JNC, 2003) recommended that dietary restriction of sodium is beneficial in reducing antihypertensive medication requirements; in some cases, it causes left ventricular hypertrophy to regress. Diets high in potassium prevent hypertension and help improve control in patients with hypertension. A 2000-calorie diet of fruits; vegetables; and low-fat dairy foods that are high in fiber, potassium, calcium, and magnesium and low in saturated and total fat helps prevent and reduce the effects of hypertension.

Exercise

Exercise increases the metabolic activity and oxygen demand of the body. The rate and depth of respiration increase, enabling the person to inhale more oxygen and exhale excess carbon dioxide. A physical exercise program has many benefits. People who exercise for 30 to 60 minutes daily have a lower pulse rate and blood pressure, decreased cholesterol level, increased blood flow, and greater oxygen extraction by working muscles. Fully conditioned people increase oxygen consumption by 10 to 20% because of increased cardiac output and increased efficiency of the myocardial muscle (JNC, 2003).

Smoking

Cigarette smoking and second-hand smoke are associated with a number of diseases, including heart disease, COPD and lung cancer. Cigarette smoking worsens peripheral vascular and coronary artery diseases (McCance and Huether, 2010). Inhaled nicotine causes vasoconstriction of peripheral and coronary blood vessels, increasing blood pressure and decreasing blood flow to peripheral vessels.

Women who take birth control pills and smoke cigarettes have an increased risk for thrombophlebitis and pulmonary emboli. Smoking during pregnancy can result in low-birth-weight babies, preterm delivery, and babies with reduced lung function (LungUSA, 2010). Even exposure to second-hand smoke can be a risk for low-birth-weight babies, preterm delivery and miscarriages (ACS, 2010).

The risk of lung cancer is 10 times greater for a person who smokes than for a nonsmoker. In the United States, the use of tobacco accounts for 30% of all cancer deaths. This includes 87% of the deaths from lung cancer and cancer of the larynx, mouth, pharynx, esophagus and bladder. Smoking has been linked to the development of other cancers, including kidney, cervix and leukemia (ACS, 2010). Nicotine patches, gum, and lozenges are available over-the-counter and nicotine nasal spray and inhalers can be obtained by prescription. Prescription drugs such as bupropion (Zyban) and varenicline (Chantix) are also available to help people quit smoking (LungUSA, 2010).

Exposure to environmental tobacco smoke (second-hand smoke) increases the risk of lung cancer and cardiovascular disease in the nonsmoker. Children with parents who smoke have a higher incidence of asthma, pneumonia and ear infections. Babies exposed to second-hand smoke are at higher risk for sudden infant death syndrome (ACS, 2010).

Substance Abuse

Excessive use of alcohol and other drugs impairs tissue oxygenation in two ways. First, the person who chronically abuses substances often has a poor nutritional intake. With the resultant decrease in intake of iron-rich foods, hemoglobin production declines. Second, excessive use of alcohol and certain other drugs depresses the respiratory center, reducing the rate and depth of respiration and the amount of inhaled oxygen. Substance abuse by either smoking or inhaling substances such as crack cocaine or fumes from paint or glue cans causes direct injury to lung tissue that leads to permanent lung damage. The report on inhalant abuse (huffing) by teenagers to get a euphoric effect includes use of a wide variety of substances such as paint thinner, nail polish remover, glue, spray paint, nitrous oxide and other common household products. Sudden death can occur from cardiac arrhythmias; or chronic abuse can cause damage to heart, lungs, and kidneys (Stoppler, 2005).

Stress

A continuous state of stress or severe anxiety increases the metabolic rate and oxygen demand of the body. The body responds to anxiety and other stresses with an increased rate and depth of respiration. Most people adapt; but some, particularly those with chronic illnesses or acute life-threatening illnesses such as an MI, cannot tolerate the oxygen demands associated with anxiety.

Environmental Factors

The environment also influences oxygenation. The incidence of pulmonary disease is higher in smoggy, urban areas than in rural areas. In addition, a patient's workplace sometimes increases the risk for pulmonary disease. Occupational pollutants include asbestos, talcum powder, dust and airborne fibers. For example, farm workers in dry regions of the southwestern United States are at risk for coccidioidomycosis, a fungal disease caused by inhalation of spores of the airborne bacterium *Coccidioides immitis*. Asbestosis is an occupational lung disease that develops after exposure to asbestos. The lung with asbestosis often has diffuse interstitial fibrosis, creating a restrictive lung disease. Patients exposed to asbestos are at risk for developing lung cancer, and this risk increases with exposure to tobacco smoke.

Critical Thinking

Successful critical thinking requires a synthesis of knowledge, experience, information gathered from patients, critical thinking attitudes, and intellectual and professional standards. Clinical judgments require you to anticipate information, analyze the data, and make decisions regarding your patient's care. During assessment consider all elements that build toward making an appropriate nursing diagnosis.

Knowledge
- Cardiopulmonary anatomy and physiology
- Cardiopulmonary pathophysiology
- Clinical signs and symptoms of altered oxygenation
- Developmental factors affecting oxygenation
- Impact of lifestyle
- Environmental impact

Experience
- Caring for patients with impaired oxygenation, activity intolerance, and respiratory infections
- Personal experience with how a change in altitude or physical conditioning affects patient's respiratory patterns
- Experience observing patient's response to oxygenation therapies
- Personal experience with respiratory infections or cardiopulmonary alterations

Assessment
- Identify recurring and present signs and symptoms associated with impaired oxygenation
- Determine the presence of risk factors for alterations
- Ask the patient about use of medications
- Determine the patient's normal and current activity status
- Determine the patient's tolerance to activity

Standards
- Apply intellectual standards of clarity, precision, specificity, and accuracy when obtaining a health history for the patient with cardiopulmonary alterations
- Apply relevant standards from American Cancer Society, American Heart Association, American Thoracic Society

Attitudes
- Carry out the responsibility of obtaining correct information about the patient
- display confidence while assessing extent of patient's respiratory alterations
- Be creative in assessing cultural factors influencing patient's risk factors

Critical thinking for clinical judgement.

Alterations in Respiratory Functioning

Illnesses and conditions affecting ventilation or oxygen transport cause alterations in respiratory functioning. The three primary alterations are hypoventilation, hyperventilation and hypoxia.

The goal of ventilation is to produce a normal arterial carbon dioxide tension ($PaCO_2$) between 35 and 45 mm Hg and a normal arterial oxygen tension (PaO_2) between 80 and

100 mm Hg. Hypoventilation and hyperventilation are often determined by arterial blood gas analysis (McCance and Huether, 2010). Hypoxemia refers to a decrease in the amount of arterial oxygen. Nurses monitor arterial oxygen saturation (SpO_2) using a noninvasive oxygen saturation monitor pulse oximeter. Normally SpO_2 is greater than or equal to 95%.

Hypoventilation

Hypoventilation occurs when alveolar ventilation is inadequate to meet the oxygen demand of the body or eliminate sufficient carbon dioxide. As alveolar ventilation decreases, the body retains carbon dioxide. For example, atelectasis, a collapse of the alveoli, prevents normal exchange of oxygen and carbon dioxide. As more alveoli collapse, less of the lung is ventilated, and hypoventilation occurs.

In patients with COPD, the administration of excessive oxygen results in hypoventilation. These patients have adapted to a high carbon dioxide level so their carbon dioxide–sensitive chemoreceptors are essentially not functioning. Their peripheral chemoreceptors of the aortic arch and carotid bodies are primarily sensitive to lower oxygen levels, causing increased ventilation. Because the stimulus to breathe is a decreased arterial oxygen (PaO_2) level, administration of oxygen greater than 24% to 28% (1 to 3 L/min) prevents the PaO_2 from falling to a level (60 mm Hg) that stimulates the peripheral receptors, thus destroying the stimulus to breathe (McCance and Huether, 2010). The resulting hypoventilation causes excessive retention of carbon dioxide, which can lead to respiratory acidosis and respiratory arrest.

Signs and symptoms of hypoventilation include mental status changes, dysrhythmias and potential cardiac arrest. If untreated, the patient's status rapidly declines, leading to convulsions, unconsciousness and death.

Hyperventilation

Hyperventilation is a state of ventilation in which the lungs remove carbon dioxide faster than it is produced by cellular metabolism. Severe anxiety, infection, drugs or an acid-base imbalance induces hyperventilation. Acute anxiety leads to hyperventilation and exhalation of excessive amounts of carbon dioxide. Increased body temperature (fever) increases the metabolic rate, thereby increasing carbon dioxide production. The increased carbon dioxide level stimulates an increase in the patient's rate and depth of respiration, causing hyperventilation.

Hyperventilation is sometimes chemically induced. Salicylate (aspirin) poisoning and amphetamine use result in excess carbon dioxide production, stimulating the respiratory center to compensate by increasing the rate and depth of respiration. It also occurs as the body tries to compensate for metabolic acidosis. For example, the patient with diabetes in ketoacidosis produces large amounts of metabolic acids. The respiratory system tries to correct the acid-base balance by over breathing. Ventilation increases to reduce the amount of carbon dioxide available to form carbonic acid. This can also result in the patient developing respiratory alkalosis. Signs and symptoms of hyperventilation include rapid respirations, sighing breaths, numbness and tingling of hands/feet, light-headedness, and loss of consciousness (Ackley and Ladwig, 2011).

Hypoxia

Hypoxia is inadequate tissue oxygenation at the cellular level. It results from a deficiency in oxygen delivery or oxygen use at the cellular level. It is a life-threatening condition. Untreated it produces possibly fatal cardiac dysrhythmias.

Causes of hypoxia include (1) a decreased hemoglobin level and lowered oxygen-carrying capacity of the blood; (2) a diminished concentration of inspired oxygen, which occurs at high altitudes; (3) the inability of the tissues to extract oxygen from the blood, as with cyanide poisoning; (4) decreased diffusion of oxygen from the alveoli to the blood, as in pneumonia; (5) poor tissue perfusion with oxygenated blood, as with shock; and (6) impaired ventilation, as with multiple rib fractures or chest trauma.

The clinical signs and symptoms of hypoxia include apprehension, restlessness, inability to concentrate, decreased level of consciousness, dizziness and behavioral changes. The patient with hypoxia is unable to lie flat and appears both fatigued and agitated. Vital sign changes include an increased pulse rate and rate and depth of respiration. During early stages of hypoxia the blood pressure is elevated unless the condition is caused by shock. As the hypoxia worsens, the respiratory rate declines as a result of respiratory muscle fatigue.

Cyanosis, blue discoloration of the skin and mucus membranes caused by the presence of desaturated hemoglobin in capillaries, is a late sign of hypoxia. The presence or absence of cyanosis is not a reliable measure of oxygen status. Central cyanosis, observed in the tongue, soft palate, and conjunctiva of the eye where blood flow is high, indicates hypoxemia. Peripheral cyanosis, seen in the extremities, nail beds, and earlobes, is often a result of vasoconstriction and stagnant blood flow.

Effect of Airway Diseases on Respiration

Chronic respiratory diseases (CRDs) affect the airways and other structures of the lungs. Some of the most common are chronic obstructive pulmonary disease (COPD), asthma, occupational lung diseases and pulmonary hypertension. In addition to tobacco smoke, other risk factors include air pollution, occupational chemicals and dusts, and frequent lower respiratory infections during childhood. CRDs are not curable; however, various forms of treatment that help open the air passages and improve shortness of breath can help control symptoms and improve daily life for people living with these conditions. The WHO Global Alliance against CRDs (GARD) vision is "a world in which all people breathe freely". GARD focuses on the needs of people with CRDs in low- and middle-income countries.

The "airways" are the bronchial tubes that conduct air from the mouth to the alveoli of the lungs where oxygen is taken up into the blood stream and carbon dioxide is removed. Thus the term "airway disease" or "airway condition" refers to a disorder that narrows the airways and interferes with the smooth passage of air in and out of the lungs.

There are many types of airway conditions, cancerous and noncancerous, and they can be caused by disease, structural abnormalities, injury, and factors such as infection, allergies and medical treatments. Issues can be acute or chronic and can arise in both the upper and lower portions of the airway.

Types of Airway Conditions

Airway conditions include:

❖ **Asthma:** A chronic lung condition that causes inflammation and narrowing of the airway
❖ **Benign airway tumors:** Noncancerous masses that arise in the airway
❖ **Lung diseases:** Including chronic obstructive pulmonary disease (COPD) and cystic fibrosis
❖ **Airway stenosis:** A narrowing of the airway
❖ **Airway cancer:** A rare cancer that occurs in the airway
❖ **Airway fistulas:** Holes that occur in the membranes that separate the airway from adjacent structures

Airway Cancer

Airway cancers are uncommon cancers that originate in the airway, or windpipe (trachea). They include primary cancers, such as squamous cell carcinomas, adenoid cystic carcinomas, tracheal carcinoid tumors and mucoepidermoid carcinomas.

Causes and symptoms

Airway cancers are most commonly related to smoking. Human papillomavirus (HPV) can also lead to airway tumors.

Often the first sign of airway cancer is difficulty breathing, which occurs as a tumor grows and obstructs the airway.

Diagnosis

If a doctor suspects airway cancer, he or she will conduct a physical examination and order tests to confirm the diagnosis. Further tests might be needed to help determine the cancer's stage and precise location.

Imaging techniques used to diagnose airway cancer might include:
* **Advanced endobronchial staging equipment:** This equipment includes linear endobronchial ultrasound, which visualizes airway tissue that can be sampled by instruments passed through the bronchoscope, and electromagnetic navigational bronchoscopy to evaluate harder-to-reach lesions.
* **Chest X-ray:** X-rays help physicians visualize abnormalities in the airway.
* **Contrast enhanced or multidetector computed tomography (CT) scan:** CT technology helps physicians visualize the location and extent of airway cancer.
* **Magnetic resonance imaging (MRI):** MRI helps physicians identify suspicious areas that could indicate airway cancer and learn if, and how far, it has spread.
* **Positron emission tomography (PET):** Cancer cells absorb large amounts of radioactive sugar that are used in this technique, and a special camera creates images of that radioactivity, enabling physicians to identify cancerous cells.
* **Endoscopic ultrasonography:** This technology maps sound waves to show physicians if cancer is present in the airway.

Additional testing also might include a tissue sample (biopsy) of the airway tissue to determine the presence of cancer.

Treatment

Airway cancer treatment options depend on the cancer's precise location and stage; the patient's overall health, goals, and preferences; and other factors.

UT Southwestern's thoracic cancer specialists might consider these therapies for treating airway cancer:
* **Endotracheal treatments:** These minimally invasive therapies include thulium (versus holmium) laser resection and laser therapy in which blood-thinning drugs are taken prior to using a low-current laser that destroys cancerous cells. Endotracheal therapies typically are used to treat superficial malignancies, dysplasias and early-stage cancers.
* **Medical treatment (chemotherapy):** Chemotherapy drugs, taken orally or intravenously, might be used to target and kill airway cancer cells. Chemotherapy also might be used in conjunction with radiation therapy (chemoradiation) to treat airway cancer.

❖ **Radiation therapy:** Radiation therapy uses high-energy radiation to destroy cancer cells in the airway. UT Southwestern is a recognized leader in the development and use of cancer-fighting radiation therapies.

❖ **Surgery:** Highly precise surgery to remove cancerous tissue might be used in some cases of airway cancer.

Support services

Harold C Simmons Comprehensive Cancer Center offers an array of support services to people undergoing treatment at UT Southwestern for airway cancer—and even for those who have been treated in the past. These services range from survivorship seminars to nutrition counseling to support groups.

Benign Airway Cancers

Benign (noncancerous) airway tumors are rare and include papillomas (HPV-related), granular cell tumors, hamartomas, carcinoid tumors, hemangiomas, neurogenic tumors, cartilaginous tumors or chondromas, and others.

These tumors are managed by a variety of interventional pulmonary and surgical techniques. In some cases, the tumor can be treated minimally invasively by a combination of advanced interventional bronchoscopic procedures.

When surgery is the most appropriate option, our surgeons work closely with UT Southwestern's interventional pulmonologists, chest radiologists, and otolaryngologists to deliver comprehensive care—all in one location, and usually on the same day.

Symptoms

Symptoms are related to the presence of the tumor causing irritation of the airway and obstruction of the airflow:

❖ Cough
❖ Frequent bouts of upper respiratory infections or pneumonia
❖ Hemoptysis or coughing up blood
❖ Shortness of breath
❖ Wheezing

Diagnosis

Airway tumors can be difficult to diagnose because they are so rare, and in most cases, slow growing. They may be misdiagnosed as another problem such as asthma, chronic bronchitis, or COPD.

If we suspect that you have a benign airway tumor, we will conduct a physical examination and order tests to confirm the diagnosis.

Tests and imaging techniques used to diagnose benign airway tumors might include:

❖ Chest X-rays (radiographs)
❖ Computed tomography (CT) with 3-D reconstruction
❖ Flexible and rigid bronchoscopy, endobronchial ultrasound (EBUS), and other interventional pulmonary procedures
❖ Magnetic resonance imaging (MRI)
❖ Pulmonary function tests (PFT)

Treatments

Our team of highly specialized thoracic surgeons and interventional pulmonologists treat these tumors with a variety of techniques, including:

- ❖ **Bronchoscopic tumor removal (resection):** To open up the airway
- ❖ **Airway reconstructive surgery:** To remove the tumor and reconstruct the airway to maintain airflow to the lungs
- ❖ **Laser surgery and other advanced bronchoscopic procedures:** Includes thermal ablation or mechanical modalities to remove the tumor
- ❖ **Stenting:** A hollow tube to maintain the airflow to the lungs
- ❖ **Tracheotomy:** Surgery to bypass the airway obstruction

Related conditions

Our thoracic surgery team treats thoracic (chest) conditions that can be associated with benign airway tumors, including airway stenosis and cancerous airway tumors.

Asthma

Asthma is marked by recurring episodes of reversible airway narrowing (caused by contraction of muscle in the airway wall, or "bronchospasm") manifested by shortness of breath, cough, wheezing and chest tightness.

Chronic Obstructive Pulmonary Disease

Chronic obstructive pulmonary disease (COPD) is another name for emphysema and chronic bronchitis, most often (but not always) associated with smoking. COPD is a chronic condition in that the airway narrowing is not fully reversible as it can be in asthma. Patients with mild COPD may experience shortness of breath only in association with respiratory infections or when performing strenuous exercise. Patients with more advanced COPD commonly experience persistent shortness of breath, cough, and frequent sputum or phlegm production.

Cystic Fibrosis

Cystic fibrosis is a hereditary disease usually (but not always) apparent in childhood and is marked by recurrent bouts of lung infections, difficulty breathing due to mucus accumulation, faulty digestion, and excessive loss of salt in sweat.

All of these conditions are treatable. Current medical therapy can reverse airway narrowing, improve symptoms and reduce the frequency of attacks. But no known treatment will cure any of these conditions. This is why the Airway Clinical Research Center was created—to develop better therapies, and eventually cures, for these common and important causes of impairment and distress.

Movement of Air

Atmospheric Pressure

Pressure is conventionally measured as millimeters (mm) of mercury (Hg). 'Millimeters of mercury' (mm Hg) refers to the height of a column of mercury attached to an instrument that detects pressure (e.g., a sphygmomanometer). Other units of pressure, such as that used in Video 7, include bar, pounds per square inch (psi) and pascals (Pa). All units of pressure can be interconverted, so 1 bar = 14.5 psi, 1 psi = 51.7 mm Hg and 1 mm Hg = 133 Pa.

At sea level, the atmospheric pressure (i.e., the pressure exerted by the gases in the Earth's atmosphere) is about 760 mm Hg. During inhalation, the volume of the lungs increases and the pressure inside the lungs decreases below that of atmospheric pressure. This creates a pressure gradient that draws air into the lungs. During exhalation, the lungs return to their original size, pressure in the lungs rises compared with the atmospheric pressure and air moves out.

Partial Pressure

Pressure is an important factor in O_2 and CO_2 exchange in the alveoli. The pressure of each individual gas in the atmosphere is described as its **partial pressure**.

Partial pressure is calculated by multiplying the percentage of the particular gas in the atmosphere by the total atmospheric pressure. For example, O_2 accounts for about 21% of the Earth's atmosphere so the partial pressure of O_2 (PO_2) in the atmosphere is 0.21×760 mm Hg = 160 mm Hg. CO_2 is present only in trace amounts, so the partial pressure of CO_2 (PCO_2) in the atmosphere is roughly 0.3 mm Hg.

Diffusion of Gases in Respiration

Diffusion

The rate of gas diffusion through the alveolar-capillary membrane is determined by several factors, including (1) the pressure difference of each gas between both sides of the membrane, (2) the solubility of the gas, (3) the surface area of the membrane, (4) the distance through which the gas must diffuse, and (5) the molecular weight of the gas.

Diffusing capacity is a measure of how well oxygen and carbon dioxide are transferred (diffused) between the lungs and the blood, and can be a useful test in the diagnosis and to monitor treatment of lung diseases. Diffusing capacity can also be important prior to lung surgery as a predictor of how well the surgery will be tolerated. Diffusing capacity may be reduced in a few ways, and healthcare providers usually use the measure along with other pulmonary function tests to diagnose and determine the severity of either restrictive or obstructive lung diseases.

Diffusion Barrier

The diffusion barrier in the lungs consists of the following layers:
* Alveolar **epithelium**
* Tissue **fluid**
* Capillary **endothelium**
* **Plasma**
* **Red cell** membrane

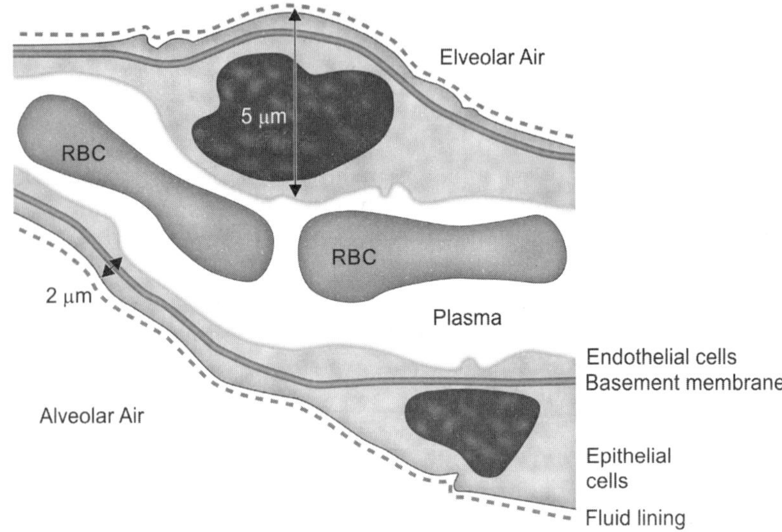

Diffusion of gases in respiration.

Meaning of a Low Diffusing Capacity

Oxygen and carbon dioxide both need to pass through a thin layer in the lungs called the alveolar-capillary membrane. This is the layer between the small air sacs in the lung (the alveoli) and the smallest blood vessels that travel through the lungs (capillaries).

How well oxygen that is inhaled can pass (diffuse) from the alveoli into the blood, and how well carbon dioxide can pass from the blood capillaries into the alveoli and be exhaled, depends on how thick this membrane is, and how much surface area is available for the transfer to take place.

There are two separate mechanisms by which diffusing capacity may be reduced:
1. Diffusing capacity may be low if lung disease is present that causes the membrane to be thicker, for example, in diseases such as pulmonary fibrosis and sarcoidosis.
2. Diffusing capacity may also below if there is less surface area available for the transfer of oxygen and carbon dioxide, for example, with emphysema or if a lung or part of a lung is removed for lung cancer.

Diseases Associated With a Low Diffusing Capacity

Understanding a low diffusing capacity requires looking at the differences between obstructive and restrictive lung diseases and how these affect lung function.

Restrictive Lung Diseases Causing Thickening of the Alveolar-Capillary Membrane

* Pulmonary fibrosis
* Sarcoidosis

Obstructive Lung Diseases and Diseases Causing Less Surface Area in the Lungs

* Emphysema
* Lung cancer
* Lung surgery

Other Conditions Which Decrease the Surface Area of the Alveoli-Capillary Membrane

❖ Pulmonary embolism
❖ Primary pulmonary hypertension

Causes of High Diffusing Capacity

This may occur with asthma, polycythemia vera (a disease with an elevated hemoglobin level), and congenital diseases that cause blood to be shunted from the left side of the heart to the right side of the heart. With these conditions, however, there are often other signs, symptoms, and testing abnormalities that lead to the diagnosis.

Oxygenation (the delivery of oxygen to the body's tissues and cells), is necessary to maintain life and health. Clients with compromised oxygenation status need careful assessment and thoughtful nursing care to achieve an adequate and comfortable level of oxygenation function.

PHYSIOLOGY OF OXYGENATION

The delivery of oxygen to the body's cells is a process that depends upon the interplay of the pulmonary, hematologic and cardiovascular systems. Specifically, the processes involved include ventilation, alveolar gas exchange, oxygen transport and delivery, and cellular respiration.

ASSESSMENT

Health History

The health history of the individual experiencing oxygenation deficits is important in the development of the plan of care. The health history should begin with a thorough exploration of the presenting problem, including how long it has been present and whether it has recently gotten worse, then should proceed to explore the medical history, impact of the illness on activities of daily living, and the client's knowledge level and coping abilities.

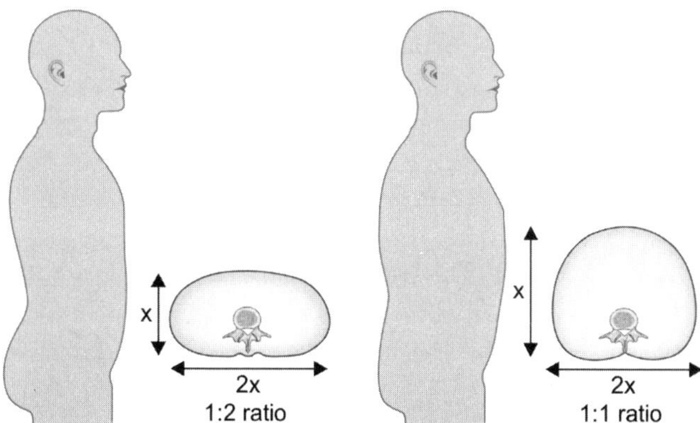

Changes in chest configuration and posture. The normal ratio of the anterior posterior diameter to the lateral diameter is 1:2. With a barrel chest, the ratio between the diameters is 1:1.

Physical Examination

Inspection will begin when the nurse first encounters the client. This is a time to make general notes of the client's efforts at ventilation, especially anxious or distressed appearance, flaring of nostrils, position preferences and general chest configuration. While counting the respiratory rate, also note the rhythm or pattern of the breathing for regularity or irregularity. The signs and symptoms of hypoxia are relative to the onset. Early clinical manifestations of hypoxia include restlessness, apprehension, anxiety, dizziness, inability to concentrate, confusion, agitation, increased pulse rate, increased rate and depth of respiration, and elevated blood pressure (unless the hypoxia is caused by shock). If the hypoxia goes untreated, the respiratory rate may decline and changes in the level of consciousness progress to stupor, or coma indicating ischemia of neuronal cells resulting from oxygen deprivation. Perfusion deficits resulting in poor circulation can be visually noted in mottled skin, cyanosis (bluish coloration of the skin) and edema. The bluish discoloration of cyanosis is the result of the presence of desaturated hemoglobin in capillaries that may occur from either hypoxia or stagnant blood flow. When cyanosis is observed in the tongue, soft palate, and conjunctiva of the eye, it indicates hypoxemia, whereas cyanosis of the extremities, nail beds, and earlobes is often a result of vasoconstriction and stagnant blood flow. Clubbing of the fingers, which manifests as a flattened angle of the nail bed and a rounding of the fingertips, is a sign of chronic hypoxia.

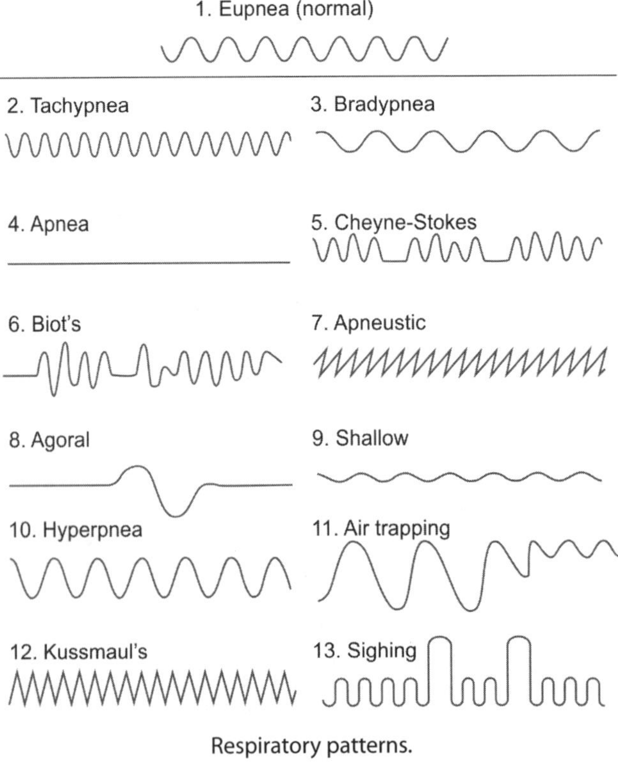

Respiratory patterns.

Health History Related to Oxygenation

Presenting problem	Qualifiers
Cough	**Onset:** Sudden or gradual, how long ago **Nature:** Dry, moist, barking, hacking, productive, nonproductive **Pattern:** Continuous, occasional, related to time of day, position or activity, weather severity **Associated symptoms:** Pain, shortness of breath, wheezing **Alleviating factors:** Vaporizers, OTC medications
Sputum	Amount, color, odor, presence of blood in sputum
Shortness of breath	**Onset:** Sudden or gradual **Nature:** Precipitated by choking or gagging **Pattern:** Associated with activity or position; continuous or intermittent **Associated symptoms:** Pain, cough, diaphoresis
Pain	**Location/radiation nature:** Stabbing, dull, aching, burning, squeezing, crushing **Associated symptoms:** Dizziness, nausea, diaphoresis, palpitations

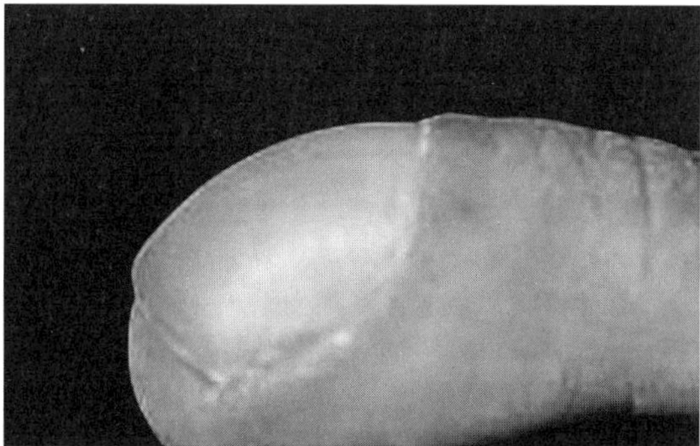

Clubbing of the finger as a result of chronic hypoxia. (*Courtesy:* Robert A. Silverman, M.D., Clinical Associate Professor, Department of Pediatrics, Georgetown University.

Nursing Tip

Percussion Hint

Sound waves travel better through a solid medium than through an air-filled medium. Therefore:

- The more solid a structure, the higher its pitch, the softer its intensity, and the shorter its duration.
- The more air-filled a structure, the lower its pitch, the louder its intensity, and the longer its duration.

Characteristics of Adventitious Breath Sounds

Breath Sound	Respiratory Phase	Description	Conditions
Fine crackle	Predominantly inspiration	Dry, high-pitched crackling, popping: short duration; roll hair by ears between your fingers to simulate this sound	Chronic obstructive pulmonary disease, congestive heart failure, pneumonia, pulmonary fibrosis, atelectasis
Coarse crackle	Predominantly inspiration	Moist, low-pitched crackling, gurgling; long duration	Pneumonia, pulmonary edema, bronchitis, atelectasis
Sonorous wheeze	Predominantly expiration	Low-pitched; snoring	Asthma, bronchitis, airway edema, tumor, bronchiolar spasm, foreign body obstruction
Sibilant wheeze	Predominantly expiration	High-pitched; musical	Asthma, chronic bronchitis, emphysema, tumor, foreign body obstruction
Pleural friction rub	Inspiration and expiration	Creaking, grating	Pleurisy, tuberculosis, pulmonary infarction, pneumonia, lung abscess
Stridor	Predominantly inspiration	Crowing	Croup, foreign body obstruction, large airway tumor

Auscultation may reveal adventitious breath sounds such as rales (crackles) or wheezes (rhonchi), pleural friction rub, or stridor, all indicators or alterations in ventilation. Circulation deficits will be noted upon auscultation by gallops, or extra heart sounds, and murmurs, or sounds produced by blood flowing through a malfunctioning valve.

Diagnostic and Laboratory Data

There are many tests to measure oxygenation status. Pulse oximetry uses light waves to measure oxygen saturation (SaO_2) noninvasively. Arterial blood gases (ABGs) measure a number of indicators that can affect oxygenation status. Sputum collection is another valuable tool in assessing a client's oxygenation functioning; and common findings and their indications. Measurements of lactic acid, hemoglobin, and hematocrit are also useful in determining the effectiveness of the body's oxygen delivery to tissues. Clients undergoing these tests are often apprehensive and need nursing care and education directed at their knowledge levels.

Arterial Blood Gases

Measurement	Normal arterial values	Clinical significance
pH	7.35–7.45	Indicates acid-base balance
Pco_2	35–45 mm Hg	Partial pressure of carbon dioxide; indicates adequacy of alveolar ventilation; represents respiratory component of acid-base balance
HCO_3^-	22–26 mEq/L	Bicarbonate level; indicates metabolic component of acid-base balance
PaO_2	80–100 mm Hg	Partial pressure of oxygen; represents oxygen dissolved in plasma
SaO_2	96–98%	Saturation of hemoglobin with oxygen

Protocol: Assisting a Client with Sputum Collection	
Purpose	To collect an adequate sample of sputum for laboratory analysis and/or culture; to minimize contamination of the sample with oral or other secretions
Level	Independent
Supportive data	Increasing the client's knowledge promotes cooperation and increases the diagnostic value of the sample obtained
Assessment	• Verify the type of test to be performed (cytology studies should be collected into a cup containing a preservative solution; cultures must be collected into a sterile container). • Assess the client's level of consciousness and ability to follow instructions. • Assess the client's breath sounds; coarse rales indicate the presence of sputum in the airways
Interventions	• Obtain correct specimen container • Wash hands and don clean gloves • Assist the client to rinse the mouth with water (not mouthwash) • Instruct client to raise sputum from the lungs, not the throat or nose • Instruct client to expectorate sputum into the cup without touching the inside of the container • Replace cap on container as soon as sample is obtained. Label container and wash the outside if indicated • Place in a bag with a biohazard label for transport • Provide mouth care for the client and assist to a comfortable position • Remove gloves and wash hands. Send specimen to lab immediately
Documentation	Document amount, color, character, and odor of sputum obtained and time the specimen was sent to the lab

Pathologies Associated with Different Colors of Sputum	
Sputum color	*Pathology*
Mucoid	Tracheobronchitis, asthma
Yellow or green	Bacterial infection
Rust or blood-tinged	Pneumonia, pulmonary infarction, tuberculosis
Black	Black lung disease
Pink	Pulmonary edema

Selected Tests for Oxygenation Status	
Test	*Indications/possible findings*
Ventilatory function tests	• Volume of air in the lungs at various phases of the ventilatory cycle • Speed and ease of airflow through the airways • Strength of the respiratory muscles
Chest X-ray	• Areas of fluid accumulation (infiltrates) • Solid masses (suggestive of tumors) • Abnormal accumulations of calcium, areas of necrosis (as seen in tuberculosis) • Excessive air trapping (suggestive of emphysema) • Abnormal accumulations of air or fluid in the pleural space (suggestive of pleural effusion or pneumothorax) • Gross abnormalities in size, shape, position of thoracic structures

Contd...

Contd...

Test	Indications/possible findings
Computerized tomography (CT) scan, magnetic resonance imaging (MRI)	• Detailed pictures of thoracic structures
Ventilation scan	• Areas of impaired airflow (suggestive of pulmonary emboli)
Bronchoscopy	• Sputum collection • Examination of tissue
Thoracentesis	• Tissue sample collection
Echocardiography	• Size and motion of cardiac structures • Accumulation of fluid in the pericardial sac (suggestive of pericardial effusion)
Electrocardiography	• Heart rate and rhythm • Abnormal sites of impulse formation (ectopic pacemakers) • Areas of blocked or delayed impulse transmission • Chamber enlargement (as seen in heart failure) • Areas of ischemia, injury or infarction
Stress test	• Changes in ECG tracings (may indicate ischemic heart disease)

Improving oxygenation involves promoting ventilation, assisting diffusion of gases, and facilitating the perfusion of oxygen throughout the body.

GENERAL RESPIRATORY HEALTH AND POLICY

Promoting respiratory health begins with promoting healthy lifestyles. Respiratory health is maintained by exercise, clean air, and a competent cough reflex. Exercise is an important part of promoting respiratory and cardiovascular health. During exercise, ventilation improves as the lungs expand more fully, and perfusion is enhanced by the increased cardiac output.

Facilitating Respiratory Health

❖ Exercise regularly—30 minutes, three to four times per week.
❖ Do not smoke or use tobacco products.
❖ Avoid secondhand smoke.
❖ Support legislation to control and eliminate pollution.
❖ Ensure adequate ventilation of wood stoves and furnaces.
❖ Reduce exposure to noxious fumes at home and at work.

When a patient's health is compromised by age, lifestyle, surgery, or disease, respiratory functioning may be disrupted. Advanced interventions to improve oxygenation require a collaborative approach. Nurses, physicians, and respiratory therapists work together to enhance ventilation, diffusion, and oxygenation through a variety of approaches. The following strategies for improving oxygenation will be reviewed:

❖ Improving physical mobility
❖ Breathing and coughing exercises
❖ Mobilizing secretions
❖ Maintaining airway patency
❖ Closed chest drainage

* Oxygen therapy
* Mechanical ventilation

IMPROVING PHYSICAL MOBILITY

When a patient's ability to move is compromised, maintaining physical and respiratory functioning becomes an important nursing intervention. Pain, surgical incision, medications, and age may make it difficult for the patient to move and breath. Chest expansion and alveolar inflation are diminished during immobility and may result in atelectasis, inadequate gas exchange, or even pneumonia.

The best position for maximum chest expansion is upright. Encourage able patients to ambulate three times a day to enhance ventilation and maintain cardiovascular conditioning. Patients undergoing surgery should be ambulated postoperatively as soon as allowed by the surgeon and at least three times a day thereafter. Premedication of the postoperative patient with an analgesic (30 to 45 minutes before the activity) will improve mobility and depth of inhalation. For the bedridden patient, the semi-Fowler's or high-Fowler's position allows maximum chest expansion. In the patient with chronic airflow limitation (CAL), the orthopnea position or tripod position may provide relief from dyspnea and enhance ventilation. The tripod position involves having the patient sit at the bedside with a table in front of him or her, allowing for propping of the elbows on the table while compressing the lower chest.

If the patient is bedridden, he or she should be turned from side to side every 2 hours to improve chest expansion on the upward side and increased perfusion of the lung on the dependent side. Occasionally the prone position is used to improve oxygenation in ventilated patients who continue to deteriorate despite other interventions.

Patients with chronic respiratory disorders such as emphysema may have an impaired ability to oxygenate their blood and a decreased capacity to exert themselves. With less oxygen in the blood, less is available for the cells when activity increases the oxygen demands of the tissues. Deep breathing and coughing exercises (discussed later in this chapter) may be used to increase oxygenation and maintain airway patency.

Respiratory diseases such as emphysema or chronic bronchitis change the structure and the functioning of the respiratory tract. The diaphragm becomes flattened, reducing the ability of the chest to expand. Air becomes trapped in distal alveoli and the bases of the lungs. Air trapping causes a ventilation/perfusion (V/Q) mismatch with resultant hypoxemia. Even normal activities, such as walking and eating, can be exhausting to a patient with a chronic respiratory disorder. Nursing care for these patients includes teaching ways to reduce oxygen demand, such as:

* Pace activities with rest periods.
* Eat frequent, light meals to decrease metabolic demands and gastric fullness, which might press the diaphragm upward.
* Avoid holding the breath during activities, which will further diminish the Po_2 and increase dyspnea.
* Avoid the Valsalva maneuver, which increases intrathoracic pressure and decreases blood return into the thorax, resulting in dizziness.
* Decrease temperature if febrile, as each degree (Fahrenheit) elevation results in a 7% increase in metabolic demand.
* Use energy conservation exercises such as performing the work part of an activity during exhalation and using pursed-lip breathing during exertion.

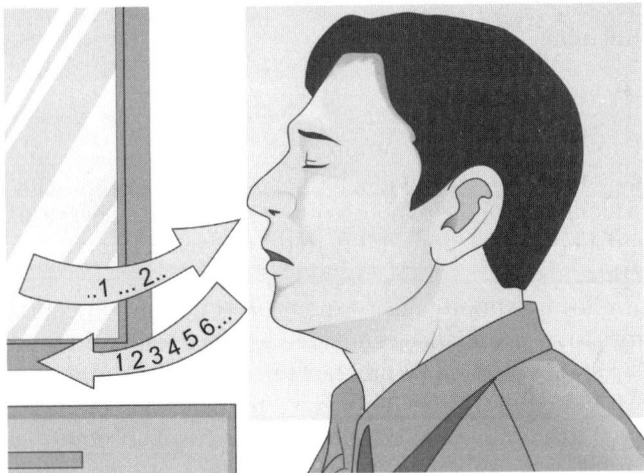

Preoperative teaching is important in providing patients with information regarding the risks of developing respiratory problems postoperatively. General anesthesia, postoperative pain, immobility, and pain medications can alter normal ventilation and put patients at risk for atelectasis, pneumonia, thrombophlebitis, and pulmonary embolism. Interventions to improve ventilation, oxygenation, and mobility postoperatively include the following:

- ❖ Encourage breathing exercises and incentive spirometry every 1 to 2 hours to maximize lung expansion.
- ❖ Promote early ambulation and leg exercises to improve venous circulation.
- ❖ Maintain airway patency with coughing to clear secretions and, if necessary, suctioning.
- ❖ Administer pain medication prior to ambulation or chest physical therapy and use splinting to support surgical incisions.

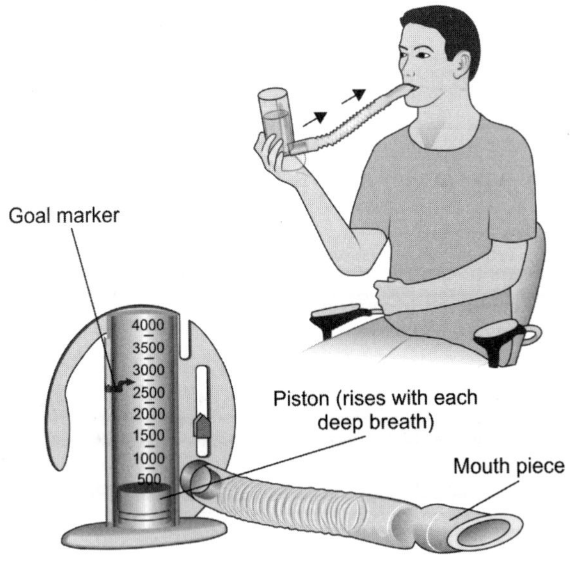

Incentive spirometry.

BREATHING EXERCISES

Breathing exercises may help patients control breathing, improve ventilation, decrease anxiety, and increase activity levels. Some exercises are more suited to patients with chronic airflow limitations (CAL), and others are more useful with anxious patients or those with postoperative pain.

Diaphragmatic Breathing

Diaphragmatic breathing is indicated for patients with CAL or anxiety because it allows for slow, deep breaths. Slow deliberate breaths using the abdomen and chest muscles may slow the frequency of the ventilations and help the patient focus.

❖ Place the patient in a sitting position on the side of the bed or in the semi- or high-Fowler's position.

❖ Have the patient place one hand on his or her chest and the other on his or her upper abdomen above the umbilicus. Another method that may be useful is to place a light object (e.g., tissue box) on the patient's abdomen so he or she can see abdominal movement during diaphragmatic breathing.

❖ Teach the patient to inhale slowly through the nose, feeling the abdomen rise up under his hands but with little movement in the chest.

❖ Instruct the patient to exhale through pursed lips using the abdominal muscles (see next section on pursed-lip breathing).

❖ Assess the patient's response (e.g., dizziness and lightheadedness may indicate hyperventilation and necessitate slowing the frequency of the ventilations).

❖ Repeat for three breaths and rest for 1 minute.

Pursed-Lip Breathing

The **pursed-lip breathing** technique is especially useful in patients with diseases of chronic airway limitation because it slows the collapse of the small airways by maintaining a higher bronchiole pressure and prolonging expiration. It can also be used to control breathing in the dyspneic patient, to prevent holding the breath during activity (a common problem in patients with CAL), and to reduce air trapping in the alveoli.

❖ Assist the patient into a sitting or high, semi-Fowler's position.

❖ Instruct the patient to purse his or her lips as if to whistle with lips slightly open.

❖ Have the patient inhale through the nose to a count of two and slowly exhale through pursed lips to a count of four or until he or she has completely exhaled.

❖ Repeat this technique for 10 minutes, increasing the frequency to four to five times a day.

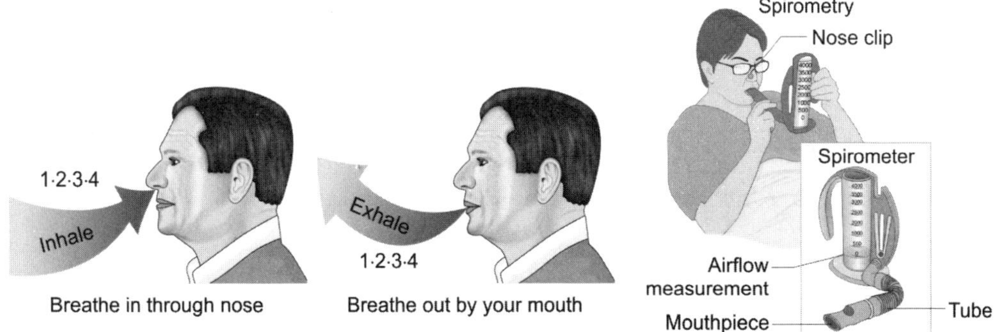

Pursed lip breathing.

Breathing technique using spirometer.

Incentive Spirometry

Incentive spirometry or sustained maximal inspiration devices (SMI) are tools that help maximize ventilation by increasing lung volume, flow, and alveolar inflation. The device measures respiratory volume and provides a visual stimulus via a colored, plastic float to induce the patient to breath deeply. Incentive spirometry can be combined with breathing exercises to maximize ventilation.

Incentive spirometers are usually plastic, disposable units that patients may take home after discharge from a facility. They are useful in patients who have the diminished ability to breathe deeply and during the postoperative period, especially after thoracic or abdominal surgery when deep inhalation may be limited by pain. During the postoperative period, general anesthesia, incisional pain, and narcotic medications all diminish alveolar inflation. The incentive spirometer provides visual cues of preoperative functioning and postoperative goals. The preoperative levels are marked on the spirometer and can be used to monitor recovery after surgery. Flow incentive spirometers are useful for patients at low risk for developing postoperative atelectasis. Volume spirometers are useful with higher risk patients because they measure lung inflation more precisely.

MOBILIZING SECRETIONS

Clearing respiratory secretions promotes patent airways and easier ventilation of the lungs, and prevents mucus stasis. Secretions are easier to cough up if they are thin, rather than thick and tenacious. Therefore, adequate fluid intake, humidification of inspired air, and possibly expectorant medication (e.g., guaifenesin) are important interventions in mobilizing secretions. Other medications that can be used before breathing exercises are inhaled bronchodilators such as albuterol or systemic bronchodilators such as theophylline. These medications allow the airways to relax and dilate so that the breathing and coughing exercises are more effective.

Patients with chronic respiratory disorders such as COPD and cystic fibrosis may require more aggressive interventions to remove mucous from the respiratory passages. A **mucus clearance device** or a *flutter* can help patients mobilize secretions. This handheld device has a ball valve that vibrates when the patient exhales, causing vibrations to be transmitted in the airways and loosen secretions. The device is held by the patient with the stem parallel to the floor. The patient exhales with flattened cheeks followed by huffing to remove the secretions.

Coughing

Coughing is the most effective and natural way to clear the airways. A good coughing technique allows for adequate mobilization and expulsion of pulmonary secretions. Normally a cough is an involuntary response, but it can be controlled consciously. In healthy patients, a cough begins with inhalation, followed by glottic closure, and then the rapid opening of the glottis and rapid expulsion of the air. Sometimes the air is expelled at speeds up to 100 miles per hour. In patients with some respiratory disorders, the normal cough reflex may be diminished or there may be excessive secretions. Three techniques that can be used to help patients clear secretions are cascade coughing, huff coughing (huffing), and quad coughing.

Cascade Coughing

Cascade coughing is a useful technique during the postoperative period with patients who have CAL or neuromuscular diseases or those who are bedridden. Cascade coughing allows the patient to increase chest expansion during inhalation and more forcefully expel secretions with coughing.

❖ Have the patient in an upright position such as sitting or semi-Fowler's position.

❖ Teach the patient to inhale and exhale slowly and deeply.

❖ Then, have the patient inhale deeply and exhale, closing his throat and using small coughs without inhaling again, pause, and then inhale again very slowly (to decrease the cough stimulus). If paroxysmal coughing starts, instruct the patient to use slow deep breaths or pursed-lip breathing until the coughing urge passes.

❖ Rest and repeat for a total of three cycles.

❖ Assess ability to expel secretions and/or auscultate the lungs.

❖ Try to set up a regular coughing schedule for patients with CAL to keep airways patent.

Huff or Open Glottis Coughing

Huff or open glottis coughing (**huffing**) is a useful technique in patients with chronic airway limitation such as COPD.

❖ Have the patient in the sitting or semi-Fowler's position with arms crossed below the rib cage (hugging a pillow may be more comfortable).

❖ Instruct the patient to inhale slowly, hold for 2 seconds, tighten the abdominal, leg, and gluteal muscles (to increase intrathoracic pressure), and then exhale in short huffs, actually saying the word *huff.*

❖ Repeat and try to cough on exhalation.

❖ Assess the patient's response and ability to expel secretions.

❖ Auscultate the lungs.

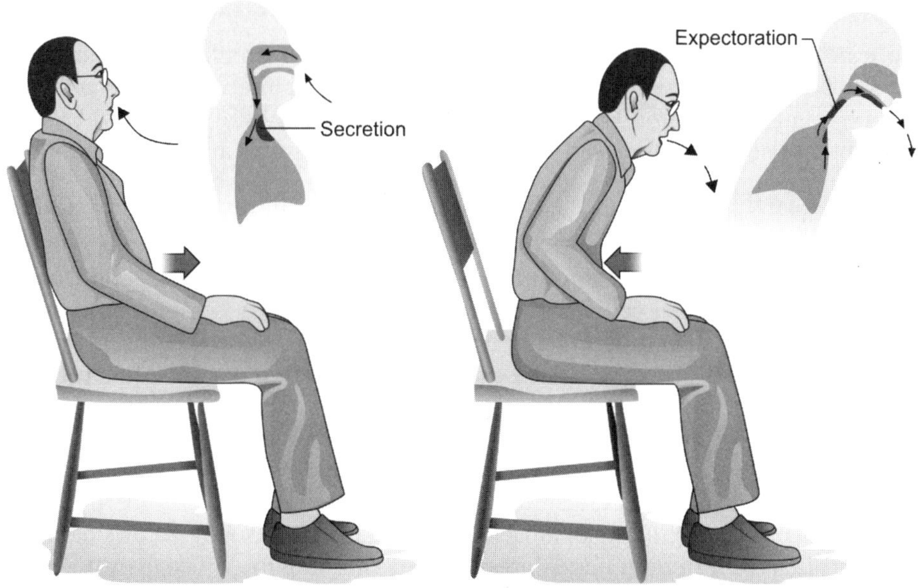

Huff coughing.

Quad Coughing

Quad coughing may assist patients with muscle weakness such as multiple sclerosis to expel secretions. Using a modified Heimlich maneuver, the patient places the heels of both hands between the umbilicus and the xiphoid process, pressing inward and upward during coughing or huffing to clear secretions.

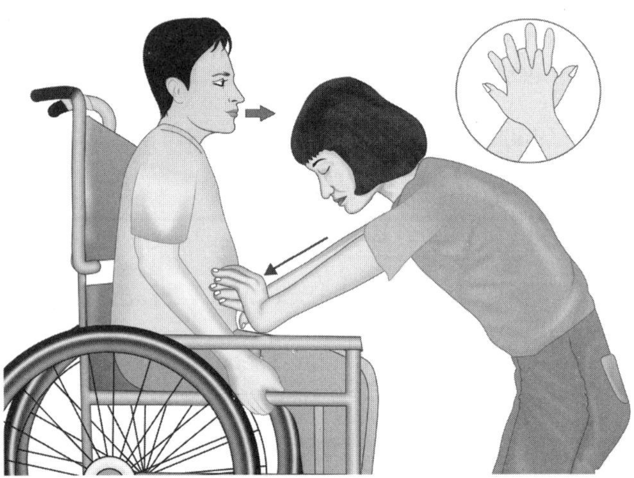

Quad coughing.

Chest Physical Therapy

Chest physical therapy (CPT) is another method to mobilize secretions and maintain airway patency and alveolar expansion. It may be combined with other interventions such as incentive spirometry, inhaled bronchodilators, and suctioning. Outcomes of successful CPT include improved breath sounds, increased PaO_2, expulsion of sputum, and improved airflow on spirometry.

Chest physical therapy is composed of three techniques that may be used individually or in combination. These techniques—percussion, vibration, and postural drainage—are performed by respiratory therapists or nurses. **Percussion** is performed by applying cupped hands in a rhythmic sequence over a part or the entire lung. It is useful in patients with cystic fibrosis and bronchiectasis and may be combined with vibration. Using the percussion technique, a hollow sound is produced as the cupped hand creates an air pocket when applied to the chest wall. It is used to loosen secretions. Percussion may be combined with postural drainage positions to optimize drainage of particular lung segments. Percussion is contraindicated in patients with cardiac conditions, osteoporosis, pneumothorax, hemopneumothorax, or pleural effusion.

Vibration is another technique of loosening secretions that usually follows percussion. It involves the placement of both hands pressing and vibrating the rib cage over the affected lung. The arm and shoulder muscles contract isometrically, producing a small vibration that is transmitted through the patient's chest wall and airways. This vibration is thought to increase the turbulence of the air in the lung and to loosen secretions. Vibration is useful in patients with cystic fibrosis and bronchiectasis.

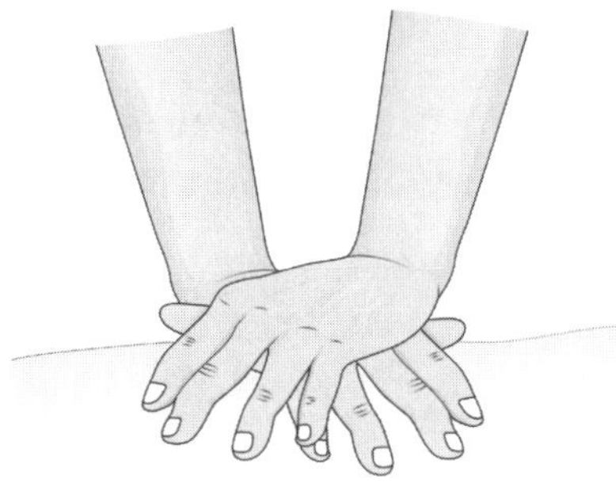

Hand position for vibration of the chest wall.

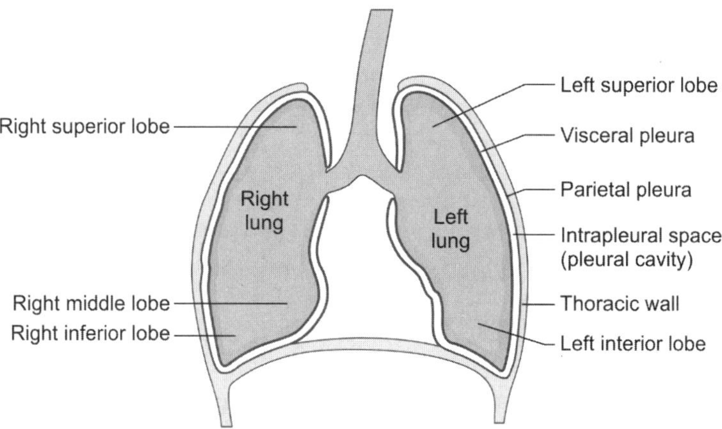

Lobes of the lungs.

Postural drainage involves positioning the patient in such a way as to allow gravity to drain particular segments of the lungs. Several positions may not be tolerated by the patient because the head is lower than the torso. The positions can be adapted by raising the head of the bed so that the patient is comfortable and can breathe easily. Postural drainage may be contraindicated if the patient has cardiac conditions or increased intracranial pressure. Particular positions can be combined with percussion and vibration to further mobilize secretions.

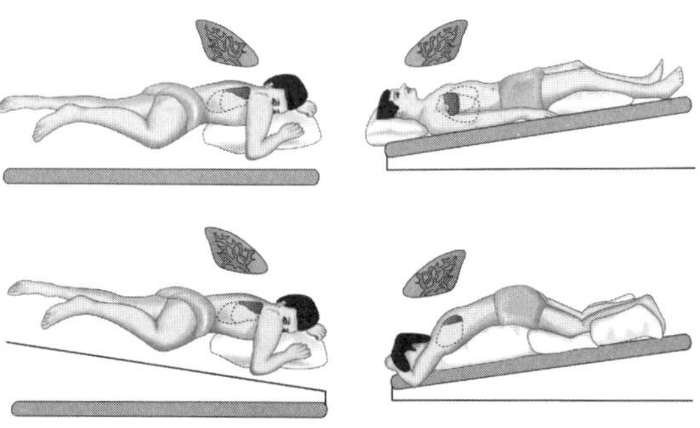

Postural drainage.

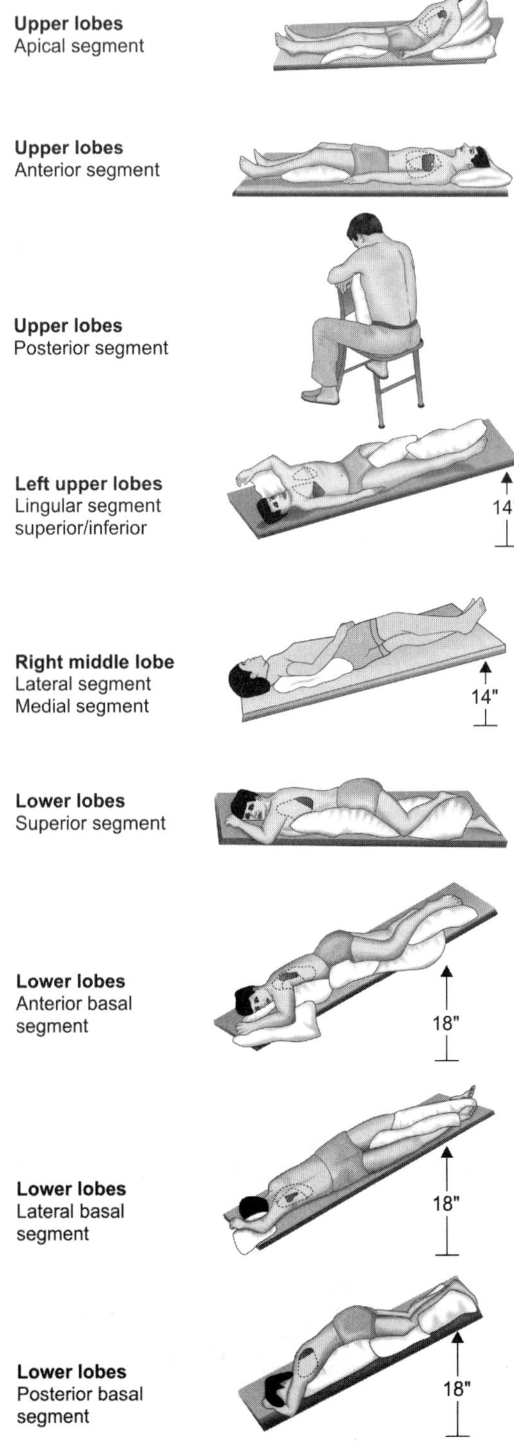

Postural drainage positions.

Vibratory PEP Therapy

Vibratory Positive Expiratory Pressure (PEP) therapy uses handheld devices such as "flutter valves" or "Acapella" devices for patients who need assistance in clearing mucus from their airways. These devices (see Figure) require a prescription and are used in collaboration with a respiratory therapist or advanced health care provider. To use Vibratory PEP therapy, the patient should sit up, take a deep breath, and blow into the device. A flutter valve within the device creates vibrations that help break up the mucus so the patient can cough it up and spit it out. Additionally, a small amount of positive end-expiratory pressure (PEEP) is created in the airways that helps to keep them open so that more air can be exhaled.

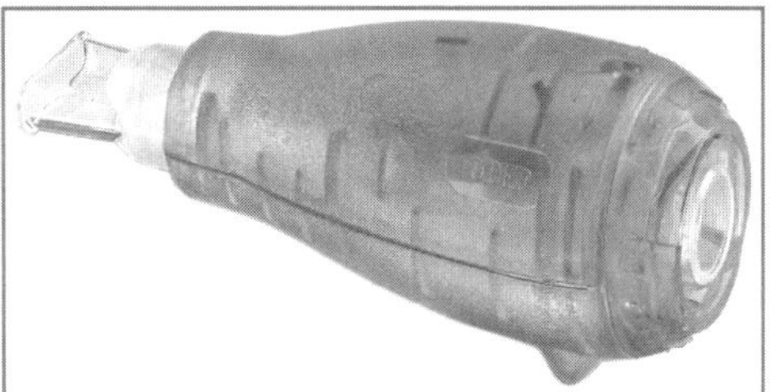

Flutter valve device.

MAINTAINING A PATENT AIRWAY

In all patients, maintaining a patent airway is the most important intervention to improve oxygenation. Airway patency is especially important if the patient is unconscious, anesthetized, or obtunded. In these conditions, the airways may collapse and secretions may accumulate, impeding the passage of air into the lungs. For example, patients who are semiconscious after anesthesia may not be able to maintain a patent airway because the tongue falls back and may occlude the posterior oropharynx. Artificial airways may be placed to maintain patency of the airway, allow for suctioning of secretions, and permit mechanical ventilation. The most common types of artificial airways are oral airways, nasopharyngeal airways, endotracheal tubes, and tracheostomy tubes.

Oral airways are rigid, plastic devices used to maintain the normal structure of the oropharynx. They are used for short-term airway maintenance, such as in postanesthesia units while the patient recovers from anesthetic agents. Oral airways are curved to follow the normal anatomy of the oropharynx from the lips, over the tongue, and into the posterior oropharynx. The opening allows for air passage through as well as around the airway and permits suctioning of secretions in the posterior oropharynx. Once the patient is alert enough to maintain the airway and clear secretions, the oral airway is removed as it can be very irritating.

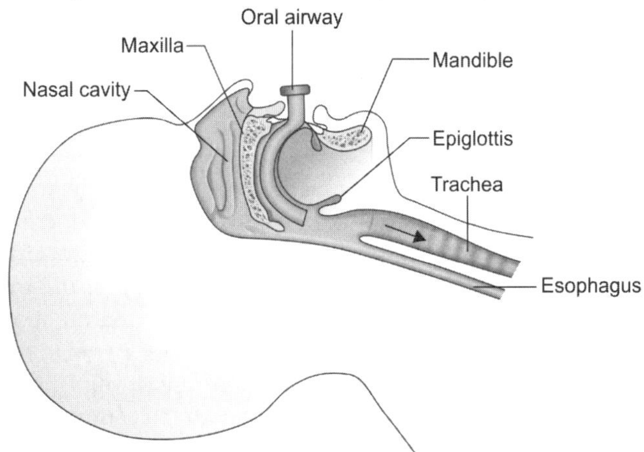

Insertion of oral airways.

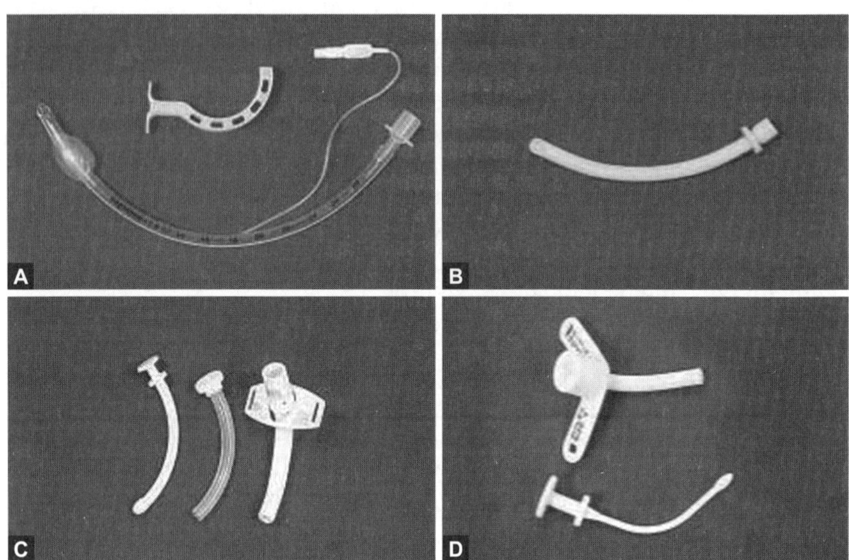

Types of artificial airways: A. Oral airway and endotracheal tube; B. Nasal trumpet;
C. Tracheostomy tube; D. Pediatric tracheostomy tube.

Insertion of an Oral Airway	
1.	Measure the oral airway along the patient's jaw with the open end of the curve facing the patient's neck to ensure that the airway is the correct size. The curve of the airway should follow the angle of the patient's jawline.
2.	Check that dentures are removed and that there are no loose teeth before inserting the airway.
3.	Place the patient in the supine position and open the mouth using the "cross-finger technique," using the thumb and forefinger on the upper and lower teeth to open the mouth.
4.	Gently put the airway in upside down until past the teeth and then rotate it over the tongue to follow the curve of the oropharynx.
5.	Tape the airway in place and position the patient on his side to prevent aspiration of secretions or vomitus.
6.	Suction at least hourly to remove secretions.
7.	Evaluate respiration and adequacy of the airway frequently.

OXYGEN ADMINISTRATION

Oxygen administration is a therapy to maintain adequate tissue oxygenation while minimizing cardiopulmonary work. There are a variety of reasons that cause doctors to initiate oxygen administration, that includes maintenance of oxygenation while providing anesthesia, increased metabolic demand, CO (carbon monoxide) exposure, treatment of headaches, supplementation due to affected oxygen exchange during the treatment of lung illnesses, and more are included in the reasons for its initiation.

The atmosphere consists of approximately 21% oxygen at sea level. This percentage decreases in a near-linear fashion with an increase in altitude. O_2 mask (non-rebreather, venti-mask, simple), or nasal cannula is used to deliver supplemental oxygen to the patient. In some cases, oxygen is added into BiPAP (bilevel positive airway pressure) or CPAP (continuous positive airway pressure) system. To deliver oxygen to intubated patients, ventilators are used.

Oxygen is required by all tissues to support cell metabolism; in acute illness, low tissue oxygenation (hypoxia) can occur due to a failure in any of the systems that deliver and circulate oxygen. Hypoxia is an indication to start oxygen therapy; this can be a life-saving intervention, but given without appropriate assessment and ongoing evaluation, it can also be detrimental to patients' health.

Physiology and Anatomy

The optimal oxygenation of the patients depends upon their airway anatomy. For instance, a trauma patient whose nasal passages are impeded by blood would be provided supplemental oxygen suboptimally using a nasal cannula while it might be hard to achieve oxygenation goals using CPAP or BiPAP system (i.e., sealed masks) for a patient with micrognathia.

The patient's position must be upright while being provided with supplemental oxygen unless there is a contraindication to such positioning such as level of sedation, patient risk, anatomy, and trauma before the c-spine clearance.

Indications of Oxygenation

Hypoxemia (decreased level of oxygen in the blood) is the most readily accepted indication for supplemental oxygenation. Oxygen saturation targets are 92 to 98% in a healthy patient. Values under 90% are considered to be low. Normal arterial oxygen is around 775–100 mm Hg, or 95–100%. Low levels of oxygen in blood or hypoxemia show symptoms, such as tiredness, confused behavior, SOB (shortness of breath), and others that can even damage your body.

For patients with chronic hypercapnic conditions, the values for oxygen saturation can be as low as 80%. These values are measured by pulse oximetry. In the critical care setting, pulse oximetry is far and widely used for monitoring oxygenation. Respiratory status of patients in ICU is also monitored by pulse oximetry. But in cases of CO (carbon monoxide) or cyanide poisoning and anemia, pulse oximeter gives falsely elevated readings and is not an adequate indicator of perfusion.

Chronic

Chronic indications include:
- **COPD** (chronic obstructive pulmonary disease). It refers to a group of diseases that cause breathing-related problems and airflow blockage. It has no cure but it can be treated.
- Pulmonary fibrosis (which is caused by scarred tissues present deep in lungs. They become stiff and thick which can make it harder for the person to catch a breath and as result blood does not get properly oxygenated). Its symptoms include SOB, fatigue, clubbing, dry cough, aching muscles, and joints, etc.
- **Cystic fibrosis** (It is an inherited disease in which sticky, thick mucus buildup that can damage many of the organs of the body). Its symptoms include continuous damage to the respiratory system and chronic digestive system problems.
- **Sarcoidosis** (It is a disease characterized by the growth of a tiny group of inflammatory cells in different parts of the body. Most commonly in lymph nodes and lungs. But it can also affect the heart, skin, eyes, and other organs).

Acute

These acute indications refer to medical emergencies that require high concentrations of oxygen in all cases. These cases include:

- **Shock**
- **Sepsis** (i.e., a possibly life-threatening condition caused by the body's response to an infection)
- **Major trauma, cardiac arrest and during resuscitation** (to provide adequate arterial oxyhemoglobin saturation)
- **Anaphylaxis** (which is a potentially life-threatening and severe allergic reaction)
- **Cyanide and carbon monoxide (CO) poisonings**
- **TRALI** (transfusion-related acute lung injury) which is a rare but serious syndrome characterized by sudden acute respiratory distress following transfusion.

These acute indications refer to medical emergencies that may or may not require oxygen administration. These cases include:

- **Asthma:** It causes repeated attacks of early morning or nighttime coughing, breathlessness, wheezing, and chest tightness.
- **Bronchitis:** It is caused when the airway of the lungs swell and produce mucus in the lungs.
- **Acute heart failure, or heart failure exacerbations**
- **Pulmonary embolism:** It is a sudden blockage in the lung artery.

Contraindications

Common herbicide paraquat is harmful to people, and because of its redox activity, oxygen therapy exacerbates the effects of paraquat poisoning.

High oxygen exposure can cause vision loss or blindness in newborns through the development of neovascularization of the retinas, which puts them at risk for retinopathy of prematurity, or ROP. Antioxidants in adults and vitamin E given to premature neonates may offer some protection for babies who need extra oxygenation.

Because dry (non-humidified) air is used, oxygen delivery can increase insensible losses, especially at high flow rates. Furthermore, giving cool or even cold oxygen to susceptible patients can raise their risk of hypothermia; however, this can be readily avoided by warming and humidifying the patient prior to administration.

Exposure to elevated FIO_2 during oxygen therapy can result in oxygen poisoning, an iatrogenic disease. When patients are receiving extra oxygen, their oxygen saturation levels should be watched. Some chemicals change into superoxide anions, also referred to as hydroxyl radicals, during the metabolism of oxygen. These radicals are harmful to human tissue. PaO_2 levels, diffusing capacity, and lung compliance all decline as a result of the pathophysiological alterations that occur at the alveolar level. High partial pressures of oxygen can cause toxicity to the central nervous system (CNS). Proteinaceous exudates, alveolar haemorrhages, and alveolar and interstitial edoema are among the acute alterations in the lungs brought on by oxygen intoxication. Extended exposure to oxygen induces a proliferative phase characerised by the growth of type II epithelial cells and fibroblasts, succeeded by the formation of collagen deposits.

Exposure to FIO_2 greater than 0.60 for as little as 24 to 48 hours can lead to severe irreversible pulmonary fibrosis.

OXYGENATION EQUIPMENT

There are several types of equipment a nurse may use when providing oxygen therapy to a patient. Each device is described in detail below:

Pulse Oximeter

A pulse oximeter is a commonly used portable device used to obtain a patient's oxygen saturation level at the bedside or in a clinic. The pulse oximeter, commonly referred to as a "Pulse Ox," is an electronic device that measures the oxygen saturation of hemoglobin in a patient's red blood cells, referred to as SpO_2. The normal range for SpO_2 for an adult without an underlying respiratory condition is above 92%. The pulse oximeter analyzes light produced by the probe as it passes through the finger to determine the saturation level of the hemoglobin molecule.

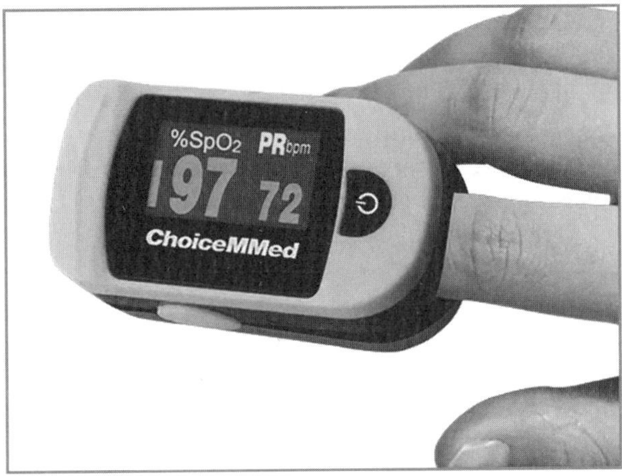

Portable pulse oximeter.

Portable Pulse Oximeter

Pulse oximetry readings can be inaccurate for several reasons and must be interpreted using the nurse's clinical judgment. The most common cause of inaccuracy with pulse oximeters is motion artifact. Patient movement can cause pulsatile venous flow to be incorrectly measured as arterial pulsations, thus producing false oximetry and pulse-rate readings. Another common cause of inaccuracy is poor peripheral perfusion. Poor peripheral perfusion can be caused by conditions such cardiac and vascular disease. In these situations, use a specific pulse oximeter probe for the forehead, bridge of nose or earlobe to obtain the reading. In any clinical situation where the client's fingertips are cool or cold, attempt to warm them by using moist heat or a warm blanket, then apply the pulse oximetry probe when the fingers are warmed for a more accurate reading. Nail polish can also cause an inaccurate pulse oximetry reading and must be removed before placing the probe. Finally, in emergency situations such as carbon monoxide poisoning, other molecules besides oxygen can attach to hemoglobin and cause a falsely high SpO_2 reading even though the patient does not have enough oxygen to meet metabolic demands.

Oxygen Flow Meter

In inpatient settings, rooms are equipped with wall-mounted oxygen supply outlets that are nationally standardized in a green color, whereas air outlets are standardized with a yellow color. Oxygen flow meters are attached to the green oxygen outlets, and then the oxygenation device is attached to the flow meter. See for an image of an oxygen flow meter. An oxygen flow meter consists of a glass cylinder containing a steel ball with an opening through which oxygen from the supply source is injected through an adapter. This adapter is commonly referred to as a "tree" because of its appearance. Oxygen is turned on, and the flow rate of oxygen is controlled by turning the green valve on the side of the glass cylinder. The flow rate is set according to the location of a steel ball inside the cylinder and the numbered lines on the glass cylinder, flow rate is currently set at two liter per minute (L/min). It is essential to implement safety precautions whenever oxygen is used. Read more about "Safety with Oxygen Therapy" later in this section.

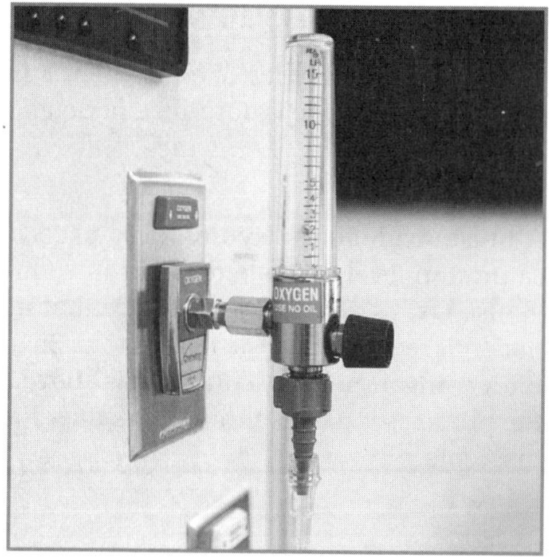

Oxygen flow meter.

Portable Oxygen Supply Devices

Portable oxygen tanks are commonly used when transporting a patient to procedures within the hospital or to other agencies. Oxygenation devices are connected to the tank in a similar manner as the wall-mounted oxygen flow meter. It is crucial for nurses and transporters to ensure the tank has an adequate amount of oxygen for use during transport, is turned on, and the appropriate flow rate is set.

Portable Oxygen Tank

Instead of oxygen tanks, oxygen concentrators are commonly used by patients in their home environment. Oxygen concentrators are also produced in portable sizes that are lightweight and easy for patient use while travelling and mobile in the community. Oxygen concentrators work by taking the 21% concentration of oxygen in the air, running it through a molecular sleeve to remove the nitrogen and concentrating the oxygen to a 96% level, thus producing between 1 and 6 liters per minute of oxygen. Oxygen concentrators may provide pulse flow or continuous flow. Pulse flow only occurs on inhalation, whereas continuous flow delivers oxygen throughout the entire breath cycle. Pulse versions are the most lightweight because oxygen is provided only as needed by the patient.

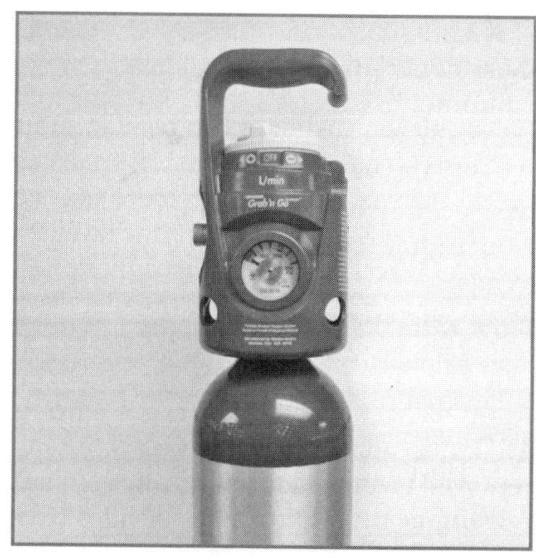

Portable oxygen tank.

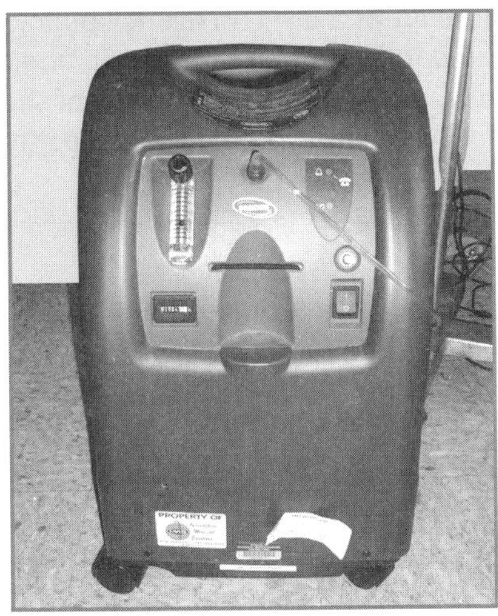

Home oxygen concentrator.

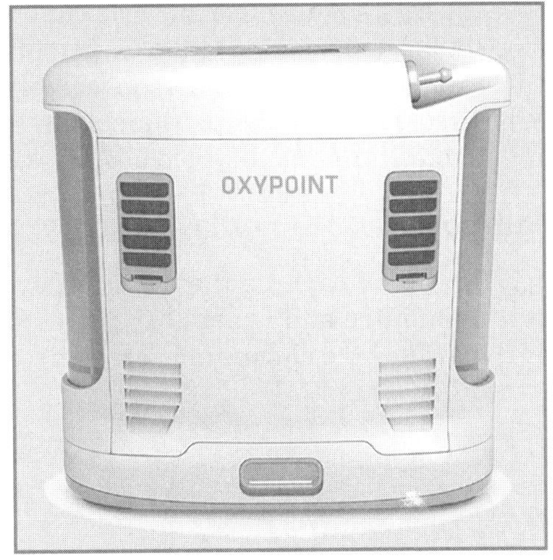

Portable oxygen concentrator.

Nasal Cannula

A nasal cannula is the simplest oxygenation device and consists of oxygen tubing connected to two short prongs that are inserted into the patient's nares. The tubing is connected to the flow meter of the oxygen supply source. To prevent drying out the patient's mucus membranes, humidification may be added for hospitalized patients receiving oxygen flow rates greater than 4 L/minute or for those receiving oxygen therapy for longer periods of time.

Nasal cannulas are the most common type of oxygen equipment. They are used for short- and long-term therapy (i.e., COPD patients) and are best used with stable patients who require low amounts of oxygen.

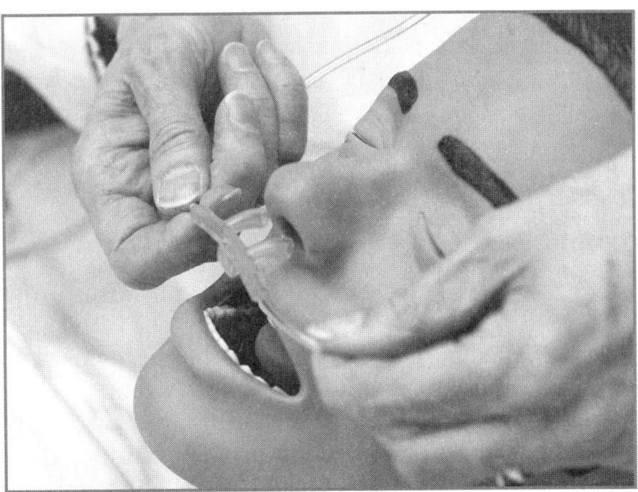

Nasal cannula.

Flow rate: Nasal cannulas can have a flow rate ranging from 1 to 5 liters per minute (L/min), with a 4% increase in FiO_2 for every liter of oxygen, resulting in range of fraction of inspired oxygen (FiO_2) levels of 24–44%.

Advantages: Nasal cannulas are easy to use, inexpensive, and disposable. They are convenient because the patient can talk and eat while receiving oxygen.

Limitations: The nasal prongs of nasal cannula are easily dislodged, especially when the patient is sleeping. The tubing placed on the face can cause skin breakdown in the nose and above the ears, so the nurse must vigilantly monitor these areas. Based on agency policy, the nurse should add padding to the oxygen tubing as needed to avoid skin breakdown and may apply a water-based lubricant to prevent drying. However, petroleum-based lubricant should not be used due to the risk of flammability. Nasal cannulas are not as effective if the patient is a mouth breather or has blocked nostrils, a deviated septum, or nasal polyps.

High-flow Nasal Cannula

High-flow nasal cannula therapy is an oxygen supply system capable of delivering up to 100% humidified and heated oxygen at a flow rate of up to 60 liters per minute. Patients with high-flow nasal cannulas are generally in critical condition and require advanced monitoring.

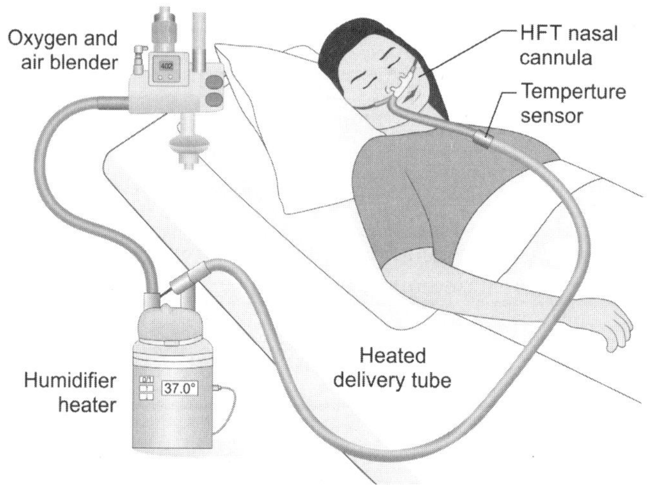

High-flow nasal cannula system.

Simple Mask

A simple mask fits over the mouth and nose of the patient and contains exhalation ports (i.e., holes on the side of the mask) through which the patient exhales carbon dioxide. These holes should always remain open. The mask is held in place by an elastic band placed around the back of the head. It also has a metal piece near the top that can be pinched and shaped over the patient's nose to create a better fit. Humidified air may be attached if the oxygen concentrations are drying for the patient.

Simple Face Mask

Flow rate: Simple masks should be set to a flow rate of 6 to 10 L/min, resulting in oxygen concentration (FiO_2) levels of

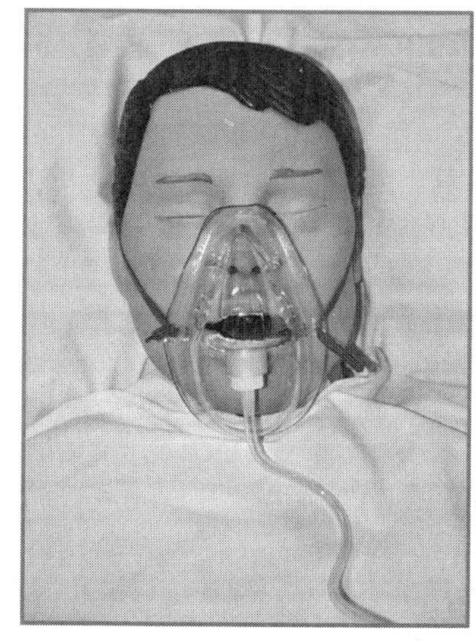

Simple face mask.

35–50%. The flow rate should never be set below 6 L/min because this can result in the patient rebreathing their exhaled carbon dioxide.

Advantages: Face masks are used to provide moderate oxygen concentrations. Their efficiency in oxygen delivery depends on how well the mask fits and the patient's respiratory demands.

Disadvantages: Face masks must be removed when eating, and they may feel confining for some patients who feel claustrophobic with the mask on.

Non-rebreather Mask

A non-rebreather mask consists of a mask attached to a reservoir bag that is attached with tubing to a flow meter. See image of a non-rebreather mask. It has a series of one-way valves between the mask and the bag and also on the covers on the exhalation ports. The reservoir bag should never totally deflate; if the bag deflates, there is a problem and immediate intervention is required. The one-way valves function so that on inspiration, the patient only breathes in from the reservoir bag; on exhalation, carbon dioxide is directed out through the exhalation ports. Non-rebreather masks are used for patients who can breathe on their own but require higher concentrations of oxygen to maintain satisfactory blood oxygenation levels.

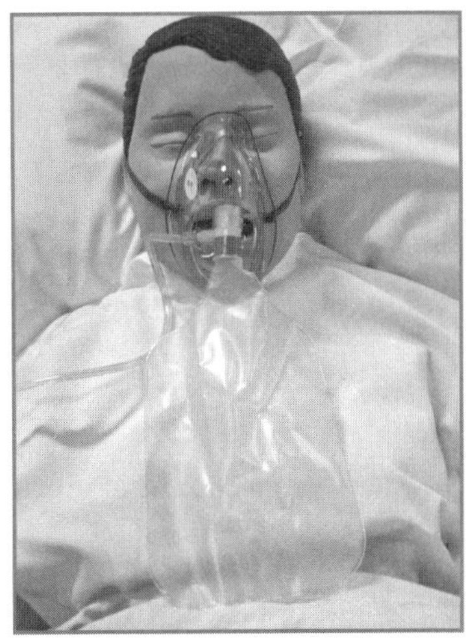
Non-rebreather mask.

Flow rate: The flow rate for a non-rebreather mask should be set to deliver a **minimum** of 10 to 15 L/minute. The reservoir bag should be inflated prior to placing the mask on the patient. With a good fit, the non-rebreather mask can deliver between 60% and 80% FiO_2.

Advantages: Non-rebreather masks deliver high levels of oxygen noninvasively to patients who can otherwise breathe unassisted.

Disadvantages: Due to the one-way valves in non-rebreather masks, there is a high risk of suffocation if the gas flow is interrupted. The mask requires a tight seal and may feel hot and confining to the patient. It will interfere with talking, and the patient cannot eat with the mask on.

Partial Rebreather Mask

The partial rebreather mask looks very similar to the non-rebreather mask. The difference between the masks is a partial rebreather mask does not contain one-way valves, so the patient's exhaled air mixes with their inhaled air. A partial rebreather mask requires 10–15 L/min of oxygen, but only delivers 35–50% FiO_2.

Venturi Mask

Venturi masks are indicated for patients who require a specific amount of supplemental oxygen to avoid complications, such as those with chronic obstructive pulmonary disease (COPD). Different types of adaptors are attached to a face mask that set the flow rate to achieve a specific

FiO_2 ranging from 24% to 60%. Venturi adapters are typically set up by a respiratory therapist, but in some facilities, they may be set up by a nurse according to agency policy.

Flow rate: The flow rate depends on the adaptor and does not correspond to the flow meter. Consult with a respiratory therapist before changing the flow rate.

Advantages: A specific amount of FiO_2 is delivered to patients whose breathing status may be affected by high levels of oxygen.

Oxymask

Oxygen delivery device that has an open design that eliminates the need for valves and reservoirs. O_2 flow is directed towards the nose and mouth. Large openings in mask allows CO_2 to escape, decreases claustrophobia, increases ability to communicate and allows for delivery of PO fluids and meds without removing mask.

Flow rate: Can deliver 24–90% oxygen concentration on 1–15 LPM oxygen which increases flexibility and safety of product.

Advantages: Increased flexibility and safety due to variable oxygen flow rates. Decreased claustrophobia and increased ability to communicate without removing mask.

Oxymizer

A special nasal cannula that provides a larger luminal diameter in combination with an oxygen reservoir. Oxymizer is designed as either a moustache or pendant style. Some patients do not like the weight of the device which is greater due to the oxygen reservoir and tubing size.

Flow rate: 1/4 to 1/2 of the previous flow rate required. The oxymizer can deliver up to 15 LPM.

Advantages: The oxymizer is able to help maintain adequate O_2 saturations in hypoxic patients with a lower flow rate resulting in reduced O_2 costs, portable O_2 sources last longer, decreased nasal irritation and dryness.

Continuous Positive Airway Pressure (CPAP)

A continuous positive airway pressure (CPAP) device is used for people who are able to breathe spontaneously on their own but need help in keeping their airway unobstructed, such as those with obstructive sleep apnea. The CPAP device consists of a special mask that covers the patient's nose, or nose and mouth, and is attached to a machine that continuously applies mild air pressure to keep the patient's airways from collapsing.

A prescription is required for a CPAP device in the hospital or patient's home environment. In the hospital, the FiO_2 is set up with the CPAP mask by the respiratory therapist. In a home setting, an adapter is added so that oxygen is attached using a flowmeter with preprogrammed settings so the patient and/or nurse are only required to turn the machine on before sleeping and off upon awakening. It is important to keep the mask and tubing clean to prevent infection, so be sure to follow agency policy for cleaning the equipment regularly. If a humidifier is attached, distilled water or sterile water should be used to fill it, but never tap water. A patient wearing a CPAP device while sleeping.

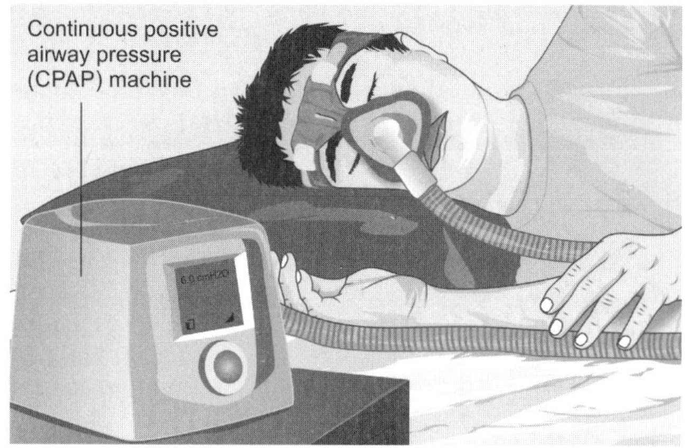

CPAP machine.

BiPAP

A bilevel positive airway pressure (BiPAP) device is similar to a CPAP device in that it is used to prevent airways from collapsing, but BiPAP devices have two pressure settings. One setting occurs during inhalation and a lower pressure setting is used during exhalation. Patients using BiPAP devices in their home environment for obstructive sleep apnea often find these two pressures more tolerable because they do not have to exhale against continuous pressure. In acute-care settings, BiPAP devices are also used for patients in acute respiratory distress as a noninvasive alternative to intubation and mechanical ventilation and are managed by respiratory therapists. BiPAP devices in home settings are set up in a similar manner as CPAP machines for ease of use.

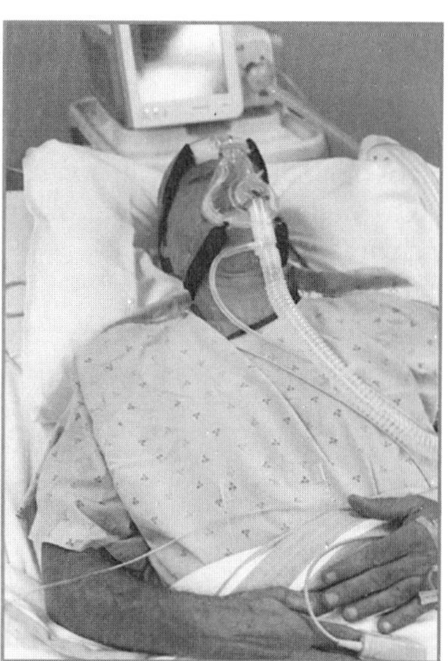

Simulated patient wearing a BiPAP mask.

Bag Valve Mask (Ambu Bag)

A bag valve mask, commonly known as an "Ambu bag," is a handheld device used in emergency situations for patients who are not breathing (respiratory arrest) or who are not breathing adequately (respiratory failure). In this manner, this device is different from the other devices because it assists with **ventilation**, the movement of air into and out of the lungs, as well as oxygenation. Bag valve masks are produced in different sizes for infants, children, and adults to prevent lung injury, so it is important to use the correct size for the patient.

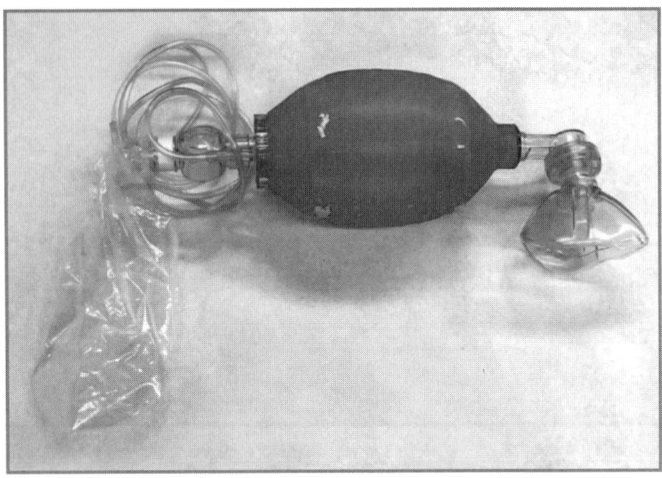

Bag valve mask (Ambu bag).

Use of Bag Valve Mask

When using a bag mask valve, the rescuer manually compresses the bag to force air into the lungs. Squeezing the bag once every 5 to 6 seconds for an adult or once every 3 seconds for an infant or child provides an adequate respiratory rate. In inpatient settings, the bag mask valve is attached to an oxygen supply to increase the concentration of oxygenation provided with each breath.

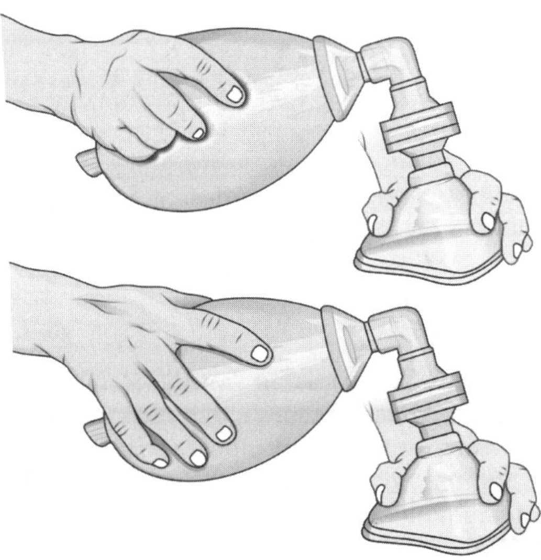

Use of a bag valve mask.

It is vital to obtain a tight seal of the mask to the patient's face, but this is difficult for a single rescuer to achieve. Therefore, two rescuers are recommended; one rescuer performs a jaw thrust maneuver, secures the mask to the patient's face with both hands, and focuses on maintaining a leak-proof mask seal, while the other rescuer squeezes the bag and focuses on the amount and the timing.

Flow rate: The flow rate for a bag valve mask attached to an oxygen source should be set to 15 L/minute, resulting in FiO_2 of 100%.

Advantages: A bag valve mask is portable and provides immediate assistance to patients in respiratory failure or respiratory arrest. It also can be used to hyperoxygenate patients before procedures that can cause hypoxia, such as tracheal suctioning.

Disadvantages: The rate and depth of compression of the bag must be closely monitored to prevent injury to the patient. In the event of respiratory failure when the patient is still breathing, the bag compressions must be coordinated with the patient's inhalations to ensure that oxygen is delivered and asynchrony of breaths is prevented. Complications may also result from overinflating or overpressurizing the patient. Complications include lung injury or the inflation of the stomach that can lead to aspiration of stomach contents. Additionally, rescuers may tire after a few minutes of manually compressing the bag, resulting in less than optimal ventilation. Alternatively, an endotracheal tube (ET) can be inserted by an advanced practitioner to substitute for the mask portion of this device.

Endotracheal Intubation

When a patient is receiving general anesthesia prior to a procedure or surgery or is experiencing respiratory failure or respiratory arrest, an endotracheal tube (ET) is inserted by an advanced practitioner, such as a respiratory therapist, paramedic, or anesthesiologist, to maintain a secure airway. The ET tube is sealed within the trachea with an inflatable cuff, and oxygen is supplied via a bag valve mask or via mechanical ventilation.

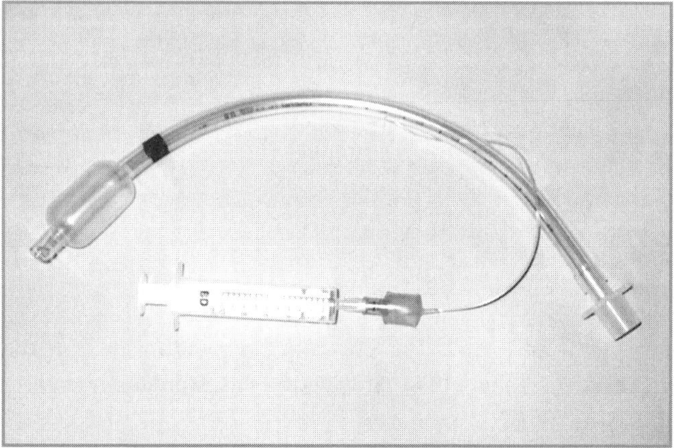

An endotracheal tube.

Mechanical Ventilator

A mechanical ventilator is a machine attached to an endotracheal tube to assist or replace spontaneous breathing. Mechanical ventilation is termed invasive because it requires placement of a device inside the trachea through the mouth, such as an endotracheal tube. Mechanical ventilators are managed by respiratory therapists via protocol or provider order. FiO_2 can be set from 21–100%. Nurses collaborate with respiratory therapists and the health care providers regarding the overall care of the patient on a mechanical ventilator.

Tracheostomy

A tracheostomy is a surgically-made hole called a stoma that goes from the front of the patient's neck into the trachea. A tracheostomy tube is placed through the stoma and directly into the trachea to maintain an open (patent) airway and to administer oxygen. A tracheostomy may be performed emergently or as a planned procedure.

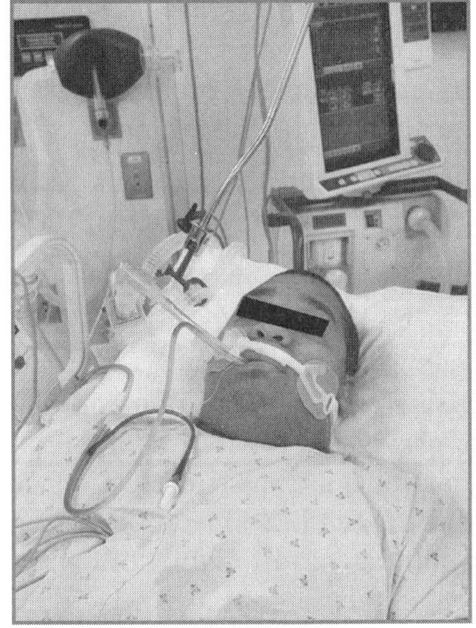

Simulated intubated patient with an endotracheal tube and attached on a mechanical ventilator.

Flow Rates and Oxygen Percentages

When administering oxygen to a patient, it is important to ensure that oxygen flow rates are appropriately set according to the type of administration device.

Settings of Oxygenation Devices

Device	Flow Rates and Oxygen Percentage
Nasal cannula	Flow rate: 1-6 L/min FiO_2: 24% to 44%
High-flow nasal cannula	Flow rate: up to 60 L/min FiO_2: Up to 100%
Simple mask	Flow rate: 6–10 L/min FiO_2: 28% to 50%
Non-rebreather mask	Flow rate: 10–15 L/min FiO_2: 60–80% Safety Note: The reservoir bag should always be partially inflated
CPAP, BiPAP, venturi mask, mechanical ventilator	Use the settings provided by the respiratory therapist and/or provider order
Bag valve mask	Flow rate: 15 L/min FiO_2: 100% Squeeze the bag once every 5 to 6 seconds for an adult or once every 3 seconds for an infant or child

Oxygen Therapy Safety Guidelines

Guideline	Additional Information
Remember that oxygen is a medication	Oxygen is a medication and should not be adjusted without consultation with a physician or respiratory therapist
Store oxygen cylinders correctly	When using oxygen cylinders, store them upright, chained, or in appropriate holders so that they will not fall. Full oxygen tanks should be stored separately from partially-full or empty oxygen tanks
Use tank holders appropriately	When transporting a patient, proper tank holders must be used per Joint Commission guidelines. Tanks should never be placed on the patient's bed
Do not allow smoking near the oxygen devices	Oxygen supports combustion. No smoking is permitted around any oxygen delivery devices in the hospital or home environment
Keep oxygen cylinders away from heat sources	Keep oxygen delivery systems at least 5 feet from any heat source
Check for electrical hazards in the home or hospital prior to use	Determine that electrical equipment in the room or home is in safe working condition. A small electrical spark in the presence of oxygen will result in a serious fire. The use of a gas stove, kerosene space heater, or smoker is unsafe in the presence of oxygen. Avoid items that may create a spark (e.g., electrical razor, hair dryer, synthetic fabrics that cause static electricity, or mechanical toys) with nasal cannula in use. Petroleum-based lubricants should not be used on the lips or around the nasal cannula
Check levels of oxygen in portable tanks	Check oxygen levels of portable tanks before transporting a patient to ensure that there is enough oxygen in the tank

Competencies Required for Delivering Oxygen Therapy

Basic

- ❖ Be aware of, and understand, local oxygen policy/guidelines
- ❖ Demonstrate a basic understanding of oxygen physiology, normal and abnormal values
- ❖ Be able to discuss the indications for oxygen and the potential risks
- ❖ Demonstrate an ability to use oxygen equipment safely, including an awareness of fire risks and cylinder use
- ❖ Demonstrate an ability to use a pulse oximeter to determine oxygen saturations
- ❖ Demonstrate accurate monitoring and recording of oxygen therapy
- ❖ Be able to recognise changes in a patient's respiratory status
- ❖ Understand how to use oxygen in emergency situations, for example, cardiac arrest

Registered Nurses (Basic Plus)

- ❖ Demonstrate an understanding of target range prescriptions and applications to different patient groups
- ❖ Demonstrate an ability to assess suitability of delivery devices for individual patients and recognize when a change of device is needed
- ❖ Be able to correctly identify and set up a range of oxygen-delivery devices
- ❖ Understand how to select appropriate oxygen/driving gas for nebulized therapy

❖ Demonstrate accurate recording of adjustments to the oxygen dose and the patient's response
❖ Recognise the need for escalation of treatment/medical review and further assessment.

<table>
<tr><td align="center">Key points</td></tr>
</table>

◀ Hypoxia is an indication that oxygen therapy should be started.
◀ If blood oxygen levels are not low, oxygen will not treat breathlessness.
◀ A target oxygen saturation range should be prescribed to guide therapy.
◀ A lower target saturation range should be prescribed for patients at risk of hypercapnia.
◀ The amount of oxygen received by the patient is dependent on the delivery device used; ensure appropriate device is selected.

SUCTIONING

Airway suctioning refers to the collective measures that are used for clearing the airway of a patient. It involves suctioning, clearing secretions, and maintaining the patency of the airway. It is of particular importance for patients with mechanical ventilators, endotracheal tube (ET) intubations, tracheostomies, or other airway adjuncts. Clearance of airway secretions is a normal process and is critical to the prevention of respiratory infections, atelectasis, and preservation of airway patency.

Clearance of airway secretions is a normal process and is critical to the prevention of respiratory infections, atelectasis, and preservation of airway patency. Patients on mechanical ventilation and intubated patients are at risk of increased secretions as they are sedated, supine, and have mechanical adjuncts that prevent spontaneous clearance of secretions. Suctioning can help maintain and establish the gas exchange, adequate oxygenation, and alveolar ventilation. Suctioning can be performed through an endotracheal tube, a tracheostomy tube, the mouth, or the nose.

There are two separate suctioning techniques, namely the closed and open system. Basic principles of suctioning are the same, and care should be incorporated during suctioning. Closed suctioning includes an inline suctioning system.

There is no consensus on the time interval for suctioning airways. It depends on the clinical picture; such as the age of the patient, the associated risk factors, and the ease of obtaining adjunct airway equipment in case of disruption or loss of the airway.

The type of suctioning involved depends on the anatomy of the region that is being suctioned.
❖ **Nasopharyngeal suctioning:** Insertion of the catheter should be on a downward slant through the nostril into the floor of the nasopharynx.
❖ **Endotracheal suctioning:** Insertion of the catheter should be into the ET tube to the appropriate depth.
❖ **Airway stoma:** Insertion of the catheter into the stoma.

Indications

❖ Suctioning of airway in mechanically intubated patients
❖ Suctioning in patients with altered mental status or under the effects of sedatives or hypnotics
❖ Suctioning for patients with neuromuscular disease, atonia, or hypotonia
❖ Suctioning of patients with copious respiratory secretions
❖ Infants and children with respiratory diseases and distress
❖ Obtaining endotracheal or tracheal samples for cell counts and cultures
❖ Monitoring efficacy of treatment

Follow agency policy regarding setting suction pressure. Pressure should not exceed 150 mm Hg because higher pressures have been shown to cause trauma, hypoxemia, and atelectasis. The following ranges are appropriate pressure according to the patient's age:

- **Neonates:** 60–80 mm Hg
- **Infants:** 80–100 mm Hg
- **Children:** 100–120 mm Hg
- **Adults:** 100–150 mm Hg

Suction only when clinically indicated and for up to 15 seconds at a time to decrease the risk of respiratory complications. Hyperoxygenation and hyperventilation should be performed prior to the nasal and tracheal procedures to avoid the most common hazards of suctioning (hypoxemia, arrhythmias, and atelectasis). For nasal suctioning, increase the amount of O_2 the patient is receiving for a few minutes prior to the procedure and instruct the patient to take several deep breaths. For tracheal suctioning, do the same. If the patient is on a ventilator, you can either hyperoxygenate and ventilate with the Ambu bag or provide a few extra machine assisted breaths prior to the procedure. Allow the patient to recover and hyperventilate and hyperoxygenate between each passing of the suction catheter. The patient should recover for 30–60 seconds between passes.

When performing nasal suctioning, have the patient lean their head backwards to open the airway. This helps guide the catheter toward the trachea rather than the esophagus.

CHEST PHYSIOTHERAPY

Chest physical therapy (CPT or chest PT) is an airway clearance technique (ACT) to drain the lungs, and may include percussion (clapping), vibration, deep breathing, and huffing or coughing.

It aims to unclog the patient's airways and help them return to physical activity and exertion. The respiratory physiotherapist employs many diverse interventions, including pulmonary rehabilitation, early mobilization, and airway clearance techniques, all having beneficial effects on the symptoms associated with respiratory diseases. For example, improved sputum clearance and cough efficacy, reduced dyspnea, and improved physical fitness. The beneficial effects are demonstrated in improved functional ability and reduced intensive care and hospital stay, with savings in associated healthcare costs. Physiotherapists specializing in respiratory care work in a variety of settings including intensive care units (ICUs), hospital wards, and primary care settings.

As well as "chest physiotherapy", which includes the management of clients with excessive airway secretions, maximising oxygenation, improving lung volume, preserving musculoskeletal function, and providing advice and education to patients and their carers–respiratory physiotherapists have an essential role in early mobilisation, exercising, and muscle retraining for clients across the spectrum of conditions. Examples being—respiratory conditions (COPD, bronchiectasis, cystic fibrosis); neuromuscular diseases (muscular dystrophy, cerebral palsy, spinal cord injury), and during peri-operative care mainly in upper abdominal surgeries.

Purposes

The purpose of chest physiotherapy are:

- To facilitate removal of retained or profuse airway secretions.
- To optimize lung compliance and the ventilation-perfusion ratio/improve gas exchange.
- To decrease the work of breathing.
- Improve exercise tolerance.
- Prevent secondary complications.

Classification

There are various physiotherapy treatments incorporated within chest physiotherapy. Chest physiotherapy techniques can be classified as **conventional, modern, or instrumental techniques** based on evolving research.

Conventional Techniques

Conventional chest physiotherapy is also known as **traditional chest physiotherapy**. It was advocated first in 1915. It involves manual handling techniques to facilitate mucociliary clearance. Postural drainage along with percussion and vibration (PDPV) was previously widely named as Chest Physiotherapy. Later, coughing exercises and forced expiratory techniques (huffing) were incorporated within it. PDPV with huffing has shown an effective outcome. It can be self-administered or performed with the assistance of another person (a physiotherapist, parent, or caregiver). PDPV works better if applied with bronchodilator therapy.

Postural Drainage

Postural drainage (see link) involves positioning a person with the assistance of gravity to aid the normal airway clearance mechanism. Postural drainage positioning varies based on specific segments of the lungs with a large amount of secretions. Postural drainage is the drainage of secretions, by the effect of gravity, from one or more lung segments to the central airways (where they can be removed by a cough or mechanical aspiration). Each position consists of placing the target lung segment(s) superior to the carina. Positions should generally be held for 3 to 15 minutes (longer in special situations). Standard positions are modified as the patient's condition and tolerance warrant. Before determining the postural drainage position, it is very important to auscultate the lungs and identify the lung segments where added sound (Crepitus, Ronchi) is heard. Postural drainage can be facilitated with percussion and vibration in the postural drainage position.

Percussion

Percussion is also referred to as **cupping, clapping, and tapotement**. The purpose of percussion is to intermittently apply kinetic energy to the chest wall and lungs. This is accomplished by rhythmically striking the thorax with a cupped hand or mechanical device directly over the lung segment(s) being drained.

Vibration

Vibration involves the application of a fine tremorous action (manually performed by pressing in the direction that the ribs and soft tissue of the chest move during expiration) over the draining area. In this technique, **a rapid vibratory impulse** is transmitted through the chest wall from the flattened hands of the therapist by isometric alternate contraction of forearm flexor and extensor muscles, to loosen and dislodge the airway secretions.

Coughing

Coughing includes directed coughing and various assisted coughing techniques.

Forced Expiratory Technique (FET)

Forced expiratory techniques involve diaphragmatic inspiration, relaxing the scapulohumeral region, and expiring forcefully from mid to low lung volumes whilst maintaining an open glottis ("huffing" exercises). It is more effective than coughing.

Indication of Conventional Techniques

Postural Drainage Positioning

❖ Inability or reluctance of the patient to change body position (e.g., mechanical ventilation, neuromuscular disease, drug-induced paralysis).
❖ Poor oxygenation associated with the position (e.g., unilateral lung disease).
❖ Potential for or presence of atelectasis.
❖ Presence of artificial airway.

PDPV

❖ Difficulty clearing secretions with expectorated sputum production > 25–30 mL/day (adult).
❖ Evidence or suggestion of retained secretions in the presence of an artificial airway.
❖ Presence of atelectasis caused by or suspected of being caused by mucus plugging.
❖ Diagnosis of diseases, such as cystic fibrosis, bronchiectasis, or cavitating lung disease.
❖ Presence of foreign body in the airway.
❖ Patient with copious sputum or with central consolidation.

Frequency

Positioning: Ventilated and critically-ill patients—as necessary with the goal of once each hour or every other hour as tolerated, around the clock. Less acute patients should be turned every two hours as tolerated.

PDPV

❖ In critical care patients, including those on mechanical ventilation, PDT should be performed every 4 to every 6 hours as indicated. PDT order should be re-evaluated at least every 48 hours based on assessments from individual treatments.
❖ In spontaneously breathing patients, frequency should be determined by assessing patient response to therapy.
❖ Acute care patient orders should be re-evaluated based on patient response to therapy at least every 72 hours or with a change of patient status.
❖ Domiciliary patients should be re-evaluated every three months and with a change of status.

Modern Techniques

Over the years, several additional noninvasive clearance methods have been developed to augment this traditional approach. Modern techniques use a variation of flow through breath control to mobilize secretions. It includes an active cycle of breathing and autogenic drainage.

Active Cycle of Breathing Technique

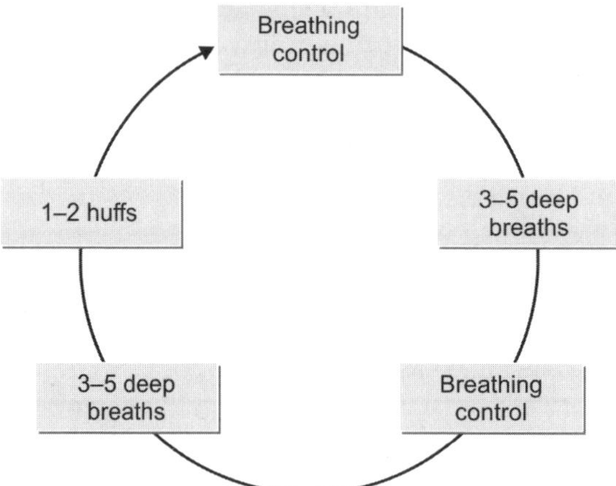

Active cycle of breathing technique (ACBT) is an active breathing technique performed by the patient, and can be used to mobilize and clear excess pulmonary secretions and to generally improve lung function. It has a series of three main phases—breathing control, thoracic expansion, and forced expiratory technique.

Autogenic Drainage

Autogenic drainage is a diaphragmatic breathing pattern used by patients with respiratory illnesses (e.g., cystic fibrosis, bronchiectasis) to clear the lungs of mucus and other secretions. Various techniques are used, all of which combine positive reinforcement of deep breathing and voluntary cough suppression for as long as possible before evacuating the airways of mucus.

Instrumental Techniques

Instrumental techniques, such as non-invasive ventilation have been considered useful as an adjunct therapy to airway clearance and to provide respiratory support. Common instrumental techniques are:

❖ **Positive expiratory pressure (PEP):** There are various positive expiratory pressure devices that provide resistance to expiration through a mouthpiece or facemask, followed by forced expirations. The inhalation is at tidal volume, and the expiration is slightly active against devices. These devices help to remove secretions by increasing functional residual capacity and thus enhancing collateral ventilation and removing secretions from collapse airways. Some of the devices are Flutter, Acapella, lung flute, etc.

❖ **Continuous positive airway pressure:** Generated by exhalation against a constant opening pressure, this produces positive end-expiratory pressure (PEEP). Continuous positive airway pressure can also be delivered by commercially available pressure drivers. These generally require tightly fitting nasal prongs or a CPAP face mask. Bubble CPAP can be used in a low resource environment and in the pediatric population. It consists of an interface (nasal cannula), inspiratory tubing, and expiratory tubing immersed in an underwater bottle system.

❖ **High-frequency chest wall oscillation (HFCWO):** An airway clearance technique in which external chest wall oscillations are applied to the chest using an inflatable vest that wraps around the chest. These machines produce vibrations at variable frequencies and intensities, helping to loosen and thin mucus and separate it from airway walls.

❖ HFCWO involves an inflatable jacket that is attached to a pulse generator by hoses that mechanically enable the equipment to perform at variable frequencies (5–25 Hz). The generator sends air through the hose, which causes the vest to inflate and deflate rapidly. The vibrations not only separate mucus from the airway walls but also help move it up into the large airways. Typically, it is paused during the 20- to 30-minute HFCWO treatment every 5 minutes to cough out loosened mucus that has moved into the large airways.

❖ **Intrapulmonary percussive ventilation (IPV):** Designed to promote mobilization of bronchial secretions and improve efficiency and distribution of ventilation, providing intrathoracic percussion and vibration and an alternative system for the delivery of the positive pressure to the lungs. Each IPV session lasted fifteen minutes and was performed twice a day (morning and afternoon). Intrapulmonary percussive ventilation uses a pneumatic device to deliver a series of pressurised gas minibursts at rates of 100 to 225 cycles per minute to the respiratory tract, by a mouthpiece. The duration of each percussive cycle is manually controlled by a thumb button. During the cycle, constant PAP is maintained at the airway. It also incorporates nebulizer for the delivery of the aerosol.

Assessment of Need and Outcome

The following should be assessed together to establish a need for chest physiotherapy:
❖ Excessive sputum production.
❖ Effectiveness of cough.
❖ History of pulmonary problems treated successfully with PDT (e.g., bronchiectasis, cystic fibrosis, lung abscess).
❖ Decreased breath sounds or crackles or rhonchi suggesting secretions in the airway.
❖ Change in vital signs.
❖ Abnormal chest X-ray consistent with atelectasis, mucus plugging, or infiltrates.
❖ Deterioration in arterial blood gas values or oxygen saturation.

The following can be used as an outcome tool to determine the effectiveness of treatment:
❖ Change in sputum production.
❖ Change in breath sounds of lung fields.
❖ Patient subjective response to therapy.
❖ Change in vital signs.
❖ Change in chest X-ray.
❖ Change in arterial blood gas values or oxygen saturation.
❖ Change in ventilator variables.
❖ Change in modified Borg Scale-dyspnea level.
❖ Change in peak expiratory flow rate.

Contraindication of Conventional Techniques

Positioning

All positions are contraindicated for:
❖ Intracranial pressure (ICP) >20 mm Hg
❖ Head and neck injury until stabilized (absolute)
❖ Active hemorrhage with hemodynamic instability (absolute)
❖ Recent spinal surgery (e.g., laminectomy) or acute spinal injury

❖ Acute spinal injury or active hemoptysis
❖ Empyema
❖ Bronchopleural fistula
❖ Pulmonary edema associated with congestive heart failure
❖ Large pleural effusions
❖ Pulmonary embolism
❖ Aged, confused, or anxious patients who do not tolerate position changes
❖ Rib fracture, with/without flail chest
❖ Surgical wound or healing tissue

Trendelenburg position is contraindicated for:
❖ Intracranial pressure (ICP) >20 mm Hg
❖ Patients in whom increased intracranial pressure is to be avoided (e.g., neurosurgery, aneurysms, eye surgery)
❖ Uncontrolled hypertension
❖ Distended abdomen
❖ Oesophageal surgery
❖ Recent gross hemoptysis related to recent lung carcinoma treated surgically or with radiation therapy.
❖ Uncontrolled airway at risk for aspiration (tube feeding or recent meal)
    Reverse Trendelenburg is contraindicated in the presence of hypotension or vasoactive medication.

External Manipulation of the Thorax

In addition to contraindications previously listed
❖ Subcutaneous emphysema.
❖ Recent epidural spinal infusion or spinal anesthesia.
❖ Recent skin grafts, or flaps, on the thorax.
❖ Burns, open wounds, and skin infections of the thorax.
❖ Recently placed transvenous pacemaker or subcutaneous pacemaker (particularly if mechanical devices are to be used).
❖ Suspected pulmonary tuberculosis.
❖ Lung contusion.
❖ Bronchospasm.
❖ Osteomyelitis of the ribs.
❖ Osteoporosis.
❖ Coagulopathy.
❖ Complaint of chest-wall pain.

Complications

❖ Hypoxemia
❖ Bronchospasm
❖ Increased intracranial pressure
❖ Acute hypotension during procedure
❖ Pulmonary hemorrhage

❖ Pain or injury to muscles, ribs, or spine
❖ Vomiting and aspiration
❖ Bronchospasm
❖ Dysrhythmias

How to Do It

With postural drainage, the person lies or sits in various positions so the part of the lung to be drained is as high as possible. That part of the lung is then drained using percussion, vibration, and gravity.

When the person with CF is in one of the positions, the caregiver can clap on the person's chest wall. This is usually done for three to five minutes and is sometimes followed by vibration over the same area for approximately 15 seconds (or during five exhalations). The person is then encouraged to cough or huff forcefully to get the mucus out of the lungs.

Cupping (percussion) by the caregiver on the chest wall over the part of the lung to be drained helps move the mucus into the larger airways. The hand is cupped as if to hold water but with the palm facing down. The cupped hand curves to the chest wall and traps a cushion of air to soften the clapping.

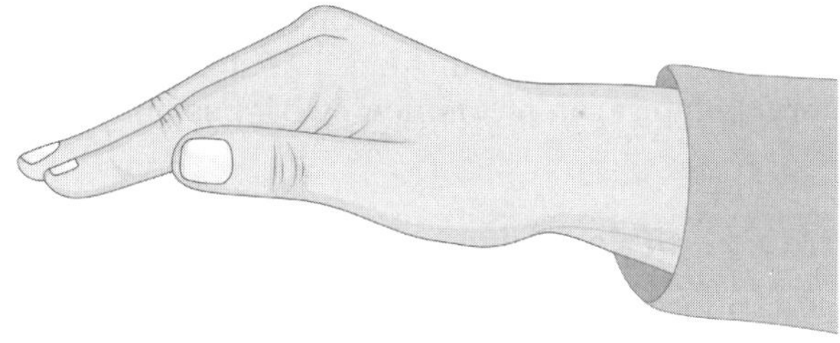

Cupping.

Percussion is done forcefully and with a steady beat. Each beat should have a hollow sound. Most of the movement is in the wrist with the arm relaxed, making percussion less tiring to do. If the hand is cupped properly, percussion should not be painful or sting.

Special attention must be taken to not clap over the:
❖ Spine
❖ Breastbone
❖ Stomach
Lower ribs or back (to prevent injury to the spleen on the left, the liver on the right and the kidneys in the lower back).

Different devices may be used in place of the traditional cupped palm method for percussion.

Vibration is a technique that gently shakes the mucus so it can move into the larger airways. The caregiver places a firm hand on the chest wall over the part of the lung being drained and tenses the muscles of the arm and shoulder to create a fine shaking motion. Then, the caregiver applies a light pressure over the area being vibrated. (The caregiver may also place one hand over the other, then press the top and bottom hand into each other to vibrate.)

Vibration is done with the flattened hand, not the cupped hand. Exhalation should be as slow and as complete as possible.

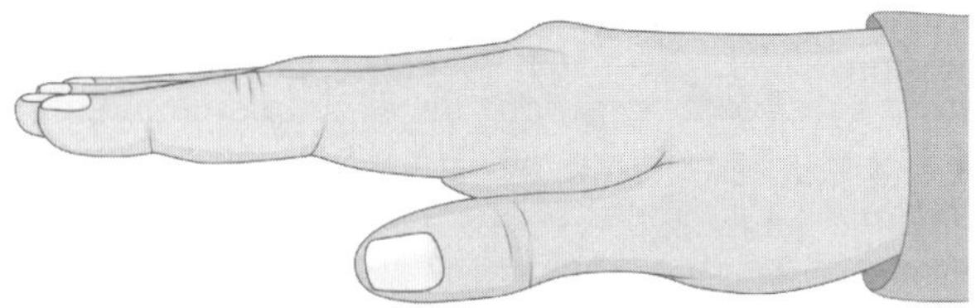

Correct hand position for vibration

Deep breathing moves the loosened mucus and may lead to coughing. Breathing with the diaphragm (belly breathing or lower chest breathing) is used to help the person take deeper breaths and get the air into the lower lungs. The belly moves outward when the person breathes in and sinks in when he or she breathes out. Your CF respiratory or physical therapist can help you learn more about this type of breathing.

Duration of Chest Physiotherapy

Generally, each treatment session can last between 20 to 40 minutes. CPT is best done before meals or one-and-a-half to two hours after eating, to decrease the chance of vomiting. Early morning and bedtimes are usually recommended. The length of CPT and the number of times a day it is done may need to be increased if the person is more congested or getting sick. Your CF doctor or respiratory therapist can recommend what positions, how often and how long CPT should be done.

Doing CPT Comfortably and Carefully

Both the person with CF and the caregiver should be comfortable during CPT. Before starting, the person should remove tight clothing, jewelry, buttons, and zippers around the neck, chest and waist. Light, soft clothing, such as a T-shirt, may be worn. Do not do CPT on bare skin. The caregiver should remove rings and other bulky jewelry, such as watches or bracelets. Keep a supply of tissues or a place to cough out the mucus nearby.

The caregiver should not lean forward when doing percussion, but should remain in an upright position to protect his/her back. The surface that the person with CF lies on should be at a comfortable height for the caregiver.

Many families find it helpful to use pillows, sofa cushions, or bundles of newspapers under pillows for support, as well as cribs with adjustable mattress heights/tilts, foam wedges, or bean bag chairs while doing CPT. Infants can be positioned with or without pillows in the caregiver's lap.

❖ Schedule CPT around a favorite TV show.
❖ Play favorite songs or recorded stories.
❖ Spend time playing, talking, or singing before, during, and after CPT.
❖ For kids, encourage blowing or coughing games during CPT, such as blowing pinwheels or coughing the deepest cough.
❖ Ask willing and capable relatives, friends, brothers, and sisters to do CPT. This can provide a welcome break from the daily routine.
❖ Minimize interruptions. Finding ways that make CPT more enjoyable can help you keep a regular routine and get maximum health benefits.

Instructions for CPT

The following diagrams describe the positions for CPT. In the diagrams, shaded areas show where the chest should be clapped or vibrated. As a reminder:

Pillows may be used for added comfort. If the person tires easily, the order of the positions can be varied, but all areas of the chest should be percussed or clapped.

Please remember to clap and vibrate only over the ribs.

Avoid clapping and vibrating over the spine, breastbone, stomach, and lower ribs or back to prevent trauma to the spleen on the left, the liver on the right, and the kidneys in the lower back. Do not clap or vibrate on bare skin.

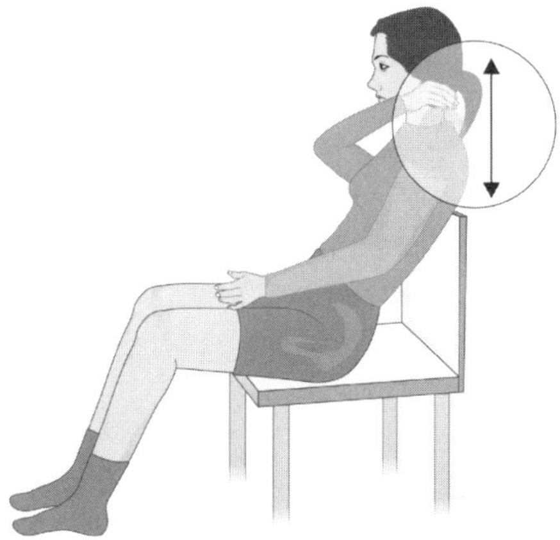

Self-percussion—upper lobes.

Your client should sit upright and reach across his/her chest to clap on front of chest over the muscular area between the collarbone and the top of the shoulder blade. Repeat on the opposite site. Your client can also clap his/her own upper back if able to reach it.

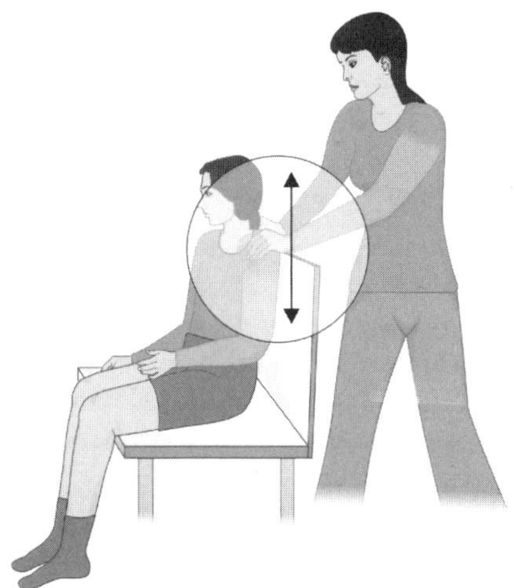

Upper front chest—upper lobes.

Have your client sit upright. Clap on both sides of the upper front chest over the muscular area between the collarbone and the top of the shoulder blade.

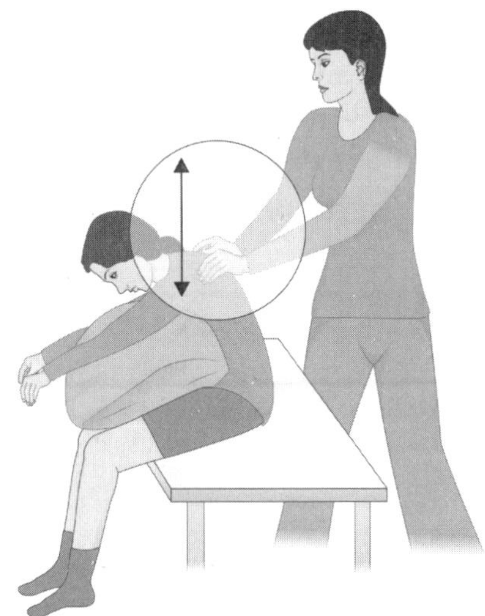

Upper back chest—upper lobes.

Have your client sit up and lean forward on a pillow over the back of a sofa or soft chair at a 30-degree angle. Stand or sit behind your client and clap both sides of the upper back. Take care not to clap on your client's backbone.

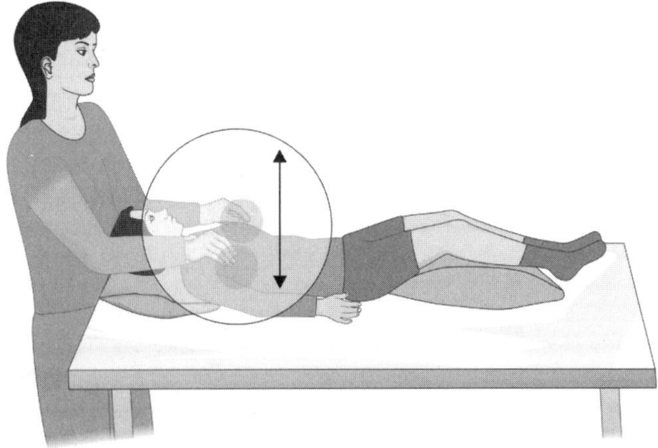

Upper front chest—upper lobes.

Have your client lie on his/her back with arms to sides. Stand behind your client's head. Clap both sides of your client's chest between the collarbone and nipple.

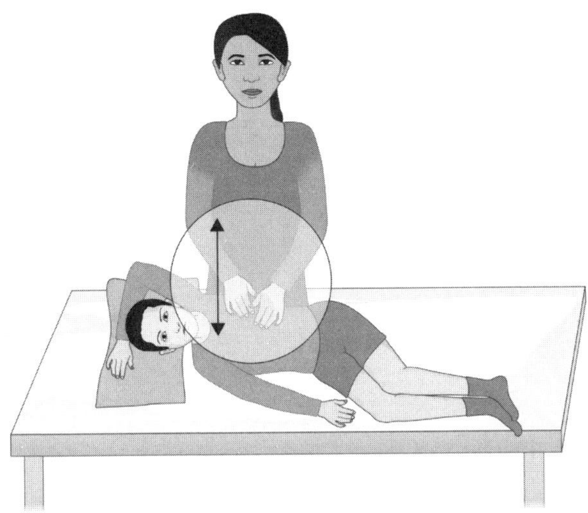

Left side front chest.

Have your client lie with left side up and raise his or her left arm overhead. Clap over the lower ribs just below the nipple area on the front side of left chest. Do not clap on your client's stomach.

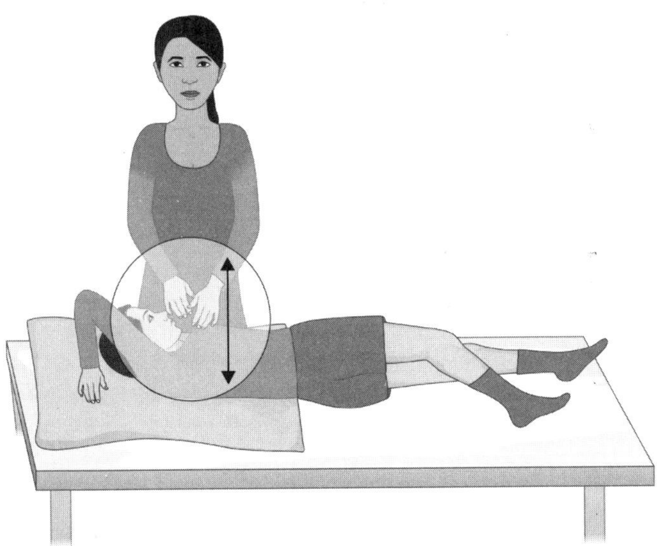

Right side front chest.

Have your client lie with right side up and raise his/her right arm overhead. Clap over the lower chest just below the nipple area on the front side of right chest. Do not clap your client's lower rib cage.

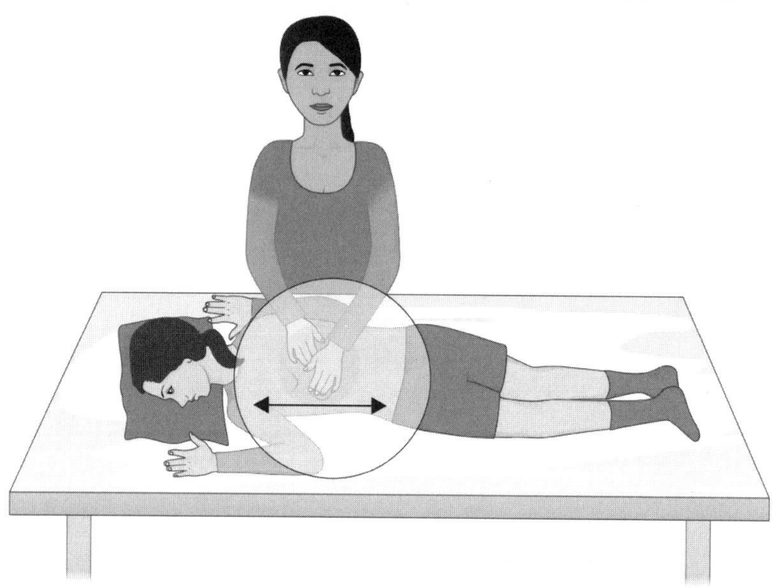

Lower back chest—lower lobes.

Have your client lie on his/her stomach. Clap both sides at the bottom of his/her chest just above the bottom edge of the rib cage. Do not clap the lower rib cage or over the backbone.

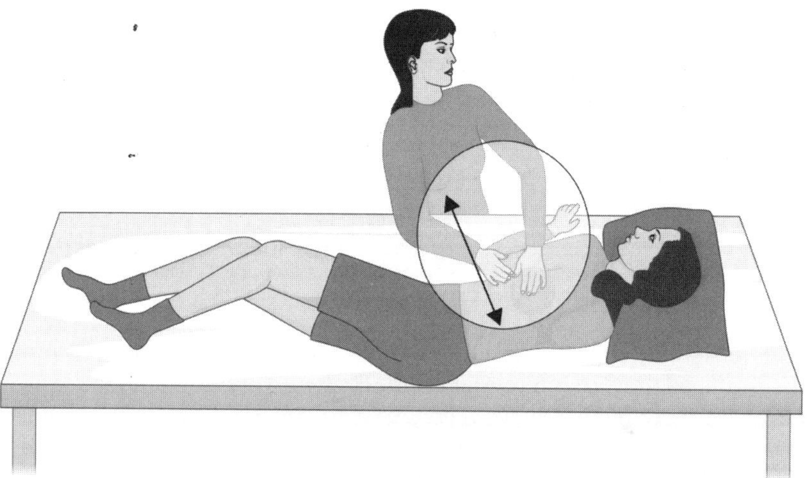

Left lower side back chest—lower lobe.

Have your client lie with left side up and roll toward you a quarter turn so you can reach your client's back. Clap on the lower left side of his/her chest just above the bottom edge of the rib cage.

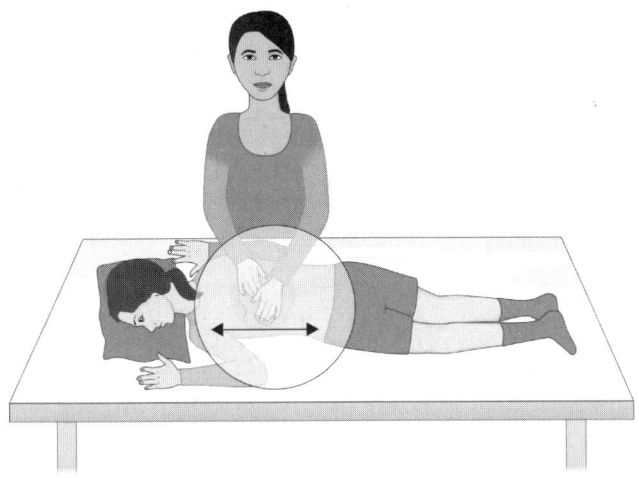

Right lower side back—lower lobe.

Have your client lie with right side up and roll toward you a quarter turn so you can reach your client's back. Clap on the lower right side of his/her chest just above the bottom edge of the rib cage.

Chest Drainage (Thoracentesis)

Introduction

Chest drains also known as under water sealed drains (UWSD) are a drainage system of three chambers consisting of a water seal, suction control and drainage collection chamber. UWSD are designed to allow air or fluid to be removed from the pleural cavity, while also preventing backflow of air or fluid into the pleural space. This allows for the expansion of the lungs and restoration of negative pressure in the thoracic cavity. Appropriate chest drain management is required to maintain respiratory function and haemodynamic stability. Chest drains may be placed routinely in theatre, PICU and NICU; or in the emergency department and ward areas in emergency situations. Some patients will have Redivac drains inserted, these are different from a UWSD.

Chest drainage is a procedure to drain fluid from the pleural space between the lung and chest wall. Inflammation, infection and traumatic injury, among other things, can cause fluid to build up in the cavity.

Chest drains, also referred to as chest tubes, under water sealed drainage (UWSD), thoracic catheter, tube thoracostomy, or intercostal drain. They provide a method of removing air and fluid substances from the pleural space. The idea is to create a one-way mechanism that will let air/fluid out of the pleural space and prevent outside air/fluid from entering into the pleural space. This is accomplished by the use of an underwater seal.

Principles of Underwater Seal Drainage

❖ The main aim of the drainage system is to remove fluid/air from pleura and preventing its re-entry into the pleural space.

❖ This is achieved when distal end of the drain tube is submerged 2 cm under the surface level of the water in the drainage (or collection) chamber. It in turn creates a hydrostatic resistance of +2 cm H_2O in the drainage chamber.

❖ Normal intrapleural pressure is negative. However, if air or fluid enters the pleural space, intrapleural pressure becomes positive. Air is eliminated from the pleural space into the drainage chamber when intrapleural pressure is greater than +2 cm H_2O. Thus, air moves from a higher to lower pressure along a pressure gradient. The drainage chamber has a vent to allow air to escape the chamber, and not build up within the chamber.

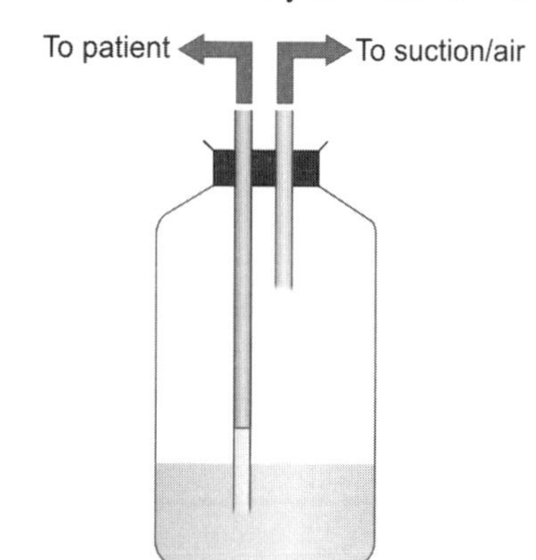

Mechanism of action of chest drain.

❖ Also, fluids will drain by gravity into the drainage chamber, and will not spill back into the pleural space if the bottle is always kept below the level of the patient's chest.

❖ To summarize the mechanism of action of UWSD by observations in tubing and drainage chamber:
  - Airflow is governed by changes in intra-pleural pressure.
  - Negative pressure during inspiration causes water level in tube to rise slightly.
  - Positive pressure during expiration pushes air and fluid out of the pleural space and into the tube and collection bottle.
  - Air bubbles out of tube into the underwater seal.
  - Fluid drains by gravity, mixing with water and raising the fluid level.

Indications for Insertion of a Chest Drain

❖ Chylothorax
❖ Pleural effusions
❖ Pneumothorax
❖ Post-cardiac surgery
❖ Hemothorax
❖ Removal of an air collection in the pleural space
  - Pneumothorax can be treated with a thoracostomy tube placement if it is preventing adequate expansion of the lung or concern exists for the future development of tension physiology, such as in a patient receiving positive pressure ventilation. Recent research has also shown that an air space measuring less than 35 mm in the largest axis can be observed. Chest tubes are usually routinely left after cardiothoracic surgery.
  - Tension pneumothorax diagnosis based on clinical suspicion should be immediately treated by thoracostomy tube placement. If unable to place a thoracostomy tube, a needle decompression or a finger thoracostomy will temporize the patient by venting the chest.
  - Hemothorax or pneumothorax may be appropriate to manage with a chest tube depending on the totality of circumstances and discretion of the treating physician.
❖ Removal of fluid collection or accumulation between visceral and parietal pleura
  - Hemothorax, generally considered, indicated if the calculated volume is greater than 300 cc.

- Pleural effusion (malignant or benign) can become symptomatic from displacement and collapse of alveolar space.
- Chylothorax, where thoracostomy is considered part of the definitive therapeutic modality, along with dietary modification.
- An empyema should almost universally be treated with surgical management (e.g., drainage, irrigation, decortication, etc.) as medical management is rarely successful.
- ❖ Use as a delivery conduit to introduce medication or fluid into the pleural space.
  - Internal warming allows warm fluid to circulate through the thoracic space to provide an external heat source for the core and circulating blood volume.
  - Pleurodesis with a talc slurry can be instilled through the chest tube to promote scarring of the visceral and parietal pleura together.
  - Hyperthermic intrathoracic chemotherapy (HITHOC) allows for the delivery of chemotherapeutic agents directly into the thoracic space for malignant pleural mesothelioma and metastatic disease.

Components and Types of Chest Drain Systems

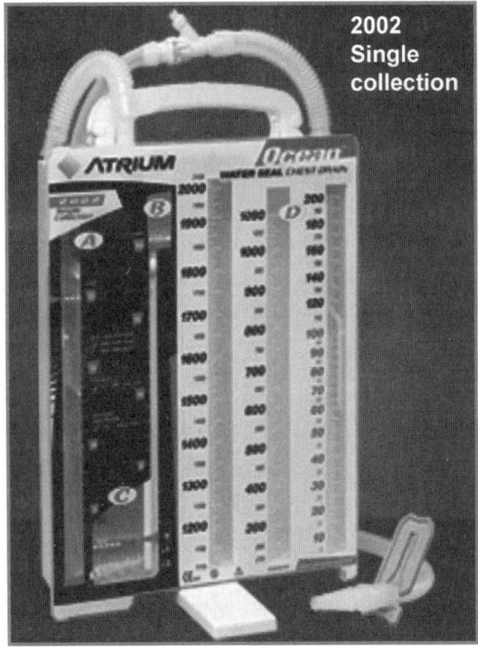

Under water seal drain system.
(OCEAN, Single Collection Water Seal Drain, A = Suction Control Chamber, B = Water Seal Chamber, C = Air Leak Monitor, D = Collection Chamber)

Unobstructed Chest Tube

It is inserted into pleural cavity/mediastinal cavity to allow air/fluid to leave the chest. Usually made of clear pliable plastic which may be radio-opaque.

Tubing

Consists of a 6 foot long flexible tubing which connects the chest tube to the chest drain system.

Water Seal Chamber

- ❖ Column B—air released from the pleural space goes into the water seal chamber. Lets the air out of the chest while preventing air from the outside getting back in. Chamber should always have 2 cm H_2O inside it (>2 cm can be too difficult to expire against and <2 cm is an ineffective seal meaning air could re-enter the pleural space). Calibrated to reflect intrapleural pressure which should be negative (in a spontaneously breathing adult approx. –8 cm H_2O on inspiration and –4 cm H_2O on expiration). Contains a ball which should be oscillating (no oscillation can mean (a) there's a kink in the system (check patient isn't lying on any tubes) or (b) the pneumothorax has healed (will show up on CXR).
- ❖ **Unnamed chamber:** Column C—records the amount of bubbling which is taking place. 1–2 bubbles is normal but >5 can be indicative of a leak somewhere in the system. Leak could be caused by (a) disconnection somewhere in the circuit or (b) a massive tear in the pleura which requires negative pressure in the form of a suction drain. Column A—should have 20 cm H_2O.
- ❖ One-way mechanism to prevent return of air/fluid (valve).
- ❖ Suction control device (optional)/usually 3–5 kPa.

UNDERWATER DETECTOR SYSTEM (UWDS)

Glass Bottle System

- ❖ **Bottle A:** The simplest form of underwater seal drainage systems. This system can drain both fluid and air. The distal end of the drainage tube must remain under the water surface level. There is always an outlet to the atmosphere to allow air to escape. It is suitable for use with a simple pneumothorax, when the vent is left open to the atmosphere, or following a pneumonectomy when the tubing is clamped and released hourly.
- ❖ **Bottle B:** This system is suitable for the drainage of air and fluid. The first chamber is for collection of fluid and the second is for the collection of air. As the two are separate, fluid drainage does not adversely affect the pressure gradient for evacuation of air from the pleural space. A separate chamber for fluid collection enables monitoring of volume and expelled matter.
- ❖ **Bottle C:** Suction is required when air or fluid needs a greater pressure gradient to move from the pleural space to the collection system. Suction may be applied via a third bottle or a suction chamber.

Plastic Bottle System

- ❖ Pleur-evac chest drainage system
- ❖ Thora-seal chest drainage unit

Indications for Chest Drain Insertion

Chest drains are inserted as an invasive procedure to; remove fluid/air from the pleural space/ mediastinum, and/or re-expand the lungs and restore negative intrapleural pressure and respiratory function.

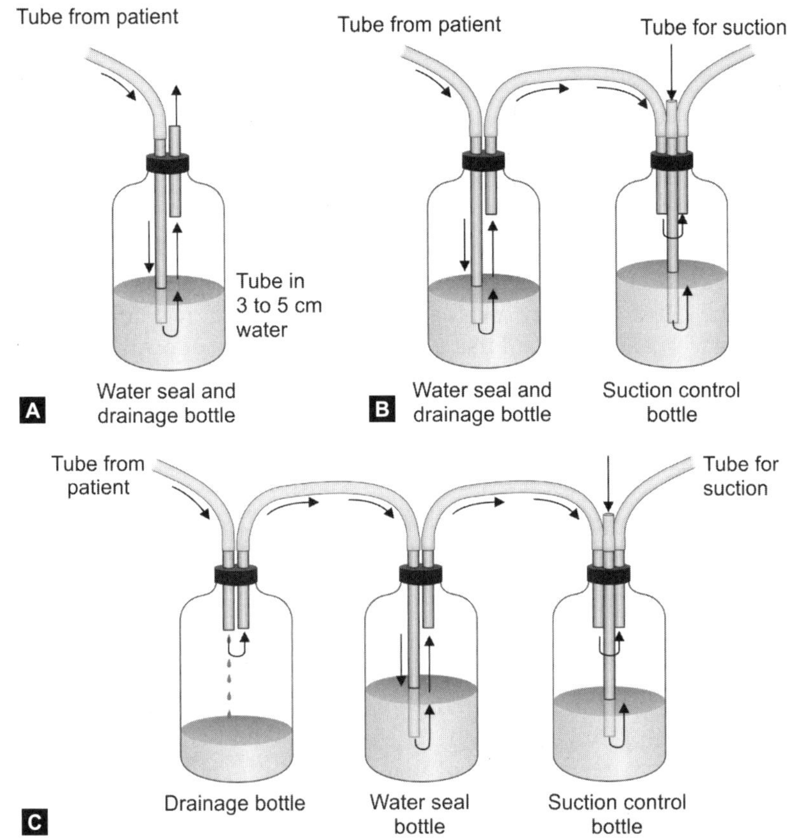

Glass bottle system of water seal drainage.

Conditions that require a chest drain include:
- **Pneumothorax:** "Air in the pleural cavity". This occurs when there is a breach of the lung surface or chest wall which allows air to enter the pleural cavity and consequently cause the lung to collapse.
- **Pleural effusion:** A collection of fluid abnormally present in the pleural space, usually resulting from excess fluid production and/or decreased lymphatic absorption.
- **Hemothorax:** The presence of blood in the pleural space. The source of blood may be the chest wall, lung parenchyma, heart, or great vessels.
- **Chylothroax:** It is a type of pleural effusion. It results from lymph formed in the digestive system called chyle accumulating in the pleural cavity due to either disruption or obstruction of the thoracic duct.
- **Empyema:** It is a collection or gathering of pus within a naturally existing anatomical cavity. For example, pleural empyema is empyema of the pleural cavity. It must be differentiated from an abscess, which is a collection of pus in a newly formed cavity.
- Postcardiac or thoracic surgery.

Chest Drainage Systems

Traditional Chest Drainage

In 1967, Deknatel introduced the first integrated disposable chest drainage unit based on the three-bottle system. Now that we have reviewed normal anatomy, physiology, and pathophysiology, let's discuss each of the three chambers in detail.

Collection Chamber

At the right side of the unit is the collection chamber. The patient tubing connects the drainage unit directly to the chest tube. Any drainage from the chest flows into this chamber. The collection chamber is calibrated and has a write-on surface to allow for easy measurement and recording of the time, date, and amount of drainage.

Water Seal Chamber

The middle chamber of a traditional chest drainage system is the water seal. The main purpose of the water seal is to allow air to exit from the pleural space on exhalation and prevent air from entering the pleural cavity or mediastinum on inhalation. When the water seal chamber is filled with sterile fluid up to the 2 cm line, a 2 cm water seal is established. To maintain an effective seal, it is important to keep the chest drainage unit upright at all times and to monitor the water level in the water seal to check for evaporation.

❖ Bubbling in the water seal chamber indicates an air leak. The patient air leak meter indicates the approximate degree of air leak from the chest cavity. The meter is made up of numbered columns, labeled from 1 (low) to 7 (high). The higher the numbered column through which bubbling occurs, the greater the degree of air leak. By documenting the number, the clinician can monitor air leak increase or decrease.

❖ The water seal chamber also has a calibrated manometer to measure the amount of negative pressure within the pleural cavity. The water level in the small arm of the water seal rises as intrapleural pressure becomes more negative. If there is no air leak, the water level should rise and fall with the patient's respirations, reflecting normal pressure changes in the pleural cavity. During spontaneous respirations, the water level should rise during inhalation and fall during exhalation. If the patient is receiving positive pressure ventilation, the oscillation will be just the opposite — the water level should fall with inhalation and rise with exhalation. This oscillation is called tidaling and is one indicator of a patent pleural chest tube. At the top of the water seal chamber is a high negativity float valve and high negativity relief chamber. These safety features maintain the water seal in the event of high negative pressures. Three situations can cause high negative pressure: 1. The patient in respiratory distress, coughing vigorously, or crying; 2. Chest tube stripping; 3. Decreasing or disconnecting suction.

❖ High negativity is indicated by rising water in the small arm of the water seal chamber. If the water rises beyond –20 cm, the high negativity float valve will rise and impede the flow of water, allowing the patient to develop as much negativity as needed for inspiration. In instances of falsely imposed high negative pressure, such as stripping chest tubes, water will continue to rise, filling the high negativity relief chamber. The relief chamber automatically vents excessive negative pressure, thus preventing respiratory compromise from accumulated negativity.

❖ Vigorous milking or stripping can create dangerously high negative pressures. Research has documented negative pressures as high as –450 cm H_2O. Pleur-evac prevents accumulation of excessive high negative pressure as discussed above; however, the transient high negative pressures created by vigorous stripping can put the patient at risk for mediastinal trauma and graft trauma. Use extreme caution and follow your hospital policy. A manual high negativity relief valve is located on top of chest drainage systems. Depressing the high negativity relief valve allows filtered air into the system, relieving negativity and allowing the water level to return to baseline in the water seal. Use the high negativity relief valve with caution. If suction is not operative, or if operating on gravity drainage, depressing the high negativity relief valve can reduce negative pressure within the collection chamber to zero (atmosphere) with the resulting possibility of a pneumothorax.

Wet Suction Control

The chamber on the left side of the unit is the suction control chamber. Traditional chest drainage units regulate the amount of suction by the height of a column of water in the suction control chamber. Note: it's the height of water, not the setting of the suction source, that actually limits the amount of suction transmitted to the pleural cavity. A suction pressure of –20 cm H_2O is commonly recommended. Lower levels may be indicated for infants and for patients with friable lung tissue, or if ordered by the physician. In a wet suction control system such as the Pleur-evac° A-7000/A-8000 series, fill the suction control chamber to the desired height with sterile fluid. Connect the short suction tubing to a suction source, and adjust the source suction to produce gentle bubbling in the suction control chamber. Increasing suction at the suction source will increase airflow through the system, but will have minimal effect on the amount of suction imposed on the chest cavity. Excessive source suction not only causes loud bubbling (which can disturb patients and caregivers), but also hastens evaporation of water from the suction control chamber. This results in a lower amount of suction applied to the patient as the level of water decreases. Self-sealing diaphragms are provided to adjust the water level in this chamber.

New Generation Chest Drains

Dry Suction

❖ The next step in the evolution of chest drainage units was the development of dry suction control chambers. Dry suction control systems provide many advantages: higher suction pressure levels can be achieved, set-up is easy, no continuous bubbling provides for quiet operation, and there is no fluid to evaporate which would decrease the amount of suction applied to the patient.

❖ Instead of regulating the level of suction with a column of water, the dry suction units are controlled by a self-compensating regulator. A dial to set the suction control setting is located on the upper left side of each unit. To set the suction setting, rotate the dial until the red stripe appears in the semi-circular window at the prescribed suction level and clicks into place. Suction can be set at –10, –15, –20, –30, or –40 cm of water. The unit is pre-set at –20 cm of water when opened.

❖ Connect the short suction tubing or suction port to the suction source. Source suction must be capable of delivering a minimum of 16 liters per minute (LPM) air flow. Increase suction source until the orange float appears in the suction control indicator window.

Site and Position

Confirm the Site for Drain Insertion

The marking of a site using thoracic ultrasound for subsequent remote aspiration or pleural drain insertion is not recommended.

Real time bedside ultrasound imaging, wherever available, should be used to select the appropriate site for pleural drain placement

A chest X-ray (CXR) must be available at the time of drain insertion unless the patient is in shock or has hemodynamic compromise from the tension pneumothorax. In this instance, an urgent CXR should be obtained after needle decompression.

A pleural drain should not be inserted without further image guidance if:

* The expected free air (in case pneumothorax) or fluid (in case of pleural effusion) cannot be aspirated with a needle at the time of inserting the local anesthesia.
* If the expected free air is not evident at the time of needle/cannula decompression of suspected tension pneumothorax.

Triangle of Safety

Insertion of a pleural drain should be made within the triangle of safety with the following potential exceptions:

* Where breast tissue covers the triangle of safety and insertion would require the drain to pass through breast tissue
* When an ultrasound assessment has defined a better position for access to a pleural effusion
* The mid clavicular line is considered more appropriate for management of pneumothorax.

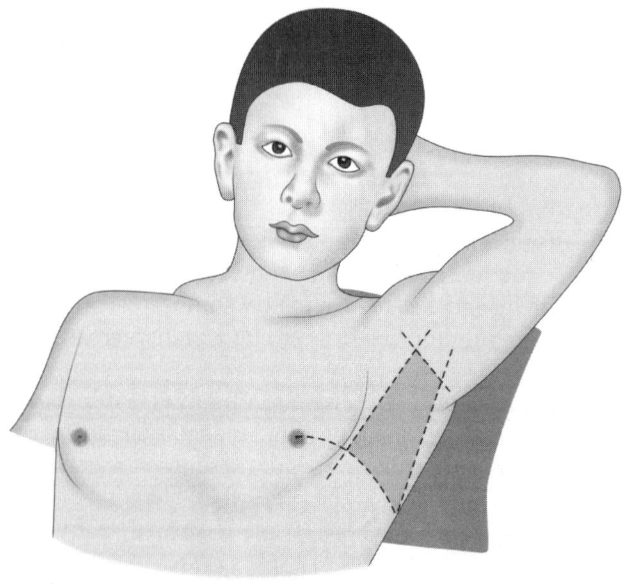

Triangle of safety.

Positions of the Patient

The preferred position for standard pleural drain insertion is on the bed, head and trunk elevated 30–45 degrees and slightly rotated, with the arm on the side of the lesion behind the patients head or on the hips to expose the lateral decubitus position.

An alternative is for the patient to sit upright leaning over an adjacent table with a pillow under the arms or in the lateral posture.

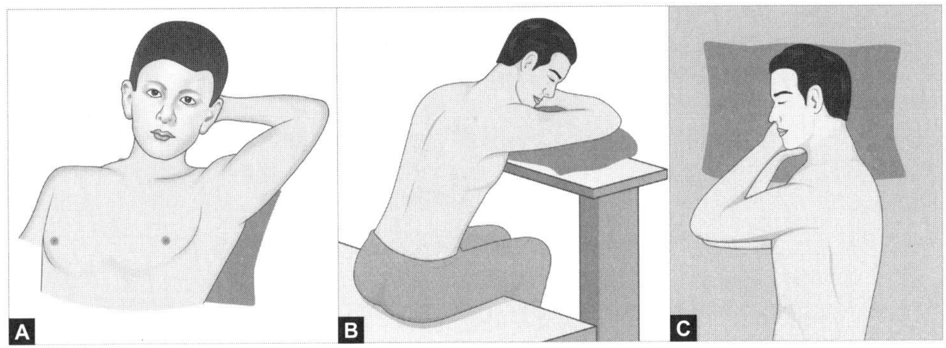

Common patient positions for chest drain insertion.

CARE OF CHEST DRAIN

Chest Drain Assessment and Management

Start of Shift Checks

- ❖ Ensure that there is emergency equipment at bedside including:
  - ◆ At least two drain clamps per drain (for use in emergency only)
- ❖ Two suction outlets—x1 chest drain and x1 for airway management
- ❖ Auscultate the chest
- ❖ Assess the chest tube and system tubing (i.e., for kinks, dislodgement, etc.) as well as the drain dressing to ensure it is intact and for any signs of infection
- ❖ Check that the drain is anchored appropriately
- ❖ Labelling of each drain tube in accordance with EMR documentation
- ❖ Drain is on suction and that the amount of suction correlates with the medical team order on EMR
- ❖ Assess for any leakages or movement in water chamber
- ❖ Check that the drain in not clamped (unless ordered by medical staff).

UWSD Labelling

It is imperative that the UWSD is labelled in a way that is clear and visible. This is extremely important when removing the drain to ensure the correct drain is removed. Please refer to the image below for the correct labelling of an UWSD. The criteria for correct labelling includes the following:

- ❖ **How:** Clear, visible writing (dark font and capital letters) on a label that can be complete stuck down
- ❖ **What:** Include the position (e.g., pleural, mediastinal, etc.) and side (e.g., right, left)
- ❖ **Where:** Top of the USWD and avoid covering any measurements/numbers

❖ **Who and when:** Labelling should be completed by the cardiac theatre nurses/surgeons post operatively prior to transfer of the patient back to the ward. Should a UWSD require changing post operatively on the ward, the responsibility of labelling lies with the direct caregiver (e.g., nurse changing the UWSD or bedside nurse).

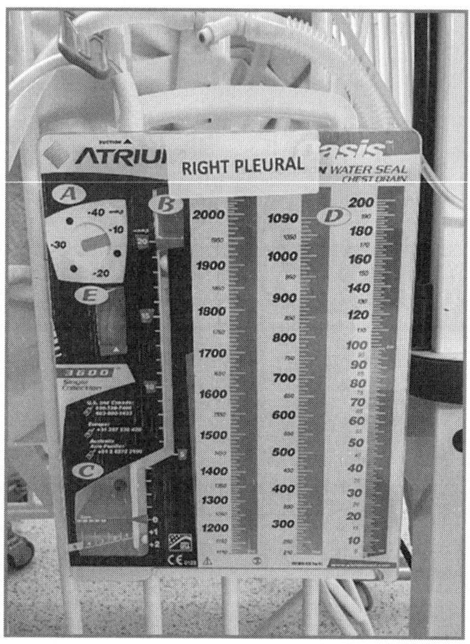

Postural drainage system.

Patient Assessment

Vital Signs

❖ Auscultate chest at shift commencement
❖ Routine four hourly observations including assessment of respiratory effort
❖ If the patient is on an opioid infusion continuous monitoring is required and hourly cardiorespiratory observations (HR, SpO_2, BP, RR) should be documented

For Ward Areas

On insertion of chest drain monitor and document on EMR flowsheets patient observations (HR, SpO_2, BP, RR, respiratory effort and temperature):

❖ 15 minutely for 1 hour
❖ 1 hourly for 4 hours then 1–4 hourly as indicated by patient condition

Drain Insertion Site and Dressing Assessment

❖ Check that the dressing is clean and intact
❖ Assess for any ooze, bleeding or signs of infection/inflammation every hour and document this within EMR: Small amounts of ooze can be a normal presentation postoperatively, however if any abnormal presentations are observed—notify the medical team, consider taking and sending swabs of the site and take a clinical photo and upload onto EMR
❖ Observe that the sutures remain intact and secure (particularly long-term drains where sutures may erode over time)

Skin Integrity

Assess skin at a minimum four hourly for pressure injuries particularly where the tubing is in contact with the skin. Effective anchoring below the insertion sites will assist with preventing this.

UWSD Unit and Tubing

- ❖ Ensure all connections between chest tubes and drainage unit are tight and secure
- ❖ Assessment of chest tube and system tubing should occur at the beginning of the shift and every hour throughout the shift. Tubing should have no kinks or obstructions that may inhibit drainage
- ❖ **Never lift drain above chest level:** The unit and all tubing should be below patient's chest level to facilitate drainage. Ensure the unit is securely positioned on its stand or hanging on the bed
- ❖ Drain tubing should always be secured to patient bed to prevent accidental removal and anchored to the patient's skin to prevent pulling of the drain
- ❖ Ensure the water seal is maintained at 2 cm at all times.

Pain

- ❖ Ensure that patients with an UWSD have appropriate and regular pain relief (IV opioid infusion, PCA, etc.). A CPMS referral should also be in place and also consider appropriate administration of pain relief prior to mobilization, physiotherapy sessions or other activities that involve movement, etc.
- ❖ Pain assessment should be conducted and documented four hourly unless more frequently warranted

Suction

- ❖ Ensure that the suction is on and ensure that the "red bellow" is all the way out
- ❖ If suction is required orders should be written by medical staff and documented within the "Orders" tab on EMR. Suction on the drainage unit should be set to the prescribed level, please see below. Suction is not always required as it may lead to tissue trauma and prolongation of an air leak in some patients.
  - ♦ 5 cm H_2O is commonly used for neonates
  - ♦ 10 cm H_2O to –20 cm H_2O is usually used for children

Drainage

- ❖ Every hour, the UWSD tubing should be "tilted and tipped" in order to ensure the fluid within the tubing accumulates within the chamber
- ❖ *Milking of chest drains using roller clamps is only to be done with written orders from medical staff. Milking drains creates a high negative pressure that can cause pain, tissue trauma and bleeding*

Volume

Document hourly the amount of fluid in the drainage chamber (for each drain if multiple present) in the fluid balance flowsheet on EMR.

Assess the cumulative total of drainage output and notify medical staff of the following:

- ❖ A sudden increase in amount of drainage:
  - ◆ Greater than 5 mL/kg in 1 hour
  - ◆ Greater than 3 mL/kg consistently for 3 hours
- ❖ Significantly reduced output over an extended length of time or if a drain with ongoing loss suddenly stops draining
- ❖ Blocked drains are a major concern for cardiac surgical patients due to the risk of cardiac tamponade

If the chamber tips over and blood has spilt into next chamber, simply tip the chamber up to allow blood to flow to original chamber.

Color and Consistency

Color and consistency of drainage should be documented hourly along with documentation of volume amounts. If there is a change (e.g., hemoserous, bright red, serous, chylous/creamy) notify medical staff immediately.

Consider taking sample of drainage to assess for chylothorax.

Air Leak (Bubbling)

- ❖ The water seal chamber should be assessed every hour for any potential air leaks. An air leak will be characterized by intermittent bubbling in the water seal chamber when the patient with a pneumothorax exhales or coughs.
- ❖ The severity of the leak will be indicated by numerical grading on the UWSD (1-small leak 5-large leak).
- ❖ Continuous bubbling of this chamber indicates large air leak between the drain and the patient. Check drain for disconnection, dislodgement and loose connection, and assess patient condition. Notify medical staff immediately if problem cannot be remedied.
- ❖ If suspected or confirmed leakage, clamp drain tubing closest to patient and escalate accordingly and document on fluid balance flowsheet on EMR.

Oscillation (Swing)

The water in the water seal chamber will rise and fall (swing) with respirations. This will diminish as the pneumothorax resolves. Assess and document on fluid balance flowsheet on EMR.

Other Considerations

- ❖ Referral to a physiotherapist should be made to enhance chest movement and prevent a chest infection and mobilization and transferring should be encourage as appropriate where possible
- ❖ Parent education on managing potential accidental dislodgement should be discussed.

Patient Positioning

Patients who are ambulant post operatively will usually have fewer complications and shorter lengths of stay. If a patient is on strict bed rest or is an infant, regular changes in position should be encouraged to promote drainage, unless the patient's clinical condition prevents doing so.

Patient Transport

* If the patient needs to be transferred to another department or is ambulant, the suction should be disconnected and left open to air
* Remember that during transport, the tubing should not be clamped and that the UWSD should remain below chest level
* Clamps must not be used on the patient for transport because of the risk of tension pneumothorax
* When transporting the patient, be weary of tubing getting caught in the bed and utilize a "cart/trolley" where possible for ease of transport especially for multiple drains. Remember to remove anchor from bed before mobilizing the patient.

Specimen Collection

Collect drainage specimens for culture through the needless sampling port located by the in-line connector.

Equipment Required

* Specimen container
* Alcohol swab
* 10 mL syringe
* Dressing pack
* Gloves
* Eye protection

Procedure

* Wait for the fluid to collect in a loop of the tubing
* Perform hand hygiene, then don gloves and eye protection
* Clean the sampling port with an alcohol wipe and leave to dry for 20 seconds
* Temporarily clamp the tubing above where the fluid has collected
* Connect a 10 mL luer lock syringe to the sampling port and aspirate the fluid out of the tubing. **Do not pierce tubing/sampling port**
* Place fluid in sterile specimen container
* Once the syringe is disconnected remove all clamps and kinks
* Perform hand hygiene

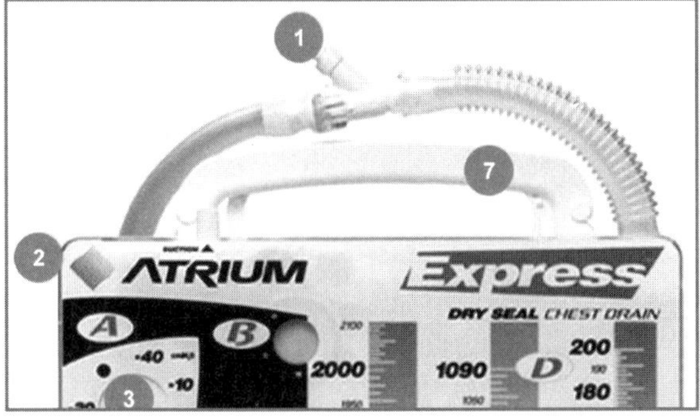
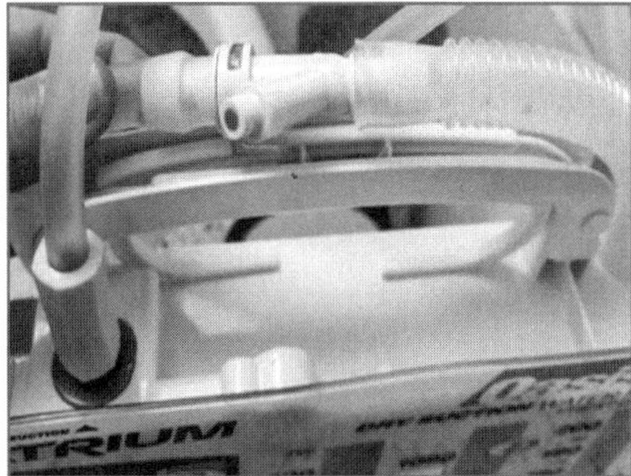

Tubing of water deal.

Chest Drain Dressings

Dressing Change

Dressings should be changed:
- Every seven days unless otherwise indicated
- If they are no longer dry and intact, or signs of infection
- Infected drain sites require daily changing, or when wet or soiled
- Changes are a risk for accidental drain removal. Avoid unnecessary changes
- Dressings should ensure drain is secure
- Dressings should allow site visibility and prevent pressure on skin

Equipment Required

- Dressing pack
- Chlorhexidine solution (yellow or blue)
- Gloves
- Two small occlusive tegaderm dressings
- Split gauze

Procedure

- Perform hand hygiene and then don gloves
- **Remove old dressing:** Preferably get someone who is not sterile to don latex gloves and remove the dressing
- Clean the drain site using the appropriate chlorhexidine solution:
  - Use standard aseptic technique with **body temperature sterile normal saline**
  - If the wound is showing signs of being infected, contaminated or soiled use the **yellow solution** (aqueous chlorhexidine 0.15% w/v cetrimide 15%)
- Once the site is dry apply two layers of split gauze in the direction where the split facing up and it wraps around the drain. Another two layers of split gauze should then be placed on top of the first layer of gauze in the opposite direction (split facing down)
- Cover gauze using hypafix™ (approx two pieces, enough to cover the gauze completely)
- Remove gloves and perform hand hygiene.

For cardiac surgical patients with drains inserted intra-operatively: Ensure dressing does not communicate with sternotomy dressing or wound.

Anchoring Drain Tubing

- Apply Comfeel™ or similar to protect fragile skin from 'tag' of tape
- Use "sleek"™ or "hypafix"™ to secure the drain tube. When securing and folding the sleek around the tubing, ensure that the tubing isn't secured flat down and that there is a "gap of tape" between the comfeel™ and tubing.

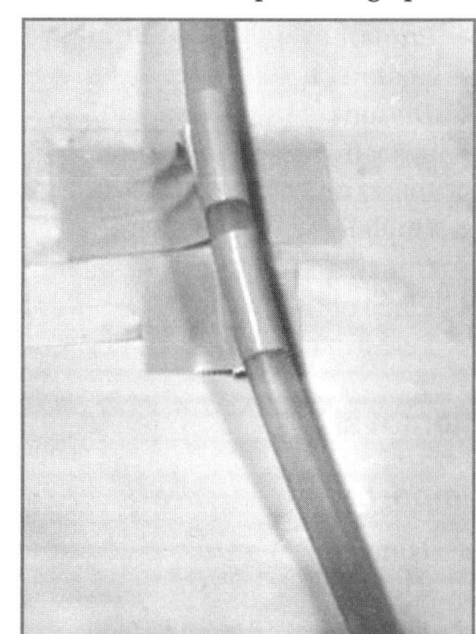

Drain tubing.

Removal of Dressings

❖ To remove dressing when placed flat against the skin—lift corner from the skin and slowly stretch the in dressing in a motion that is parallel to the skin.
❖ To remove semipermeable dressing placed in a sandwich position:
  ◆ Hold the corners of the dressing on either side of the drain and pull them away from each other; this should create a pocket around the drain
  ◆ Peel each of the dressings away from each other until you reach patient skin
  ◆ Slowly stretch the rest of the pressing in a motion that is parallel to the patient's skin to remove the rest of the dressing.

Changing the Chamber

Indications

The chest drain chamber needs to be replaced when it is ¾ full or when the UWSD system sterility has been compromised, e.g., accidental disconnection.

Equipment Required

❖ New UWSD
❖ Dressing pack
❖ Gloves
❖ Eye protection

Procedure

❖ Perform hand hygiene
❖ Use personal protective equipment to protect from possible body fluid exposure
❖ Using an aseptic technique, remove the unit from packaging and place adjacent to old chamber
❖ Prepare the new UWSD as per manufacturer's directions supplied with drain
❖ Ensure patients drain is clamped to prevent air being sucked back into chest
❖ Disconnect old chamber by holding down the clip on the in-line connector to pull the tubing away from the chamber
❖ Insert the tubing into the new chamber until you hear it click
❖ Unclamp the chest drain
❖ Check drain is back on suction
❖ Place old chamber into yellow infectious waste bag and tie
❖ Perform hand hygiene

Removal of Chest Drains

Important Considerations for Drain Removal

❖ There must be written documentation for drain removal by medical staff in EMR specifying which drain/s are to be removed
❖ The responsibility of the proceduralist removing drains is to check the patient's post-operative X-ray prior to drain removal

- ❖ Chest X-ray Must be checked by the proceduralist before any chest drain removal and after removal. The X-ray is then reviewed by surgical team to follow up if further management is required
- ❖ Drain labelling must be physically checked by proceduralist prior to removal to ensure removal of correct drain/s. Consult cardiac surgeon for further clarification.

Indications

- ❖ Drainage diminishes to little or nothing
- ❖ Absence of an air leak (pneumothorax)
- ❖ No evidence of respiratory compromise
- ❖ Chest X-ray showing lung re-expansion

Equipment Required

- ❖ Dressing trolley with yellow infectious waste bag attached
- ❖ Dressing pack (sterile towel, sterile gauze)
- ❖ Sterile gloves
- ❖ Appropriate skin cleaning solution for procedure:
  - ◆ *Neonates <1500 g:* Chlorhexidine irrigation solution 0.1% (blue solution)
  - ◆ *For all other patients:* Aqueous chlorhexidine 0.15% w/v cetrimide 15% (yellow solution)
- ❖ Steri-strips
- ❖ Suture cutter
- ❖ Band aids
- ❖ Clamps
- ❖ Eye protection
- ❖ Occlusive dressing
- ❖ Sharps container

Patient and Pre-procedure Preparation

- ❖ Ensure patient is fasted, has been administered adequate and age-appropriate pain control, sedation (fast appropriately) and distraction therapy
- ❖ Consider environment, e.g., treatment room or privacy screens if in ward area and the involvement of Child Life Therapy if required
- ❖ Ensure you have enough staff to assist with the procedure and ensure that the patient is monitored throughout the procedure
- ❖ *Heparin infusions for cardiac patients should not be discontinued prior to drain removal*
- ❖ *Always remove pacing wires (cardiac patients) before removing the drains and ensure that the drains are unclamped during the removal of wires*

Procedure

- ❖ Perform hand hygiene
- ❖ Opening dressing pack and add sterile equipment and 0.9% saline
- ❖ Don disposable gloves
- ❖ Remove all dressings around the area
- ❖ **Clamp drain tubing and ensure suction is disconnected—double check with assisting nurse. If there are multiple drains in-situ, clamp all drains before removal. Once the required drains are removed, unclamp remaining drains**
- ❖ Remove disposable gloves, perform hand hygiene and don sterile gloves

* Place sterile towel under tubes
* Clean around catheter insertion site and 1–2 cm of the tubing with age appropriate skin cleaning solution
* If purse string present (cardiac patients) unwind in preparation for assistant to tie
* Remove suture securing drain (ensuring purse string suture not cut)
* Instruct patient to exhale and hold if they are old enough to cooperate; if not, time removal with exhalation
* Pinching the edges of the skin together, remove the drain using smooth, but fast, continuous traction
* The assistant pulls purse string suture closed as soon as the drain is removed, tying 2 knots and ensuring the suture is not pulled too tight. Cut tails of suture about 2 cm from knot
* If there is no purse string present remove drain and quickly seal hole with occlusive dressing (i.e., Tegaderm™)

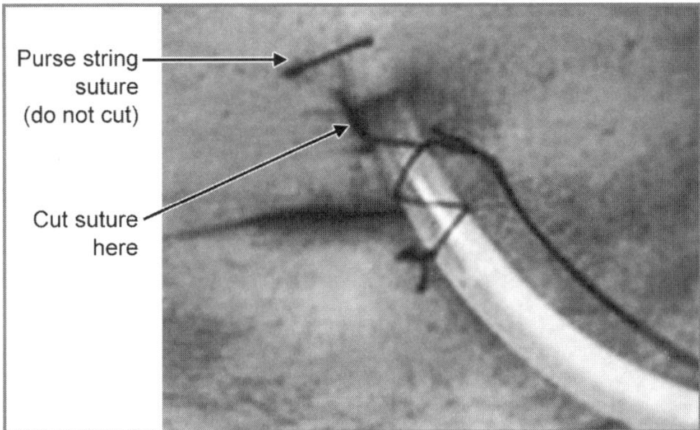

Removal of chest tube.

* Apply steristrips over insertion site if needed
* Remove and discard equipment into a yellow infectious waste bag and tie
* Perform hand hygiene

Post-Procedure Care

* Attend to patients comfort and sedation score as per procedural sedation guideline
* CXR should be performed post-drain removal, ideally 2 hours post (max 4 hours)
* Patients in PICU may wait until routine daily CXR if clinically well
* Clinical status is the best indicator of re-accumulation of air or fluid. CXR should be performed if patient condition deteriorates
* Monitor vital signs closely (HR, SpO_2, RR, respiratory effort and BP) on removal and then every hour for 4 hours post removal, and then as per clinical condition
* Document the removal of drain in the LDA flowsheet in EMR
* Remove sutures four days post-drain removal
* Dressing to remain in situ for 24 hours post removal unless contaminated

Complications and Troubleshooting

Pneumothorax: Signs and symptoms include:

* Decreased SpO_2, increased respiratory effort, diminished breath sounds, decreased chest movement, complaints of chest pain, tachycardia or bradycardia, hypotension

❖ Notify medical staff and request an urgent CXR
❖ Prepare for insertion/repositioning of chest drain
❖ Ensure drain system is intact with no leaks, or blockages, such as kinks or clamps

Bleeding at the Drain Site

❖ Don gloves
❖ Apply pressure to insertion site
❖ Place occlusive dressing over site
❖ Notify medical staff
❖ Check coagulation results
❖ Check drain chamber to ensure no excessive blood loss

Infection of Insertion Site

❖ Notify medical staff
❖ Swab wound site
❖ Consider blood cultures

Accidental Disconnection of System

❖ Clamp the drain tubing at the patient end. Clean ends of drain and reconnect. Ensure all connections are cable tied. If a new drainage system is needed cover the exposed patient end of the drain with sterile dressing while new drain is setup. Ensure clamp is undone when problem has resolved.
❖ Check vital signs and consider getting a CXR
❖ Alert medical staff

Accidental Drain Removal

❖ Apply pressure to the exit site and seal with steristrips. Place an occlusive dressing over the top
❖ Check vital signs, consider the need for a CXR and alert medical staff
❖ The incident must be documented in the VHIMS by the nurse attending to procedure.

Purse String Cut or not Present

❖ Small bore drains, such as pigtails do not require purse strings. Simply apply an occlusive dressing.
❖ **For large bore drains:**
  ♦ Pinch or apply pressure to the exit site
  ♦ Apply steristrips to close exit site and cover with an occlusive dressing
  ♦ Notify the responsible medical team to review patient and consider need for a suture
  ♦ The incident must be documented in the VHIMS by the nurse delegated to remove the drain.

Unable to Remove Chest Drain

❖ If the drain is unable to be removed with reasonable traction being applied, notify the responsible surgical team.
❖ If unsafe to be removed on the ward, the patient might have to go to theater and have it removed under general anesthetic.

Retained Drain during Removal

* If the tube fractures during drain removal and remnants of the tubing are left within the patient contact the treating team immediately (initiate MET call as needed or if patient becomes unstable).
* An urgent chest X-ray should be conducted.
* The patient should be prepared for theater, e.g., keep fasted.
* The whole drain unit should be kept in the patient's room until surgical review and will need to be kept for collection to enable quality review.
* The piece of drain tubing that remains in the patient will also be kept once surgically removed to allow for appropriate follow up of the incident's cause.
* The incident must be documented in the VHIMS by the nurse delegated to remove the drain.
* Please refer to surgical drains (non-cardiac) guideline and RCH policy for missing or non-intact drains.

Family-centered Care

* Explain purpose of chest drain to family and when it is likely to be removed
* Discuss the need for pain relief for the child to be comfortable enough to move and participate in physiotherapy
* Encourage parental involvement with mobilising, sitting out of bed and assisting with chest physiotherapy to aid faster recovery.
* Multidisciplinary care, e.g., physiotherapy referral

PULSE OXIMETER

Introduction

It is a non-invasive method of continuously monitoring the monitoring the oxygen saturation of hemoglobin SpO_2. When oxygen saturation is measured with pulse oximetry, it is referred to as SpO_2. It is a "The Fifth Vital Sign".
* Increased amplitude indicates vasodilation
* Decreased amplitude indicates vasoconstriction or hypovolemia.

Definition

Pulse oximetry is a noninvasive, continuous, and relatively inexpensive method for transcutaneous measurement of the degree to which hemoglobin in arterial blood is saturated with oxygen (SaO_2).

History

* In 1935 Karl Matthes (German physician 1905–1962) developed the first 2–wavelength ear O_2 saturation meter red and green filters.
* The original was made by Glenn allan Millikan in the 1940s.
* Further developed in 1972 by Takuo Aoyagi and Michio Kishi, bioengineers at Nihon Kohden using the ratio of red to infrared light absorption of pulsating components at the measuring site.
* By 1987, the standard of care for the administration of a general anesthetic in the US included pulse oximetery infrared light absorption.

Operating Principle

Pulse oximetry works on the principle of spectre analysis for measurement of oxygen saturation, i.e., the detection and quantification of components in solution by their unique light absorption characteristics.

Pulse oximeters combine the principle of spectrophotometry and plethysmography to noninvasively measure the oxygen saturation in arterial blood.

Plethysmography

Measurement of volume changes within an organ or whole body (usually resulting from fluctuations in the amount of blood or air it contains) or related phenomena is called plethysmography.

Spectrophotometry

All atom and molecules absorb specific wavelength of light. This property is the basis for an optical technique known as spectrophotometry.

The pulse oximeter estimates SpO_2 from differential absorption of red (660 nm) and near infrared light (940) in tissue.

Pulse Oximeter

It is used to measure oxygen saturation in the body, i.e., how much of the hemoglobin in the blood is carrying the oxygen.

Each pulse oximeter probe contains:
- LED, which emit two wavelengths of light
- A photodetector on the other side measures the intensity of transmitted light at each wavelength.

TYPES OF OXIMETERS

Pulse oximeter as part of an anesthetic machine
- A portable desktop unit
- A finger/mobile pulse oximeter

Oxygen saturation: Oxygen enters the lungs and then is passed on into blood carries the oxygen to the various organs in our body.

Equipments

Probes

- The probe sensor, transducer comes in contact with the patient.
- One or more LEDs that emit light at specific wavelengths and a photodetector.
- LEDs provide monochromatic light.
- Reusable or disposal.
- Self-adhesive probes are less likely to come off if the patient moves.
- Probes are available in different sizes.
- Contamination should be reduced.

Cable—the probe is connected to the oximeter by an electrical cable.

Console

- ❖ A microcomputer that monitors and controls signal levels, calculations, activates alarms and messages.
- ❖ Panel displays pulse rate, SpO_2 and alarm limits.
- ❖ Most instruments provide an audible tone whose pitch changes with the saturation.

DIFFERENT SITES

Sites of probe placement:
- ❖ Fingers
- ❖ Toe
- ❖ Ear
- ❖ Nose
- ❖ Tongue
- ❖ Cheek
- ❖ Forehead

Definition

Pulse oximetry is an invasive and painless test that measures your oxygen saturation level, or the oxygen levels in the blood. It can rapidly detect even small changes in how efficiently oxygen is being carried to the extremities furthest from the heart, including the legs and the arms.

The pulse oximeter is a small, clip-like device that attaches to a body part, such as toes or an earlobe. It is most commonly put on a finger, and its often used in a critical care setting, such as emergency rooms or hospitals. Some doctors, such as pulmonologists, may use it in office.

PURPOSES AND USES

The purpose of pulse oximetry is to check how well your heart is pumping oxygen through the body.

It may be used to monitor the health of individuals with any type of condition that can affect blood oxygen levels, especially while they are in the hospital. These conditions include:
- ❖ Chronic obstructive pulmonary disease (COPD)
- ❖ Asthma
- ❖ Pneumonia
- ❖ Lung cancer
- ❖ Heart failure
- ❖ Heart attack
- ❖ Congenital heart defects

There are a number of different common use cases for pulse oximetry, including:
- ❖ To assess how well a new lung medication is working
- ❖ To evaluate whether someone needs help breathing
- ❖ To evaluate how helpful a ventilator is
- ❖ To monitor oxygen levels during or after surgical procedures that require sedation
- ❖ To determine how effective supplemental oxygen therapy is, especially when treatment is new

- ❖ To assess someone's ability to tolerate increased physical activity
- ❖ To evaluate whether someone momentarily stops breathing while sleeping—such as in cases of sleep apnea—during a sleep study

There are a number of different common use cases for pulse oximetry, including:

- ❖ To assess how well a new lung medication is working.
- ❖ To evaluate whether someone needs help breathing.

How it Works

- ❖ During a pulse oximetry reading, a small clamp-like device is placed on a finger, earlobe, or toe. Small beams of light pass through the blood in the finger, measuring the amount of oxygen. It does this by measuring changes of light absorption in oxygenated or deoxygenated blood. This is a painless process.
- ❖ The pulse oximeter will thus be able to tell oxygen saturation levels along with heart rate.

Normal values are variable and must be interpreted in light of altitude, the patient's age, and cardiopulmonary function.

- ❖ Remember that the relationship between oxygen saturation and partial pressure of oxygen is nonlinear. It is prudent to commit to memory the following:
  - ◆ SpO_2 of 90% represents a PaO_2 of 60 mm Hg.
  - ◆ SpO_2 of 75% is a PaO_2 of 40 mm Hg.
  - ◆ SpO_2 of 50% is a PaO_2 of 27 mm Hg.
- ❖ Factors that can distort the normal relationship between oxygen saturation and partial pressure of oxygen must be considered.
  - ◆ With alkalosis or hypothermia, the PaO_2 may be lower than predicted by the SpO_2.
  - ◆ With acidosis or hyperthermia, the PaO_2 may be higher than predicted by the SpO_2.

Limitations of Pulse Oximetry

- ❖ Pulse oximetry is only a presumptive reflection of SaO_2 and does not provide information regarding pH, $PaCO_2$, or respiratory rate.
- ❖ **Pulse oximetry is confounded by the presence of carbon monoxide:**
  - ◆ The device will misinterpret carboxyhemoglobin as oxyhemoglobin and thereby provide a false elevation.
  - ◆ When carbon monoxide poisoning is suspected, an ABG analysis is a more reliable measurement of oxygenation.

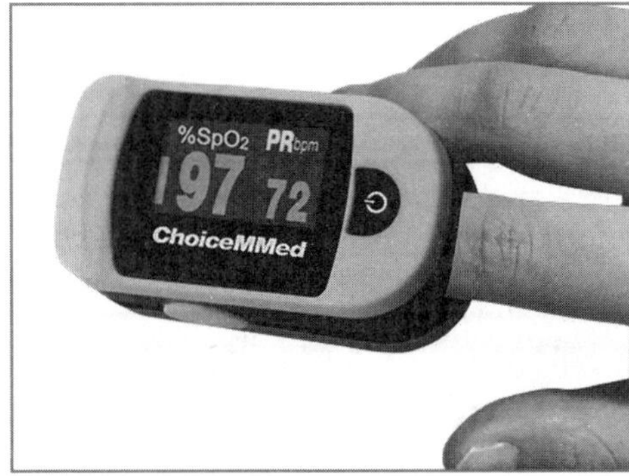

Portable pulse oximeter.

RESTORATIVE AND CONTINUING CARE

1. **Hydration**
2. **Humidification**

Introduction

Humidifiers are devices that add moisture to the air to prevent dryness that can cause irritation in many parts of the body.

Humidifiers can be particularly effective for treating dryness of the skin, nose, throat, and lips. They can also ease some symptoms caused by the flu or common cold.

But overusing humidifiers or not cleaning humidifiers properly can potentially worsen respiratory problems and cause other health conditions.

❖ A means using a device to condition the air delivered to the respiratory airways. This therapy is particularly useful for patients who are mechanically ventilated or have impaired respiratory tracts. Humidification can assist clearance of secretions when clearance mechanism is not effective or when upper airways bypassed by endotracheal tube. The main goal of humidification therapy is to maintain normal physiologic conditions in lower airways.

❖ Humidification is a method to artificially condition the gas used in respiration of a patient as a therapeutically modality. Active method is by adding heat or water or both to the device or passive which is recycling heat and humidity which is exhaled by the patient.

Respiratory humidification is a method of artificial warming and humidifying of respiratory gas for mechanically ventilated patients. The term respiratory gas conditioning stands for warming and humidification as well as purification of respiratory gas.

These three essential functions of respiratory gas conditioning serve the reparation of inspired respiratory gas for the sensitive lungs. If natural respiratory humidification fails, pulmonic infections and damage to lung tissue may be the consequence.

Mechanism of Action

In a healthy person, 75% of respiratory gas conditioning takes place in the upper respiratory tract (nasopharynx). The remaining 25% are taken over by the trachea.

The upper respiratory tract warms, humidifies and cleanses 1,000 to 21,000 liters of respiratory gas daily, depending on body size and physical capability.

Warming

Warming of breathing air is effected by many small blood vessels, net-like coating the nasal and oral mucous membrane (mucosa). Nerve impulses regulate the amount of blood flow like a body's-own heating system. Thus vessels

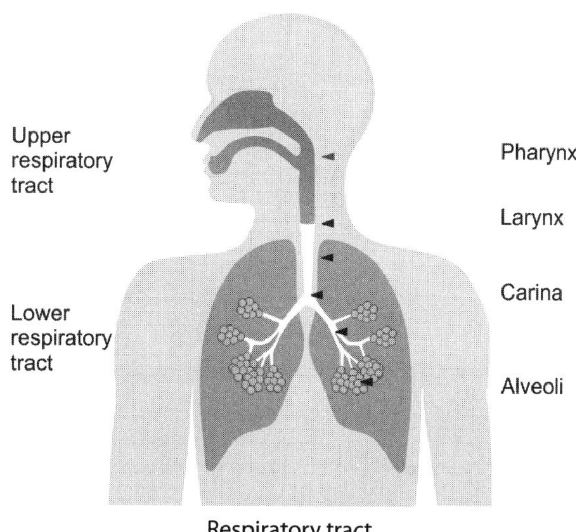

Respiratory tract.

are supplied with more blood when breathing cold air (warming of respiratory gas), and less when breathing warm air.

Humidification

During inspiration, well-vascularized mucous membranes inside the nose and mouth release moisture to the passing respiratory gas. As a result, a healthy adult person evaporates 200 to 300 mL of water per day. While inspiring through nose or mouth the mucous membranes cool down.

During exhalation this cooling effect causes a portion of moisture in the air coming from the lungs (100% relative humidity at 37°C) to condensate on the mucous membranes, whereby the mucous membranes are moisturized again.

On the way to the lower respiratory tract, the respiratory gas already humidified in the nasopharynx is conditioned further until the isothermal saturation limit is reached. Isothermal saturation limit means the maximum possible humidity at a given temperature, which amounts to 100% relative humidity and 44 mg absolute humidity at 37°C. A healthy breathing person reaches that equilibrium during nasal breathing at the bifurcation of the trachea. Hence, only water vapor-satiated and body-warm air reaches the alveoli.

Cleaning

While the removal of inhaled particles in the upper respiratory tract primarily takes place through coughing and sneezing (tussive clearance), in the deeper respiratory tracts mucociliary clearance is paramount. It is the most important cleaning mechanism of the bronchi.

Mucociliary Clearance

The main bronchi down to the alveoli are lined with a respiratory epithelium. On it, cilium is existent, bearing hair-shaped structures on its surface (cilia). The cilia are surrounded by fluid mucous layer, the periciliary liquid. This ciliary layer is covered by viscous mucus which traps foreign matter and microorganisms.

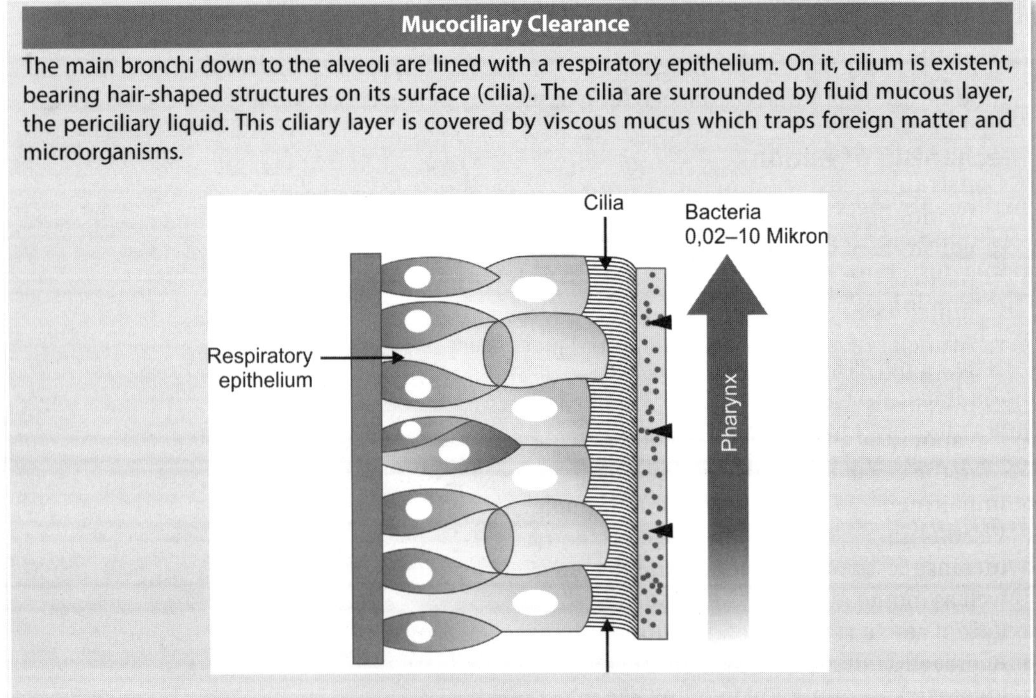

The coordinated movement of the cilia in the periciliary liquid transports the mucus together with foreign matter towards the mouth, where it can be swallowed or coughed up. The efficiency of this clearance mechanism depends on the number of cilia, their structure and motility, and the quantity and consistency of the mucus. Optimum functionality of the mucociliary clearance requires a temperature of 37°C and an absolute humidity of 44 mg/dm^3 corresponding to a relative humidity of 100%. Insufficient heat and moisture in the lower respiratory tract causes the ciliary cells to stop transporting. Under these conditions, bacterial germinal colonization is facilitated.

When is Respiratory Gas Conditioning Affected?

Natural respiratory gas conditioning can be affected by mechanical ventilation using cold and dry respiratory gas. In case of noninvasive respiration (e.g., respiratory masks), a continuous positive flow is administered (e.g., CPAP).

The resulting increased oral breathing causes undesirable accompanying symptoms.

In the long run, the upper respiratory tracts dry out caused by a permanent positive pressure supply with cool respiratory gas. The consequences are painfully inflamed nasal and oral mucous membranes as well as blockage of air passages and congestion of secretion in the respiratory apparatus. In particular, leakages at the respiratory mask may promote drying out of the nasal mucous membranes. A continuous supply of warm respiratory gas significantly reduces these clinical symptoms.

In case of invasive respiration (intubation or tracheotomy), the upper respiratory tracts are bypassed, thus prevented from exercising their natural function. Respiratory gas conditioning is transferred solely to the trachea, which cannot provide the necessary humidifying, warming and clearing performance all by itself.

The results of noninvasive and invasive respiration are:
- ❖ **Insufficient warming effect:** Insufficiently warmed up air arrives in the lungs.
- ❖ **Insufficient humidification effect:** Due to isothermal saturation limit, insufficiently warmed up air cannot carry the required amount of moisture.
- ❖ **Constrained clearance of the respiratory tract:**
  - ♦ In intubated or tracheotomized patients, the tussive clearance function is significantly constrained or failing completely. With these patients, the mechanical removal of foreign particles and germs must be taken over by mucociliary clearance—which however functions only if sufficient moisture is present.
  - ♦ Artificial respiration with cold and dry respiratory gas causes mucus on the respiratory epithelium to become more viscous, within a short time impairing the functionality of the cilia. The stroke frequency of the cilia slows down to final suspension (at <30% water vapor saturation after 3–5 minutes). After no more than one hour, damages are detectable in the cell smear. The consequences may be severe.
- ❖ Impairment of the ciliary function through
- ❖ Viscous mucus and swelling mucous membranes
- ❖ Increase in airway resistance and decrease of compliance through increasing secretion as well as incrustation
- ❖ Risk of atelectases formation due to reduced surfactant activity
- ❖ Aggravation of gas exchange in the lung
- ❖ Increased susceptibility to pulmonic infections

Respiratory Humidifier AIRcon–functional Principle

To prevent aforesaid complications, it is imperative to take measures to compensate loss of heat and moisture, if a patient is mechanically ventilated over a longer period of time.

AIRcon compensates for this heat and moisture loss. Dry and cold inspiratory air is passed from the ventilator to the humidifier chamber.

There it floats above the water surface and absorbs heat and humidity in form of water vapor (pass-over-procedure). Since water vapor cannot transport germs, the risk of contamination is considerably reduced.

Then, the conditioned inspiratory air is transported to the patient. An embedded heating wire in the breathing tube keeps the temperature constant and prevents condensation.

Thus, AIRcon keeps the respiratory epithelium mucous layer supple and cilia flexible. Foreign particles and microorganisms, which may lead to pulmonary infections or lung tissue damage, can be transported successfully.

Advantages of the Respiratory Humidifier AIRcon over HMEs

- Providing the physiological temperature of 37°C with the optimum of 100% relative humidity
- Maintaining of mucociliary clearance over long periods of time
- Secretion liquefaction reduces the risk of tube or cannula occlusion
- No increase of dead space or breathing resistance
- Applicable also for neonates of <2500 g
- No sustainable moisture losses during extraction
- Operation with heated and unheated breathing tube systems possible
- Intelligent alarm management
- Individual adjustability to patient's needs

Active Humidification—Accessories

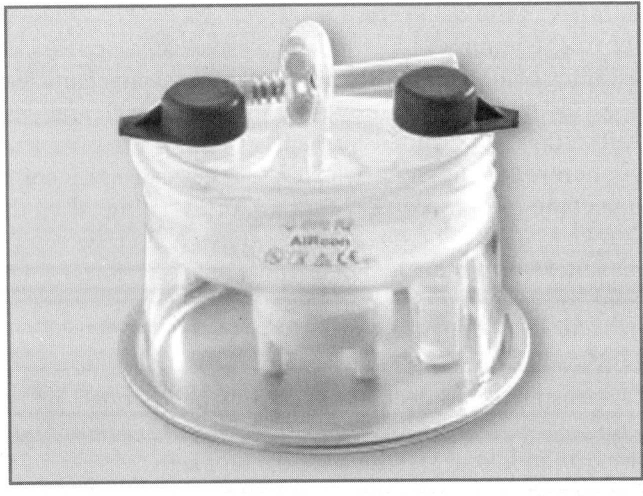

Humidifier chamber.

❖ **Practical autofill system:** An integrated floater ensures the correct water fill level.
❖ **Constant volume:** A regulated autofill mechanism ensures a constant volume in the humidifier chamber.
❖ **Economical:** Our range of products includes disposable humidifier chambers (usable for up to 7 days), and reusable humidifier chambers (autoclavable at 134°C).

Mountings

❖ **Universal application:** Our mountings are applicable with conventional and common standard rails.
❖ **Stable support:** The mountings are specifically designed for the device and ensure safe and stable support.

Breathing Tube Systems

❖ **Reduced condensate formation:** The integrated heating wire reduces condensate formation which causes increased breathing resistance, a false triggering of the respirator, or promotes the growth of germs.
❖ **High-quality materials:** Breathing tubes made of medically approved materials are used. Unless otherwise indicated, all materials are Latex, PC and DEHP free.
❖ **Individual adaptation:** Our disposable breathing tube systems (usable up to 7 days) and reusable systems (autoclavable at 134°C) can be used for neonates, children and adults. We offer configurations for clinics and for home care. In addition, we also design breathing tube systems for individual requirements.

Indications of Humidification

❖ **Primary:**
  ◆ Overcoming humidity deficit created when upper airway is bypassed.
  ◆ To humidify dry medical gases.
❖ **Secondary:**
  ◆ To manage hypothermia.
  ◆ To treat bronchospasm caused by cold air.

Clinical signs and symptoms of inadequate humidification:
❖ Dry and non-productive cough
❖ Atelectasis increased airway resistance
❖ Increased work of breathing
❖ Increased incidence of infection
❖ Thick and dehydrated secretions
❖ Complaints of substernal pain and airway dryness.

Principles of Humidifier Function

❖ **Temperature:** As the temperature of a gas increases, its ability to hold water vapor (capacity) increases and vice versa.
❖ **Surface area:** There is more opportunity for evaporation to occur with greater surface area of contact between water and gas.

❖ **Time of contact:** There is greater opportunity for evaporation to occur, the longer a gas remains in contact with water.

❖ **Thermal mass:** The higher the mass of water or core element of a humidifier, the higher its capacity to transfer or hold heat.

Advantages and Disadvantages of Nebulizer

Advantages

❖ It can carry air that fully saturated with water vapor without heated.

❖ We can increase the amount of the water vapor in the inhaled air.

Disadvantages

❖ It is very expensive.

❖ The pneumatic nebulizer needs high air flow to operate.

❖ The ultrasonic nebulizer need electric supply to operate thus it may cause electric shock.

COUGHING TECHNIQUE

Coughing is effective in maintaining a patent airway. Coughing permits the client to remove secretions from both the upper and lower airways. The series of events in cough mechanism are:

❖ **Deep inhalation:** This increases lung volume and airway diameter. Thus, air can pass to partially obstructing mucus plugs or other foreign matter.

❖ Closure of the glottis.

❖ **Active contraction of the expirations muster:** When the expiratory muscles contract against the closed glottis, high intrathoracic pressure is developed.

❖ **Opening of glottis:** With high intrathoracic pressure, glottis is opened and a large flow of air is expelled at a high speed providing momentum for mucus to move to the upper airway. After the cough mucus can be expectorated or swallowed.

The various coughing techniques include cascade, huff, quad coughing, and controlled coughing.

Cascade Cough

Ask the client to take a slow deep breath and hold it for 2 seconds, while contracting expiratory muscles. Tell the client to open the mouth and perform a series of coughs throughout exhalation, thereby coughing at lowered lung volumes. This helps for airway clearance and maintains a patent airway in clients with large volumes of sputum.

Huff Cough

In this, the client on exhalation opens the glottis by saying the word "huff". The huff cough stimulates a natural cough reflex. This method is useful for clearing central airway. Clients, who practice this regularly, inhale more air and may progress to cascade cough.

Quad Cough

This is used for client without abdominal muscle control, e.g., clients with spinal cord injuries. The client or nurse pushes inward and upward on the abdominal muscles to the diaphragm while the client breathes with maximal expiratory efforts, causing the cough.

Controlled Coughing

Ask the client to take two slow, deep breaths, inhaling through nose and exhaling through mouth. Inhale deeply third time and hold breath to count of 3. Cough fully for two or three consecutive coughs without inhaling between cough. Tell the client to push all air out of lungs. Client should be cautioned to cough properly and not just clearing the throat. Instruct the client to cough 2 or 3 times every 3 hour during walking hours.

The effectiveness of cough is determined by the amount of sputum expectorated and the client's report of swallowed sputum.

Clients with upper and lower respiratory tract infections and chronic pulmonary disease should practice coughing exercise every 2 hours while they are awake and clients with copious amount of sputum must cough hourly while awake and expectorate out sputum till the acute phase of sputum production is over.

BREATHING EXERCISES

Introduction

Breathing is an function controlled by the autonomic nervous system and is also under volitional control. Breathing exercises are a form of exercise which can improve the overall efficiency at which the lungs function (American Lung Association). They can be helpful in individulals with both healthy lungs as well as those with impaired lung function. In the absence of disease our breathing becomes altered with stress and when left unchecked over time can result in breathing pattern disorders.

Benefits of breathing exercises include a variety of health-related reasons, e.g., to enhance the respiratory system by improving ventilation; strengthening respiratory muscles; make breathing more efficient; and for relieving stress and anxiety reduction.

Diaphragmatic Breathing

Diaphragmatic breathing is a type of breathing exercise that helps strengthen the diaphragm, an important muscle that helps with breathing, as it represents 80% of breathing. Diaphragmatic exercises help to make people feel relaxed and rested.

This breathing exercise is also sometimes called belly breathing or abdominal breathing.

Technique

- ❖ **Focusing on the diaphragm:** Place one hand on the chest and the other on your stomach. Take a slow deep breath, paying attention to which hand moves. *In diaphragmatic breathing, the stomach hand should move most.*
- ❖ **Slowing breathing:** Inhale to fully inflate the lungs, then slowly exhale. Breathing out through the nose can help control exhalation rate. Pause briefly after exhaling then inhale again

Improper breathing can upset the oxygen and carbon dioxide exchange and contribute to anxiety, panic attacks, fatigue, and other physical and emotional disturbances.

Deep Breathing

Deep breathing helps to relieve shortness of breath by preventing air from getting trapped in the lungs and helps inhalation of more fresh air to the base of the lungs. It may help the client to feel more relaxed and centered.

Technique

❖ While standing or sitting, draw your elbows back slightly to allow your chest to expand.
❖ Take a deep inhalation through the nose.
❖ Retain your breath for a count of 5.
❖ Slowly release your breath by exhaling through the nose

Pursed-lip breathing is a breathing technique that consists of exhaling through tightly pressed (pursed) lips and inhaling through the nose with the mouth closed. It is a simple breathing technique that helps with making deep breaths slower and more intentional.

This technique has been found to benefit people who have anxiety-associated lung conditions, e.g., emphysema and chronic obstructive pulmonary disease (COPD).

Breathing Technique

❖ Inhale quietly through your nose for the count of four. Fill lungs completely to the point where you feel your abdomen is filled full of air like a balloon.
❖ Hold your breath for four counts.
❖ Through pursed lips, slowly exhale through your mouth making a whoosh sound for eight counts.

Box Breathing

Box breathing can be helpful with relaxation. Box breathing is a breathing exercise to assist patients with stress management and can be implemented before, during, and/or after stressful experiences. Box breathing involves visualizing a journey around the four sides of a square, pausing while traveling horizontally, and breathing in while traveling up the square and out while traveling down it. This exercise can be implemented in many environments, not requiring a calm environment to be effective.

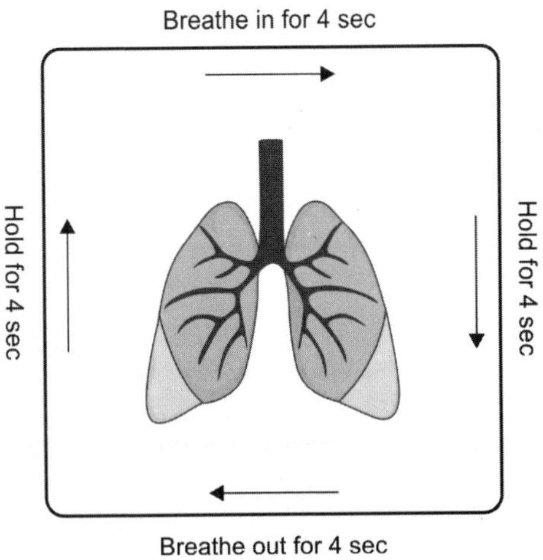

Box breathing.

❖ **Step one:** Breath in through the nose for a count of 4.
❖ **Step two:** Hold your breath for a count of 4.
❖ **Step three:** Breath out for a count of 4.

❖ **Step four:** Hold your breath for a count of 4.
❖ Repeat

MINDFUL BREATHING

Mindfulness meditation involves focusing on your breathing and bringing attention to the present without allowing your mind to drift off to the past or future.

❖ A calming focus is chosen, including a sound ("om"), positive word ("peace"), or phrase ("breathe in calm, breathe out tension") to repeat silently as the client inhales or exhales.
❖ The mind and body then let go and relax.
❖ When the client notices the mind has drifted, they take a deep breath and gently return attention to the present.

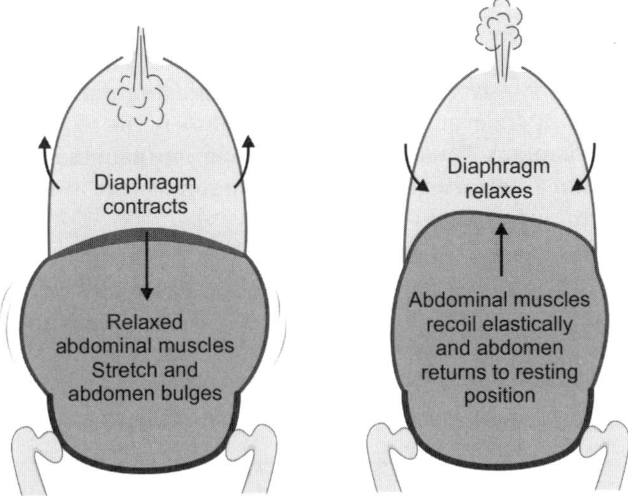

Mindful breathing.

Cardiac Coherence Breathing

Cardiac coherence corresponds to the interconnectivity reflex of the respiratory and cardiac systems, through the autonomous nervous system managing those systems' rhythms coherence, and regulation of one another. This exercise corresponds to acting on the respiratory rhythm in order to influence the cardiac one. It can be practiced at different paces for different objectives and results.

The method described by Dr David O'Hare in his book 365, meaning 3 times/day, 6 breaths/minute, for 5 minutes long is a method that had proven its immediate and residual effects as well as its long term. Such as a decrease in cortisol level, blood pressure regulation, and lower risk of heart disease, oxytocin hormone production increase, regulation of blood sugar level, increased memorization and concentration. This is made possible by a larger activation of the autonomous nervous system implying a better hormone regulation and systems managed by the autonomous nervous system.

The technique by itself: The main pace is known as 4/6; meaning 4 seconds of inhalation and 6 seconds of exhalation

This exercise does not require the use of any special equipment.

Research Findings

Breathing affects all body systems; these systems in turn influence breathing. Optimal breathing patterns help to maintain homeostasis, but when breathing is disrupted, significant issues can arise.

Examples of how breathing can help in health outcomes are:

- Breathing exercises can improve pulmonary function, respiratory muscle strength, exercise capacity, dyspnea, and health-related quality of life in patients with COPD.
- Evidence suggests that diaphragmatic breathing may decrease stress as measured by physiologic biomarkers, as well psychological self-report tools.
- Evidence exists to support the use of breathing exercises in the treatment of chronic, nonspecific low back pain.
- Breathing-based meditation decreases posttraumatic stress disorder (PTSD) symptoms in US military veterans.
- The way of breathing decisively influences autonomic and pain processing. Deep slow breathing in concert with relaxation are essential feature in the modulation of sympathetic arousal and pain perception. Thus can be useful in chronic pain management.
- Breathing exercises for adults with asthma may have some positive effects on quality of life, hyperventilation symptoms, and lung function.

UNIT

Fluid, Electrolyte and Acid-Base Balance

8

UNIT OUTLINE

- Physiological regulation of fluid, electrolyte and acid-base balances
- Factors affecting fluid, electrolyte and acid-base balances
- Disturbances in fluid volume
- Electrolyte imbalances
- Acid-base imbalances
- Intravenous therapy
- Peripheral venipuncture sites
- Types of IV fluids
- Calculation for making IV fluid plan
- Complications of IV fluid therapy
- Measuring fluid intake and output
- Administering blood and blood components
- Restricting fluid intake
- Enhancing fluid intake

LEARNING OBJECTIVES

At the end of this unit, the reader will be able to:
- Define electrolyte.
- Explain composition of body fluids.
- Describe regulation of body fluids.
- Enumerate factors affecting fluid and electrolyte.
- Describe hypovolemia, hypervolemia.
- Explain edema.
- Identify electrolyte imbalance.
- Interpret arterial blood gas.
- Define IV therapy.
- Categorize IV solutions.
- Distinguish IV solutions.
- Identify complications of IV therapy.
- Calculate intake and output.
- Practice blood transfusion.

INTRODUCTION

Between 50 and 60% of the human body by weight is water. Because fluid is the main constituent of the body, the body's fluid balance is very important. Body fluids contain other dissolved substances in the form of electrolytes, gases and nonelectrolytes. The balance or homeostasis, of water and dissolved substances is maintained through functions of almost every organ of the body. Nurses routinely care for the patients with serious and even life-threatening fluid, electrolyte and acid-base disturbances. One of nursing's important role is the prevention of these disturbances in high-risk populations, such as infants, older people, and patients with cardiac and renal disorders.

The phrase fluid and electrolyte balance implies homeostasis or consistency of fluid and electrolyte levels. It means that both the amount and distribution of fluids and electrolyte level is normal and constant. For homeostasis to be maintained body input of water and electrolyte must be balanced by output. Cell function depends not only on a continuous supply of nutrients and removal of metabolic waste, but also on the physical and chemical homeostasis of the surrounding fluids. This was recognized with great style in 1857 by the French Physiologist Claude Bernard, who said; "It is fixity of the internal environment which is the condition of free and independent life."

ELECTROLYTES

Electrolytes are compounds that separate into ions, or charged particles, in water. Electrolytes form when salts, such as sodium chloride or potassium phosphate, dissociate and form ions. For example, sodium chloride dissociates into a sodium ion and a chloride ion when dissolved in water.

There are two types of electrolytes:

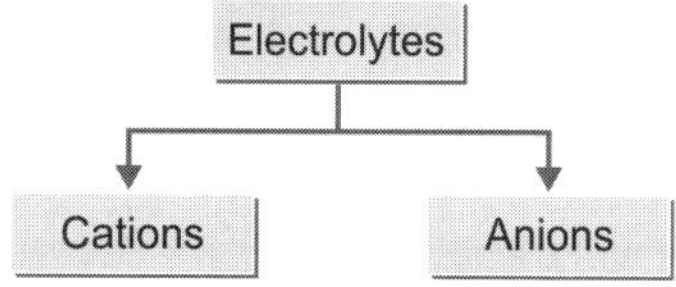

The major positively charged electrolytes are known as cations. Examples of cations include sodium, calcium, potassium, and magnesium. The major negatively charged electrolytes are anions. Examples of anions include chloride, phosphate, sulfate, and bicarbonate. If a compound dissolves in water and dissociates into an anion and a cation, then that compound is an electrolyte.

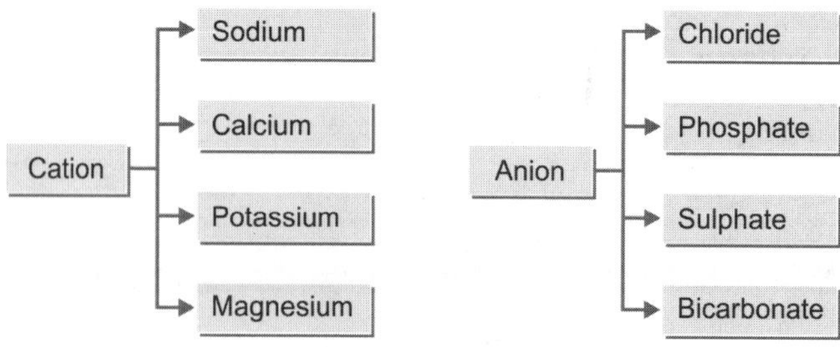

DEFINITION

❖ **Fluid:** Fluid is a substance composed of molecules which freely change their relative position without separation of mass.
❖ **Fluid balance:** A state in which the volume of body water and its solutes is within normal limits and there is normal distribution of fluids in the intracellular and extracellular.

❖ **Electrolyte:** A compound which, when dissolved in a solution will dissociate into ions. These ions are electrically charged particles and thus will conduct electricity.

❖ **Electrolyte balance:** The maintenance of the correct balance between the different elements in body tissues and fluids.

COMPOSITION OF BODY FLUID

The body fluid contains substances called electrolytes that are sometimes called mineral or salts. An electrolyte is an element or compound which, when dissolved or melted in water or another solvent, separates into ions and is capable of carrying an electric current positively charged electrolytes are called cations (Na^+, K^+, Ca^{2+} etc.) and negatively charged electrolytes are called anions(Cl^-, HCO_4^-, SO_4^- etc.)

Electrolyte distribution in body	
Electrolytes	*Serum value(in mEg/L)*
Sodium (Na^+)	135–145
Potassium (k^+)	3.5–5
Calcium (Ca^{2+})	4.5–5.5
Bicarbonate (HCO_3^-)	22–26
Chloride (Cl^-)	90–110
Magnesium (Mg^{2+})	1.5–2.5
Phosphate (PO_4^{3-})	1.7–4.6

REGULATION OF BODY FLUIDS

Fluid Intake

Fluid intake is regulated primarily through the thirst mechanism. The thirst control center is located within the hypothalamus in the brain. Thirst is the conscious desire of water and is one of the major factors that determine fluids intake. A number of stimuli trigger this center, including the osmotic pressure of body fluids, vascular volume and angiotensin. For example, a long distance runner loses significant amount of water through perspiration and breathing, increasing the concentration of solute and the osmotic pressure of fluids. This increase osmotic pressure stimulates the thirst center, causing the runner to experience the sensation of thirst and the desire to drink to replace lost fluids.

During periods of moderate activity at moderate temperature, the average adult drinks about 15,000 mL per day but needs 2,500 mL per day, an additional 1,000 mL, this added volume is required from foods.

❖ **Fluid output:** The routes of fluid output are
   • *Urine:* Urine formed by the kidneys and excreted from the urinary bladder is the major avenue of fluid output. Normal urine output for an adult is 1,400–1,500 mL per 24 hours. Urine volume automatically increases as intake increases.
   • *Insensible loss:* Insensible fluid loss occurs through the skin and lungs. It is called insensible because it is not noticeable and cannot be measured (insensible loss occurs through the skin in two ways—diffusion and perspiration which is noticeable but not measurable).

Another type of insensible loss is in the exhaled air. In adults this is normally 300–400 mL per day.

Feces: An average adult loss only 100–200 mL of fluid through feces each day.

❖ **Hormonal regulation:**
  ◆ *Antidiuretic hormone:* Antidiuretic hormone which regulates water excretion from the kidney is synthesized in the anterior portion of the hypothalamus and acts on the collecting ducts of the lobule. When serum osmolality rises, ADH is produced, causing the collecting ducts to become more permeable to water. This increase more water to be reabsorbed into the blood. As more water is reabsorbed urine output falls and serum osmolality decrease.
  ◆ *Renin-angiotensin–aldosterone system:* If blood flow or pressure to the kidney decrease, rennin is realized. Renin causes the conversion of angiotensinogen to angiotensin-I, which is then converted to angiotensin-II, by angiotensin converting enzyme. Angiotensin-II acts directly on the nephrons to promote sodium and water retention in addition it stimulates the release of aldosterone from renal cortex which also promotes sodium retention.

CATIONS

Major cations within the body fluids include sodium, potassium, calcium and magnesium. Cations interchange when one cations leave the cell and is replaced by another. This occurs because cells tend to maintain electrical neutrality.

Sodium Regulation (Na⁺)

Sodium is the most abundant cation (90%) in ECF. Sodium ions are the major contributors to maintaining water balance through their effect on serum osmolality, nerve impulse transmission, regulation of acid-base balance, and participation in cellular chemical reactions. It moves easily between intravascular and interstitial spaces and moves across cell membranes by active transport. Sodium intake is regulated by dietary intake and aldosterone secretion. The normal extracellular sodium concentration is 135–145 mEq/L.

Potassium Regulation (K⁺)

It is the major cation of ICF. It regulates many metabolic activities and is necessary for glycogen deposits in the liver and the skeletal muscle, transmission and conduction of nerve impulses, normal cardiac conduction and skeletal and smooth muscle contraction. The normal range for serum potassium concentrations is 3.5–5 mEq/L.

Calcium Regulation (Ca⁺⁺)

Calcium is the most abundant electrolyte in the body. Up to 99% of the total amount of calcium in the body is found in bones and teeth in ionized from. Calcium is necessary for bone and teeth formation, blood clotting, hormone secretion, cell membrane integrity, cardiac conduction, transmission of nerve impulses and muscle contraction. Normal serum ionized calcium is 4.5–5.5 mg/dL. Normal total calcium is 8.5–10.5 mg/dL.

Magnesium (Mg^{++})

Magnesium is the second most important cation in the ICF. Magnesium is essential for enzyme activities, neurochemical activities and cardiac and skeletal muscle excitability. Plasma concentration of magnesium range from 1.5 to 2.5 mEq/L.

ANIONS

The three major anions of body fluids are chloride, bicarbonate and phosphate.

Chloride regulation (Cl$^-$)

Chloride is the major anion in ECF. Normal concentration of chloride range from 95 to 105 mEq/L.

Bicarbonate regulation (HCO$_3^-$)

Bicarbonate is the major chemical base buffer within the body. The bicarbonate is found both in ECF and ICF. The normal arterial bicarbonate levels range between 22 and 26 mEq/L, venous: 24–30 mEq/L.

Phosphorus-Phosphate regulation (PO$_4^-$)

Phosphate is a buffer anion found primarily in ICF. It assists in acid-base balance Phosphate and calcium help to develop and maintain bones and teeth. The normal serum level is 2.8–4.5 mg/dL.

FACTORS AFFECTING FLUID AND ELECTROLYTES

Fluid and electrolyte balance is achieved by the body through the process of homeostasis. Homeostasis is the collective series of adjustments that prevent change in the internal environment of the body. Electrolytes are involved in maintaining homeostasis through the following physiologic body functions:

❖ Osmotic equilibrium
❖ Acid-base balance
❖ Intracellular and extracellular concentration differentials
❖ Acid-base balance is an equilibrium state of hydrogen ion concentration. When an acid-base imbalance occurs, the body attempts to compensate by developing an opposite acid-base imbalance to offset the effects of the primary disorder. If the acid-base balance gets disrupted and remains untreated, the effects can be electrolyte abnormalities or even death. Sodium is integral to the maintenance of acid-base balance. The sodium-potassium pump functions to balance cellular electrolytes by actively pumping sodium out of cells in exchange for potassium.

Illness, environmental factors, diet, and diuretics are all factors that affect the balance of fluids and electrolytes.

Illness can lead to water imbalance in the body. Too much water can cause water intoxication via overhydration as well as hyponatremia. Hyponatremia refers to low sodium levels in the blood.

FLUID VOLUME DEFICIT

Introduction

Fluid volume deficit (also known as hypovolemia) is a state or condition where the fluid output exceeds the fluid intake. It occurs when the body loses both water and electrolytes from the ECF in similar proportions. Common sources of fluid loss are the gastrointestinal tract, polyuria, and increased perspiration.

Risk factors for deficient fluid volume are as follows: Vomiting, diarrhea, GI suctioning, sweating, decreased intake, nausea, inability to gain access to fluids, adrenal insufficiency, osmotic diuresis, hemorrhage, coma, third-space fluid shifts, burns, ascites, and liver dysfunction. Fluid volume deficit may be an acute or chronic condition managed in the hospital, outpatient center, or home setting.

The term hypovolemia refers collectively to two distinct disorders:
1. Volume depletion, which describes the loss of sodium from the extracellular space (i.e., intravascular and interstitial fluid) that occurs during gastrointestinal hemorrhage, vomiting, diarrhea, and diuresis; and
2. Dehydration, which refers to the loss of intracellular water (and total body water) that ultimately causes cellular desiccation and elevates the plasma sodium concentration and osmolality.

Dehydration is the excessive loss of water from the body. Signs of dehydration include:
* Headache
* Fatigue
* Decreased urine output
* Poor skin turgor, or skin elasticity

Skin turgor can be tested by pinching the skin on the top of the hand. If the skin takes longer than a couple seconds to return to normal, then the skin turgor is considered poor. This is an indicator of dehydration.

Dehydration can be due to illness where fluid is lost, such as having diarrhea, emesis, or hemorrhaging,

Environmental Factors

Electrolyte imbalance can occur due to environmental factors. Environmental factors capable of inducing fluid loss through the lungs and through sweat include:
* High altitude
* Low humidity
* High temperatures
* Burns
* Cancer
* Cardiovascular disease, heart failure or high blood pressure
* Dehydration due to not drinking enough liquids or from excessive vomiting, diarrhea, sweating (hyperhidrosis) or fever.
* Overhydration or water intoxication (drinking too much water)
* Eating disorders
* Kidney disease
* Liver disease like cirrhosis
* Substance use disorder

Certain medications can also affect electrolyte levels. These include:

❖ Antibiotics
❖ Chemotherapy drugs
❖ Corticosteroids
❖ Diuretics and laxatives

Fluid volume deficit also known as dehydration can be a common occurrence and nursing diagnosis for many patients. Dehydration is when there is a loss of too much fluid from the body. This leads to a lack of water in the body's cells and blood vessels. It is due to more fluids being expelled from the body than the body takes in.

Causes

There are several reasons an individual may become dehydrated. Below is a brief list of some potential causes:

❖ Vomiting
❖ Diarrhea
❖ Excessive sweating
❖ Fever
❖ Frequent urination
❖ Lack of oral fluid intake
❖ Medications (i.e., diuretics)
❖ Other medical conditions (i.e., diabetes)
❖ Pregnancy and breastfeeding

Symptoms

There are several signs and symptoms that may be present for an individual suffering from dehydration. Some symptoms can be vague and a sign for other conditions as well so it is important the nurse is completing a full assessment and brining all the pieces of the assessment together in making clinical decisions. A brief list of signs and symptoms includes:

❖ Headache
❖ Confusion
❖ Fatigue
❖ Dizziness/light-headedness
❖ Weakness
❖ Dry mouth/dry cough
❖ Tachycardia with hypotension
❖ Decreased appetite
❖ Muscle cramps
❖ Constipation
❖ Concentrated urine
❖ Dry skin
❖ Feeling of thirst

For very young children or infants who are unable to verbalize, additional signs and symptoms may be present that include:

❖ Crying without tears
❖ No wet diapers for 3 hours or longer

❖ High fevers
❖ Irritability
❖ Sunken eyes
❖ Unusually drowsy

At Risk Population

Some individuals and populations are more at risk of developing dehydration than others.
These populations include:
❖ Elderly patient
❖ Infants and children
❖ Individuals with chronic conditions
❖ Individuals with complex medication regimens (especially those including the use of
   diuretics)
❖ Active individuals who may not be rehydrating after exercising

Expected Outcomes

❖ Patient's vital signs will remain stable and/or return to patient's baseline
❖ Patient's intake and output will stabilize
❖ Patient's lab values will return to baseline
❖ Patient will verbalize measures to take at home to maintain hydration/prevent dehydration

Nursing Assessment for Fluid Volume Deficit

❖ **Complete a thorough head-to-toe assessment:** This will allow the nurse to assess the entire
   person and put all data together when making clinical decisions and assist in identifying the
   cause of dehydration.
❖ **Assess intake and output:** This will allow the nurse objective data in determining the
   patient's net loss of fluid.
❖ **Assess vital signs:** Vital signs may be abnormal if dehydrated (i.e., tachycardia and/or
   hypotension).
❖ **Assess laboratory values:** Patients may have abnormal blood work levels due to dehydration
   (i.e., abnormal electrolyte levels or renal function).
❖ **Assess skin turgor:** Loss of skin elasticity can be a sign of dehydration.
❖ **Assess urine color and concentration:** Dark and concentrated urine can be a sign of
   dehydration; patients should produce at least 30 mL of urine/hour.
❖ **Auscultate cardiac sounds:** Abnormal cardiac sounds may be heard with severe dehydration
   and dysrhythmias can develop.
❖ **Assess cardiac rhythm:** Dysrhythmias may develop if severely dehydrated and if electrolyte
   abnormalities are present.
❖ **Assess mental status:** Severe dehydration may cause alteration in mentation.

Nursing Interventions for Fluid Volume Deficit

❖ **Encourage/remind patient of the need for oral intake:** As individuals age sometimes,
   there is a loss of thirst, reminding and encouraging individuals may help them to remember
   the need to continue drinking fluids even if they do not feel they are thirsty.

❖ **Administer intravenous hydration if needed:** Severely dehydrated patients or patients unable to take oral hydration may require IV hydration to maintain appropriate hydration level.

❖ **Educate patient and family on possible causes of dehydration:** Education will help allow the patient and family to have a better understanding of the diagnosis and preventative measures they can take in the future to avoid dehydration.

❖ **Administer electrolyte replacements as needed/as ordered:** Dehydration can lead to electrolyte abnormalities; it is important the nurse monitors for this and provides supplemental replacements when needed.

❖ **Educate patient and family on how to monitor intake and output:** Patients and family members will need to know how to monitor intake and output once discharged home to ensure they are maintaining appropriate hydration level.

❖ **Weigh patient daily:** Daily weight measurements will allow the nurse to easily monitor for potential fluid overload when rehydrating patients.

❖ **Educate patient on the importance of maintaining a proper hydration and nutrition status regularly:** Education will help the patient to become more independent upon discharge and will help them to understand what they can do to prevent further episodes of dehydration.

HYPOVOLEMIA

Hypovolemia refers to a low extracellular fluid (ECF) volume, often involving a decrease in both water and sodium levels. In order to maintain bodily functions and preserve homeostasis (i.e., a relatively equivalent state), the body requires a specific amount of blood and other bodily fluids. An imbalance caused by hypovolemia results in a decreased ECF volume, which can adversely affect several organ systems. For example, the heart may begin to beat faster in order to compensate for the low ECF.

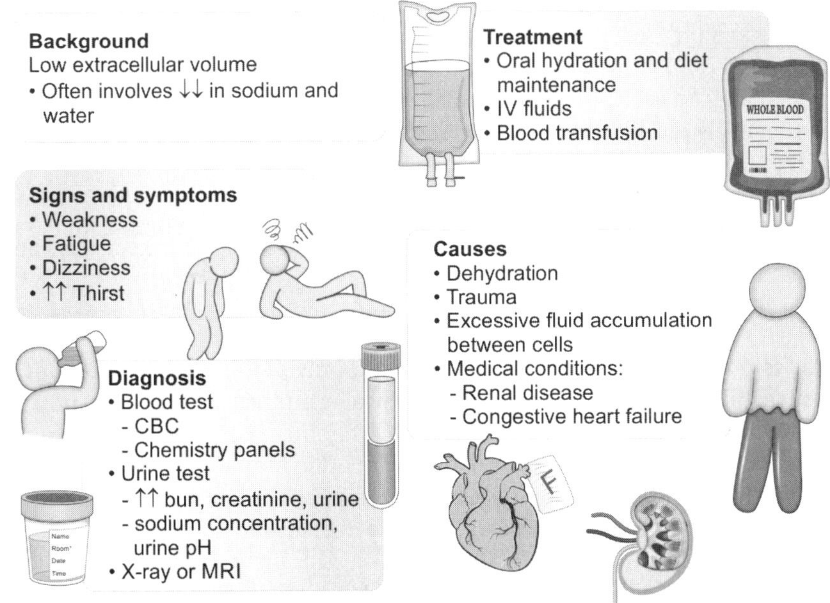

Causes

Hypovolemia is commonly caused by dysfunction of various organs, such as congestive heart failure or kidney failure. Rarely, neurological disorders, particularly those affecting the hormones that regulate kidney functioning can also cause hypovolemia.

Another common cause of hypovolemia is dehydration, which may result from excessive water evaporating from the skin in extreme heat or when experiencing a fever. Dehydration can also result from continuous vomiting or diarrhea without sufficient fluid intake, usually associated with infections that cause gastroenteritis.

Hypovolemia may also result from excessive accumulation of fluids within the interstitial space, between cells. For instance, when an infection becomes severe, sepsis can occur, which is a life-threatening condition in which the individual's response to the infection leads to organ dysfunction and systemic inflammation. In turn, fluids begin to leak out into the interstitial space, thereby causing hypovolemia. Other conditions that can cause fluids to exit blood vessels include pancreatitis, pericarditis, burns, and nutritional hypoalbuminemia.

Finally, hypovolemia may also be caused by sudden blood loss due to a trauma, like a motor vehicle accident or a fall from a height. External or internal bleeding may occur and, if not identified quickly, can be life-threatening.

Signs and Symptoms

The general symptoms of hypovolemia include weakness, fatigue, dizziness, and increased thirst. Other more severe symptoms may also be present, including low urine output (i.e., oliguria), cyanosis characterized by blue discoloration of the skin from poor circulation, pain in the abdominal region or chest, and confusion or a decreased level of consciousness.

Many clinical signs can be found upon examination. Some more reliable indicators include an increase in heart rate by more than 15–20 beats per minute upon standing (i.e., orthostatic tachycardia) or a decrease in blood pressure by more than 10–20 mm Hg when standing (i.e., orthostatic hypotension). Additionally, a decreased jugular venous pressure (JVP) can indicate hypovolemia.

Severe cases can lead to hypovolemic shock, which occurs once there's not enough fluid for the heart to effectively pump. This condition requires emergent medical care as organ damage can occur if they do not receive enough blood to function. Hypovolemic shock is characterized by tachycardia, hypotension, peripheral hypoperfusion, and peripheral vasoconstriction. When hypovolemic shock occurs as a result of blood loss, it is referred to as hemorrhagic shock and when it occurs due to sepsis, it is called septic shock.

Diagnoses

Hypovolemia is diagnosed after a medical evaluation involving an assessment of signs and symptoms, medical and family history, and a physical examination. Subsequently, blood and urine tests, including a complete blood count and chemistry panels (i.e., a blood test that includes electrolytes, liver, and kidney function), are often conducted. Individuals with renal causes of hypovolemia often show an increased BUN, creatinine, urine sodium concentration, and urine pH. Blood tests can also indicate possible development of acid-base disorders, like metabolic acidosis for individuals with diarrheal illnesses. Individuals in hypovolemic shock may also experience hepatic or cardiac ischemia, often revealed by the chemistry panel and cardiac biomarkers (e.g., myocardial lactate extraction). Additional diagnostic tests, such as X-ray, CT, or MRI, may be conducted depending on the suspected underlying cause.

Management

Treatment for hypovolemia varies based on the underlying cause, but the goal is always aimed at restoring fluid balance and replacing any continued fluid loss. In mild cases, individuals are typically treated by oral hydration and a maintenance diet, which increases their intake of sodium and vitamins. In more severe cases, intravenous fluids, modified based upon the underlying condition, are administered. Typically, individuals receive isotonic saline, which is a mixture of sodium chloride and water that contains the same concentration of sodium chloride as found normally in the human body. However, other choices vary by the nutrient composition of the specific individual's blood. For example, an individual who has elevated sodium levels (i.e., hypernatremia) and has lost both water and salts will typically receive hypotonic saline, which is a mixture of sodium chloride and water that contains less sodium chloride than what is found normally in the human body. Additionally, individuals who have lost blood from hemorrhage often receive a blood transfusion. Other treatments may be required to treat the underlying cause, such as medications for heart failure or dialysis for kidney failure.

FLUID OVERLOAD (HYPERVOLEMIA)

Fluid overload (FO) is characterized by hypervolemia, edema, or both. In clinical practice it is usually suspected when a patient shows evidence of pulmonary edema, peripheral edema, or body cavity effusion. FO may be a consequence of spontaneous disease or may be a complication of intravenous fluid therapy. Most clinical studies of the association of FO with fluid therapy and risk of harm define it in terms of an increase in body weight of at least 5–10%, or a positive fluid balance of the same magnitude when fluid intake and urine output are measured. Numerous observational clinical studies in humans have demonstrated an association between FO, adverse events, and mortality, as have two retrospective observational studies in dogs and cats. The risk of FO may be minimized by limiting resuscitation fluid to the smallest amount needed to optimize cardiac output and then limiting maintenance fluid to the amount needed to replace ongoing normal and pathological losses of water and sodium.

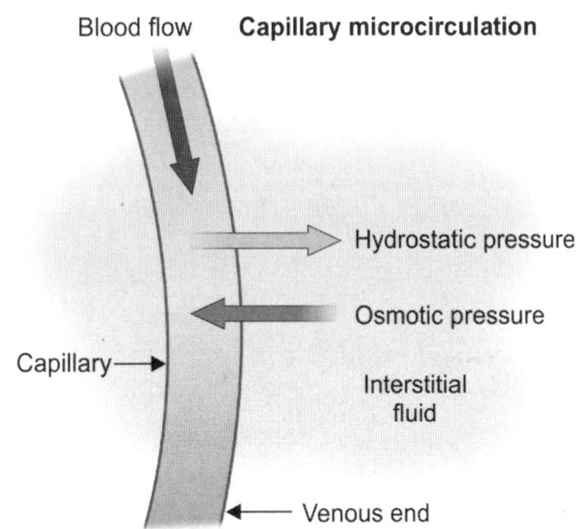

Hypervolemia, also known as fluid overload, is the medical condition where there is too much fluid in the blood.

Signs and Symptoms

The excess fluid, primarily salt and water, builds up in various locations in the body and leads to an increase in weight, swelling in the legs and arms (peripheral edema), and/or fluid in the abdomen (ascites). Eventually, the fluid enters the air spaces in the lungs (pulmonary edema) reduces the amount of oxygen that can enter the blood, leading to anemia and causes shortness of breath (dyspnea) or enters pleural space by transudation (pleural effusion which also causes dyspnea), which is the best indicator of estimating central venous pressure is increased. It can also cause swelling of the face. Fluid can also collect in the lungs when lying down at night, possibly making nighttime breathing and sleeping difficult (paroxysmal nocturnal dyspnea).

Complications

Congestive heart failure is the most common result of fluid overload. Also, it may be associated with hyponatremia (hypervolemic hyponatremia).

Causes

Excessive sodium and/or fluid intake:

❖ IV therapy containing sodium
❖ As a transfusion reaction to a rapid blood transfusion
❖ High intake of sodium

Sodium and water retention:

❖ Heart failure
❖ Liver cirrhosis
❖ Nephrotic syndrome
❖ Corticosteroid therapy
❖ Hyperaldosteronism
❖ Low protein intake

Fluid shift into the intravascular space:

❖ Fluid remobilization after burn treatment
❖ Administration of hypertonic fluids, e.g., mannitol or hypertonic saline solution
❖ Administration of plasma proteins, such as albumin

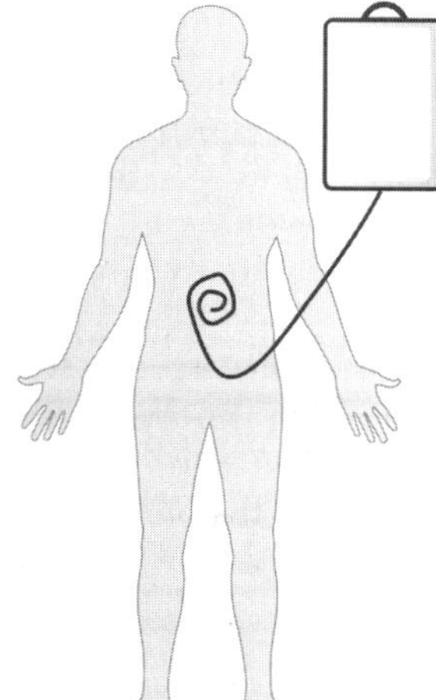

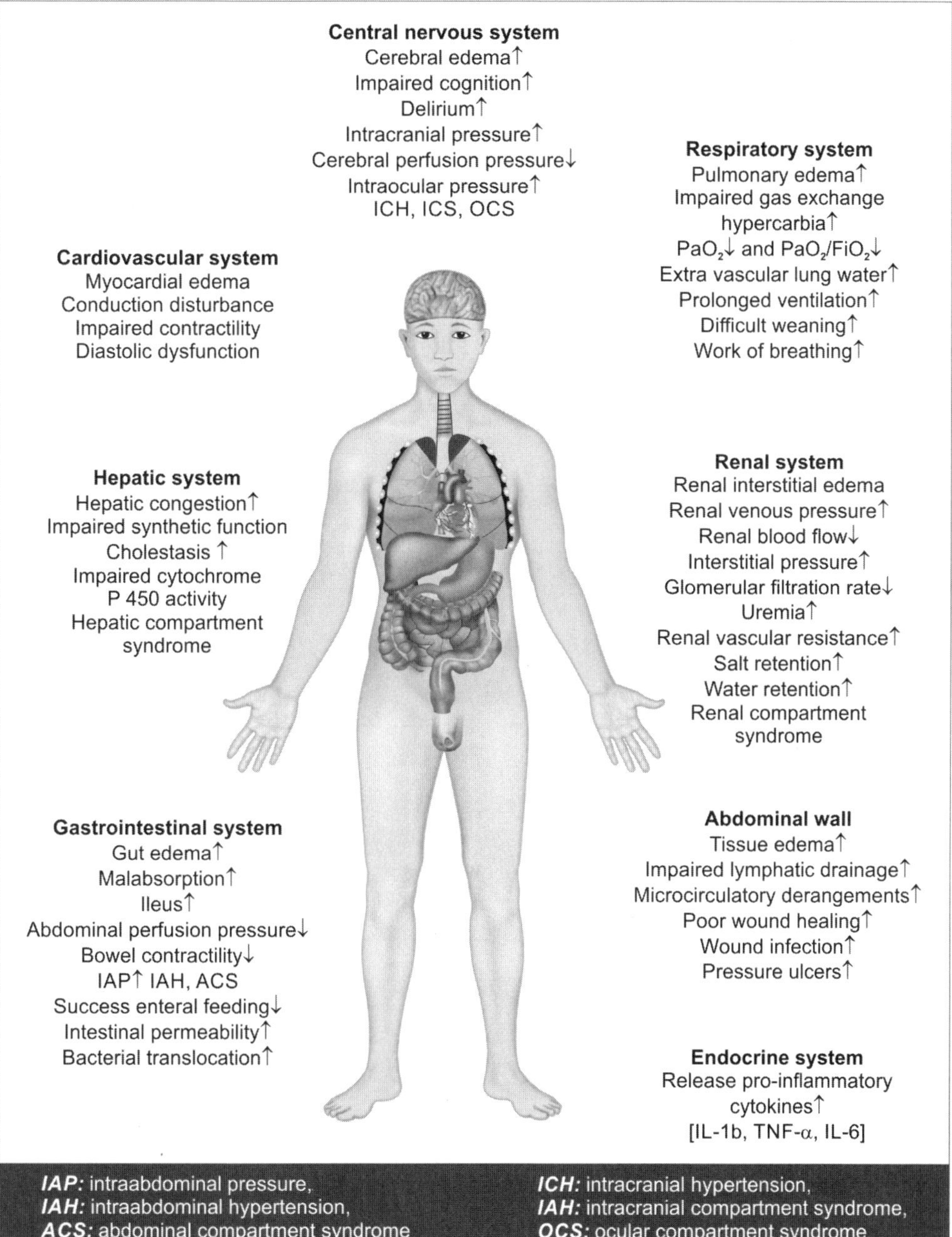

EDEMA

Edema, also spelled oedema, and also known as fluid retention, dropsy, hydropsy and swelling, is the buildup of fluid in the body's tissue.

Mechanism

Six factors can contribute to the formation of edema:
1. Increased hydrostatic pressure;
2. Reduced colloidal or oncotic pressure within blood vessels;
3. Increased tissue colloidal or oncotic pressure;
4. Increased blood vessel wall permeability (such as inflammation);
5. Obstruction of fluid clearance in the lymphatic system;
6. Changes in the water-retaining properties of the tissues themselves. Raised hydrostatic pressure often reflects retention of water and sodium by the kidneys.

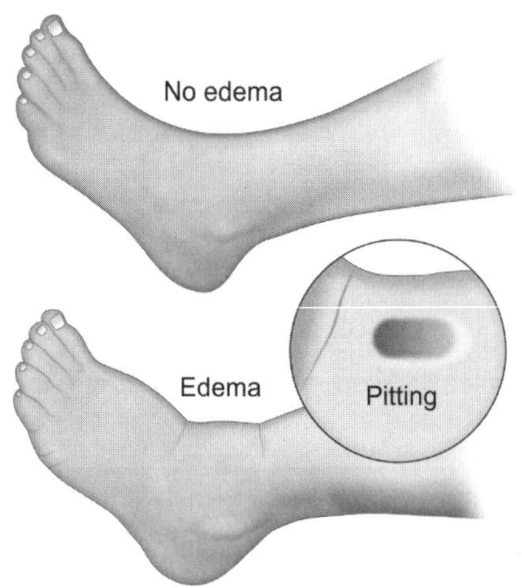

Symptoms

Symptoms depend on the underlying cause, but swelling, tightness, and pain are common.

A person with edema may also notice:
* Swollen, stretched, and shiny skin
* Skin that retains a dimple after a few seconds of pressure
* Puffiness of the ankles, face, or eyes
* Aching body parts and stiff joints
* Weight gain or weight loss
* Decreased urine production
* Fuller hand and neck veins
* Visual anomalies

Types

There are many types of edema. Each one can indicate a range of further health conditions.

Types Include

Peripheral edema: This affects the feet, ankles, legs, hands, and arms. Symptoms include swelling, puffiness, and difficulty moving certain parts of the body.

Pulmonary edema: This occurs when excess fluid collects in the lungs, making breathing difficult. This can result from congestive heart failure or acute lung injury. It is a serious condition, it can be a medical emergency, and it can lead to respiratory failure and death.

Cerebral edema: This occurs in the brain. It can happen for a range of reasons, many of which are potentially life threatening. Symptoms include:
* Headache
* Neck pain or stiffness
* Whole or partial vision loss
* Changes in consciousness or mental state

❖ Nausea
❖ Vomiting
❖ Dizziness

Macular edema: This is a serious complication of diabetic retinopathy. Swelling occurs in the macula, which is the part of the eye that enables detailed, central vision. The person may notice changes to their central vision and how they see colors.

Pitting edema: With this type, which can occur in peripheral edema, pressure applied to the skin leaves an indent or pit in the skin.

Pitting edema can be demonstrated by applying pressure to the swollen area by depressing the skin with a finger. If the pressing causes an indentation that persists for some time after the release of the pressure, the edema is referred to as pitting edema. Any form of pressure, such as from the elastic in socks, can induce pitting with this type of edema. This type of edema may be normal depending on the severity. Almost everyone who wears socks all day will have mild pitting edema by the end of the day.

Grade Pitting Edema

A grading system is often used to determine the severity of the edema on a scale from +1 to +4. It is assessed by applying pressure on the affected area and then measuring the depth of the pit (depression) and how long it lasts (rebound time).

Grade +1: up to 2 mm of depression, rebounding immediately.

Grade +2: 3–4 mm of depression, rebounding in 15 seconds or less.

Grade +3: 5–6 mm of depression, rebounding in 60 seconds.

Grade +4: 8 mm of depression, rebounding in 2–3 minutes.

In nonpitting edema, which usually affects the legs or arms, pressure applied to the skin does not result in a persistent indentation. Nonpitting edema can occur in certain disorders of the lymphatic system such as lymphedema, which is a disturbance of the lymphatic circulation that may occur after a mastectomy, lymph node surgery, radiation therapy, morbid obesity, venous insufficiency, or be present from birth (congenitally).

Another cause of nonpitting let edema is called pretibial myxedema, which is a swelling over the shin that occurs in some people with hypothyroidism. Nonpitting leg edema is difficult to treat. Diuretic medications are generally not effective, although elevation of the legs periodically during the day and compressive devices may reduce the swelling.

Pitting edema measurement scales.		
	S.B. O'Sullivan and T.J. Schmitz **Physical rehabilitation: assessment and treatment**	
1+	Barely detectable impression when finger is pressed into skin	2 mm depression, barely detectable. Immediate rebound
2+	Slight indentation. 15 seconds to rebound	4 mm deep pit. A few seconds to rebound
3+	Deeper indentation. 30 seconds to rebound	6 mm deep pit. 10–12 seconds to rebound
4+	>30 seconds to rebound	8 mm: very deep pit. >20 seconds to rebound

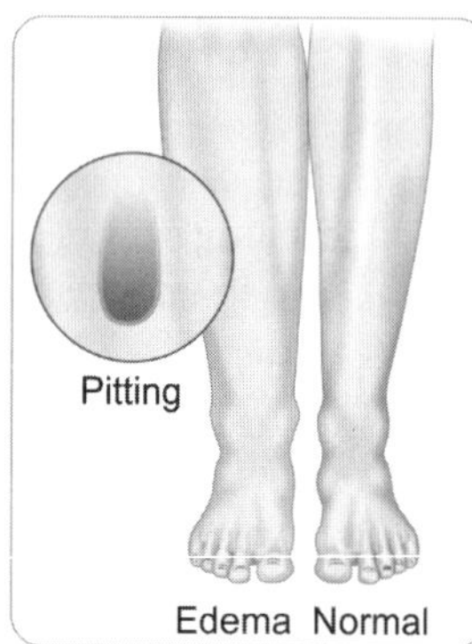

Pitting edema
Indentation in the affected area

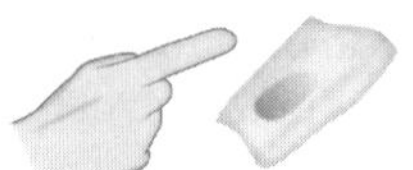

Excess fluid mainly composed of water

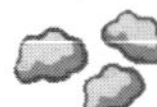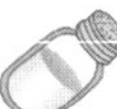

Nonpitting edema
Associated with conditions affecting the thyroid of lymphatic system

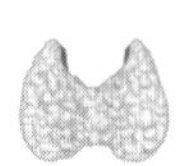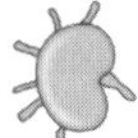

Build-up composed of proteins, salts, and water

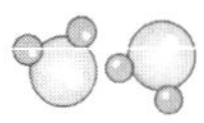

Grading scale

Grade +1
Up to 2 mm of depression, rebounding immediately

Grade +2
3–4 mm of depression, rebounding in 15 seconds or less

Grade +3
5–6 mm of depression, rebounding in 60 seconds

Grade +4
8 mm of depression, rebounding in 2–3 min

Common risk factors

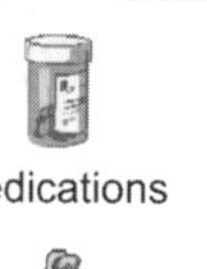
Medications

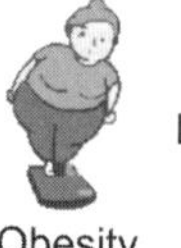
Obesity

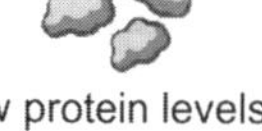
Low protein levels

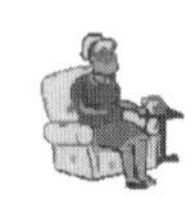
Sitting/Standing in same position too long

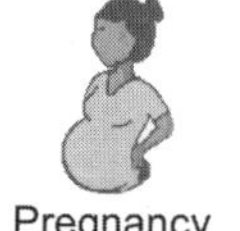
Pregnancy

Treatment
Important to diagnose and treat underlying cause

Mild cases
• Resolve on its own
• Facilitated by elevating affected limb

Severe cases
Diuretic prescribed to help eliminate excess fluid through urine

Chronic cases
Compression socks to promote circulation

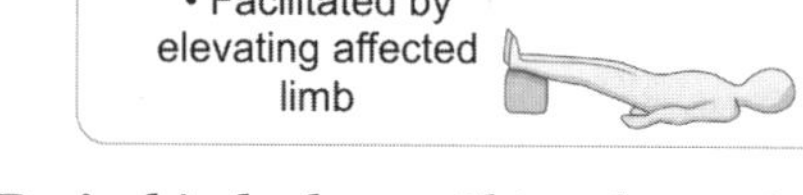

Periorbital edema: This refers to inflammation and puffiness around the eye or eyes. The puffiness is due to fluid buildup and is usually temporary.

Edema can occur in other locations as well, but those mentioned above are the most common.

Edema can indicate one of many serious health conditions. It is important for a person to check with a doctor if they are concerned about any kind of swelling.

Causes

Edema can result from circulatory problems, infection, tissue death, malnutrition, total body fluid overload, and electrolyte problems.

There are many other possible causes of edema, including the following.

Heart Failure

If one or both of the lower chambers of the heart cannot pump blood properly, blood can accumulate in the limbs, causing edema.

Kidney Disease or Kidney Damage

The body of a person with a kidney disorder may not be able to eliminate enough fluid and sodium from the blood. This puts pressure on the blood vessels, which causes some of the liquid to leak out. Swelling can occur around the legs and eyes.

Damage to the glomeruli, which are the capillaries in the kidneys that filter waste and excess fluids from the blood, can result in nephrotic syndrome. One symptom of this is a low level of the protein albumin in the blood. This can lead to edema.

Liver Disease

Cirrhosis affects liver function. It can lead to changes in the secretion of hormones and fluid-regulating chemicals and reduced protein production. This causes fluid to leak out of the blood vessels into surrounding tissue.

Cirrhosis also increases pressure within the portal vein, which is the large vein that carries blood from the intestines, spleen, and pancreas to the liver. Edema can occur in the legs and abdominal cavity.

Certain Medications

Certain medications can also increase the risk of edema these include:

* Vasodilators, which are drugs that open blood vessels
* Calcium channel blockers
* Nonsteroidal anti-inflammatory drugs
* Estrogens
* Some chemotherapy drugs
* Some diabetes drugs, such as thiazolidinediones

Pregnancy

During pregnancy, the body releases hormones that encourage fluid retention and the body to retain more sodium and water than usual. The face, hands, lower limbs, and feet may swell.

When a person is resting in a reclined position during pregnancy, the enlarged uterus can press on a vein known as the inferior vena cava. This can obstruct the femoral veins, leading to edema.

During pregnancy, the blood clots more easily. This can increase the risk of deep vein thrombosis (DVT), which is another potential cause of edema.

Eclampsia, which results from pregnancy-induced hypertension, or high blood pressure, can also cause edema.

Dietary Factors

A number of dietary factors can also affect the risk of edema, such as:

* Consuming too much salt (in people who are susceptible to developing edema)
* Malnutrition, wherein edema can result from low protein levels in the blood
* A low intake of vitamin B1, B6, and B5

Diabetes

Some complications of diabetes include:

- ❖ Cardiovascular disease
- ❖ Acute renal failure
- ❖ Acute liver failure
- ❖ Protein-losing enteropathy, which is an intestinal condition that causes protein loss.
- ❖ These complications, and certain medications for diabetes, can result in edema.
- ❖ Diabetic macular edema is the swelling of the retina in diabetes.

Conditions Affecting the Brain

Some causes of swelling in the brain include:

a. **Head injuries:** A blow to the head may result in an accumulation of fluids in the brain.
b. **Stroke:** A major stroke can result in brain swelling.
c. **Brain tumors:** A brain tumor will accumulate water around itself, especially as it builds new blood vessels.

Allergies

Some foods and insect bites may cause edema of the face or skin in people who have allergies or sensitivities to them. Severe swelling can be a symptom of anaphylaxis.

Swelling in the throat can close a person's airway, so they cannot breathe. This is a medical emergency.

Problems with the Extremities

Some extremity-related causes of edema include:

A blood clot: Any blockage, such as a clot in a vein, can prevent the blood from flowing. As pressure increases in the vein, fluids start to leak into the surrounding tissue, causing edema.

Varicose veins: These usually occur because valves become damaged. Pressure increases in the veins, and they start to bulge. The pressure also increases the risk of fluids leaking into the surrounding tissue.

A cyst, growth, or tumor: Any lump can cause edema if it presses against a lymph duct or vein. As pressure builds up, fluids can leak into the surrounding tissue.

Lymphedema: The lymphatic system helps remove excess fluid from tissues. Any damage to this system—from a surgical procedure, an infection, or a tumor, for example—can result in edema.

Miscellaneous Conditions

Some other possible causes of edema include:

Prolonged immobility: People who are immobile for a long time can develop edema in their skin. This can be due both to fluid pooling in gravity dependent areas and the release of antidiuretic hormone from the pituitary.

High altitude: This, combined with physical exertion, can increase the risk of edema. Acute mountain sickness can lead to high-altitude pulmonary edema or high-altitude cerebral edema.

Burns and sunburn: The skin reacts to burns by retaining fluid. This causes localized swelling.

Infection or inflammation: Any tissue that is infected or inflamed can become swollen. This is usually most noticeable in the skin.

Menstruation and premenstruation: Hormone levels fluctuate during the menstrual cycle. During the days before menstruation, levels of progesterone are lower, and this may cause fluid retention.

Birth control pills: Any medication that contains estrogen can cause fluid retention. It is not uncommon for people to gain weight when they first start using birth control pills.

Menopause: Around menopause, hormone fluctuations can cause fluid retention. Hormone replacement therapy can also trigger edema.

Thyroid disease: Hormonal imbalances associated with thyroid problems can lead to edema.

Complications

Untreated edema can lead to:
* Painful swelling, with pain that gets worse
* Stiffness and difficulty walking
* Stretched, itchy skin
* Infection in the area of swelling
* Scarring between the layers of tissue
* poor blood circulation
* Loss of elasticity in the arteries, veins, and joints
* Ulcerations on the skin

Prevention

Wearing compression stockings can help reduce the swelling and discomfort associated with edema.

Some self-care techniques can help reduce or prevent edema.

These include:
* Reducing salt intake
* Losing weight, if appropriate
* Getting regular exercise
* Raising the legs when possible to improve circulation
* Wearing supporting stockings, which are available to purchase online
* Not sitting or standing still for too long
* Getting up and walking about regularly when traveling
* Avoiding extremes of temperature, such as hot baths, showers, and saunas
* Dressing warmly in cold weather

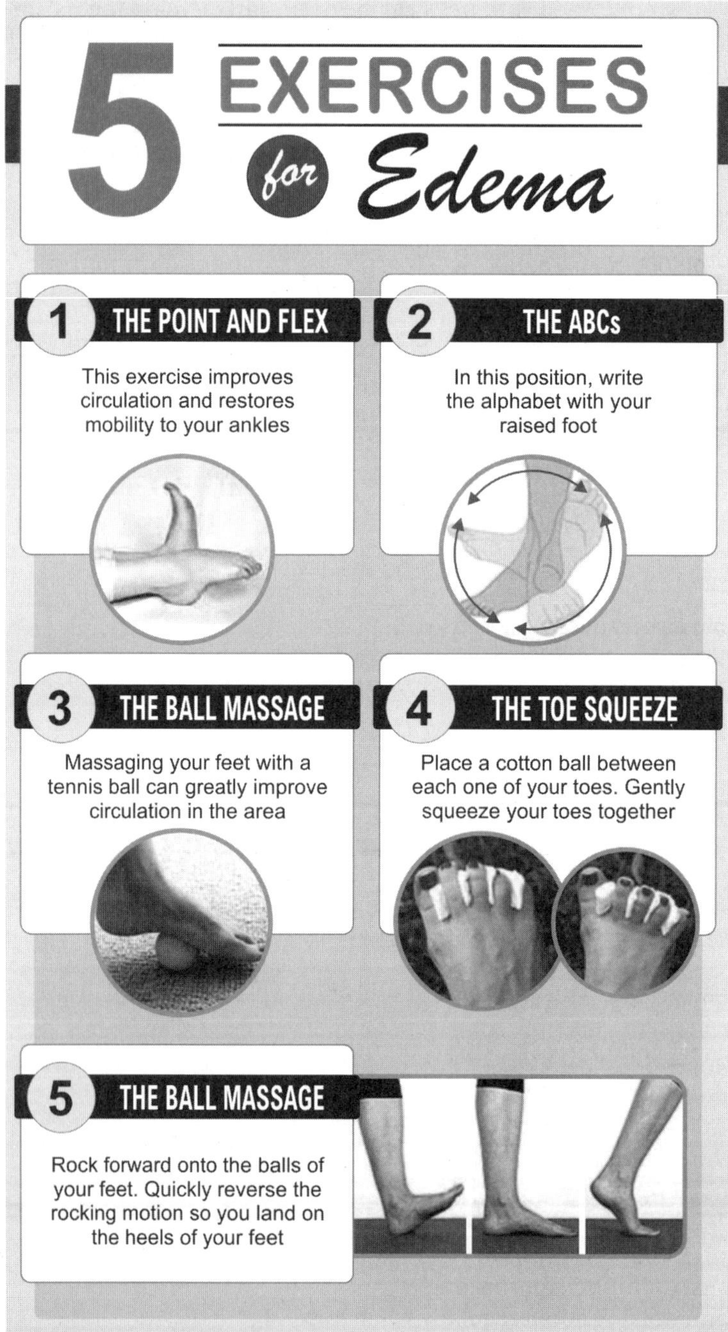

ELECTROLYTES IMBALANCES

❖ **Hyponatremia:** Hyponatremia is a serum sodium level below 135 mEq/L

Etiology:
- Occur when total body water is decreased
- Kidneys inability to excrete sufficiently diluted urine
- Diuresis (increased urine excretion)
- Diuretics
- GI suction
- Excessive perspiration followed by increased water intake.

Clinical manifestation:
- *Gastro intestinal:* Nausea, vomiting, diarrhea, bowel sounds, abdominal cramps.
- *Cardiovascular:* Decrease in diastolic pressure tachycardia, orthostatic hypotension weak pulse.
- *Pulmonary:* Changes in rate of respirations
- *Neurologic:* Headache, lethargy, confusion slowed problem solving, diminished muscle tone on extremities, weakness and tremor.
- *Integumentary:* Dry skin, pale, dry mucous membrane.

Medical management
◊ Determine cause of hyponatremia and to correct it.
◊ Correct body water osmolarity
◊ If client has hyponatremia due to fluid volume excess, intake of fluids will be restricted to allow the sodium to regain balance.
◊ If the serum sodium level falls below 125 mEq/L, sodium replacement is needed.

Pharmacologic management:
◊ For client with moderate hyponatremia 125 mEq/L IV saline solution (0.9% Nacl) or lactated ringers solution may be ordered.
◊ When the serum sodium level is 115 mEq/L or less, a concentrated saline solution such as 3% Nacl is indicated.

Dietary Management:
◊ A balanced diet is usually adequate for mild hyponatremia (126–135 mEq)
   – More severe hyponatremia may require sodium replacement
◊ If the clients have hyponatremia due to excess fluids, a fluid restricted diet may be prescribed.
◊ Fluids may be restricted 800–1000 mL/day.

❖ **Hypernatremia:** Hypernatremia is a serum sodium level over 145 mEq/L

Etiology:
- Diabetes insipidus
- Excess Nacl IV fluid intake
- Accidental or international salt intake
- Hypertonic feedings
- Canned vegetables
- Renal losses

Clinical manifestations:
- *Gastro intestinal:* Anorexia, nausea and vomiting
- *Integumentary:* Dry skin and flushed, mucous membranes dry and sticky, thirst

- *Neurologic:* Restlessness, agitation, irritability, lethargy, coma, tremor, seizures
- *Cardiovascular:* Tachycardia, hypotension or hypertension
- *Renal:* Oliguria

Laboratory findings:

Serum sodium >145 mEq/L

Medical management:

- To decrease total body sodium and replace fluid loss either a hypo-osmolar electrolyte solution (0.2% or 0.45% Nacl) or D5W is administered.
- Hypernatremia caused by sodium excess can be treated with D5W and diuretic such as furosemide.

Dietary management:

- Dietary restrictions on sodium are useful to prevent hypernatremia in high-risk clients.
- Clients with renal disease may need to have their sodium intake restricted to 500–2,000 mg/day.

❖ **Hypokalemia:** Hypokalemia is a serum potassium level of less than 3.5 mEq/L

Causes:

- Diarrhea vomiting, nasogastric suctioning
- Malnutrition, starvation potassium free diet
- Potassium wasting diuretics
- Diabetic acidosis

Clinical Manifestations:

- *Gastro internal:* Anorexia, vomiting, diarrhea.
- *Musculoskeletal:* Muscle weakness, paralysis, leg cramps.
- *Cardiovascular:* Dysrhythmia, vertigo, postural hypotension, flattened T wave.
- *Respiratory:* Shallow respiration shortness of breath.
- *Neurologic:* Fatigue, lethargy, decreased tendon reflexes, confusion.

Laboratory findings: Serum potassium <3.5 mEq/L.

Medical Management

❖ Determining and correcting the cause of the imbalance.
❖ Extreme hypokalemia requires cardiac monitoring.

Pharmacologic Management

❖ Oral potassium replacement therapy is usually prescribed for mild hypokalemia (serum potassium 3.3–3.5 mEq/L)
❖ Potassium is extremely irritating to gastric mucosa, therefore the drug must be taken with Glass of water or juice or during meals.
❖ Potassium chloride can be administered intravenously for moderate or severe hypokalemia and must be diluted in IV fluids.
❖ Administration of potassium by IV push may result in cardiac arrests. Potassium can be given in doses of 10–20 mEq/hour diluted in IV fluid if the client is on heart monitor.
❖ High concentration of potassium is irritating to heart muscle. Thus correcting a potassium deficit may take several days.

Dietary Management

The administration of foods that are high in potassium help to correct the problem as well as prevent further potassium looses. The adult recommended allowance of potassium is 1,875–5,625 mg.

Common sources of food containing potassium—cabbage, carrot, cucumber, mushrooms, spinach, tomato, fruits—banana, guava, orange.

Nursing Diagnosis

- Hypokalemia R/T vomiting, diarrhea, cushings syndrome, or decreased intake.
- Risk for injury R/T muscle weakness and hypotension.
- Altered nutrition less then body requirement R/T insufficient intake of foods rich in potassium.

HYPERKALEMIA

Hyperkalemia is an elevated potassium level over 5.0 mEq/L.

Etiology

- Retention of potassium—renal insufficiency, renal failure, decreased urine output, potassium sparing diuretics.
- Excessive release of cellular potassium—severe traumatic injuries. Severe burns, severe infection, metabolic acidosis.
- Excessive IV infusions or oral administration of potassium.

Clinical Manifestations

- **Cardiovascular:**
  - First tachycardia then bradycardia
  - Electrocardiographic changes
  - Peaked narrow T waves, wide QRS complex, depressed ST segment, widened PR interval.
- **Gastrointestinal:** Nausea, diarrhea, hyperactive bowel sounds.
- **Neuromuscular:** Muscle weakness, muscle cramps, tingling sensation (paresthesia)
- **Renal:** Oliguria and later anuria

Laboratory Findings

- Serum potassium >5.0 mEq/L
- Serum osmolality >295 mOsm/kg
- Serum creatinine >1.5 mg/dL
- BUN >25 mg/dL

Medical Management

- When serum potassium level is 5.0–5.5 mEq/L restriction of dilatory potassium intake.
- If potassium excess is due to metabolic acidosis, correcting the acidosis with sodium bicarbonate promotes potassium uptake into the cells.
- Improving urine output decreases elevated serum potassium level.

* When hyperkalemia is severe, immediate actions are needed to be taken to avoid severe Cardiac disturbances.
* Intravenous calcium gluconate infusions to decrease the antagonistic effect of potassium excess on the myocardium.
* Infusion of insulin and glucose or sodium bicarbonate to promote potassium uptake into the cells.

Nursing Diagnosis

* Hyperkalemia R/T renal dysfunction, shock from traumatic injuries or burns.
* Dysrhythmias R/T hyperkalemia.

Hypocalcemia

Hypocalcemia is a serum calcium below 4.5 mEq/L or 8.5 mg/dL

Etiology

* Inadequate dietary calcium intake, vitamin D deficiency.
* Malabsorption of fat in intestine.
* Metabolic alkalosis (less ionized calcium)
* Renal failure with hyperphosphatemia, acute pancreatitis. Burns, Cushing's disease, hypoparathyroidism.
* Medications—magnesium sulfate.

Clinical Manifestation

* Neuromuscular—tetany symptoms: Twitching around mouth, tingling and numbness of fingers, facial spasm, convulsions.
* Respiratory—dyspnea, laryngeal spasm.
* Gastrointestinal—increased peristalsis, diarrhea.
* Cardiovascular—dysrhythmias, palpitations
* Hematologic—prolonged bleeding time.

Medical Management

* Determining and correcting the cause of hypocalcemia.
* Asymptomatic hypocalcemia is usually corrected with oral calcium gluconate calcium lactate or calcium chloride.
* Administer calcium supplements 30 minutes before meals for better absorption and with glass of milk because vitamin D is necessary for absorption of calcium from the intestine.
* Intravenous calcium chloride or calcium gluconate (10%) is given slowly to avoid hypertension, bradycardia and other arrhythmias.

Dietary Management

* Chronic or mild hypocalcemia can be treated in part by having the client consume a diet high in calcium, e.g., cheese, milk, spinach.
* If hypocalcemia is secondary to parathyroid deficiency the client must avoid high phosphate foods (e.g., milk products, carbonated beverages).

Nursing Diagnosis

❖ Hypocalcemia R/T diarrhea, pancreatitis, renal failure or decrease intake.
❖ Risk for injury R/T increase neuromuscular irritability resulting from hypocalcemia.
❖ Altered healthy maintenance R/T knowledge deficit regarding foods high in calcium.

Hypercalcemia

Hypercalcemia is a serum level over 5.5 mEq/L or 11 mg/L

Etiology

❖ Metastatic malignancy—lung, breast, ovarian, prostatic, bladder, leukemia, kidney
❖ Hyperparathyroidism
❖ Thiazide diuretic therapy
❖ Prolong immobilization
❖ Excessive intake of calcium supplements and vitamin D
  ◆ **Clinical manifestations**
      Gastrointestinal
  ◆ Anorexia, vomiting, constipation, decreased peristalsis
  ◆ Neuromuscular
  ◆ Mild to moderate hypercalcemia-weakness, fatigue, depression, difficulty to concentrate.
  ◆ Severe hypercalcemic state-extreme lethargy, confusion and coma
  ◆ Cardiovascular
  ◆ Dysrhythmias, heart block
  ◆ Electrocardiographic changes
  ◆ Shortened ST segment and lengthened QT interval
  ◆ Renal
  ◆ Polyuria, kidney stones, renal failure
  ◆ Musculoskeletal
  ◆ Bone pain, fracture

Laboratory Findings

❖ Serum calcium >5.5 mEq/L (>11.5 mg/dL)
❖ Arterial blood gasses–PH <7.45
$$HCO_3 > 26 \text{ mEq/L}$$

Medical Management

Treatment consists of correcting the underlying cause.
❖ Intravenous normal saline (0.9% Nacl) given rapidly with furosemide to prevent fluid overload, promote urinary calcium excretion.
❖ Calcitonin decreases serum calcium level by inhibiting the effects of PTH on the osteoclasts and increasing urinary calcium excretion.
❖ Corticosteroid drugs decrease calcium levels by competing with vitamin D thus resulting in decreased intestinal absorption of calcium.
❖ If the cause is excessive use of calcium or vitamin D supplements or calcium containing antacids these agents should be either avoided or used in reduced dosage.

❖ A newer form of drug therapy is etidronate disodium. This drug reduces serum calcium by reducing normal and abnormal bone reabsorption of calcium and secondarily by reducing bone formation.

Dietary Management

Forcing fluids will assist in adequately hydrating the client and flushing excess calcium through the kidney.

❖ Nursing diagnosis
❖ Hypercalcemia R/T metastatic lesions hyper parathyroidism
❖ Thiazide therapy or increased intake of calcium
❖ Health maintenance altered R/T excessive ingestion of calcium supplements and calcium-containing antacids.
❖ Risk for injury R/T potential pathologic fractures, mental confusion and immobility.

ARTERIAL BLOOD GAS

Arterial blood gas (ABG) sampling is a test often performed in an inpatient setting to assess the acid-base status of a patient. A needle is used to draw blood from an artery, often the radial, and the blood is analyzed to determine parameters such as the pH, pCO_2, pO_2, HCO_3, oxygen saturation, and more. This allows the physician to understand the status of the patient better. ABGs are especially important in the critically ill. They are the main tool utilized in adjusting to the needs of a patient on a ventilator. The following are the most important normal values on an ABG:

❖ pH = 7.35–7.45
❖ pCO_2 = 35–45 mm Hg
❖ pO_2 = 75–100 mm Hg
❖ HCO_3^- = 22–26 mEq/L
❖ O_2 Sat = greater than 95%

The ability to quickly and efficiently read an ABG, especially in reference to inpatient medicine, is paramount to quality patient care.

❖ Look at the pH
❖ Decide whether it is acidotic, alkalotic, or within the physiological range
❖ $PaCO_2$ level determines respiratory contribution; a high level means the respiratory system is lowering the pH and vice versa.
❖ HCO_3^- level denotes metabolic/kidney effect. An elevated HCO_3^- is raising the pH and vice versa.
❖ If the pH is acidotic, look for the number that corresponds with a lower pH. If it is a respiratory acidosis, the CO_2 should be high. If the patient is compensating metabolically, the HCO_3^- should be high as well. A metabolic acidosis will be depicted with an HCO_3^- that is low.
❖ If the pH is alkalotic, again, determine which value is causing this. A respiratory alkalosis will mean the CO_2 is low; a metabolic alkalosis should lend an HCO_3^- that is high. Compensation with either system will be reflected oppositely; for a respiratory alkalosis the metabolic response should be a low HCO_3^- and for metabolic alkalosis, the respiratory response should be a high CO_2.
❖ If the pH level is in the physiological range but the $PaCO_2$ and/or bicarb are not within normal limits, there is likely a mixed disorder. Also, compensation does not always occur; this is when clinical information becomes paramount.
❖ Sometimes it is difficult to ascertain whether a patient has a mixed disorder.

Increased Anion Gap Metabolic Acidosis

A primary metabolic acidosis, that is, one which is the primary acid-base disorder, has many causes. These are separated into those which cause a high anion gap and those that do not. The plasma anion gap is a way to help clinicians determine the cause of a metabolic acidosis. When there is a metabolic acidosis present, certain ions in the blood are measured that help determine the etiology of an acidemia. The anion gap increases whenever bicarbonate is lost due to it combining with a hydrogen ion that was previously attached to a conjugate base. When bicarbonate combines with a hydrogen ion, the result is carbonic acid (H_2CO_3). The conjugate base can be any negatively charged ion that is not a bicarbonate or a chloride.

The formula for anion gap is:
$[Na]^-([Cl]^+[HCO_3])$

Humans are electrically neutral, but all cations and anions are not being measured. The normal anion gap is equal to 8 +/– 4. Most of this number is due to albumin; this anion is not accounted for in the formula which is a large reason why the gap is not closer to zero. Albumin is normally 4 mg/dL. Because of the large effect of albumin on anion gap, if a patient's albumin level is abnormal, their expected anion gap will not be accurate. This can be corrected using simple math. The normal anion gap and albumin level differ by a factor of three (normal anion gap of 12, normal albumin of 4 mg/dL). If a patient has an anion gap of 24, that means there are 12 units of the conjugate base present that normally would not be due to the combination of hydrogen ions with bicarbonate. If this same patient has an albumin level of 3 mg/dL, their expected anion gap should actually be about 9. This means that, rather than 12 units of the conjugate base present, there are really 15 units.

A more complex method of analyzing ion contribution to pH alterations is the strong ion difference/strong ion gap. This method emphasizes the effect of other ions on acid-base balance and is useful for learning about acid-base balance. However, this approach is more burdensome than the standard anion gap and involves more calculations. Many therefore believe that its use in clinical practice is limited.

The mnemonic MUDPILES has classically been used about the causes of high anion gap metabolic acidosis. MUDPILES stands for methanol, uremia, diabetic ketoacidosis, paraldehyde, infection, lactic acidosis, ethylene glycol, and salicylates. A new mnemonic, GOLDMARK, has been suggested to be an improvement. GOLDMARK is an anagram for glycols (ethylene and propylene), oxoproline, lactate, methanol, aspirin, renal failure, and ketones. If a patient has an anion gap over 12, these mnemonics are helpful to remember the possible causes of the disorder.

Narrow Anion Gap Metabolic Acidosis

If the acidosis involves a normal anion gap, there is a loss of bicarbonate rather than an increased amount of hydrogen ions, with a concomitant increase in chloride ions. To keep a physiological neutral state, chloride ions migrate out of the cells and into the extracellular space. This causes the patient's serum chloride to increase and keeps the anion gap at a normal level. This means that a metabolic acidosis without an abnormal anion gap is also a hyperchloremic metabolic acidosis. A metabolic acidosis without an increased anion gap results from many processes including severe diarrhea, type 1 renal tubular acidosis (RTA), long-term use of carbonic anhydrase inhibitors, and suctioning of gastric contents. When a patient has a narrow ion gap hyperchloremic acidosis, the provider can calculate the urine anion gap (UAG) to help determine etiology.

The following is the equation for urine anion gap where Na is sodium, K is potassium, and Cl is chloride:

$(Na + K) - Cl$

The renal system attempts to ameliorate the effects of pathological metabolic acidosis by excreting ammonium (NH_4^+) into the urine. A UAG between 20–90 mEq/L denotes low or normal $NH4^+$ secretion. One between –20 mEq/L and –50 mEq/L suggests the main cause of the metabolic acidosis is prolonged severe diarrhea.

Another important formula to use with metabolic acidosis is the Winter formula. This equation provides the clinician with the expected pCO_2 value. This is important because there could be another acid-base disorder present.

The winter formula is:

Expected $pCO_2 = (1.5 \times HCO_3) + 8 +/- 2$

If the pCO_2 value is within range of the expected pCO_2, there is no mixed disorder, just respiratory compensation. When the value is lower or higher than expected, there is a mixed disorder; lower would mean a respiratory alkalosis and higher a respiratory acidosis. A shortcut for the Winter formula is that the last two digits of the pH +/– 2 is about equal to the expected pCO_2.

Respiratory Acidosis

During exhalation, carbon dioxide produced by cellular respiration is projected into the environment. In the human body, carbon dioxide combines with water via carbonic anhydrase and forms carbonic acid which dissociates into a hydrogen ion and bicarbonate. This is why a reduced respiratory rate will lead to a decreased pH; the more carbon dioxide is exhaled, the less carbon dioxide present for this reaction.

Respiratory acidosis as a primary disorder is often caused by hypoventilation. This can be due to multiple causes including chronic obstructive pulmonary disease, opiate abuse/overdose, severe obesity, and brain injury. When respiratory acidosis occurs, the metabolic response should be to increase the amount of bicarbonate via the renal system. This does not always occur, and renal pathology can easily hinder the appropriate physiological response, leading to increased danger for the patient.

Metabolic Alkalosis

Metabolic alkalosis also can be divided into two main categories that help ascertain the cause: chloride responsive vs. nonchloride responsive. In nonchloride-responsive metabolic alkalosis, the urine chloride is <20 mEq/L. Some causes include vomiting, hypovolemia, and diuretic use.

Respiratory Alkalosis

Any pathology that leads to the increased expiration of carbon dioxide can result in respiratory alkalosis. When excess CO_2 is expired, the pH of the human body is increased due to less carbonic acid being created. Physiologically, the appropriate compensation is a decreased amount of bicarbonate being created by the renal system. Some causes of respiratory alkalosis include panic attacks with hyperventilation, pulmonary embolism, pneumonia, and salicylate intoxication.

IV THERAPY

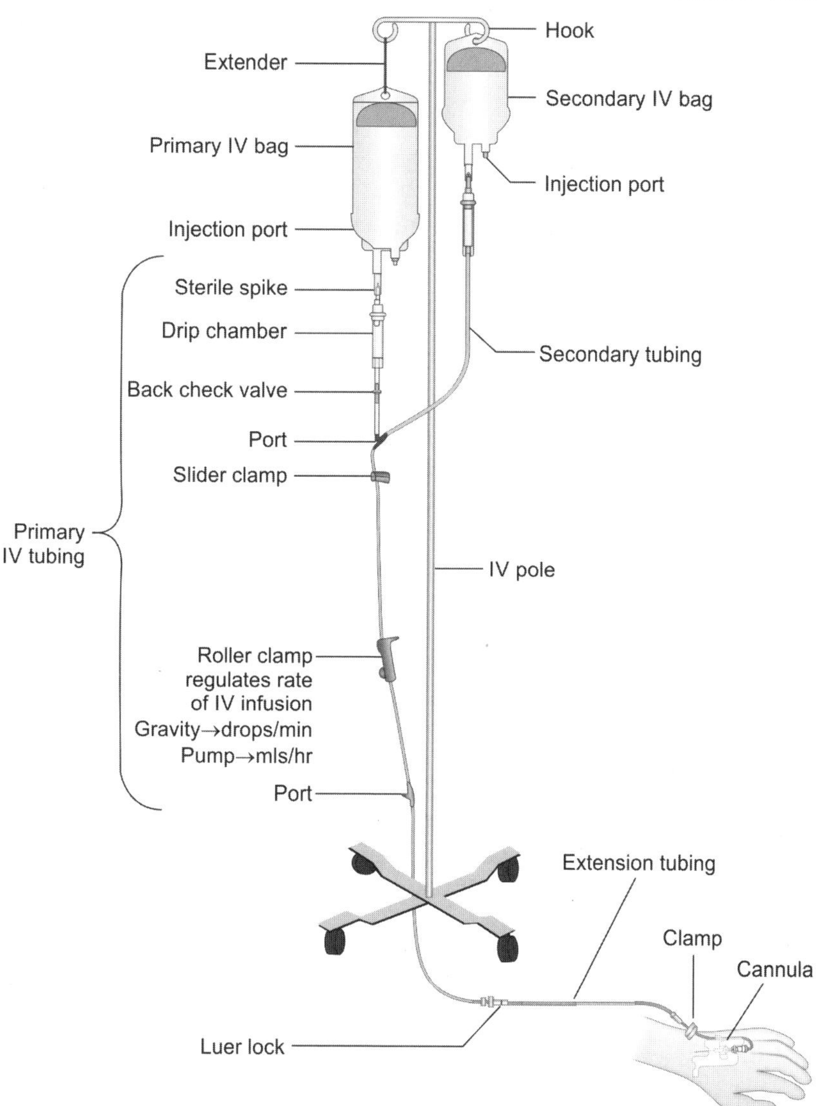

INTRAVENOUS ADMINISTRATION EQUIPMENT

When a peripheral vein has a cannula inserted, extension tubing is connected to the hub on the cannula and flushed with normal saline to maintain patency of the cannula. Most peripheral intravenous cannulas will have extension tubing, a short, 20 cm tube with a positive fluid displacement/positive pressure cap attached to the hub of the cannula for ease of access and to decrease manipulation of the catheter hub (Vancouver Coastal Health, 2008). The extension tubing must be changed each time the peripheral catheter is changed. When the peripheral cannula is not in use, the extension tubing attached to the cannula is called a saline lock.

Intravenous fluids are administered through thin, flexible plastic tubing called an infusion set or primary infusion tubing/administration set (Perry et al., 2014). The infusion tubing/administration set connects to the bag of IV solution. Primary IV tubing is either a macro-drip solution administration set that delivers 10, 15, or 20 gtts/mL, or a micro-drip set that delivers 60 drops/mL. Macro-drip sets are used for routine primary infusions. Micro-drip IV tubing is used mostly in pediatric or neonatal care, when small amounts of fluids are to be administered over a long period of time (Perry et al., 2014). The drop factor can be located on the packaging of the IV tubing.

Primary IV tubing is used to infuse continuous or intermittent fluids or medication. It consists of the following parts:

Backcheck valve: Prevents fluid or medication from travelling up the IV

Access ports: Used to infuse secondary medications and give IV push medications

Roller clamp: Used to regulate the speed of, or to stop or start, a gravity infusion

Secondary IV tubing: Shorter in length than primary tubing, with no access ports or backcheck valve; when connected to a primary line via an access port, used to infuse intermittent medications or fluids. A secondary tubing administration set is used for secondary IV medication.

IV solution bags should have the date, time, and initials of the health care provider marked on them to be valid. Add-on devices (e.g., extension tubing or dead-enders) should be changed every 96 hours, if contaminated when administration set is replaced, or as per agency policy. Intravenous solution and IV tubing should be changed if:

❖ IV tubing is disconnected or becomes contaminated by touching a nonsterile surface
❖ Less than 100 mL is left in the IV solution bag
❖ Cloudiness or precipitate is found in the IV solution
❖ Equipment (date and time) is outdated
❖ IV solution is outdated (24 hours since opened)
❖ Primary and secondary administration sets should be changed regularly to minimize risk and prevent infection (CDC, 2011; Fraser Health Authority, 2014). Change IV tubing according to agency policy.

Frequency of IV tubing changes	
safety considerations: All IV tubing must be changed using sterile technique. IV tubing is changed based on the type of tubing, time used, and the type of solution. If possible, coordinate IV tubing changes with IV solution changes.	
Frequency of IV tubing change	*Type of IV tubing and solution*
Every 72–96 hours	Primary tubing with hypotonic, isotonic, or hypertonic continuous solution, when insertion site is changed, or when indicated by the type of solution or medication being administered
Every 24 hours	Secondary or intermittent IV solution or medication. Rationale: When an intermittent infusion is repeatedly disconnected and reconnected for infusion, there is increased risk of contamination at the catheter hub, needleless connector, and the male Luer end of the administration set, potentially increasing risk for CR-BSI

Contd...

Contd...

Every 24 hours	Infusions containing fat emulsions (IV solutions combined with glucose and amino acids infused separately or in a 3 in 1 admixture). Example: Total parenteral nutrition (TPN)
4 hours or 4 units, whichever comes first, or between products	Blood and blood products

INFUSING IV FLUIDS BY GRAVITY OR AN ELECTRONIC INFUSION DEVICES (EID)

To ensure therapeutic effectiveness of IV fluids, a constant, even flow is necessary to prevent complications from too much or too little fluid. A physician must order a rate of infusion for IV fluids or for medications. The rate of infusion for medications (given via a secondary or primary infusion) can be found in the parenteral drug therapy manual (PDTM). If an order for IV fluids is "to keep vein open" (TKVO), the minimum flow rate is 20–50 mL per hour, or according to physician's orders.

A health care provider is responsible for regulating and monitoring the amount of IV fluids being infused. IV fluid rates are regulated in one of two ways:

Gravity: The health care provider regulates the infusion rate by using a clamp on the IV tubing, which can either speed up or slow down the flow of IV fluids. An IV flow rate for gravity is calculated in gtts/min.

Electronic infusion device: The infusion rate is regulated by an electronic pump to deliver the fluids at the correct rate and volume. All IV pumps regulate the rate of fluids in mL/hr. An IV pump (EID) is used for many types of patients, solutions, and medications.

❖ An IV pump must be used for:
❖ All CVC devices
❖ All opioid infusions (use a patient-controlled analgesia)
❖ All pediatric patients
❖ All medication as described in the PDTM
❖ Infusion rates below 60 mL/hr

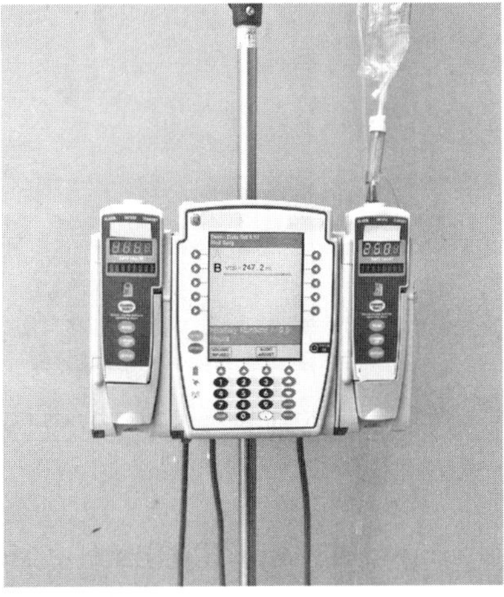

Electronic infusion device (EID).

To calculate the drops per minute for an infusion by gravity, follow the steps in below Table.

Calculating the drops per minute (gtts/min) for an infusion by gravity.	
Steps	**Additional information**
1. Verify the physician order	An order may read: Example 1. Give NS IV 125 mL/hr Example 2. Give 1,000 mL of NS IV over 8 hours
2. Determine the drop factor on the IV administration set	The drop factor is the amount of drops (gtts) per minute. IV tubing is either macro tubing (10, 15, or 20 gtts/min) or micro tubing (60 gtts/min). The drop factor (or calibration of the tubing) is always on the packaging of the IV tubing
3. Complete the calculation using the formula	Use the formula: $$\frac{\text{Infusion rate (mL/hr)} \times \text{IV drop factor (gtts/min)}}{60 \text{ (Administration time is always in minutes)}} = \text{drops per minute}$$ To calculate mL/hr, divide $1{,}000 \div 8 = 125$ mL/hr Example: Infuse IV NS at 125 mL/hr. IV tubing drop factor is 20 gtts/min $$\frac{125 \times 20}{60} = 41.6 \text{ gtts/min, round up to 42 gtts/min (Round down or up to the nearest whole number)}$$
4. Regulate IV infusion using the roller clamp	Observe and count the drips in the drip chamber and regulate for 42 gtts/min (one full minute). Alternatively, divide 42 by 4 (rounded down from 10.4 to 10 gtts/min) to count for 15 seconds. The gtts/min should be assessed regularly to ensure the IV is infusing at the correct rate (e.g., every 1 to 2 hours, if the patient accidentally bumps the IV tubing, or if a patient returns from another department) Regulate IV tubing by using a roller clamp.

Assessing an IV System

All patients with IV fluid therapy (PIV and CVC) are at risk for developing IV-related complications. The assessment of an IV system (including the IV site, tubing, rate, and solution) often depends on what is being infused, the patient's age and medical condition, type of IV therapy (PIV or CVC), and agency policy.

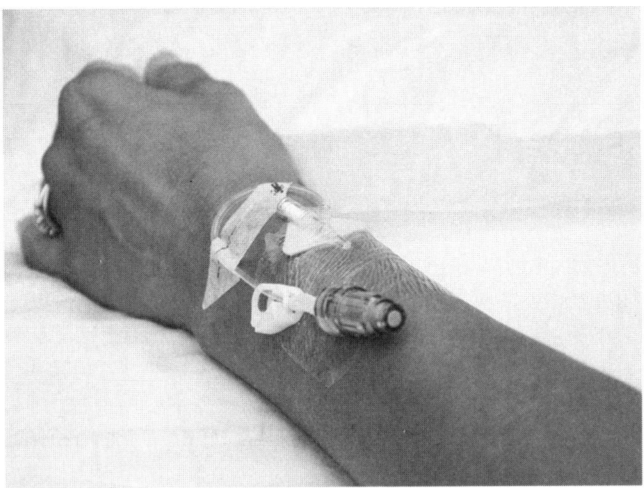

Assess IV site prior to use.

Checklist: Assessing an IV system.
Disclaimer: Always review and follow your hospital policy regarding this specific skill
Safety considerations: • IV systems must be assessed every 1–2 hours or more frequently if required • An IV system should be assessed at the beginning of a shift, at the end of a shift, if the electronic infusion device alarms or sounds, or if a patient complains of pain, tenderness, or discomfort at the IV insertion site • Review the patient's chart to determine insertion date and type of solution ordered • A peripherally inserted catheter is usually replaced every 72–96 hours, depending on agency policy • If the peripheral catheter or central venous catheter is not in use, or is being used intermittently, flushing is required to keep the site patent. Refer to agency policy for flushing guidelines • A not-in-use peripheral IV site is generally flushed every 12 hours with 3–5 mL of normal saline • Review the in-and-out sheet to determine expected amount in the IV solution bag • Patients with cardiac or renal disease, as well as pediatric patients, are at a higher risk for IV-related complications • Elderly patients often have fragile veins and may require closer monitoring

Steps	*Additional Information*
1. Perform hand hygiene	This step reduces the transmission of microorganisms
2. Introduce yourself and explain the purpose of the assessment	This builds trust with patient and allows time for the patient to ask questions
3. Confirm patient ID using two patient identifiers (e.g., name and date of birth), and compare the MAR printout with the patient's wristband	This step ensures you have the correct patient and complies with agency standard for patient identification

Contd...

Contd...

Steps	Additional information
	Compare MAR with patient wristband
4. Apply nonsterile gloves (optional)	This reduces the transmission of microorganisms
5. Assess the IV insertion site and transparent dressing on IV site	Check IV insertion site for signs and symptoms of phlebitis or infection. Check for fluid leaking, redness, pain, tenderness, and swelling. IV site should be free from pain, tenderness, redness, or swelling Ensure patient is informed to alert the health care provider if they experience pain or notice swelling or redness at the IV site. If patient is unable to report pain at IV site, more frequent checks are required
6. Inspect the patient's arm for streaking or venous cords; assess skin temperature	Assess complications on hand and arm for signs and symptoms of phlebitis and infiltration/extravasation
7. Assess IV tubing for kinks or bends	Kinks or bends in tubing may decrease or stop the flow of IV fluids. Ensure tubing is not caught on equipment or side rails on bed Tubing should be properly labeled with date and time
8. Check the rate of infusion on the primary and secondary IV tubing. Verify infusion rate in physician orders or medication administration record (MAR)	If IV solution is on gravity, calculate and count the drip rate for one minute If solution is on an IV pump, ensure the rate is correct and all clamps are open as per agency protocol If secondary IV medication is infusing, ensure clamp on secondary IV tubing is open. The EID is unable to distinguish if the primary bag or secondary bag is infusing
9. Assess the type of solution and label it on bag. Check volume of solution in bag	IV solutions become outdated every 24 hours Ensure the correct solution is given If 100 mL of solution or less is left in the bag, change the IV solution and document on in-and-out sheet If an IV pump is used, ensure it is plugged into an outlet Ideally, the IV solution should be 90 cm above patient heart level

Contd...

Contd...

Steps	**Additional information**
10. Assist patient into comfortable position, place call bell in reach, and put up side rails on bed as per agency policy	These precautions prevent injury to the patient
11. Perform hand hygiene	This step prevents the spread of microorganisms
12. Document procedure and findings as per agency policy	Timely and accurate documentation promotes patient safety

INTRAVENOUS SOLUTIONS

When patients experience deficient fluid volume, intravenous (IV) fluids are often prescribed. IV fluid restores fluid to the intravascular compartment, and some IV fluids are also used to facilitate the movement of fluid between compartments due to osmosis. There are three types of IV fluids.

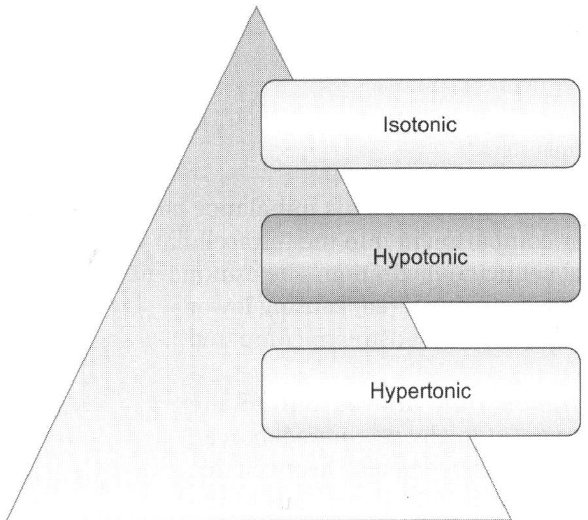

Isotonic Solutions

Isotonic solutions are IV fluids that have a similar concentration of dissolved particles as blood. An example of an isotonic IV solution is 0.9% normal saline (0.9% NaCl). Because the concentration of the IV fluid is similar to the blood, the fluid stays in the intravascular space and osmosis does not cause fluid movement between compartments. Isotonic solutions are used for patients with fluid volume deficit (also called hypovolemia) to raise their blood pressure. However, infusion of too much isotonic fluid can cause excessive fluid volume (See Figure on next page).

Hypotonic Solutions

Hypotonic solutions have a lower concentration of dissolved solutes than blood. An example of a hypotonic IV solution is 0.45% normal saline (0.45% NaCl). When hypotonic IV solutions are infused, it results in a decreased concentration of dissolved solutes in the blood as

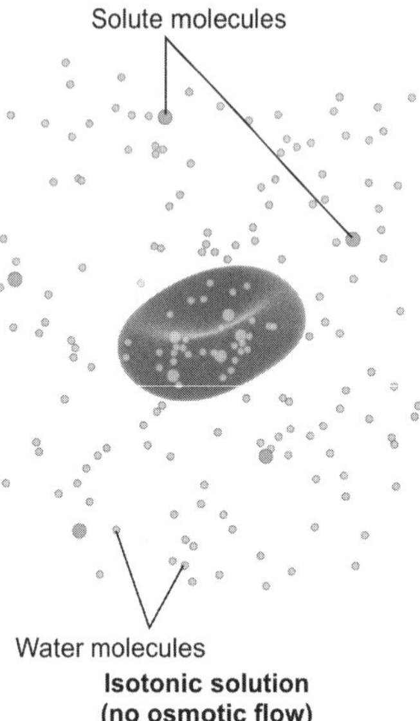

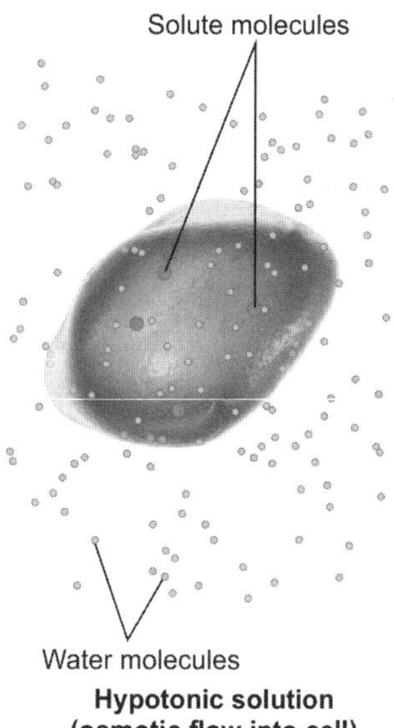

**Isotonic solution
(no osmotic flow)**

Lack of fluid movement when isotonic IV
solution is administered.

**Hypotonic solution
(osmotic flow into cell)**

Hypotonic IV solution causing osmotic
movement of fluid into cell.

compared to the intracellular space. This imbalance causes osmotic movement of water from the intravascular compartment into the intracellular space. For this reason, hypotonic fluids are used to treat cellular dehydration. The osmotic movement of fluid into a cell when a hypotonic IV solution is administered, causing lower concentration of solutes in the bloodstream compared to within the cell.

However, if too much fluid moves out of the intravascular compartment into cells, cerebral edema can occur. It is also possible to cause worsening hypovolemia and hypotension if too much fluid moves out of the intravascular space and into the cells. Therefore, patient status should be monitored carefully when hypotonic solutions are infused.

Hypertonic Solutions

Hypertonic solutions have a higher concentration of dissolved particles than blood. An example of hypertonic IV solution is 3% normal saline (3% NaCl). When infused, hypertonic fluids cause an increased concentration of dissolved solutes in the intravascular space compared to the cells. This causes the osmotic movement of water out of the cells and into the intravascular space to dilute the solutes in the blood. Osmotic movement of fluid out of a cell when

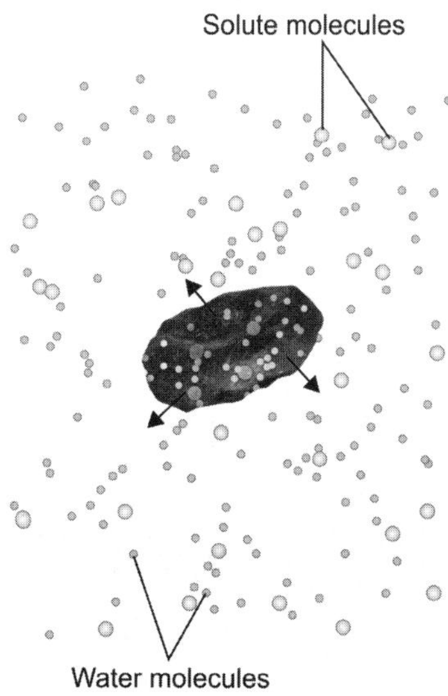

**Hypertonic solution
(osmotic flow out of cell)**

Hypertonic IV solution causing osmotic
fluid movement out of a cell.

hypertonic IV fluid is administered due to a higher concentration of solutes (pink molecules) in the bloodstream compared to the cell.

When administering hypertonic fluids, it is essential to monitor for signs of hypervolemia such as breathing difficulties and elevated blood pressure. Additionally, if hypertonic solutions with sodium are given, the patient's serum sodium level should be closely monitored. See below Table for a comparison of types of IV solutions, their uses, and nursing considerations.

See Figure on next page for an illustration comparing how different types of IV solutions affect red blood cell size.

Comparison of IV solutions.			
Type	**IV solution**	**Uses**	**Nursing considerations**
Isotonic	0.9% normal saline (0.9% NaCl)	Fluid resuscitation for hemorrhaging, severe vomiting, diarrhea, GI suctioning losses, wound drainage, mild hyponatremia, or blood transfusions	Monitor closely for hypervolemia, especially with heart failure or renal failure
Isotonic	Lactated Ringer's solution (LR)	Fluid resuscitation, GI tract fluid losses, burns, traumas, or metabolic acidosis. Often used during surgery	Should not be used if serum pH is greater than 7.5 because it will worsen alkalosis. May elevate potassium levels if used with renal failure
Isotonic	5% dextrose in water (D5W) *starts as isotonic and then changes to hypotonic when dextrose is metabolized	Provides free water to help renal excretion of solutes, hypernatremia, and some dextrose supplementation	Should not be used for fluid resuscitation because after dextrose is metabolized, it becomes hypotonic and leaves the intravascular space, causing brain swelling. Used to dilute plasma electrolyte concentrations
Hypotonic	0.45% sodium chloride (0.45% NaCl)	Used to treat intracellular dehydration and hypernatremia and to provide fluid for renal excretion of solutes	Monitor closely for hypovolemia, hypotension, or confusion due to fluid shifting into the intracellular space, which can be life-threatening. Avoid use in patients with liver disease, trauma, and burns to prevent hypovolemia from worsening. Monitor closely for cerebral edema
Hypotonic	5% dextrose in water (D5W)	Provides free water to promote renal excretion of solutes and treat hypernatremia, as well as some dextrose supplementation	Monitor closely for hypovolemia, hypotension, or confusion due to fluid shifting out of the intravascular space, which can be life-threatening. Avoid use in patients with liver disease, trauma, and burns to prevent hypovolemia from worsening. Monitor closely for cerebral edema

Contd...

Contd...

Type	IV Solution	Uses	Nursing Considerations
Hypertonic	3% sodium chloride (3% NaCl)	Used to treat severe hyponatremia and cerebral edema	Monitor closely for hypervolemia, hypernatremia, and associated respiratory distress. Do not use it with patients experiencing heart failure, renal failure, or conditions caused by cellular dehydration because it will worsen these conditions
Hypertonic	5% dextrose and 0.45% sodium chloride (D50.45% NaCl)	Used to treat severe hyponatremia and cerebral edema	Monitor closely for hypervolemia, hypernatremia, and associated respiratory distress. Do not use it with patients experiencing heart failure, renal failure, or conditions caused by cellular dehydration because it will worsen these conditions
Hypertonic	5% dextrose and lactated Ringer's (D5LR) D10	Used to treat severe hyponatremia and cerebral edema	Monitor closely for hypervolemia, hypernatremia, and associated respiratory distress. Do not use it with patients experiencing heart failure, renal failure, or conditions caused by cellular dehydration because it will worsen these conditions

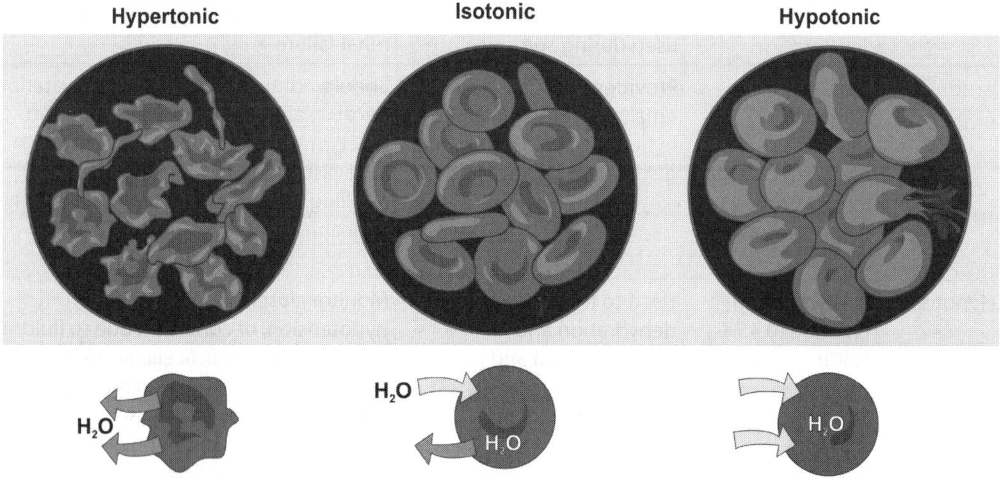

Comparison of osmotic effects of hypertonic, isotonic, and hypotonic IV fluids on red blood cells.

Osmolarity

Osmolarity is defined as the proportion of dissolved particles in an amount of fluid and is generally the term used to describe body fluids. As the dissolved particles become more concentrated, the osmolarity increases. Osmolality refers to the proportion of dissolved particles in a specific weight of fluid. The terms osmolarity and osmolality are often used interchangeably in clinical practice.

Osmolarity: The concentration of solutes per unit volume of solvent (mOsm/L); often used interchangeably with osmolality in clinical practice. It is the preferred term to describe the osmotic pressure of parenteral fluids as it takes into account all osmotically active particles, including those that enter cells (e.g., glucose, urea).

Tonicity: The capacity of extracellular fluid to create an osmotic gradient that will cause water to move into or out of the intracellular compartment; cannot be measured and has no units. It reflects the osmotic effect of particles that cannot easily pass cell membranes, i.e., the effective osmotic pressure gradient.

Osmolarity vs Tonicity		
Solution	**Osmolarity**	**Tonicity**
Isoosmolar	Equivalent to the intracellular compartment	Can be isotonic or hypotonic
Hyperosmolar	Higher than the intracellular compartment	Can be hypertonic, isotonic or hypotonic
Hypoosmolar	Lower than the intracellular compartment	Can only be hypotonic

PERIPHERAL PUNCTURE SITES

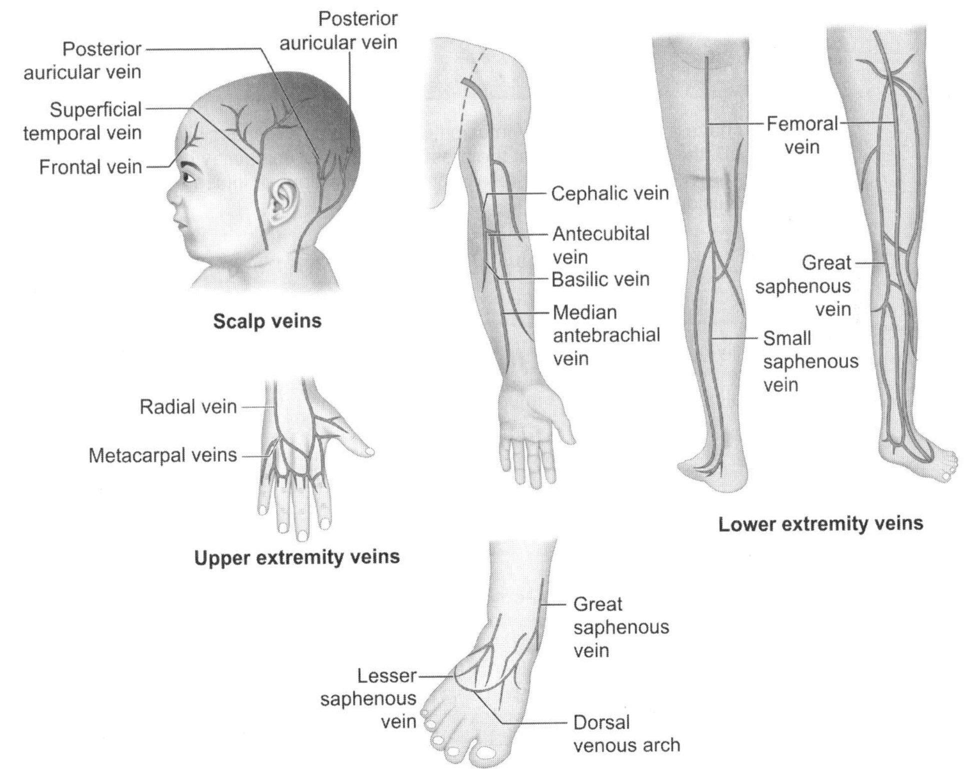

CALCULATION FOR IV FLUID PLAN

An addition to the baseline fluid requirements for adults, sometimes additional replacement fluid is needed to quickly replace lost fluid volume (hypovolemia) and restore proper fluid balance. This is most commonly seen in dehydration due to a gut problem such as vomiting or diarrhea. Blood loss, as from an injury, is another common cause. For patients with substantial blood loss, the priority will be to stop the bleeding and replace the loss with a blood transfusion, but IV fluid replacement often has a role in treatment, as well.

When a patient needs fluid replacement, there are two primary routes of administration: oral and intravenous (IV). As a simple guideline: if the gut works, use it! When it can be given safely and well-tolerated, oral rehydration is just as effective and may be safer and more comfortable for the patient. Particularly in cases of diarrhea, oral rehydration is strongly recommended. The correct solution for oral rehydration will include glucose, which helps with the absorption of fluid and electrolytes, but not a high amount of sugar, as is often included in sports drinks. Recipes for adding sugar and electrolytes to drinking water are available from the World Health Organization. These simple treatments are often lifesaving.

Many patients cannot tolerate oral rehydration, and guidelines indicate a need for IV fluid replacement. These would include individuals with diagnoses such as vomiting, bowel obstruction, and coma. Patients who cannot sit up, cannot swallow safely, cannot stop vomiting, or may have surgery soon may not be allowed to have anything by mouth. This is often designated NPO, which stands for the Latin nil per os, or NBM, meaning "nothing by mouth." These patients will all require intravenous fluid (IVF).

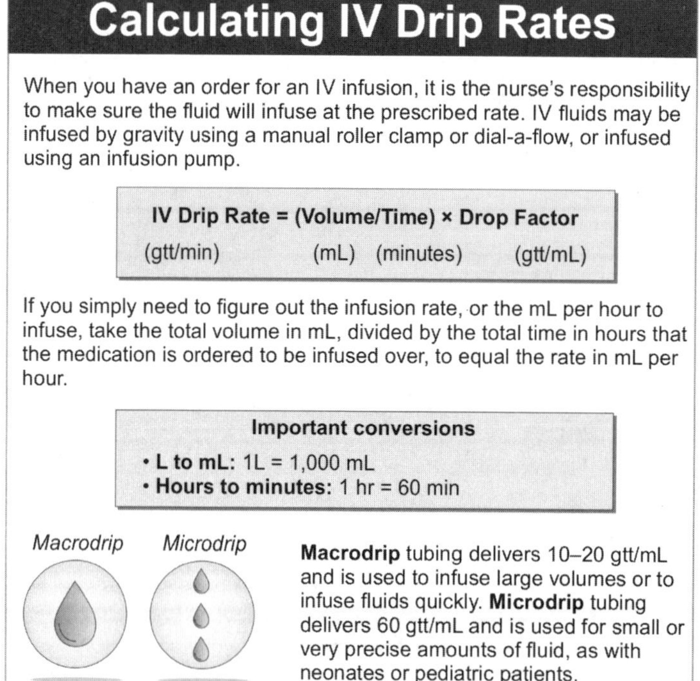

Fluid management is an essential aspect for any patient admitted to the hospital. If possible, patients should take fluids enterally since this is the natural route of fluid intake. However, many patients who are sick enough to need admission to the hospital might have a reason they cannot tolerate oral intake. Alternative routes of administration such as intravenous access can deliver fluids directly to the vascular system.

There are many ways to assess a patient's volume status to determine their fluid needs. Often, one can determine the patient's fluid status clinically based on a variety of physical exam findings and objective data from their vital signs. Laboratory markers are helpful as adjunctive data. The following is a list of findings that can help determine whether a patient is fluid-depleted or volume overloaded.

Vital Signs

* **Weight:** One of the most sensitive indicators of patient volume status changes is their body weight. Patient weight changes approximate a gold standard to determine fluid status. Unfortunately, due to differences in scales available to hospital staff, this can be a challenging target to measure. It is ideal to weigh a patient daily on the same scale to determine trends in weight changes. One can see weight gain in states of fluid excess and weight loss in states of fluid deficit. It is also helpful to look at patient records to see any recent outpatient visits before hospitalization, which might indicate a patient's normal baseline weight.
* **Heart rate:** Tachycardia can represent a compensatory physiologic response to maintain perfusion in the setting of hypovolemia. This can be an early finding in compensated hypovolemic shock. However, there are many other reasons for tachycardia, such as pain, fever, and anxiety.
* **Blood pressure:** Falling blood pressure is an ominous finding in the setting of tachycardia, indicating that the cardiovascular system can no longer compensate adequately for hypovolemia. Conversely, elevated blood pressures can be seen in hypervolemia.
* **Orthostatic vital signs:** A drop of at least 20 mm Hg systolic blood pressure or 10 mm Hg diastolic blood pressure within 2–5 minutes of quiet standing after 5 minutes of supine rest indicates orthostatic hypotension. Dehydrated or elderly patients who have lost sensitivity in their baroreceptors in their blood vessels might display these findings.
* **Respiratory rate:** Increased respiratory rate indicates a compensatory response to metabolic acidosis from lactic acidosis due to poor tissue perfusion. This is an early finding in hypovolemic shock.
* **Urine output:** Expect a minimum of 1.5 mL/kg per hour in children and greater than 1 mL/kg per hour in adults. Special situations such as administering nephrotoxic medications such as acyclovir warrant higher thresholds for urine output to minimize renal toxicity.

Physical Exam Findings

* **Capillary refill:** Normally less than 2 seconds. Easy to test on fingertips and toes.
* **Fontanelle:** Sunken fontanelle on the skull of an infant suggests hypovolemia.
* **Edema:** Peripheral edema can be a sign of volume overload or third spacing of intravascular fluid.
* **Tear production:** Relevant in infants and children; important to ask parents for their observations and evaluate the child while in the exam room.
* **Peripheral pulses:** Check brachial and femoral pulses in infants; check radial or dorsalis pedis pulses in older patients; can see fast and thready pulses in dehydration states.
* **Skin turgor and eyeball appearance:** Severe cases of dehydration might present with flaccid or tented skin; eyeballs might also appear sunken back into orbital cavities.

- ❖ **Tactile temperature of skin:** Classically find cool and clammy skin found in hypovolemic shock due to peripheral vasoconstriction causing hypoperfusion of skin, especially at the extremities (i.e., hands or feet).
- ❖ **Mucous membranes:** Appreciate dry, sandpaper-like texture of the oral mucosa or tongue in states of dehydration.
- ❖ **Jugular vein appearance:** Appreciate a distended jugular vein in volume overload state; can also be found in patients with congestive heart failure who are euvolemic but not pumping blood appropriately.

Laboratory Findings

- ❖ **BUN/creatinine:** Can be elevated secondary to prerenal acute kidney injury from decreased renal blood flow due to decreased intravascular volume.
- ❖ **Transaminases:** Can see an elevation in AST or ALT due to hypoperfusion of hepatic tissue and subsequent tissue hypoxia causing hepatocyte injury, also known as "shock liver."
- ❖ **Hemoconcentration:** Can see elevated hematocrit due to a relative abundance of red blood cells relative to intravascular fluid volume.

Equipment

- ❖ Intravenous (IV) fluid solutions
- ❖ 5% dextrose in 0.9% sodium chloride (normal saline) +/– potassium additive
- ❖ 5% dextrose in 0.45% sodium chloride (half normal saline) +/– potassium additive
- ❖ Lactated Ringer's

Enteral Tubes

- ❖ Nasogastric tube
- ❖ Orogastric tube
- ❖ Gastric tube
- ❖ Nasoduodenal tube
- ❖ Gastrojejunal tube

Enteral Fluid Solutions

- ❖ Commercial rehydration solutions
- ❖ WHO rehydration solution
- ❖ Infant feeds (breastmilk or formula)
- ❖ Commercially available sports drinks

Preparation

The pediatric population demands careful consideration of a child's size in determining their rate of fluid maintenance. A 3-month-old infant has much different fluid needs than those of a more fully grown 8-year-old child. In many cases, a simple calculation called the 4–2–1 rule can determine the hourly rate of fluid maintenance required for a child based on weight. The following example shows an application of this formula.

> **First 10 kg = 4 mL/kg per hour**
> **Next 10–20 kg = 2 mL/kg per hour**

Any remaining weight over 20 kg = 1 mL/kg per hour.

For example, a 22 kg child would have the following maintenance fluid requirements.

First 10 kg = 4 mL/kg per hour × 10 kg = 40 mL per hour

Next 10–20 kg = 2 mL/kg per hour × 10 kg = 20 mL per hour

Remaining 2 kg = 1 mL/kg per hour × 2 kg = 2 mL per hour

Total hourly rate = 40 + 20 + 2 = 62 mL per hour

Another commonly used formula predicts fluid needs over a 24-hour period. The following example shows an application of this formula.

First 10 kg = 100 mL/kg per day

Next 10–20 kg = additional 50 mL/kg per day

Any remaining weight over 20 kg = additional 20 mL/kg per day

For example, a 70 kg man would have the following maintenance fluid requirements.

First 10 kg = 100 mL/kg/day × 10 kg = 1000 mL per day

Next 10–20 kg = 50 mL/kg/day × 10 kg = 500 mL per day

Remaining 50 kg = 20 mL/kg/day × 50 kg = 1,000 mL per day

Total fluids per day = 1,000 + 500 + 1,000 = 2,500 mL per day

Hourly fluid rate = 2,500/24 = 104 mL per hour

IV Drip Rate

No pump = rate will be gtt/min-also known as gravity drip

Formula for gtt/min: $\dfrac{\textbf{mL/hr} \times \textbf{drop factor}}{\textbf{60 (minutes)}} = \textbf{gtt/min}$

Example of calculating gtts/min:

Order: 1,000 mL of D5/W to infuse 130 mL/hr.

Drop factor of tubing is 20 gtts = 1 mL

Formula:

$$\frac{mL/hr \times drop\ factor}{60\ minutes} = gtt/min$$

130 mL/hr × 20 gtt/min = 2,600 = 43 gtt/min

60 minutes = 1 hr

Manually would have to count drops as you watch the clock for one minute

HINT: Count for 15 seconds and multiply by 4 = 60 seconds

Electronic Volumetric Pumps

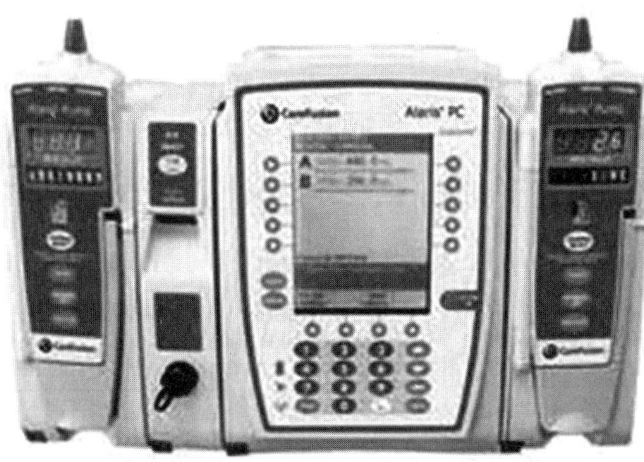

❖ Infuse fluids into the vein under pressure and against resistance
❖ Do not depend on gravity
❖ Pumps are programmed to deliver a set amount of fluid per hour
❖ Milliliters per hour (mL/hr)
  Milliliter calculation that results in a decimal fraction round to a whole milliliter
  IV Pump = rate will be mL/hr

Formula

Total number of milliliters ordered = mL/hour
Number of hours to run

Order: 2,000 mL LR to infuse in 10 hours
Using formula for setting up calculation:
Determine the amount of IV fluid ordered and divide this by the number of hours

$$\frac{2,000 \text{ mL}}{10 \text{ hr}} = 200 \text{ mL/hr}$$

Answer: Set the IV pump controller at 200 mL/hr

Determining the Number of Hours an IV will Run

Formula:

Number of milliliters ordered = Number of hours to run
Number of milliliters per hour
Example of how to calculate how long IV will run

Q. How many hours will 500 mL of D5½ NS run at 125 mL/hour?

Number of milliliters ordered = Number of hours to run
Number of milliliters per hour

$$\frac{500 \text{ mL}}{125 \text{ mL/hour}} = 4 \text{ hours}$$

COMPLICATION OF IV THERAPY

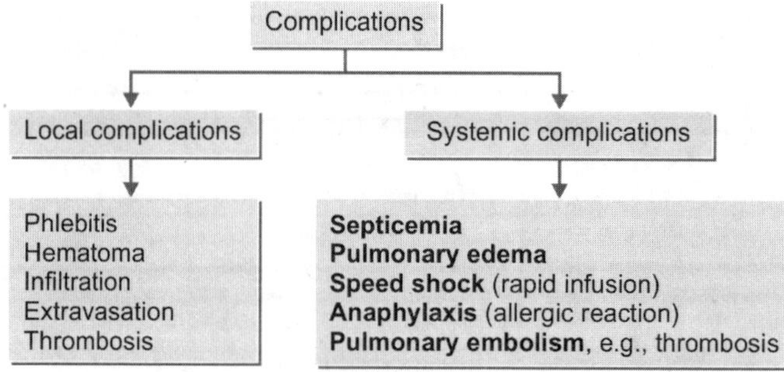

Complication of IV Therapy

Complication	Signs and symptoms	Prevention	Nursing interventions/treatment
Occlusion is the partial or complete obstruction of a catheter, which obstructs the infusion of solutions or medications. Occlusions can result from the coagulation of blood (thrombotic) or from obstruction due to catheter problems or buildup of infusion precipitates and residue (mechanical)	Electronic pump "occlusion" alarm is activated frequently Noticeable slowing of infusion rate Difficulty aspirating from catheter Visible clots in the catheter Pain upon infusion	Flush the access device according to facility guidelines Correct any obvious signs of mechanical occlusion Use in-line, air eliminating filters Monitor infusions of possible precipitate-forming solutions Monitor three in one parenteral infusions Avoid temperature fluctuations during parenteral nutrition infusions	Identify type of occlusion (thrombolytic or mechanical). Notify the physician immediately if occlusion is thrombolytic (or cause of occlusion can not be determined). Obtain orders for thrombolytic agent and catheter clearance. If mechanical occlusion, troubleshoot the catheter line (e.g., observe for kinks, clogged in-line filter, sutures causing occlusion). If occlusion cannot be resolved, notify physician If occlusion is due to precipitates (drug or mineral), notify physician and obtain orders for catheter clearance and catheter clearing agent If occlusion is due to lipid residue, notify physician and obtain orders for catheter clearance and catheter clearing agent. Notify the physician immediately if pinch-off, catheter rupture, or migration is suspected Document observations, interventions, resident's response and outcome in the resident's medical chart
Phlebitis is inflammation of the vein. It is a common complication associated with intravenous therapy. It may occur up to 48 hours after catheter removal	Warmth, redness and inflammation Resident complains of heat, stinging Discomfort at access site Pain and tenderness along pathway of afflicted vein Induration of vein, palpable venous cord Purulent drainage		Assess degree of phlebitis using the phlebitis scale Discontinue infusion and remove catheter Disinfect the access site. **Note:** If purulent drainage is present, obtain a culture sample prior to disinfection Apply pressure to removal site to prevent bleeding Apply intermittent warm, moist heat for 20 minutes TID, per physician's order If infection is suspected, culture catheter tip Notify physician of phlebitis Document the observations, interventions, resident's response and outcome in resident's medical chart **Note:** When inserting a new catheter, use the nonaffected extremity if possible

Contd...

Contd...

Complication	Signs and symptoms	Prevention	Nursing interventions/treatment
Infiltration occurs when the catheter dislodges from the vein and nonvesicant solution or medication is administered into the surrounding tissue	Edema, blanching, cool, stretched and/or firm skin Mild to moderate pain; numbness Pitting edema Circulatory impairment No blood return from IV access	Confirm patency of catheter prior to administering medications or solutions Once infusion begins, observe the access site for 1–2 minutes Do not pull or tug on the catheter or administration set Use a syringe barrel size of 10 mL or greater when flushing	Assess degree of infiltration using the infiltration scale Discontinue infusion and remove catheter Apply pressure at removal site to prevent bleeding Apply warm compress to help absorb infiltrate If leaking of the tissue is present, apply sterile dressing. Notify physician of infiltration grade 3 or 4 Complete an incident report Document observations, interventions, resident's response and outcome in resident's medical chart **Note:** When inserting a new catheter, use the nonaffected extremity if possible
Extravasation occurs when the catheter dislodges from the vein and a vesicant solution or medication is administered into the surrounding tissue, leading to tissue necrosis	Blisters, tissue necrosis, sloughing of tissue Edema, blanching, stretched, firm and/or cool skin Pain, heat, stinging at access site	Confirm patency of catheter prior to administering medications or solutions Once infusion begins, observe the access site for 1–2 minutes Do not pull or tug on the catheter or administration set Administer vesicant solutions with extreme caution. Use a syringe barrel size of 10 mL or greater when flushing	Discontinue infusion immediately. Do not remove catheter unless instructed to do so by physician Notify physician and obtain orders to treat extravasation Administer antidote as ordered, either through existing catheter or by injection If ordered to remove catheter, aspirate as much infiltrate as possible before removing and apply pressure to access site to prevent bleeding Apply ice to affected area Elevate affected extremity Encourage normal ROM of affected extremity **Note:** When inserting a new catheter, do not use the affected extremity Document in resident's medical record: date and time of extravasation; catheter type and size, date, and time of catheter insertion; solution or medication infused, method of administration, time and rate of infusion, and estimated amount infused; appearance of site; physician notification; treatment/antidote measures; and resident's response and outcome Photograph the access site at time of injury, at 24 hours postinjury, at 48 hours post-injury, and at one week postinjury Complete incident report

Contd...

Contd...

Complication	Signs and symptoms	Prevention	Nursing interventions/treatment
Allergic reaction is a generalized hypersensitivity reaction to a solution, medication, or additive Allergic reactions can be immediate or delayed, mild or severe. Severe allergic reactions (anaphylaxis) can be life threatening	Chills and fever Urticaria Erythema 4 Pruritis Shortness of breath Respiratory distress Anaphylactic shock Cardiac arrest	Obtain a thorough history of drug allergies Place ID bracelet on resident noting allergies Flag medical record and alert other providers of resident's allergies Re-check resident identification and blood type during blood transfusion procedures	Stop infusion immediately Discontinue any suspected medication or substance causing the reaction Maintain vascular access Notify physician immediately Administer treatment as ordered Do not use the same administration tubing used to administer the suspected allergen Monitor vital signs Document observations, interventions, resident's response and outcome in the resident's medical chart Complete an incident report
Catheter-related Infections (CRIs) can be local, systemic or both. Local infections are limited to the catheter insertion site, exit site of tunneled catheters, or implanted port pocket. Systemic infections are characterized by the presence of >10–15 times the colony forming units of bacteria per mL of blood drawn from the vascular access device. CRIs can be life threatening. Prompt assessment and intervention are essential	Inflammation or purulence at catheter site Tenderness Erythema Induration Sudden onset of symptoms Onset or worsening of symptoms upon start or increased rate of infusion Febrile episode Necrosis of skin over reservoir of implanted port	Use aseptic technique during initiation and care of IV catheters Follow the CDC guidelines for proper hand antisepsis Assess access site and administration set at established intervals. (see policies entitled peripheral IV and midline IV dressing changes and central venous catheter dressing and extension set or injection/ access port changes. Change administration set and rotate IV access site at established intervals (see policy entitled administration set changes)	If local infection is suspected: notify physician immediately; obtain site culture, per physician order and report results; apply warm compresses, as ordered; administer anti-infective therapy, as ordered; and remove VAD, as ordered If systemic infection is suspected: notify physician immediately; obtain blood cultures from vascular access device and from a peripheral vascular site; culture infusion solution of medication, if contamination is suspected; administer anti-infective therapy, as ordered; and remove VAD, as ordered Document observations, interventions, physician notification, resident's response and outcomes Complete an incident report

Contd...

Contd...

Complication	Signs and symptoms	Prevention	Nursing interventions/treatment
Septicemia is a systemic infection characterized by the presence of pathogens and their toxic metabolites in the circulating blood	Septicemia: Fever Headache Chills Diarrhea Hypotension Vomiting Backache Flushing Nausea Late Stage Septicemia: Cyanosis Shock Hyperventilation Death Vascular collapse	Use aseptic technique during initiation and care of IV catheters Follow the CDC guidelines for proper hand antisepsis Inspect medications and solutions prior to administration Assess access site and administration set and established intervals Change administration set and rotate IV access site at established intervals	Notify physician immediately Administer interventions and treatment as ordered Obtain cultures of catheter, infusate, blood, as ordered Obtain cultures prior to administration of anti-infectives Remove VAD, as ordered Document observations, interventions, resident's response and outcome in the resident's medical chart Complete an incident report
Catheter-related venous thrombosis (CRVT) is the formation of a thrombus (fibrin) along the venous wall. CRVT is a potentially life-threatening complication. Prompt assessment and intervention are essential	Pain or burning in neck, chest, or shoulders Swelling of face, neck, arm, or at catheter exit site Numbing or tingling in extremities Superficial collateral veins on the chest Periorbital edema Tachycardia Shortness of breath	Flush catheters routinely Administer low-dose anticoagulant therapy, as ordered Use a syringe barrel size of 10 mL or greater when flushing.	Notify physician immediately Initiate anticoagulant and/or thrombolytic therapy as ordered Prepare resident for radiographic studies, as ordered Document observations, interventions, resident's response and outcome in the resident's medical chart Complete an incident report

Contd...

Contd...

Complication	Signs and symptoms	Prevention	Nursing interventions/treatment
Air embolism is characterized by the entry of an air bolus into the vascular system. If the air bolus enters the cardiac circulation, it blocks the ejection of blood from the right ventricle into the pulmonary artery	Chest pain Shortness of Breath Cyanosis Hypotension Weak pulse Tachycardia Syncope Loss of consciousness Shock Cardiac arrest	Use air-eliminating filters Clamp catheter and tubing during administration set changes Use luer-lock connections for infusion equipment and piggy-backs Prime infusion sets and tubing prior to connecting to VAD Place resident in supine position and have them perform Valsalva maneuver when removing CVCs After catheter removal, apply pressure to exit site Apply occlusive dressing to exit site and change every 24 hours until site is epithelialized	Notify physician immediately Place resident in left trendelenburg's position If embolism is due to open or leaking administration set, clamp line close to VAD and change administration set and tubing If embolism is due to disconnected or damaged central venous access device, clamp catheter and repair, if appropriate Remove CVC, as ordered after new catheter has been inserted Administer interventions and treatment, as ordered Monitor resident closely Document observations, interventions, resident's response and outcome in the resident's medical chart Complete an incident report
A catheter embolism occurs when a catheter piece becomes dislodged and enters the general circulation. Major vessel blockage results in loss of circulation, cardiac irritability, and/or cardiac arrest	Cyanosis Hypotension Tachycardia Syncope/loss of consciousness	Inspect catheters for defects before using When using through-the-needle catheters, never pull catheter back through the needle When using over-the-needle catheters, never withdraw or reinsert once threaded Use appropriate size syringe and technique when flushing catheter	Notify physician immediately Place tourniquet above venipuncture site. Do not occlude arterial flow Place resident on bed rest Monitor resident closely for signs of distress Administer interventions and treatment, as ordered Document observations, interventions, resident's response and outcome in resident's medical chart Complete incident report

Contd...

Contd...

Complication	Signs and symptoms	Prevention	Nursing interventions/treatment
Pulmonary edema is a result of fluid overload within the circulatory system. Pulmonary edema can lead to congestive heart failure, shock and cardiac arrest	Restlessness Increased pulse rate Headache Shortness of breath Nonproductive cough Flushed skin Hypertension Dyspnea with gurgle, rales upon auscultation Frothy sputum Engorged neck veins Pitting edema Edematous eyelids	Assess resident prior to infusion therapy for history of complications related to IV therapy, cardiac or respiratory problems, present fluid status, ability to tolerate fluid volume Monitor closely for signs and symptoms of fluid intolerance	Place resident on strict bed rest in high Fowler's position (HOB elevated 90°) Slow infusions, maintain venous patency Notify physician immediately Monitor vital signs/intake and output Administer interventions and treatments per physician orders: oxygen; pain medication; diuretic; and/or vasodilators Document observations, interventions, resident's response and outcome in resident's medical chart Complete incident report
Speed shock occurs when a foreign substance is too rapidly introduced into the body. Speed shock can occur even when the amount introduced is small in volume. Speed shock can be identified when sudden onset of symptoms is associated with infusion therapy	Dizziness Flushed skin Headache Irregular heart rate	Monitor administration sets and electronic pumps to ensure correct flow-rate Use electronic pumps to ensure accurate rate of flow	Stop the infusion immediately Maintain vascular access Notify physician immediately Administer interventions and treatments as ordered Document observations, interventions, resident's response and outcome in resident's medical chart Complete incident report

MONITORING FLUID INTAKE AND OUTPUT

Introduction

Normally, the amount of total body water should be balanced through the ingestion and elimination of water: Ins and Outs. To ensure this balance, as a nurse, you may need to track and record all fluid intake and output on an intake and output sheet, commonly known as an I and O sheet. This is particularly important for certain groups of clients, like those on special fluid orders, including "encourage fluids" and "restrict fluids;" those who are at risk of developing dehydration, or losing too much body fluid, which impairs normal body functions; or those who might develop edema where swelling occurs in tissues due to excess fluid buildup.

High-risk of dehydration exists for those who may not be drinking an adequate amount of fluids throughout the day or those who might be losing too much due to receiving certain medications, like diuretics, or through vomiting, diarrhea, bleeding, burns, excessive sweating, fever, or vigorous exercise. Common signs include dry mouth, excessive thirst, and dark urine.

Likewise, clients at risk of developing edema include those receiving intravenous fluids or those with heart or kidney disease, where the body has trouble eliminating excess fluid. The fluid builds up and causes swelling, especially in the lower extremities.

Nurses should check with the plan of care to find out if their clients' intake and output should be monitored. So, every time one of these clients receives or loses fluids in any way, the exact volume can be recorded. These volumes are then totaled at the end of every shift and then at the end of a 24-hour period.

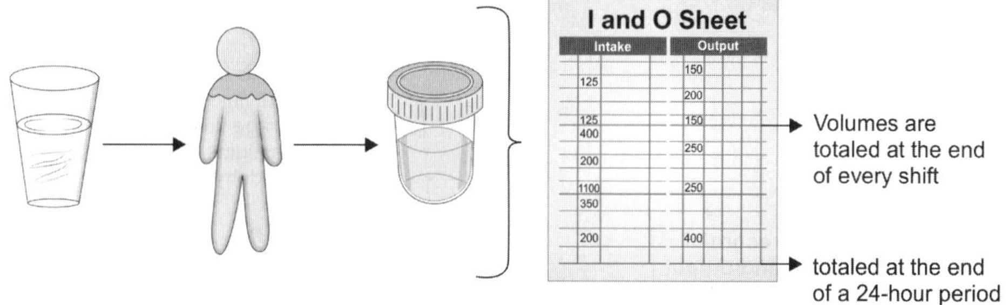

Track and record all fluid intake and output on an intake and output sheet, commonly known as an I and O sheet.

MEASURING FLUID INTAKE

For fluid intake, you'll need to count:
- ❖ Anything the client drinks, including water and beverages.
- ❖ All foods that are liquid at room temperature, like ice cream, gelatin, sherbert, pudding, custard, ice chips, and popsicles.
- ❖ The fluids provided through intravenous therapy, enteral, or total parenteral nutrition.
- ❖ Fluid intake is typically measured in milliliters (mL). But some containers use different units, so, you may need to be able to make the appropriate conversions.
  - ◆ 1 mL = 1 cubic centimeter (cc) = 0.001 liters (L)
  - ◆ 1 fluid ounce = 30 mL
  - ◆ 1 pint = ~ 500 mL
  - ◆ 1 quart = ~ 1,000 mL

It's also important to know the usual serving sizes in your facility. As a rule of thumb,

- 1 teaspoon = 5 mL
- 1 tablespoon = 15 mL
- 1 cup = 250 mL

But for other containers, like mugs, glasses, or bowls, the volume of fluid contained may vary. Keeping in mind any necessary conversions, gather the supplies you will need, including:

- Gloves
- A graduated measuring container

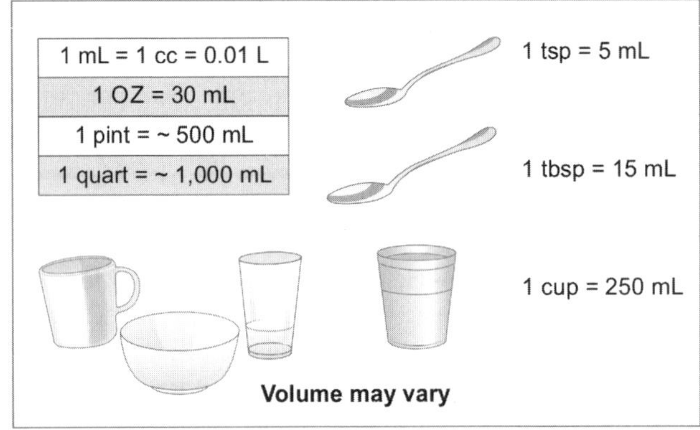

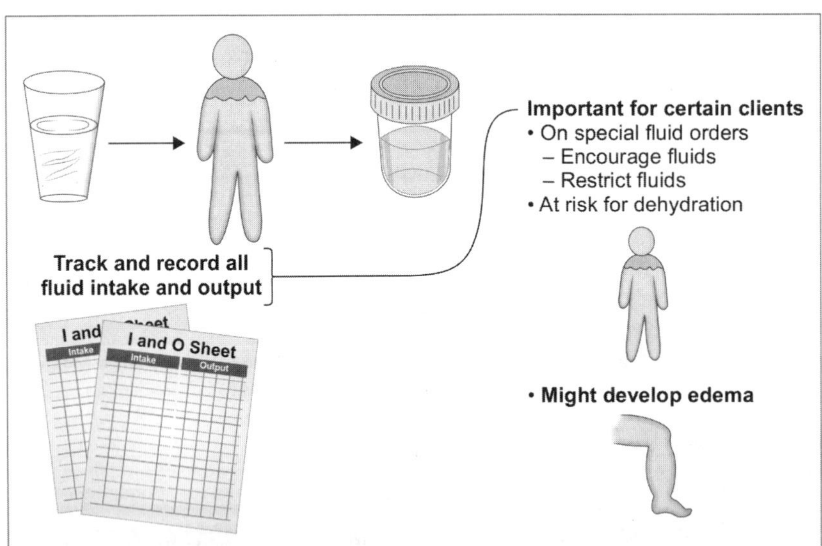

Unit conversions when measuring volume.

Procedure

Add all fluid volumes served to that client. For example, during your shift, the client could have been served with 200 mL of water, 360 mL of soda, and 140 mL of milk. All together, these equal 700 mL.

Put on your gloves and transfer whatever has remained from each liquid into a graduated measuring container. Remember to keep the graduate even and at eye level to ensure precise measurements.

Subtract the volume in the graduate from the total volume of fluid served to the client. For example, if the volume left in the graduate is 80 mL, this is subtracted from the full serving amount of 700 mL, giving us a total fluid intake of 620 mL.

Remove your gloves and practice hand hygiene.

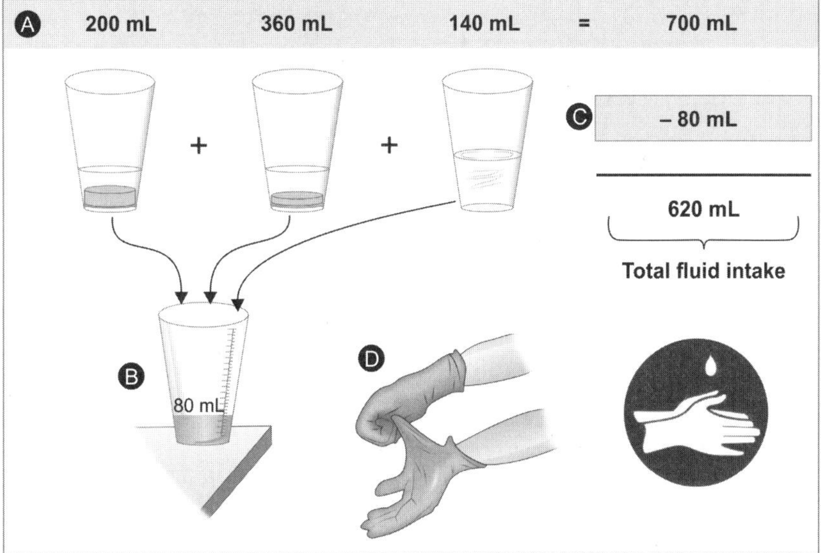

How to measure fluid input. (A) Add all fluid volumes served to the client; (B) Transfer remainder of liquids into a graduated measuring container; (C) Subtract the volume in the graduate from the total volume of fluid served; (D) Remove gloves and practice hand hygiene.

MEASURING FLUID OUTPUT

Fluid output includes:

❖ Urine
❖ Vomitus
❖ Wound drainage
❖ Diarrhea
❖ Blood

Special precautions are required for certain clients, like those undergoing chemotherapy, because their urine, stool, and vomit can contain the chemotherapy agent.

Once again, your supplies include:

◆ Gloves
◆ A graduated container
◆ If there is a possibility of splashing, personal protective equipment, such as a gown, goggles or face shield, and a mask.

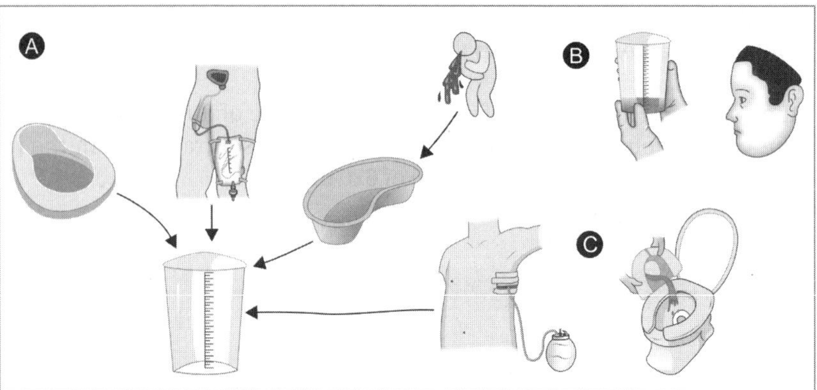

Some key steps in measuring fluid output. (A) Collect all forms of the client's fluid output into a receptacle with volume marks; (B) Hold the receptacle or graduate at eye level to measure the fluid volume; (C) Empty the contents into the toilet.

Procedure

- Provide these clients with urine receptacles specifically labeled with their name and bed location. Tell them to only urinate in these receptacles and notify you when they are finished before discarding the contents.
- Commonly used urine receptacles are specimen "hats" that can be positioned under the toilet seat or a bedside commode to collect urine.
- Collect all forms of the client's fluid output into a receptacle with volume marks. Most receptacles already have volume marks, but not all of them.
- If the client is using a bedpan or catheter drainage bag, empty their contents into a graduated container.
- If the client vomits, collect it in an emesis basin. Blood and wound drainage might be collected in drainage pouches. If the emesis basin and drainage pouch do not have volume marks, pour the contents of both receptacles into a graduate.
- Hold the receptacle or graduate at eye level to measure the fluid volume.
- Empty the contents into the toilet and clean, rinse, and disinfect both the receptacle or graduate as well as the toilet
- You may also have to assess the volume of fluid losses outside of containers. This could be the case if a client has vomited out of the emesis basin, if there's blood or wound drainage not contained in a drainage pouch, as well as in the case of diarrhea.
- Remove your gloves and practice hand hygiene.

Documentation

When measuring a client's fluid intake and output, be sure to report the following to the healthcare provider:

- Changes in the usual amount of intake; for example, a client refusing to drink the served fluids
- Changes in the color, clarity, or odor of the output
- If the intake and output is not balanced
- If you observe edema, especially in the lower extremities, or signs of dehydration, such as dark urine or a dry mouth

After that, document:

❖ The date and time

❖ Your observations

❖ The measured amounts of fluid intake and output on the client's paper or electronic I and O record

❖ A typical I and O sheet has a column with time and two separate sections for intake and output.

❖ Intake is divided into oral intake, which you will need to fill with the amount you measured, and parenteral intake, where you will add fluid intake coming from intravenous therapy, enteral, or total parenteral nutrition.

❖ For the output, there's usually one section for urine and one for everything else.

❖ Document the amount measured as well as how the fluid was collected, such as through voiding or a urinary catheter. Make sure all amounts are in milliliter.

Blood Transfusion

Blood transfusions are a relatively common medical procedure, and while typically safe, there are multiple complications that practitioners need to be able to recognize and treat. This activity reviews the indications for blood transfusion, including for special patient populations, the pre-transfusion preparation, and the potential complications of blood transfusions. In addition, this activity highlights the role of the interprofessional team in caring for patients undergoing blood transfusions.

PATIENT INSTRUCTION/PREPARATION

Transfusion Service personnel will notify patient unit personnel by telephone when ordered blood is ready for transfusion. The risks of transfusion, including adverse symptoms and alternatives to homologous (allogeneic) transfusion, must be discussed with the patient well before transfusion. This discussion should be documented by the physician/practitioner in the patient's electronic medical record and signed consent form. Patient education materials are available to assist in this process (see patient information materials). The patient's blood pressure, pulse, respirations, and temperature must be taken and recorded within 60 minutes prior to the transfusion. The pretransfusion vital signs provide a baseline for comparison data obtained during and after transfusion. If a patient is febrile, consideration should be given to postponement of blood transfusion, since the fever may mask the development of a febrile reaction to the blood component itself.

Release and Transport of Blood

Before requesting that a blood component be delivered to the patient care unit, verify the provider's order to transfuse, administer any pretransfusion medication, record the patient's vital signs and initiate or verify patency of an intravenous line. This will allow the blood transfusion to be initiated as soon as the component arrives on the patient unit. The Transfusion Service will transport blood components via pneumatic tube or the blood component may be picked up at the transfusion service/blood bank by patient care unit personnel (CSA, RN, LPN) in a cooler. Patient care personnel must present transfusion service personnel with a release Form. The form must contain the recipient's full name, registration number, and blood component ordered. Only one unit of blood will be released at a time for a patient unless two intravenous lines are in place for that patient, allowing two units of blood to be transfused simultaneously. To avoid delay, notify the transfusion service personnel of this situation in advance. Multiple blood units will be released only to patient care units with monitored blood refrigerators (surgery) or if issued in transfusion service coolers.

Receipt of Blood Components

Only nursing personnel or physicians may accept blood or blood components when delivered to a patient unit. Immediately upon receipt, the component should be inspected for abnormal appearance and for patient identification at the patient bedside, using the patient's attached medical record number wrist or ankle band. If the name and identification number recorded on the unit tag attached to the unit do not correspond with that of the intended recipient, the component must be returned to the transfusion service. Consult with the transfusion service if there is any question. If a blood component cannot be transfused shortly after being received from the transfusion service, immediately return it to the transfusion service by messenger or pneumatic tube. To avoid waste, notify the transfusion service that blood is being returned.

An untransfused unit must be returned to the Transfusion Service within 20 minutes from the time it is received on the patient care unit. Blood components that have been out of controlled storage temperatures for more than 30 minutes cannot be safely reissued to another patient. Refrigerated blood components cannot be stored in medication refrigerators. Platelets, cryoprecipitate, and granulocytes must not be stored at refrigerator temperatures. These components have special storage requirements and cannot be stored properly on the patient unit or in the operating room.

Note: If components are no longer needed—To avoid unnecessary waste of blood resources, notify the transfusion service staff immediately if components are no longer needed for a patient, as the component may be suitable for transfusion to another patient.

Steps that Must be Taken Prior to Blood Transfusion

Verify provider's orders for transfusion and premedication.

Verify patient/component identification at the bedside. Before transfusion, the identification of the patient, using the unit tag on the bag, must be checked by two people at the patient's bedside against the identification of the intended blood recipient using the patient wristband. This step must never by bypassed. This is to be performed by qualified individuals (provider and registered nurse, two registered nurses, or by a registered nurse and a licensed practical nurse), one being the transfusionists.

If possible, ask the patient to state his or her name, and correlate this information with available identification.

Verify the blood to the provider's order for component, volume and special preparation.

Verify the blood type, donor number, component name, compatibility, and outdate match between the unit tag and the blood unit label.

Both persons must sign the unit tag. The person who hangs the blood must record the date and time of transfusion was started. The date, time, component, and unit number must be recorded on the appropriate sheet in the patient's medical record.

Immediately before transfusion, mix the unit of blood thoroughly by gentle inversion.

Follow the manufacturer's instruction for the use of filters and ancillary devices. Additional administration instructions for selected components are printed at the end of this document. If a unit of blood or a blood component has been entered for any reason by personnel not working in the transfusion service and the unit has not been transfused, the unit must be discarded and the unit tag must be completed. Note the volume transfused (indicate "NONE", if none administered). The completed unit tag must be returned to the transfusion service.

Flow Rates

Start the infusion slowly to allow for recognition of an acute adverse reaction. Complete the transfusion within 2-hours unless the patient can tolerate only gradual expansion of the intravascular volume. The infusion time should not exceed 4 hours.

Standard Infusion Rates

* Red blood cells 2–5 mL/kg/hour
* Platelets 10 minutes/unit OR 5 mL/minute
* Plasma 1–2 mL/minute
* Cryoprecipitate 1–2 mL/minute
* Granulocytes slowly

Medications

Do not add medications directly to a unit of blood during transfusion. Medications that can be administered "IV PUSH" may be administered by stopping the transfusion, clearing the line at the medication injection site with 5–10 mL of normal saline, administering the medication, reflushing the line with saline, and restarting the transfusion.

Filters

Follow manufacturer's instructions for priming.
* Do not twist the filter when attaching it to the IV tubing cannula.
* Do not use an infusion pump or suction (to fill a syringe) unless the manufacturer's instructions indicate that infusion pumps may be used. Inappropriate use of such pumps may result in filter material being infused.
* Filters must be changed every 4–6 hours or every 2–4 units.
* Administer all blood products not received in a syringe through a standard blood infusion set.

Platelets

Do not refrigerate platelets as platelet activity is reduced if cooled below room temperature.
* Platelets should be transfused immediate after they are available since platelet activity diminished rapidly during storage.
* Platelets should be administered at a rapid rate for maximum effectiveness. A rate of 5 mL/ minute is frequently used.

CRYOPRECIPITATED ANTIHEMOPHILIC FACTOR

When multiple units of cryoprecipitated antihemophilic factor (CRYO) are ordered, the transfusion service will pool the product in a single bag.
* The component must be administered within 4 hours of pooling.
* Do not refrigerate CRYO as this causes reprecipitation and loss of factor VIII activity.

❖ The component must be transfused immediately after it arrives on the patient care unit because factor VIII activity diminishes at room temperature.

❖ For maximum effectiveness, transfuse the product rapidly. The usual flow rate is 1–2 mL/minute.

❖ CRYO does not contain red blood cells. CRYO from Rh-positive donors may be given to patients who are Rh negative.

FRESH FROZEN PLASMA (FFP), FROZEN PLASMA (FP), THAWED PLASMA

The transfusion of plasma should be initiated as soon as it arrives on the patient unit. The usual flow rate is 1–2 mL/minute. Do not store at room temperature or in nonmonitored refrigerators.

❖ Thawed plasma must be transfused within 5 days.

❖ Previously frozen plasma does not contain red blood cells. Plasma from Rh-positive donors may be given to patients who are Rh negative.

GRANULOCYTE, PHERESIS OR WBC CONCENTRATES

Do not refrigerate granulocytes:

❖ Administer through a standard blood filter. Do not use a microaggregate filter or filter designed to remove white blood cells.

❖ Isotonic saline (90%) is the only intravenous solution recommended for use with this blood component.

❖ Infused slowly over 4 hours. The rate of infusion is ultimately dictated by the recipient's ability to tolerate the component volume and by adverse reactions.

❖ Premedication is recommended to avoid the need to discontinue transfusion due to a severe reaction.

❖ Document vital signs every 15 minutes during the entire procedure, every 30 minutes for 4 hours after the transfusion and then every 4 hours for 24 hours. Monitor the patient closely for moderate to severe symptoms such as urticaria, hives, wheezing, dyspnea, severe headache, cyanosis, hypotension, agitation and tachycardia. If such symptoms develop, stop the transfusion, keep the IV line open and notify the patient's physician and the transfusion service pathologist on-call for further instructions.

❖ In general, transfusion of granulocytes should be terminated only for such complication as severe flank pain, chest pain, hemoglobinemia, hypotension, laryngospasm, or acute pulmonary injury.

Managing a blood or blood product transfusion reaction
Disclaimer: Always review and follow your hospital policy regarding this specific skill.
Safety considerations: • Always review your agency's algorithm for managing mild to severe reactions. If a reaction is mild (e.g., fever), and without any other complications, a patient may continue the transfusion if monitored closely. Most other transfusion reactions require the transfusion to be stopped immediately.   • A blood transfusion reaction may occur 24–48 hours post-transfusion.   • Each separate unit presents a potential for an adverse reaction.

- Follow emergency transfusion guidelines when dealing with an emergency blood or blood product transfusion.
- Be aware of which types of blood or blood products cause the most types of transfusion reactions.
- Be aware of the types of patients at high-risk for blood or blood product transfusion reactions.
- Always have emergency equipment and medications available during a transfusion. For example, epinephrine IV should always be readily available.

Steps	*Additional information*
1. Stop transfusion immediately	The severity of a blood transfusion reaction is related to the amount of product infused and the amount of time it has been infusing
2. Keep IV line open with 0.9% saline	Keeps IV site patent for emergency medications if required
3. Complete cardiovascular and vital signs assessment	Assessment monitors the type and severity of reaction. In addition to assessment: Maintain good urinary output Avoid fluid overload Manage DIC (disseminated intravascular coagulation) or hemorrhage if clinically indicated Provide supportive measures as required (oxygen, etc.)
4. Contact physician for medical assessment and to inform about reaction	The physician responsible for the patient must be informed of all transfusion reactions
5. Check vital signs every 15 minutes until stable	Vital signs must be monitored to identify improving or worsening condition
6. Obtain blood and urine samples as soon as possible	Blood and urine samples can help identify the type of blood transfusion reaction
7. Check all labels, tags, forms, blood order, and patient's identification band to determine if there is a clerical discrepancy	Clerical errors account for the majority of blood transfusion reactions
8. Keep all blood and IV tubing for further testing by the blood bank for verification of blood product and patient identification	All blood products and IV tubing are investigated by the transfusion services and reported to Canadian Blood Services and Public Health Agency of Canada. These professional bodies are responsible for reporting and recording incidents of reactions
9. Notify blood bank	Notify blood bank when an adverse reaction occurs, even if transfusion is continued
10. Document as per agency policy	Document time, date, signs and symptoms, type of product, notification to the physician and management of reaction, and patient response to management of reaction Documentation includes, but is not limited to: Transfusion reaction form Patient chart Report for transfusion services (blood bank) Adverse event form patient safety learning system (PSLS)

TRANSFUSION OF BLOOD AND BLOOD PRODUCTS

Disclaimer: Always review and follow your hospital policy regarding this specific skill.

Safety considerations:
- No medications may be added to blood units or through IV tubing.
- Specific blood administration tubing is required for all blood transfusions. Blood tubing is changed every 4 hours or 4 units, whichever comes first.
- See agency policy for using EID for the administration of blood products.
- Intravenous immunoglobulin (IVIG) is only compatible with D5W.
- All blood products taken from the blood bank must be hung within 30 minutes and administered (infused) within 4 hours due to the risk of bacterial proliferation in the blood component at room temperature.

Steps	*Additional information*
1. Verify physician orders and all preparation steps	
2. Assess or initiate venous access	Appropriate needle gauge is based on clinical status of patient, urgency of transfusion, and venous access: #18 gauge for trauma/surgery #20–#22 for elective medical/geriatric Transfusion set must be Luer-locked to a 2.0 mL maximum extension tubing, either directly to cannula or through a Max Plus positive pressure cap. Saline lock
3. Initiate primary infusion at TKVO	Prime an IV line following checklist 66: 0.9% NS for RBC D5W for IVIG Refer to blood product fact sheets for all other products Normal saline IV solution

Contd...

Contd...

Steps	Additional information
4. Complete and document cardiovascular assessments and initial vital signs	Document any clinical sign or symptom that may be confused with a transfusion reaction (e.g., existing fever)
5. Obtain products from the transfusion areas within 30 minutes of planned transfusion	Plan for pickup or delivery of blood and blood products. Do not request blood or blood products if steps 1–4 are not complete
6. Complete visual inspection of product	Assess blood bag for any signs of leaks or contamination, such as clumping, clots, gas bubbles, or a purplish discoloration. Return to blood bank if blood bag contains any of the above signs

Visual inspection of the blood bag

Steps	Additional information
7. Initial verification: a. Compare the **transfusion medical services** (TMS) documentation with the patient record to verify: ♦ Patient first and last name and unique identifier number ♦ Physician order ♦ Consent ♦ Patient ABO grouping (G and S) b. Compare the TMS documentation with the product label attached to the product tab and verify: ♦ Patient first and last name and unique identifier number ♦ Type of blood product and ABO blood grouping ♦ 11-digit serial number ♦ Product expiry date and time ♦ Special requirements (e.g., irradiated) ♦ G and S expiry date	All verification numbers/information must match exactly Must be completed by two trained staff members competent in blood transfusion administration process as set out by the agency Confirm the patient blood type and Rh are compatible with the donor blood type and Rh If there are any discrepancies, stop the process and contact the TMS for resolution and direction. Do not proceed Ensure the blood product matches the physician's orders (red blood cells or platelets)

TMS record

Contd...

Contd...

Steps	Additional information
8. Administer premedications as ordered	Medications must be administered through an IV infusion set, and the IV site cleared with 0.9% NS
9. Final verification (must be completed by the same two staff members as noted in Step 7) Compare the patient's first and last name and unique identifier number using all of the following: Patient identification band or equivalent ID process as approved by the TMS (ask the patient to spell first and last name and state date of birth) TMS documentation Compatibility tag and label attached to blood product Only after recipient identification and product check is confirmed, invert product 5–10 times and insert spike of the blood administration set into the blood product container	All verification numbers must match exactly. If there are any discrepancies, stop the process and contact the TMS for resolution and direction. Do not proceed Identify patient Patients who are alert and oriented should be asked to: Spell first and last name State their date of birth All identifying information attached to the blood bag must remain attached at least until completion of transfusion
10. Perform hand hygiene. Prime the blood product administration set: Close clamp. Completely cover the filter with product A straight blood administration set is used for all transfusions A Y-type blood administration set should only be considered in clinical situations where additional fluid volume may be required	Do not remove the product from the presence of the patient; prime at bedside. If product is removed from bedside, the final verification process must be completed again Prime blood tubing
11. Initiate transfusion: Obtain vital signs immediately prior to transfusion, then 15 minutes after initiation, then every hour until transfusion is complete	Adults: Initiate red cells slowly (25 mL in the first 15 minutes). For all other blood transfusions, refer to the blood and product sheet as per your agency policy Some agencies use an EID to administer blood transfusions. Always check agency policy prior to transfusion For each and every unit:

Contd...

Contd...

Steps	Additional information
Maintaining asepsis, disconnect the NS infusion and connect blood administration set and start transfusion Advise patient on the signs and symptoms of transfusion reaction and what and when to report	Remain with the patient for the first 5 minutes and assess for clinical signs of transfusion reaction Complete transfusion within 4 hours of removal from the blood bank Most transfusion reactions occur within first 15 minutes of a transfusion. Infusing small amounts of blood component initially minimizes volume of blood to which patient is exposed, thereby minimizing severity of reaction Infusion of packed red blood cells
12. Monitor: Assess and observe for clinical signs and symptoms of reactions up to 24 hours post-transfusion Complete all appropriate clinical documentation	Vital signs must be monitored: Immediately prior to infusion Within 10–15 minutes Every hour until transfusion is complete Vital signs
13. In the event of a transfusion reaction, stop the infusion	Manage transfusion reactions as per protocol Complete required transfusion reaction form Return remaining blood to blood bank for further investigation
14. For additional units, repeat steps 6–12	Follow the same process to ensure patient safety
15. Flush administration set with maximum of 50 mL of normal saline and re-establish IV or SL as per physician orders	Flushing displaces any blood or blood product from the administration set. It is not necessary to flush between units of the same blood product

Contd...

Contd...

Steps	Additional information
16. Discard waste in biohazard waste container	This prevents the spread of biohazard waste
17. Complete all documentation as required by agency	Documentation may include: Transfusion record form All vital signs and reactions Any significant findings, initiation and termination of transfusion Record of transfusion on the in-and-out sheet

Fluid Restriction

The National Academies of Sciences, Engineering, and Medicine recommend that females consume close to 2.7 liters (L), or 91 ounces (oz), of fluid per day. Males should consume about 3.7 L, or 125 oz.

For people restricting fluid, the standard recommended intake is 1.5–2 L per day. The exact amount will depend on how much a person weighs, their basal metabolic rate, Trusted Source, and the severity of their heart failure.

Fluid restriction means that person can only have a certain amount of liquid each day. Fluid restriction is needed if your body is holding water. This is called fluid retention (edema or if localized to abdomen = ascites). A fluid restriction limits the amount of fluids patients are allowed to consume from food and beverages. Patients may have been put onto fluid restriction due to having a certain condition, for example:

❖ Heart failure
❖ Kidney disease
❖ Liver disease
❖ Endocrine and adrenal gland disorders
❖ Conditions that cause the release of stress hormones
❖ Treatment with medications called corticosteroids
❖ Low levels of sodium in the blood (hyponatremia)

Keep a record of the amount of every liquid a patient have each day.

Liquids can be measured in milliliters (mL), liters (L), ounces (oz), or cups (c). Choose a measurement that is familiar to you. A healthcare provider or dietitian should change units of measurement if needed.

Soup needs to be separated into liquids and solids before given to it. Write down the amount of liquid before giving.

Some tips for how to restrict fluid intake include:
❖ Using small glasses, such as juice glasses
❖ Limiting salt intake
❖ Sucking on hard candy, frozen fruit, or ice cubes
❖ Chewing gum
❖ Sipping, rather than gulping, liquid
❖ Spacing out fluid intake
❖ Controlling sugar intake
❖ Measuring out daily fluid intake in a large bottle
❖ Making a note of fluid intake through the day

- Using a refreshing mouthwash when the mouth feels dry
- Ice cubes, ice-lollies, cubes of frozen squash or fizzy drinks may be more satisfying than a drink – but remember to include these in fluid allowance.
- Try sucking boiled sweets or lemon slices.
- Eat mints or chew chewing gum.
- Try using a mouth wash or rinse mouth with ice cold water.
- Try eating frozen grapes or pineapple chunks (unless patient have been advised to restrict these foods).

Treatment Considerations and Tips

In addition to following a low-sodium diet and taking diuretics ("water pills") as prescribed by your healthcare provider, a fluid restriction can help to achieve your health goals. Depending on the fluid limit outlined for your condition and prescribed by your healthcare provider the following are strategies to help manage your daily fluid intake:

Plan out the amount of liquid you will have during the day: How much will you drink to take your medications? How much will you drink with your meals? In order to decide what works best for you, it is helpful to sit down with a nutritionist or nurse and talk with friends and family who may be able to support you. By identifying preferred drinks and your drinking pattern, you will more easily be able to decide how to adjust to your fluid restriction.

Use small cups: Using a small cup can give the perception of a full glass.

Use a designated container: Some people find it helpful to measure out their daily fluid allowance in one large container and drink only from there throughout the day.

Maintain good oral care: By brushing your teeth after meals, rinsing with alcohol free mouthwash, chewing sugarless gum or sucking on hard candy you may be able to decrease dry mouth and urges to drink.

Avoid foods with high levels of sodium (salt): These types of foods will increase your thirst.

Weigh yourself daily: It is important to use the same scale around the same time each day to get the most accurate information and report any weight gain of 2 pounds or more in one day to your physician;

Record your fluid intake: Recording your fluid intake will help make sure that you are not taking in more fluids than expected. It is a good idea to write this information on a tracking log/calendar (a sample is attached).

You will need to learn the number of cubic centimeters (cc's) or milliliters (mL's) in common servings. Some sample measurements are included below.

Soups, food prepared with water, and semi-solids such as popsicles, and jello, should count toward your total daily fluid intake.

Helpful Tips to Remember

- Food that melts at room temperature is considered a liquid.
- Include liquid amounts when taking medications.
- Maintain a daily log and track all fluid intake.
- Satisfy thirst by sucking on an ice cube, hard candy, chewing gum, or rinsing mouth with water—but do not swallow.

Fluid Measurements

1 ounce = 30 cc
8 ounces = 240 cc
1 cup = 8 ounces = 240 cc

Sample Measurements

Coffee cup = 200 cc
Clear glass = 240 cc
Milk carton = 240 cc
Small milk carton = 120 cc
Juice, JJelly for ice cream cup = 120 cc
Soup bowl = 160 cc
Popsicle half = 40 cc

Administration of Medications

UNIT

9

Unit Outline

- Medication
- Medication orders and prescriptions
- Systems of measurement
- Medication dose calculation
- Principles, 10 rights of medication administration
- Errors in medication administration
- Routes of administration
- Storage and maintenance of drugs and nurses responsibility
- Parenteral administration of drugs
- Cannulas, infusion sets–parts, types, sizes
- Types of vials and ampules
- Topical administration
- Inhalation
- Other parenteral routes

LEARNING OBJECTIVES

At the end of this unit, the reader will be able to:
- Introduce medication administration.
- Outline pharmacy abbreviations and symbols.
- State drug nomenclature.
- Define pharmacokinetic and pharmacodynamics.
- Classify forms of medication.
- Enumerate factors influencing medication action.
- Recognize prescription and orders.
- Interpret metric system.
- Define apothecary system.
- Explain household system.
- Estimate drug calculation.
- Calculate IV flow rate.
- Enumerate principles and rights of drug administration.
- Outline factors influencing errors in drug administration.
- List out types of medication error and its preventive measures.
- Describe routes of drug administration.
- Illustrate equipment for drug administration.
- Differentiate ampules and vials.
- Practice safe handling of vials.
- Define needle stick injuries and preventive measures.
- Explain irrigations: Eye, ear, bladder, vaginal, rectal.
- Other parenteral routes.

TERMINOLOGIES

- ❖ **Allergic reaction:** A reaction caused by an unusual hypersensitivity to a medication (allergic reactions can also occur with foods, animals and other environmental substances).
- ❖ **Counter indicative:** A condition or factor that increases the risks involved in using a particular drug or engaging in a particular activity (e.g., smoking).
- ❖ **Drug:** A word often used interchangeably with the word medication.
- ❖ **Generic name:** The name given by the federal government to a drug.
- ❖ **Medication:** Substance taken into (or applied to) the body for the purpose of prevention, treatment, relief of symptoms, or cure.
- ❖ **Medication administration:** The direct application of a prescribed medication—whether by injection, inhalation, ingestion, or other means—to the body of the individual by an individual legally authorized to do so.
- ❖ **Medication assistance:** Assistance with self-administration of medication rendered by a nonpractitioner to an individual receiving supported living residential services and supports.
- ❖ **Interactions:** The result, either desirable or undesirable, of drugs interacting with themselves, other drugs, foods, alcohol, or other substances (e.g., herbs or nutrients).
- ❖ **Medication error:** Any time the right medication is not taken as prescribed.
- ❖ **Delegation:** The procedure following a specific set of guidelines and standards that allow staff with a prescribed training and certification to perform medical tasks.
- ❖ **Ophthalmic:** Referring to the eyes.
- ❖ **Otic:** Referring to the ears.
- ❖ **Over-the-counter (OTC) medications:** All nonprescription medications including aspirin, antihistamines, vitamin supplements, and herbal remedies.
- ❖ **Pharmacist:** Licensed individual who prepares and dispenses drugs and is knowledgeable about their contents.
- ❖ **Physician/Doctor:** An individual licensed to practice medicine; for the purpose of prescribing medications only, the term is interpreted to mean any healthcare professional authorized by law to prescribe drugs: physician, dentist, optometrist, podiatrist, and nurse practitioner or physician's assistant (who write prescriptions is acting under the supervision of the individual's physician).
- ❖ **Prescription medications:** Medications that must be ordered by a physician or other licensed healthcare professional with authority to write prescriptions, such as a dentist or nurse practitioner.
- ❖ **PRN (pro re nata) medications:** Means that the medication is taken as needed to treat a specific symptom; PRN medications include both prescription and over-the-counter (OTC) medications. [Note: all PRN's must be documented on the Medication Administration Record (MAR)].
- ❖ **Psychoactive:** Possessing the ability to alter mood, anxiety level, behavior, cognitive processes, or mental tension; usually applied to pharmacological agents.
- ❖ **Psychoactive medications:** Refers to medications prescribed to treat a mental illness, improve functioning, or reduce challenging behaviors.; psychoactive medications include antipsychotics/neuroleptics, atypical antipsychotics, antidepressants, anticonvulsants, stimulants, sedatives/hypnotics, and antimania and antianxiety drugs; anticonvulsants and other classes of drugs are included in this category when they are prescribed for behavioral purposes. [Note: If a psychoactive medication is used solely to treat a physical condition

(e.g., sleep aid, seizures) or dementia, and is not also used to treat a mental illness or for challenging behavior, it is not considered a psychoactive medication].

❖ **Side effects:** Unintended effects produced by medication other than those for which it was prescribed; sometimes side effects, such as a severe allergic reaction, can be deadly.

❖ **Topical:** Applied to a certain area of the skin.

❖ **Trade name/brand name:** The name given by the manufacturer to a medication.

❖ Drug is any substance or product that is used or intended to be used to modify or explore physiological systems or pathological status for the benefit of the recipient.

MEDICATION

A medication (also called medicament, medicine, pharmaceutical drug, medicinal drug or simply drug). A medication is a drug used to diagnose, cure, treat, or prevent disease.

Medication is a medicine or a chemical compound used to treat or cure illness. According to *Encyclopædia Britannica*, medication is "a substance used in treating a disease or relieving pain".

As defined by the National Cancer Institute, dosage forms of medication can include tablets, capsules, liquids, creams, and patches.

Any substance or combination of substances which may be used in or administered to human beings either with a view to restoring, correcting or modifying physiological functions by exerting a pharmacological, immunological or metabolic action or to making a medical diagnosis.

Medication Administration

Medication administration means the direct application of a medication or device by ingestion, inhalation, injection or any other means, whether self-administered by a resident, or administered by a guardian (for a minor), or an authorized healthcare provider.

The giving or application of a pharmacologic or other therapeutic agent.

Medication administration means the physical act of giving medication to a client by the prescribed route.

Pharmacy Abbreviations and Symbols

The following abbreviations and symbols are commonly used on medication labels. In order to read and understand medication labels, you should be familiar with these abbreviations and symbols:

❖ Rx = Prescription
❖ OTC = Over-the-counter
❖ PRN = when necessary, or as needed
❖ Qty = quantity
❖ q (Q) = every
❖ qd = daily
❖ bid (BID) = twice a day
❖ tid (TID) = three times a day
❖ qid (QID) = four times a day
❖ h = hour
❖ hs (HS) = hour of sleep (bedtime)

❖ tsp = teaspoon (or 5 mL)
❖ Tbsp = tablespoon (3 tsps or 15 mL)
❖ oz = ounce
❖ gr = grains
❖ mg = milligrams
❖ GM, gm = grams (1,000 mg)
❖ Cap = capsule
❖ Tab = tablet
❖ AM = morning
❖ PM = afternoon/evening
❖ D/C or d/c = discontinue

	Latin term	*Common abbreviation*	*Translation*
A…			
	Ad	Ad	to, up to
		ad lib	at pleasure
	Adde	Add	add (thou)
	Agita	Agit	shake, stir
	alternis horis	alt. h	every other hour
	Ana	aa or aa	of each
	Ante	a	before
	ante cibum	ac	before food, before meals
	ante meridian	am	morning
		amp	ampule
	Aqua	aq	water
	aqua ad	aq ad	water up to
		ag dest; aqua dist	distilled water
	Auris	aur; a	ear
	auris dexter	ad	right ear
	aurix laevus	al	left ear
	auris sinister	as	left ear
	auris utro	au	each ear
	Auristillae	Aorist	ear-drops
		atc	around the clock
B…			
	Bis	b	twice
	bis in die	bid	twice a day
	Brachium	brach	the arm
		BSA	body surface area
C…			
	Capsula	Caps	a capsule
		cc	cubic centimeter
	Chartulae	Charts	powder papers; divided powders
	Cibus	cib; c	food
	Collunarium	Collun	a nose wash
	Collutorium	collut	a mouthwash
	Collyrium	collyr	an eyewash
	Compositus	comp	compound
	Congius	cong; C	gallon
	Cum	c or c	with
	cum cibus	cc	with food; with meals
D…			
	Denture	d	give (thou); let be given

Contd…

Contd...

	Latin term	Common abbreviation	Translation
	dentur tales doses	dtd	give of such doses
	Dexter	d	right
	diebus alternis	dieb. alt	every other day
	Dilutes	dil	dilute, diluted
		disp	dispense
		div	divide
		DW	distilled water
E...			
		elix	elixir
	Emulsum	emuls	emulsion
	Et	Et	and
	ex modo prescripto	emp	in the manner prescribed; as directed
F...			
	fac, fiat, fiant	f; ft	let it be made; make
		f; fl	fluid
G...			
		g; G; gm	gram
	Granum	gr	grain
	Guttae	gtt	a drop
H...			
	Hora	H	at the hour of
	hora somni	hs	at bedtime
I...			
		im	intramuscular
	Injection	inj	injection
		iv; IV	intravenous
		ivp; IVP	intravenous push
		IVPB	intravenous piggyback
L...			
	Laevus	l	Left
	Linimentum	lin	Liniment
	Liquor	liq	a solution
		lot	Lotion
M...			
	Minimum	min; Mx	Minim
	Misce	m; M	Mix
		mcg	Microgram
		mEq	Milliequivalent

Contd...

Contd...

	Latin term	Common abbreviation	Translation
		mg	Milligram
		mL	Millilitre
N...			
	Nocte	n	at night
	Naristillae	narist	nasal drops
	Nebule	neb	a spray
		NF	National Formulary
	non repetatur	non.rep.	do not repeat
		NS	normal saline
O...			
	Octarius	O	Pint
	Oculentum	occulent	eye ointment
	Oculus	o	Eye
	oculus dexter	od	right eye
	oculus laevus	ol	left eye
	oculus sinister	os	left eye
	oculus utro	ou	both eyes, each eye
	omni mane	om	every morning
P...			
	parti affectae applicandus	paa	to be applied to affected part
	per os	po	by mouth
	post cibum	pc	after meals
		pr	per rectum
	pro re nata	prn	as needed
	Pulvis	pulv	Powder
Q...			
	quater in die	qid	four times a day
	Quaque	q	each, every
	quaque die	qd	every day
	quaque hora	qh	every hour
	quantum sufficiat	qs	a sufficient quantity
	quantum sufficiat ad	qs ad	a sufficient quantity to make
R...			
S...			
	secundum artem	sa	according to the art
		SC; subc; subq	Subcutaneously
	Semis	Ss	one-half
	Signa	Sig	write, label

Contd...

Contd...

	Latin term	*Common abbreviation*	*Translation*
	Sine	S	Without
	si opus sit	sos	if necessary
		sol	Solution
	Statim	stat	Immediately
	Suppositorum	supp	Suppository
	Syrupus	syr	Syrup
T...			
	Tabella	tab	Tablet
		tbsp	Tablespoonful
	ter in die	tid	three times a day
		tinc; tr	Tincture
	Trochiscus	Troche	Lozenge
	Tussis	tuss	a cough
U...			
	Ungentum	ung.	an ointment
	ut dictum	ut dict; ud	as directed

❖ Oral medications (capsules or tablets) are usually prescribed in mg (milligrams) or gm (grams).

❖ Liquid medications are usually prescribed in mL (milliliters), cc (centimeters), or oz (ounces).

❖ Liquid medications may also be prescribed in tsp (teaspoon), or Tbsp (tablespoon).

DRUG NOMENCLATURE

Introduction

Drug nomenclature is a systematic approach to naming the active component of a drug product for the purposes of identification, standardization, and unequivocal differential characterization.

The term drug nomenclature implies to the systematic and scientific naming of drugs. A drug generally has three different categories of names: chemical name, non-proprietary name and proprietary name.

This is the system that puts drugs into classification. Drugs are classifies into convenient groups for the sake of conformity, standardization, esoteric values of manufactures, research and replication and quality assurance.

A drug generally has three categories of names:

1. **Chemical name:** It describes the chemical structure of a drug, e.g., acetylsalicylic acid is the chemical name of aspirin. And N-acetyl-p-aminophenol is the chemical name of paracetamol. Chemical name is cumbersome and not suitable for use in prescription.

2. **Nonproprietary name:** It is the name accepted by a competent scientific body/authority, e.g., The United States Adopted Name (USAN) council. Commonly the term generic name is used in place of nonproprietary name. It is uniform throughout the world and denotes the active pharmaceutical ingredient. Ideally generic name should be used in prescriptions because it is generally uniform all over the world than the branded counterparts.

3. **Proprietary name (brand name):** It is the name given by the drug manufacturers. Brand names are designed to be catchy, short, easy to remember and often suggestive (e.g., LOPRESOR suggesting drug for lowering BP) One drug may have multiple brand names. It may have different names within a country and in different countries. Brand names can also be used in prescriptions, e.g., DISPRIN is a brand name of ASPIRIN. CROCIN is a brand name of PARACETAMOL.

A chemical name is given when a new chemical entity (NCE) is developed and it describes the substance chemically, e.g., 7-chloro-1, 3-dihydro-1-methyl-5-phenyl-2H-1,4-benzodiazepin-2-one for diazepam. It is the name given to drug in accordance with rules of chemical nomenclature established by International Union of Pure and Applied Chemistry (IUPAC).

It is useful for chemists or technical personals as it provides the precise arrangement of atoms and atomic groups in the molecule. It is difficult and not used to identify the drug in a clinical (prescribing) or marketing situation. A code name, e.g., RO15-1788 (later named flumazenil) is the name given by the manufacturer for convenience and simplicity before an approved name. A nonproprietary name of a drug, after its regulatory approval, is the accepted name by a competent scientific body/authority, e.g., British Approved Name (BAN), Japanese Accepted Name (JAN) and United States Adopted Name (USAN), etc.

The nonproprietary names of newer drugs are kept uniform by an agreement to use the Recommended International Nonproprietary Name (rINN) in all member countries of World Health Organization (WHO).

A proprietary name or brand name is the name assigned by the manufacturer(s) and is the property or trade mark of the concerned pharmaceutical farm. Thus a single drug may be sold under different proprietary names by different manufacturers. For example, haloperidol is marketed under the brand names of Bezydol-P, Brain-Rest, Cizoren, Depidol, Gendol and Dolcin etc. The INN name or more popularly known as generic name identifies a pharmaceutical substance by a unique name that is globally recognized to varying extent and is public property. We will be restricting our discussion on the different aspects of INN nomenclature.

The INN nomenclature system: The system of INN was initiated by WHO through the World Health Assembly resolution and began operating in 1953. The first list of international nonproprietary names for pharmaceutical substances was published in the same year. Since then, thousands of pharmaceutical substances have been designated as INNs so far and continuously updated. WHO works in close collaboration with the major national nomenclature commissions, e.g., British Approved Name (BAN), Japanese Accepted Name (JAN), United States Adopted Name (USAN) etc. An International Nonproprietary Name (INN) identifies a pharmaceutical substance by a unique name that is globally recognized and is public property. INNs help to reduce confusion in drug nomenclature and allow us an understanding of the drug even when that individual drug is not known. They are the vital piece of information that is compulsory on medicine labels. INNs are nonproprietary in nature, which implies that the same INN can be used by all manufacturers of that pharmaceutical substance, irrespective of the brand name under which the drug is marketed by each manufacturer. These names are intended to be used in pharmacopoeias, labeling, advertising, drug regulation and scientific literature. The term approved name is used until the drug is included in an official pharmacopoeia. The approved name becomes official name after its appearance in the official pharmacopoeia. The procedure of INN selection

Any person or company proposing and requesting for an INN needs to apply to WHO online at http://www.who.int/medicines/services/inn/en/index.html. Applications are also accepted by WHO made through the national nomenclature committee from the applicants where national nomenclature commissions exist. Members of the WHO expert panel on International Pharmacopoeia and Pharmaceutical Preparations or sometimes other panel examine with a formal procedure and select a nonproprieatary, agreed name based on the information provided. A four month window period is kept thereafter for any comments or formal objection to the proposed name by any person. If no objection is raised within that period, this agreed name is published as the recommended INN. WHO has strictly recommended in 1993 that pharmaceutical companies should not derive trade names from INNs as such practice may frustrate the rational selection of INNs and compromise the patient safety by confusing the drug nomenclature. In India, the trademark registration of words that are declared as INNs or those that are deceptively similar to INNs is prohibited under Section 13 (b) of the Trade Marks Act, 1999.

INN stems: The root of the nonproprietary naming system is the collection of short name fragments called stems. They define the pharmacologically related group to which the INN belongs. Each stem has a meaning connected to a particular drug class or mode of action. The stems and their definitions have been selected by WHO experts and are used when selecting new international nonproprietary names. The naming process itself "is an evolving type of science and therefore the nomenclature process is ongoing and constantly under revision". Definitions of older stems are modified as and when newer information becomes available. An INN generally includes the "common stem" expressing the pharmacologically-related group to which the substance belongs. Names conveying anatomical, physiological, pathological or therapeutic suggestions are avoided while devising an INN. International connotations are also considered while selecting an INN. A name that sounds perfectly fine in English might have bad or even obscene connotations elsewhere. Therefore, to make pronunciation possible in various languages, the letters "h" and "k" are avoided; "e" is used instead of "ae" and "oe", "i" instead of "y", "t" instead of "th" and "f" instead of "ph". Stems are generally used as suffixes but sometimes they are also used as prefixes.

Classification System used by the INN Programme

The WHO stem classification system used by the INN Programme follows a core list to categorize the main activity of pharmaceutical substances while devising an INN. Each category included in the list has an appropriate code consisting of a capital letter and three digits, category, specific stem and appropriate information. When INNs for substances belonging to a given category include a specific stem, appropriate information is included in the list.

Pharmacokinetics

Pharmacokinetics is the quantitative study of drug movement in, through and out of the body. The overall scheme of pharmacokinetic processes is depicted in Figure on next page. The intensity of response is related to concentration of the drug at the site of action, which in turn is dependent on its pharmacokinetic properties. Pharmacokinetic considerations, therefore, determine the route(s) of administration, dose, latency of onset, time of peak action, duration of action and frequency of administration of a drug.

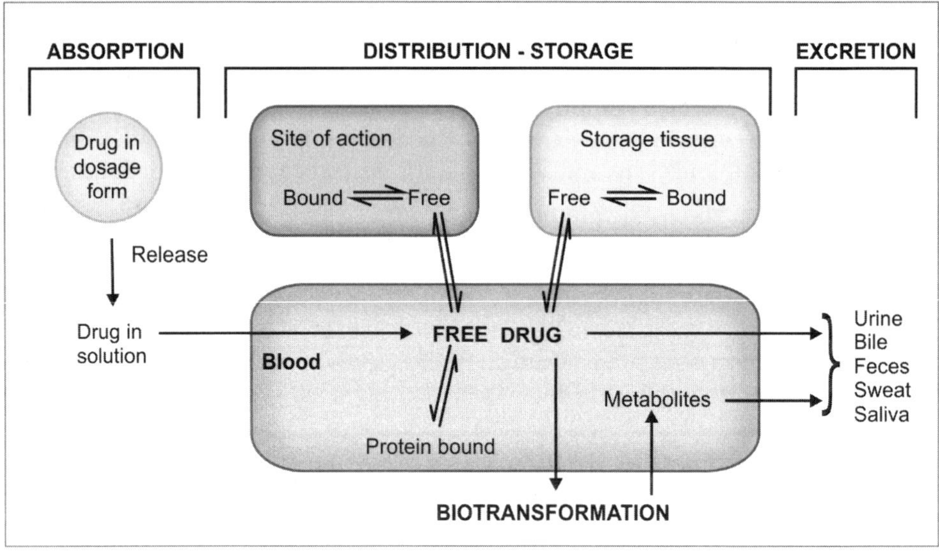

Schematic depiction of pharmacokinetic processes.

All pharmacokinetic processes involve transport of the drug across biological membranes.

Biological Membrane

This is a bilayer (about 100 Å thick) of phospholipid and cholesterol molecules, the polar groups (glyceryl phosphate attached to ethanolamine/choline or hydroxyl group of cholesterol) of these are oriented at the two surfaces and the nonpolar hydrocarbon chains are embedded in the matrix to form a continuous sheet. Extrinsic and intrinsic protein molecules are adsorbed on the lipid bilayer.

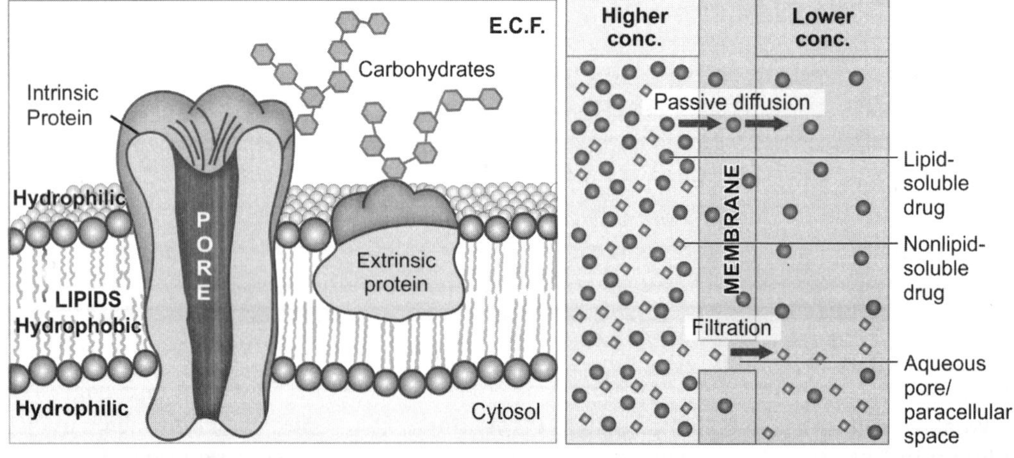

Glycoproteins or glycolipids are formed on the surface by attachment to polymeric sugars, aminosugars or sialic acids. The specific lipid and protein composition of different membranes differs according to the cell or the organelle type. The proteins are able to freely float through the membrane: associate and organize or vice versa. Some of the intrinsic ones, which extend through the full thickness of the membrane, surround fine aqueous pores. Paracellular spaces or channels also exist between certain epithelial/endothelial cells. Other adsorbed proteins have enzymatic, carrier, receptor or signal transduction properties. Lipid molecules also are capable of lateral movement. Thus, biological membranes are highly dynamic structures.

Drugs are transported across the membranes by:
- Passive diffusion and filtration
- Specialized transport

Passive Diffusion

The drug diffuses across the membrane in the direction of its concentration gradient, the membrane playing no active role in the process. This is the most important mechanism for majority of drugs; drugs are foreign substances (xenobiotics), and specialized mechanisms are developed by the body primarily for normal metabolites.

Lipid soluble drugs diffuse by dissolving in the lipoidal matrix of the membrane the rate of transport being proportional to the lipid: water partition coefficient of the drug. A more lipid soluble drug attains higher concentration in the membrane and diffuses quickly. Also, greater the difference in the concentration of the drug on the two sides of the membrane, faster is its diffusion.

Influence of pH: Most drugs are weak electrolytes, i.e., their ionization is pH dependent (contrast strong electrolytes that are nearly completely ionized at acidic as well as alkaline pH). The ionization of a weak acid HA is given by the equation:

$$pH = pKa + \log\frac{[A^-]}{[HA]} \qquad \ldots(1)$$

pKa is the negative logarithm of acidic dissociation constant of the weak electrolyte. If the concentration of ionized drug $[A^-]$ is equal to concentration of unionized drug $[HA]$, then

$$\frac{[A^-]}{[HA]} = 1$$

Since log 1 is 0, under this condition

$$pH = pKa \qquad \ldots(2)$$

Thus, pKa is numerically equal to the pH at which the drug is 50% ionized.

If pH is increased by 1 scale, then—log $[A–]/[HA] = 1$ or $[A^-]/[HA] = 10$

Similarly, if pH is reduced by 1 scale, then— $[A^-]/[HA] = 1/10$

Thus, weakly acidic drugs, which form salts with cations, e.g., *sod.* phenobarbitone, *sod.* sulfadiazine, *pot.* penicillinV, etc. ionize more at alkaline pH and 1 scale change in pH causes 10 fold change in ionization.

Weakly basic drugs, which form salts with anions, e.g., atropine *sulfate*, ephedrine *HCl*, chloroquine *phosphate,* etc. conversely ionize more at acidic pH. Ions being lipid insoluble, do not diffuse and a pH difference across a membrane can cause differential distribution of weakly acidic and weakly basic drugs on the two sides.

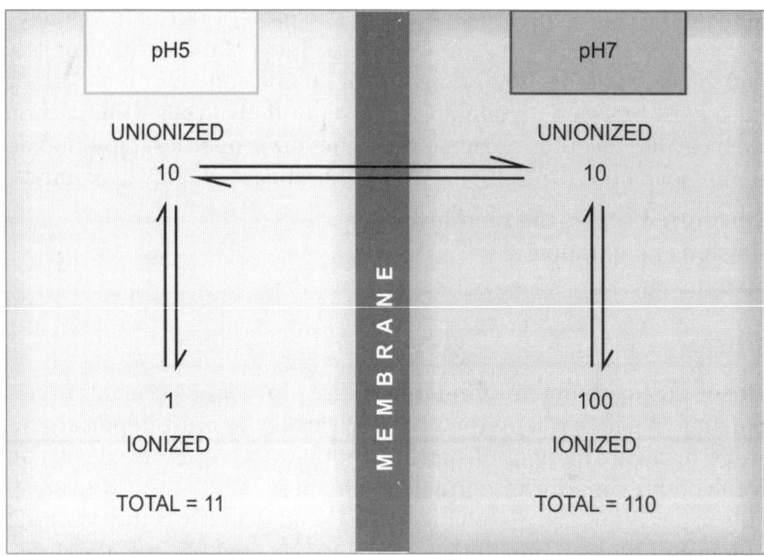

Influence of pH difference on two sides of a biological membrane on the steady-state distribution of a weakly acidic drug with pKa = 6.

Implications of this consideration are: Acidic drugs, e.g., aspirin (*pKa* 3.5) are largely unionized at acid gastric pH and are absorbed from stomach, while bases, e.g., atropine (*pKa* 10) are largely ionized and are absorbed only when they reach the intestines.

The unionized form of acidic drugs which crosses the surface membrane of gastric mucosal cell, reverts to the ionized form within the cell (pH 7.0) and then only slowly passes to the extracellular fluid. This is called *ion trapping*, i.e., a weak electrolyte crossing a membrane to encounter a pH from which it is not able to escape easily. This may contribute to gastric mucosal cell damage caused by aspirin.

Basic drugs attain higher concentration intracellularly (pH 7.0 *vs* 7.4 of plasma).

Acidic drugs are ionized more in alkaline urine—do not back diffuse in the kidney tubules and are excreted faster. Accordingly, basic drugs are excreted faster if urine is acidified.

Lipid soluble nonelectrolytes (e.g., ethanol, diethylether) readily cross biological membranes and their transport is pH independent.

Filtration

Filtration is passage of drugs through aqueous pores in the membrane or through paracellular spaces. This can be accelerated if hydrodynamic flow of the solvent is occurring under hydrostatic or osmotic pressure gradient, e.g., across most capillaries including glomeruli. Lipid insoluble drugs cross biological membranes by filtration if their molecular size is smaller than the diameter of the pores. Majority of cells (intestinal mucosa, RBC, etc.) have very small pores (4 Å) and drugs with MW >100 or 200 are not able to penetrate. However, capillaries (except those in brain) have large paracellular spaces (40 Å) and most drugs (even albumin) can filter through these. As such, diffusion of drugs across capillaries is dependent on rate of blood flow through them rather than on lipid solubility of the drug or pH of the medium.

Specialized Transport

This can be carrier mediated or by pinocytosis.

A. Carrier Transport

All cell membranes express a host of transmembrane proteins which serve as carriers or transporters for physiologically important ions, nutrients, metabolites, transmitters, etc., across the membrane. At some sites, certain transporters also translocate xenobiotics, including drugs and their metabolites. In contrast to channels, which open for a finite time and allow passage of specific ions, transporters combine transiently with their substrate (ion or organic compound)—undergo a conformational change carrying the substrate to the other side of the membrane where the substrate dissociates and the transporter returns back to its original state. Carrier transport is specific for the substrate (or the type of substrate, e.g., an organic anion), saturable, competitively inhibited by analogues which utilize the same transporter, and is much slower than flux through channels. Depending on requirement of energy, carrier transport is of two types:

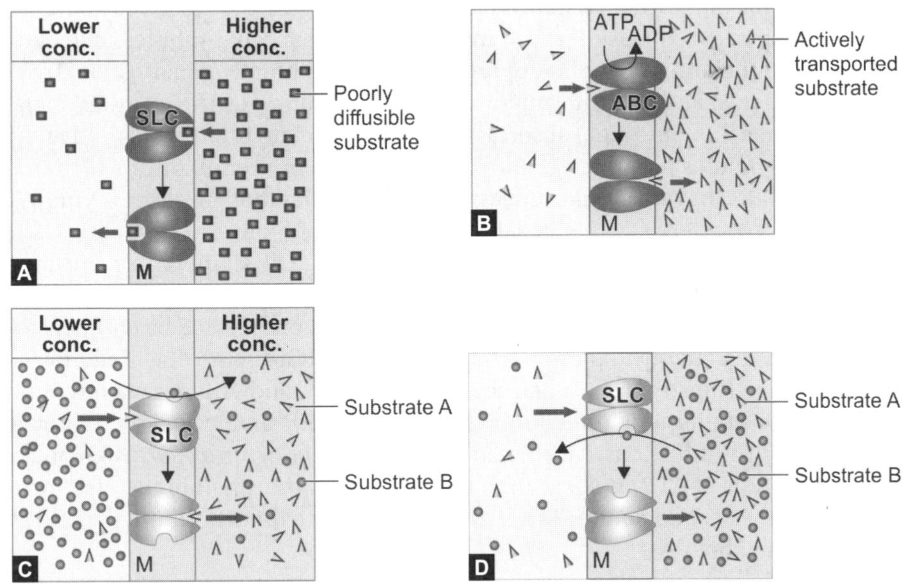

Illustration of different types of carrier mediated transport across biological membrane.

ABC: ATP-binding cassette transporter; SLC: solute carrier transporter; M: membrane

A. Facilitated diffusion: The carrier (SLC) binds and moves the poorly diffusible substrate along its concentration gradient (high to low) and does not require energy

B. Primary active transport: The carrier (ABC) derives energy directly by hydrolyzing ATP and moves the substrate against its concentration gradient (low to high)

C. Symport: The carrier moves the substrate 'A' against its concentration gradient by utilizing energy from downhill movement of another substrate 'B' in the same direction

D. Antiport: The carrier moves the substrate 'A' against its concentration gradient and is energized by the downhill movement of another substrate 'B' in the opposite direction.

a. **Facilitated diffusion:** The transporter, belonging to the superfamily of *solute carrier* (SLC) transporters, operates passively without needing energy and translocates the substrate in the direction of its electrochemical gradient, i.e., from higher to lower concentration. It nearly facilitates permeation of a poorly diffusible substrate, e.g., the entry of glucose into muscle and fat cells by GLUT 4.

b. **Active transport:** It requires energy, is inhibited by metabolic poisons, and transports the solute against its electrochemical gradient (low to high), resulting in selective accumulation of the substance on one side of the membrane. Drugs related to normal metabolites can utilize the transport processes meant for these, e.g., levodopa and methyl dopa are actively absorbed from the gut by the aromatic amino acid transporter. In addition, the body has developed some relatively nonselective transporters, like *P-glycoprotein* (Pgp), to deal with xenobiotics. Active transport can be primary or secondary depending on the source of the driving force.

   i. *Primary active transport:* Energy is obtained directly by the hydrolysis of ATP. The transporters belong to the superfamily of *ATP-binding cassette* (ABC) transporters whose intracellular loops have ATPase activity. They mediate only efflux of the solute from the cytoplasm, either to extracellular fluid or into an intracellular organelli (endoplasmic reticulum, mitochondria, etc.)

   Encoded by the multidrug resistance 1 (MDR1) gene, Pgp is the most well known primary active transporter expressed in the intestinal mucosa, renal tubules, bile canaliculi, choroidal epithelium, astrocyte foot processes around brain capillaries (the bloodbrain barrier), testicular and placental microvessels, which pumps out many drugs/metabolites and thus limits their intestinal absorption, penetration into brain, testes and fetal tissues as well as promotes biliary and renal elimination. Many xenobiotics which induce or inhibit Pgp also have a similar effect on the drug metabolizing isoenzyme CYP3A4, indicating their synergistic role in detoxification of xenobiotics.

   Other primary active transporters of pharmacological significance are multidrug resistance associated protein 2 (MRP 2) and breast cancer resistance protein (BCRP).

   ii. *Secondary active transport:* In this type of active transport effected by another set of SLC transporters, the energy to pump one solute is derived from the downhill movement of another solute (mostly Na^+). When the concentration gradients are such that both the solutes move in the same direction, it is called *symport* or *cotransport*, but when they move in opposite directions, it is termed *antiport* or *exchange transport*. Metabolic energy (from hydrolysis of ATP) is spent in maintaining high transmembrane electrochemical gradient of the second solute. The SLC transporters mediate both uptake and efflux of drugs and metabolites.

The organic anion transporting polypeptide (OATP) and organic cation transporter (OCT), highly expressed in liver canaliculi and renal tubules, are secondary active transporters important in the metabolism and excretion of drugs and metabolites (especially glucuronides). The Na^+,Cl^- dependent neurotransmitter transporters for serotonin and dopamine (SERT and DAT) as well as the vesicular transporter for biogenic amines are active SLC transporters that are targets for action of drugs like tricyclic antidepressants and reserpine, etc. The absorption of glucose in intestines and renal tubules is through secondary active transport by sodium glucose transporters (SGLT1 and SGLT2).

As indicated earlier, carrier transport (both facilitated diffusion and active transport) is saturable and follows the Michaelis Menten kinetics. The maximal rate of transport is dependent on the density of the transporter in a particular membrane, and its rate constant

(Km), i.e., the substrate concentration at which rate of transport is half maximal, is governed by its affinity for the substrate. Genetic polymorphism can alter both the density and affinity of the transporter protein for different substrates and thus affect the pharmacokinetics of drugs. Moreover, tissue specific drug distribution can occur due to the presence of specific transporters in certain cells.

B. Pinocytosis

It is the process of transport across the cell in particulate form by formation of vesicles. This is applicable to proteins and other big molecules, and contributes little to transport of most drugs.

PHARMACOKINETICS

Pharmacodynamics is the study of a drug's molecular, biochemical, and physiologic effects or actions. It comes from the Greek words "pharmakon," meaning "drug," and "dynamikos," meaning "power."

All drugs produce their effects by interacting with biological structures or targets at the molecular level to induce a change in how the target molecule functions in regard to subsequent intermolecular interactions. These interactions include receptor binding, postreceptor effects, and chemical interactions. Examples of these types of interactions include:

❖ Drugs binding to an active site of an enzyme
❖ Drugs that interact with cell surface signaling proteins to disrupt downstream signaling, and
❖ Drugs that act by binding molecules like tumor necrosis factor (TNF).

Pharmacodynamics and pharmacokinetics are the two branches of pharmacology, with pharmacodynamics studying the action of the drug on the organism and pharmacokinetics studying the effect the organism has on the drug.

Pharmacodynamic actions include:

❖ Stimulating activity by directly inhibiting a receptor and its downstream effects
❖ Depressing activity by direct receptor inhibition and its downstream effects
❖ Antagonistic or blocking a receptor by binding to it but not activating it
❖ Stabilizing action, where the drug apparently behaves as neither an agonist nor antagonist
❖ Direct chemical reactions (beneficial in therapy and also as an adverse event)

Any of these factors can work both therapeutically as well as precipitate an adverse event.

Pharmacodynamics places particular emphasis on dose-response relationships, which are the relationships between the concentration of a drug and its effect, whether negative or positive, upon the organism.

Negative/undesirable effects include the increased probability of cell mutation (otherwise known as carcinogenic activity), induced physiological damage, abnormal chronic conditions, adverse reproductive effects, and lethality. Therefore, knowledge of a drug's behavior is absolutely vital in drug development studies.

Pharmacodynamics (sometimes described as what a drug does to the body) is the study of the biochemical, physiologic, and molecular effects of drugs on the body and involves receptor binding (including receptor sensitivity), postreceptor effects, and chemical interactions. Pharmacodynamics, with pharmacokinetics (what the body does to a drug, or the fate of a drug within the body), helps explain the relationship between the dose and response, i.e., the drug's effects. The pharmacologic response depends on the drug binding to its target. The concentration of the drug at the receptor site influences the drug's effect.

A drug's pharmacodynamics can be affected by physiologic changes due to:

- ❖ A disorder or disease
- ❖ Aging process
- ❖ Other drugs

Disorders that affect pharmacodynamic responses include genetic mutations, thyrotoxicosis, malnutrition, myasthenia gravis, Parkinson disease, and some forms of insulin-resistant diabetes mellitus. These disorders can change receptor binding, alter the level of binding proteins, or decrease receptor sensitivity.

Aging tends to affect pharmacodynamic responses through alterations in receptor binding or in postreceptor response sensitivity.

Pharmacodynamic drug–drug interactions result in competition for receptor binding sites or alter postreceptor response.

Multicellular Pharmacodynamics

Recently, pharmacodynamic concepts have been expanded to include multicellular pharmacodynamics (MCPD). MCPD concepts help researchers to understand the dynamic and static relationships between drugs and multicellular four-dimensional organization in organisms. In this way, a drug's action upon a minimal multicellular system can be studied both *in vivo* and *in silico*.

Networked multicellular pharmacodynamics extends the MCPD concept to include accurate modeling of regulatory genomic networks in combination with signal transduction pathways. With these concepts, the complex interacting components within a cell and how drugs affect them can be studied more effectively.

Forms of Medication

A medical professional may choose a particular dosage form to target a specific area or body organ without the systemic or side effects of oral or injectable medications. For instance, skin treatments such as topical creams, ointments, lotions, patches, or other dosage forms such as nasal sprays, eye drops, and suppositories to deliver medication to the affected area without causing systemic (body-wide) side effects. Liquid forms of medicine typically contain the same active ingredient as solid forms, and they are the more optimal option for children and adults with difficulty swallowing tablets.

Different Forms of Oral Medication

Oral medications start working once they reach the digestive tract and are absorbed into the bloodstream. Other medication forms, such as topical treatments and injections, bypass the digestive tract and enter the bloodstream directly.

Tablets

This solid dosage form is the most common form of oral medication. The active pharmaceutical ingredient is bound into a solid form (pill) with one or more inactive substances. Tablets or pills are available in different shapes and sizes.

Some of the advantages of administering medication in pill form include:

- ❖ Affordability (they are mass-produced and generally inexpensive)
- ❖ Stable dosage form (they have a long shelf-life)

❖ Accurate dosing (you don't need to measure the dose, but keep in mind, sometimes, you will have to split the scored tablet into smaller doses based on the prescribed dosage)
❖ Ease of use (you can swallow a pill with a glass of water)
❖ Light and compact (they are easy to travel with)
❖ The convenience of combination products (some pills contain more than one active substance)
❖ Bitter medicines can be coated to make them more palatable

The disadvantages of tablets include:
❖ Aftertaste (may leave a bad taste in the mouth after swallowing)
❖ Slower acting (may take longer to work)
❖ More likely to irritate the gastrointestinal tract causing nausea, vomiting, and diarrhea

There are different types of oral tablets, such as:

a. **Enteric coated tablets:** These are coated with special polymers that prevent them from dissolving in stomach acid and allow them to be absorbed in the small intestine. Examples include certain antibiotics and proton pump inhibitors to treat gastroesophageal reflux disease.

b. **Sublingual tablets:** A sublingual tablet is placed under the tongue, where it dissolves and is absorbed into the blood via the oral mucosa. Examples include sublingual nitroglycerine used to treat angina chest pain.
   This method of administration is useful when you want the drug to work quickly. In addition, it is suitable for people who cannot swallow tablets. It's also useful for medications that are not well absorbed in the stomach or if their effectiveness is decreased by digestion.
   The disadvantages of sublingual tablets are that eating, drinking, and smoking can affect how well they work. Also, they can irritate the mouth.

c. **Chewable tablets:** This form of medicine is chewed and then swallowed. It is often considered the best form of oral medication for children and elderly people. Advantages of chewable tablets include:
   ◆ Quick action
   ◆ Come in various flavors
   ◆ You don't need water to swallow them, so you can take them anytime.

   Disadvantages include:
   ◆ It may not taste pleasant to some people
   ◆ It may need special storage and careful handling
   ◆ Can interfere with dental appliances

d. **Orally disintegrating tablets:** These pills dissolve on the tongue, become liquified, are swallowed subconsciously, and then the tiny pieces of the drug travel to the stomach and intestines, where the absorption occurs. Pros of this method of administering medication include ease of use and quick onset of action. Cons are that they may be more expensive and not as stable as other solid dosage forms.

e. **Effervescent tablets:** These are dissolved in water and then drunk. Pros are ease of use, better absorption, and a reasonably quick action onset.
   Cons: They are relatively more expensive, depending on the type of drug. You should pay attention to what type of liquid this tablet can be dissolved in, as water and juice are acceptable depending on the type of medication.

f. **Lozenges:** Also called troches, pastilles, or cough drops, lozenges are medicated tablets that dissolve slowly in the mouth and lubricate or soothe irritated tissues in patients with sore throats. They offer local pain relief and ease of use for children and adults who have difficulty swallowing pills.

Capsules

This solid form contains the medicine in a soft or hard gelatin shell. The shell breaks down in the digestive tract and releases the active substance.

Advantages include a possibly palatable taste for some and relatively fast action. Disadvantages of a capsule are that it is more expensive to manufacture, less stable with unfavorable storage conditions, and has a shorter shelf life. These products may contain animal products.

Spansules

These are a type of advanced drug delivery system. Spansules deliver the drug at a steady rate over a fixed period of several hours. For example, a doctor may prescribe Dexedrine Spansules to treat ADHD symptoms.

Softgels

These are similar to capsules except that the active substances are in the form of liquids contained in a gelatin shell.

Liquid Form

Liquid medications are in solution form, making them easy to swallow. In addition to the tasty flavor, they are ideal for the pediatric population. The dosing is more flexible than a pill, as it comes in various concentrations such as milligram/milliliter (mg/mL). Also, they are absorbed faster compared to a solid dosage form.

However, you need to measure the dose of a liquid medicine precisely with a medicine-measuring spoon or syringe. Liquids are also less stable and generally have a shorter shelf life. Some liquid medications may need to be refrigerated, which can be inconvenient with transport and travel.

GRANULES AND POWDERS

These often come in pre-measured packets and are taken by mixing in water or soft foods like applesauce, pudding, or yogurt.

The benefits of powder medication are ease of swallowing after being mixed, and the apple sauce or pudding may mask the unpleasant taste. Powders and granules are generally stable, have a long shelf life, and are easily transported. Also, it's possible to give larger doses of medication that would be uncomfortable to swallow in compressed tablet form.

The disadvantages of powders and granules are that not all drugs can be manufactured in this form. Also, the taste and consistency of the final product after mixing might not be appealing to some people.

Different Drug Forms

1. **Liquids:** Drugs can be delivered in two liquid forms. The first is an aqueous solution of one or more active drug ingredient dissolved in water or a saline solution (a solution of sodium chloride). These liquids are intended for injection and are shipped in appropriate

sterile containers. Small quantities for injection are supplied in vials or glass ampules. For administering via intravenous drips, the solutions of drugs are typically metered into a saline solution.

It is possible, in the case of drug compounds that are not soluble or poorly soluble in water, to create a suspension of the drug in an aqueous solution. Suspensions are more commonly used for medicines that are intended for oral administration.

Suspensions can be provided in the following forms:

- *Emulsions:* A suspension of oil or fat in water can be prepared with the aid of emulsifying agents, often an anionic surfactant—a material whose molecule is hydrophobic at one end and hydrophilic at the other. An example surfactant commonly used in pharmaceutical preparations is sodium stearate. In an emulsion, the sub-microscopic oil particles are coated by the emulsifying agents to create what chemists call a micelle. Unlike an oil globule which tends to separate out from water on account of a massive difference in surface tension of the two liquids, a micelle of oil is stable in water. Using emulsifying agents therefore helps stabilize the suspension of oil in water. Suspensions are often used for oral medications.
- *Gels:* Gels are quasi-solid materials that have a large number of cross-linked molecules usually holding aqueous solutions of the active pharmaceutical ingredient. Gels are commonly used for topical application as ointments or lotions.
- *Magmas:* Magmas are a combination of bulky suspension of poorly soluble substances in an aqueous liquid. Magmas are also known as "milks" due to their resemblance to conventional dairy milk. An example of a pharmaceutical magma is milk of magnesia. Magmas and gels are somewhat similar except that the particles suspended in magmas are generally larger and bulkier. Due to this, magma suspensions require shaking before administration.
- *Mixtures* are usually aqueous liquid preparations which contain suspended, insoluble, solid substances/drugs and are intended for internal use. The insoluble particles may be held in suspension by suitable suspending or thickening agents. The insoluble substance must be in a very finely divided states and it must be uniformly distributed throughout the preparation. This is accomplished by using a colloid mill, special methods of precipitation and suspending agents. There are three main reasons for having the insoluble substance as finely divided as possible:
  1. If the mixture approaches the colloidal state by including kaoli, magnesium trisilicate, or magnesium phosphate, the more active the particles become when in contact with inflamed surfaces.
  2. Finely divided particles suspend more easily than large particles, enabling the mixture becoming more homogenous. This is especially desirable when administering medication to form an evenly distributed, soothing, protective coating on the gastrointestinal tract.
  3. The palatability of many preparations is enhanced by using colloidal suspending agents.
- **Tinctures:** A tincture is typically an alcoholic extract of plant or animal material or solution of such, or of a low volatility substance (such as iodine and mercurochrome).

2. **Solids:** Below are the different solid dosage forms available in the market today.
   - Powder is the most common solid form; most drugs can be dried and divided into portions that can be used in internal and external applications. Effervescent powders are popular

as oral medications as when the powders are dissolved in water, they release gaseous carbon dioxide, which makes the medicine palatable.

- Another solid form is that of capsules made from gelatin or a non-animal substitute. Capsules may contain dry materials, oil or liquid ingredients. The thin capsule material dissolves fast enabling the drug to be absorbed quickly by the body. Some capsules are coated to prevent them from dissolving immediately when exposed to the stomach's acid. Such capsules are said to have an enteric coating–they disintegrate and release the drug once when pH of the surrounding fluids reaches a certain value, typically above pH 5, in the small intestines. Capsules are usually taken orally, though in certain instances they can be administered through the rectum or vagina.

- Tablets are another popular solid form of drug delivery. In this form the drug is mixed with various other ingredients such as binders, diluents and lubricants that enable the material to be moulded and compressed into the desired shape. Binders are agents that help the material particles to stick together. Depending on the size, weight and shape of a particular tablet, diluents may or may not be added. Lubricants are necessary to prevent the granules from sticking to the mixing machine and the pill or tablet press. Tablets, like capsules, may also be coated to improve their palatability or to create enteric tablets.

- **Pellets:** Pellets are sphere-shaped drugs formed through compression.

- **Pills:** Pills were powdered drugs that featured the active ingredients mixed with adhesive substances to create small dosage forms for oral administration; capsules and tablets have generally replaced pills nowadays.

- **Lozenges and troches:** These forms are usually provided in flat, round shapes that can be dissolved by saliva in the mouth.

Other External Forms of Drug Administration

- ❖ **Liniment:** Liniments are liquid forms of drug that are applied by rubbing into the skin. These forms often contain anodyne compound to alleviate pain and a rubefacient, which reddens the skin, e.g., by causing dilation of the capillaries and an increase in blood circulation.

- ❖ **Ointments:** These drug forms are often semi-solid preparations in which the drug is incorporated into a base material. Ointment bases fall into four general classes: (1) hydrocarbon bases (oleaginous ointment bases)—these keep medicaments in prolonged contact with the skin, act as occlusive dressings, and are used chiefly for emollient effects; (2) absorption bases that either permit the incorporation of aqueous solutions with the formation of a water-in-oil emulsions, or are water-in-oil emulsions that permit the incorporation of additional quantities of aqueous solutions; such bases permit better absorption of some medicaments and are useful as emollients; (3) water-removable bases (creams)—these are oil-in-water emulsions containing petrolatum (petroleum jelly), anhydrous lanolin, or waxes; they may be washed from the skin with water and are thus more acceptable for cosmetic reasons; they favor absorption of serous discharges in dermatologic conditions; and (4) water-soluble bases (greaseless ointment bases) containing only water-soluble substances.

- ❖ **Lotions:** Lotions are liquid forms, which are applied to the skin to protect, cool, cleanse, act as emollient and even provide antipruritic treatment.

❖ **Paste:** Pastes are ointment-like type of form where drugs and other solid substances (e.g., zinc oxide) are mixed together with an adhesive fatty base (e.g., petroleum jelly). Pastes are semi-solid preparations intended for topical application affected areas of the skin. Usually they are thick (contain 25% of solids by weight) and do not melt at normal temperature. Remain on the area for longer duration than ointments and are therefore generally more effective.

❖ **Suppositories:** A form where drugs are mixed together and molded into the desired shape to be inserted into the body cavity.

❖ **Sprays:** Sprays contain drugs in liquid form and are administered using an atomizer.

❖ **Inhalants:** These devices contain drugs and are administered by inhaling the vapor sent out from the inhalant and directly to the patient's nasal passage.

Other Types and Forms of Medicine

Related Words

Amphetamine

A drug that increases energy and excitement and makes you less hungry.

Anabolic Steroid

A drug that increases muscles, used illegally by some sports people to make themselves stronger.

Anesthesia

An anesthetic that is given to someone before they have a medical operation, or the use of anesthetics.

Anesthetic

A drug or gas that is given to someone before a medical operation to stop them feeling pain. An anesthetic that affects the whole of your body by making you unconscious is called a general anesthetic and an anesthetic that affects only a part of your body is called a local anesthetic.

Analgesic

A drug that reduces pain.

Antacid

A medicine that reduces the amount of acid in your stomach.

Antibiotic

A drug that cures illnesses and infections caused by bacteria. Doctors often give people a course of antibiotics, when they have to take a fixed amount of medicine each day for several days.

Anticoagulant

A substance that prevents blood from coagulating (=becoming more solid).

Antidepressant

A drug used for treating someone who is depressed (=so unhappy that they are considered ill).

Antidote

A substance that prevents a poison from having bad effects.

Antihistamine

A drug used to treat an allergy (=a bad reaction to something you swallow or touch).

Anti-inflammatory

A drug taken to reduce inflammation (=swelling, heat, and pain).

Antiretroviral (Adjective)

Antiretroviral drugs are used to treat certain types of virus, especially HIV (=the virus that causes aids).

Antiviral

A drug or treatment that is used to treat an infection or disease caused by a virus.

Barbiturate

A strong drug that doctors give to people to make them calm or help them sleep.

Beta-blocker

A drug that makes your heart work more slowly, used for treating high blood pressure.

Booster

Medical a small extra amount of a medical drug that you are given so that a drug you had before will continue to be effective.

Caplet

A pill shaped like an oval (=a long narrow circle).

Capsule

A small round container filled with medicine that you swallow whole.

Contraceptive

A drug, method, or object used for preventing a woman from becoming pregnant.

Cough Drop

A type of sweet containing medicine that you suck when you have a cough or a sore throat.

Cough Mixture

British a liquid medicine that you take to help to cure a cough.

Cough Sweet

British a cough drop.

Cough Syrup

Cough mixture.

Decongestant

A drug that helps you breathe more easily when you have a cold.

Depressant

A drug or substance that makes you feel relaxed and makes your body work and react more slowly.

Draught

Literary a liquid medicine that you drink.

Drops

Liquid medicine that you put into your eyes, ears, or nose.

Ear Drops

Liquid medicine that you put in your ear to treat an ear infection

Emetic

A substance that makes you vomit.

Enema

A liquid used to give someone an enema.

Expectorant

A medicine that you use for helping you to cough liquid up from your lungs.

Fertility Drug

A drug given to a woman to improve her fertility.

Gas

A gas given to people before an operation to make them sleep, or during medical treatment so that they will feel less pain

General Anesthetic

A substance that a doctor puts into your body so that you will sleep and not feel any pain during an operation.

Herbal Medicine

Medicine made from plants.

Hypnotic

A drug that makes you go to sleep.

Inhalant

A medicine or drug that you breathe into your lungs.

Injection

A drug or another substance that is injected into your body.

Jab

British an injection (=amount of medicine given through a needle) that is intended to stop you from getting a disease.

Laxative

A medicine, food, or drink that helps you to make solid waste leave your body when you use the toilet.

Legal High

A psychoactive drug that was not or is not illegal.

Linctus

British a thick liquid medicine used for curing coughs.

Local Anesthetic

A type of anesthetic (=a drug to stop you feeling pain) that affects only one part of your body.

Lozenge

Medicine shaped like a sweet that you suck if you have a cough or sore throat.

Magic Bullet

A medicine designed to cure an illness quickly and completely, without affecting other parts of the body.

MMR Vaccine

A drug given to young children by injection to protect them against measles, mumps, and rubella.

Multivitamin

A pill that some people take to make them healthier, containing various vitamins and minerals.

Narcotic

Medical a drug that people use when they are very ill in order to feel less pain and sleep better.

Opiate

Medical a drug that contains opium and is used for reducing pain and making you go to sleep.

Opioid

A substance that is similar to the illegal drug opium in its effects and the way it can cause addiction.

Painkiller

A medicine that reduces pain.

Pastille

A round sweet that contains medicine, for example, for a sore throat.

Patent Medicine

A medicine that you can buy from a shop without a doctor's prescription.

Pessary

A solid medicine or chemical substance put into a woman's vagina to cure an infection or to prevent her becoming pregnant.

Pill

A small piece of solid medicine that you swallow with water.

Prescription Drug

A drug that you can only get if you have a prescription from your doctor.

Prophylactic

Medical a medicine or treatment used for preventing disease or infection.

Purgative

A food or drug that makes you go to the toilet.

Relaxant

Something, especially a drug, that relaxes you.

Sedative

A drug that makes someone calmer, or makes them sleep.

Serum

A liquid that is put into someone's blood to help them to fight an infection or a poison.

Sleeping Pill

A pill that you take to help you to sleep.

Sports Supplement

A food substance or drug that people can take to increase their energy or to become more healthy.

Statin

A drug that is used to reduce the amount of cholesterol in the blood.

Steroid

A chemical that is produced in the body or made as a drug. Steroids can act as hormones or be used for treating conditions such as swelling, or, illegally, by athletes to improve their performance.

Supplement

A pill or special food that you take or eat when your food does not contain everything that you need.

Suppository

A drug in the form of a small block that is put inside the rectum or vagina to treat a medical condition.

Suppressant

A drug that stops or limits the effects of something.

Syrup

A sweet liquid that contains medicine.

Tablet

A small hard round piece of medicine that you swallow.

Tincture

A medicine made by mixing a small amount of a drug with alcohol.

Tonic

A medicine that you take to get more energy and feel healthier, especially after you have been ill or working too hard.

Tranquillizer

A drug that makes people calmer when they are very worried or nervous.

Truth Drug

A drug used for trying to make someone tell the truth.

Vaccine

A substance put into the body, usually by injection, in order to provide protection against a disease.

FACTORS INFLUENCING MEDICATION ACTION

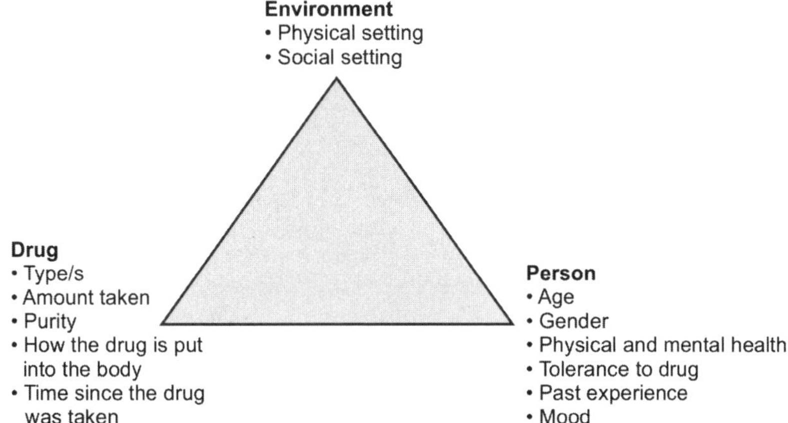

A multitude of host and environmental factors influence drug response. Understanding of these factors can guide choice of appropriate drug and dose for individual patient.

Variation in response to the same dose of a drug between different patients and even in the same patient on different occasions will occur. The range of variability may be marked or limited depending on the pharmacokinetic and Pharmacodynamic characteristics of the drug. Drugs mostly disposed by metabolism are most effected (e.g., propanolol) while those excreted by the kidneys are least effected (e.g., atenolol).

❖ Physiological factors
❖ Pathological factors (diseases)
❖ Genetic factors
❖ Environmental factors
❖ Interaction with other drugs

There exists no specific dose. The decision lies with the doctor. Giving optimum dose is mandatory for desired results. Pharmacopoeia gives the guidelines and ranges. All factors affecting absorption and biotransformation may influence the outcomes of drug actions.

Physiological Factors

Age

The adult dose is for people between 18 and 60 years of age. The tissues of an infant and child are highly sensitive to large number of drugs. Children under 12 years require fraction of adult dose because:

❖ Drug metabolizing enzyme system is inefficient in them (glucuronidation takes 3 months to develop)
❖ Their barriers are not fully developed (BBB, blood aqueous barrier), thus are more sensitive to CNS stimulants. All parts of the body are affected by the drug.
❖ Infants have an immature renal tubular transport system. Penicillin, streptomycin and amino glycosides are not administered. After one year of age, elimination by kidneys is increased.
❖ Hepatic metabolizing capacity is also under developed. Chloramphenicol may cause gray baby syndrome.

The dose for a child is calculated from the adult dose up to 8 years of age. The average adult dose is for an individual of medium built. For very thin or obese individual the dose may be modified using either the body surface area or body weight, i.e.,

Surface area is found from height and weight, and is around $1.7–1.8/m^2$.

$$\text{Dose to be prescribed} = \frac{\text{Body surface area (m}^2) \times \text{adult dose}}{1.7}$$

$$\text{Dose to be prescribed} = \frac{\text{Wt in kg} \times \text{AD}}{70}$$

$$\text{Child dose} = \frac{\text{Body surface area in m}^2 \text{ of child} \times \text{AD}}{1.7 \text{ (average body surface area in AD)}}$$

Newborns

The drug dosage of newborn is decreased because:

❖ Gastric acid secretion are not adequate, e.g., GIT absorption of ampicillin and amoxicillin is greater in neonates due to decreased gastric acidity
❖ Liver microsomal enzymes (glucuronyl transferase) are deficient. Administration of chloramphenicol may lead to gray baby syndrome because of inadequate glucuronidation of chloramphenicol resulting in drug accumulation.
❖ Plasma protein binding is less.
❖ Glomerular filtration rate (GFR) and tubular secretions are not adequate.
❖ There is immaturity of blood brain barriers in neonates.
    Sulfonamides may lead to hyperbilirubinemia and kernicterus.

Children

❖ In children tetracyclines may cause permanent teeth staining.
❖ Corticosteroids may lead to growth and development retardation.
❖ Antihistaminics may cause hyperactivity.

Geriatric Age Group (>60 Years)

Patient requires special consideration because physiological changes occur with age are to be kept in mind such as:

❖ Reduced body weight
❖ Reduced body fat
❖ Reduced intestinal motility and mesenteric blood flow.
❖ Reduced renal and hepatic functions
❖ Altered mental functions
    Elderly often require lesser doses than adults because they are prone to suffer from adverse drug reactions. If liquid preparations are available, they should be preferred as are convenient for absorption.
❖ **Liver functions are impaired:** Drugs like diazepam, theophylline having lower therapeutic index, may have much larger half lives (2 hrs in normal 90 hrs in old)
❖ **Kidney functions are also impaired:** Drugs like digoxin, lithium and amino glycosides have decreased excretion
❖ Plasma protein binding is decreased leading to greater amounts of active drugs.
❖ Increased sensitivity to CNS depressants like diazepam, morphine also occurs

Sex

❖ Testosterone increases the rate of biotransformation of drugs.

❖ Decreased metabolism of some drugs in female (diazepam) occurs. Females are more susceptible to autonomic drugs (estrogen inhibits choline esterase). Drugs used for ulcer may cause increased prolactin.

❖ During menstruation, salicylates and strong purgatives should be avoided as they may increase bleeding.

Pregnancy

In pregnancy following are to be considered:

❖ Cardiac output

❖ GFR and renal elimination of drugs.

❖ Volume of distribution

❖ Metabolic rate of some drugs

Lipophilic drugs cross placental barrier and are slowly excreted. During pregnancy, uterine stimulants, strong purgatives and drugs likely to have teratogenic effects should be avoided, especially during first trimester no drug should be given unless absolutely necessary.

During labor, morphine should be avoided as it crosses placental barrier and depresses respiration in newborn.

Plasma Protein Binding

Malnutrition causes decreased amino acids, decreased proteins leading to decreased binding sites for drugs.

Body Weight

Dose is given per kg body weight. Average muscular weight is between 50 and 100 kg, with 70 kg being the average.

Lactation

During lactation, drugs may be excreted through milk and may affect the infant, e.g., some purgatives, penicillin, chloramphenicol and oral anticoagulants.

Food

Drugs are better absorbed in empty stomach. To prevent gastric irritation most drugs are taken after or between foods, which affects the outcomes. Antimotion drugs are taken on empty stomach. Helminthes (for evacuation of worms) are also taken on empty stomach.

Allergy

Allergy is the abnormal response of drug resulting from antigen-antibody reaction, leading to liberation of histamine and histamine-like substances; therefore, there may be skin rashes, urticaria, bronchoconstriction and fall of blood pressure. Allergic reactions may occur immediately or may be delayed for many days.

Immediate and acute allergic reactions lead to acute anaphylactic shock which is dangerous for patient and may even be fatal, e.g., penicillin, sera, vaccines. Steps which can be taken include:

* History taking of previous allergic reactions.
* Test dose should be given first.
* Drugs required to deal with emergency should be kept ready.

Sometimes skin rashes or urticaria along with fever and pain in joints and swelling of lymph nodes may occur after a few days. This is delayed type of allergy called serum sickness type reaction.

Drug Dependence (Drug Addiction)

Drug dependence is a state of periodic or chronic intoxication which is detrimental to person and society. It becomes almost impossible to carry out normal physical functions without the drug.

Components of phenomenon of addiction include:

* Euphoria—sense of happiness and forgetfulness
* Tolerance—due to increased production of enzymes
* Psychic dependence (habituation)—person desires but in absence of drug no harm occurs
* Physical dependence
* Withdrawal symptoms (abstinence syndrome)—symptoms opposite pharmacological actions of drug develop in absence of drug.

Pathological Factors

Diseases cause individual variation in drug response

Liver Disease

In liver diseases, prolong duration of action occurs because of increased half-life. Plasma protein binding for warfarin, tolbutamide is decreased leading to adverse effects.

If hepatic blood flow is reduced, clearance of morphine—propranolol may be affected.

Impaired liver microsomal enzymes may lead to toxic levels of diazepam, rifampicin and theophylline.

Renal Disease

GFR, tabular function and plasma albumin may be affected leading to abnormal effects of digoxin, lithium, gentamicin and penicillin.

Malnutrition

Plasma protein binding of drugs is reduced along with the amount of microsomal enzymes, leading to increased portion of free, unbound drug, e.g., warfarin

Genetic Factors

Genetic abnormalities influence the dose of a drug and response to drugs. It affects the drug response in individuals at 2 levels.

1. At the level of receptors
2. At the level of drugs metabolizing enzyme

Thus, interfering with the functions such as rate of plasma drug clearance.

Pharmacogenetics is the study of the relationship between genetic factors and drug response.

Idiosyncrasy

Idiosyncrasy is the abnormal drug reaction due to genetic disorder. It is the unpredictable response seen on first dose of drug on hereditary basis. This may be due to:

- Acetylation
- Oxidation
- Succinylcholine apnea
- Glucose 6-phosphate dehydrogenase deficiency.

  All individuals do not respond in similar way to same drug. Idiosyncrasy is used to describe abnormal drug response on administration of first dose.

Genetic Polymorphism

The existence in a population of two or more phenotypes with respect to the effect of a drug, e.g., acetylation enzymes deficiency.

Acetyl transferase (non-microsomal) affects Isoniazid, sulfonamides, etc.

Slow acetylator phenotype may show peripheral neuropathy.

Rapid acetylator phenotype may show hepatitis.

Pseudocholinesterase Deficiency

Succinylcholine is a skeletal muscle relaxant. Succinylcholine apnea may occur due to paralysis of respiratory muscles.

Malignant Hyperthermia

Occurs by succinylcholine due to inherited inability to chelate calcium by sarcoplasmic reticulum resulting in Ca release, muscle spasm and rise in temperature.

Oxidation Polymorphism

In case of debrisoquine

- Extensive metabolizers (EM) need larger dose.
- Poor metabolizers (PM)—need smaller dose.

Deficiency of Glucose-6 Phosphate Dehydrogenase (G-6-PD)

G-6-PD deficiency in RBCs leads to hemolytic anemia upon exposure to some oxidizing agents like:

- Antimalarial drug, primaquine
- Long acting sulfonamides
- Fava beans (favism).

Environmental Factors

Route of Administration

Some drugs are incompletely absorbed after oral intake, when given intravenously; their dose has to be reduced. Examples include morphine and magnesium sulfate. Magnesium sulfate when given orally is osmotic purgative, but its 20% solution is injected intravenously to control the convulsions in eclampsia of pregnancy.

Time of Administration

Hypnotics (producing sleep) act better when administered at night and smaller doses are required. Aminoglycosides like streptomycin when given intravenously cause neuromuscular blockage, which is not observed after intramuscular injection.

Effect of Climate

Metabolism is low in hot and humid climate. Purgatives act better in summer while diuretics act better in winters. Oxidation of drugs is low at higher altitudes.

Racial Differences

Castor oil, a purgative, is ineffective in Chinese. The dilating effect of ephedrine in fair people on pupil is absent in Negroes.

Preparation of Drug

Drugs in solid forms disintegrate slowly. Onset of action is rapid when drug is given in liquid form.

Age of Drug

Action may be modified if kept for longer durations. Outdated tetracyclines give rise to excretion of amino acids in urine. Chloroform and carbon tetrachloride become toxic if kept for long durations.

Acidic or Basic Medium

If GIT has decreased acidity, acidic drugs like benzyl penicillin are not effective orally.

Effect of Disease

Certain drugs are only effective in disease conditions. These include antipyretics like aspirin and paracetamol, which do not reduce temperature in case of healthy individuals.

Iron is better absorbed in iron deficiency anemia. As the anemia improves, it has less response.

Hypersusceptibility to Drugs

Variations in individuals leading to prolonged effects of drugs. Examples include diazepam, 2 mg of which are used as antianxiety producing no hang overs. In hypersusceptible individuals, the drug has prolonged action causing hangovers and hypnotic actions.

Opioids like morphine cause analgesia and sedation in 10 mg dose effective for 4–6 hours. In hypersusceptible individuals, effect might be prolonged to 10–12 hours. These are individual based variations.

Hypersensitivity

Hypersensitivity is the quantitatively abnormal response with certain groups of drugs. Response is seen in subtherapeutic doses not capable of producing pharmacological actions. This has immunological basis, e.g., allergy. 25% of the drugs show hypersensitivity.

Hematological disorders can occur more pronounced in atopic individuals, who are already exposed to antigens, e.g., ashthemics are more prone to allergic reactions.

Nearly all drugs show hypersensitivity in some category, which might be self-limiting or even life-threatening. Penicillin when administered may cause anaphylactic shock. High molecular weight drugs have a greater tendency to show hypersensitivity. History taking is helpful in predicting hypersensitivity. Test dose can be given intradermally and localized reactions can be seen.

Tolerance

Resistance to normal therapeutic dose of drug, producing lesser response to normal therapeutic dose is known as tolerance. This is acquired character. Examples include morphine, person is initially responsive, if continued, changes occur at cellular and pharmacokinetic level, reducing the action. Thus one has to increase the dose of drug to overcome.

Alcoholics do not respond to hypnotics and analgesics, dose of which has to be increased many folds. In fact they may even tolerate toxic levels.

Cross Tolerance

A person tolerant to drugs resembling in chemical structure is known as cross tolerance. Those drugs resembling in chemical structures show cross tolerance. If a person is tolerant to morphine, he also shows tolerance to pethidine (synthetic derivative) and codeine.

Complete cross tolerance is observed in cases like diazepam and flurazepam.

Incomplete cross tolerance occurs with the drugs sharing the same pharmacological properties. Examples include barbiturates and general anesthetics, site of action is CNS, incomplete cross tolerance may be observed although they are not resembling chemically, but having same pharmacological properties.

Tachyphylaxis

Repeated administration of a drug at short intervals of time leads to a rapidly developing tolerance. This occurs with indirectly acting drugs. On repeated administration, depletion of endogenous receptors occurs. It is also known as acute tolerance. Example includes ephedrine, which acts by releasing noradrenaline from adrenergic stores. After repeated administration, these stores are exhausted and pharmacological action is not restored even on increasing the dose.

Interactions of Drugs

Synergism

Synergism is the facilitation/potentiation of pharmacological response by concomitant use of two drugs.

Potentiation

The total effect will be more than the sum of their individual effects. Examples are:
- Acetylcholine + physostigmine. Physostigmine inhibits the action of esterase prolonging the effect of acetylcholine.
- Levodopa (Parkinsonism) + carbidopa/benserazide. Levo dopa is decarboxylated peripherally, carbidopa inhibits the decarboxylase.
- Sulfonamide (effective against some microorganisms) when combined with trimethoprim is effective against a wider range of microorganisms.
  The action is more than the normal therapeutic effect.

Additive Effect (Summation)

In this case the total pharmacological action of two drugs will be equal to the sum of their individual effect on simultaneous administration. The response is not more than their total algebraic sum, e.g.:

1. Aspirin + paracetamol as analgesic/antipyretic
2. Ephedrine + theophylline as bronchodilator
3. Nitrous oxide + ether as general anesthetic
4. Antihypertensive drugs
5. Cardiac stimulants

Antagonism

When two drugs, administered simultaneously, oppose the action of each other on the same physiological system, the phenomenon is called antagonism. It can be of following types:

Chemical Antagonism

It involves reduction of the biological activity of a drug by a chemical reaction with another agent, e.g., between acids and alkalies: BAL and arsenic. Antacids, used for dyspepsia involve administration of sodium bicarbonate to react with hydrochloric acid. In cases of heavy metal poisoning chelating agents are used like dimerzapam.

In iron poisoning deproxamine is given which binds sulfhydryl groups forming insoluble complexes which can be easily detoxified.

Pharmacological Antagonism

Pharmacological antagonism is of two types:

I. *Competitive or reversible antagonism:* In this type of antagonism the agonist and antagonist compete with each other for the same receptors. The extent of antagonism will depend on the relative number of receptors occupied by the two compounds. Other features are:
   - Antagonist has chemical resemblance with agonist.
   - Antagonism can be overcome by increasing the concentration of the agonist at receptor site. It means the maximal response to agonist is not impaired.
   - Antagonist shifts the dose response curve to right
   - Emax of agonist is obtained with high concentration of agonist
   - Duration of action is short. It depends on drug clearance

   Example is of acetylcholine and atropine antagonism on muscarinic receptors. In presence of antagonist, log dose response curve of agonist shifts to right, indicating a higher concentration of agonist is required for same response. Maximum height of the curve can be attained by overcoming the action of antagonist. This leads to a parallel shift of log dose response curve towards right.

II. *Noncompetitive antagonism:* Here an antagonist inactivates the receptor in such a way so that the effective complex with agonist cannot be formed irrespective of the concentration of the agonist. This can happen by various ways:
   - The antagonist might combine at the same site in such a way that even higher concentration of the agonist can not displace it.
   - The antagonist might combine at a different site in such a way that agonist is unable to initiate characteristic biological response

♦ The antagonist might itself induce a certain change in R so that the reactivity of the receptor site where agonist should interact is abolished.

Other features of this antagonism are:

♦ Antagonist has no chemical resemblance with agonist.
♦ Maximum response is suppressed
♦ Although antagonist shifts the dose response curve to right, the slope of the curve is reduced.
♦ The extent of antagonism depends on the characteristics of antagonist itself and agonist has no influence upon the degree of antagonism or its reversibility.
♦ Emax of agonist is decreased even with high concentration of agonist.
♦ Duration of action is long which depends upon new receptor synthesis.

Example is of phenoxybenzamine and adrenaline at alpha adrenergic receptors.

III. *Physiological antagonism:* In this interaction of two drugs, both are agonists, so they act at different receptor sites. They antagonize the action of each other because they produce opposite actions. Classical example of physiological antagonism is adrenalin and histamine. Former causes bronchodilatation while later bronchoconstriction. So adrenalin is a life-saving drug in anaphylaxis.

Clinical significance of drug antagonism

♦ It helps to correct adverse effects of a drug, e.g., ephedrine and phenobarbitone.
♦ It is useful to treat drug poisoning, e.g., morphine with naloxone
♦ It guides to avoid drug combinations with reduced drug efficacy such as a penicillin and tetracycline combination.

❖ **Patients are not taking medications exactly as directed.**

While most Americans recognize the importance of taking prescribed medication as directed, those who skip or forget doses are less likely to understand the health consequences of nonadherence.

Nearly three-quarters of Americans report that they do not always take their medication as directed, despite knowing that they should. This problem causes more than one-third of medicine-related hospitalizations and nearly 125,000 deaths in the United States each year, and it adds $290 billion in avoidable costs to the healthcare system annually.

Beyond general adherence issues, medications can also sometimes interact with other prescription drugs, vitamins, or supplements. Pharmacists should encourage patients to read labels in order to avoid this issue.

❖ **A patient's diet may be interfering with medications.**

There is a dynamic relationship between the foods we eat and the medications we take. Many foods can substantially interfere with therapeutic goals and change the absorption of a medication into the bloodstream.

For example, high-fat, high-cholesterol foods can sharply reduce the effect of angiotensin-converting enzyme inhibitors like enalapril, as well as statins and some other cholesterol medications.

However, not all negative interactions between medications and diet stem from poor nutrition. Patients may not recognize that otherwise healthy foods can have severe consequences when they're mixed with certain drugs.

As medication experts, pharmacists should clearly communicate the risk of possible food-drug interactions for both prescription and OTC medications.

Examples of potentially dangerous food-drug interactions include:

- Calcium-rich foods + antibiotics
- Pickled, curd, and fermented foods + monoamine oxidase inhibitors
- Vitamin K-rich foods + warfarin
- Grapefruit and grapefruit juice + statins

❖ **A patient's lifestyle habits may be interfering with medications.**

Negative lifestyle factors such as excess weight, smoking, physical inactivity, and binge drinking can affect the health of patients taking certain medications.

With smoking, for instance, the most consistently observed effect of cigarettes on drug metabolism is an increase in the clearance of drugs that are substrates of CYP1A2, which include clozapine, fluvoxamine, olanzapine, tacrine, and theophylline.

Meanwhile, alcohol intake can have both short and long-term effects in patients with diabetes, including interactions with diabetes medications and worsening of pre-existing complications. For example, mixing insulin and oral hypoglycemic with alcohol may increase the risk of hypoglycemic reactions, while mixing metformin with chronic alcohol use may predispose a patient to lactic acidosis.

❖ **A patient may have comorbid conditions.**

Approximately 50% of all patients with chronic conditions have comorbidities.

Because current health care practice focuses on diagnosing and prescribing, the need to taper, reduce, or discontinue inappropriate medication therapy receives relatively little attention.

PRESCRIPTION AND ORDER

Typically, the term medication order refers to a written request on a physician's order form or a transcribed verbal or telephone order in an inpatient setting. This order becomes part of the patient's medical record. The term prescription refers to a medication order on a prescription blank to be filled in an outpatient or ambulatory care setting. The two serve essentially the same purpose. They both represent a means of communication for the prescriber to give instruction to the dispenser of the medication or to those who will be administering the medication.

A prescription is a lawful order of a practitioner for a *drug* or *device* for a specific patient. In a more specific sense, it means a written request for the preparation and administration of any medication for an outpatient. A prescription may order a manufactured drug product or a compounded drug product. It may order a wheelchair or a walker.

A medication order, drug order or physician's order is a request for a drug product for inpatients in institutional settings.

BASICS OF PRESCRIPTIONS AND MEDICATION ORDERS

Although different states may vary slightly in their requirements for what information needs to be contained on a prescription, in general, it must contain the following information:

❖ Name of the patient
❖ Drug name
❖ Drug strength
❖ Drug dosage form, quantity prescribed

* Directions for use
* And the name, address, and
* Signature of the prescriber.

Additional information that may be included is the:
* Date of issue
* Number of refills authorized
* Address and/ or date of birth of the patient
* And prescriber's drug enforcement administration (DEA) registration number.

There are stricter regulations for prescriptions written for scheduled or controlled substances. Additional information would be present on a prescription for a pediatric patient, such as patient age and weight, or a prescription from a veterinarian, which would include the animal species.

Medication orders typically contain similar information that would be included on a prescription. This includes the patient's name and a secondary identifier such as the patient's date of birth, medical record number, or social security number (less commonly used now); the patient's location and room number; date and time of the order; the drug name, dose, route, frequency, and duration; and the prescriber's name and signature, as shown below:

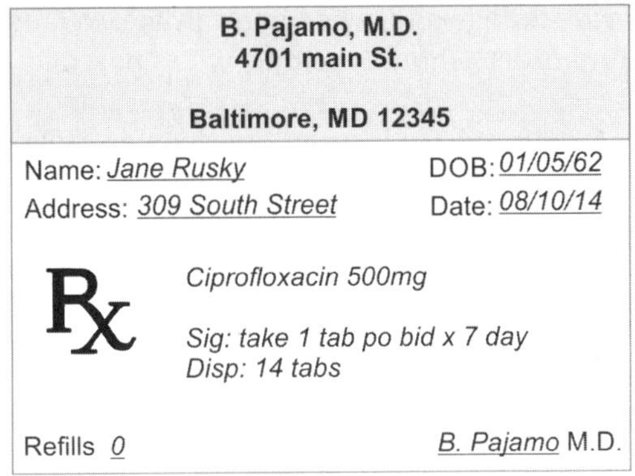

Providers who prescribe controlled substances must register with the DEA to do so. They are provided with a DEA registration number that must be indicated on prescriptions and orders for controlled substances.

The **DEA number** is a unique number that contains two letters and seven numbers. This number can be verified to help identify fraudulent registration numbers and prescriptions. Let's use DEA number AF1234563 as an example.

For prescribers, the first character in their DEA number should be the letter A or B. For mid-level practitioners (i.e., physician's assistant [PA], nurse practitioner [NP], etc.), the first character is the letter M. The second character of the DEA number is the first letter of the prescriber's last name, unless, for example, the prescriber recently got married and changed their last name after receiving a DEA number. Our prescriber's last name should start with the letter F. The seven digits that follow the letters can be verified mathematically as well. First, add the odd numbers, the first, third, and fifth digits (1 1 3 1 5 5 9). Second, add the even numbers, the second, fourth, and sixth digits, and multiply the sum by 2 (2 1 4 1 6 5 12; 12 3 2 5 24). Finally, add the results from the first two steps (9 1 24 5 33). The far right digit of this number (3) should be the same as the seventh digit of the DEA number (3).

Writing a Prescription

Prevention of medication errors is of utmost importance, and it must start at the time a prescription is written and transcribed/read. Some general recommendations by the USP and NABP to prevent medication errors:

* Written prescriptions/medication orders must be legible.
* Prescribers should avoid the use of certain abbreviations (e.g., abbreviations of drug names or combinations of drugs; OD for once daily since OD also stands for right eye; U for units, which may be mistaken for a zero when poorly handwritten).
* Prescriptions/medication orders should always be written using the metric system.
* Prescriptions/medication orders should include the drug name, metric weight or concentration, and dosage form. In addition, when transcribing verbal orders or typing medication names keep *one space apart* each the drug, the units, and the weights.
* A leading zero should always precede a decimal point in quantities less than one (e.g., 0.5 mg, not .5 mg) and a trailing zero should never be used after a decimal point (1 mg, not 1.0 mg).
* Numbers above 999 should have properly placed commas (e.g., 500,000 and not 500000).
* Prescribers should provide the age and, when appropriate, weight of the patient.
* Prescriptions/medication orders should include, when possible, a notation of purpose of the medication.
* Prescribers should not use imprecise instructions such as "Take as directed" or "Take as needed". Orally transmitted directions may be forgotten or misinterpreted. There is also the legal aspect for controlled substances (overdose, mishandling).
* Phoned prescriptions (and voice orders) should be reduced to writing and/or computer data entry immediately. In addition, the dose and drug strength should be checked by individual numbers as they may sound alike (e.g., "one-five" for fifteen and "five-zero" for fifty).

Examples of Prescriptions and Medication Orders

According to the National Association of Boards of Pharmacy, the minimal recommended legal requirements for outpatient prescriptions are:

* **Prescriber information:** Name, degree, address, phone number, signature, DEA registration number.
* **Patient information:** Name, address, other.
* **Date:** Date of prescription or date of issue.
* **Superscription:** R_x symbol = "take thou", "you take", "recipe".
* **Inscription:** The drug product prescribed = name, strength, dosage form of drug product prescribed (manufactured product), or name and quantity of each ingredient (compounded product).
* **Subscription:** Dispensing instructions to the pharmacist.
* **Signa (Sig.):** Directions for use by the patient.
* **Special instructions:** Refills, generic product substitution. For refills, the common interpretation for absence of information is that zero refills are authorized.
  In addition to commonly used abbreviations that should be avoided because of the potential for misinterpretation, ISMP suggests the following when writing numbers for doses on a prescription:

Do not use trailing zeros for doses expressed as whole numbers: If the dose on a prescription is 1 milligram, it should be written as "1 mg" and not "1.0 mg". The decimal point could be missed, and the strength could be misinterpreted as 10 milligrams.

- *Use a zero before a decimal point when the dose is less than a whole unit:* If the dose on a prescription is one half milligram, it should be written as "0.5 mg" and not ".5 mg". The decimal point before the number could be missed, and the strength could be misinterpreted as 5 milligrams.

- *Use commas for dosing units at or above 1,000 or use words such as "100 thousand" or "1 million" to improve readability:* If the dose on a prescription is ten thousand units, it should be written as "10,000 units" or "10 thousand units" and not "10000 units". The incorrect number of zeros could be miscounted and misinterpreted as the wrong strength.

- *Place adequate space between the dose and unit of measure:* If the dose on a prescription is 10 milligrams, it should be written as "10 mg" and not "10mg". The lack of space between the dose and strength makes the numbers and letters run together and could be misinterpreted as additional numbers.

- *Place adequate space between the drug name, dose, and unit of measure:* If the prescription is for Tegretol 300 milligrams, it should be written as "Tegretol 300 mg" and not "Tegretol300mg" or "Tegretol300 mg." The lack of space between the drug name and strength makes the numbers run together and could be interpreted as Tegretol 1,300 milligrams.

Commonly used abbreviations in prescription writing, along with their definitions

Abbreviation	*Definition*	*Abbreviation*	*Definition*
Aa	Affected area	BW	Body weight
ac	Before meals	C	Centigrade
ABW	Actual body weight	c or c̄	With
Ad	Up to	Cap	Capsule
ad*	Right ear	CC*	Cubic centimeter
am	Morning	cr, crm	Cream
Amp	Ampule	D	Day
APAP*	Acetaminophen	disc, DC*, d/c*	Discontinue
Aq	Water	Disp	Dispense
as*	Left ear	Div	Divide
ASA	Aspirin	DOB	Date of birth
ATC	Around the clock	DS	Double strength
au*	Each ear	d.t.d.	Give as such doses
bid	Twice a day	DW	Distilled water

Contd...

Contd...

Abbreviation	Definition	Abbreviation	Definition
biw	Twice a week	D5NS	Dextrose 5% in normal saline
BMI	Body mass index	D5½NS	Dextrose 5% in ½ normal saline (0.45% NaCl)
BSA	Body surface area	D5W	Dextrose 5% in water
EC	Enteric coated	OTC	Over the counter
elix.	Elixir	o.u.*	Each eye
emp	As directed	oz	Ounce
F	Fahrenheit	p or per	By
fl or fld	Fluid	p.c.	After meals
ft	Make	PCN	Penicillin
g or Gm	Gram	p.m.	Afternoon or evening
gr	Grain	p.o.	By mouth
gtt, gtts	Drop, drops	post	After
h, hr, or °	Hour	PPM	Parts per million
HCTZ*	Hydrochlorothiazide	pr	Rectally
h.s.*	At bedtime	pre-op	Before surgery
IBW	Ideal body weight	prn	As needed
ID	Intradermal	pulv	Powder
IM	Intramuscular	q	Every
inj.	Injection	qd*	Every day
IU*	International units	qid	Four times a day
IUD	Intrauterine device	qod*	Every other day
IV	Intravenous	qs	Sufficient quantity
IVP	Intravenous push	qs ad	A sufficient quantity to make
IVPB	Intravenous piggy back	s or s̄	Without
jt or j-tube	Jejunostomy tube	sc*, sq*, subq*, or subcut	Subcutaneous

Contd...

Contd...

Abbreviation	Definition	Abbreviation	Definition
KVO	Keep vein open	Sig.	Write on label
L	Liter	SL	Sublingual
LE	Lower extremities	sol.	Solution
LR	Lactated Ringer's injection	ss*	One half
M^2 or m^2	Square meter	stat.	Immediately
mcg or µg*	Microgram	supp.	Suppository
MDI	Metered dose inhaler	susp.	Suspension
mEq	Milliequivalent	syr.	Syrup
mg	Milligram	tab	Tablet
min	Minute	tal. dos.	Such dose
ml or mL	Milliliter	tbsp.	Tablespoon
MOM	Milk of magnesia	t.i.d.	Three times a day
mOsm or mOsmol	Milliosmole	tinc	Tincture
MR	May repeat	tiw*	Three times a week
MRX_	May repeat _ times	top	Topically
NG or NGT	Nasogastric or nasogastric tube	tsp	Teaspoon
No. or no.	Number	U* or u*	Unit(s)
noct.	Night	ud* or utdict	As directed
non rep. or N.R.	Do not repeat or no refills	UE	Upper extremities
NPO	Nothing by mouth	ung	Ointment
NS	Normal saline (0.9% NaCl)	vag	Vaginally
½ NS	Half-strength normal saline (0.45% NaCl)	vol	Volume
NTG	Nitroglycerin	w/	With
od*	Right eye	wa	While awake
oint	Ointment	w/o	Without
os*	Left eye	x	Times

SYSTEM OF MEASUREMENT

The systems of medication measurement are the apothecary, metric, and household systems. Nurses should be proficient in the use of these systems of medication measurements to administer medications safely.

Incorrect measurements, conversions, or drug calculations will affect the dose of medication a patient receives. Mistakes in calculating medications often lead to fatal errors. These mistakes in measuring and calculating medications could cause harm to the patient.

THE METRIC SYSTEM

The **metric system** is a decimal system of weights and measures based on units of ten in which gram, meter, and liter are the basic units of measurement. However, gram and liter are the only measurements from the metric system that are used in medication administration. The meter is a unit of distance, the gram (abbreviated g or gm) is a unit of weight, and the liter (abbreviated L) is a unit of volume.

The most frequently used metric units of weight and their equivalents are summarized:

Metric System Units of Weight and Equivalents

1 kilogram (kg)
1 gram (g)
1 milligram (mg)
1 microgram (mcg)
1 kg = 1,000 g
1 g = 1,000 mg
1 mg = 1,000 mcg

Another way to understand the metric units of weight and their equivalents is to visualize the relationship between the measurements and equivalents displayed below.

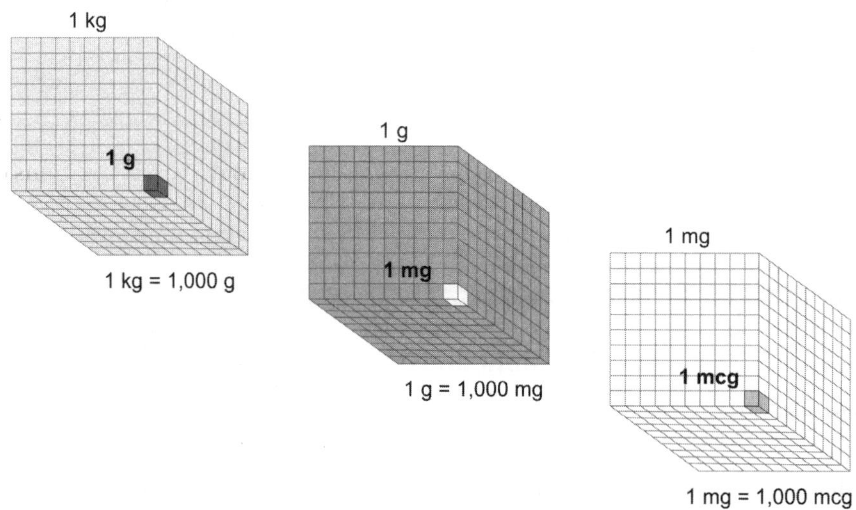

Metric system units of weight and equivalents.

The most frequently used metric units for volume and their equivalents are summarized:

Metric System Units of Volume and Equivalents

1 liter (L)
1 milliliter (mL)
1 cubic centimeter (cc)
1 L = 1,000 mL
1 mL = 1 cc

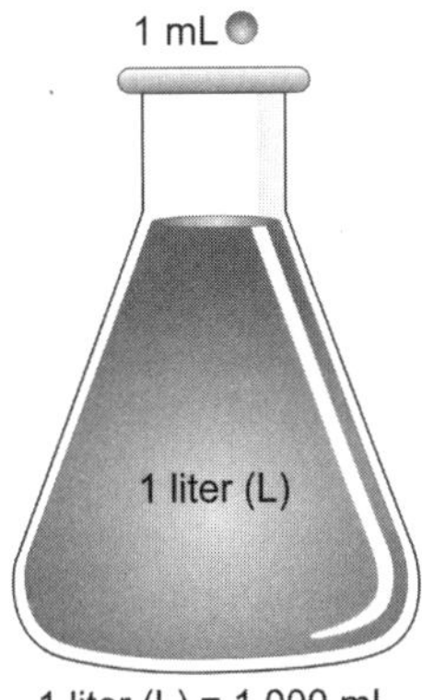

Metric system unit of volume.

APOTHECARY SYSTEM

The **apothecary system** is a system of measuring and weighing drugs and solutions in which fractions are used to identify parts of the unit of measure. The basic units of measurement in the apothecary system include weights and liquid volume. Although this may be replaced by the metric system, it is still necessary to understand it because some physicians continue to order medications using this system, and they also may include Roman numerals in the medication order.

The apothecary system originated as a system for dispensing medications using weights and measures. In, using this conversion system, grains convert to milligrams, minims (m) and drams (dr) convert to milliliter (mL), and ounces (oz) convert to milliliters.

The most frequently used measurements and equivalents within the apothecary system's units of weight are summarized below, and the most frequently used measurements and equivalents within the apothecary system's units of volume are also summarized.

Apothecary System Units of Weight and Equivalents

1 pound (lb)
1 ounce (oz)
1 dram (dr)
1 grain (gr)
1 lb = 16 oz

1 oz = 8 dr
1 dr = 60 gr

Apothecary System Units of Volume and Equivalents

1 gallon (gal)
1 quart (qt)
1 pint (pt)
1 fluid ounce (fl oz)
1 fluid dram (fl dr)
1 minim (M)
1 gal = 4 qt
1 qt = 2 pt
1 pt = 16 fl oz
1 fl oz = 8 fl dr
1 fl dr = 60 M
1 fl oz = 1 oz
1 fl dr = 1 dr

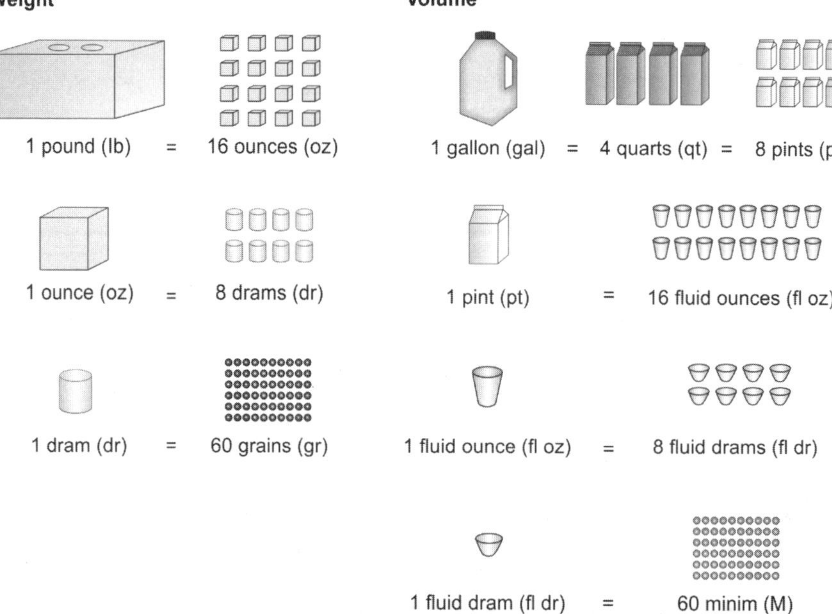

Apothecary system of equivalents for weight and volume. Please note that the figures are not shown to scale.

THE HOUSEHOLD SYSTEM

The use of household measurements is considered inaccurate because of the varying sizes of cups, glasses, and eating utensils, and this system generally has been replaced with the metric system. However, as patient care moves away from hospitals, which use the metric system, and into the community, it is once again necessary for the nurse to have an understanding of the household measurement system to be able to use and teach it to clients and families.

The most frequently used measurements and equivalents within the household measurement system are summarized below:

Household Measurement System and Equivalents

1 cup
1 tablespoon (tbsp or T)
1 teaspoon (tsp or t)
1 drop (gtt)

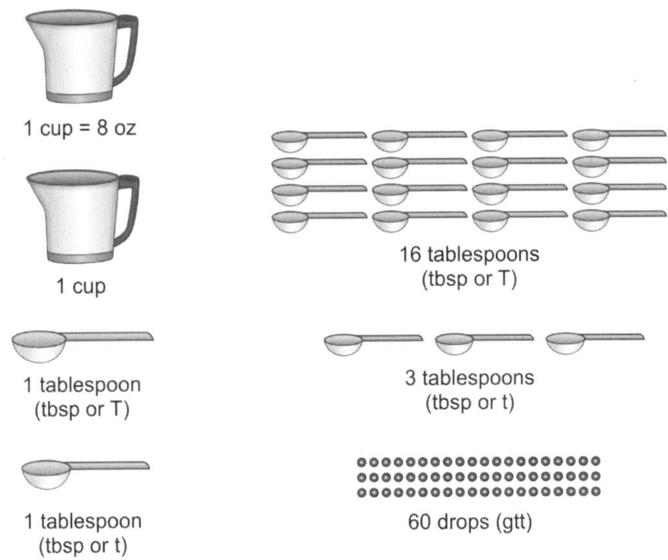

Household measurement system and equivalents for volume.

1 cup = 8 ounces (oz)
2 Tbsp = 1 oz
3 tsp = 1 tbsp
1 tsp = 60 gtt

Temperature

Clients and families are required to monitor temperature changes associated with various medical conditions. Two thermometers may be used for monitoring temperature: a Fahrenheit thermometer or a Celsius thermometer.

DRUG CALCULATION

Methods for Drug Dosage Calculations

Standard Method

The commonly used formula for calculating drug dosages.

Where in:

- ❖ D = desired dose or dose ordered by the primary care provider.
- ❖ H = dose on hand or dose on the label of bottle, vial, ampule.
- ❖ V = vehicle or the form in which the drug comes (i.e., tablet or liquid).

Standard Formula
Formula = Desired (D) × Vehicle (V)/on hand = amount to administer

Example
Order: Acetaminophen 500 mg **On hand:** Acetaminophen 250 mg in 5 mL Desired (D) = 500 mg On hand (H) = 250 mg Vehicle (V) = 5 mL **Computation:** 500 mg/250 mg × 5 mL = 10 mL **Answer:** 10 mL

Ratio and Proportion Method

- ❖ Considered as the oldest method used for drug calculation problems.
- ❖ For the equation, the known quantities are on the left side, while the desired dose and the unknown amount to administer are on the right side.

Where in:

- ❖ D = desired dose or dose ordered by the primary care provider.
- ❖ H = dose on hand or dose on the label of bottle, vial, ampule.
- ❖ V = vehicle or the form in which the drug comes (i.e., tablet or liquid).
- ❖ X = amount to administer
- ❖ Once the equation is set up, multiply the extremes (H and *x*) and the means (V and D). Then solve for *x*.

Ratio and Proportion Method
$H : V = D : x$

Example

Order: Erythromycin 750 mg
On hand: Erythromycin 250 mg capsules
Desired (D) = 750 mg
On hand (H) = 250 mg
Vehicle (V) = 1 capsule
Computation: 250 (H) : 1 (V) = 750 (D) : x
Multiply the extremes and the means:
250x = 750
x = 3 capsules
Answer: 3 capsules

Fractional Equation Method

A method similar to ratio and proportion but expressed as fractions.

Where in:
- ❖ D = desired dose or dose ordered by the primary care provider.
- ❖ H = dose on hand or dose on the label of bottle, vial, ampule.
- ❖ V = vehicle or the form in which the drug comes (i.e., tablet or liquid).

Fractional Equation Method

H/V = D/X

Example

Order: Digoxin 0.25 mg
On hand: Digoxin 0.125 mg tablets
Desired (D) = 0.25 mg
On hand (H) = 0.125 mg
Vehicle (V) = 1 tablets
Computation: 0.125 mg/1 = 0.25 mg / x
Answer: 2 tablets

IV FLOW RATE CALCULATION

To calculate IV flow rates, the nurse must know the total volume of fluid to be infused and the specific time for the infusion.
- ❖ Intravenously administered fluids are prescribed most frequently based on milliliters per hour to be administered. The volume per hour prescribed is administered by setting the flow rate, which is counted in drops per minute.
- ❖ There are three commonly used ways on how to indicate flow rates:
    1. **Milliliters per hour (mL/h):** Calculated by dividing the total infusion volume by the total infusion time in hours

2. **Number of drops per one (1) minute (gtts/min):** Calculated by multiplying the total infusion volume to the *drop factor* and then dividing by the total infusion time in minutes.
3. **Infusion time:** Total volume to infuse divided by milliliters per hour being infused.

Drop factor (sometimes called drip factor): The total number of drops delivered per milliliters of solution. This rate varies by brand and types of infusion sets and are printed on the package of the infusion set.

❖ Generally, **macrodrops** have a drop factor of **10, 12, 15,** or **20 drops/mL**.
❖ **Micro drip** sets, on the other hand, have a drop factor of **60 drops/mL**.

Formula for calculating milliliters per hour (mL/hour)

mL/h = total infusion time(h)/total infusion volume (mL)

Example: Your patient needs 2,000 mL of saline IV over 4 hours for a patient with deficient fluid volume. How many milliliters per hour will you set on a controller?

Where:
Total infusion volume (mL) = 2,000 mL
Total infusion time = 4 hours

Computation: 2,000 mL/4 hours = 500 mL/hour

Answer: 500 mL/hour

Formula for calculating drops per minute (gtts/min)

Drops per minute (gtts/min) = total time of infusion in minutes/total infusion volume × drop factor

Example: A patient is receiving 250 mL normal saline IV over 4 hours, using tubing with a drip factor of 10 drops/mL. How many drops per minute should be delivered?

Where:
Total infusion volume = 250 mL
Drop factor = 10 gtts/mL
Total infusion time = 4 hours or 240 minutes

Calculate: 250 mL × 10 gtts/mL L240 min = 10.42 gtts/min

Answer:
10 gtts/min (rounded off)
Fun fact: gtts is an abbreviation of the latin word "guttae" meaning drops.

Formula for infusion time (H)

Infusion time (hour) = milliliters per hour being infused (mL/hour)/total volume to infuse (mL)

Example: A patient is ordered to received 1,000 mL of NSS to be administered at 125 mL/hour. How many hours will pass before you change the IV bag?

Where:
Total volume to infuse = 1,000 mL
mL infused per hour = 125 mL/hour

Calculate: 1,000 mL/125 mL/h = 8 h

Answer: 8 hours

Factors affecting IV Infusion

The following factors affect the infusion rate if an infusion pump is not used:
- **Size of the catheter:** A catheter with a larger bore allows solution to flow faster.
- **Height of the IV bag:** The higher the IV bag, the faster the infusion will flow.
- **Position of the insertion site:** A change in the position of the client's arm may decrease the flow, while elevation on a pillow may increase flow rate. If the IV is inserted into the antecubital area, the solution can flow freely if the client extends the arm and can be obstructed if the client bends the arm at the elbow.
- Monitoring and regulating the rate of the infusion is a responsibility of the nurse.
- A slower rate is usually necessary for older adults or those who are at risk of fluid overload (e.g., heart disease or client with head injury).
- A faster IV flow rate is therapeutic for patients who have lost large amounts of body fluids and those who are severely dehydrated.
- Never increase the rate of infusion if it is running behind schedule. Check for obstructions and collaborate with primary care providers to determine the patient's ability to tolerate an increased flow rate.
- Flow rate is regulated by tightening or releasing the IV tubing clamp and counting the drops for 15 seconds then multiplying the number 4 to get drops per minute.
- Sometimes, the IV rate order will say "to keep open" (TKO) or "keep vein open" (KVO). This order does not specify the Milliliters per hour. Generally, KVO is infused at 50 mL/h.

PRINCIPLES AND RIGHTS OF DRUG ADMINISTRATION

Principles of Drug Administration

The administration of mediation is an essential aspect of nursing care. Safe practice is essential and the nurse must be aware of their professional and legal responsibilities in relation to all aspects of medication management. In relation to children's and young people's nursing practice, the nurse also needs to consider the child's developmental stage, their ability to consent to treatment and the role of parents/carers.

Key principles associated with good practice in the administration of medication are:
- The nurse should be able to demonstrate an understanding of the plan of treatment for the child.
- The prescription should be legible, unambiguous and it should be legal.
- The prescription should be checked for date prescribed, drug prescribed, dose prescribed, route prescribed, duration of treatment, any additional required information, e.g., blood levels required after second dose, and it must be signed.
- Any contraindications to the prescribed drug must be identified by the nurse and appropriate action taken.
- Allergies must be checked and noted on the prescription chart.
- The nurse needs to be aware of the effects that the medication will have on the patient and also be aware of the side effects. The child and their family should be advised accordingly so as to avoid alarm and concern.
- The pediatric formulary must be available and referred to prior to the administration of the medication.
- Medication should be prepared in a quiet area and interruption should be avoided during this period.

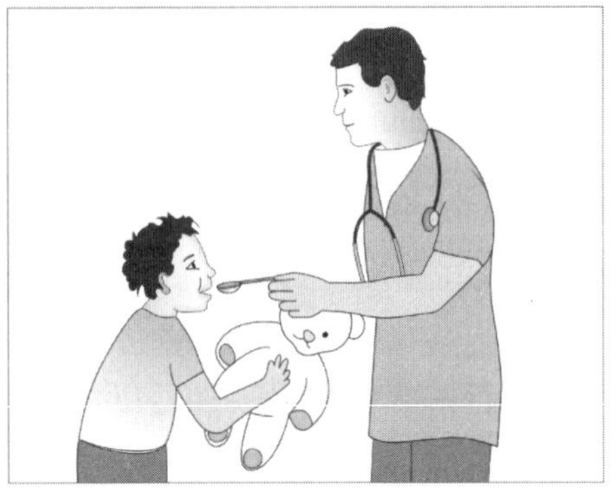

Distraction techniques are important

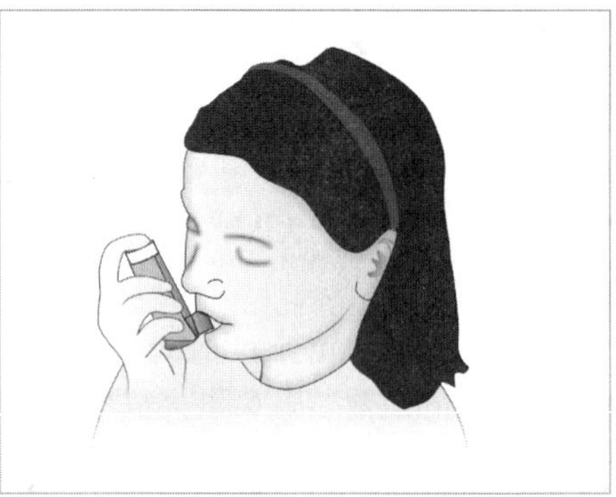

Encourage children to administer their
own medication

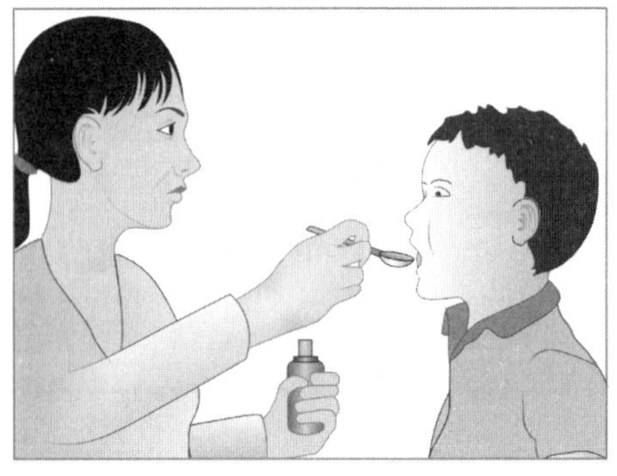

Involve parents in the administration of
their child's medicine

The 5 'Rs'

- Right drug

- Right dose

- Right patient

- Right route

- Right frequency

Fundamental principles of safe
drug administration

- ❖ The correct equipment should be collected initially.
- ❖ The nurse should check the prescription for date, time, frequency, dose, additional information and signature as part of the initial preparation process.
- ❖ The medicine container should be checked for drug name, dose, expiry date and that the content is clear and not contaminated.
- ❖ Local policy will determine the number of staff required to administer medication. Student nurses should be involved in this process.
- ❖ Consent must be obtained before administer the medication.
- ❖ The nurse administering the medication must ensure they observe the client taking the medication.
- ❖ The medication chart should only be signed once the client has swallowed/inhaled the medication. If the client refuses the medication or is unable to receive the medication as prescribed, for whatever reason, then this must also be documented on the prescription chart.
- ❖ Involve the play therapist and employ distraction techniques as required.
- ❖ Safely dispose of all equipment used in accordance with local policy.
- ❖ Discuss any required clinical holding techniques with the client before the first dose of mediation is required.
- ❖ Adhere to any additional requirements, e.g., if the medication is required to be taken on an empty stomach, then ensure this happens.

❖ If therapeutic serum levels are required, then ensure the child has the required blood sampling performed and that the results are available, scrutinized and acted on before any subsequent administration of the medication occurs.
❖ Remember the five 'Rs' of safe drug administration:
   1. Right drug
   2. Right dose
   3. Right patient
   4. Right route
   5. Right frequency.
Talk with the individual and explain what you are doing before you give medications. Answer any questions that the individual has.
❖ Help the individual to be as involved as possible in the process.
❖ Provide privacy for the individual.
❖ Give medication administration your complete attention.
   ♦ Give medications in a quiet area, free from distractions.
   ♦ Never leave medications unattended, even for a moment!
❖ Wash your hands! You must wash your hands before giving medications and then again after you have given medication to each individual.
❖ Education of the client should happen early in the admission process.

Rights of Drug Administration

10 Rights of medication administration: Understanding the 10 Rights of Drug Administration can help prevent many medication errors. Nurses, who are primarily involved in the administration of medications, benefit from this simplified memory aid to help guide them to administer medications safely.

1. **Right drug:** The first right of drug administration is to check and verify if it's the right name and form. Beware of look-alike and sound-alike medication names. Misreading medication names that look similar is a common mistake. These look-alike medication names may also sound alike and can lead to errors associated with verbal prescriptions. Check out The Joint Commission's list of look-alike/sound-alike drugs.
2. **Right patient:** Ask the name of the client and check his/her ID band before giving the medication. Even if you know that patient's name, you still need to ask just to verify.
3. **Right dose:** Check the medication sheet and the doctor's order before medicating. Be aware of the difference between an adult and a pediatric dose.
4. **Right route:** Check and verify the order (i.e., per oral, IV, SQ, IM)
5. **Right time and frequency:** Check the order for when it would be given and when was the last time it was given.
6. **Right documentation:** Make sure to write the time and any remarks on the chart correctly.
7. **Right history and assessment:** Secure a copy of the client's history to drug interactions and allergies.
8. **Right drug approach and right to refuse:** Give the client enough autonomy to refuse the medication after thoroughly explaining the effects.
9. **Right drug-drug interaction and evaluation:** Review any medications previously given or the diet of the patient that can yield a bad interaction to the drug to be given. Check also the expiry date of the medication being given.
10. **Right education and information:** Provide enough knowledge to the patient of what drug he/she would be taking and what are the expected therapeutic and side effects.

MEDICATION ERROR

"Any preventable event that may cause or lead to inappropriate medication use or patient harm while the medication is in the control of the health care professional, patient, or consumer. Such events may be related to professional practice, health care products, procedures, and systems, including prescribing, order communication, product labelling, packaging, and nomenclature, compounding, dispensing, distribution, administration, education, monitoring, and use".

Medication administration error (MAE) is defined as "any difference between what the patient received or was supposed to receive and what the prescriber intended in the original order". Medication administration errors are typically thought of as a failure in one of the five "rights" of medication administration (right patient, medication, time, dose, and route).

Factors that may Influence Medication Errors

A. Factors associated with health care professionals
- Lack of therapeutic training
- Inadequate drug knowledge and experience
- Inadequate knowledge of the patient n Inadequate perception of risk
- Overworked or fatigued health care professionals
- Physical and emotional health issues
- Poor communication between health care professional and with patients

B. Factors associated with patients
- Patient characteristics (e.g., personality, literacy and language barriers)
- Complexity of clinical case, including multiple health conditions, polypharmacy and high-risk medications

C. Factors associated with the work environment
- Workload and time pressures
- Distractions and interruptions (by both primary care staff and patients)
- Lack of standardized protocols and procedures
- Insufficient resources
- Issues with the physical work environment (e.g., lighting, temperature and ventilation)

D. Factors associated with medicines
- Naming of medicines
- Labeling and packaging Factors associated with tasks
- Repetitive systems for ordering, processing and authorization
- Patient monitoring (dependent on practice, patient, other health care settings, prescriber)

E. Factors associated with computerized information systems
- Difficult processes for generating first prescriptions (e.g., drug pick lists, default dose regimens and missed alerts)
- Difficult processes for generating correct repeat prescriptions
- Lack of accuracy of patient records
- Inadequate design that allows for human error Primary-secondary care interface
- Limited quality of communication with secondary care
- Little justification of secondary care recommendations

Types of Medication Error

The different types of medication errors include (but are not necessarily limited to):

- **Prescribing errors:** Wherein the selection of a drug is incorrect based on the patient's allergies or other indications. Additionally, the wrong dose, form, quantity, route (oral vs intravenous), concentration, or rate of admission could be used.
- **Omission errors:** In which there is a failure to give a medication dose before the next one is scheduled.
- **Wrong time errors:** Wherein a medication is given outside the predetermined interval from its scheduled time.
- **Improper dosing errors:** Wherein a greater or lesser amount of a medication is delivered than is required to manage the patient's condition.
- **Wrong dose errors:** Wherein the correct dosage was prescribed, but the wrong dose was administered.
- **Improper administration technique errors:** Such as administering a medication intravenously instead of orally.
- **Wrong drug preparation errors:** wherein a medication is incorrectly formulated (i.e., too much or too little diluting solution added when a medication is reconstituted).
- **Fragmented care errors:** wherein a lack of communication exists between the prescribing physician and other healthcare professionals.

PREVENTIVE MEASURES

Know the Patient

This includes the patient's name, age, date of birth, weight, vital signs, allergies, diagnosis, and current lab results. If patients have a barcode armband use it. The added administration times of using arm band systems have led some nurses to create potentially dangerous "workarounds" to avoid scanning barcodes. Don't make this potentially dangerous mistake—use all of the information at your disposal to ensure patient safety, and avoid shortcuts.

Know the Drug

Nurses need access to accurate, current, readily available drug information, whether the information comes from computerized drug information systems, order sets, text references, or patient profiles. If you have any questions or concerns about a drug, don't ignore your instincts-ask. Remember that you are still culpable, even if the physician prescribed the wrong medication, the wrong dose, the wrong frequency, etc.

Keep Lines of Communication Open

Breakdowns in communication among physicians, nurses, pharmacists, and others in the healthcare system can lead to medication errors. The "SBAR" method can help alleviate miscommunications. SBAR (Situation, Background, Assessment, Recommendation) works like this:

- **Situation:** "The situation is that Mr Smith is complaining of chest pain."
- **Background:** "He had hip surgery yesterday. About two hours ago he began complaining of chest discomfort. His pulse is 115, and he is short of breath and agitated."

❖ **Assessment:** "My assessment is that Mr Smith may be having a cardiac event."

❖ **Recommendation:** "My recommendation is that you see him immediately, and that we start him on O$_2$ and administer an analgesic immediately. Do you agree?"

Communication is vitally important, as it is the root cause of many sentinel events, according to the Joint Commission (TJC).

Double Check High Alert Medicines

High-alert medicines such as heparin can have devastating consequences if not administered properly. A tragic case involving the death of three infant patients after receiving massive heparin overdoses happened as a result of misleading packaging. Since this incident, the drug manufacturer now uses larger font sizes, tear-off cautionary labels, and different colors to distinguish drug doses. Medications often look alike and sound alike-this can be a source of errors. Double check high alert medications with another nurse to prevent accidental overdoses and other medication errors.

Document Each Drug Administered

Accurate documentation is essential and should include accurate recording of the drug information, the name of the drug, the dose, route, time, patient response, and any refusal of the drug by the patient.

Take an Active Role in Correcting Issues you Identify

If you see that look-alike or sound-alike medications are stored next to each other, ask your supervisor to correct the problem, emphasizing the increased risk of medication errors. Request that medications be reconciled (i.e., that the names, dosages, and administration routes of all medications are compared to identify conflicts). Request that a bar coding system be implemented that allows for the verification of the six medication rights (right individual, right medication, right dose, right time, right route, right documentation).

Inform the Patient of the Drugs they are Receiving

Make sure your patients know the names of the medications they are taking, what they look like, what they are for, how to take them or how they will be administered, the dosage, and the potential side effects and interactions.

Ask for Continuing Education

Ask for mandatory training sessions about medications that are introduced to facility. Training should include medication-related policies, procedures, and protocols. Updates like these, along with comprehensive nurse CE programs that include healthcare videos, empower nurses and can help prevent medication errors.

Nurse educators and continuing education providers should include all of these prevention tips, and more, in nurse education programs to help nurses avoid medication errors that could have detrimental or even deadly consequences for patients, and significant consequences for nurses, including disciplinary action, job dismissal, criminal charges, and mental anguish.

Nurses Responsibility in the Administration of Medications

- Assess gag reflex and patients ability to swallow.
- Do not touch tablets.
- Head end of the bed should be elevated at least by 90 degrees to administer oral medications.
- Make sure the patient as swallowed the medication.
- It is essential to hand wash before preparation of drugs.
- Always check for patient's history for allergies.
- Check the expired dates of drugs and before administering.
- Never administer medications prepared by another staff member.
- Before administering unfamiliar drugs try to know the route of administration, dose or combination of medications.
- Explain the procedure to the client discuss the need for medication.
- Before administering the anti-hypertensive medication check BP.
- Before administering an analgesics assess the type of pain its intensity, and location.
- Report on error in medication immediately to the charge nurse and the physician.
- Record the date, time, name of the drug administered. The dose of the medicine and the strength immediately after the medicine.

ROUTES OF DRUG ADMINISTRATION

Modes or routes of drug administration differ from the extensively administered oral route to parenteral and inhalational routes. There are also some specialized routes and modes of drug delivery, for example, the liposomal delivery, prodrug delivery, and others. Each of these routes of administration has its own advantages and disadvantages, which must be considered and compared to each other before selecting the same.

Factors determining route of administration are as follows:
- Drug characteristics like state of drug (solid/liquid/gas), and other properties of drug such as its solubility, stability, pH, and irritancy.
- Clinical scenarios such as emergency or regular treatment.
- Patient conditions like unconscious state, or if patient is experiencing diarrhea or vomiting.
- Age
- Comorbid diseases
- Patient/doctor choice
- Rate and extent of absorption of the drug from different routes.
- Effect of digestive enzymes and first pass metabolism on the drug.

Routes of drug administration can be divided broadly into two categories

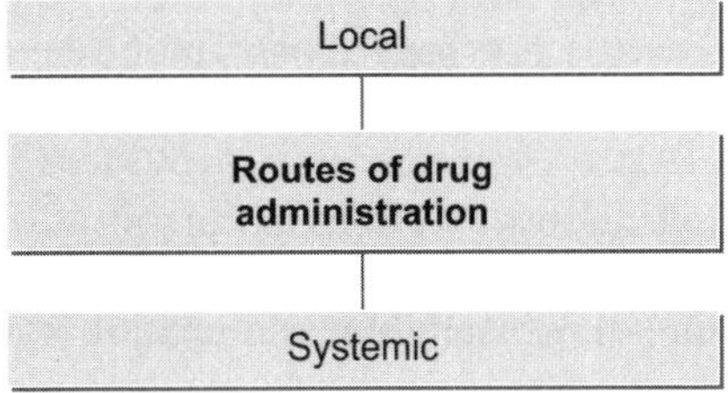

Local and systemic route includes enteral route which further comprises oral and rectal (drug is directly administered into the gastrointestinal tract [GIT]), whereas parenteral route comprises sublingual (under the tongue), inhalation (into bronchi) and injection. Further, injection includes intravenous (IV, into the vein), intramuscular (IM, into the muscle), and subcutaneous (SC, under the skin).

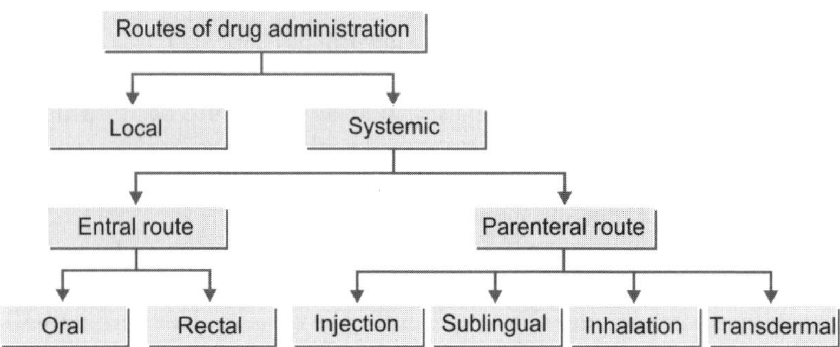

Local Route

It is one of the simplest routes of drug administration, wherein the drug can be given at the desired site of action. Systemic absorption of drugs is minimal; hence systemic side effects can be avoided. Following are some of the local routes:

Topical

The drugs applied to skin/mucous membrane for local actions. A few examples are as follows:

- **Oral cavity:** Drugs can be delivered only to oral mucosa in the form of lozenges or rinse, for example, clotrimazole troche for oral conditions.
- **GIT:** Nonabsorbable drug can be used to have local effect only, for example, neomycin for gut sterilization before surgery.
- **Rectum and anal canal:** Drug in liquid/solid form is used through this route for various actions.
  - *Evacuant enema:* Through this route, drugs are used for bowel evacuation, for example, soap water enema. Soap acts as lubricant and water stimulates the rectum.
  - *Retention enema:* For example, methylprednisolone in ulcerative colitis.
  - Suppository solid dosage form drug is inserted in rectum, for example, bisacodyl for bowel evacuation.
- **Eye, ear, and nose:** Drugs can be delivered to nasal mucosa, eyes, or ear canal in the form of drops, ointments, and sprays. This route can be employed for allergic/infective conditions of these organs.
- **Bronchi (inhalational):** This route of drug administration is used for conditions like bronchial asthma and chronic obstructive pulmonary disorder (COPD), wherein drug is absorbed by bronchial mucosa through inhalation, for example, salbutamol.

❖ **Vagina:** Drugs can be applied/inserted in the form of tablet, cream, or pessary to vagina. This route is mainly used for vaginal candidiasis.

❖ Urethra—Medication in the form of solution/jellies can be applied to urethra, for example, lignocaine.

Deeper Areas

These are, for example, intra-articular tissue or retrobulbar region. They can be reached by using syringe and needle. However, in order to reduce systemic absorption of drug, only slowly absorbed drugs should be used, for example, lidocaine for local anesthesia can be given as intrathecal injection. Also, hydrocortisone acetate is given as an intra-articular injection.

Systemic Route

Through this route, drug reaches the blood, is distributed across the body, and produces systemic effects. Broadly, this route can be divided into enteral, parenteral, and specialized drug delivery.

Enteral Route

This route includes oral and rectal.

Oral

This is the most common and accepted route of drug administration. Following oral administration, drug reaches the systemic circulation and is widely distributed across all tissues. Oral route has advantages of being safe, painless, and convenient for repeat and long-term use. Moreover, through this route, drug can be self-administered and does not require professional assistance. However, oral route has few limitations like slow onset of action, and thus cannot be given in emergencies, unpalatable/irritant drugs (e.g., chloramphenicol), unabsorbable drugs (e.g., neomycin), drugs with high first pass metabolism (e.g., lignocaine), medications destroyed by digestive juices (e.g., insulin). Other drawbacks included are they cannot be given in unconscious/uncooperative/unreliable patients and those having vomiting and diarrhea. Many dosage forms are available for oral administration; for example, solid forms like tablets, capsules, and liquid preparations such as syrups, elixirs, and suspensions. Tablets are made by compressing powdered drug along with binding agents and excipients, whereas capsules contain shell of gelatin, which is a tasteless natural substance. Two types of capsules are available—hard gelatin capsule (contain drug in solid form) and soft gelatin capsule (drug as an oily liquid form). In case of pediatric patients, swallowing of tablets/capsules is often problematic; in such cases, oral liquid preparations can be used.

Some of the above mentioned limitations of this route can be overcome by enteric coating of tablets and/or sustained/controlled release formulation. Enteric coating of tablets is done by cellulose and acetate. This has advantages like it prevents gastric irritation, protects drug from gastric acid, and retards drug absorption, thus increasing its duration of action. On the other hand, sustained/controlled release formulations have different coatings which dissolve at different time intervals. Advantages of this formulation are increase in duration of action, thus decreasing dosing frequency and increasing patient compliance, for example, sustained release nifedipine.

Sublingual

Drug which is lipid soluble is kept under the tongue or crushed and applied to buccal mucosa. Drug is absorbed into veins surrounding oral mucosa; later, it enters superior vena cava and heart and eventually reaches systemic circulation, for example, buprenorphine and nitroglycerin (used to terminate anginal attack). Advantages of this route is that drugs with high first pass liver metabolism are readily available in systemic circulation when given by this route. Other advantages include rapid onset of action, drug can be self-administered, and action can be terminated by spitting out tablet. Limitations of this route is that it is irritant, lipid insoluble, and unpalatable; hence, it cannot be given. Additionally, it cannot be used in children.

Rectal

This route can be used for systemic effects apart from local effects. Drugs are absorbed by hemorrhoid veins, and to some extent, they bypass liver metabolism. This route possesses certain advantages like irritant/unpleasant drug can be administered through this route. It can be used as suppository as well as in uncooperative/recurrent vomiting patients. Nevertheless, it has limitations like being embarrassing to patients, having erratic drug absorption, and leading to rectal inflammation in case of irritant drugs, for example, diazepam for febrile convulsions in children.

Parenteral Route

This is route of drug administration other than the enteral route. It includes drugs administered by injection, inhalation, and transdermal route. It has advantages like rapid onset, thus can be used in emergency; also, it can be used in uncooperative patients and patients with vomiting/diarrhea. This route is suitable for irritant drugs, drugs with high first pass metabolism, orally nonabsorbable drugs, and medication destroyed by digestive juices. The disadvantages of this route are that it is expensive and not easy for self-administration.

Inhalation

Volatile liquids and gases are administered by this route, for example, general anesthetics. Inhaled drug is absorbed through vast surface of alveoli; hence action is rapid.

Transdermal Route (Adhesive Patches)

Patches deliver drug into circulation for systemic effects. Patches have multilayers like backing film, drug reservoir, rate controlling micropore membrane, and adhesive layer with priming dose, for example, scopolamine for motion sickness, nitroglycerin for angina, estrogen for hormone replacement therapy (HRT), and fentanyl for analgesia. Few advantages of this route include self-administration, good patient compliance, prolonged action, minimal side effects, and constant plasma concentrations of drug. However, this route has drawbacks like being expensive, local irritation (itching, dermatitis), and patch may fall without being noticed.

Intradermal

Drug is injected into dermal layer of skin, for example, bacillus Calmette–Guerin (BCG) vaccination and drug sensitivity testing.

Subcutaneous (SC)

Drug is injected into SC tissue which has nerve supply but less vascular supply, for example, insulin and adrenaline. Self-administration is also possible; depot preparations for prolonged action can be used, for example, Norplant for contraception. This route is unsuitable for irritant drugs as well as has slow onset, thus cannot be used in emergency.

Intramuscular (IM)

Drug is injected into large muscles, deltoid, gluteus maximum, and lateral aspect of thigh in children. With this route, rapid onset of action can be achieved compared to oral route; also, depot preparations (used to prolong drug action), mild irritants, soluble substances, and suspensions can be given. Nonetheless, IM route requires aseptic condition, administration by professionals, can be painful, and may lead to abscess and local tissue injury.

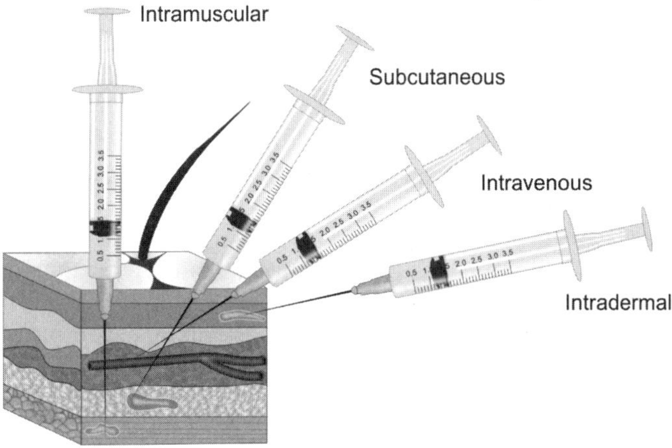

Intravenous (IV)

Direct injection of drug into vein. Drug can be given as bolus administration as well as slow IV infusion. Bolus administration is single, large dose rapidly/slowly injected as single unit, for example, furosemide, whereas slow IV injection involves addition of drug into a bottle containing dextrose/saline, for example, dopamine infusion in cardiogenic shock. With this route, 100% bioavailability and rapid onset of action can be achieved; hence it is suitable for emergencies. For example, when sedative drug midazolam is IV administered, sedation occurs in 2 to 4 minutes. Moreover, large volumes of fluids, for example, dextrose and highly irritant drugs, for example, anticancer drugs can be given through this route. Constant plasma concentration can be maintained using this route of administration. However, once drug is injected, drug action cannot be terminated. Administration of drug through this route can cause local irritation, thrombophlebitis, and necrosis.

Requirement of strict aseptic conditions and impossibility of self-administration are its other drawbacks. Also, depot preparations cannot be given. Caution in the form of ensuring tip of needle is in vein as well as slow administration of drug should be exercised while giving drugs through IV route.

Intra-arterial

This route is used when localized effect of a drug in a particular tissue or organ is desired. For example, in the treatment of renal tumor or head/neck cancer, drug is injected into renal artery or carotid artery, respectively.

Intrathecal

Injection of drug into subarachnoid space (into cerebrospinal fluid [CSF]). This route can be used as a method for direct delivery of a drug into the central nervous system (CNS), for example, spinal anesthesia (lignocaine) and antibiotics (in meningitis).

Epidural Injection

This is injection into epidural space, which is an area outside dura mater. It is different from intrathecal as drug is not directly administered into CSF. Local anesthetic drugs are given by this route to provide analgesia during childbirth.

Intra-articular

Drug is injected into joint space, for example, hydrocortisone for rheumatoid arthritis. This route requires aseptic condition and can cause damage to cartilage on repeated use.

Specialized Drug Delivery

Ocusert

Drug is kept beneath lower eyelid, for example, pilocarpine in glaucoma. Major advantage is single application releases drug for 1 week.

Progestasert

It is intrauterine contraceptive device which releases progesterone for 1 year.

Liposomes

Drug incorporated in minute phospholipid vesicles, for example, liposomal amphotericin for fungal infection.

Monoclonal Antibiotics

These are immunoglobulins which react with specific antigen. These can be used for targeted delivery, for example, anticancer drugs.

Storage and Handling of Medication

Medicines must be stored securely in an environment that will not affect their potency. All healthcare organizations should have Standard Operating Procedures and policies in place to ensure compliance with the manufacturer's storage recommendations and the relevant legislation, for example the storage of controlled drugs. Drugs must be stored in a locked cupboard or medical fridge according to the manufacturer's recommended temperature range. The appropriate temperature range should be monitored and both a room thermometer and fridge thermometer is required to enable this. Organizational policies should be available to ensure that medicines requiring storage within a medical fridge, for example, Syntocinon, are stored appropriately when used within the community setting. Midwives must also follow organizational policy for the supply, storage, administration and disposal of controlled drugs that may be used in hospital and community settings.

Steps should be taken to prevent human error and potential harm. Drugs should be stored to minimize mix-ups between medications of a similar appearance, for example intravenous (IV) solutions bags and vials of sterile water, normal saline and lidocaine. Measures should also be in place to reduce distractions that may occur in a busy care environment during drug rounds and the making up of IV infusions. Midwives should never prepare substances for injection in advance of immediate use or administer medication drawn into a syringe or container by another practitioner when not in their presence.

Storage

- ❖ Drugs and biological are kept in secure areas, and locked when appropriate.
- ❖ Stored in pharmacy and other areas to support patient care.
- ❖ Medications are properly and safely stored throughout the organization according to manufacturer recommendations and pharmacists instructions.
- ❖ Controlled substances must be locked within a secure area.
- ❖ Only authorized personnel have access locked drug storage areas
  - ◆ L and D and critical care is secure if access is limited.
  - ◆ OR suite is secure if actively providing care, otherwise non-mobile carts are locked and mobile carts are in a locked room.
  - ◆ Mobile carts are locked in a secure room.
  - ◆ Bedside medications—need to address security
- ❖ Under competent supervision
- ❖ Medication security

Examples of non-compliance:
- ❖ Medications left unattended on top of medication carts
- ❖ Medication carts unlocked secretary
- ❖ Housekeeping staff have access to drugs
- ❖ Extra break away locks available
- ❖ No policy addressing storage of drugs between receipt and administration carts stored in hallways > 15 minutes

Refrigerator

- ❖ Keep drugs separate (no food)
- ❖ Track temperatures on an ongoing basis (alarm, daily checks). Document action taken when out of range.
- ❖ Assure integrity of drug storage when the area is closed (such as over a weekend).
- ❖ 36–46°F (2–8°C) per USP/NF standards (Dietary refrigerators are colder 34–40°F)

Examples of non-compliance:
- ❖ Refrigerator deviated from recommended range and disposition of medications not defined in policy or no action documented.

- ❖ Vaccine refrigeration temperature checks documented twice daily (CDC recommendation)
- ❖ Freezer—temperatures for drug storage are kept between –20 and –10°C (–4 and –14°F).
- ❖ Controlled room temperature for drug storage is kept between 68 and 77°F. Warmer temperatures according to hospital policy. Refer to manufacturer for expiration date guidelines.
- ❖ For example, IV solution, irrigation solutions and water or saline pour bottles are dated when placed in the warmer and stock is rotated so the oldest product is always in front.
- ❖ Warmers are kept < 104°F. When the expiration date is reached these products are removed from the warmer and identified as being warmed. They are used or discarded within 24 hours.

Good Practices

- ❖ Store externals separate from internals
- ❖ Store flammables, hazardous drugs and chemicals separately
- ❖ Cabinets under sinks only contain cleaning products—No drugs
- ❖ Cleanliness of mortar and pestles

Should have policy on medication cart keys and keyless locks

- ❖ Drug samples—not recommended in hospital, particularly controlled substances. Follow regulations for clinic use.
- ❖ Outdated drugs–quarantine area

Example of non-compliance:
- ❖ Expired medications found in nuclear medicine department
- ❖ Pharmacy does not have labeled quarantine area
- ❖ Using date opened for expiration date
- ❖ Controlled drugs–Standard is to keep locked or controlled through automated dispensing technology (such as Omnicell, AcuDose, Pyxis). May double lock according to hospital policy. Address access privileges.

Life safety procedures: No cardboard boxes stored on floor and no storage within 18 inches of ceiling (from sprinkler head).
- ❖ Medication storage areas are periodically inspected
- ❖ Concentrated electrolytes are present in patient care areas only when necessary and precautions are used to prevent errors
- ❖ Policy addresses medication storage from time of receipt to time of administration
  - ◆ Safe storage
  - ◆ Safe handling
  - ◆ Security of medications
  - ◆ Disposition—returned to approved drug storage location or the pharmacy by end of shift

Home Medications

- ❖ Disposition (sent home or locked in pharmacy?)
- ❖ Circumstances when they can be used

* Pharmacist must visually inspect and approve
* Notify physician if not authorized
* Should not be liquid (including eye drops)

Temperature

The temperature in the store should not be above 25°C.

Storage temperatures are defined by European pharmacopoeia as follows:
* **Freezer:** –15 to 0°C
* **Refrigerator:** +2 to +8°C
* **Cool:** +8 to +15°C
* **Ambient temperature:** +15 to +25°C

Air and Humidity

In a store, relative humidity should not be above 65% (there are several devices for humidity measurement).

Air is a factor of deterioration due to its content of oxygen and humidity. All containers should remain closed. In airtight and opaque containers (hospital type), drugs are protected against air and light. Opening containers long before the use of drugs should be avoided.

Patients should be informed that tablets should not be removed from blisters until immediately before administration.

Light

Drugs should be protected from light, particularly solutions. Parenteral forms should be preserved in their packaging. Colored glass may give illusory protection against light.

ORAL, SUBLINGUAL, BUCCAL ROUTES

Prior to oral administration of medications, ensure that the patient has no contraindications to receiving oral medication, is able to swallow, and is not on gastric suction. If the patient is having difficulty swallowing (dysphagia), some tablets may be crushed using a clean mortar and pestle for easier administration. Verify that a tablet may be crushed by consulting a drug reference or a pharmacist. Medications such as enteric-coated tablets, capsules, and sustained-release or long-acting drugs should never be crushed because doing so will affect the intended action of the medication. Tablets should be crushed one at a time and not mixed, so that it is possible to tell drugs apart if there is a spill.

Position the patient in a side-lying or upright position to decrease the risk of aspiration. Offer a glass of water or other oral fluid (that is not contraindicated with the medication) to ease swallowing and improve absorption and dissolution of the medication, taking any fluid restrictions into account.

Remain with the patient until all medication has been swallowed before signing that you administered the medication.

- Perform hand hygiene
- Check room for additional precautions
- Introduce yourself to patient
- Confirm patient ID using two patient identifiers (e.g., name and date of birth)
- Check allergy band for any allergies
- Complete necessary focused assessments and/or vital signs, and document on MAR
- Provide patient education as necessary
- Plan medication administration to avoid disruption
- Dispense medication in a quiet area
- Avoid conversation with others
- Follow agency's no-interruption zone policy
- Prepare medications for one patient at a time
- Follow the seven rights of medication administration

Steps	Additional information
1. Check MAR against doctor's orders	• Check that MAR and doctor's orders are consistent 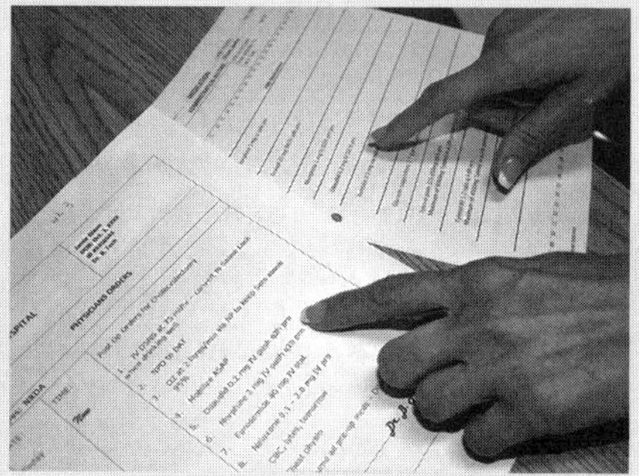 • Compare physician orders and MAR • Night staff usually complete and verify this check as well

2. Perform the seven rights x 3 (must be done with each individual medication):
  ➢ The right patient
  ➢ The right medication (drug)
  ➢ The right dose
  ➢ The right route
  ➢ The right time
  ➢ The right reason
  ➢ The right documentation
Medication calculation: D/H x S = A
(D or desired dosage/H or have available x S or stock = A or amount prepared)
	• **The right patient:** Check that you have the correct patient using two patient identifiers (e.g., name and date of birth).
	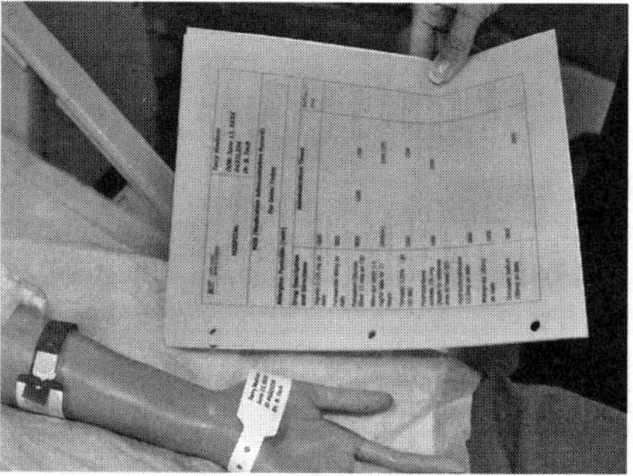
	• Compare MAR with patient wristband
	• **The right medication (drug):** Check that you have the correct medication and that it is appropriate for the patient in the current context.

Contd...

Contd...

<table>
<tr>
<td></td>
<td>

- **The right dose:** Check that the dose makes sense for the age, size, and condition of the patient. Different dosages may be indicated for different conditions
- **The right route:** Check that the route is appropriate for the patient's current condition
- **The right time:** Adhere to the prescribed dose and schedule
- **The right reason:** Check that the patient is receiving the medication for the appropriate reason
- **The right documentation:** Always verify any unclear or inaccurate documentation prior to administering medications

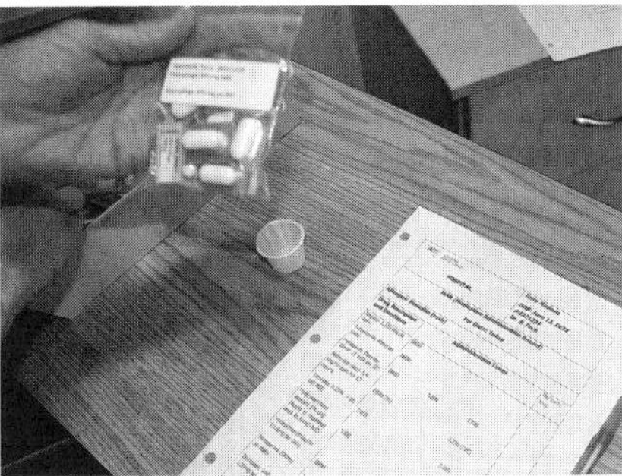

- Check the right patient, medication, dose, route, time, reason, documentation
- Never document that you have given a medication until you have actually administered it

</td>
</tr>
<tr>
<td>

3. The label on the medication must be checked for name, dose, and route, and compared with the MAR at three different times:
   - When the medication is taken out of the drawer
   - When the medication is being poured
   - When the medication is being put away/or at bedside

</td>
<td>

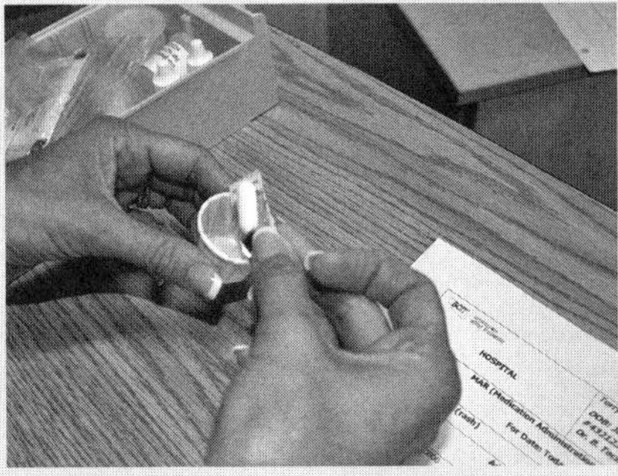

- Perform seven checks three times before administering medication
- These checks are done before administering the medication to your patient.
- If taking drug to bedside (e.g., eye drops), do third check at bedside.

</td>
</tr>
</table>

Contd...

Contd...

4. Place all medications that patient will receive in one cup, except medications that require pre-assessment (e.g., blood pressure or pulse rate). Place these in a separate cup and keep wrapper intact	Keeping medications that require pre-assessment separately acts as a reminder and makes it easier to withhold medications if necessary
5. Do not touch medication with ungloved hands. Use clean gloved hands if it is necessary to touch the medication	Using gloves reduces contamination of the medication.
6. Circle medication when poured	• Pour medication. Circle MAR to show that medication has been poured 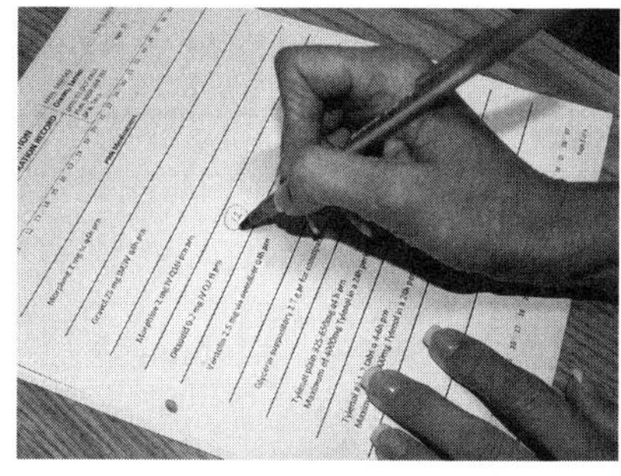 • Circle medication once it has been poured

7. Patient education
  ➤ Discuss purpose of each medication, action, and possible adverse effects
  ➤ Ask patient if they have any allergies
	• The patient has the right to be informed and provided with reasons for medication, action, and potential adverse effects. Giving this information will likely improve adherence to medication therapy and patient reporting of adverse effects
	• Confirms patient's allergy history

Important: If patient expresses concerns over medications, do not give medication. Verify doctor's order and explore patient concerns before administering medication	

8. Positioning
  ➤ Help patient to sitting position. If patient is unable to sit, use the side-lying position
  ➤ Have patient stay in this position for 30 minutes after administering medication
  ➤ Offer patient water or desired oral fluid.
  ➤ Ensure proper body mechanics for health care provider
	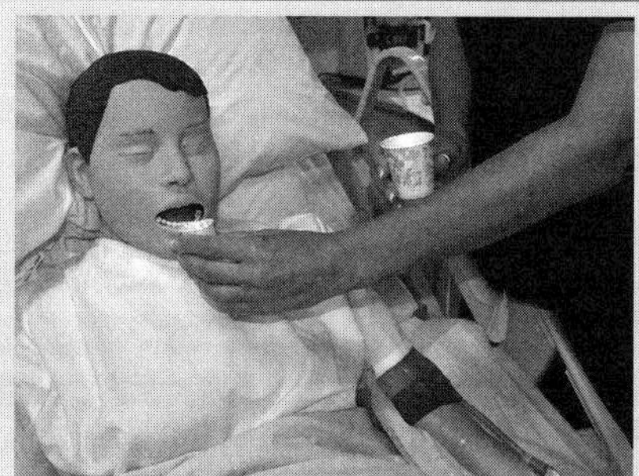
	• Position patient appropriately for medication administration
	• Correct positioning reduces risk of aspiration during swallowing

Contd...

Contd...

	• Water or other oral fluids will help with swallowing of medication • Proper body mechanics reduces risk of injury to health care provider

9. Administer medication orally as prescribed.
  ➢ **Tablets:** Place in mouth and swallow using water or other oral fluids
  ➢ **Orally disintegrating medications:** Remove carefully from packaging. Place medication on top of patient's tongue, and have patient avoid chewing the medication. Water is not needed
  ➢ **Sublingually:** Place medication under patient's tongue and allow to dissolve completely. Ensure patient avoids swallowing the medication
  ➢ **Buccal:** Place medication in mouth and against inner cheek and gums and allow to dissolve completely
  ➢ **Powdered medication:** Mix at bedside with water to avoid thickening of medication that may occur with time
	• Follow any specific descriptions for administration of the medication
	• Wear gloves if placing the medication inside the patient's mouth

10. Post-medication safety check
  ➢ Stay with patient until all medications are swallowed or dissolved
  ➢ Perform post-assessments and/or vital signs if applicable
  ➢ Sign MAR and place in appropriate chart
  ➢ Perform hand hygiene
  ➢ Document any additional information, such as patient education, reasons why medication not administered, and adverse effects, as per agency policy
	• Do not sign for any medications if you are not sure the patient has taken them
	• Post-assessments determine effects and potential adverse effects of medications

11. Return within appropriate time to evaluate patient's response to the medications and to check for possible adverse effects
 	
If patient presents with any adverse effects:
  ➢ Withhold further doses
  ➢ Assess vital signs
  ➢ Notify prescriber
  ➢ Notify pharmacy
  ➢ Document as per agency policy
	Most sublingual medications act in 15 minutes, and most oral medications act in 30 minutes

Buccal Route

The word buccal (pronounced "buckle") comes from the Latin "**bucca**," which means cheek. When administering a medication via this route, the medication is generally placed between the gums and cheek, which will allow it to be absorbed in the mucous membrane in the mouth and delivered into the bloodstream.

When a medication is placed between the gums and inner lips (instead of cheek), it is referred to as the **sublabial route** (labial refers to lips). The **buccal route** or **sublabial route** should not be confused with the **sublingual route**, which involves placing a medication under the tongue.

An example of some medication types that use the buccal route include the following:
- Certain opioid/Pain medications (example: some forms of Fentora/fentanyl)
- Smoking cessation medications
- Nitroglycerin
- Anti-seizure medications
- Hormone therapy medications and more

Medications administered via the buccal route may come in a solid form (such as a quick dissolve tablet or lozenge), a liquid form (spray, syringe, or droplets), or as a buccal film that can be placed along the gums or cheek.

Buccal Administration Preparation

- Before administering a medication via the buccal route, you should first perform medication rights to ensure that you have the right patient, right medication, right dose, given at the right route, right time, and so forth.
- Next, you'll perform hand hygiene and don gloves.
- You'll quickly assess the patient's mouth using a tongue blade. Make sure that there is not excess food or debris on the teeth or gums, and if there is, it may be a good time to perform mouth care for the patient.
- Inspect the mucous membranes for any sores or lesions, and avoid placing the medication over those areas unless you are instructed to do so.

Read the Medication Instructions

- Before administering the medication, it is important to read the medication's instructions. Some medications will be very specific on the buccal placement. For example, the medication may instruct you to place the tablet above the 3rd maxillary molar or above an incisor tooth.
- In addition, the medication instruction will dictate how soon the patient can eat, drink, or smoke once the medication has been placed, possible side effects, and so on. You should educate your patient about those details.
- Furthermore, most medications will instruct the patient to avoid splitting, crushing, swallowing, or chewing the medication while it dissolves. However, some medications may allow swallowing once it has dissolved for a certain period. For example, one buccal form of fentanyl (Fentora) instructs the patient to allow the medication to dissolve for up to 25 minutes. However, after 30 minutes, the patient may swallow any remainder of the tablet with a glass of water.

❖ Therefore, be sure to read the instructions because medications differ on these important details.

❖ If the patient has already received a prior dose of the medication, refer to the nursing documentation for your patient, as these medications sometimes require an alternate placement for additional doses.

How to Administer Medication: Buccal Route

❖ Make sure your gloves remain dry before handling any tablets, as they are made to dissolve when they contact moisture. Use the tongue blade to open the cheek when you are ready to administer the medication. Place the tablet (or film/liquid) in the area specified in the medication's instructions. For the example below, I placed the tablet above the maxillary left 2nd molar.

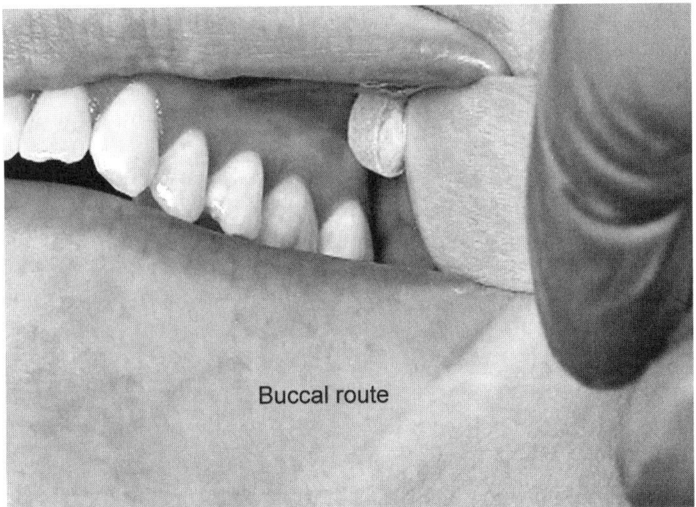

❖ Once you place the medication, release the tongue blade and allow the cheek to close against the medication to help it dissolve into the mucous membrane. You may want to use your finger to gently hold the medication in place for a moment as it starts to dissolve, unless instructed otherwise.

❖ Some medications can dissolve quickly in the buccal route, while some are meant to stay in place for several hours.

❖ Once you are finished, doff your gloves, perform hand hygiene, and document.

Tips for Nurse Documentation

When you document, you'll want to note the specific placement of the medication. For example, you might note that you placed the medication at the maxillary arch above the left second molar. This is important because some medications will require an alternate placement for additional doses, and the other nurses will need to know the last placement before administering another dose.

Equipment

IV set

An infusion set that is used to administer intravenous therapy, wherein a liquid substance is delivered directly into the patients' vein. It provides medical personnel with a brisk and effective means to deliver fluids and medication during medical conditions such as dehydration, electrolyte imbalances, specialized medication delivery, or for blood transfusions. However, the type of administration depends upon the rate and type of infusion, and the kind of solution container used. An IV infusion set should always be tailored to the patient and the planned treatment procedure.

Most infusion sets are made up of PVC material to ensure high strength, ease of sealing, resistance to sterilization procedures, and are relatively more economical. Based on the purpose of usage, the IV infusion set is divided into two types:

1. **Micro drip set:** This infusion set is used for pediatric patients and specific adult patients who require a small, closely-regulated dose of IV solution as it delivers a small quantity with each drop.
2. **Macro drip set:** This set infuses large quantities of IV solution at rapid rates as it delivers a large quantity with each drop.

IV infusion sets are divided into two main categories based on the fluid type. One is for transferring blood and the other for giving non-blood products such as saline. There are multiple variations of these two core types. But, the basic components of an IV infusion set that remain constant across all its variations are:

❖ Long sterile tube
❖ Connector
❖ Drip chamber
❖ V-track controller
❖ Spike

The spike is punctured/fitted into a sterile bottle containing a pre-filled IV solution. The drip chamber allows the fluid to flow one drop at a time and makes it easy to see the flow rate. The long sterile tube with a V-track controller helps control the flow rate. The IV set has a connector that can be attached to the access device. The Y-sets, T-sets, and V-sets are differently shaped three-way connectors that allow an additional infusion set to be connected onto the same line for delivery of antibiotics or other continuous fluid drips.

IV infusion sets are an integral part of intravenous therapy, which is one of the most commonly used treatment alternatives for various health conditions.

Ultrafusion

❖ Sharp air vented spike
❖ Bacteria retention air inlet with snap cap

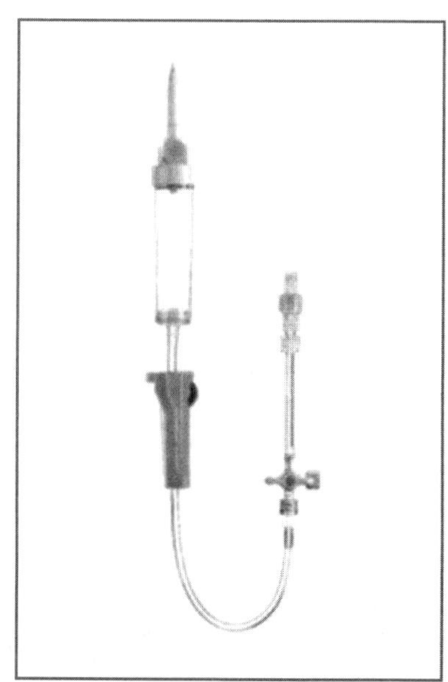

IV Set with three way stop cock and priming filter.

* ❖ "Y" injection port (latex free) designed for multiple injections
* ❖ Available with Back Check Valve to prevent back flow

Photofusion Set

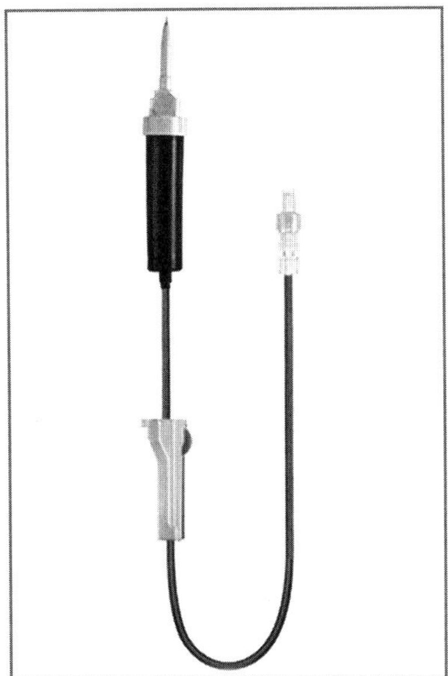

Priming Filter

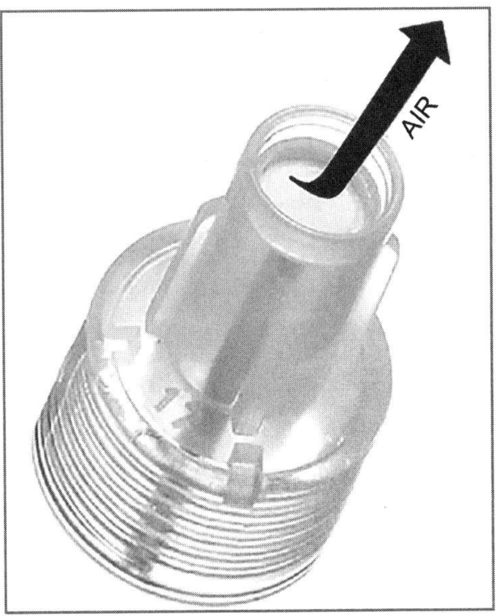

IV Infusion set for photosensitive drugs.

❖ Protects light sensitive drugs from UV exposure
❖ UV resistant tubing minimizes decomposition of the active ingredients of various drugs
❖ Hydrophobic priming filter cap to prevent fluid leakage
❖ Latex free
❖ DEHP free

Polyflo Novo

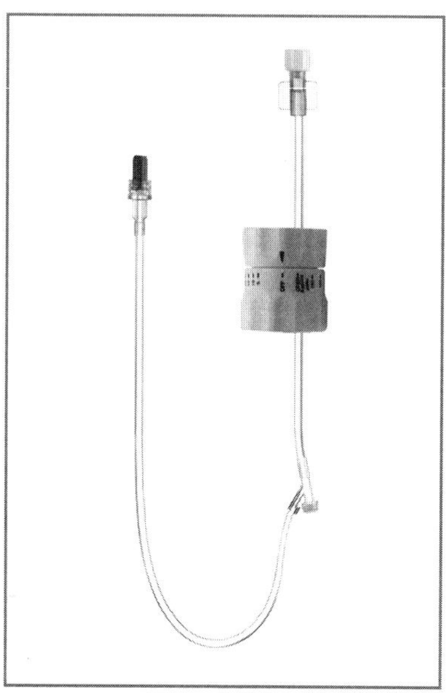

Also Available with Dual Scale

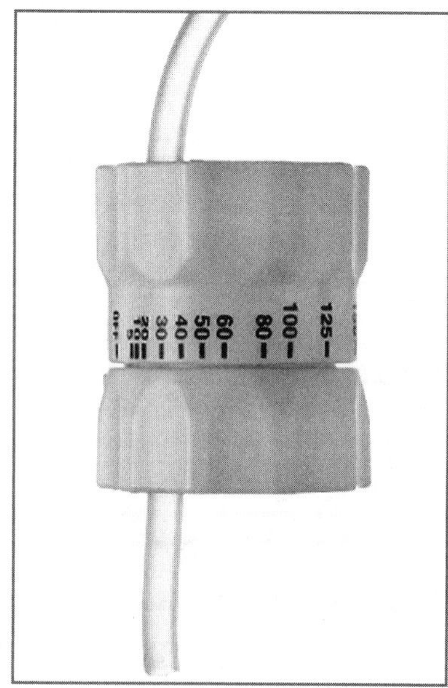

Polytrol–Micro Set

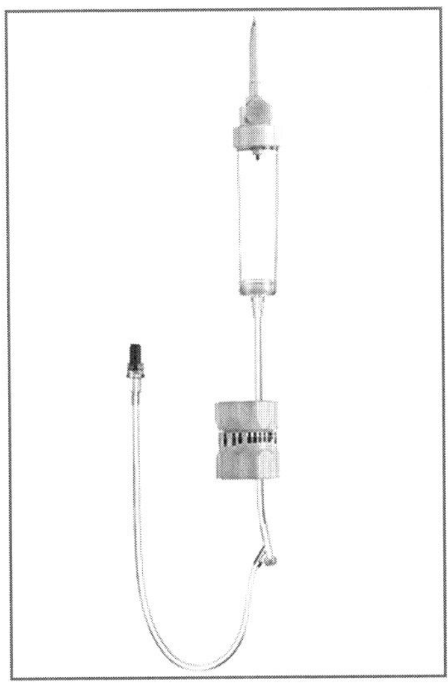

Needle Free Y-Site

- ❖ Flow regulator integrated into IV infusion set for precise flow control
- ❖ Flow rate 5 mL/hr to 250 mL/hr
- ❖ Approximately 60 drops/mL
- ❖ Also available with standard drip chamber (20 drops/mL)
- ❖ Latex free

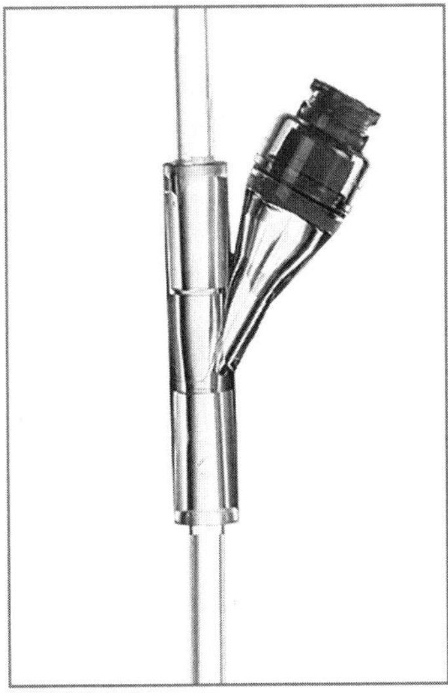

IV Infusion set with microdrip and flow regulator.

Common Features

- ❖ For gravity feed only
- ❖ 15 micron fluid filter in drip chamber
- ❖ Soft and kink resistant DEHP free PVC tubing ensures uniform flow rate
- ❖ Smooth roller clamp facilitates easy, safe control and adjustment of fluid rates
- ❖ Standard tube length: 150 cm
- ❖ Tube dia: I Ø 3 mm and O Ø 4.1 mm

Microfusion Set

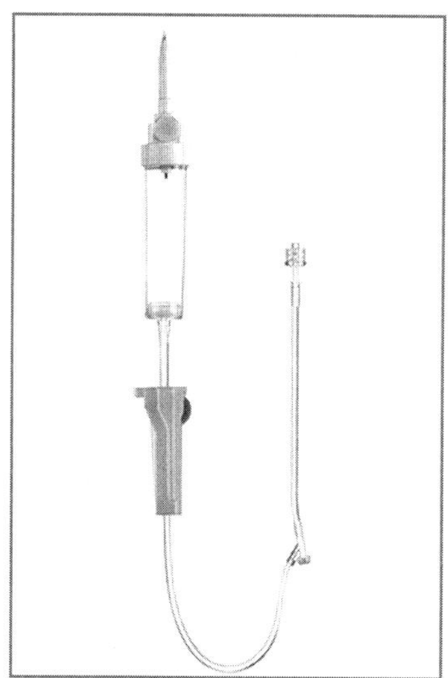

Micro Dipper

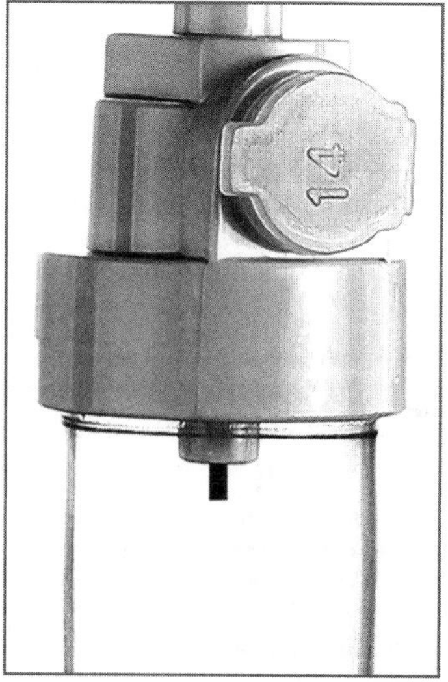

IV Infusion set with microdrip.

❖ Micro IV infusion set for pediatric use
❖ Approximately 60 drops/mL

Polyfusion W

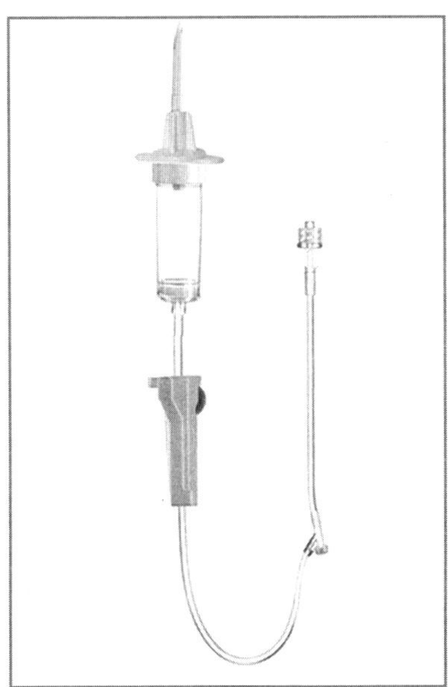

Rotating Luer Lock

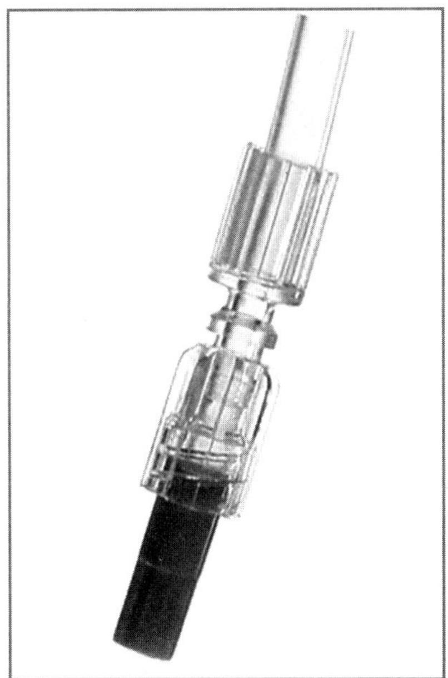

Luer Lock

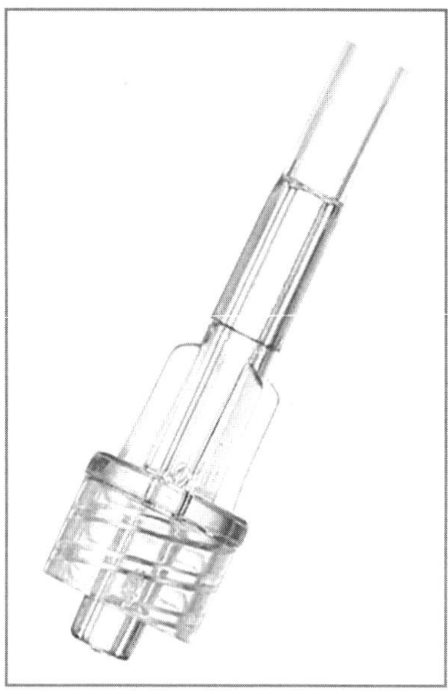

Needle Free Y-Site

❖ Sharp and winged spike for easy insertion
❖ Approximately 10 drops/mL

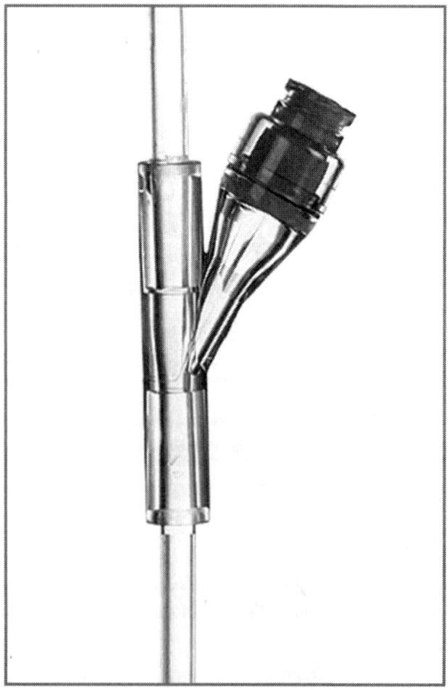

IV Infusion set with winged spike.

Common Features

❖ Transparent and flexible drip chamber
❖ 15 micron fluid filter in drip chamber
❖ Soft and kink resistant PVC tubing
❖ Smooth roller clamp facilitates easy and controlled adjustment of fluid rates
❖ Standard tube length: 150 cm
❖ "Y" injection port (latex free) designed for intermittent medications
❖ Tube dia: I Ø 3 mm and O Ø 4.1 mm
❖ DEHP free,
❖ Latex free

Novofusion Set

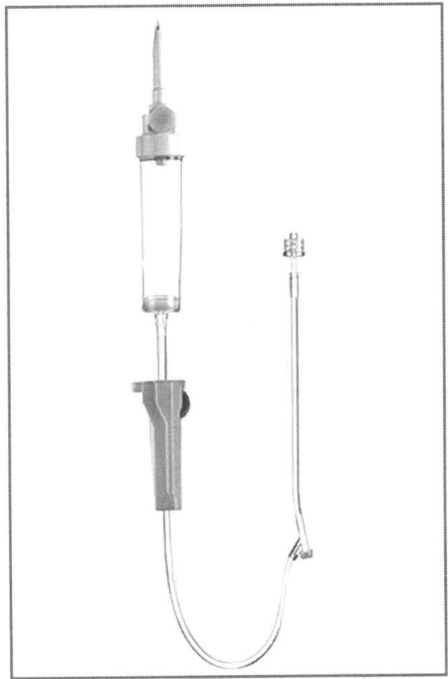

IV Infusion set with air vent.

❖ Sharp air vented spike
❖ Bacteria retention air inlet with snap on cap
❖ "Y" injection port (latex free) designed for multiple injections
❖ Suitable for pressure and gravity infusions
❖ Latex free
❖ DEHP free

CANNULA

A cannula refers to a small tube that is inserted into a body cavity, duct, or vessel for medical purposes. There are two main types of cannulas: intravenous (IV) cannulas and nasal cannulas. IV cannulas consist of short, flexible tubing that are placed into a vein and are usually used for blood transfusions, blood draws, administration of medication, and providing fluids. On the other hand, nasal cannulas are a simple yet effective device for delivering oxygen. They consist of a flexible tube with two protruding tips that sit inside the nostrils to deliver oxygen. They can be useful if the individual is experiencing difficulty breathing as nasal cannulas can decrease the work required to breathe and the strain on the heart, therefore treating hypoxia or hypoxemia.

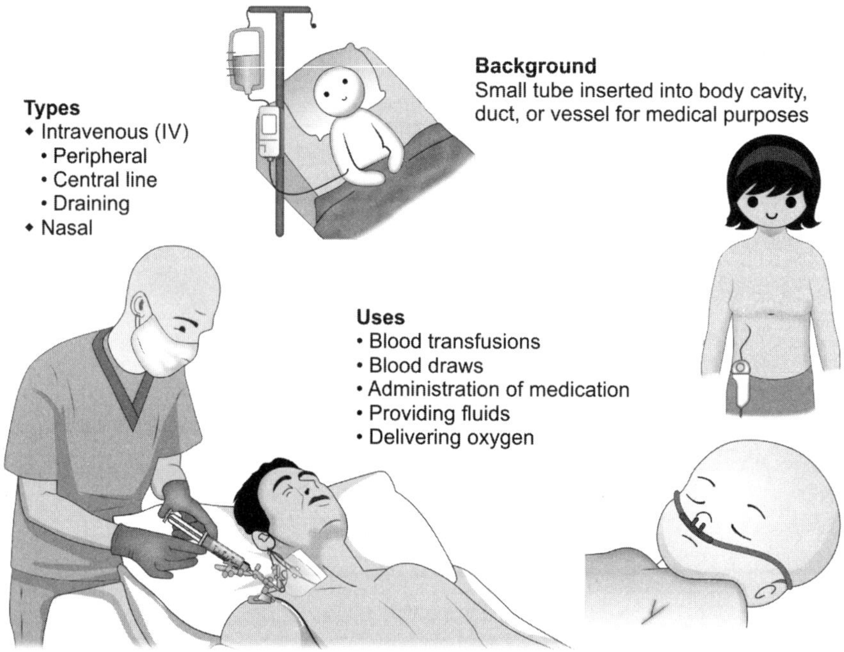

Common reasons for inserting a cannula include:
- ❖ Administration of intravenous fluids to maintain hydration.
- ❖ To treat dehydration in patients who are unable to tolerate sufficient oral fluid.
- ❖ To administer intravenous medication.
- ❖ To transfuse blood or blood products.
- ❖ To assist close observation and monitoring of a deteriorating patient.
- ❖ 'Just in case' cannulation

IV cannula subtypes include the peripheral IV cannula, the central IV cannula, and the draining cannulas. There are also several sizes of intravenous cannulas. The most common sizes range from 14 to 22 gauge. The higher the gauge number, the smaller the cannula. Different sized cannulas move liquid through them at different rates.

Peripheral IV Cannulas

Medical professionals typically use peripheral IV cannulas in the emergency room and during surgery in order to provide necessary fluids or to insert contrast when taking a radiological image. These cannulas are for short-term use and may be taped to the skin to prevent them from moving.

Sizes of the IV Cannula

Size	Color	Length	Flow rate (mL/min)	Uses	Nursing consideration
14G	ORANGE	45	250–300	• Used for adolescent and adult major surgery and trauma • Infusion of large amount of fluids or colloids	• Painful insertion • Required large insertion
16G	GREY	45	150–240	• Adolescent and adult major surgery and trauma • Infusion of large amount of fluids or colloids	• Painful insertion • Required large insertion
18G	GREEN	45	100–120	• Adolescent and adult major surgery and trauma • Infusion of large amount of fluids or colloids	Commonly used
20G	PINK	32	55–80	• Older children, adolescent and adult • Ideal for IV infusion and blood infusion • Medication administration • Emergency management	• Easy to insert into small, thin, fragile veins • Difficult to insert into though skin
22G	BLUE	25	22–50	• Older children, adolescent and elderly adult • IV infusion with moderate flow rates • Medication administration	• Insertion to though skin is difficult
24G	YELLOW	19	23	• Infant toddler, older children • Major surgery and trauma among children • Can administer fluids and medication	Less painful insertion to though skin is difficult
26G	VIOLET	19	10–15	• Neonate, infant and elderly adults • Suitable for infusion but infusion rate is low	Insertion to though skin is difficult and less painful

Flow rate calculation: When calculating the flow rate of IV solutions, remember that the number of drops required to deliver 1 mL varies with the type of administration set.

Administration sets are of two types:
1. **Macro drip set (delivers 10–20 drops/mL)**
2. **Micro drip set (60 drops/mL)**

$$\text{Flow rate} = \frac{\text{Volume of infusion in mL}}{\text{Time of infusion in minutes}} \times \text{Drip factor (in drops/mL)}$$

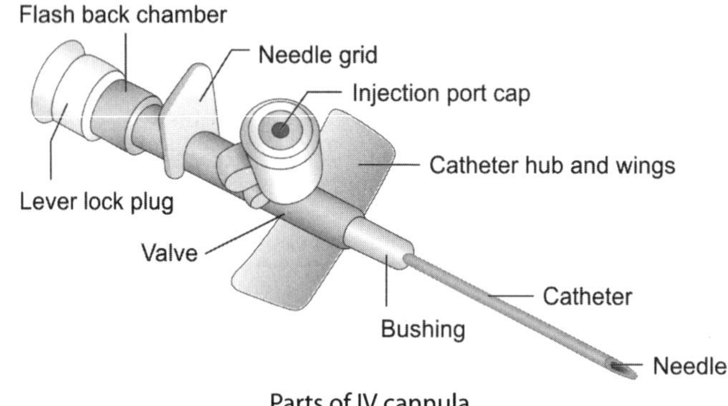

Parts of IV cannula.

Central IV Cannulas

Medical professionals may use a central line cannula for an individual who needs long-term treatments that require weeks or months of IV medication or fluids. For example, an individual receiving chemotherapy might require a central IV cannula for the intravenous infusion of the drugs. Central IV cannulas can quickly deliver medication and fluids into the body via the jugular, femoral, or subclavian vein. They can get easily infected; therefore, if any signs of infection (e.g., erythema, swelling, induration, fever) occur, they are typically removed.

Draining Cannulas

Health care providers use draining cannulas to drain fluids or other substances from the body. They can be used in procedures such as extracorporeal membrane oxygenation (ECMO), which is typically only used in critically ill patients with severe pulmonary and/or cardiac failure. In ECMO, blood is drained from the venous system, oxygenated, and then returned to the body. Sometimes draining cannulas might be used during liposuction. In that case, the cannula is connected to a trocar, which is a sharp metal or plastic instrument that can puncture tissue and remove fluid from or insert fluid into a body cavity or organ.

IV Cannula Insertion

When inserting an IV cannula in an individual's vein (usually in their arm), the patient is asked to lie or sit down with one of their arms exposed and extended by their side. The healthcare professional performing the procedure will choose the insertion point, which is usually in the individual's non-dominant arm or hand. Then, the area is thoroughly cleaned with an antiseptic while a tourniquet is tied above the desired insertion point. When ready, the healthcare professional will insert the IV cannula into a vein. The needle is only required to puncture the skin and vein. Once the cannula is placed in the vein, the needle is withdrawn as the cannula slides over the needle and into the vein. The cannula is then secured in place with medical tapes, such as a wrap or a special bandage.

Types of Nasal Cannulas

A standard nasal cannula consists of lightweight plastic tubing that is inserted just inside an individual's nostrils. The oxygen flow in a standard nasal cannula is lower than in other types, such as high flow nasal cannula (HFNC). The nasal cannula allows breathing through the mouth or nose, is available for all age groups, and is adequate for short or long-term use. Unlike the numbered sizes of intravenous cannulas, nasal cannulas are available in sizes for adults, children, and infants. Regular flow nasal cannulas provide only up to 4–6 liters per minute of supplemental oxygen. The delivered oxygen percentage varies, depending on the rate and depth of the individual's breathing. When cannulas are used at higher flow rates (i.e., greater than 4 L/min), the airway mucosa may dry, so a humidifier may be used to help prevent drying of the nasal and oral mucous membranes.

High-flow Nasal Cannula (HFNC)

High-flow nasal cannula therapy systems (HFNCs) offer an increased flow rate of oxygen compared to standard nasal cannulas. HFNCs deliver oxygen at a flow rate of up to 60 liters per minute. The latest models of HFNCs can also heat the gas to 98.6°F (37°C) to ensure the individual can breathe easily. Some individuals prefer the HFNC because it is lighter, more comfortable, and does not irritate their airways as much as a standard nasal cannula. In fact, HFNC was highly effective for individuals with COVID-19 who experienced respiratory distress.

At-home Nasal Cannulas

Nasal cannulas can be portable to give an individual the independence of receiving oxygen therapy at home. The procedure for fitting a nasal cannula for home is very similar to insertion of a nasal cannula at the hospital; however, a home nasal cannula will attach to a portable oxygen supply. The healthcare provider may instruct the individual on how to use the equipment and how often to refill the oxygen supply.

Nasal Cannula Insertion

When inserting a nasal cannula, the individual may be asked to sit up straight (if possible) to expand their lungs fully. The flow meter is then inserted into a power source and attached to a nozzle. The flow meter is turned on and assessed to ensure oxygen is coming through properly. The healthcare provider may then place the nasal cannula into the individual's nose with the two prongs of the cannula placed just inside the individual's nostrils. The extended tubes are then looped around the individual's ears and a plastic slider is set under the chin so it stays in place. Finally, the flow rate may be evaluated every 4–8 hours in order to assess the individual's oxygen levels and how they are responding to oxygenation.

Oral Route

The drug is administered to or by way of the mouth. A drug given via this route is absorbed into the systemic circulation from the gastrointestinal tract. The oral route is the most frequently used route for drug administration.

Oral Dosage Forms

- Solid dosage forms, e.g., tablets (immediate-release, enteric-coated, modified-release), capsules, granules, powders
- Liquid dosage forms, e.g., syrups, elixirs, suspensions

Advantages of the Oral Route

- Cheap
- Generally safe route of drug administration
- Simple and convenient for the patient
- The patient can self-administer
- Non-invasive.

Disadvantages of the Oral Route

- Drug absorption may vary. Examples of factors affecting drug absorption are gastro-intestinal motility, gastric emptying rate and the presence of food in the gastrointestinal tract
- Subject to first-pass metabolism
- Oral route not possible in unconscious patients
- Unsuitable in patients who are vomiting
- Slow onset of action
- The drug may be destroyed by digestive enzymes and/or stomach acid

Sublingual Route

A dosage form designed for the sublingual (SL) route is administered under the tongue. The drug is absorbed from the blood vessels that lie under the tongue and enters the systemic circulation directly, thus avoiding first-pass metabolism.

Sublingual Dosage Forms

- Sublingual tablets, e.g., glyceryl trinitrate SL tablet
- Sublingual films, e.g., suboxone SL film
- Sublingual sprays, e.g., glyceryl trinitrate SL spray

Advantages of the Sublingual Route

- Rapid drug absorption
- Quick onset of action
- Avoids first-pass metabolism
- The patient can self-administer

- ❖ Convenient for the patient
- ❖ Can be quickly terminated by spitting out the sublingual tablet if required
- ❖ This route can be used by people who have difficulty in swallowing tablets

Disadvantages of the Sublingual Route

- ❖ Most drugs are not available as sublingual formulations
- ❖ The taste of the sublingual dosage form may not be liked by the patient
- ❖ Placing the sublingual dosage form under the tongue until it dissolves may be considered inconvenient by some patients.
- ❖ Irritation to the oral mucosa.

Buccal Route

The buccal route is administered by placing the buccal dosage form between the gum and the inner cheek. The drug is rapidly absorbed from the buccal mucosa and enters the systemic circulation, thus avoiding first-pass metabolism. In addition, this route can also be used for a local effect (e.g., hydrocortisone muco-adhesive buccal tablet for the treatment of aphthous ulceration of the mouth).

Buccal Dosage Forms

- ❖ Buccal tablets, e.g., prochlorperazine maleate
- ❖ Chewing gum, e.g., nicotine gum

Advantages of the Buccal Route

- ❖ Rapid drug absorption
- ❖ Avoids first-pass metabolism
- ❖ Convenient for the patient

Disadvantages of the Buccal Route

- ❖ The taste of the buccal dosage form may not be liked by the patient
- ❖ Irritation to the oral mucosa

Intravenous Route

A drug administered by the intravenous (IV) route is given directly into a vein as direct injection or infusion.

Intravenous Dosage Forms

- ❖ Injection
- ❖ Emulsion injection
- ❖ Solution for injection
- ❖ Solution for infusion

Advantages of the Intravenous Route

- ❖ Immediate effect (suitable for emergencies)
- ❖ Can be given to unconscious patients

- ❖ Avoids first-pass metabolism
- ❖ Achieves predictable and precise control over drug plasma levels compared to other routes

Disadvantages of the Intravenous Route

- ❖ Possible anaphylaxis
- ❖ Risk of infection
- ❖ Inconvenient to the patient
- ❖ Painful
- ❖ Expensive compared to other routes
- ❖ Risk of phlebitis or extravasation
- ❖ Requires trained medical/nursing staff to administer
- ❖ Once injected, the drug cannot be recalled
- ❖ Labor intensive and time-consuming, e.g., may require calculating the dose, looking up the diluents to be used, checking for IV drug compatibilities, preparation of IV drug and administering the injection.

Intramuscular Route

The intramuscular (IM) route is given directly into the muscle (e.g., gluteus medius and deltoid).

Intramuscular Dosage Forms

Solution for intramuscular injection

Advantages of the Intramuscular Route

- ❖ Immediate onset
- ❖ Depot or sustained release
- ❖ Avoids first-pass metabolism
- ❖ Easier to administer compared to the intravenous route

Disadvantages of the Intramuscular Route

- ❖ Expensive
- ❖ Requires trained medical/nursing staff
- ❖ Irritating drugs may be painful
- ❖ Slower onset than IV route
- ❖ Variable drug absorption dependent upon the muscle group used and the blood flow to the muscle

Subcutaneous Route

The subcutaneous (SC) route is injected into the subcutaneous tissue. It can be given as direct injection or infusion.

Advantages of the Subcutaneous Route

- ❖ Can be self-administered by the patient
- ❖ Some drugs have a long duration of action, e.g., flupentixol
- ❖ Low risk of systemic infection

Disadvantages of the Subcutaneous Route

- Variable drug absorption dependent on blood flow
- Only a small volume of the drug can be administered.

Pulmonary/Inhalation Route

The inhalation route is used for a local effect or systemic effect. The drug is inhaled through the mouth and delivered into the lungs.

Pulmonary Dosage Forms

- Metered-dose inhalers (MDIs)
- Dry powder inhalers

Advantages of Inhalation Route

- Rapid onset of action
- Systemic side effects minimized
- Reaches the site of action

Disadvantages of Inhalation Route

- Proper inhaler technique required for the drug to work maximally
- Only a small number of drugs can be given via this route
- May stimulate the cough reflex

Nasal Route

Administration of a drug directly into the nose.

Nasal Dosage Forms

- Nose spray
- Nose drops

Advantages of Nasal Route

- Can be self-administered by the patient
- Rapid onset of action
- Minimal side effects

Disadvantages of Nasal Route

Some nasal drops or sprays may lead to an unpleasant taste in the mouth

Rectal Route

Administration into the rectum for a localized effect or a systemic effect.

Rectal Dosage Forms

- Suppositories
- Enemas

Advantages of Rectal Route

- ❖ The patient can self-administer
- ❖ Can be used for a local effect
- ❖ Can be used in patients unable to swallow, vomiting or unconscious
- ❖ Reduced first-pass metabolism

Disadvantages of Rectal Route

- ❖ Uncomfortable and messy to use
- ❖ Inconvenient for the patient
- ❖ Absorption can be slow and erratic
- ❖ Not well accepted by the patient

Vaginal Route

Administered into the vagina.

Vaginal Dosage Forms

- ❖ Vaginal pessaries
- ❖ Vaginal creams
- ❖ Vaginal rings

Advantages of Vaginal Route

- ❖ The patient can self-administer
- ❖ Can be used for a local effect
- ❖ Avoids first-pass metabolism

Disadvantages of Vaginal Route

- ❖ Uncomfortable and messy to use
- ❖ Patient compliance
- ❖ Local irritation
- ❖ Inconvenient to the patient
- ❖ Not well accepted by the patient

Cutaneous Route

Administration to the skin.

Cutaneous Dosage Forms

Dermatological preparations, e.g., ointments, creams, liquids, powders, solutions, shampoos.

Advantages of Cutaneous Route

- ❖ The patient can self-administer
- ❖ Can be used for a localized effect
- ❖ Systemic side effects/drug interactions avoided or reduced

Disadvantages of Cutaneous Route

* Some preparations may be messy or difficult to apply
* Some dermatological preparations are time-consuming to apply
* Adverse drug reactions to excipients contained in the dosage form

Otic/Ear Route

Administration to or by way of the ear.

Otic Dosage Forms

Ear drops

Advantages of the Otic Route

Produce a local effect

Disadvantages of the Otic Route

* May be difficult for some patients to administer themselves
* This route may be considered time-consuming by the patient as they need to remain on their side/tilt the ear for a few minutes after instillation of ear drops

Ocular/Eye Route

Administration of drug into the eye.

Ocular Dosage Forms

* Eye ointment
* Eye drops

Advantages of the Ocular Route

* Convenient for the patient
* Systemic side effects reduced

Disadvantages of the Ocular Route

* May cause temporary blurring of vision upon instillation of eye drops/ointment
* Barriers to administration, e.g., poor manual dexterity, poor vision
* Not all ocular dosage forms can be used with contact lenses

Transdermal Route

Absorption of the drug through the skin and into the systemic circulation.

Transdermal Dosage Forms

* Transdermal patches
* Transdermal gels

Advantages of the Transdermal Route

❖ Convenient for the patient
❖ Long duration of drug action
❖ Usually requires less frequent application, e.g., 24 hours/72 hours
❖ The patient can self-administer
❖ Avoids first-pass metabolism
❖ Steady plasma concentration
❖ Slow absorption

Disadvantages of the Transdermal Route

❖ Can be expensive
❖ Local irritation

SYRINGES

Syringes are used to administer parenteral medications. A disposable syringe is a sterile device that is available in various sizes ranging from 0.5 to 60 mL. A syringe consists of a plunger, a barrel, and a needle hub. Syringes may be supplied individually or with a needle and protective cover attached.

Syringes and needles have an essential role as injection devices, fluid or biopsy collection (sampling), irrigation, or suction. Syringes consist of different types of tips.

A syringe consists of a barrel, a plunger, and a needle. The plunger is used to control the dosage of liquid through the needle or the tube. The barrel is mostly made up of polypropylene with obvious markings of different measurements. Some of the syringes are made up of glass and even metal but are not as common as plastic ones. Syringes come in various types depending on the purpose that they are being used for. Their different types are defined according to their capacity, syringe tips, needle sizes, and needle gauges.

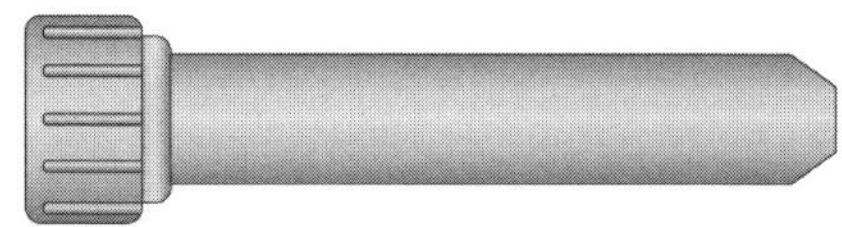

Disposable syringe and needle (parts labelled)

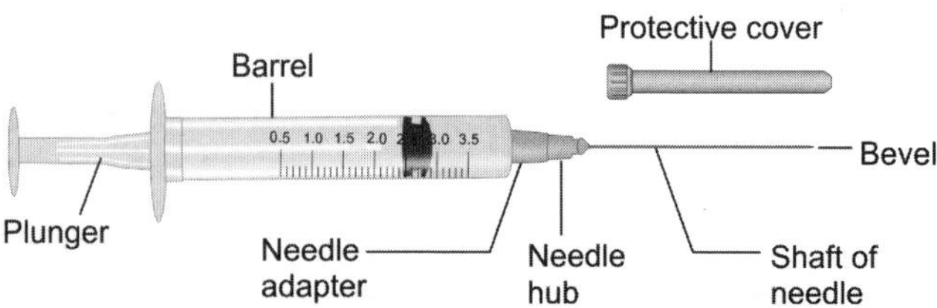

Types of Syringes

There are five common types of syringe tips are:

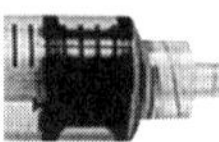 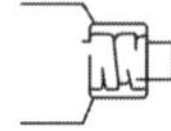

1. Luer lock tip: "Locking fit" secure screw type connection

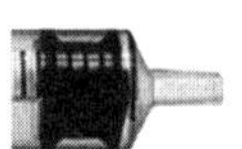 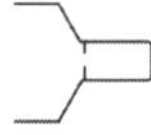

2. Luer slip tip: Friction-fit conection, slip connection

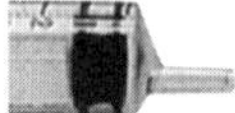 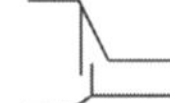

3. Eccentric tip: Off center tip, perfect for injecting into a vein

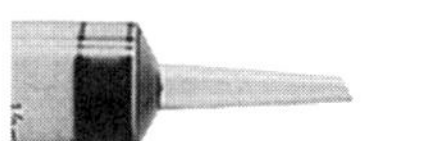 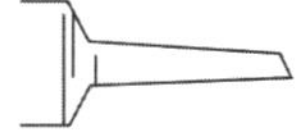

4. Catheter tip: Longer slip tip, used for irrigation or with medical tubing

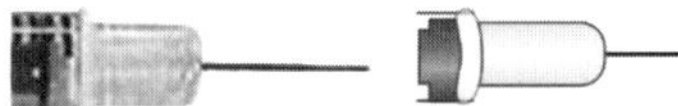

5. Permanently attached: Syringe with permanently attached needle

Types of syringe tips.

1. Luer Lock Tip

Luer lock syringes have threads in the needle hub that provide a secure connection of needles, tubing, or other devices. A luer lock syringe with a barrel and a readable scale. This image shows a syringe that holds 12 cc, also referred to as 12 mL. When withdrawing medication, match up the top of the plunger and the line on the barrel scale with the amount of medication you need to administer. In this image, 3 mL of medication is contained in the syringe.

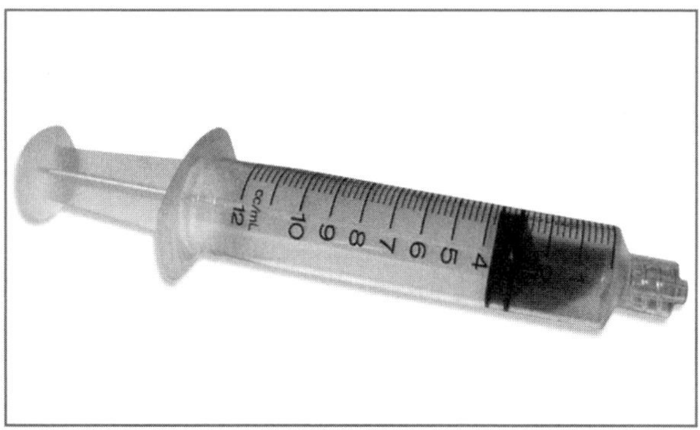

Luer lock syringe.

Insulin is administered using a specific insulin syringe. Insulin syringes are marked in units, not milliliters (mL), because insulin is prescribed by providers in units, not mL. A regular syringe marked in milliliters should never be used to administer insulin. All insulin syringes have orange caps for quick identification, but verify the markings are in units to prevent a medication error. A 50-unit insulin syringe with a white safety shield attached.

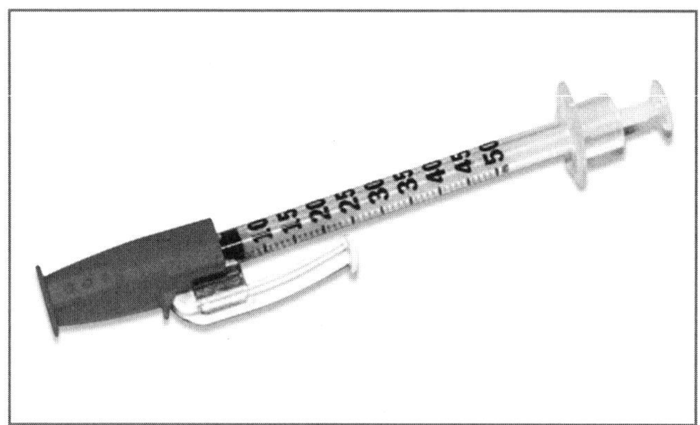

2. Luer Slip Tip

Luer slip tip has a slip connection and has a friction-fit connection. Insert the syringe tip of Luer slip into the needle hub or other attaching device into push manner. Due to simple sliding, the attaching device into syringe tip, not ensure to secure fitting.

Luer slip tip syringe sizes: 1 mL, 3 mL, 5 mL, 10 mL, 20 mL, 30 mL, 60 mL

3. Eccentric Tip

Eccentric tip syringe has an off-center tip, used for surface vein or artery injection. This syringe is perfect for injecting into a vein.

Eccentric tip size: 10 mL, 20 mL, 60 mL

4. Catheter Tip

Catheter tip type of syringe used for irrigation, or with medical tubing, or flushing (clearing) catheter or injecting through a tube.

Catheter tip size: 2 oz only

5. Permanently Attached

The permanently attached syringe is a syringe with a permanently attached needle.

For example:
- ❖ Tuberculin syringe: Permanently attached needle
- ❖ Disposable syringe: Attached with needle

Types of Syringes Based on Barrel Sizes

Figuring out the syringe size is very important for injecting the dosage of medicine in the patient. When choosing the syringe, it is required to make sure that the syringe's size is according to the volume of the drugs. For a larger volume dosage of medicines, you must choose the larger capacity syringes accordingly. Another essential factor that should be kept in mind when choosing the right syringe is the desired pressure flow. Larger capacity syringes have lower pressure flow and vice versa.

Syringe sizes are specified based on the amount of liquid that they can hold. The syringe size or capacity can be measured in two ways: milliliters (mL) and cubic centimeters (cc). The milliliter measurement is used for the liquid volume, whereas cubic centimeters measurement is used for the volume of solids. One cubic centimeter (cc) is approximately equal to 1 milliliter (mL).

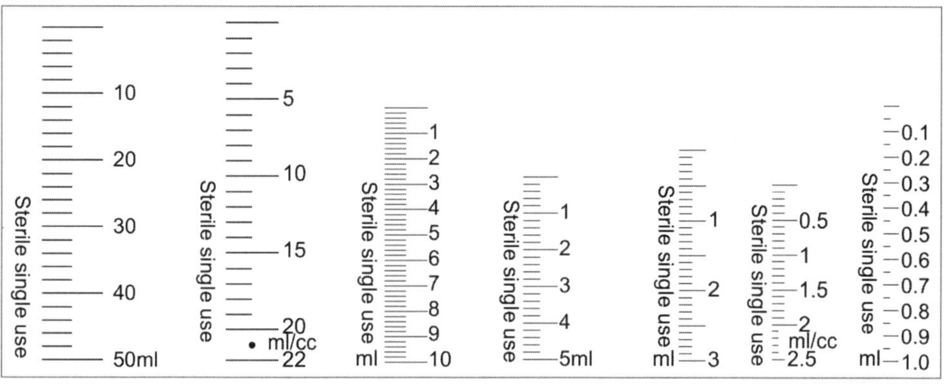

Barrel sizes.

The syringe barrel has markings on it according to the milliliter (mL) scale to let the user know the exact dosage of the medication that is being injected. Another vital thing to consider while reading from the syringe is precisely measuring the plunger's top ring.

Most Commonly used Syringe Sizes

The different syringes are based on their capacity in milliliter (mL) or cubic centimeter (cc). The volume of the syringe should be enough to fulfill the medication that is to be injected. The syringe sizes can range from 0.25 mL to 450 mL. The size of the syringe is also used to determine the needle size and needle gauge. Below we will discuss some of the most commonly used syringe sizes.

1 mL or Less than 1 mL Syringes

1 mL syringes are commonly used for diabetic and tuberculin medication, as well as intradermal injections. The tuberculin syringes have greater than half inches of needle length and have needle gauge between 26G and 27G. We can use 1 mL syringes with needle gauge size between 25G and 26G as an intradermal injection.

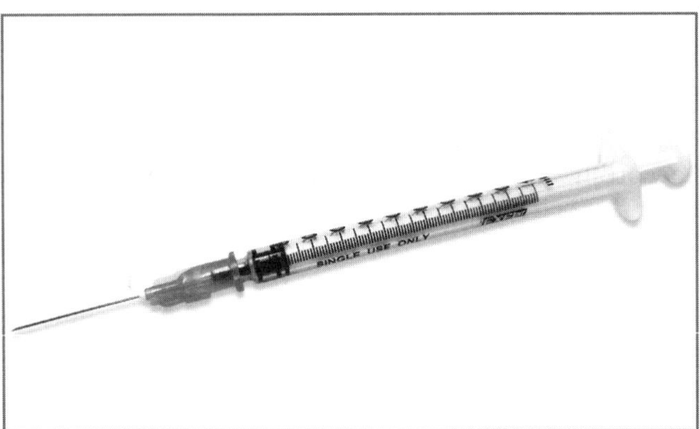

Tuberculin syringe.

The insulin syringes have mostly three different sizes because they are injected in a lower dose than other medications. If you have to inject the insulin dose of 30 units or lesser than 30 units, you have to use a 0.3 mL syringe. Similarly, if you have to inject a dose between 31 to 50 units, you have to use a 0.5 mL syringe, and if the recommended dosage is between 51 to 100 units, you have to use the 1mL syringe. Their needles are not greater than half inches and have needle gauge between 29G and 31G.

Insulin Syringe

2 mL–3 mL Syringes

The syringes between 2 and 3 mL are mostly used for vaccine injections. The syringe size must be determined according to the vaccine dose. The needle gauge for vaccine injections is mostly between 23G and 25G, and the needle length can vary according to the patient's age and other factors. Choosing the right length needle is very important in terms of avoiding any risk of injection site reactions.

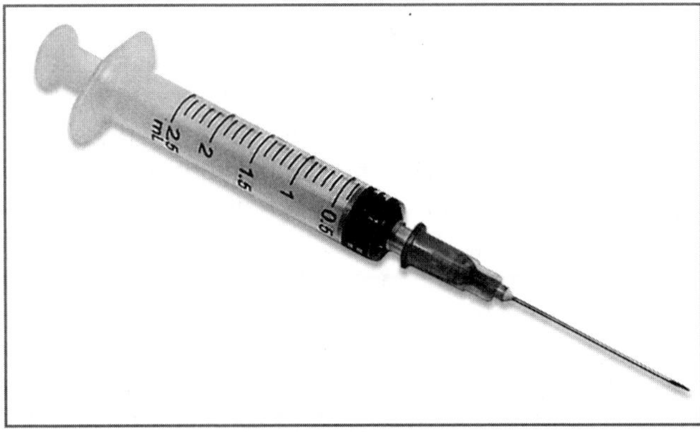

2.5 mL syringe.

5 mL Syringes

The syringes with a capacity of 5 mL can measure doses of liquid medication up to 5 ccs. These syringes are used for intramuscular injections or only the injections that are given directly into the muscles. Intramuscular injections should be given at an angle of 90°, and the gauge size of the needle should be between 22G and 23G.

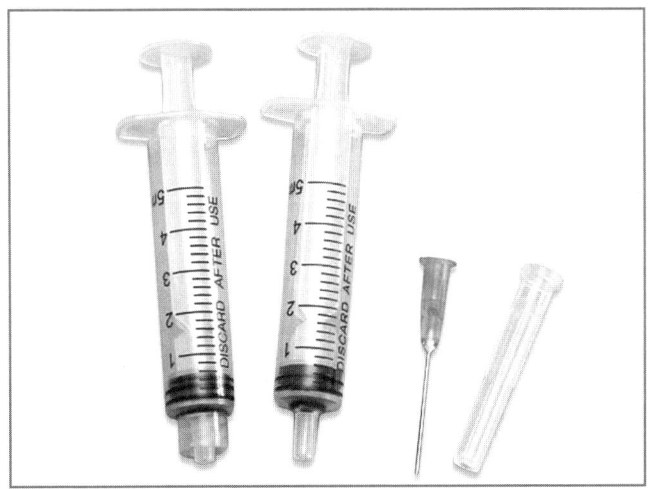

5 mL syringe.

10 mL Syringes

The 10 mL syringes are used for large volume intramuscular injections, which require higher doses of medication to be injected. The needle length for intramuscular injections should be between 1 and 1.5 inches for adults, and the needle gauge should be between 22G and 23G.

20 mL Syringes

The 20 mL syringes have a larger capacity, which makes them ideal for mixing different medicines. For instance, taking multiple drugs and fusing them in a syringe and then injecting them in an infusion set before finally injecting it into the patient.

50–60 mL Syringes

The larger 50–60 mL syringes are commonly used with scalp vein set for intravenous injections. We can choose a wide range of scalp vein sets (from 18G to 27G) according to the diameter of the vein and the viscosity of the aqueous solution.

NEEDLE

Needles are made out of stainless steel. They are sterile and disposable and are available in various lengths and sizes. A needle is made up of the hub, shaft, and bevel. The hub fits onto the tip of the syringe. All three parts must remain sterile at all times. The bevel is the tip of the needle that is slanted to create a slit into the skin.

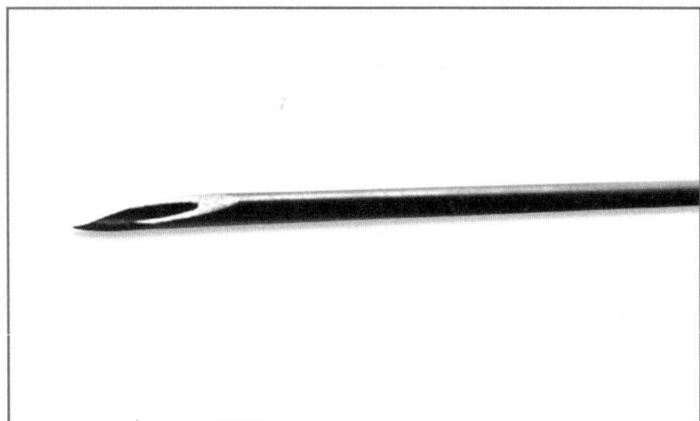

Bevel of a needle.

Gauge and Length

The **gauge** of a needle refers to its diameter. Needles range in various sized gauges from small diameter (25 to 29 gauge) to large diameter (18 to 22 gauge). Note that the larger the diameter of a needle, the smaller the gauge number. Larger diameter needles (18–22 gauge) are typically used to administer thicker medications or blood products.

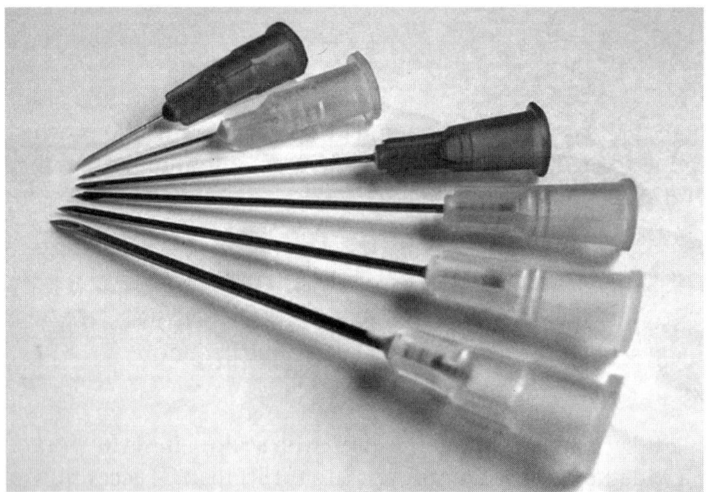

Needle lengths and gauges.

Gauge and length are marked on the outer packaging of needles. Needle length varies from 1/8 inches to 3 inches and is selected based on the type of injection. Nurses select the appropriate gauge and length according to the medication ordered, the anatomical location selected, and the patient's body mass and age. For example, an intramuscular injection requires a longer needle to reach muscle tissue than an intradermal injection that is inserted just under the epidermis.

Injection types	Locations	Needle gauge and length	Total amount of injectable fluid	Degree of angle when injecting	Considerations
Intradermal	• Upper third of the forearm • Outer aspects upper arms • Between scapula	• 25–27G • 3/8"–5/8"	0.1 mL	5–15°	The forearm is the recommended site for tuberculosis (TB) testing for all ages. Allergy testing may be performed between the scapulae. Older adults have decreased skin elasticity, so the skin should be held taut to ensure the medication is administered properly.
Subcutaneous	• Outer upper arms • Anterior thighs • Upper outer gluteal area • Upper back • Abdomen	• 25–31G • 1/2"–5/8"	Up to 1 mL Up to 0.5 mL in infants and small children	45–90°	The older patient's skin is less elastic, and subcutaneous tissue may be reduced in the skinfolds. The upper abdomen should be used for patients with less subcutaneous tissue.
Intramuscular	• Ventrogluteal • Vastus lateralis • Deltoid	• 18–25G • 1/2"–1 1/2" (based on age/size of patient and site used)	0.5–1 mL (infants and children) 2–5 mL (adults)	90°	The ventrogluteal site is recommended in adults. The vastus lateralis site is preferred for infants because that muscle is most developed. The deltoid site is recommended for vaccinations in adults

AMPULES

An ampule, or ampule, is a tiny single dosage vial with a sealed neck. Ampules could be of glass or plastic. Mostly, they are of glass. The neck of an ampule is sealed using an open flame in order to prevent contamination. This leads to an airtight obstruction for prevention of air, moisture and water from contaminating the liquid inside the ampule.

The seal is unfastened by cracking the top off the neck that causes a tidy and hassle-free break without any additional glass shards or slivers. Ampules cannot be reused and once the sealed neck is snapped off to have access to the pharmacy drug or any other stored liquid or solid, it is thrown away. However, once opened, the content can be stored into a sealed sterile vial or into slim pins.

Parenteral medications are supplied in sterile vials, ampules, and prefilled syringes. **Ampules** are small glass containers containing liquid medication ranging from 1 mL to 10 mL sizes. They have a scored neck to indicate where to break the ampule.

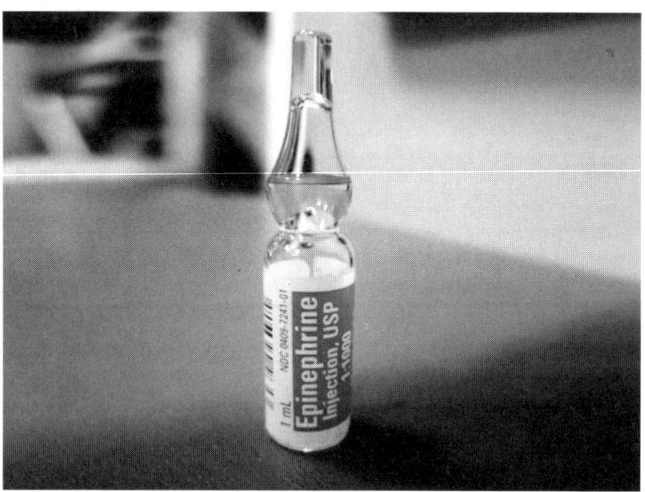

When breaking open an ampule, it is important to use appropriate steps to avoid injury. First, tap the ampule while holding it upright to move fluid down out of the neck. Place a piece of gauze around the neck, and then snap the neck away from your hands.

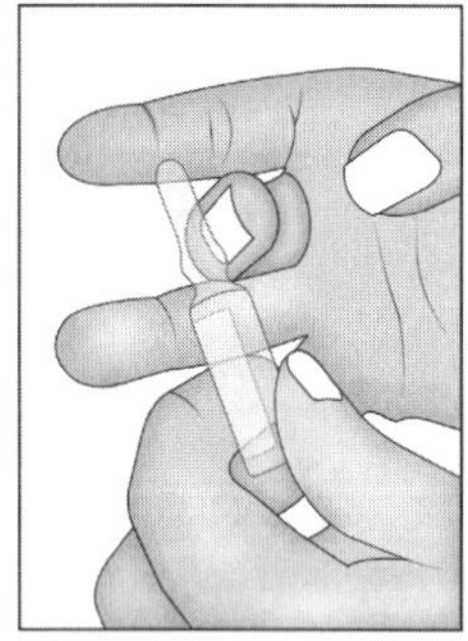
Tapping moves fluid down neck

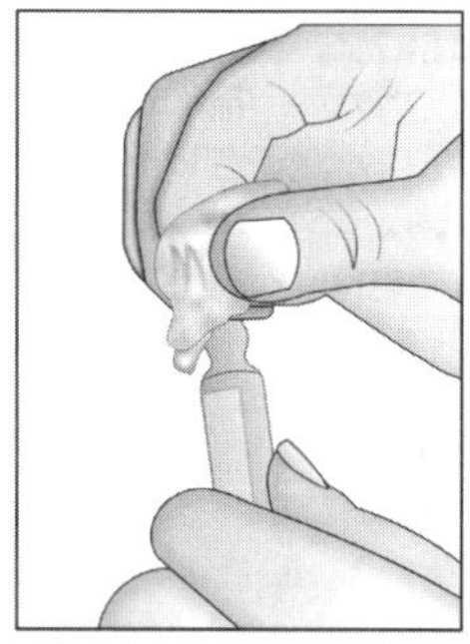
Gauze pad placed around neck of ampule

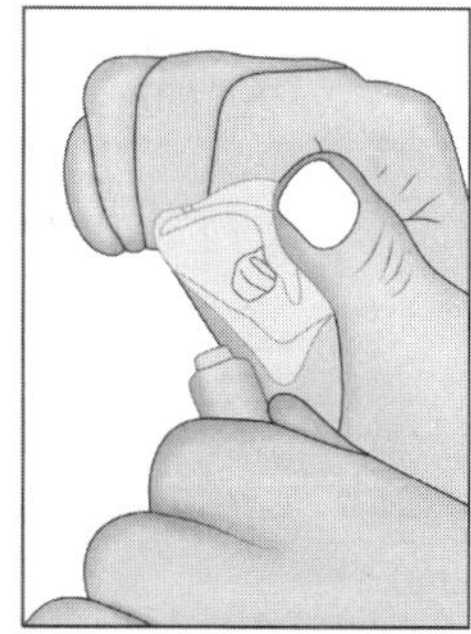
Neck snapped away from hands

Opening an ampule.

Types of Glass Ampules

Prescored Ampules

These prescored medical glass ampules offer excellent biological product preservation and extended shelf-life for injectable content. Ampule stems can be flame sealed to provide tamper evidence and are prescored for easy opening.

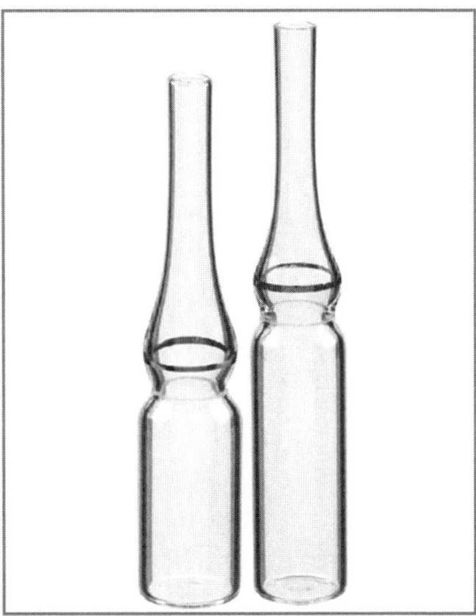

Cryule(™) Cryogenic Ampules

These prescored glass ampules offer excellent preservation of biological content and are suitable for sterilization and gas-phase liquid nitrogen cold storage applications. Ampule stems can be flame sealed to provide tamper evidence and are prescored for easy opening.

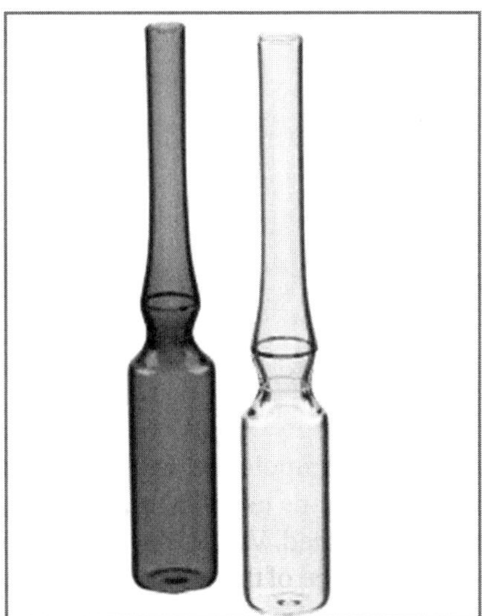

Vacule (™) Lyophilization Ampules

These glass ampules are commonly used for small volume lyophilization samples. Prescored for easy opening.

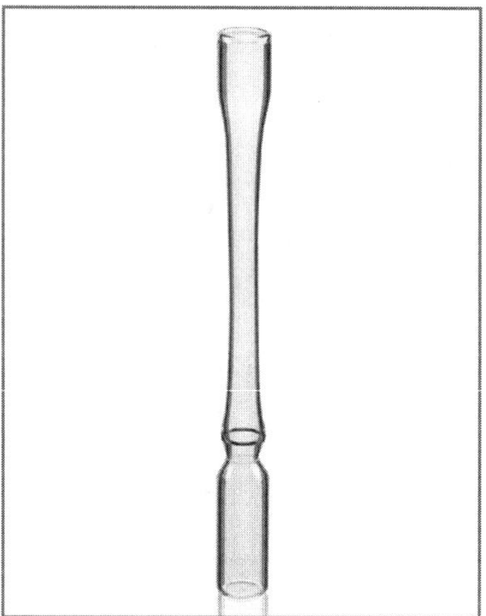

Standard Ampules

Commonly used for packaging of certified standards.

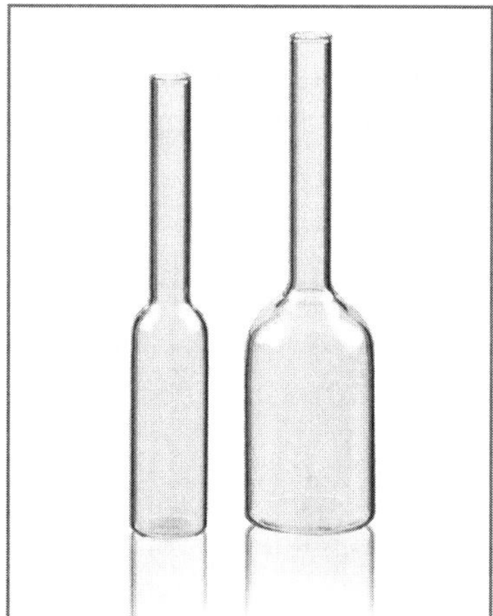

VIALS

Vial is a broader term as compared to an ampule. Vial is a small multidose container that can hold serums, liquid drugs and other compounds used mostly in the medical industry. It is typically made of glass and may or may not be sealed. Vial, in the form of container possesses a screw on cap or a rubber plug. In some cases, the top of the vial possesses dropper to estimate the liquid to retrieve. Vial has a flat base so that it can be rested on a flat surface or on the counter.

Closure systems are of different types. For glass vials, screw cap is used. For lip vials, cork or plastic stopper and for crimp vials, a rubber stopper and a metal cap are usually used. In case of a plastic vial, hinge caps (flip-flops or snap caps), are used.

A vial is a single- or multidose plastic container with a rubber seal top. Most rubber seals are covered by a plastic cap. A single-use vial must be discarded after one use. Multidose vials are used for medications like insulin and must be labeled with the date it was opened. Refer to agency policy regarding how long an open vial may be used and how it should be stored. For example, insulin is typically refrigerated until the vial is opened, and then it can be stored at room temperature for 28 days.

A vial is a closed system. Air must be injected prior to medication withdrawal to maintain a pressure gradient so that solution can be removed from the vial. It is also important to closely observe and maintain the tip of the needle within the level of medication inside the vial as it is removed.

To remove medication from a vial, pull air into the syringe to match the amount of medication you plan to remove. Hold the syringe like a pencil and insert the needle into the rubber stopper on the top of the vial. Push the plunger down until all of the air is in the bottle. This helps to keep the right amount of pressure in the bottle and makes it easier to draw up the medication. With the needle still in the vial, turn the bottle and syringe upside down (vial above syringe). Pull the plunger to fill the syringe to the desired amount. Check the syringe for air bubbles. If you see any large bubbles, push the plunger until the air is purged out of the syringe. Pull the plunger back down to the desired dose. Remove the needle from the bottle. Be careful to not let the needle touch anything until you are ready to inject.

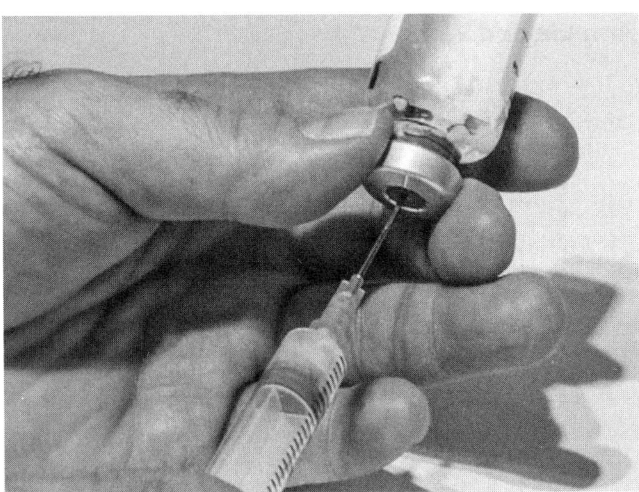

Removing medication from a vial.

Prefilled Syringes

Prefilled syringes can provide greater patient safety by reducing the potential for inadvertent needle sticks and exposure to toxic products that can occur while withdrawing medication from vials. Prefilled syringes, with premeasured dosage, can reduce dosing errors and waste. They are especially useful during emergent situations that require rapid administration of medication.

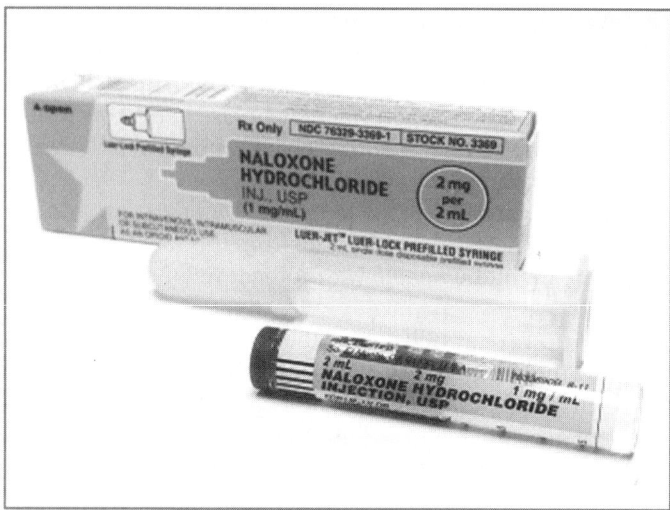

Prefilled syringe.

Difference between Ampule and Vial

1. Definition of Ampule and Vial

Ampule

An ampule is also known as ampul, **ampule**, or ampulla. It is a sealed vial that contains or stores a sample, usually liquid or solid.

Vial

A vial is also called as a phial or flacon. It is a small cylindrical container made of glass typically for holding liquid medications.

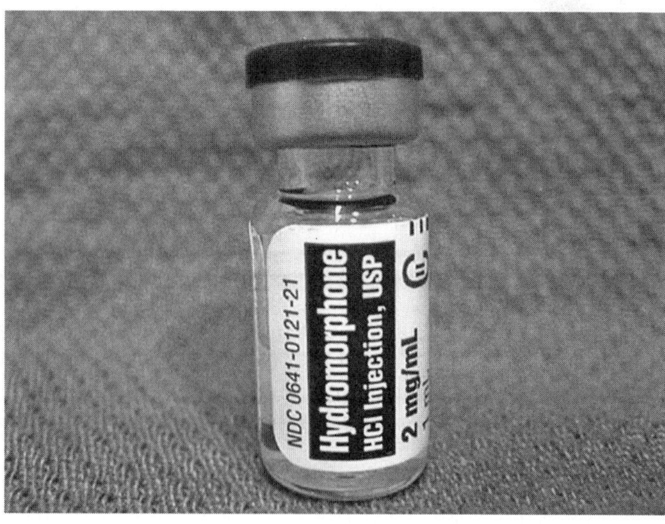

2. Applications of Ampule vs Vial

Ampule

- ❖ Pharmaceuticals
- ❖ Retail industry
- ❖ Diagnostics
- ❖ Veterinary
- ❖ Spa items
- ❖ First Aid
- ❖ Cosmetics
- ❖ Dental
- ❖ Health and beauty aids
- ❖ Toiletries

Vial

- ❖ Pharmaceutical applications (liquids, powders or capsules)
- ❖ Autosampler devices in analytical chromatography.
- ❖ Scientific sample vessels
- ❖ Research applications
- ❖ Industrial applications

3. Potency Protection of Ampule and Vial

Ampule

Unstable chemical compounds that, in the presence of oxygen or any other element keep themselves intact, remain potent when stored in an ampule. Typically, medical drug manufacturers suck out the air from the ampule before sealing it in order to prevent any contamination or degradation of the content within the container.

Vial

A vial is not typical hermetic types and is known to best store the stable elements.

4. Reuse of Ampule and Vial

Ampule and Vial

Both Ampules and vials require reconstitution. Ampules and vials can be seen on the shelves of pharmaceutical laboratories or chemistry-based laboratories. Both categories of vessels play a significant role in storing and preserving liquids, medicinal fluids, medicinal capsules and other similar contents, typically for pharmaceutical purposes. These are used to mix medicines in order to be delivered to a patient. Although both the storage containers refer

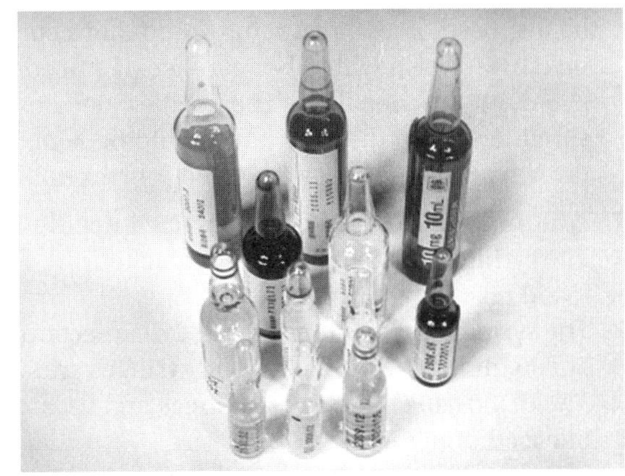

to glass or sometimes plastic containers, they benefit from several different designs and serve different purposes.

Difference between ampule and vial.	
Ampule	*Vial*
They possess hermetically sealed neck	They may be sealed or not
Ampules cannot be reused	Vials can be sterilized and used again
Oddly shaped	Flat shape
Temporary storage vehicle	Content can be stored for a longer period
It is something which doesn't have a rubber stopper and you need to break it to have access to medication	It has a rubber stopper that you put your needle into for getting access to the liquid or the compound mixture
Ampules require complicated machinery for manufacturing purposes	Vials are mostly manufactured in a home basement where the top is simply crimped on the glass vial
These are made by melting the thin top of the glass to form a small twisted capillary and is then closed and sealed	These are transfusion bottles that are sealed by rubber closures on to which aluminum seals are crimped
Laser sealing system or conventional gas flame	Rubber stoppered vials.

SAFE HANDLING OF SHARPS

- ❖ Auto-inoculation should be avoided at all costs.
- ❖ Glassware that has been broken or chipped should be disposed of properly.
- ❖ Use a brush and a pan to collect broken glass. You must never use your hands.
- ❖ Never manipulate, break, bend, recap, or remove the disposable needles from the syringes.
- ❖ Each member of the healthcare team ought to get rid of his or her own sharps; used knives should never be transmitted straight from a single individual to another. A kidney tray could potentially used for this. Only used needles that have been cleansed with freshly manufactured sodium hypochlorite solutions containing 0.5–1% (common bleach) should be disposed of using puncture-proof hard containers made of plastic or cardboard. Don't mix this rubbish with other garbage. If a needle shredder is available, it may be possible to shred only the needles or the needles, needles, and syringe tip, depending on what kind of shredder. Sharp disposal jars should be kept near to the place of use, and they should be thrown away when they are three-fourths full.

Decontamination/disinfection of used needles and syringes:
- ❖ The syringe and needle are still attached.
- ❖ Avoid recapping the needle.
- ❖ The syringe receives the aspirated disinfectant.
- ❖ For 30 minutes, the needles and syringes are submerged in a flat pan of disinfection.
- ❖ The disposable needles or syringes are discarded when any disinfecting solution has been released from them.
  The reused syringes and needles undergo a 30-minute autoclave or boil.

Do's

* Pass a tray with syringes and needles. Ideally, use a needle cutter to cut it.
* If a needle cutter does not exist, place the needle and the syringes in a solution of 2% hypochlorite.
* Remove the needle's cap close to where it was used.
* Use forceps to remove an open needle from a tray or drum.
* If cutters are not accessible, burn the tips of the syringes to destroy them.

Don'ts

* Never hand a needle or syringe to the next individual.
* Never break, bend, or recap a used needle with your hands.
* Never use bare or gloved hands to evaluate the needle's fineness before usage.
* Never handle an open needle.
* Never smash it with a stone or hammer to rid of it.

Definition of Needle Stick Injuries

A needle thrust injury is a percutaneous accidental puncture often brought on by a needle tips or other sharp object. Among the blood-borne diseases that might be disseminated by such an injury are the human immunodeficiency virus (HIV), hepatitis B virus (HBV), and hepatitis C virus (HCV).

RISK FACTORS

The Practice of Recapping the Needle

Most of the time healthcare workers have the habit to recap the needles to keep inside the tray but this is a wrong practice.

Unsafe Needle Devices

Healthcare organization should supply slandered needle devices if the quality of the device is not satisfactory there are chances for needle stick injury.

Improper Disposal of Sharps

All healthcare workers should follow universal waste segregation system and color coding, all sharps should be disposed in the sharp boxes.

Improper Techniques/Procedure

Every healthcare practitioner should follow safe technique and hospital should have written protocol for invasive procedures.

Unsafe Handling of Sharps

While handling sharps one should see their own safety and other safety.

Lack of Legislative Process/Policies

All hospital should have written policies for infection control and management of sharps needle.

Unexpected Movement of the Patient

Prevention

- ❖ Never recap needles/ avoid recapping.
- ❖ Plan for safe handling and proper disposal before beginning any procedure using needles or sharp instruments/objects.
- ❖ Always use devices with safety feature.
- ❖ Follow organizations policies, protocol and report promptly (immediately) in case of any exposure.
- ❖ Prepare the patient, environment and equipment prior to any invasive procedure.
- ❖ Provide a supportive and safe hospital environment for the employee.
- ❖ Let the wound bleed; you can tell whether it is bleeding by holding it over running water. Using lots of soap and running water, clean the wound.

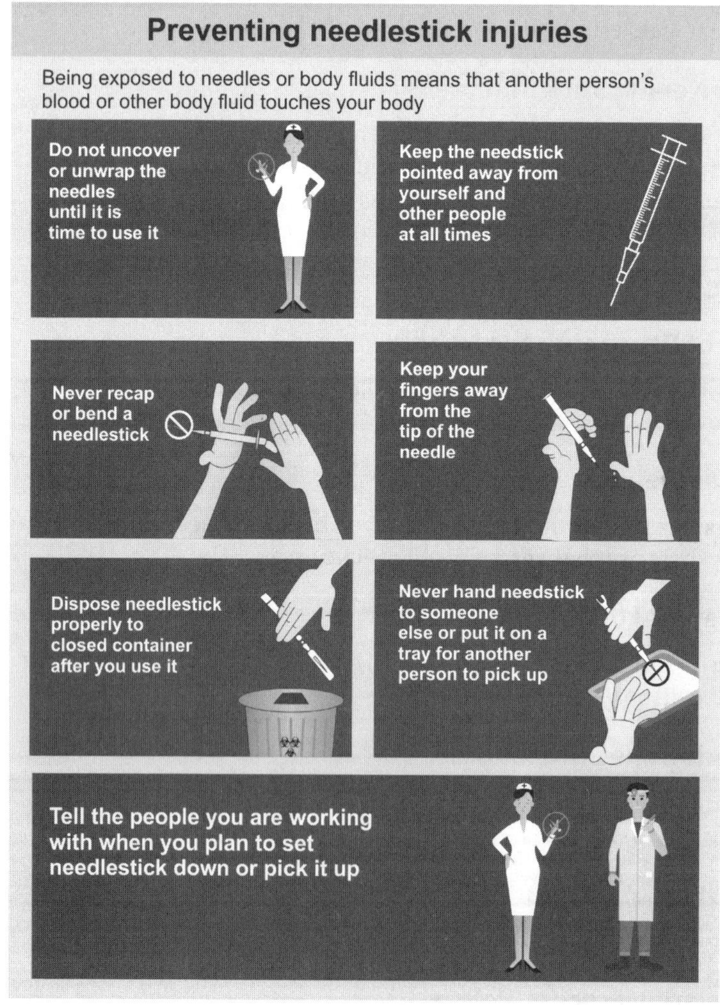

❖ Avoid sucking or scrubbing the wound.

❖ After the wound has dried, apply a waterproof dressing or plaster. As recommended by as per hospital, seek medical advice.

❖ Follow the written guidelines of hospital and the immediate supervisor/head of the department shall be informed soon after the exposure.

❖ Fill an electronic incident reporting form (sprint) at the same day and notify IPAC team, staff clinic physician and quality.

❖ The staff health clinic shall manage the exposed health care personal (HCP) on an urgent basis.

❖ Ensure proper management and facilitate post exposure treatment and vaccination.

❖ The treating physician (staff clinic) shall perform immunology and serology blood samples of source patient.

TOPICAL DRUG ADMINISTRATION

Medication may enter the body via the skin through mucous membranes when applied topically. Topical medicine is a term for medication that is applied in this manner. Additionally, it may be utilized to treat inflammation or other issues in certain body areas.

The skin may also be nourished and safeguarded using topical medications. Some topical drugs are used for localized therapy, while others, which are absorbed via the skin, are intended to have an impact on the whole body.

Pastes, Ointments and Oils

Ointments are blends of different fats that are simple to apply. They are constructed of wax, oil, or a mixture of these materials. Examples include healing ointments and fatty antiseptic ointments.

Fat, which is liquid at normal temperature, is the base of oils. They might be massage oils, essential oils like peppermint oil, or additions for oil baths.

Pastes are special ointments that include numerous powder ingredients together with a high fat content. They get quite thick as a result, making it difficult to massage them in. Zinc paste is one example.

Creams, Lotions and Foams

Creams are water and fat combinations that spread readily. An emulsifier is utilized to integrate and stabilize the two components since water and fats don't typically mix well. Emulsion is another name for the outcome. Lotions or milk are more liquid emulsions that are based on water. A topical foam is created as an emulsion contains air.

Oil-in-water emulsions (O/W emulsion) and water-in-oil emulsions (W/O emulsion) are two types of water-and-oil emulsions that may be distinguished by their primary constituent.

O/W emulsions have more water in them. Light treatments that are simple to absorb, cool, and hydrate the skin are some examples.

W/O emulsions, in contrast, have more fat in water. They serve as a barrier to keep liquids from penetrating the skin. They are used in creams that are thicker and created especially for dry skin conditions like eczema.

Gels, Tinctures and Powders

A special form of cream with a water basis are called gels. The main components of them are thickeners like starch, which can bind large amounts of water while retaining the active chemicals that are present in it.

Gels are easy to apply to the skin, have no oil, and may include a range of active ingredients. Examples include anti-itch gels and pain relief gels. Gels create a coating on the epidermis and cool the skin by causing water to evaporate there.

Powders are applied and remain on the skin. They may also include carrier materials (like talc) in addition the solid active component. Powders dry the skin and create a layer that protects it. For instance, there are powders to cure fungus infections or itching.

Topical drugs in liquid form are called tinctures. They are produced by dissolving or emulsifying dry extracts, often from plants. The most frequent solvent is alcohol. Iodine tincture, which is used to treat wounds, is one such example.

Shake lotions are skin care products that include both fluid and solids. They might be regarded as "liquid powder" since they have no fewer than 50% solids in it. They contain extremely little or no fat. In situations of chickenpox and shingles, zinc-infused white shake lotion is used to treat the skin blisters. Before using, shake the liquid and powder mixture in these lotions into suspension since they will ultimately separate.

Sprays and Patches

Some medications may be sprayed directly onto mucous membranes or the skin. Sprays are used, for instance, to clean surfaces, treat injuries, and reduce swelling of nasal mucous membranes.

A patch may be used to distribute a number of pharmaceuticals that are intended to enter the body's tissues gradually. A patch might give medication for a predetermined period of time. In along with medical patches, there are patches for nicotine and hormones.

Numerous advantages come with this technique of medication administration, including very even drug absorption and no gastrointestinal adverse effects. Furthermore, applying patches is practical. The term "transdermal therapeutic systems" (TTS) is another name for these kinds of patches. It is essential to delete the old patch before applying the new one. Also, take care not to leave it there once again.

APPLYING A TRANSDERMAL PATCH

Disclaimer: Always review and follow your hospital policy regarding this specific skill.

Safety considerations:
- Perform hand hygiene.
- Check room for additional precautions.
- Say hello to the patient.
- Verify the patient's identity by utilizing two identifiers (such as name and birthdate).
- Look for allergies on the allergy band.
- Complete necessary focused assessments and/or vital signs, and document on MAR.
- As required, provide patients patient education.
- Arrange the distribution of medications in a calm place to minimize disturbance.
- Steer clear of social interactions.

Contd...

Contd...

• Adhere to the agency's no-interruptions policy. • Make pharmaceutical preparations for ONE client at a time. • Comply with the seven rights of administering medicine.	

Steps	Additional information
1. Check MAR against doctor's orders.	• Check that MAR and doctor's orders are consistent. 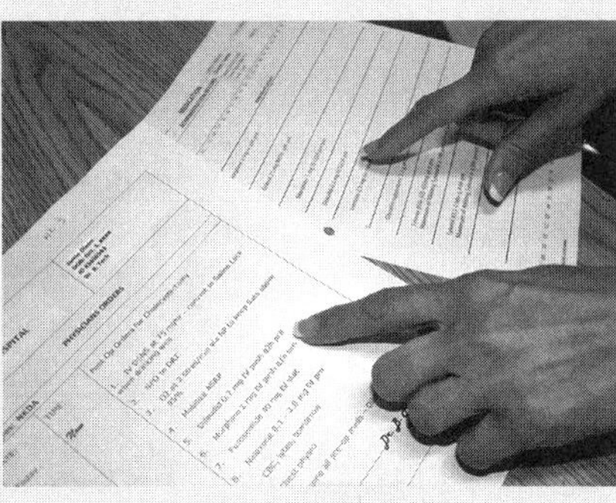 • Compare physician orders and MAR • This inspection is often completed and verified by night employees as well.

2. Perform the seven rights × 3 (must be done with each individual medication):
  ➢ The right patient
  ➢ The right medication (drug)
  ➢ The right dose
  ➢ The right route
  ➢ The right time
  ➢ The right reason
  ➢ The right documentation
Medication calculation: D/H × S = A (desired dosage/have available × stock = amount prepared)
	The right patient: Verify that the patient you have is the right one by utilizing two patient identifiers, such as name and birthdate.
	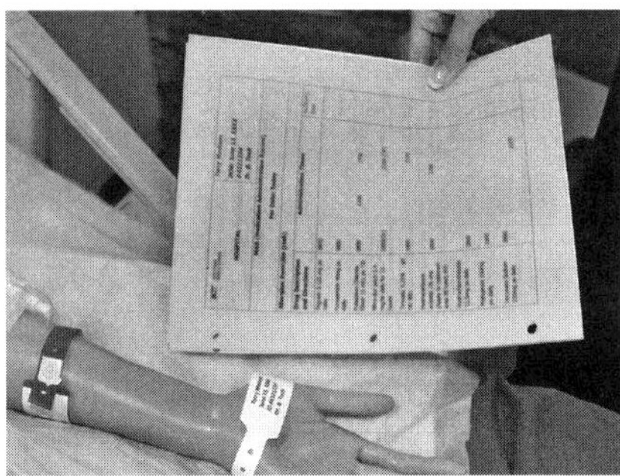
	• Compare MAR with patient wristband
	• Make sure you get the proper medication along with that it is suitable for the patient receiving care in the specific situation before you start taking it.
	• A dose that is suitable for someone's age, size, overall condition is the right dosage. Varied dosages may be suggested for varied situations.
	• The ideal path is one that takes into account the patient's existing state.
	The appropriate moment: Follow the timetable and dosage instructions.
	• Verify sure the patient is getting the drug for the proper purpose before prescribing any prescription.

Contd...

Contd...

	• **The correct paperwork:** Before giving medicine, always double-check any ambiguous or incorrect documentation. 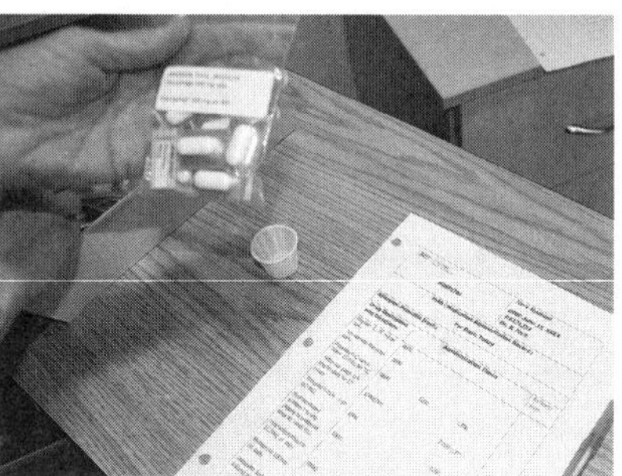 • Verify the appropriate patient, dosage, route, time, cause, and documentation. • Never record the administration of a drug until you actually do so.

3. The drug's name, dose, and route must be checked three times against the MAR on the label:
  ➢ Upon removal of the drug from the drawer
  ➢ During the pouring of the drug
  ➢ When the medicine is being stored or placed beside the bed
	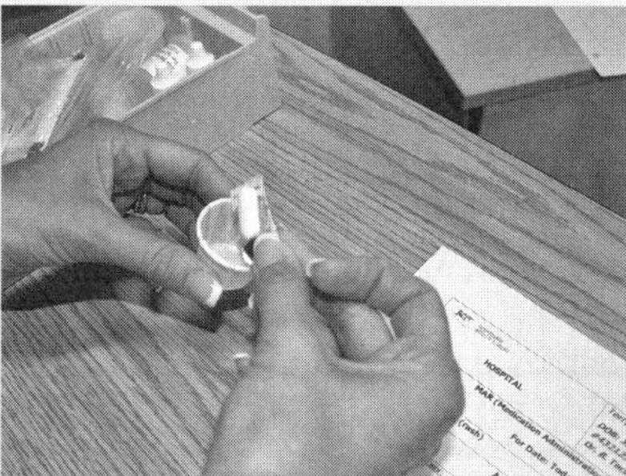
	• Seven checks should be made three times before medicine is given.
	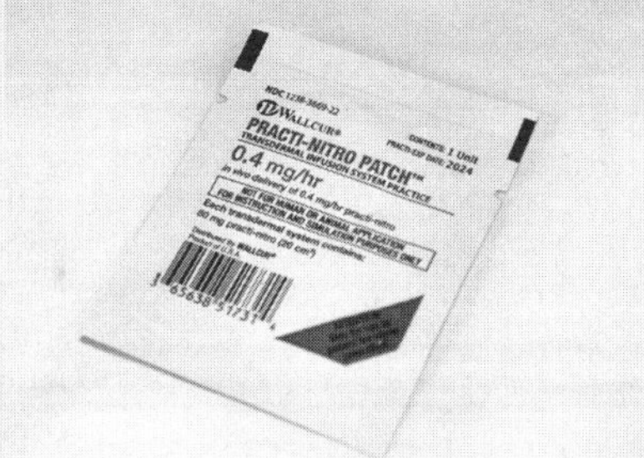Transdermal patch
	• Before giving your patient their medicine, these checks are performed. Do a third checkup before delivering a drug to the patient's bedside, for instance eye drops.

Contd...

Contd...

4. Remove the old patch if it's still on your skin before applying the transdermal patch. Completely purge the area. Check the old patch for any symptoms of skin sensitivity and note them as required by agency policy.	Not removing the prior patch might lead to a pharmaceutical overdose. Look for an ancient spot in the creases of the skin. 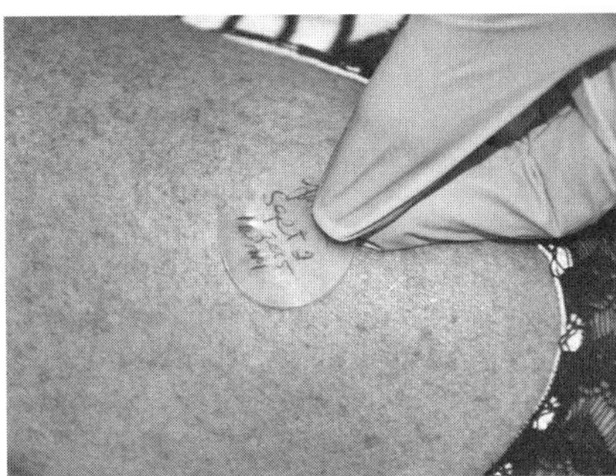 Remove previous patch
5. The previous patch should be torn or folded in half with the adhesive sides together and disposed of in accordance with agency policy (often in a biohazard trash bag).	By doing this, inadvertent medicine exposure is avoided.
6. Use a felt-tip or soft-tip pen to inscribe the date, the duration, and your initials on the outside of the new patch. A ballpoint pen should not be used.	Other medical professionals are informed of the software's date and time via patch initialization. 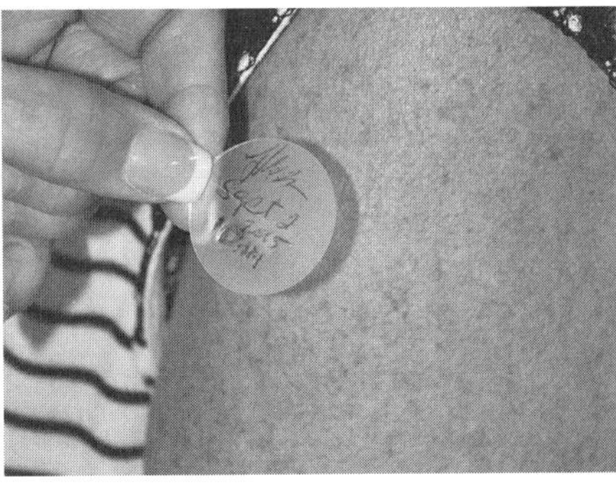 Use a felt-tip or soft-tip pen to inscribe the date, the duration, and your initials on the outside of the new patch. Ballpoint pens may harm patches, affecting how well they distribute medications.
7. Apply the fresh patch to a clean, dry, hairless, and skin irritation-free area.	If hair removal is required, clip the hair rather than shaving to prevent skin discomfort. Even distribution of the drug is ensured by a constant surface.

Contd...

Contd...

Note: When the dressing is removed, there should typically be a "patch-free period" of 10–12 hours since wearing the patch constantly might lead to the development of resistance to the drug. To find out whether the patch has to be removed overnight, see the doctor's instructions.	
8. When gently removing the support from the patch, be cautious to grasp the insert at the four ends and avoid contacting the medication with your fingers.	This avoids drug interference and maintains the patch's stickiness.
9. When applying a patch, one hand is placed over the patch's surface and held there for ten seconds. To ensure that the patch is properly secured to the skin, push firmly all the way around its edges.	This guards against patch loss and guarantees that the drug is delivered effectively. 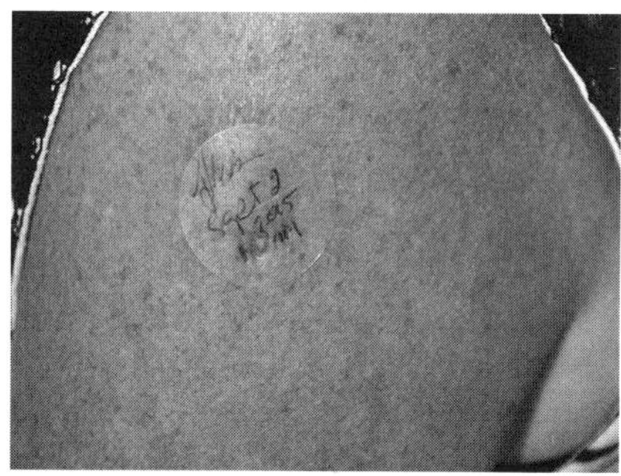 Apply new transdermal patch
10. Perform hand hygiene.	This prevents the transfer of microorganisms. 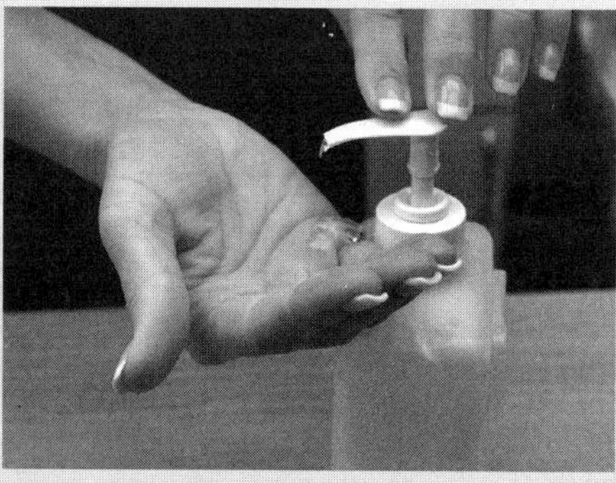 Hand hygiene with ABHR
Note: To prevent skin irritability, wait at least one week before applying a fresh patch to previously applied areas. Don't ever cut a transdermal patch in half; if the dosage changes, a new patch is needed. Avoid placing a heating pad on top of the patch since doing so can slow down absorption, which might have dangerous consequences.	
11. Document in accordance with agency guidelines, making careful to include the administrative site on the MAR.	Accurate and timely documentation improves patient safety.

APPLYING TOPICAL CREAMS, LOTIONS, AND OINTMENTS

Disclaimer: Always review and follow your hospital policy regarding this specific skill.	

Safety considerations:
- Perform hand hygiene.
- Check room for additional precautions.
- Say hello to the patient.
- Verify the patient's identity by utilizing two identifiers (such as name and birthdate).
- Look for allergies on the allergy band.
- Complete necessary focused assessments and/or vital signs, and document on MAR.
- As required, provide patients patient education.
- Arrange the administration of medications to prevent disruption.
- Hand out medicine in a calm setting.
- Steer clear of social interactions.
- Adhere to the agency's no-interruptions policy.
- Make pharmaceutical preparations for ONE patient in a time.
- Comply with the seven rights of administering medicine.

Steps	Additional Information
1. Check MAR against doctor's orders.	• Check that MAR and doctor's orders are consistent. 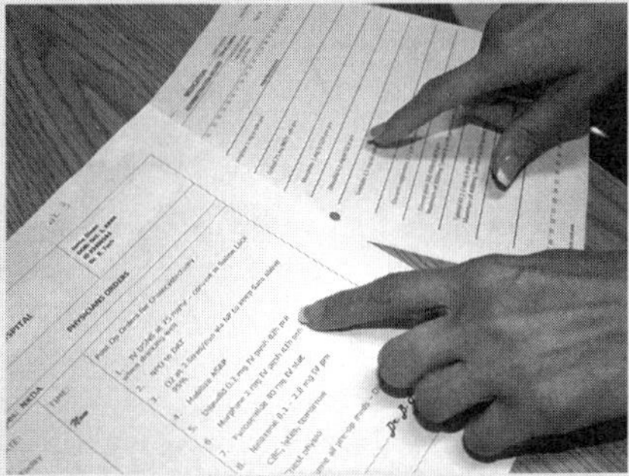 • Compare physician orders and MAR • This inspection is often completed and verified by night employees as well.
2. Perform the seven rights × 3 (must be done with each individual medication): ➢ The right patient ➢ The right medication (drug) ➢ The right dose ➢ The right route ➢ The right time ➢ The right reason ➢ The right documentation Medication calculation: D/H × S = A (**D** or desired dosage/**H** or have available × **S** or stock = **A** or amount prepared)	• **The right patient:** Verify that the patient you have is the right one by utilizing two patient identifiers, such as name and birthdate. 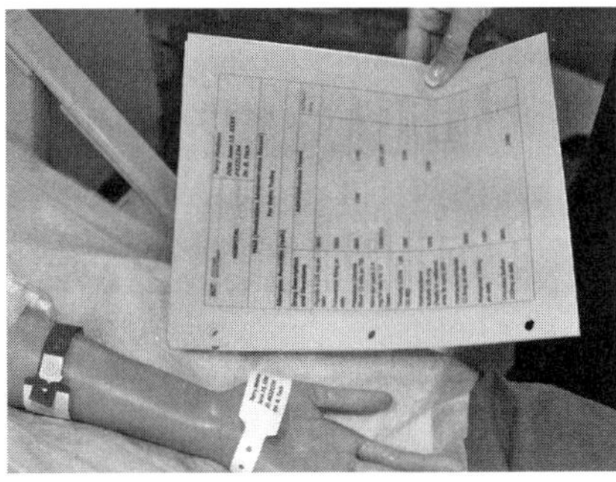

Contd...

Contd...

	• Compare MAR with patient wristband • The proper medicine (medication): Verify that you are using the right drug to ensure it is suitable for the individual receiving treatment in the given situation. • The patient's ages, size, and health should all be taken into consideration while determining the right dose. Different dosages could be suggested for certain circumstances. • The ideal path is one that takes into account the patient's existing state. • **The appropriate moment:** Follow the timetable and dosage instructions. • Verify sure the patient is getting the drug for the proper purpose before prescribing any prescription. • **The correct paperwork:** Before giving medicine, always double-check any ambiguous or incorrect documentation. 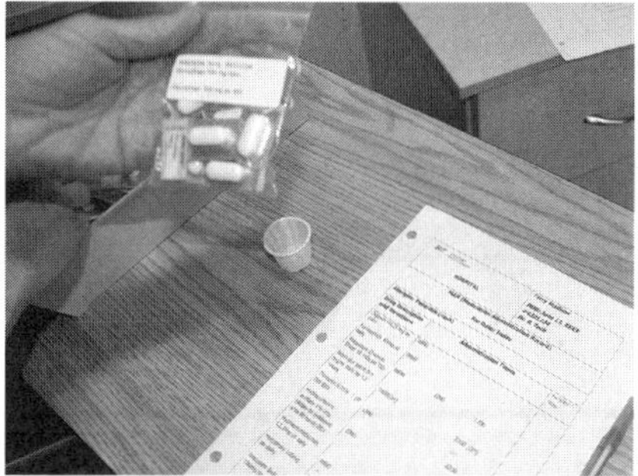 • Verify the appropriate patient, dosage, route, time, cause, and documentation. • NEVER record the administration of a drug until you actually accomplished so.
3. The drug's name, dose, and route must be checked three times against the MAR on the label: ➤ Upon removal of the drug from the drawer ➤ During the pouring of the drug ➤ When the medicine is being stored or placed beside the bed	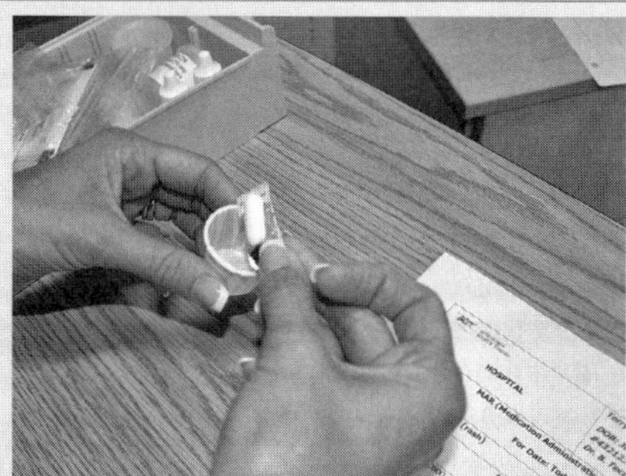 • Seven checks should be made three times before medicine is given. • Before giving your patient their medicine, these checks are performed. When bringing a medication to the bedside, such as eye drops, do a third check.

Contd...

Contd...

4. Unless the skin is damaged, use non-sterile gloves; after that, use sterile gloves.	• Gloves protect medical professionals from coming into touch with drugs. 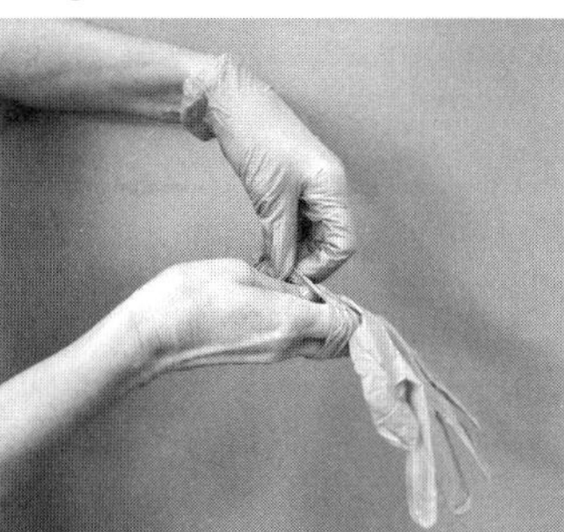 • Put non-sterile gloves on. • Sterile gloves will stop the spread of pathogens in the event that skin is damaged.
5. With water and a fresh cloth, wash, rinse, and pat dry the afflicted area.	Previous topical drugs are eliminated by this.
6. When the skin is still moist, administer a topical medicine if it is really dry and flaky.	Applying to wet skin helps the skin's layers maintain moisture.
7. Hand hygiene should be practiced in between glove changes.	To stop the spread of microbes, handle open skin lesions using sterile gloves. 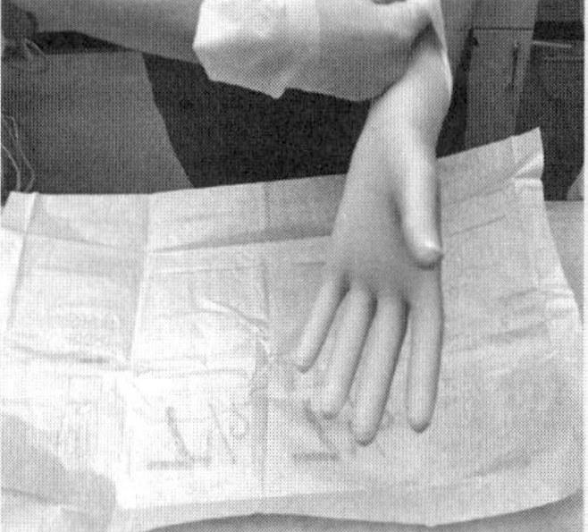 Whenever a patient has open lesions, use sterile gloves.
8. Put the necessary dosage of medicine in your palms and soften it by rubbing them together.	Spreading topical medicine is made simpler by softening. 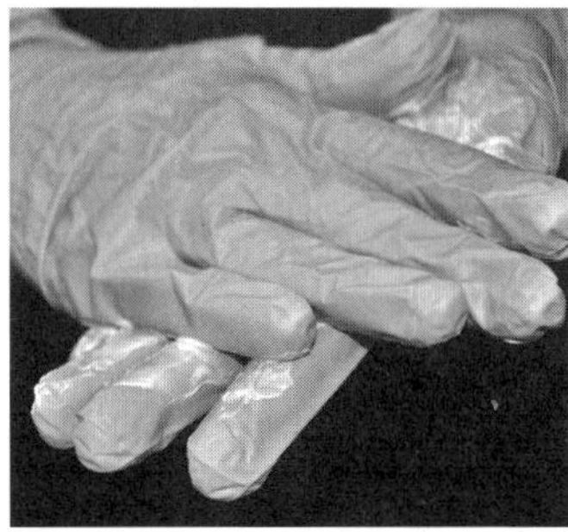 To soften and toast the hands, massage the drug

Contd...

Contd...

9. Inform the patient that the first application could feel chilly. Apply medicine using long, steady strokes that correspond to the hair's natural direction. Avoid forceful rubbing.	By doing this, hair follicle inflammation is avoided.
10. Inform the patient that their skin can feel oily following application.	Oils are used in certain topical treatments.
11. Document in accordance with agency guidelines, making careful to include the administrative site on the MAR.	Improved patient safety results from accurate and timely recording.
12. Perform hand hygiene.	This procedure stops the spread of germs. Hand hygiene with ABHR

APPLYING TOPICAL POWDER

Disclaimer: Always review and follow your hospital policy regarding this specific skill.

Safety considerations:
- Perform hand hygiene.
- Check room for additional precautions.
- Say hello to the patient.
- Verify the patient's identity by utilizing two identifiers (such as name and birthdate).
- Look for allergies on the allergy band.
- Complete necessary focused assessments and/or vital signs, and document on MAR.
- As required, provide patients patient education.
- Arrange the distribution of medications in a calm place to minimize disturbance.
- Steer clear of social interactions.
- Adhere to the agency's no-interruptions policy.
- Make pharmaceutical preparations for one patient at a time.
- Comply with the seven rights of administering medicine.

Contd...

Contd...

Steps	Additional Information
1. Check MAR against doctor's orders.	• Check that MAR and doctor's orders are consistent. 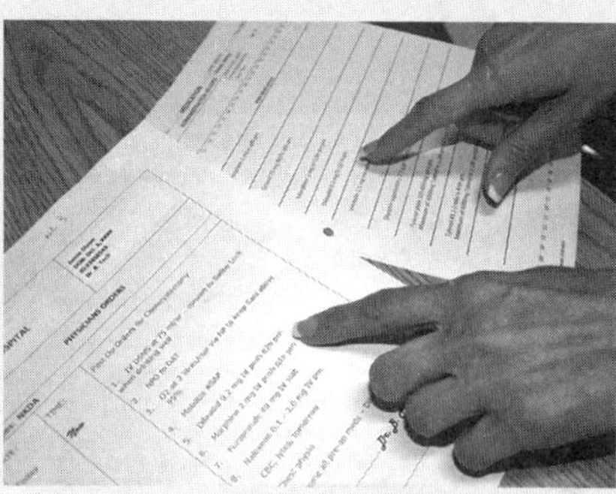 • Compare physician orders and MAR • This inspection is often completed and verified by night employees as well.

2. The seven rights must be carried out three times for each medication:
  ❯ The right patient
  ❯ The right medication (drug)
  ❯ The right dose
  ❯ The right route
  ❯ The right time
  ❯ The right reason
  ❯ The right documentation
Medication calculation: D/H x S = A
(**D** or desired dosage/**H** or have available x **S** or stock = **A** or amount prepared)
	• **The ideal patient is:** Use two patient indicators, such as the patient's name and birthday, to confirm that the patient we have is the correct one.
	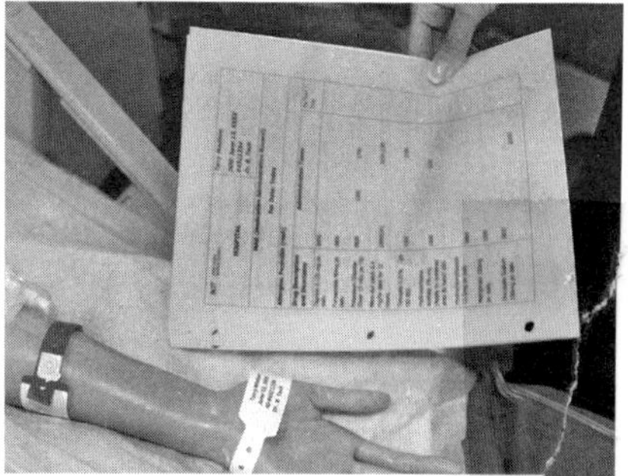
	• Compare MAR with patient wristband
	• **The proper medicine (medication):** Verify that you are using the right drug as well as whether it is suitable for the individual being treated in the given situation.
	• A dose that is suitable for the person's age, size, plus condition is the right dosage. varied dosages may be suggested for varied situations.
	• The ideal path is one that takes into account the patient's existing state.
	• **The appropriate moment:** Follow the timetable and dosage instructions.
	• Verify sure the patient is getting the drug for the proper purpose before prescribing any prescription.
	• **The correct paperwork:** Before giving medicine, always double-check any ambiguous or incorrect documentation.

Contd...

Contd...

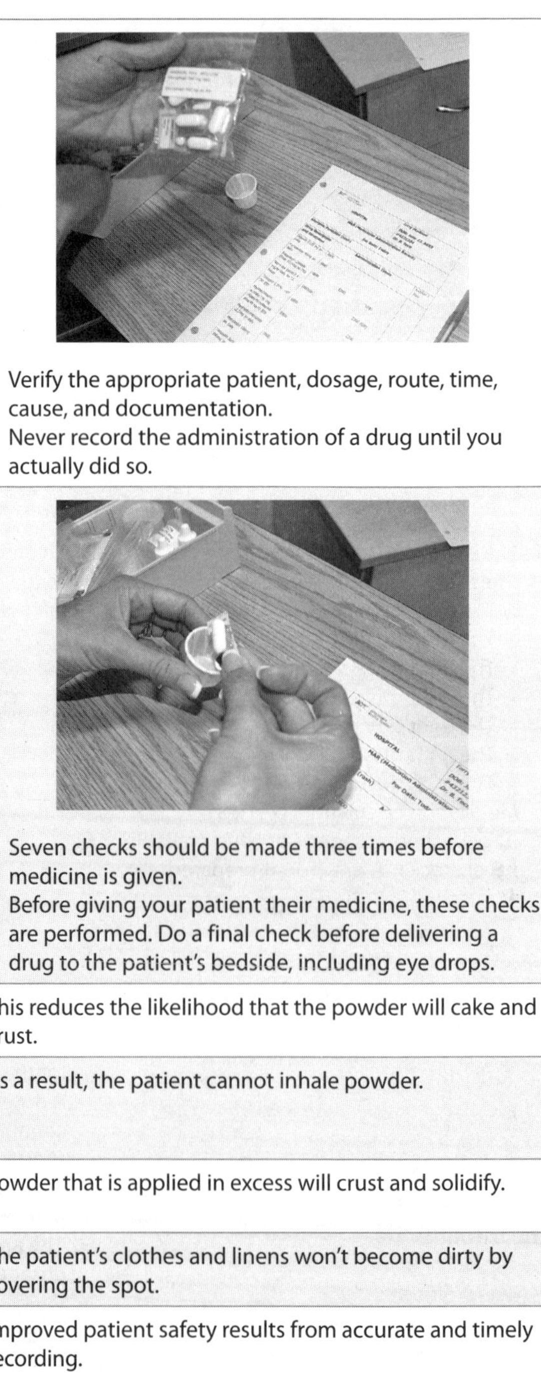

	<ul><li>Verify the appropriate patient, dosage, route, time, cause, and documentation.</li><li>Never record the administration of a drug until you actually did so.</li></ul>
3. The drug's name, dose, and route must be checked three times against the MAR on the label: <ul><li>Upon removal of the drug from the drawer</li><li>During the pouring of the drug</li><li>When the medicine is being stored or placed beside the bed</li></ul>	<ul><li>Seven checks should be made three times before medicine is given.</li><li>Before giving your patient their medicine, these checks are performed. Do a final check before delivering a drug to the patient's bedside, including eye drops.</li></ul>
4. Before applying, make sure the skin is absolutely dry and clean.	This reduces the likelihood that the powder will cake and crust.
5. If the patient is applying the powder near to their face, ask them to move away from it or briefly cover it with a clean towel.	As a result, the patient cannot inhale powder.
6. Apply a thin coating of powder to the skin.	Powder that is applied in excess will crust and solidify.
7. Dress the afflicted area with the recommended dressing, as directed.	The patient's clothes and linens won't become dirty by covering the spot.
8. Document in accordance with agency guidelines, making careful to include the administrative site on the MAR.	Improved patient safety results from accurate and timely recording.

Contd...

Contd...

9. Perform hand hygiene	• Prevents transfer of microorganisms. 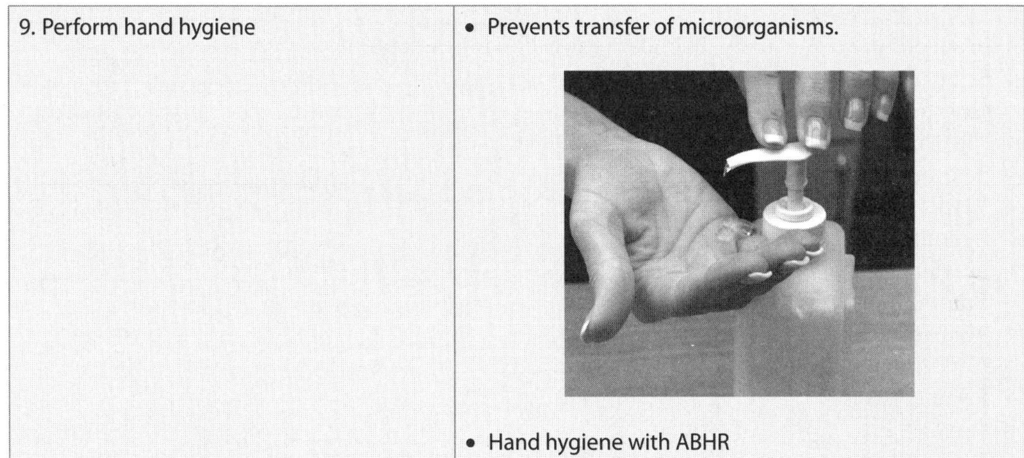 • Hand hygiene with ABHR

SWABBING THE THROAT

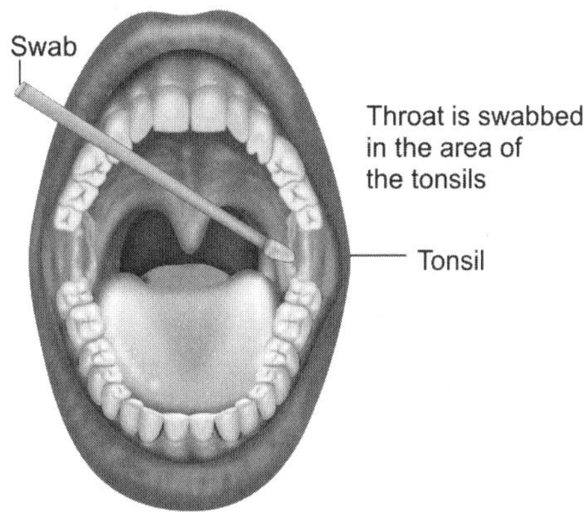

To find the bacteria that might infect the throat, a throat swab culturing is a laboratory test. The most frequent application is for diagnosis strep throat.

A throat culture, sometimes referred to as a throat swab, is laboratory testing used primarily to identify the presence of bacteria in the mouth's posterior region that are likely causing one to get ill. These germs may cause bacterial or viral diseases such as whooping cough and strep throat, pneumonia, tonsillitis, and meningitis.

For instance, the presence of the team A streptococcus bacteria (*Streptococcus pyogenes*) in the throat swab is a strong indication that someone may have strep throat.

Before Swabbing

Before using the swab, refrain from eating, drinking, or brushing teeth. Since the tests are cognizant of acid, patient should avoid eating or drinking for approximately 30 minutes before to taking the sample since doing so might result in a false positive.

Indications

A throat culture test usually diagnoses the following infections:

* Strep throat
* Gonorrhea (gonococcal pharyngitis)
* Thrush
* Scarlet and rheumatic fever
* Pertussis
* Diphtheria
* Scarlet fever
* Pneumonia
* Abscess
* Abdominal pain
* Fever
* Headache
* Loss of appetite
* Pain and difficulty swallowing
* Red spots on the roof of mouth (petechiae)
* Swollen lymph nodes
* Tonsils that looks red with white spots

If patient also have a skin rash and a swollen tongue, health provider may suspect scarlet fever.

Patients are far more likely to sustain an infection caused by viruses than a bacterial or fungal infection if they have a sore throat along with any of the diseases that follow:

* Cough
* Hoarseness
* Pink eye (conjunctivitis)
* Runny nose
* Sneezing

Instructions for collecting a throat swab

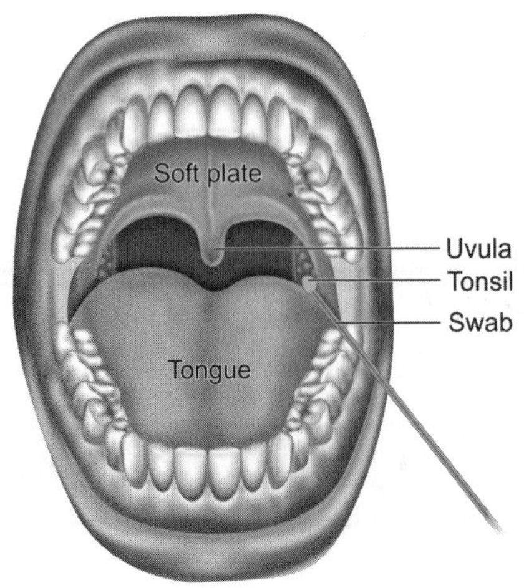

1. Wash hands with soap and water.
2. Remove the swab from the package holding it at the end of the stick
3. Position yourself in front of the mirror, or in front of the person you will be swabbing.
4. Tilt the head back slightly, open the mouth wide to expose the tonsils and back of the throat.
5. Use the tongue depressor to hold the tongue away from the back of the throat.
6. Locate the areas of redness and white spots on the tonsils.
7. Rub the swab over the area, back and forth, avoid touching the tongue or roof of the mouth.
8. While holding the swab, remove the cap from the accompanying tube. **Do not lay the swab down.**
9. Place the swab in the tube.
10. Wash your hands with soap and water.

GARGLING

Gargling is a crucial component of daily oral hygiene regimen. It aids in the removal of germs from areas of the mouth that are difficult to clean with a toothbrush or floss. Additionally, if a person currently have an upper respiratory infection, it helps hasten recovery.

Method 1

1. **Find a clean glass:** You now own a "gargling cup." Even if you aren't required to use a special cup, doing so tends to be safer since it prevents the spread of germs, instead of to, instance, sipping directly from a bottle the mouthwash.
2. **Fill your gargling cup with your gargling liquid of choice:** A little amount is OK; it's preferable to start off with less than too much.
3. **Put a small amount of the liquid in mouth and swish it around:** During this first sweep, the front and sides the mouth should be targeted since gargling won't reach those regions.
   - Swish the liquid used for gargling in mouth back and forth by moving tongue and cheeks in and out.
   - Some individuals like to slightly reheat the liquid used for gargling before using it. Warm water with a little salt in it feels good at the back regarding the mouth, but using mouthwash will probably not be pleasant.
4. **Tilt head back, and without swallowing the liquid, try to open your mouth and make an "ahhh" sound:** To prevent mistakenly swallowing any of the liquid, keep your epiglottis, a little flap located at the back of the throat, closed.
   - It could take some getting accustomed to, but if done properly, the vibrations in your mouth's back will cause the liquid you're gargling to swirl around, almost as if it were boiling.
   - By coating the back of your teeth with the liquid of your choice while gargling, you may reduce some bacterial growth and ease sore throat symptoms.
5. **Spit the gargling liquid out into the sink:** Continue with your oral health routine by brushing your teeth or flossing.

Method 2

- ❖ **Gargle with a simple salt water (saline) solution for respiratory health:** Warm water and a half-teaspoon (3 g) of salt are combined in a cup (240 mL). To get the salt to dissolve, stir the mixture. To help prevent infection of the respiratory tract, gargle three times each day with saline solution.
  - One study found that a simple salt solution gargled three times daily resulted in a 40% decrease in upper respiratory tract infections.
  - Gargling with saltwater not only seems to help with symptoms of the cold, but it also helps to stay healthy throughout the flu and cold season.
  - According to other research, saline solutions may help treat congestion and sore throats.
- ❖ **Try a commercial or homemade mouthwash for fresh breath:** Mouthwash aids in infection prevention, oral hygiene, and breath freshening all at once. Millions of individuals use mouthwash every day, every day of the week, as a component to their oral hygiene regimen.
  - Mouthwashes containing alcohol tends to be a bit more strong but come with a number of risky side effects, such as increased risk of cancer, mouth ulcers, corrosion fillings, and other dental problems. Use them sparingly.

- Persons may even prepare own mouthwash. In actuality, it's really simple. The following dishes are fast and hydrating:
    ◊ Peppermint and tea tree mouthwash
    ◊ Angelica mouthwash
    ◊ A host of other simple mouthwashes
- ❖ **Use a simple baking soda and water combination to ease mouth sores:** Baking soda, often known as sodium bicarbonate, is a well-known cleanser with several domestic uses.

1 teaspoon (5 g) of baking soda should be dissolved in 5 cups (120 mL) of warm water to form a mouthwash. To enhance the taste and give a breath freshener, you may choose to add some drops of peppermint oil.

According to studies, rinsing mouth with baking soda may help maintain a healthy pH level and deter germs that thrive in acidic environments. Canker sores as well as mouth ulcers benefit greatly from its excellent pain relief properties.

- ❖ **Try adding lemon and honey to hot water for a soothing gargle:** Both honey and lemon are effective throat relaxants. This liquid's ability to be really consumed after gargling, in contrast to other alternatives, is another benefit. Try combining 1 tablespoon (15 mL) of each lemon and honey juice with 6 fluid ounces (180 mL) of water. Gargle the mixture, then swallow it if you have throat discomfort or need a way to get rid of a little mucus.
- ❖ **5 Swish some chamomile tea to ease a scratchy throat:** You may consume tea after gargling it in the same manner as the honey and lemon. Make a cup of tea made with chamomile for yourself and let it warm up to a comfortable temperature not scorching. Before swallowing, take a sip then gargle for a bit.
    - If you have a hoarse voice, chamomile tea is extremely beneficial for soothing your throat.
    - When your throat is painful or swollen, other herbal teas, such peppermint and raspberry, are also calming.
    - Be careful not to gargle with too much saltwater as it is possible to choke.
    - It is advisable to gargle with mouthwash or water after brushing teeth since doing so on its own is ineffective for preventing cavities.
    - Select a mouthwash with a scent your like; it helps

SUPPOSITORY/MEDICATED PACKING IN RECTUM/VAGINA

A kind of medicine that is placed into the rectum is a rectal suppository. When you are unable to take drugs orally, you may use rectal suppositories. These techniques may be particularly beneficial for small children and elderly people who are unable to take oral drugs.

If you have nausea or another condition that makes it impossible for people to swallow beverages or tablets, you may need to take medications that decrease fever, such as acetaminophen, intravenously. Fever-lowering medications used orally may help lessen the risk of gastric and small intestine side effects.

Rectal suppositories have traditionally been used to provide drugs such as laxatives and hemorrhoid treatments in addition to these medications. Other drugs that can be injected into the rectum.

- ❖ Hydrocortisone
- ❖ Mesalazine for the treatment of inflammatory bowel disease (IBD)
- ❖ Bisacodyl or glycerol for constipation
- ❖ Promethazine or ondansetron for nausea and vomiting
- ❖ Certain pain medications, such as ibuprofen or oxycodone

In rare circumstances, patients who may be asleep may also be administered drugs rectally,

Positions

Overall, lying on side is the suggested posture for administering a rectal suppository. This may also make it easier to deliver the drug to a receiver and makes it feasible to administer its suppository to oneself easily. For the best results, lie on your left side, your knees bent inward toward your chest.

If the first position is painful for any reason or if insertion the suppository appears to be difficult, try laying on your lower back, your hips lifted up your skull parallel to the floor (knee chest position).

Insertion Depth Limits

Age group	Suppository insertion
Adults	About 3 inches
Children	2 inches or less
Infants	½ inch

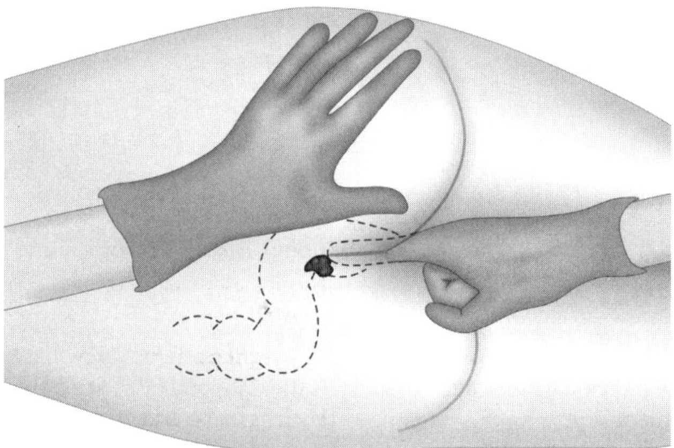

Administering medication rectally.

Drugs administered via PR have a faster effect than those assigned orally and have a better bioavailability, which means that more of the potent medication is available since the upper gastrointestinal digesting processes have not hampered it. Rectal absorption results in less change in the route and more drug entering the systemic circulation. In addition to more effectively delivering medication, rectal administration also reduces various side effects such as diarrhea, vomiting, or gastrointestinal discomfort.

When oral administration is not permitted, rectal medications are given for either their worldwide effects (such as analgesics) or local effects for the gastrointestinal tract (such as laxatives). When you have rectal bleeding and prolapse, after rectal especially colon surgery, or when the levels of platelets are low, rectal medications shouldn't be utilized. The process for giving rectal suppositories and enemas is outlined in Checklist.

CHECKLIST: MEDICATION ADMINISTERED RECTALLY

Safety considerations:
- Perform hand hygiene.
- Check room for additional precautions.
- Say hello to the patient.
- Verify the patient's identity by utilizing two identifiers (such as name and birthdate).
- Look for allergies on the allergy band.
- Carry out any required targeted evaluations or tests, and keep records on MAR.
- As required, provide patients patient education.
- Arrange the distribution of medications in a calm place to minimize disturbance.
- Steer clear of social interactions.
- Adhere to the agency's no-interruptions policy.
- Make pharmaceutical preparations for one patient as one time.
- Comply with the seven rights of administering medicine.

Steps	Additional Information
1. Check MAR against doctor's orders.	• Check that MAR and doctor's orders are consistent. 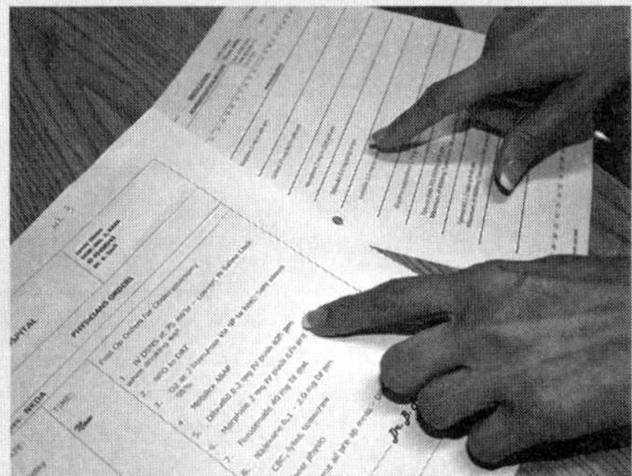 • Compare physician orders and MAR • Night staff usually complete and verify this check as well.

2. Perform the seven rights x 3 (must be done with each individual medication):
   ➤ The right patient
   ➤ The right medication (drug)
   ➤ The right dose
   ➤ The right route
   ➤ The right time
   ➤ The right reason
   ➤ The right documentation
Medication calculation: D/H x S = A
(**D** or desired dosage/**H** or have available x **S** or stock = **A** or amount prepared)
	• **The right patient:** Verify that the patient you have is the right one by utilizing two patient identifiers, such as name and birthdate.
	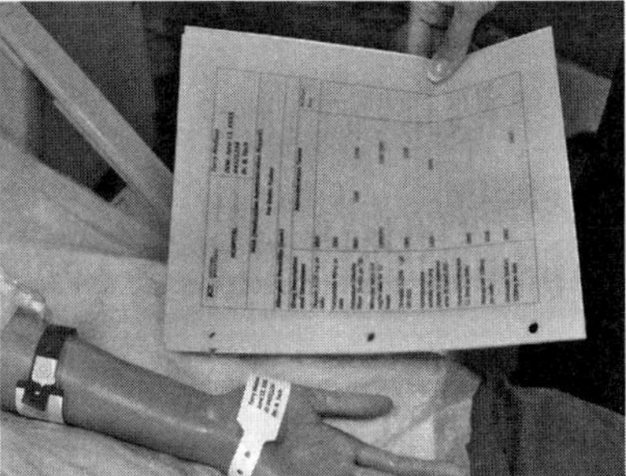
	• MAR and patient wristband comparison
	• **The proper medicine (medication):** Verify that you are using the right drug as well as that it is suitable for the individual being treated in the given situation.

Contd...

Contd...

	<ul><li>A dose that is suitable for the person's age, size, plus condition is the right dosage. varied dosages may be suggested for varied situations.</li><li>The ideal path is one that takes into account the patient's existing state.</li><li>**The appropriate moment:** Follow the timetable and dosage instructions.</li><li>Verify sure the patient is getting the drug for the proper purpose before prescribing any prescription.</li><li>**The correct paperwork:** Before giving medicine, always double-check any ambiguous or incorrect documentation.</li></ul>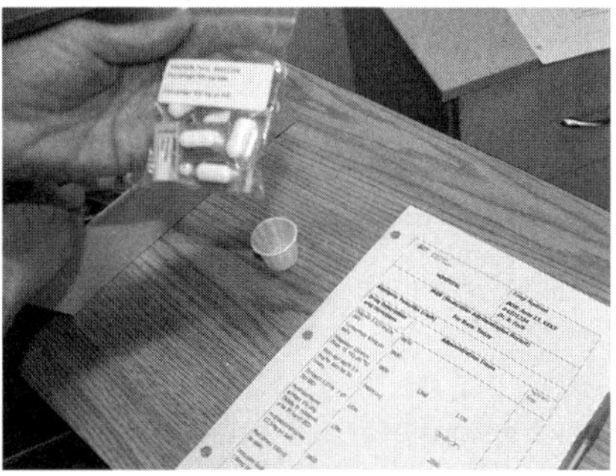<ul><li>Verify the appropriate patient, dosage, route, time, cause, and documentation.</li><li>Never record the administration of a drug till you have actually done so.</li></ul>
3. The drug's name, dose, and route must be checked three times against the MAR on the label: Upon removal of the drug from the drawer During the pouring of the drug When the medicine is being stored or placed beside the bed	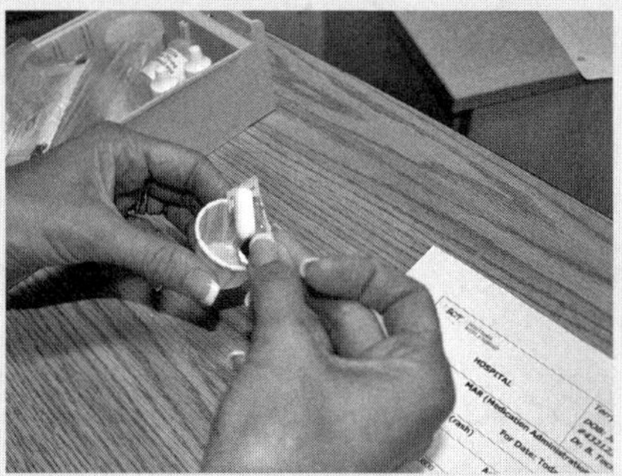<ul><li>Seven checks should be made three times before medicine is given.</li><li>Before giving your patient their medicine, these checks are performed.</li><li>Do a third examination before delivering a drug to the patient's bedside, especially eye drops.</li></ul>
4. Prior to giving the patient a rectal drug, if at all feasible, have the patient urinate.	Injecting medication into excrement is not advised.

Contd...

Contd...

5. Before giving any drugs, make sure you have a water-soluble lubricant on hand.	Suppository penetrates rectal canal with less friction because to lubricant.
6. To the patient: Describe the process. Give the patient explicit instructions on how to administer the suppository or enema correctly if they want to do so.	The patient might feel more at ease applying the suppository themselves.

Note: Certain individuals may have bradycardia as a result of accidental vagal activation. Be advised that the rectal route may not be acceptable in certain cases due to cardiac issues. Inform the physician.

7. Lift the mattress to working height. ➢ Laying on their left side having the upper leg stretched over the lower leg, the patient is placed in the Sims position. ➢ Offer the patient seclusion and drape them so that just their anal region and buttocks are visible. ➢ Lay a cloth over the patient's buttocks.	• Positioning a nurse when they are providing medicine helps avoid damage. This promotes relaxation and preserves patients' privacy. • Linens are shielded by drapes from probable fecal discharge.
8. Put on some fresh, non-sterile gloves.	The wearer of gloves avoids coming into touch with body fluids and mucosal membranes. Don't use sterile gloves.
9. Look for signs of active rectal bleeding or diarrhea in the patient.	In these circumstances, rectal medicines are contraindicated.
10. If the preceding gloves were contaminated, use clean, non-sterile gloves.	Nurses are shielded from body fluids and pores by gloves. Apply non-sterile gloves
11. The rounded tip of the medication and the big finger on your dominant hand should both be lubricated once the wrapper has been removed off the tablet or enema tip. If using an enema, merely moisten the tip.	When an enema or suppository enters the rectal canal, lubricant lessens friction.

Contd...

Contd...

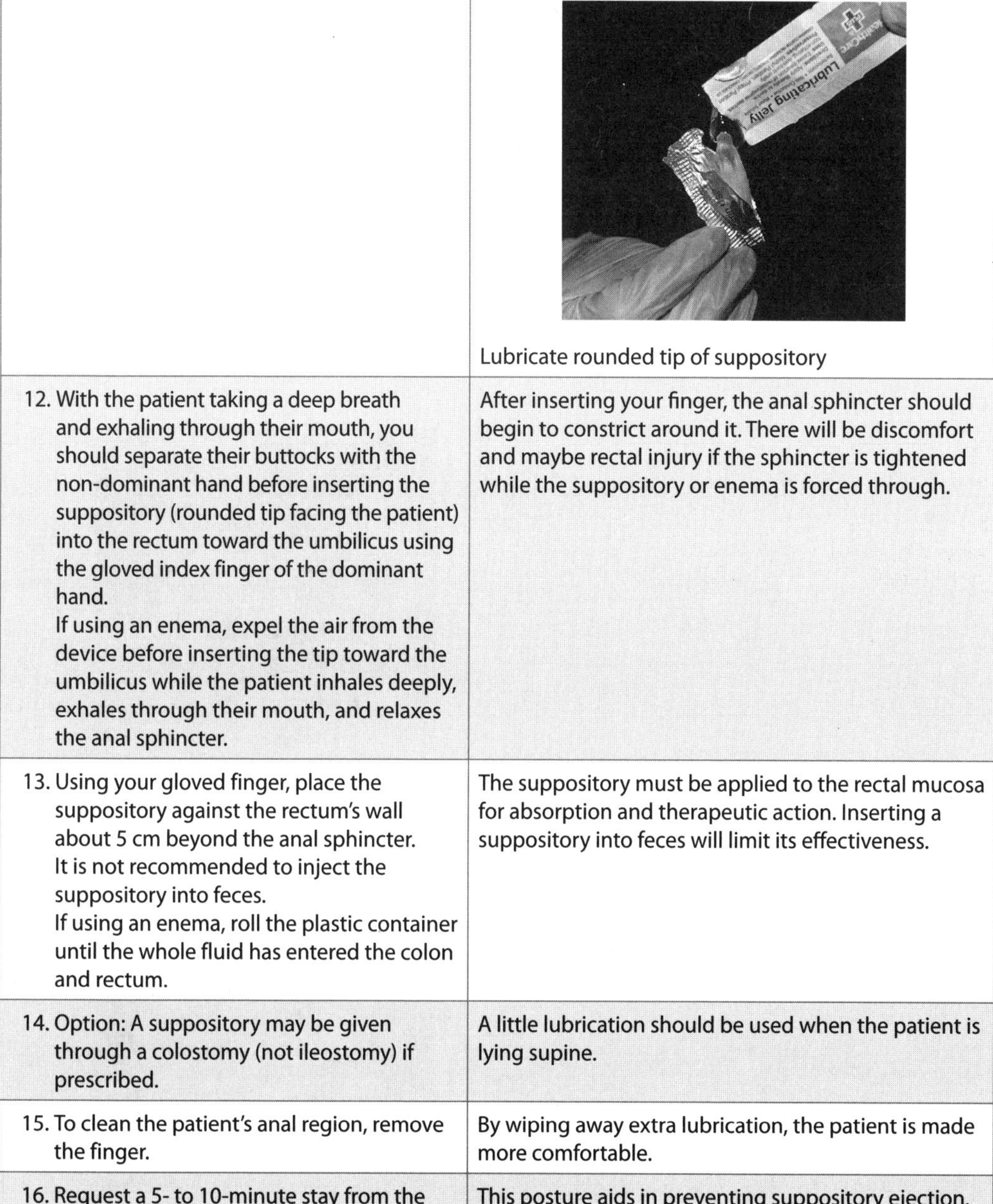

Lubricate rounded tip of suppository

12. With the patient taking a deep breath and exhaling through their mouth, you should separate their buttocks with the non-dominant hand before inserting the suppository (rounded tip facing the patient) into the rectum toward the umbilicus using the gloved index finger of the dominant hand. If using an enema, expel the air from the device before inserting the tip toward the umbilicus while the patient inhales deeply, exhales through their mouth, and relaxes the anal sphincter.	After inserting your finger, the anal sphincter should begin to constrict around it. There will be discomfort and maybe rectal injury if the sphincter is tightened while the suppository or enema is forced through.
13. Using your gloved finger, place the suppository against the rectum's wall about 5 cm beyond the anal sphincter. It is not recommended to inject the suppository into feces. If using an enema, roll the plastic container until the whole fluid has entered the colon and rectum.	The suppository must be applied to the rectal mucosa for absorption and therapeutic action. Inserting a suppository into feces will limit its effectiveness.
14. Option: A suppository may be given through a colostomy (not ileostomy) if prescribed.	A little lubrication should be used when the patient is lying supine.
15. To clean the patient's anal region, remove the finger.	By wiping away extra lubrication, the patient is made more comfortable.
16. Request a 5- to 10-minute stay from the patient.	This posture aids in preventing suppository ejection.

Contd...

Contd...

17. Turning gloves inside out can let you get rid of them, along with any discarded materials, according to agency guidelines. Perform hand hygiene.	Gloves help to stop the spread of pathogens. 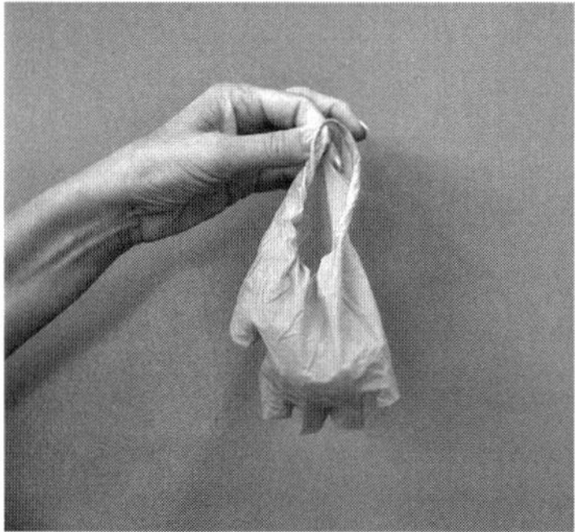 Dispose of gloves 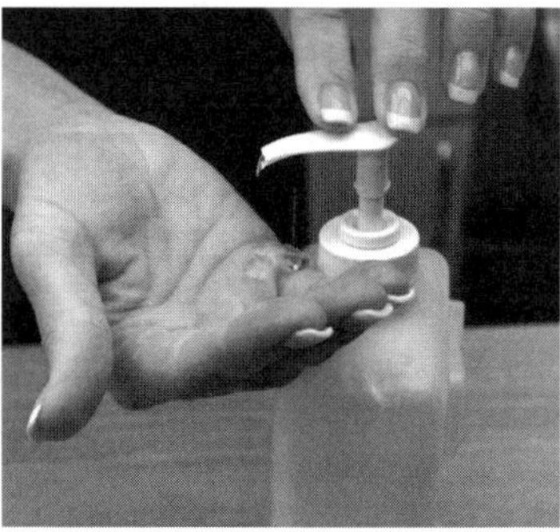 Hand hygiene with ABHR
18. Make sure a call bell is handy and that a bedpan or toilet is accessible and nearby.	Patient will need a bedpan, toilet, or access to one within close vicinity if the suppository contains a laxative and stool softener. 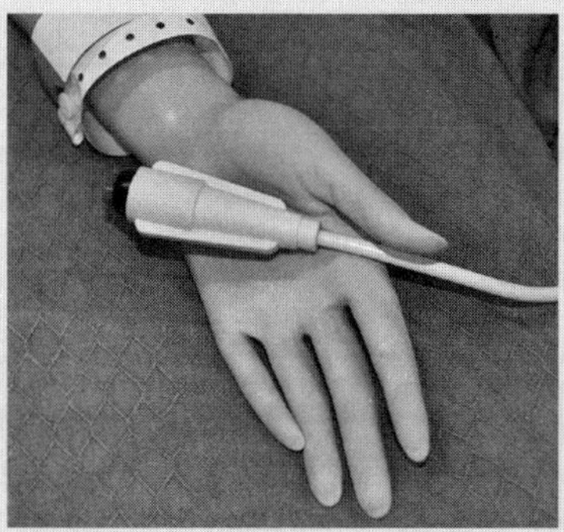 Ensure call bell is available to patient
19. Include the patient's tolerance for administration in the procedural documentation as per agency policy.	Patient safety is enhanced by timely and precise recording.

MEDICATION ADMINISTERED VAGINALLY

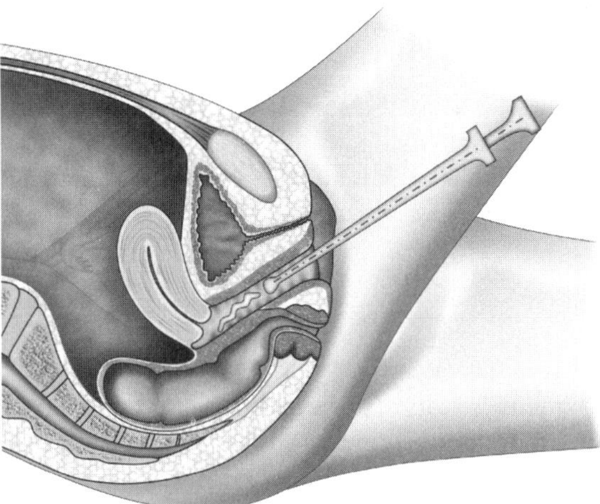

Administering medication vaginally using an applicator.

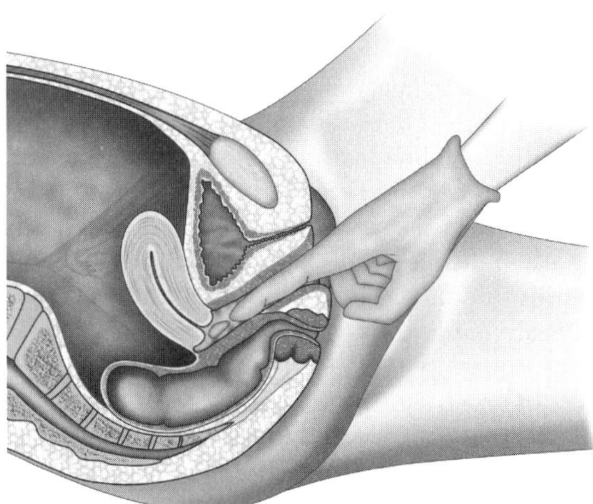

Administering medication vaginally without an applicator.

To treat infections that occur in female patients, vaginal suppositories may be necessary. Vaginal suppositories are inserted either by hand or using an applicator. They are bigger and more oval then rectal suppositories.

Definition

Topical medications designed exclusively for placement in a woman's vagina are known as vaginal drugs. They are made up and absorbed via the vaginal mucosa as a cream, bubbles, gel, pill, or suppository. An exclusive applicator supplied by the supplier is used to dispense vaginal medication in the form of a lotion, foam, gel, or tablet. Suppositories are formed like little bullets and contain medication suspended in wax. The index finger is used to put them into the vagina. The most frequent time to deliver vaginal medications is before bed since the reclining posture improves drug absorption.

Purpose

The most typical uses of vaginal medications are to treat infections, inflammation, and dryness within the vaginal mucous membrane. Chemotherapy, which is used to treat cancer, spermicides, and aborticides, which are used to induce labor, are some additional categories of vaginal medications.

Precautions

Drug should be delivered into the vagina softly since vigorous use of applicators and fingernails during drug administration might traumatize vaginal tissue. Relaxing the patient will help them be less resistant to the manner of insertion. When someone is agitated and aggressive, it is not advisable to try to implant vaginal medicine.

If a medication is not intended for vaginal use, it should not be administered that way. Oral use of vaginal medication is not recommended.

Description

With her legs bent, a patient should be lying on her back. Her heels should be level on the mattress and her thighs should be bent up toward her hips. The patient's sense of vulnerability may be lessened by placing a sheet over the belly and upper legs that ends just above the knees. You should adhere to the filling instructions for the applicator. The client should be instructed to spread her knees at this stage. The nurse has to cleanse their hands before donning disposable gloves. The nurse should split the labia and reveal the vaginal entrance with one hand. The nurse should use cotton balls or a fresh washcloth to wipe the area with soapy, warm water if there's any drainage or exudate. After rinsing, the vaginal entrance should be let to air dry. The labia should next be spread and the applicator or a sup placed into the vaginal entrance with a tiny quantity of water-soluble lubrication on the tip. Once resistance is encountered, the tablet or brush should be slowly pushed down 2–4 inches (5–10 cm) into the posterior (i.e., rear) wall of the vagina and toward the spine. Next, tilt the medication or applicator upward. The plunger of an applicator should be carefully pressed in order to release the medication while applying cream or gel. After then, the nurse should take their finger as well as the applicator out of the vagina. It is important to properly dispose of the disposable latex gloves.

Preparation

To maintain privacy, the door to the bedroom should be closed before to starting to give vaginal medications (If the nurse is a man, there must already be a female staff member present). Just before to administration, the patient should urinate. Every time a drug is administered, the nurse should examine the pharmaceutical label to prevent medication mistakes. The medication has to be examined to ensure that it is the appropriate drug, dosage (i.e., strength), timing, patient, and administration technique. Check the label's expiry date; using expired medicine is never advised. If the nurse hasn't put on disposable protective gloves already, they should be done now. He or she should wash their hands and put on gloves.

Aftercare

To stop the spread of microorganisms, the used applicator need to be set down on a fresh piece of paper towel. For at least 10 minutes (30 minutes after a suppository), the patient should be covered and urged to remain in a reclining posture with their knees raised. This will give the drug time to absorb. If the applicator being used is reused, it must be cleaned in warm, soapy water, completely rinsed, allowed to air dry, and then reinserted into the medication container or a bag made of plastic until the next usage. Put the used gloves then throwaway applicator in a garbage bag, seal it, and throw it away. The nurse has to wash their hands. To shield the patient's underwear from potential medication leaks, offer her a mini-pad (or little sanitary napkins).

After receiving vaginal medication, the patient should be advised not to use skirts since they can absorb the medication faster than the vaginal mucus, preventing the drug's full effects from being felt.

Complications

Vaginal medicines may cause tissue irritation or adverse responses. The following dosage of medication should not be administered until the doctor has been contacted if there is obvious irritation, swelling, of red of the tissue or if the individual complains of discomfort or burning.

CHECKLIST: MEDICATION ADMINISTERED VAGINALLY

Safety considerations:
- Perform hand hygiene.
- Check room for additional precautions.
- Say hello to the patient.
- Verify the patient's identity by utilizing two identifiers (such as name and birthdate).
- Look for allergies on the allergy band.
- Carry out any required targeted evaluations or tests, and keep records on MAR.
- As required, provide patients patient education.
- Arrange the distribution of medications in a calm place to minimize disturbance.
- Steer clear of social interactions.
- Adhere to the agency's no-interruptions policy.
- Make pharmaceutical preparations for one patient at a time.
- Comply with the seven rights of administering medicine.

Steps	*Additional information*
1. Check MAR against doctor's orders.	Students must check that MAR and doctor's orders are consistent.

Contd...

Contd...

	• Compare physician orders and MAR • This inspection is often completed and verified by night employees as well.

2. Perform the seven rights x 3 (must be done with each individual medication):
  ➢ The right patient
  ➢ The right medication (drug)
  ➢ The right dose
  ➢ The right route
  ➢ The right time
  ➢ The right reason
  ➢ The right documentation
Medication calculation: D/H x S = A (**D** or desired dosage/**H** or have available x **S** or stock = **A** or amount prepared)
	• **The right patient:** Verify that the patient you have is the right one by utilizing two patient identifiers, such as name and birthdate.
	
	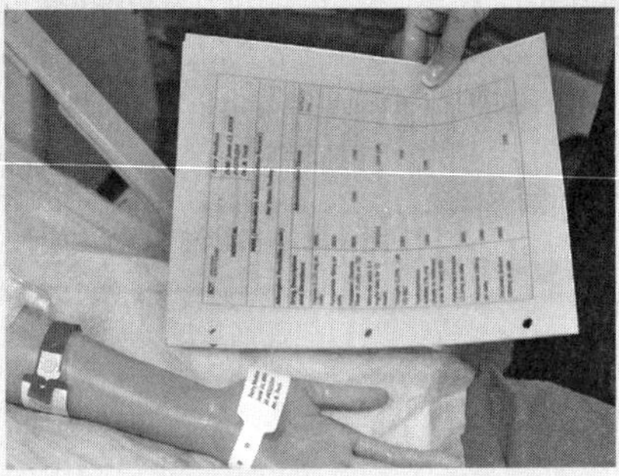
	
	• Compare MAR with patient wristband
	• **The proper medicine (medication):** Verify that you are using the right drug as well as whether it is suitable for patients in the given situation.
	• A dose that is suitable for the person's age, size, plus condition is the right dosage. varied dosages may be suggested for varied situations.
	• The ideal path is one that takes into account the patient's existing state.
	• **The appropriate moment:** Follow the timetable and dosage instructions.
	• Verify sure the patient is getting the drug for the proper purpose before prescribing any prescription.
	• **The correct paperwork:** Before giving medicine, always double-check any ambiguous or incorrect documentation.
	
	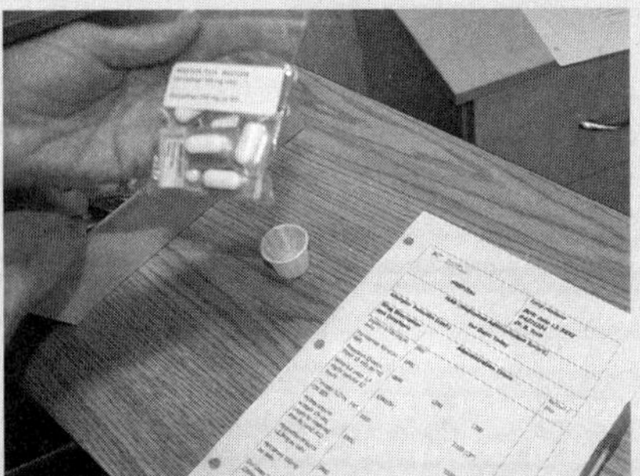
	
	• Verify the appropriate patient, dosage, route, time, cause, and documentation.
	• Never record the administration of a drug until you've have actually done so.

Contd...

Contd...

3. The drug's name, dose, and route must be checked three times against the MAR on the label:
  ➢ Upon removal of the drug from the drawer
  ➢ During the pouring of the drug
  ➢ When the medicine is being stored or placed beside the bed
	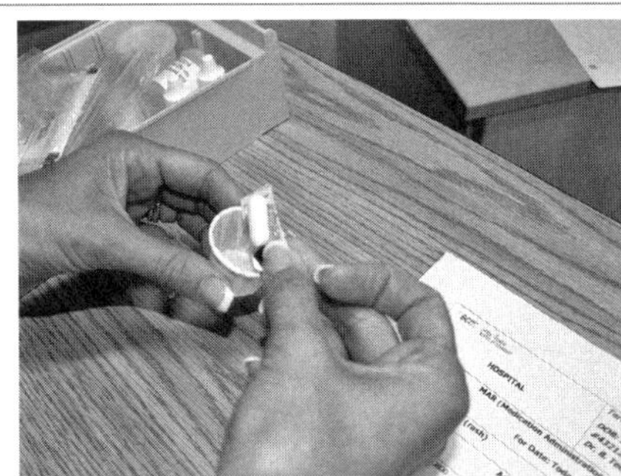
	
	• Seven checks should be made three times before medicine is given.
	• Before giving your patient their medicine, these checks are performed. Do a third examination before delivering a drug to the patient's bedside, for example eye drops.

4. Inform the patient about the technique before putting the drug vaginally. Give the patient detailed advice on how to administer the vaginal drug correctly if they want to do so.	The patient could feel more at ease giving themselves the vaginal medicine.
5. Make sure you have dissolved in water lubricant on hand before administering any medications.	Lubricant lessens friction while medicine is placed against the vaginal mucosa.
6. Have patient void prior to procedure.	During a process, voiding stops the passage of urine.

7. Lift the mattress to working height.
  ➢ Lay the patient down on the bed with their legs bent somewhat and their feet facing up.
  ➢ Provide privacy, and drape patient so that vaginal area is exposed.
	The nurse's position when providing medicine helps avoid injuries.
	Draping promotes relaxation and preserves patients' privacy.

8. Put on some fresh, non-sterile gloves.	Gloves protect the healthcare worker from contact with bodily fluids and mucous membranes. 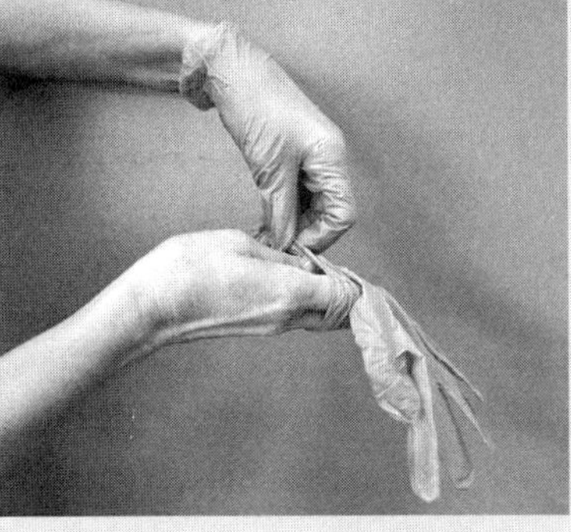 Apply non-sterile gloves

Contd...

Contd...

9. With the dominant hand's index finger, generously lubricate the suppository after removing it from its container. Suppository is most effective at room temperature.	Lubricant lessens friction while medicine is placed against the vaginal mucosa. 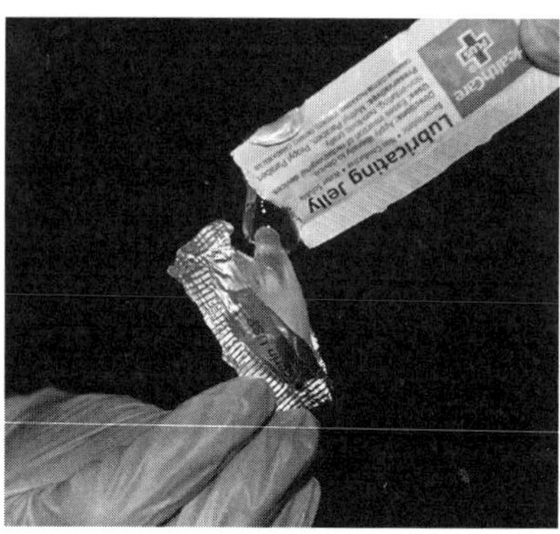 Lubricate suppository
10. Make a little separation between the labial folds with your non-dominant hand. Using the median finger of the glove on the dominant hand, insert the lubricated suppository about 8–10 cm up the rear vaginal.	Exposes the vaginal opening and aids in distributing medicine evenly.
11. Remove finger, then wipe off extra lubrication.	Patient comfort is maintained by wiping.
Note: Vaginal medicine may be inserted using an applicator. Follow the steps outlined above and any particular manufacturer instructions.	
12. Turning gloves inside out can let you get rid of them, along with any discarded materials, according to agency guidelines. Keep your hands clean.	Gloves help to stop the spread of pathogens. 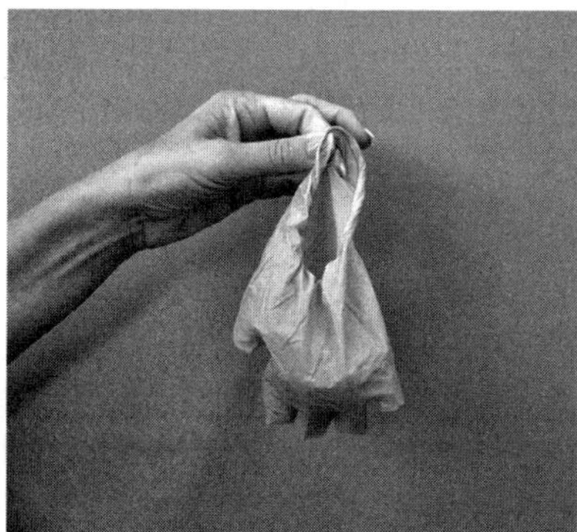 Dispose of gloves

Contd...

Contd...

	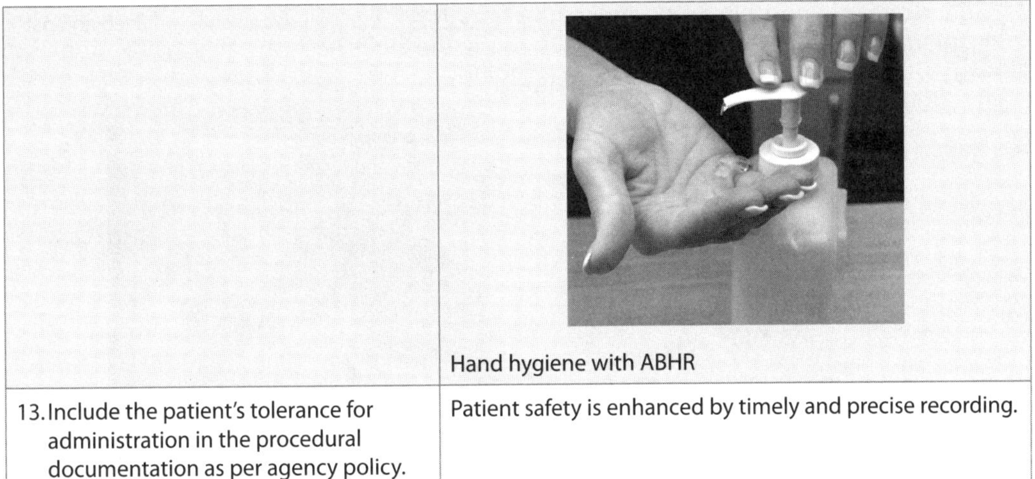 Hand hygiene with ABHR
13. Include the patient's tolerance for administration in the procedural documentation as per agency policy.	Patient safety is enhanced by timely and precise recording.

INSTILLATIONS

Ear

This treatment is used to reduce wax buildup, treat ear infections, and inject medicine into the auditory canal.

Preparation

- ❖ Examine the resident's care plan to see whether they have any unique requirements.
- ❖ Assemble the tools and materials as necessary.
- ❖ Provide privacy.

Equipment and Supplies

The following tools and materials are required to complete this process.
- ❖ Medicine dropper
- ❖ Cotton balls
- ❖ Solution (as prescribed)
- ❖ Bowl (one-half full of warm water)
- ❖ Cotton applicators; and
- ❖ Personal protective equipment (e.g., gowns, gloves, mask, etc., as needed).

Steps in the Procedure

- ❖ Med warmed to room temperature.
- ❖ Child should be placed prone or supine w/affected side upward.
- ❖ Infant → pinna is pulled downward and back
  Ages 3 or older:
  Pinna is pulled up and back

❖ Dropper should be held near entrance of ear canal w/o touching it
❖ Child remains in position for several minutes to allow full coverage
  If patient is an adult, place a cotton ball loosely in the outermost ear canal for 15 minutes to absorb excess medication (choking hazard in children)

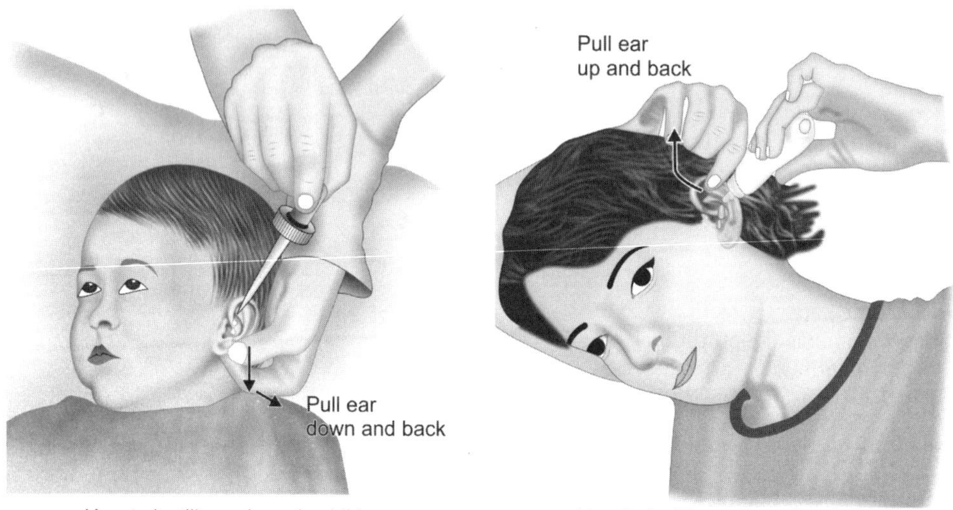

How to instill ear drops in children How to instill ear drops in adults

❖ Put the necessary equipment on the overbed table or nightstand. Place the items in a convenient location for access.
❖ Wash and thoroughly dry hands.
❖ Don gloves.
❖ In a dish of warm water, put the bottle containing the ear solution. Warm the solution slightly. Unless specifically instructed to do so by a doctor, NEVER put a cold remedy on the ear.
❖ Instruct the person in question to tilt his or her head up on the afflicted side if they are sitting up.
❖ Place the resident's head on a mattress pillow with the afflicted side facing up if they are bedridden.
❖ Use cotton swabs to gently clean the external auditory canal.
❖ Fill the dropper with the medicine. Make sure it's heated by testing it on your wrist.
❖ Drop the drug into ear with care. (Note: Avoid touching ear or a different surface with the ear dropper's tip.) In order to keep the bottle firmly closed, replace the cap.
❖ To straighten the canal's alignment and enable the drug to enter the ear, clasp an auricle (flap of the ear).
❖ If the person residing complained of pain, halt the procedure and contact the nurse management.
❖ The canal on the outside should be filled with a tiny quantity of cotton. (Note: This is to cover any potential medicine runs. Don't, however, obstruct the ear canal. Keep cotton within ear's bottom portion.)
❖ Tell the resident to stay in this posture for ten to fifteen minutes.

* If there is leaking, gently dry their ears with cotton balls. Note: Only one ball of cotton should be used each wipe.
* Place used cotton swabs in the appropriate container.
* Put your gloves in the proper container after removing them. Wash, them completely dry, your hands.
* After cleaning, put equipment back where it belongs—for example, on a nightstand or in the restroom.
* Place discarded tools and materials in the appropriate bins.
* Clean up the over-the-bed table and put it back where it belongs.
* As specified in the resident's care plan, lower the bed to its lowest setting and arrange the siderails and bed's head in the proper locations.
* Adjust the bed linens. Ensure the resident is at ease.
* Put the call light in the resident's line of sight.
* Thoroughly wash and pat dry hands.
* If the person requests it, reopen the door and curtains.

Documentation

The resident's medical record has to include the following details:
* When and on what day the ear injections were administered.
* The name and position of the person or people who administered the ear drops.
* The kind of remedy injected into the ear.
* All evaluation information gathered about the resident's ear.
* The resident's reaction to the surgery.
* The reason(s) for the resident's refusal of the therapy, together with any subsequent actions.
* The name and signature of the person who entered the data.

EAR

Description of Drugs

Miotics

Miotics are medications that make the pupil constrict. These are used in the treatment of esotropia, accommodation insufficiency, and glaucoma control.

A direct-acting parasympathomimetic medication called pilocarpine. Sterile eye drops containing pilocarpine nitrate are available in concentrations of 1%, 2%, or 4%. Pilocarpine works to cure glaucoma by reducing aqueous secretion and increasing outflow capacity (by contracting the ciliary muscle). Following topical treatment, rhinosis begins within 10–30 minutes and endures for 4–8 hours.

Carbachol

A cholinergic called carbachol is made into a sterile cosmetic ophthalmic solution. When allergy and tolerance to pilocarpine develop, carbachol, a direct-acting parasympathomimetic, may be utilized.

Iodide of phosphorus: The concentrations of phospholine iodide are 0.03%, 0.06%, 0.125%, and 0.25%. The iris, ciliary muscle I, along with other parasympathetically innervated components of the eye are enhanced by the effects of endogenously generated acetylcholine when used topically with phospholine iodide, a long-acting cholinesterase inhibitor.

Mydriatics

Mydriatics are medications that enlarge the pupil.

Phenylephrine hydrochloride, available as a 5% and 10% ocular solution, is mostly a direct-acting drug that stimulates the alpha receptors in the areas that the recipient's ganglionic pathetic nerve fibers have innervated. Additionally, it induces the veins in the conjunctiva to blanch. It is a mydriatic and does not have any cycloplegic effects.

Cyclopentolate Hydrochloride

Anticholinergic cyclopentolate 1% is manufactured as a neutral ophthalmic solutions. Additionally offered in solutions at 5% and 2% concentrations.

The eye is the most sensitive organ to which medication may be given (Perry et al., 2014). The conjunctive sac is the optimal area to give eye (ophthalmic) medications since the surface of the cornea is exceptionally sensitive. Eye drops are sterile variations of water-and-oil solutions, emulsions, or lysates of one or more active substances that may also include preservatives. Therefore, eye drops are characterized as liquid drops that are administered directly to the area of the eye, often in little quantities, such as one or a few drops.

The administration of ophthalmic medications into a patient's eye is known as eye drop instillation.

Objectives

* ❖ To combat infection
* ❖ To relieve pain and discomfort
* ❖ To dilate or constrict the pupil

Indications

Eye examination treatment of disease.

Contraindications

Allergies to the medications.

Equipment

* ❖ Sterile solution of medication
* ❖ Small gauze squares or cotton balls
* ❖ Gloves

Procedure

Instilling eye (ophthalmic) medications

Disclaimer: Always review and follow your hospital policy regarding this specific skill.	

Safety considerations:
- Perform hand hygiene.
- Check room for additional precautions.
- Say hello to the patient.
- Verify the patient's identity by utilizing two identifiers (such as name and birthdate).
- Look for allergies on the allergy band.
- Complete necessary focused assessments and/or vital signs, and document on MAR.
- As required, provide patients patient education.
- Arrange the distribution of medications in a calm place to minimize disturbance.
- Steer clear of social interactions.
- Adhere to the agency's no-interruptions policy.
- Make pharmaceutical preparations for ONE person at time.
- Comply with the SEVEN RIGHTS of administering medicine.

Steps	*Additional information*
1. Check MAR against doctor's orders.	• Check that MAR and doctor's orders are consistent. • Compare physician orders and MAR • This inspection is often completed and verified by night employees as well.
2. The following three SEVEN RIGHTS must be carried out with each unique medication: ➤ The right patient ➤ The right medication (drug) ➤ The right dose ➤ The right route ➤ The right time ➤ The right reason ➤ The right documentation Medication calculation: D/H × S = A (D or desired dosage/H or have available × S or stock = A or amount prepared)	• The right patient: Verify that the patient you have is the right one by utilizing two patient identifiers, such as name and birthdate. • Compare MAR with patient wristband • Verify you and your doctor are utilizing the correct medication to make sure it is appropriate for the person getting therapy in the specific circumstance. • The appropriate dosage is one that is appropriate for the patient's age, size, and condition. For various circumstances, different doses could be advised. • The ideal path is one that takes into account the patient's existing state. • The appropriate moment: Follow the timetable and dosage instructions. • Verify sure the patient is getting the drug for the proper purpose before prescribing any prescription. • The correct paperwork: Before giving medicine, always double-check any ambiguous or incorrect documentation. • Verify the appropriate patient, dosage, route, time, cause, and documentation. • NEVER record the administration of a drug until you actually accomplished so.

Contd...

Contd...

3. The drug's name, dose, and route must be checked three times against the MAR on the label: a. Upon removal of the drug from the drawer	• Seven checks should be made three times before medicine is given. • Before giving your patient their medicine, these checks are performed.
b. During the pouring of the drug c. When the medicine is being stored or placed beside the bed	Do a third test before delivering a drug to the patient's bedside, for example eye drops.
4. Give the patient a tissue before administering eye medicine.	When administered, drops may leak from the eye.
5. Put on sterile, clean gloves.	• Gloves protect the nurse from potential contact with patient body fluids and medications. • Apply non-sterile gloves
6. Use a warm towel or piece of gauze to remove any discharge or crusting from the eyelashes and eyelids. Move from the inner to the outside eye region while using each section of the cleaning surface just once.	Cleaning clears the ocular region of particles.
7. If the patient is laying down, put a cushion under their neck or tilt their head backwards if they are sitting up.	Reaching the conjunctival sac to administer drops is made simpler by tilting the head back.
8. Turn the eye drop bottle over and give the patient instructions to look up and focus on something in the air.	If the patient suffers a cervical spine injury, do not tilt their head back.
9. Use your thumb or a couple of fingers to gently pull the patient's lower lid down, exposing the conjunctival sac.	It will be easier to keep the eye motionless if it is focused.
10. Eye drops: Avoid touching the eye, eyelids, or hair while holding the eye-drop container above the eye. Apply one drop or two to the conjunctival sac, depending on the dose.	• The drug might get contaminated if the container's tip is touched to anything. • Instill eye drops in left eye
11. After injection, open the lower lid and advise the patient to softly shut their eyes. While the patient's eyes are closed, ask them to move their eye.	• This process enables the drug to be applied evenly across the eye. • Have patient close eyes after drop is instilled
12. When administering eye drops, apply light pressure to the inner canthus for thirty to sixty seconds only to prevent medication from entering the lacrimal duct.	As a result, the medication's systemic effects are reduced.
13. Tell the client not to touch their eyes.	This guards against eye discomfort and damage.
14. Take off the gloves and help the patient find a secure posture.	• Patient comfort and safety are therefore guaranteed. • Dispose of gloves
15. Perform hand hygiene.	• The transmission of bacteria is stopped by good hand hygiene. • Hand hygiene with ABHR
16. Follow the agency's instructions while putting together the paper. Include the procedure's date, time, dose, method, the eye or eyes that got the medication, and the patient's response.	The safety of the patient is supported by timely and accurate recording.

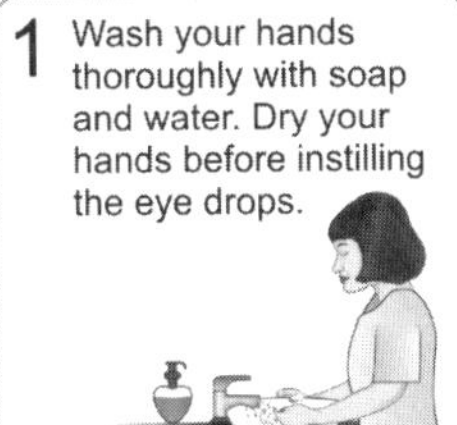

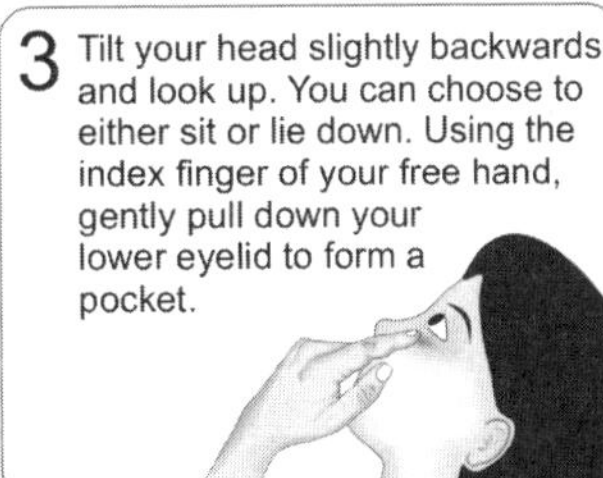

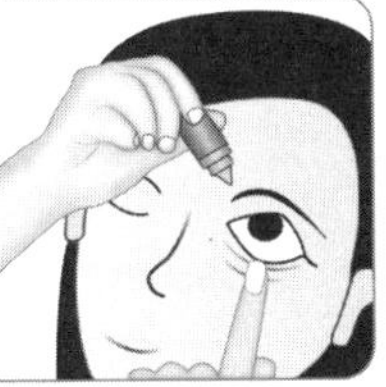

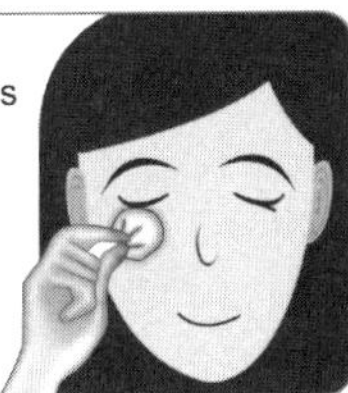

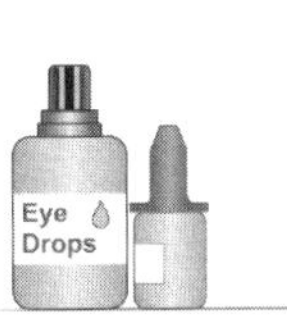

NASAL INSTILLATIONS

Introduction

Allergies, sinus infections, and nasal congestion are all treated by nasal instillations. Although the nose is not typically sterile, due to its proximity to the sinuses, clinical asepsis should be closely monitored when employing nasal instillation.

Definition

A medication solution prepared for inhalation into the nose is known as a nasal installation. Nasal sprays or drops are used to provide nasal medication.

A nasal installment is a process in which a medication solution is injected directly into the nose as nasal sprays or drops.

Drop by drop introduction of a liquid into the nostrils is known as nasal instillation.

Purposes

❖ To shrink swollen mucus membrane of nasal cavity (astringent effect)
❖ In order to assist drainage and loosen secretions.
❖ In order to cure sinus or nasal infections.
❖ To give local anesthesia.
❖ To combat infection.

- ❖ To provide astringent effect.
- ❖ To relieve inflammation and congestion in case of rhinitis.
- ❖ To diagnose nasal conditions
- ❖ To reduce swelling and congestion in the event of rhinitis
- ❖ To prevent and control bleeding

General Instructions

- ❖ Clean procedures are used.
- ❖ Avoid touching your nose's tip with a dropper since it might be contaminated.
- ❖ Refrain from using a dropper to contact the inside of the nose as this might make the patient sneeze.
- ❖ Adjust the patient's position as required to allow the afflicted region to receive medication.
- ❖ Avoid using oily solutions as drops for the nasal passages since they disrupt the natural function of the cilia.
- ❖ Avoid using decongestants excessively or regularly since they lose their effectiveness and may make the patient's congestion worse.
- ❖ After the medication has been administered, tell the patient to stay in the same posture for a while so that it may work on the anterior nares' mucous membrane and subsequently drain into the lower nares.

Equipment

- ❖ Medication with a clean dropper
- ❖ A medication chart.
- ❖ A handkerchief/facial tissue/small towel.
- ❖ Pillow
- ❖ Kidney tray
- ❖ Paper bag
- ❖ Gloves

Instilling Nasal Medications

Safety considerations:
- Perform hand hygiene.
- Check room for additional precautions.
- Say hello to the patient.
- Verify the patient's identity by utilizing two identifiers (such as name and birth date).
- Look for allergies on the allergy band.
- Complete necessary focused assessments and/or vital signs, and document on MAR.
  - ➢ As required, provide patients patient education.
  - ➢ Arrange the distribution of medications in a calm place to minimize disturbance.
  - ➢ Steer clear of social interactions.
  - ➢ Adhere to the agency's no-interruptions policy.
  - ➢ Make pharmaceutical preparations for ONE client at once.
  - ➢ Comply with the SEVEN RIGHTS of administering medicine.

Contd...

Contd...

Steps	Additional information
1. Check MAR against doctor's orders.	• Check that MAR and doctor's orders are consistent. 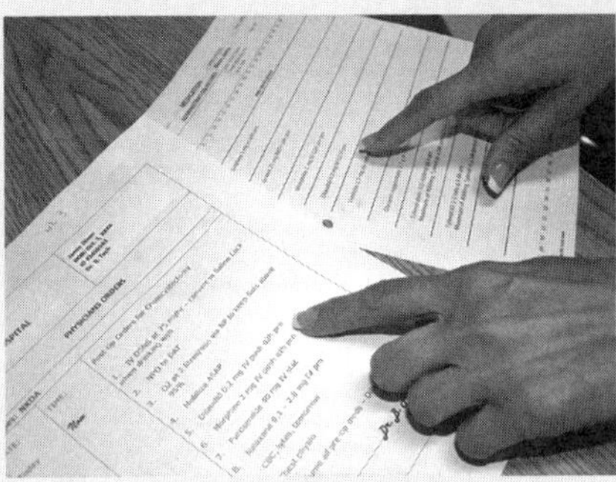 • Compare physician orders and MAR • Night staff usually complete and verify this check as well.
2. The Seven rights must be carried out three times for each medication: 1. The right patient 2. The right medication (drug) 3. The right dose 4. The right route 5. The right time 6. The right reason 7. The right documentation Medication calculation: D/H x S = A (**D** or desired dosage/**H** or have available x S or stock = **A** or amount prepared)	• The right patient: Verify that the patient you have is the right one by utilizing two patient identifiers, such as name and birthdate. 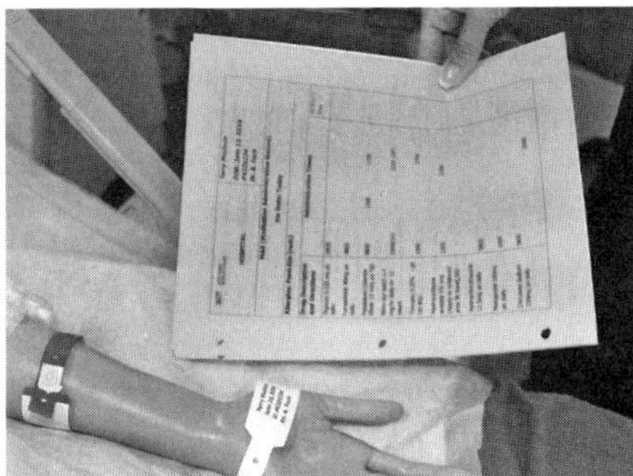 • MAR and patient wristband comparison • The correct medication: Ensure that the substance you are employing is appropriate for the patient receiving care in the particular circumstance. • A dose that is suitable for someone's age, size, plus condition is the right dosage. Varied dosages may be suggested for varied situations. • The ideal path is one that takes into account the patient's existing state. • The appropriate moment: Follow the timetable and dosage instructions. • Verify sure the patient is getting the drug for the proper purpose before prescribing any prescription. • The correct paperwork: Before giving medicine, always double-check any ambiguous or incorrect documentation.

Contd...

Contd...

	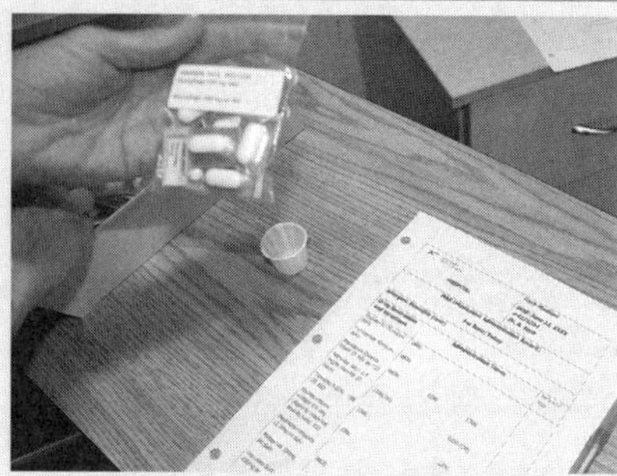 • Verify the appropriate patient, dosage, route, time, cause, and documentation. • Never record the administration of a drug until you actually did so.

3. Name, dosage, and route on the medication's label must be verified and compared the MAR three times:
  1. Upon removal of the drug from the drawer
  2. During the pouring of the drug
  3. When the medicine is being stored or placed beside the bed
	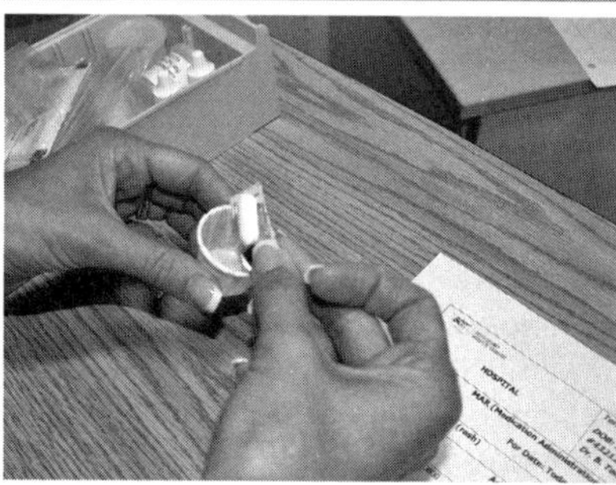
	• Seven checks should be made three times before medicine is given.
	• Before giving your patient their medicine, these checks are performed.
	• When bringing a medication to the bedside, such as eye drops, do a third check.

4. Put on clean, non-sterile gloves before administering nasal medicine.	• The nurse is shielded from possible contact with patient bodily fluids and drugs by wearing gloves. 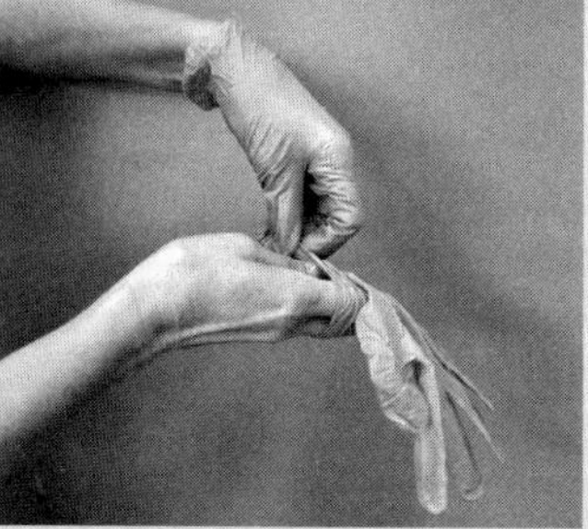 • Apply non-sterile gloves
5. Ask the patient to blow their nose and give them some tissues.	Prior to administering medicine, this helps cleanse the nostrils.

Contd...

Contd...

6. Position patient with head over a headrest (under the neck) when seated back or laying down.	• Medication may now flow back into the nasal cavity in this position. • If the patient suffers a cervical spine injury, do not tilt their head back.
7. Draw fluid into the prescription dropper until there is plenty for both nares. Don't put extra liquid back in the stock bottle.	The danger of medicine contamination rises when liquids is returned to the stock bottle.
8. Request mouth breathing from the patient. ➢ Drop medicine into each naris one at a time, holding the dropper approximately 1 cm above the naris. ➢ Have the patient breathe gently through the other nostril while using a spray for the nasal cavity, keeping one nostril closed. ➢ Avoid using the spray bottle's dropper on your naris.	• Place the dropper approximately 1 cm above the naris. • Aspiration of the drug may be avoided by mouth breathing. • The drug and the dropper/spray bottle will get contaminated if you touch your nares with them.
9. Place the patient in this position for two to three minutes.	The drug cannot escape from this place.
10. Take off the gloves and help the patient find a secure posture.	Patient comfort and safety are therefore guaranteed.
11. Perform hand hygiene.	The transmission of bacteria is stopped by good hand hygiene. Hand hygiene with ABHR
12. Follow the agency's instructions while putting together the paper. Include the following information: date, time, dose, route, its naris the medication was injected into (or both nares, if necessary), and the patient's response to the medication.	To guarantee patient safety, timely and correct documentation is essential.

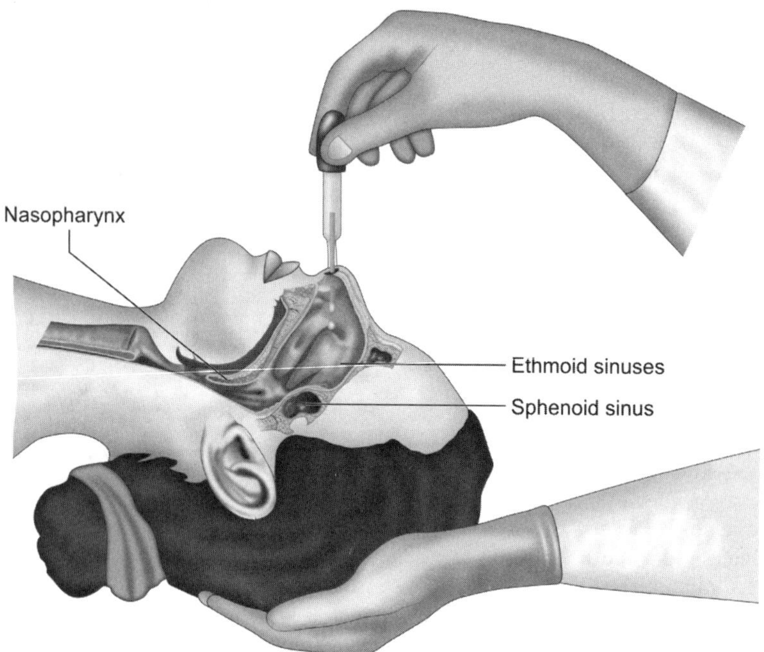

Installation of nasal drops.

BLADDER INSTILLATION

When diet changes, stress reduction techniques, and over-the-counter medications are ineffective, bladder installations are recommended in the American Urological Association's clinical recommendation for IC/BPS. Instillations of various medications straight into the bladder are known as bladder cocktails or bladder instillations. Some examples of installations are:

* Alkalinized lidocaine and heparin
* Dimethylsulfoxide (DMSO)
* Sodium hyaluronate
* Heparin
* Bladder cocktails
* New instillations under development

Procedure

Check the practitioner's order and obtain medication/solution from pharmacy.

Gather Supplies

* Disposable bladder irrigation tray (if catheter is indwelling)
* Sterile catheter tray (if catheter is straight catheter)
* Appropriate PPE—gloves, mask and shield
* Sterile gloves
* One or two sterile catheter plugs (if required)
* Luer lock catheter adapter

* 60 mL Luer lock syringe (if required)
* IV tubing (if required)
* Medication or prescribed solution.

Steps

* Get an order for installation with the reason of instillation if the patient doesn't have a catheter.
* Make sure all urine has been fully expelled from the bladder.
* Keep your hands clean.
* Put on the proper PPE.
* If the patient has an inside catheter, use an alcohol swab to wipe the drainage tube and catheter at the connection point. Join the catheter and the drainage tube. Placing the catheter side in a clean, graded glass basin after sealing the tube end's exit via a sterile catheter plug. It is not essential to detach while using a 3-way catheter to clamp the drainage lumen.
* Prepare the medicine for injection. To avoid bladder spasms, medications should be at the temperature of the body or at the very least at room temperature.

If medication is drawn up or supplied in a 60 mL syringe:
* Attach Luer lock catheter adapter to the end of the syringe
* Connect adapter to the catheter.

If the medication is supplied in a minibag:
* Attach IV tubing to minibag.
* Attach Luer lock catheter adapter to end of IV tubing
* Prime IV tubing and adapter with the medication
* Connect adapter to the catheter.
  * Using the catheter, drip medicine into the bladder gradually using gravity or light, equal pressure. Slowing the instillation may be essential if the patient complains of pain.
  * If cather is currently in place, keep it there or put in another catheterization plug throughout the necessary period. Remove the catheter if it is intermittent and ask the person in question to hold the urine for the appropriate amount of time.
  * After the prescribed indwelling time.
  * Allow the medicine to drain out naturally if the catheter has to be removed. Next, deflate the balloon before removing the catheter.
  * Reconnect the drainage tube to the catheter if it will stay in place, and then let gravity take its course in letting the medicine out.
  * Instruct the patient to urinate if the intermittent catheters has already been taken out.

Document

On patient progress record
* Catheterization of patient (if required)
* Medication instilled
* Indwelling time
* Solution, color, and consistency returns
* Patient response: Medication on medication administration record

In case of traumatic catheterization, inability to hold for the required amount of time, or any other patient's concerns, notify MRP.

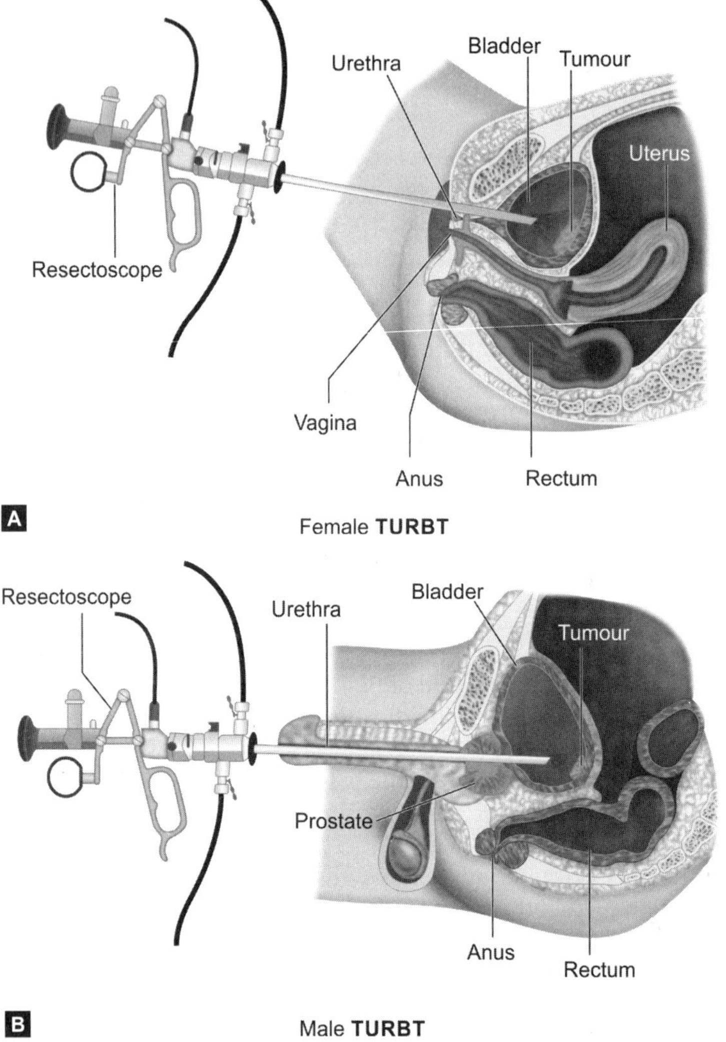

(A) Female transurethral resection of bladder tumor (TURBT); **(B)** Male TURBT.

RECTAL INSTILLATION

Rectal suppositories are smaller and fashioned like bullets. During insertion, the rounded end reduces anal trauma. The drugs in rectal suppositories may have local effects like encouraging urination or systemic ones like easing nausea. They are kept in the fridge to keep their form.

The suppository has to be placed on the rectal mucosa after passing the internal anal sphincter. If not, the patch can be thrown up before it dissolves and is absorbed by the mucosa. It is better to provide a cleaning enema in the event of a loaded rectum before administering the suppository.

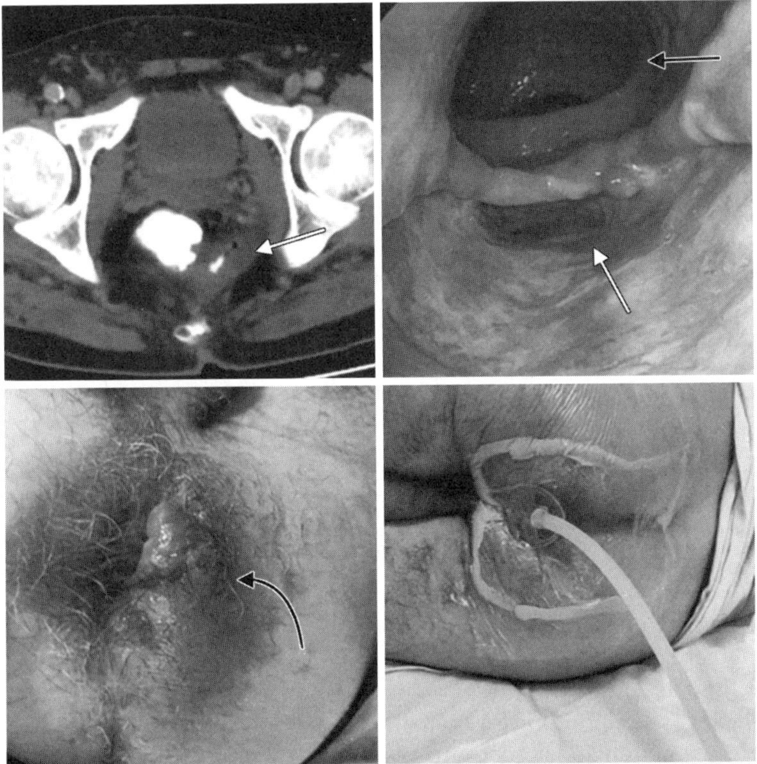

Rectal instillation.

Administration of Rectal Suppositories

Procedure

❖ Check the physician's order, client's name, drug name, route and time of administration.
Rationale: Ensure safe and correct administration of medication.
❖ Review the medical record for any history of rectal surgery or bleeding.
Rationale: These conditions are contraindications for suppository.
❖ Wash hands.
Rationale: Reduces the chance of infection.
❖ **Prepare articles:**
  ◆ Rectal suppository.
  ◆ Lubricating jelly.
  ◆ Clean disposable gloves.
  ◆ Rag pieces.
❖ Put on gloves.
Rationale: Prevents contact with fecal matter.
❖ Identify the patient.
Rationale: Avoid errors in medication.

* Explain the procedure, if the patient want, allow self-administration.
  Rationale: Promote better IPR (inter personal relationship) and cooperation.
* Arrange supplies at bedside and provide privacy.
  Rationale: Ensure smooth procedure.
* Drape the patient, exposing only the anal area. Give Sims position.
  Rationale: Prevent embarrassment and promote relaxation.
* Examine the external condition of the anus and palpate the rectal walls. Change the gloves if soiled.
  Rationale: Helps to detect any active rectal bleeding. Palpation helps to find out if the rectum is loaded with feces.
* Remove the suppository from the wrapper and lubricate the rounded end. Lubricate the index finger of right hand.
  Rationale: Lubrication reduces friction.
* Instruct the patient to take slow deep breaths through mouth and relax the anal sphincter.
  Rationale: Relaxation of anal sphincter prevents pain on introduction of suppository.
* Retract buttocks with gloved left hand. Insert suppository gently through anus past internal sphincter and against rectal wall, 10 cm (4 in) in adults and 5 cm (2 in) in children and infants.
  Rationale: For adequate absorption and therapeutic action suppository must be placed against the rectal mucosa.
* Withdraw finger and wipe anal area.
  Rationale: Provide comfort.
* Discard the gloves into appropriate container.
  Rationale: Prevent transfer of microorganisms.
* Tell the patient to remain flat or adopt side-lying position for 5 minutes.
  Rationale: Prevents expulsion of suppository.
* Wash hand.
  Rationale: Prevents infection.
* Check after 5 minutes to determine whether the suppository is expelled.
  Rationale: Reinsertion may be needed.
* Document name of the drug, route, time of administration and effect.
  Rationale: Reduce errors.
* Observe the effect of suppository (bowel movements) after 30 minutes of administration.
  Rationale: To ascertain whether the required result is obtained.

IRRIGATIONS

Eye Irrigation

Purpose

The objectives of this technique are to clear the eye of foreign objects, irrigate the eye after eye injection, clear the eye of discharge or chemicals, clear your eye of congestion or discomfort, and disinfect the eye.

To irrigate the lens of the eye with water in a way that any foreign objects, trash, rapid removal of chemicals or mucus from the eye, eyes, or socket.

To minimize harm and possible vision loss to the eye(s)

Should make sure patients who have had CS gas in their eye or eyes are not irrigated since this would make the situation worse.

General Guidelines

- ❖ The irrigation solution should not be heated over 100°F (37.7°C) in either water or a prescribed solution. (Caution: Applying a cold solution can make the discomfort worse. Unless otherwise indicated, use warm solutions.)
- ❖ The resident becomes anxious when their eyesight is impaired or lost. Tell the resident what will happen during the surgery and what to expect. To stop injuries and the propagation of illnesses, the resident's cooperation is crucial.
- ❖ Give the person who lives as much solitude as you can.
- ❖ The cornea is very sensitive and contains a lot of nerves. Don't use any force while doing this technique. Allow a continuous stream of the solution to run.
- ❖ If both eyes need to be irrigated, wash and completely dry your hands before doing so.
- ❖ Place your palm on the resident's forehead or nasal bridge to stabilize the syringe while the resident is being irrigated.
- ❖ Don't rush the process. Take your moment and treat the person with kindness.

Supplies and Equipment

The following tools and materials are required to complete this process.

- ❖ Sterile irrigating syringe
- ❖ Emesis basin
- ❖ Small basin for solution
- ❖ Solution (as prescribed)
- ❖ Sterile 4 × 4 gauze pads
- ❖ Cotton balls
- ❖ Towel
- ❖ Plastic cape (optional)
- ❖ Personal safety gear (such as gowns, gloves, masks, etc., if required)
- ❖ One liter of ordinary saline 0.9% times three, or six if each of the eyes are damaged
- ❖ Providing set for intravenous infusion
- ❖ Drip stand
- ❖ Suitable light source
- ❖ Minims® oxybuprocaine 0.4%–local anesthetic for adults
- ❖ Minims® proxymetacaine 0.5%–local anesthetic for children
- ❖ Protective cape, apron and paper towels or terry towels.

Procedure

Action

The following step is to cross-reference the patient's title, address, and other personal data with the case notes on casualty card. Verify the necessary steps.

Rationale: To confirm the patient's actual identity and the veracity of the required inquiry.

Step: Ask the patient about any relevant past events, including the incident's nature, timing, and location.

Rationale: To identify the kind of medicines or foreign substances that were used in the occurrence.

Step: Describe the technique and the goal of the investigation to the patient.

Rationale: To acquire patients' cooperation and informed consent as well as to assuage any worries or anxiety.

Step: Place the patient on a chair or the floor and support their head.

Rationale: To protect the security and comfort of the nurse and the patient.

Step: One is to wash your hands according to trust rules.

Rationale: To lower the possibility of cross-infection.

Step: Ask the person in pain to raise his or her head. Insert a pH indicator testing sheet at the intersection of the lower lid's center and outer third by gently drawing the lower lid down. When the strip is wet, compare the score to the pH indication (following 30 seconds).

Rationale: To lessen the patient's suffering and determine the chemical mixture's Ph.

Step: Put a single teaspoon of local anesthetic (see equipment) into the inferior fornix of the afflicted eye or eyes.

Rationale: To make patients feel better and encourage cooperation from them

Step: Put the giving set together and verify the fluid flow before using. Position all equipment on the impacted side.

Rationale: To guarantee the security of the tools and remedy. Assure a sufficient irrigation solution flow. The necessary tools are nearby.

Step: Wrap a blanket or towel across the patient's shoulder blades and neck on the affected side.

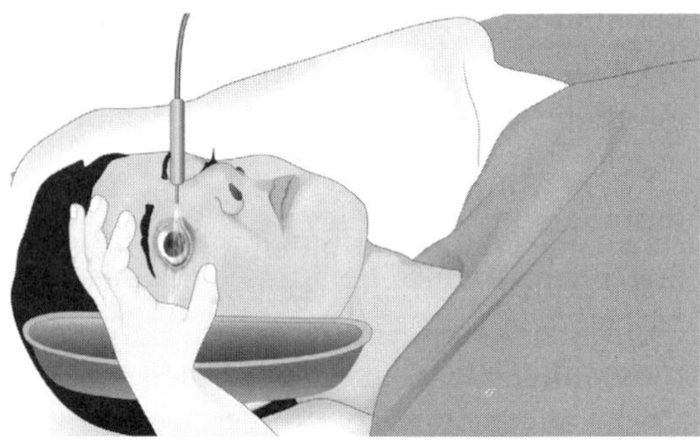

Irrigate the eye from the inner canthus to the outer canthus.

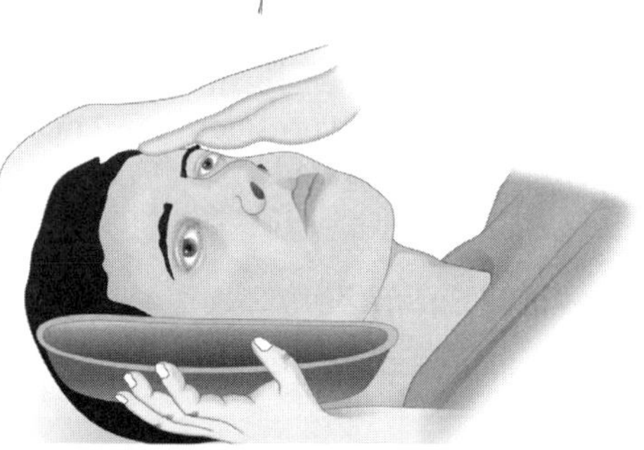

Position the patient with their head well supported and place a kidney dish against their cheek on the affected side.

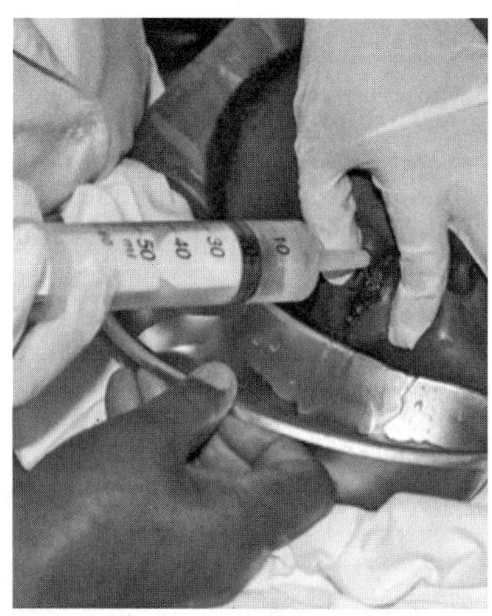

Rationale: To keep the patient's clothes safe.

Step: One is to provide the patient with an irrigation fluid receiver or dish. Next, you should tell them to tilt their heads to the afflicted side while holding the receiver against their cheek.

Rationale: To guarantee proper technique and less spillage.

Step: Place yourself behind the patient's side that is ill. Verify that the receiver is positioned properly. Keep the providing nozzle in place.

Rationale: To make it simple to do the method.

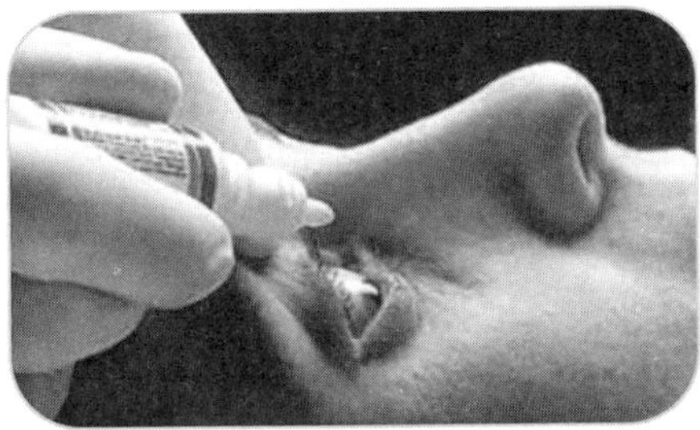

Insertion
Instill topical ocular anesthetic, if available

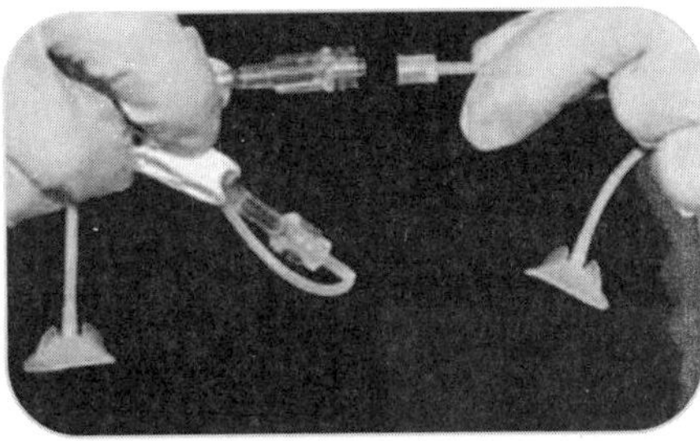

Attach a Morgan Lens Delivery Set (or a syringe or an I.V. set-up) using solution and rate of choice*; **Start flow**

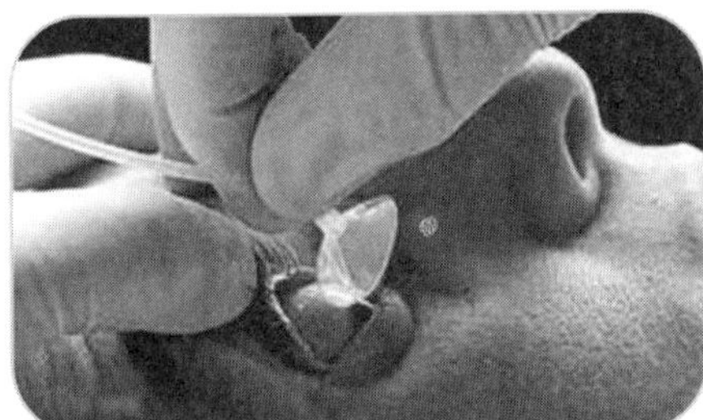

Have patient look down, insert Morgan Lens under upper lid. Have patient look up, retract lower lid, drop lens in place

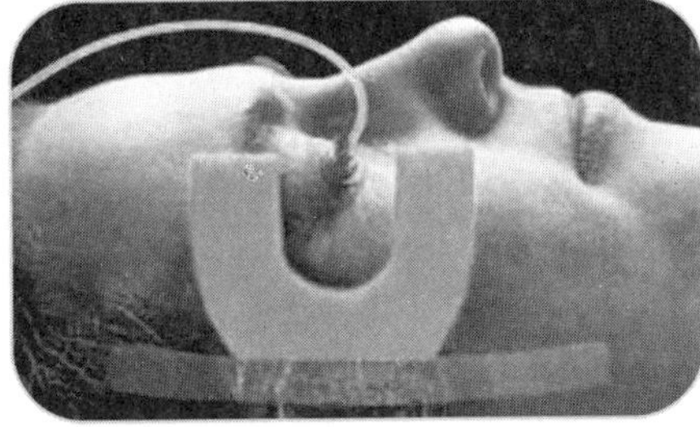

Release the lower lid over Morgan Lens; adjust flow. tape tubing to patient's forehead to prevent accidental lens removal. Absorb outflow with the Medi-duct (for best results, tape to head as shown). **Do not run dry**

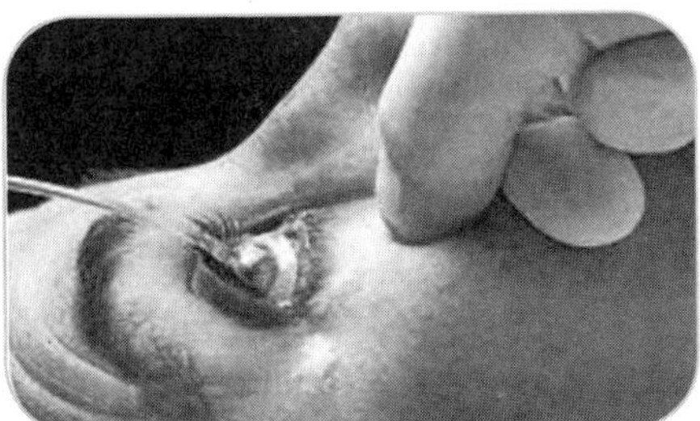

Removal
Continue flow.
Have patient look, retract lower lid—hold position

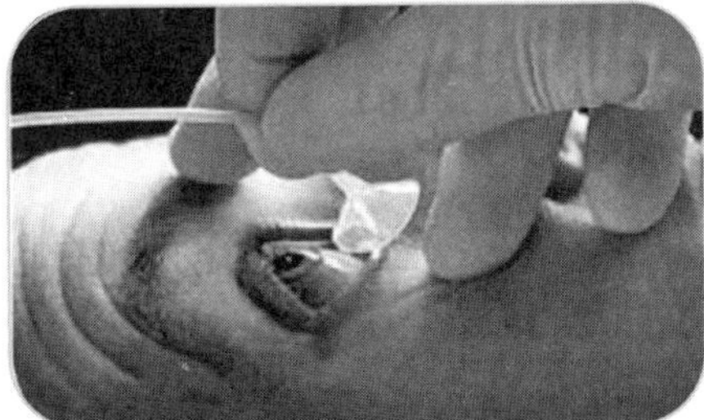

Side Morgan Lens out.
Terminate flow

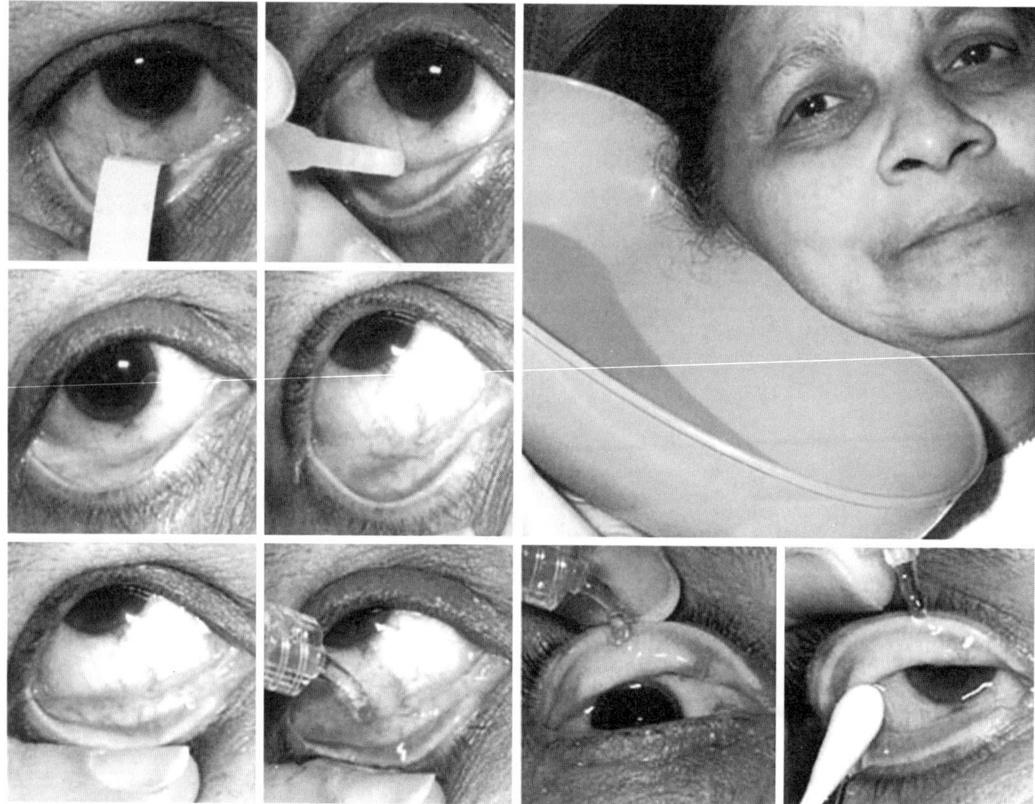

Imaging the eye after a chemical burn.

Ear Irrigation

The EAM typically contains a little quantity of wax, therefore its absence may indicate that infections, frequent bathing or dry skin conditions have hampered wax development. The only time removal could be required is when wax has accumulated. Older persons, those with learning disabilities, those who are hearing aid clients, people who push objects into their ears, and people with small EAM all have an increased risk of developing a wax build-up.

Nurses perform a process known as ear irrigation in which they cleanse the ear canal of a patient with sterilized water or a saline solution. A foreign body may need to be removed from a patient's ear, impacted ear wax may need to be softened and removed, or the ear canal may need to be cleaned of any discharge.

Purposes

- ❖ Increase the tympanic membrane's ability to carry sound because wax has obstructed it.
- ❖ Proper treatment for otitis externa when material blocks the meatus.
- ❖ To enable testing of the EAM with the power supplier tympanic membrane, remove her release, keratin, or debris.

❖ To make it simpler to create mold imprints for hearing aids, remove wax.
❖ Make it easier to remove wax and other foreign objects from the EAM that are not hygroscopic. It will be more challenging to remove hygroscopic debris (such peas and lentils) since they would expand after absorbing the water.

Contraindications

❖ This technique has previously resulted in difficulties for the patient.
❖ An infection of the middle ear in the previous six weeks has a history.
❖ There has been any kind of ear surgery performed on the patient (other than grommets being extruded no less than 18 months ago and it has been confirmed that the tympanic membrane, which surrounds the ear is intact).
❖ There is a perforation on the patient.
❖ A mucous discharge has been reported in the preceding 12 months.
❖ The pinna is painful and sensitive, suggesting acute otitis externa.
❖ A history with cleft palate, whether or not it has been corrected.

Precautions: Ear irrigation should be carried out on a low setting
❖ The patient has tinnitus
❖ The patient has a healed perforation
❖ The patient suffers from dizziness
❖ The patient is taking anticoagulants or high dose steroids
❖ The patient is immunocompromised.
❖ The patient has had radiotherapy of the head or neck.

Equipment

❖ Otoscope
❖ Head mirror and light or headlight and spare batteries
❖ Electronic irrigator
❖ Tap water at 38°C–40°C or temperature comfortable for the patient, avoiding cool water
❖ Noots trough/receiver
❖ Jobson Horne probe/carbon curette or an appropriate cotton wool carrier and good quality cotton wool or ear mop/ear canal wick
❖ Tissues and receivers for dirty swabs and instruments
❖ Disposable waterproof cape and paper towels
❖ Disposable apron and gloves

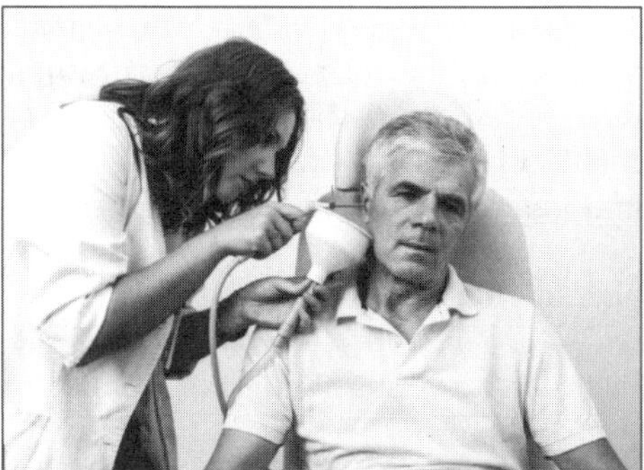

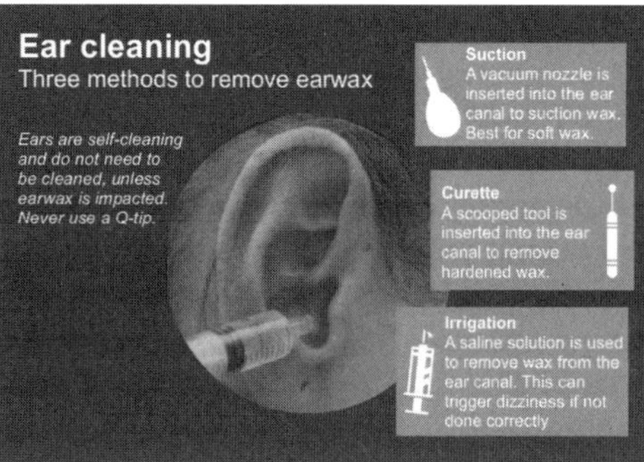

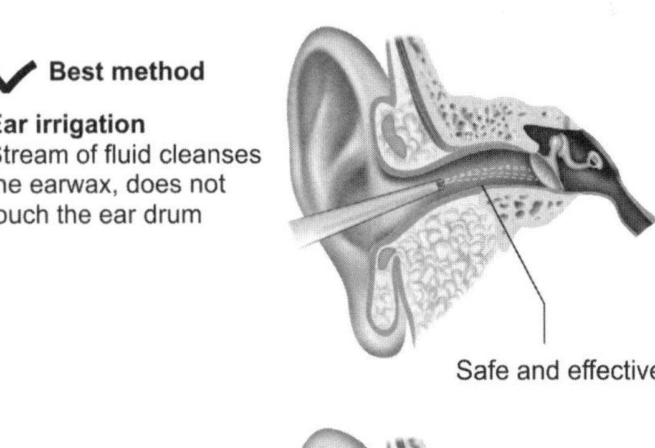

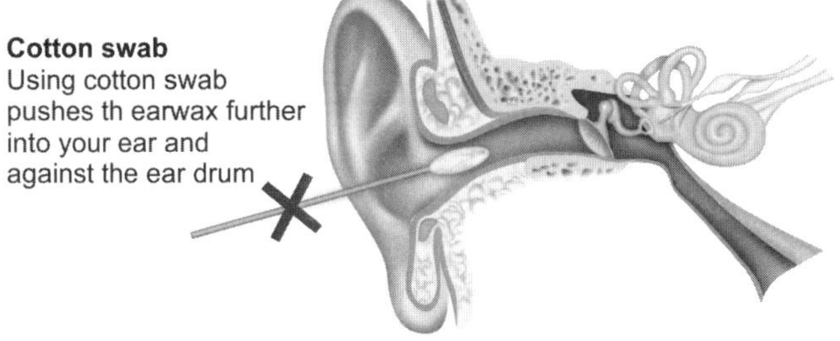

Procedure

- ❖ It is important to document the findings of the first examination as well as the patient's presenting concerns. Valid authorization should be requested and documented before proceeding.
- ❖ Examine the ears by first using direct light to examine the pinna and the scalp. After looking for any skin flaws or scars from prior surgery, examine the EAM using the otoscope.
- ❖ Check to see whether the patient has had ear irrigation in the past and if there are any contraindications to filtration.
- ❖ Ask the patient to sit on a medical chair after enduring the stages with them (a child may sit on an adult's knee as lengthy as the adult maintains their head steady).
- ❖ Verify that the headlight or other light source is installed and operating as it should.
- ❖ Place the paper cloth and safety cape on the client's shoulder and under the irrigating ear. Ask the patient to hold the receiver to their or their ear.
- ❖ Fill the irrigation system's reservoir and make sure the water is between 38 and 40°C. Minimum pressure should be set.
- ❖ Firmly 'push/twist' a fresh tip applicator into the machine's tube. Push until you hear a "click".
- ❖ Turn on your gadget for 10–20 seconds after noting the receiver, to circulate the liquid and remove any air or cold water that may have been trapped in the system. The patient will have the chance to adjust to the machine's sounds in this way. Any static water that was still within the tube is eliminated by discarding the original water flow. Check the water's temperature once again.
- ❖ Twist the end to direct the water toward the patient's head's rear along the EAM's posterior wall.
- ❖ To correct the EAM (which is facing directly backward in youngsters), gently pull it upward and outward.

❖ Inform the patient you are going to begin irrigating and that you will halt the process if they begin to feel lightheaded or in discomfort. Make sure the light is shining down the EAM. Use the foot control to aim a water jet straight at the back for the patient's head, against the posterior wall, and down the EAM ceiling. Place the tip of the water nozzle into the EAM entrance. If the wax is difficult to remove, gradually increase the pressure control. It is advised to use no more than one water reservoir per ear at a time while doing irrigation.

❖ There is research that suggests increasing the canal's water level for a period of fifteen minutes will enhance success rates. If both ears need to be irrigated with water, it would be helpful to do so and then resume the operation after a 15-minute break.

❖ Check the liquid reaching the receiver and periodically inspect the EAM through an otoscope.

❖ Make use from the Jobson Horne probe, the carbon curette, the ear canal wick, or a suitable fiber carrier and excellent quality cotton wool to dry mop any remaining water out of the meatus beneath direct view after removing any wax or debris. Infection is made more likely during the process by water stagnation and any skin damage. Infection risk is decreased by removing the pus with the cotton wool-tipped probe.

❖ Inspect the ear, including the meatus you tympanic membrane, you treat as necessary using predetermined recommendations, or seek medical attention if necessary.

❖ Share any pertinent information and tips on ear care. Tell the patient to come back if their ear begins to discharge or hurts. Encourage the patient to inquire about further guidance in accordance with local policy if the wax removal doesn't help their hearing, which was their first complaint.

❖ Describe the findings in both hearing, the technique used, the state of the external hearing meatus and tympanic membrane, and the therapy administered. The NMC guidelines for accountability and record keeping should be followed by nurses, and results should be reported. If any aberration is found, a referral for treatment at the ENT Surgical Department should be issued in compliance with local laws.

Risk Factors

Potential complications following procedure:
❖ Trauma
❖ Infection
❖ Dizziness
❖ Tinnitus

Bladder Irrigation

A treatment called bladder irrigation is used to clean the bladder's inside. It may be necessary to flush the augmented, neobladder to get rid of extra mucus the gut has produced and is now storing in the bladder. This promotes free urine flow via the catheter, prevents mucus buildup, and lessens the risk of infections and kidney stones.

The procedure of cleaning out or flushing out the bladder's contents is known as bladder irrigation.

OR

By forcing a solution of water into the bladder and promptly emptying it, the method known as bladder irrigation is used to clear blood clots or other material from the bladder.

Purposes

- To purge the bladder of germs, extra mucus, blood clots, pus, and decomposing urine.
- To reduce inflammation-related discomfort and congestion.
- To aid in recovery.
- To avoid the development of clots after bladder operations.
- To remove clots and debris from the bladder.
- To provide medicine to the bladder's lining.
- To get the catheter's patency back.
- To either treat or prevent infection.
- To stop bleeding.

Types of Bladder Irrigation

- Close continuous bladder irrigation
  - Calculating true urine output: Subtract the total amount of drainage to the amount of irrigant infused= urine output hang
- Close intermittent bladder irrigation
  - Need to clamp drainage tubing below port
  - Instill irrigant through port
- Open/manual bladder irrigation
  - Disconnect catheter from drainage bag
  - Instill irrigating solution through the connecting port

Continuous Bladder Irrigation

Continuous bladder irrigation (CBI) minimizes the danger of blood clots and preserves the patency of a urinary catheter that is implanted (IUC) by continuously irrigating the bladder using a three-way catheter.

The three-way catheter allows for simultaneous fluid input into the bladder and exit from it. The use of an IUC with a large diameter promotes debris and clot drainage.

Equipment

- Alcohol-based hand rub
- Personal protective equipment (PPE): Protective eyewear, plastic apron and gloves
- Dressing trolley
- Dressing pack
- 2x Sodium chloride 0.9% (normal saline) irrigation bags (volume as per facility procedure)
- 70% isopropyl alcohol wipes
- CBI set
- IV pole
- 6x 70% alcohol swabs
- Sterile gloves
- Waste bag
- Disposable underpad

Procedure

Constant bladder irrigation (CBI) minimizes the risk of blood clots and preserves the patency of a urinary catheter that is embedded (IUC) by continuously irrigating the bladder using a three-way catheter.

The three-way catheter permits concurrent fluid input into the bladder and exit from it. To allow for debris and clot drainage, a large diameter IUC is employed.

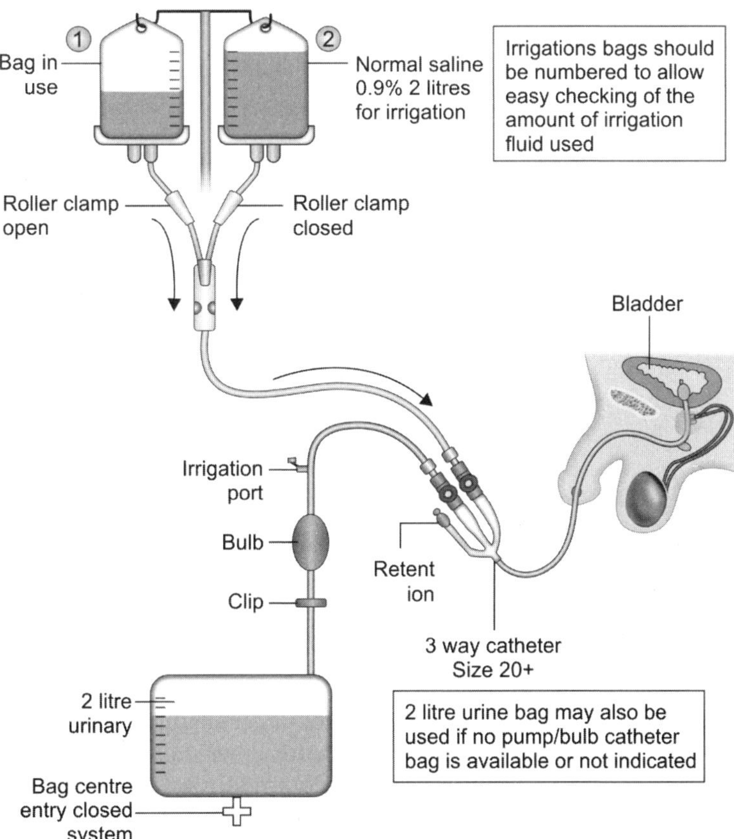

Continuous irrigation.

- ❖ Adjust the IV pole's height and lock it in place. Reminder: Only open one water flask during priming since fluid might leak from the other to the opposite side.
- ❖ Discard gloves and place a reusable underpad beneath the sprinkler port to catch any spills.
- ❖ Take care of your hands.
- ❖ Remove the sterile gloves and open the dressing's pack before adding the wipes with 70% alcohol.
- ❖ Use sterile gauze to hold the infusion port with your non-dominant hand.
- ❖ To establish the sterile field, cover the disposable sheet with the sterile paper towel using your dominant hand.

- Discard the spigot attached to the irrigation port if it is not connected using sterile gauze and your dominant hand.
- Use 70% alcohol swabs to clean the IUC irrigated arm and port properly. Permit to dry.
- Disconnect the sealing tube from the irrigation tubing's connection and firmly attach it to the watering port while using aseptic method.
- Unclamp the irrigation tube and adjust the roller clamp to determine the rate of infusion.
- Take away the washable sheet and make sure the patient is at ease.
- Get rid of garbage in accordance with facility policies.
- Take away PPE.
- A tidy cart.
- Practice good hand hygiene.
- Describe the operation carried out and the results in the patient's clinical progress records.

Intermittent Bladder Irrigation Via Closed System

In order to use a contemporary indwelling two-way catheter for intermittent bladder irrigation, a particular urine drainage system featuring a bladder irrigation port is necessary. The closed lumen technology is still in use to lower the risk of catheter-associated UTI (CAUTI).

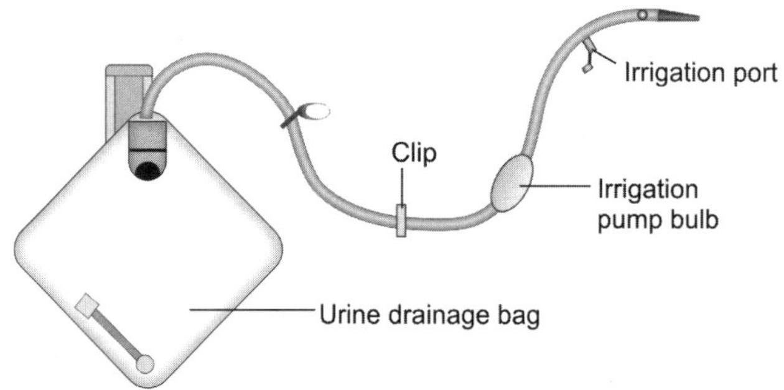

Bard irrigation pump bag.

This intermittent irrigation system can be used for:
- A two-way catheter was used in a patient with moderate hematuria; this system may be used as the first line of therapy. It is not necessary to switch the catheter from a two-way after the hematuria has reduced, to a three-way setup for continuous watering, then back again.
- Patients with end-of-life conditions whose catheters regularly get clogged with clots or other material; this method will lessen their agony while changing their catheters.
- A problematic suprapubic catheter should be avoided in favor of manual irrigation, which is constantly damaging to closed catheter systems.

Equipment

- Irrigation set (single spike)
- **Irrigation fluid:** 1–2 L sodium chloride 0.9% for irrigation (use IV sodium chloride 0.9% if not available)
- Bard irrigation pump bag (2 L urine collection bag with T irrigation port and hand pump bulb)
- Underpad (bluey)
- Chlorhexidine 0.5% with 70% alcohol wipes
- Non-sterile gloves

- ❖ PPE
- ❖ IV pole
- ❖ Irrigation chart/fluid balance chart

Procedure

- ❖ Wash your hands according to the five hand hygiene moments.
- ❖ Check for allergies, confirm the treatment, validate the patient's identification, and get permission. Assess the patient's health literacy (knowledge of the operation) as a component to this process.

  Inquire about the patient's identification as an Aboriginal or Torres Strait Islander. If yes, give the Aboriginal Interface Officer access so they may assist with health literacy. Provide patients who need one with an interpreter.
- ❖ Maintain patient comfort while positioning the patient for simple access to the catheter.
- ❖ Prime the drip irrigation set, add irrigation fluid to the irrigation fluid bags, and maintain the treatment set aseptic. Verify that the clamp on the irrigation set is closed.
- ❖ Put on protective eyewear, a gown, and non-sterile gloves.
- ❖ Put the catheter connector underneath the underpad.
- ❖ Use chlorhexidine swabs to clean the catheter drainage and T irrigation ports, then let them air dry.
- ❖ After removing the port's cap with sterile gauze, attach the irrigation to the T irrigation port.
- ❖ Attach irrigation pumped bag to catheter (remove spigot or used urine bag with cleaned gauze).
- ❖ Secure the irrigation system to the bag with a clamp (the clamp is above the urine bag's drip chamber).
- ❖ Begin watering the plants. The roller clamp may be adjusted to determine the administration rate. Dose the bladder with 50–100 mL of sodium chloride.
- ❖ Stop using the irrigation liquid.
- ❖ Apply mild pressure while pumping the hand pump to cleanse the bladder (If you're unclear how to operate the hand pump, try squeezing the tube above the pump).
- ❖ Release the catheter's clamp to let urine, dirt, and blood clots drain into the waste bag.
- ❖ Include the following information in the patient's clinical progress notes:
  - ◆ The procedure's date, time, and indication, incorporating the patient's indicators of sickness and symptoms
  - ◆ The outcome, which may include the kind and quantity of elimination, the presence or absence of clots, including the patient's response to the procedure
- ❖ The volume return of the fluid balance chart.

Manual bladder therapy is used to dissolve coagulation from the urethra and catheter and reinstate catheter patency.

To physically flush out any clots, a three-way kidney catheter is filled with sterile sodium chloride fluid at 0.9% (normal saline). This is accompanied by continuous bladder irrigation to lower the possibility of developing new clots and having an overly distended bladder.

The ideal result is the elimination of the bladder clots with free-flowing urine. Below-optimal results include:

- ❖ Inability to unblock the IUC, resulting in the need for a new catheter, overdistention of the bladder, development of a CAUTI as a result of contamination during the treatment, and more.
- ❖ A break in the closed urinary drainage system.

Equipment

- ❖ Alcohol-based hand rub
- ❖ 1 catheter pack
- ❖ 1 catheter tip 50 mL syringe 70% alcohol swabs
- ❖ 1 bottle 500 mL sterile sodium chloride 0.9% (normal saline)
- ❖ Sterile kidney dish
- ❖ 1 sterile urinary drainage bag
- ❖ Disposable underpad (bluey)
- ❖ Non-sterile jug/receptacle on bottom of trolley
- ❖ Sterile gloves
- ❖ Personal protective equipment

Procedure

- ❖ Wash your hands according to the five hand hygiene moments. Maintain cleanliness at all times throughout the treatment.
- ❖ Check for allergies, confirm the treatment, validate the patient's identification, and get permission. Assess the patient's health literacy (knowledge of the operation) as an aspect of this process.

  Inquire about the patient's identification as an Aboriginal or Torres Strait Islander. If yes, give the Aboriginal Liaison Officer access so they may assist with health literacy. Provide patients who need one with an interpreter.
- ❖ Wipe off the dressing table with 70% isopropyl alcohol, let it dry, assemble the necessary supplies, verify the cleanliness and integrity of the sterile objects, and then bring it to the patient's bedside.
- ❖ Ensure patient confidentiality.
- ❖ To make it simpler for staff to access the IUC and cut down on the time they has to invest twisting, bending, or holding challenging static postures, lie the patient down in a supine position. Obtain assistance if required.
- ❖ A single-use sheet should be placed under a person's buttocks.
- ❖ Put a blue biodegradable underpad underneath the catheter and drainage bag connector.
- ❖ Put a non-sterile container or jug at the bottom of the selected operation trolley.
- ❖ Take care of your hands.
- ❖ Open the tube pack and add the sterile drainage bag, alcohol swabs, and 50 mL syringe.
- ❖ Fill the kidney dish with sterile chloride, 0.9%.
- ❖ Practice good hand hygiene.
- ❖ Put on PPE, including sterile gloves, a disposable gown or plastic apron, and eye protection.
- ❖ Draw 50 mL of chlorine dioxide 0.9%.
- ❖ Place the gauge cubes round the tube's drainage port and the connection to the drainage bag using both hands.
- ❖ To establish a sterile area, detach the catheter out of the bag of drainage and throw away the gauze covering the catheter port and drainage bag.
- ❖ To produce a sterile area, lay the sterile newspaper towel beneath the catheter port and over the waste sheet with the dominant hand.
- ❖ Using the 70% alcohol swabs, thoroughly clean the catheter's drainage port and throw it away.

❖ Inform the individual that the next procedure will be difficult or painful. Irrigate the catheter with 50 mL volumes if sodium chloride at 0.9% flushing while drawing up on the plunger to get rid of any clots or debris. Be careful not to splash throughout the process since this might expose you to bodily fluids. If resistance is observed, appropriate pressure may be used (apart from after a bladder or renal transplant). Each syringe should be injected directly into the jug or non-sterile container at the bottom of the trolley.

❖ Apply irrigation in 50ml amounts continuously until the return is clear or clot-free.

❖ Keep the syringe in place and attach a new drainage bag.

❖ Introduce the idea of daily bladder irrigation.

❖ Remove the disposable sheets, then check to see whether the patient is comfortable.

❖ Take off PPE.

❖ Dispose of rubbish in accordance with local laws.

❖ Practice good hand hygiene.

❖ Find the difference between the transmitted and received volumes.

❖ Include the following details regarding the operation's outcome in the person's clinical recovery notes:

  ◆ The procedure's date and time.

  ◆ The rationale for the procedure, including the patient's signs and symptoms

  ◆ The volume in the fluid balance diagram in the volume the future, the kind and color of drainage, the presence from clots, plus the patient's level of toleration of the procedure are among the outcomes.

Vaginal Irrigation

Vaginal irrigation, sometimes referred to as vaginal douching or rubbing, entails the low-pressure injection if fluid into the vaginal canal to help keep the vaginal tract clean.

Gynecological therapy known as vaginal irrigation involves cleaning the vagina with huge amounts of mineral water (up to 25 L). Water has mechanical, thermal, and chemical effects. It replenishes all types of metabolism and normalizes redox processes.

Mineral water alters organism reactivity, inhibiting the inflammatory process, alleviating pelvic discomfort, restoring metabolism, and restoring normal ovarian-menstrual function of the ovaries.

In addition, water encounters a tonic impact that accelerates ovarian activity, negates late effects, and dissolves pelvic organ sticky processes. It restores tubal patency and enhances the trophic activity of the celiac plexus. Infertility is assisted by it.

Vaginal irrigation restores the coordination function that exists in the pituitary-hypothalamic area, which enhances a patient's quality and sleep and helps to solve climatic issues.

Indications for Vaginal Irrigation

Inflammatory Diseases

❖ Chronic adnexitis

❖ Chronic parametritis

❖ Pelvic peritoneal adhesions

❖ Intrauterine adhesions

❖ Vaginitis and vulvovaginitis

❖ Colpitis

- ❖ Chronic endometritis
- ❖ Uterus deviation with reduced mobility after previous inflammatory diseases
- ❖ Erosions.
- ❖ Unexplained infertility
- ❖ Tubal infertility
- ❖ Uterine infertility

Disorders of Menstrual Function

- ❖ Premenstrual syndrome
- ❖ Amenorrhea
- ❖ Dysfunctional uterine bleedings in reproductive period
- ❖ Pathologic climacteric syndrome

Contraindications

- ❖ Acute exacerbations of chronic diseases.
- ❖ Pregnancy.
- ❖ Metrofibroma (on the 8th week of pregnancy).
- ❖ Postabortion period till the first menstruation.
- ❖ Moderately severe and most severe uterine neck dysplasia.
- ❖ Acute inflammatory diseases.
- ❖ Ovary endometriosis (before operative therapy).

Purposes

- ❖ Mechanical cleaning of the cervix and vaginal tract, as in leukorrhea
- ❖ Assist in removing any unpleasant odor that might have been present.
- ❖ To irrigate and clean the cervix following cauterization in order to speed healing and decrease edema.
- ❖ Preoperative procedure on most patients having the type of gynecologic surgery.

Points to Remember

- ❖ Never perform vaginal irrigation or douching without doctor's order.
- ❖ Never give during pregnancy or menstruation.
- ❖ The patient should be considered at every step of the operation.
- ❖ Ensure complete secrecy.
- ❖ Before usage, check the douche nozzle for chips.
- ❖ After and before the surgery, wash your hands.
- ❖ When administering to patients with gonorrhea, use a gown, gloves, and goggles.
- ❖ For virgins, use smaller nozzles.
- ❖ Before usage, check the solution's temperature.

Equipment

- ❖ Sterile douche tray
- ❖ Irrigating can with tubing
- ❖ Bath blanket
- ❖ Irrigating stand
- ❖ Solution prescribed

* Flushing tray
* Screen
* Bedpan with cover
* Bed protector and clamp
* Two douche nozzles
* Kidney basin

General Instructions

* Only the doctor's orders are followed while providing douches.
* Douche should not used during periods, pregnancy or puerperium for concern of virus transmitted to the uterus.
* Both prior to and following the surgery, thoroughly wash your hands to avoid transferring any infections to or from the patient, particularly if they have sexual illnesses.
* Whenever feasible, put on gloves to avoid cross-contamination.
* Carefully eliminate and dispose of any patient-used pads.
* Before receiving any douches, properly clean the abdomen. To prevent colon bacilli from infiltrating the urethral meatus, clean the perineum immediately above downward and toward the rectum.
* For most patients, a "clean technique" is sufficient. However, when necessary, such as during vaginal procedures, "sterile technique" is used.
* Use the proper strength of liquid to prevent chemical sensitivity.
* Adjust the reservoir's height to regulate the medication's flow rate when it enters the vagina. A vaginal douche that uses too much force might push bacteria into the spinal canal. As a result, the irrigation system's peak may be adjusted at not more than 24 inches below the person's hips. Remember that the volume of a water-based solution in a container is fixed at ½ pound to earn every one foot of height. The vaginal irrigation fluid's pressure shouldn't be higher than one pound.
* To avoid friction and tissue stress, the douche nozzle always be maintained moist and lubricated.
* Adjust the solution's temperature in accordance with the irrigation's intended use. For most aspects of irrigation, an ambient temperature of 40.5°C is accepted by the individual being treated. A greater amount of heat is applied to reduce inflammation and stop bleeding.
* If your hips are raised and the forehead is lowered, gravity will help the solution inflow. If a person is placed in a sitting position once treatment is finished, gravity also helps the solution release.
* Along the vaginal wall's curve, the douche pump can be directed downwards and backward. To ensure that the anterior, posterior, and lateral fornices are flush, it should be rotated.
* The therapy should not be done hurriedly if the therapeutic results are to be reached. Two pints of liquid should be administered in a minimum of 20 to 30 minutes.
* To avoid damaging the wall of the vagina, a glass nozzle must be thoroughly checked for cracks before as well as following the insertion.
* If prescribed, take drugs right away after the douche.
* Perform the action in a suitable manner.

NURSE'S RESPONSIBILITY IN ADMINISTERING A VAGINAL IRRIGATION

Preliminary Assessment

- ❖ Verify the patient's name, bed amount, and other identifying information.
- ❖ Check the vaginal irrigation's diagnosis and intent.
- ❖ Check the doctor's instructions for details such as the kind of irrigation solution that ought to be used and any post-irrigation medicine that has to be administered.
- ❖ Verify the patient's contraindications for the vaginal douche, such as menstruation, pregnancy, the postpartum period, etc.
- ❖ To maintain a desirable posture, assess the patient's capabilities and limits.
- ❖ Verify the patient's knowledge of the technique and prior experience with vaginal instrumentation.
- ❖ Identify if a sterile or clean procedure is required for the patient.
- ❖ Look for any lesions by examining the perineum's state.
- ❖ Examine the items that are accessible in the patient's room.

Preparation of the Articles

Articles:

- ❖ Can of irrigating fluid inside the irrigation can plus tubing and clamp.
  Purpose: As a reservoir for irrigation usage.
- ❖ Douche nozzle.
  Purpose: The fluid should be directed into the canal of the genitals.
- ❖ Gloves 1 pair.
  Purpose: To keep asepsis in place and safeguard the nurse's hands.
- ❖ Water-filled jug for irrigation
  Toilet paper or a bedpan.
  Purpose: To take in the flow coming back.
- ❖ IV pole
  Purpose: To modify the irrigation can's height.
- ❖ Apron.
  Purpose: To safeguard the nurse's uniform.
- ❖ Forceps for holding a sponge and a bottle of moist cotton swabs.
  Purpose: To make the perineum clean.
- ❖ A jar filled with dry cotton balls.
  Purpose: To dry the perineum.
- ❖ Cotton applicators.
  Purpose: To administer the medicine, if prescribed.
- ❖ Mackintosh and towel.
  Purpose: To safeguard the clothing and bedding.
- ❖ Vaginal speculum.
  Purpose: To check the vagina and provide the medicine.
- ❖ Paper bag and kidney tray.
  Purpose: To take wastes in.
- ❖ Extra clothing and linens.
  Purpose: To alter after the treatment.

Preparation of the Patient and the Environment

❖ Describe to the patient the operation. Tell her how to participate in the operation and explain the order of the procedure.

❖ Use screens to provide privacy. As necessary, shut the windows and doors.

❖ Request the patient's urination. By doing this, bladder irritation will be lessened.

❖ Remove the backrest and any additional pillows.

❖ Position the patient near the edge of their bed to prevent reaching too far. The bed's height should be adjusted for the nurse's comfort while working.
To protect the bedding a bed linens, place each mackintosh a towel beneath the patient.

❖ Fanfold up the covers onto the foot of the bed and drape a bath towel or sheet over the patient. Only the perineum should be exposed as you would for any pelvic checkup. Remove or elevate the bottom clothing over the waist.

❖ Keep everything neatly organized in the bedside locker so the nurse can easily get it.

❖ Assist the patient onto the bed pan in a dorsal recumbent posture. To help gravity flow, the hips ought to rise higher than the shoulders. The patient will feel more comfortable with a pillow under their back.

Procedure

Steps of procedure:

❖ Wash hands
Reason: To prevent cross infection.

❖ Pour a little amount of the solution through the tube before pouring it into the can. Enforce the clamp. A maximum of 24 inches above the patient's hip level should be where you hang the can from the IV pole.
Reason: The force of the fluid depends on the can's height.

❖ To put on gloves.
Reason: To protect the nurse's hands.

❖ Using the forceps that are holding the sponge, clean your genitals with moist swabs.
Reason: This stops an infection from spreading to the uterine canal.

❖ Check a douche nozzle for cracks before attaching it to the can's tubing.
Reason: The vaginal wall might be damaged by fractures in the douche nozzle.

❖ Permit a thin layer of solution to cover the vulva. By changing the screw clamp, you can control the fluid flow.
Reason: Gross discharge may be removed by pouring solution on the vulva. Influences the patient's tolerance for the solution's temperature as well.

❖ With the left hand's thumb and fingers, separate the labia, then carefully slide the nozzle 2 to 3 inches into the vagina. Along the vaginal canal's bend, move the nozzle upward and downward.
Reason: The vaginal mucosa won't be harmed by adhering to the anatomical contour.

❖ Allow a steady stream of the liquid to flow. Take note of the return flow's nature. Make the nozzle turn.
Reason: The fornices (pouches) and the vaginal walls are thoroughly cleaned by spinning the nozzle.

❖ Pinch the tube and take the nozzle out of the vaginal canal after the desired quantity of fluid has been utilized. Tube clamping.
Place the deodorant nozzle in the kidney's tray after disconnecting it.
Reason: The irrigating can is thought to be clean, but the contaminated douche nozzle stops the illness from spreading there.

After Care of the Patient and the Articles

❖ In order to drain the drug out the vaginal canal, assist the patient in sitting down on the bedpan.
❖ Take out the bedpan, tip the patient onto their side, and pat the buttocks and perineum dry.
❖ Use a speculum within the uterus to view the cervix if any medication has to be provided, and cotton applicators to put on the medication. Apply a genital pad to avoid discoloration of the clothes by the drugs.
❖ Rearrange the bed after removing the mackintosh and towel. As needed, change the bed linens and clothes.
❖ Make the patient comfortable by adjusting her bed position.
❖ Entirely into the utility room, please. Note the features of the fluid in the bedpan. If any cotton balls or pads got stuck in the bedpan, remove it. After emptying the bedpan, clean it as usual. Rinse the shower top under both cold running water and warm, soapy water. Completely rinse it under running water, then either boil it or clean it with an appropriate disinfectant. After washing, dry each item, then store it where it belongs.
❖ Wash your hands.
❖ Add the surgery's date and time to the nurse's record. Take note of the solution type, dosage, kind of discharge present (if any), and the patient's reaction to the douche.
A douche is a stream of liquids that is aimed towards a bodily cavity to cleanse it out. Vaginal irrigation is the practice of soaking the vagina with water while applying little pressure. The procedure for irrigation of the exterior auditory canal, in which a solution is introduced and then swiftly removed, is analogous.

Purpose

❖ To eliminate an unpleasant or bothersome discharge from the vaginal canal.
❖ To reduce swelling and obstruction in the genital canal.
❖ To use an antibacterial solution that prevents the development of microorganisms before surgery.
❖ To stop a bleeding episode.
❖ To encourage exudate absorption and to increase pelvic organ circulation.

Solutions Used

❖ Sterile water
❖ Normal saline
❖ Sodium bicarbonate 2%
❖ Vinegar (acetic acid) 1%

* Savlon 1 in 1,000
* Potassium permanganate 1 in 4,000
* Boric acid 2%
* Acriflavine 1 in 4,000
* Dettol 2%
* Bichloride of mercury 1 in 4,000
  The temperature or the fluid varies depending on the purpose of the douche. Use the cleaning solution at or above body temperature, but make it at or below 40.5°C and let it cool. To provide warmth, the douche may be given at a temperature that the patient can tolerate, usually 43.3°C

Preparing the Patient

* Describe the purpose and need of the therapy to the patient.
* Before administering the douche, let the patient to void.

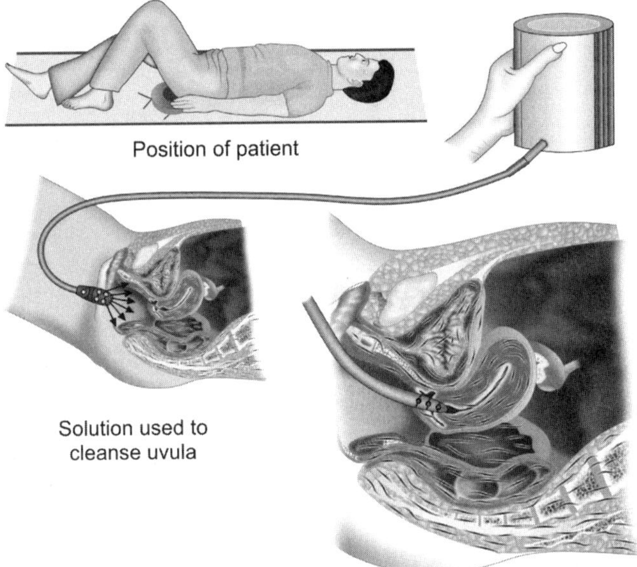

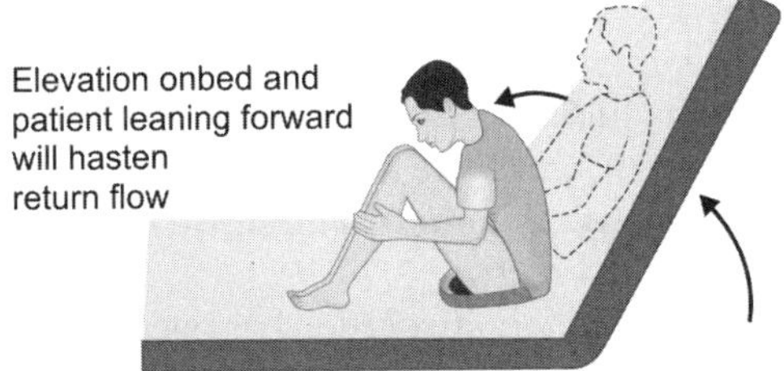

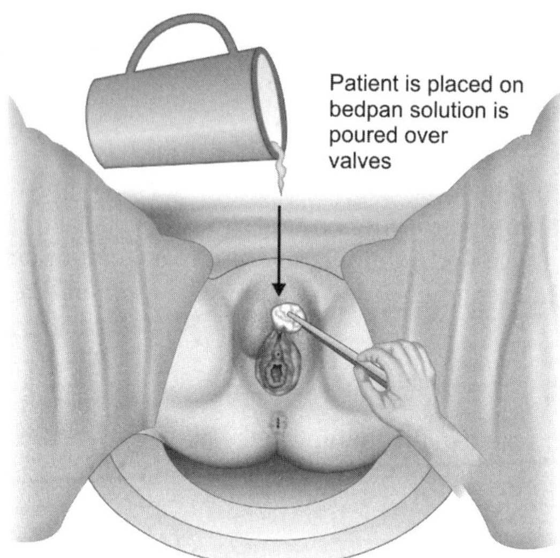

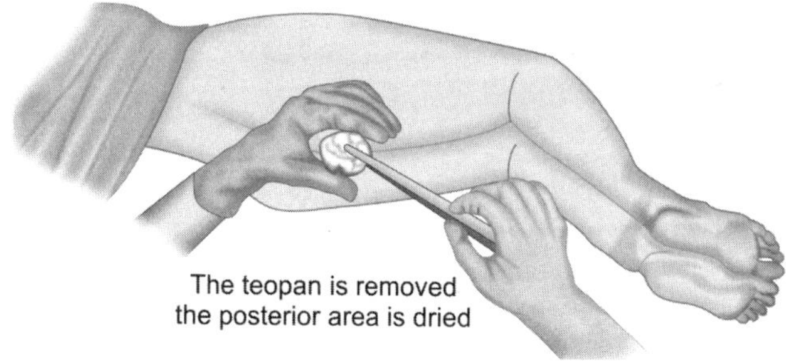

Procedure

- ❖ Bring all of your supplies to your bedside. Put on gloves and wash your hands.
- ❖ The bed's screen. Swap off the topsheet with a bathrobe.
- ❖ Place the patient's buttocks within the bed protector.
- ❖ Help the patient onto the bedpan.
- ❖ Set up and cover the patient.
- ❖ Squeeze the external genitalia.
- ❖ Hang the covered irrigation container approximately 2 feet above the bed.
- ❖ Screw the douche nozzle onto the tubing's end. Clear the air. By letting the solution pour down the back of your hand, you may check the water's temperature.
- ❖ While the brine is flowing, gently lower the nozzle and move it backward. Throughout the operation, gently jiggle the nozzle.
- ❖ Clamp and remove the nozzle before the whole solution has been used. Put the disconnected end in the kidney basin.
- ❖ Allow the patient to sit on the bedpan for a bit to let the extra solution drain.
- ❖ Take out the bedpan and completely dry the area.

- ❖ Provide comfort for the sufferer.
- ❖ Use the restroom after preparing. Before placing the contents of the bedpan in the hopper, check them. Each piece of equipment should be kept tidy and organized.

Charting and Documentation

Record the procedure, duration, volume, type, temperature, and characteristics of the reverse flow.

Rectal Irrigation

When other management strategies have failed, fecal incontinence (the involuntary spilling of solid or liquid feces) and persistent constipation are treated with rectal irrigation, also known as "anal" or "transanal" irrigation. The hot fluid is injected via the ureter (back tube) into the abdomen or lower (sigmoid) bowel to eliminate the waste.

With the aid of rectal irrigation, you may empty your lower intestine whenever it's most convenient for you. This can help you maintain regularity and lessen bloating and pain in your abdomen. For persistent constipation or incontinence, rectal irrigation can be used in conjunction with other non-surgical treatments. Many patients claim that once they begin rectal irrigation, their level of life improves.

Introduction

Rectal irrigation is often only used when less invasive bowel management techniques have failed to sufficiently address constipation and/or fecal incontinence. This can frequently involve dietary changes, modifying fluid intake, bowel habits, assuring bathroom access, evacuation methods, medication, and exercises for the pelvic floor muscles, in accordance with each individual's evaluated symptoms and needs. Most of the information provided here rests on professional opinion and real-world experience since there is currently a very little body of research supporting this technique.

Guidelines for usage neurogenic bowel dysfunction: such as multiple sclerosis, spina bifida, and spinal cord damage chronic constipation, involving obstructions during evacuation and delayed transit chronic fecal incontinence.

Equipment Necessary

- ❖ Bag for irrigation.
- ❖ Disposable gloves are optional for the patient but necessary if the healthcare provider is using irrigation
- ❖ Wipes for post-procedure skin cleansing personal safety equipment, such as disposable gloves and an apron, is required if a healthcare practitioner or caregiver is administering irrigation.
- ❖ Foley catheter made of silicone for infants: 20 French
  — Older than one year: 24 French o Catheter-tip syringe, 60 mL
- ❖ Liquid lubricant (not oil based)
- ❖ Two non-sterile troughs (such as an emesis basin) and a saline solution

Procedure

- ❖ Fill one among the basins with regular table salt.
- ❖ Draw up 20 mL of regular saline using the 60 mL catheter-tip syringe.

❖ Lubricate the catheter before inserting it.

❖ About 6 inches into the rectum, gently introduce the Foley catheter.

❖ Place the remaining end of the catheterization onto an empty container so it can drain.

❖ Let any feces or gas flow into the empty sink.

❖ Insert the catheter a little farther into the rectum to provide any remaining "pockets" of feces or gas room to release.

Administering the Saline Solution

❖ The next step is to insert catheter-tip syringe into the open end of a Foley catheter (which was in the emesis basin) and inject 20 mL of saline solution into the rectum while gently pushing on the plunger to cause the saline solution to flow through the catheter. To prevent it from falling out, maintain the catheter at exactly the same level as the anus. Don't pull on it!

❖ Allow any feces to drop into the empty nausea basin after disconnecting the catheter-tip syringe and the catheter's free end.

❖ With 20 mL, repeat this procedure. With each irrigation, move the cannula a few inches forward while advising it while twisting or spinning it. Never push the catheter. The catheter will effortlessly follow the contours of the colon as you gradually advance it.

Nasal Spray

Local drug delivery to the inside of the nose is accomplished using nasal sprays.

Types of Nasal Sprays

Pressurized canisters and pump bottles are two distinct types of containers used for nasal sprays.

Active components from four categories are found in the most popular nasal sprays:
1. Saline
2. Steroid
3. Antihistamine
4. Decongestant

Saline Sprays

A saltwater washing for the sinuses is what saline sprays for the nose are like. When you breathe, irritants and germs enter your nose. To remove them, mucus is produced in your nose. Saline sprays wash away irritants before they create irritation by acting like mucus. They may also aid in clearing out extra mucus.

The saline nasal spray contains preservatives often. These preservatives may aggravate an already inflamed or damaged nose. Saline sprays, on the other hand, may give soothing moisture if the dry winter air is irritating your nose.

Steroid Sprays

Some nasal sprays include corticosteroids in them, which assist to lessen nasal channel swelling. The best treatment for persistent congestion brought on by allergy or irritants is steroid spray. Nasacort and Flonase are examples of popular brand names. Steroid nasal sprays are safe for long-term use in adults.

Side effects include

❖ Stinging and burning of the nasal passages
❖ Sneezing
❖ Throat irritation

Antihistamine Sprays

Antihistamines are included in several nasal sprays and act to relieve congestion brought on by allergies, allergic immune response.

Azelastine-containing sprays like Astelin and Astepro have shown to be very safe. Azelastine spray for nasal use is more effective than various corticosteroid nasal sprays and oral antihistamines like Benadryl.

Possible side effects of azelastine sprays include:
❖ Bitter taste
❖ Tiredness
❖ Weight gain
❖ Muscle pain
❖ Nasal burning

Decongestant Sprays

Most DNSs (both generic and Afrin brand names) include oxymetazoline. They work by making the blood vessels in the nasal canals smaller. Short-term problems like the flu or the common cold respond better to DNSs.

Your nasal passageways are enlarged when you have congestion. They thus feel stymied. Runny nose is brought on by the edema's increased mucus production. DNSs induce blood vessel shrinking, which reduces inflammation and the subsequent mucus formation.

You could encounter any of those negative impacts if you utilize a DNS:
❖ Burning
❖ Stinging
❖ Increased mucus
❖ Dryness in the nose
❖ Sneezing
❖ Nervousness
❖ Nausea
❖ Dizziness
❖ Headache
❖ Difficulty falling or staying asleep
❖ Common cold
❖ Sinusitis
❖ Hay fever, and allergies
❖ Narrowing the blood vessels in the nose area, reducing swelling and congestion.

Steps for Using a Pressurized Canister

1. Before taking the prescription, gently blow your nose to clear out any mucus.
2. Check to make sure the canister is firmly seated in the holder. Give the canister a vigorous shake just before using it.

3. Maintain an erect posture. Exhale gradually.
4. Hold the nasal spray bottle as it is seen in the illustration to the right. On the side not getting the medication, use the tip of your finger to cover the nose.
5. Begin inhaling softly via your nose and depress the canister. Repeat the same steps on the other nostril. If you're spraying several times in each nostril, keep doing steps 2 through 5.
6. Refrain from sneezing or blowing your nose immediately after using the spray.

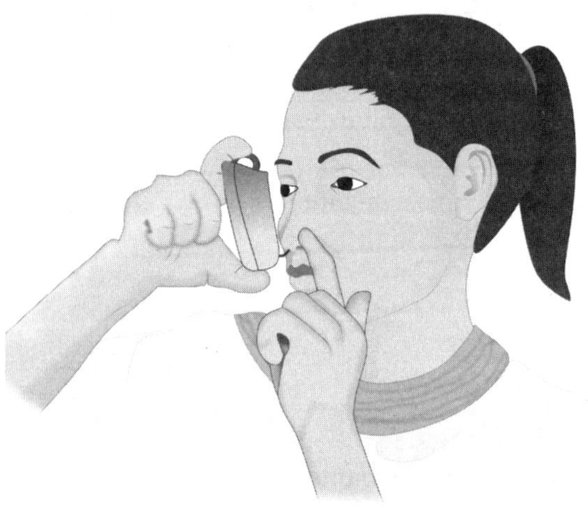

Steps for Using a Pump Bottle

1. Before taking the prescription, gently blow your nose to clear out any mucus.
2. Take away the cap. Shake the container. You may need to "prime" the pump sprayer each day before using it by squirting several times in the air then a fine mist emerges.
3. Lean your head slightly forward. Exhale gradually.

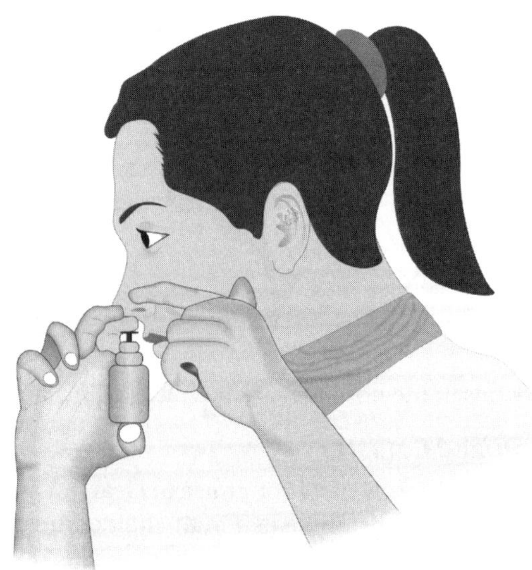

4. Place your index or middle finger on top of the pump bottle while holding it with your middle finger at the bottom. To shut the nose on the side that does not get the medication, use a finger from your other hand (see the illustration below).
5. Squeeze the pump as you begin to take slow, deep breaths using your nose. Repeat the same steps on the other nostril. If you're blasting more than once into each nostril, repeat steps two through five.
6. Refrain from sneezing or blowing your nose immediately after using the spray.

Helpful Hints

❖ Keep in mind that it can take a maximum of two weeks of nasal spray use before you feel the full results.
❖ If you use a pressure canister, wash it at least one each week.
❖ Before spraying, make sure you can breathe through each nostril; otherwise, the medication will be ineffective since it won't penetrate all the way into your nose.
❖ Aim directly. The nasal spray bottle's nozzle should be directed towards the back of the forehead. Should you don't blow straight, you risk wasting the medication and aggravating your nose worse.
❖ If you use the pump spray properly, there shouldn't be any dripping from the tip of your nose or at the back or your throat.
❖ Use of the spray should be discontinued for a day or two if your nose starts to pain, bleed, or sting. Before taking your usual medication, it might sometimes be helpful to use a generic saline nasal spray like SalineX, Ocean Nasal Mist, or NaSal.
❖ If you get nosebleeds, skip the prescription for a few days and use a sterile spray for the nose in its place. You may use a cotton swab to put a thin layer of petroleum jelly into your nose after using the saline spray. See your doctor if your bleeding or discomfort persists.
❖ Always take your medications as prescribed by your doctor. Most nasal sprays function best when used consistently and on a regular basis.
❖ Keep your medications out of the sun.

Throat Sprays

Throat sprays are used locally to irritated throat tissues by spraying them directly into the mouth, as their name suggests. The patient spits out any extra medicine after the spray has been in their throat for the allotted amount of time. It's totally safe to accidentally consume a little quantity of these drugs, so don't be concerned if you do. Scientific research has shown that throat spraying is a potent antiseptic that can get rid of many different kinds of dangerous microbes, including bacteria, viruses, and fungus.

The wide spectrum antimicrobial povidone-iodine (Betadine) found in Povidone-Iodine (Betadine) throat spray preserves all the benefits of elemental iodine while without staining or sensitizing. Similar to cough drops, throat sprays include a number of distinct active substances that give them their calming effects:

Phenol: Phenol is often mixed with other chemicals, such as menthol, and used of its local anesthetic properties. It serves as the main component in ChlorasepticTM throat sprays.

Glycerin: Glycerin coats the back of the throat to reduce inflammation, just as pectin does. It may be found in many throat spray products and is used as a sweetener.

Benzocaine: As previously mentioned, sprays with larger concentrations than cough drops are often seen. The FDA issued a warning against improper benzocaine throat spray usage because, while being rare, the abuse using benzocaine mists has been scientifically linked to a blood condition called methemoglobinemia.

Types

There are many types of throat antiseptic sprays. Natural ingredients used in antiseptic throat sprays include radial radix, propolis, and silver essential oil. Antibiotics included in lemon balm oil are believed to often aid to stop the development of germs. Products with chemicals that kill infections, viruses, and fungus, and limit bacterial development include throat antiseptic sprays, their development, such as benzalkonium, dequalinium, povidone iodine, and antibiotics like neomycin and tyrothricin. Oropharyngeal infections are often treated with these products. Nonsteroidal anti-inflammatory medications, corticosteroids, and other substances are often added to the antiseptic components of the medicine to assist treat concomitant symptoms such inflammation, edema, or swelling of his oropharyngeal mucosa, among others.

Indications

* Therapy for acute mouth and pharynx infections, such as tonsillitis, pharyngitis, gingivitis, aphthous ulcers, stomatitis, monilial infections, common colds, and influenza.
* Before to, during, and after dental or oral surgery for oral hygiene.
* To quickly and painlessly relieve a sore throat.

Contraindication

Before and during radioiodine chemotherapy for hyperthyroidism, after a permanent cure is achieved; for 4 weeks prior to radioactivity scintigraphy or radioactivity therapy for thyroid gland carcinoma; if a person has goiter, nodules in the thyroid, as well other thyroid diseases. Throat spray shouldn't be used in any of these situations.

Not recommended for usage in kids under the age of six.

Procedure

Throat spray is designed in three types. Specifically, how to use each type is as follows:

1. **How to use a throat spray without nozzle:** The number of sprinkles depends on the substance. The patient widens his mouth, places the spray bottle in front of his mouth at the level within his throat, and sprays it directly. Using a throat sprayer without a metered dosage pump involves placing the nozzle in the horizontal orientation, opening the nozzle cap, and bringing the nozzle near to the oropharynx. Then, depending on the product, pressing the spray button a certain number of times. Close the cap after cleaning the nozzle and putting it back in its rightful place.

2. **How to use a throat sprayer with a nozzle with a metered dose pump:** Press the pump tip five times to activate the metering dosage pump before spraying the throat. With your thumb and index finger, hold the spout upright so that the dropper is at the top. When used, insert the breathing line (white tube) into your mouth to seal it shut, and then bring it to your head while taking a deep breath.

Other Routes of Drug Administration

Epidural

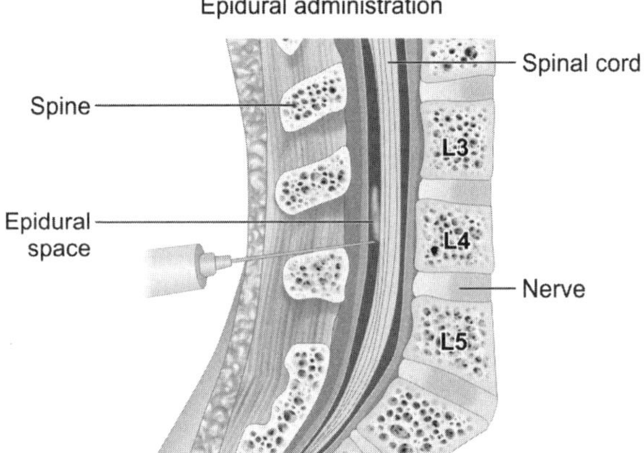

An epidural is a technique in which an anesthetic or steroid is injected into the epidural space, the region around spinal nerves. An epidural technique aims to offer an area of your body, including your legs or abdomen, with pain alleviation (analgesia) or a total loss of sensation (anesthesia).

An epidural is commonly called the following terms:
- Epidural anesthesia
- Epidural block
- Epidural steroid injection (ESI)
- Regional anesthesia
- Neuraxial anesthesia

Epidural administration (from Ancient Greek επι, upon" + *dura mater*) is a method of medication administration in which a medicine is injected into the epidural space around the spinal cord. The epidural route is used by physicians and nurse anesthetists to administer local anesthetic agents, analgesics, diagnostic medicines such as radiocontrast agents, and other medicines such as glucocorticoids. Epidural administration involves the placement of a catheter into the epidural space, which may remain in place for the duration of the treatment.

Examples of applications for epidural block.

Specialty	Surgical procedure
Orthopedic surgery	Major hip and knee surgery, pelvic fractures
Obstetric surgery	Cesarean delivery, labor analgesia
Gynecologic surgery	Hysterectomy, pelvic floor procedures
General surgery	Breast, hepatic, gastric, colonic surgery
Pediatric surgery	Inguinal hernia repair, orthopedic surgery
Ambulatory surgery	Foot, knee, hip, anorectal surgery
Cardiothoracic surgery	Thoracotomy, esophagectomy, thymectomy, coronary artery bypass grafting (on and off pump)
Urologic surgery	Prostatectomy, cystectomy, lithotripsy, nephrectomy
Vascular surgery	Amputation of lower extremity, revascularization procedures

Contd...

Contd...

Specialty	Surgical procedure
Medical conditions	Autonomic hyperreflexia, myasthenia gravis, pheochromocytoma, known or suspected malignant hyperthermia

Examples of vascular procedures performed with epidural block.

Abdominal aortic aneurysm repair (neuraxial technique seldom adequate as sole anesthetic)
Aortofemoral bypass
Renal artery bypass
Mesenteric artery bypass
Infrainguinal arterial bypass with saphenous vein or synthetic graft
Embolectomy
Thrombectomy
Endovascular procedures (intraluminal balloon dilation with stent placement; aneurysm repair)

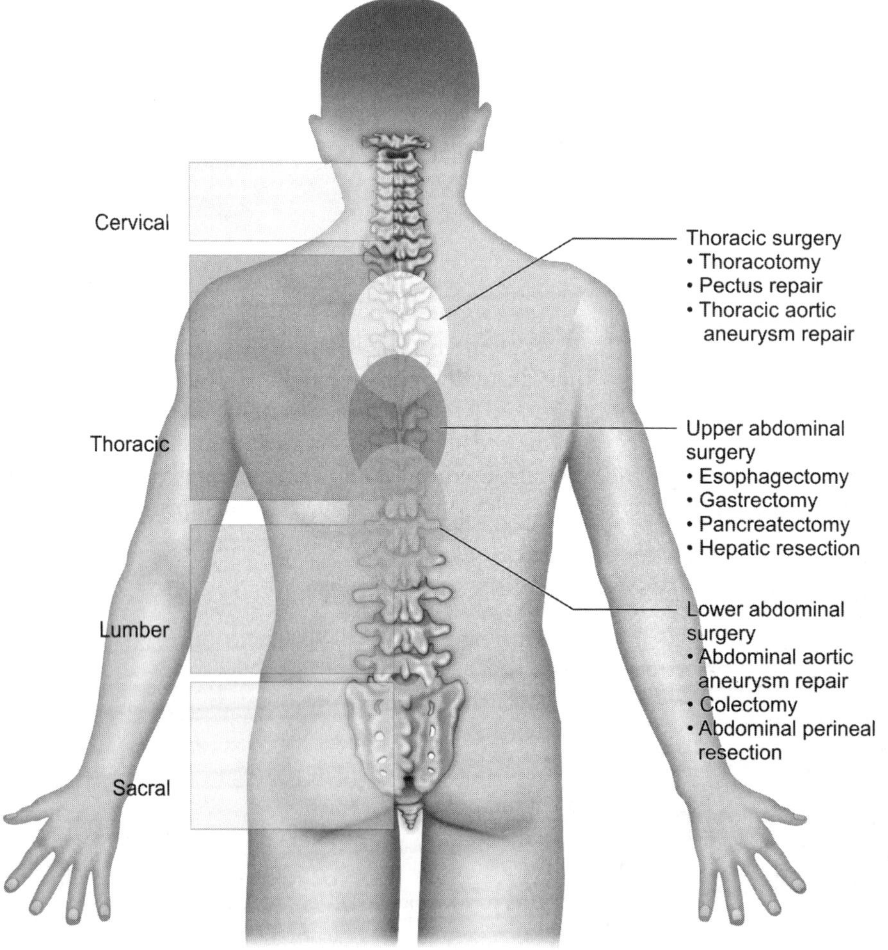

Level of placement in surgeries performed with thoracic epidural anesthesia and analgesia.

Indications for thoracic epidural anesthesia and analgesia.

Anatomic region	Procedure
Thorax	• Thoracotomy • Pectus repair • Thoracic aneurysm repair • Thymectomy • Video-assisted thoracic surgery
Upper abdomen	• Esophagectomy • Gastrectomy • Pancreatectomy • Cholecystectomy • Hepatic resection
Lower abdomen	• Abdominal aortic aneurysm repair • Colectomy • Bowel resection • Abdominal perineal resection
Urogenital/gynecologic	• Cystectomy • Nephrectomy • Ureteral repair • Radical abdominal prostatectomy • Ovarian tumor debulking • Pelvic exenteration • Total abdominal hysterectomy

Epidural Medication Delivery Options

Healthcare practitioner may provide medicine while clients are under an epidural in a number different methods, including as:

❖ **Epidural with a single injection:** In this operation, a steroid or anesthetic is administered into the epidural region around spine. The sensation in afflicted region often recovers after a single epidural anesthetic injection within just a few hours. A single epidural anesthetic injection provides momentary pain relief. The majority of injections of epidural steroid are one-time procedures.

❖ **Epidural use of a catheter:** During the majority of epidural operations, a catheter is inserted into epidural area to allow doctor to provide a continuous stream of anesthetic medicine, numerous dosages, or both. A catheter is a small, flexible tube than is inserted via a tiny hole into a body cavity. In this situation, healthcare professional inserts a catheter into spinal region that opens over the epidural space. Doctor may provide many injections of medicine this way. This kind of epidural is often recommended by medical professionals for lengthier procedures, for delivering pain alleviation throughout labor and delivery as well as for many days.

❖ **Epidural with patient-controlled analgesia (PCA):** Healthcare practitioner may let you manage how much pain relief you get via your epidural catheter while you recuperate from certain types of surgery. Patient-controlled analgesia (PCA) is the term used for this. The PCA pump's settings are configured for the painkiller your doctor provides depending on your age, weight, and the kind of operation you had. These parameters are established by your healthcare provider. The PCA pumping is simple to use since you just need to push a button to get medicine when you have pain; however, the pump won't deliver the drug if it is not yet time for another dosage.

Intrathecal

Intrathecal drug administration means the introduction of a therapeutic substance by injection into the subarachnoid space of the spinal cord.

Intrathecal administration refers to administering medication into the subarachnoid space around the spinal cord. An anesthetic is first injected into the top layer of skin to numb the area. A needle is then inserted into the lower spine between two vertebrae. Medications are injected into the subarachnoid space, filled with cerebrospinal fluid (CSF), to allow for rapid effects on the central nervous system, including the brain, spinal cord, and the meninges. Medications, such as opioids, may be administered intrathecally when individuals have intractable pain that fails to respond to other treatments; or pain that responds to analgesia, but the dose required would result in extreme adverse side effects. Pain medications are often administered intrathecally for end-of-life hospice care patients and for chronic cancer-related pain or chemotherapeutic agents.

Parenterally administered nutrition includes Kabiven and Perikabiven, combinations of amino acids, dextrose, lipids, and electrolytes.

Drugs that treat certain infections are also administered by this route, especially post-neurosurgically. The drug needs to be given this way to avoid being stopped by the blood–brain barrier. The same medication that is taken orally has enter the circulation of blood in order to reach the brain; it could end up being able to do so. Because ordinary injectable medication preparations can include preservatives or other potentially dangerous inactive substances, drugs administered through the intrathecal route sometimes need to be carefully prepared by a healthcare professional or technician.

Sometimes the route for use can simply be referred to as "Intrathecal," but the word also serves as an adjective to describe anything that occurs in or is administered into the anatomic space or potential space inside a sheath, most commonly the arachnoid membrane of the brain or spinal cord (under which is the subarachnoid space). In the spinal cord, for instance, the creation of antibodies is known as intrathecal immunoglobulin production.

Intraosseous

This 1940s-era access method has been used again in the last ten years as a quick alternative to intravenous access when it is not possible. The high rate of attainment (about 80%) of IO access being its main benefit.

All resuscitation medications may be administered intravenously (IO), albeit ceftriaxone, chloramphenicol, phenytoin, tobramycin, or vancomycin administration may cause their peak blood concentrations to be lower. Extravasation, the most typical side effect associated with IO usage, has been documented in 12% of participants.

For within vascular access, a specially developed hollow-bore needle is placed between the neural cortex and medullary region of a bone. This allows for the infusion of medically necessary medications and laboratory testing.

Indications

- ❖ IO access is the recommended method for gaining circulatory circulation during cardiac arrest.
- ❖ If arterial access is not quickly attained (if prior efforts at vein access give up, or if they take more than 90 seconds to complete), IO access should be obtained in decompensated shock.
- ❖ The infant is the exception, for whom access via the umbilical vein is still the recommended method.

Contraindications

* Proximal ipsilateral fracture
* Ipsilateral vascular injury
* Osteogenesis imperfecta

Complications

* Extravasation or subperiosteal infusion, which prevents a substance from entering the bone marrow
* Osteomyelitis (rare when used briefly): Damage to the physeal plate, complete bone penetration, local an infection, tissue necrosis, pain, compartmentalization, and bone and lipid microemboli have all been seen, notwithstanding their rarity.

Equipment

* Alcohol swabs
* 18G needle with trochar (at least 1.5 cm in length)
* 5 mL syringe
* 20 mL syringe
* Infusion fluid

Analgesia, Anesthesia, Sedation

Local anesthesia may be required if the patient is conscious.

Procedure

* Identify the appropriate site
    * *Proximal tibia:* Anteromedial surface, 2–3 cm below the tibial tuberosity
    * *Distal tibia:* Proximal to the medial malleolus
    * *Distal femur:* Midline, 2–3 cm above the external condyle
* Prepare the skin.
* Screw the needle perpendicular to or slightly away from the chondral plate into the femur after passing it through the skin. As the marrow hollow is approached, there is a give.
* Take out the trocar and use a 5-mL syringe to aspirate bone marrow to verify the location.
* Marrow should flush freely but cannot always be aspirated.
* Securing the needle and beginning the infusion (which must be supplied manually using boluses from the 20 mL syringe)

Laboratory Tests

* Aspirated bone marrow cannot be used for the majority of laboratory procedures because the particle materials might clog up and harm the testing apparatus.
* Universal donor products (Group O blood cells, Group AB plasma) will be administered for prompt transfusion assistance in the absence of a pretransfusion blood sample (not bone marrow).
* Blood culture vials, bedside glucometers, and portable I-STAT equipment may all use aspirated bone marrow.

Post-procedure Care

Once another vein has been reached, intraosseous infusion should only be used to revive the infant in an emergency.

Intraperitoneal

Large amounts of chemicals may be quickly absorbed by intraperitoneal administration, which is also the recommended injection method for isotonic, non-irritating solutions.

Intraperitoneal injections are a way to administer therapeutics and drugs through a peritoneal route (body cavity).

It is preferred when large amounts of blood replacement fluids are needed or when low blood pressure or other problems prevent the use of a suitable blood vessel for intravenous injection.

In humans, the method is widely used to administer chemotherapy drugs to treat some cancers, particularly ovarian cancer. Although controversial, intraperitoneal use in ovarian cancer has been recommended as a standard of care. Fluids are injected intraperitoneally in infants, also used for peritoneal dialysis.

A chest tube implanted intrapleurally for drainage is used to inject an intrapleural medication through the sternum into the pleural area.

Drugs injected intraperitoneally influence the intercostal nerves by diffusing between the parietal pleura to innermost intercostal muscles. The intercostal muscles the parietal pleura are traversed by the needle during intrapleural administration of a medicament on its journey to the pleural space.

Indications

Encourage analgesia, manage pleural effusions, treat spontaneous pneumothorax, and give chemotherapy.

Drugs

Tetracycline, streptokinase, anesthetics, plus chemotherapeutic drugs (to treat malignant pleural effusion or lung adenocarcinoma) are medications that are often administered intrapleurally.

Contraindications

* Pleural fibrosis with adhesions, pleural inflammation, sepsis, and hepatitis at the puncture point are all possible complications.
* Intrapleural injections shouldn't be administered to those with bullous emphysema or those undergoing respiratory treatment that uses positive end-expiratory pressure since these conditions might be made worse by the injections.

Equipment

A #16 to #20 or a #28 to #40 chest tube is used to provide an intrapleural medication to a patient who has emphysema, an effusion of the pleura, or pneumothorax. Otherwise, it is administered via a catheter and a 16G to 18G blunt-tipped intrapleural (epidural) needle. Depending on the sort of entry device the doctor employs, there may be accessory equipment. The tools must all be sterilized.

For Intrapleural Catheter Insertion

Sterilized items include gloves, a hat, a mask, a gown, and gauze. Antiseptic solution, sterile drape, local anesthetic (1% lidocaine), 18G needle or scalpel, 3- to 5-mL glass syringe with 22G 1" and 25G 5/8" needles, sterile dressings, sutures, tape, blunt-tipped intrapleural needle, and intrapleural catheter.

For Chest Tube Insertion

Sterile towels; sterile gloves; sterile cap; sterile mask; sterile gown; sterile gauze; antiseptic solution; 3–5 mL syringe; local anesthetic, such as 1% lidocaine; 18G needle or scalpel; chest tube with or without trocar (#16 to #20 catheter for air or serous fluid; #28 to #40 for blood, pus, or thick fluid); two rubber-tipped clamps, if necessary; sutures; sterile drain dressings; tape; thoracic drainage system and tubing.

For Drug Administration

Sterile gloves; sterile gauze pads; antiseptic solution; prescribed medication; appropriate-sized needles and syringes; 1% lidocaine, if necessary; infusion pump; sterile dressings; tape; two rubber-tipped clamps, if necessary.

For Chemotherapy Administration

Nonlinting, nonabsorbent disposable gown; sterile powder-free chemotherapy gloves; face shield; National Institute for Occupational Safety and Health–approved respirator mask (if aerosolization is likely); antiseptic solution; prescribed chemotherapeutic medication; sterile gauze pads; infusion pump with programmable dosing limits; syringe with a Luer-lock connector; administration set; spill kit; hazardous waste receptacle.

Implementation

❖ Wash your hands regularly.
❖ In accordance with the policies of your institution, verify the patient's identification using a minimum of two patient IDs.
❖ To assuage the patient's concerns, explain the operation to him. Motivate him to obey directions.
❖ Verify that a permission form is duly completed and attested.
❖ Practice good hand hygiene, and, where necessary, use sterile gloves alongside other safety gear.
❖ To avoid placing the catheter into the wrong place, confirm that that the insertion point is indicated.
❖ Right before the operation begins, take a break to do a last check that the patient, location, positioning, or procedure are proper and that, if required, all pertinent data and equipment are present.

Inserting an Intrapleural Catheter

- ❖ The nurse assists the doctor in inserting the intrapleural pump at the patient's bedside.
- ❖ The patient should be positioned such that his affected side is facing up. The catheter will be inserted by the physician into the third to eighth intercostal gap, 3–4 inches (7.5–10 cm) above the hind midline. After putting on a sterile cap, gown, mask, and gloves, the doctor wraps the area with a sterile drape after washing the region around the puncture site with an antiseptic-soaked gauze pad then letting it dry. A 3- to 5-mL syringe is then used to inject the local anesthetic deeply below the tissues and into the skin. To insert the blunt-tipped intrapleural needles into the chosen interspace over the upper portion of the lower rib, the doctor creates a tiny hole in the skin using an 18G needle or scalpel. The needle's tip is pointed medially at a 30- to 40-degree angle to the skin while the bevel is kept angled upward. At the time of the puncture, tell the patient to hold his breath (or momentarily turn off artificial ventilation) until the piercing instrument is taken out.
- ❖ As the needle tip punctures the posterior intercostal a membrane, the stylet is withdrawn, and the needle hub is then fitted with a glass syringe lubricated with saline and containing 2–4 mL of air.
- ❖ In order to mitigate the possibility of damaging the lung tissue, the doctor moves the needle slowly. Negative intrapleural pressure causes the plunger to migrate outward when the puncturing instrument punctures the parietal pleura. The intrapleural tubing is then inserted into the space between the pleura, which measures approximately 2 inches (5 cm), after the syringe is removed from the needle. He gently removes the needle without removing the catheter.
- ❖ Restart mechanical ventilation or let the patient know he can breathe naturally once again.
- ❖ The presence of aspirated air suggests a catheter is likely located inside the lung, and the presence of blood in the needle shows that the lumen is probably in an artery. A chest X-ray will then be ordered by the doctor to confirm the placement and check for issues like pneumothorax.
- ❖ Cover the catheter's insertion site by using a sterilized occlusive bandage to prevent it from coming undone. W Mark the dressing with the time, the date, and your initials. Take vital signs of the individual every 15 minutes in the first day after surgery and then as needed.

Use methods relevant to the patient's current age, health, and ability to comprehend and respond appropriately to conduct a complete examination of the patient's discomfort.

Inserting an Intrapleural Catheter

During intrapleural administration, the physician uses a catheter to provide a medication into the pleural cavity.

Assist the patient to lay on one side, afflicted side facing up. A 3" to 4" (7.5 to 10 cm) long posterior midline needle is inserted by the physician into the fourth through eighth intercostal gap. The needle is then medially advanced across the patient's superior rib and through the muscles of the intercostal region until it tangentially enters the pleura on the parietal side (as in the illustration). The needle is withdrawn once the catheter has been inserted into the pleural area.

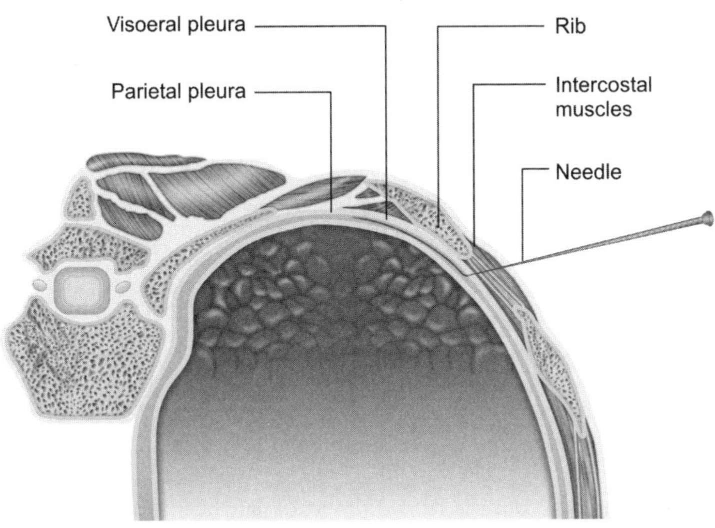

INTRA-ARTERIAL

Direct injection into an artery, usually to affect irrigated organs or tissues locally. For instance, antineoplastics administered around the tumor with less systemic side effects are an example. It may also be used to provide vasodilators to treat arterial emboli or contrast material for angiography.

Definition

Intraarterial drug injection or infusion is a method of delivering a drug directly into artery or arteries to localize its effect to a particular organ/body region, while minimizing the exposure of the body to potentially toxic effects of the agent.

UNIT

Sensory Needs

10

UNIT OUTLINE

- Components of sensory experience
- Arousal mechanism
- Factors affecting sensory functions
- Assessment of sensory alterations
- Promoting meaningful communication (patients with aphasia, artificial airway and visual and hearing impairment)
- Care of unconscious patients

LEARNING OBJECTIVES

At the end of this unit, the reader will be able to:
- Introduce sensory organs.
- Define components of sensory experience.
- Explain arousal mechanism.
- Enumerate factors affecting sensory function.
- Practice sensory alteration assessment.
- Perform assessment of sensory function.
- Define aphasia.
- Describe types of aphasia.
- Explain artificial airway.
- Illustrate types of artificial airway.
- Generate communication with visual impairment patient.
- Define care of unconscious patient.

INTRODUCTION

In a biological sense, sensory organs correspond to those that are active and have a sense of touch. As the sensory organs react to their surroundings by delivering signals to the brain, the brain participates in signal interpretation.

A human body is embodied with five sensory or sense organs:
1. Eyes—gives the sense of sight,
2. Nose—gives the sense of smell,
3. Skin—gives the sense of touch,
4. Tongue—gives the sense of taste,
5. Ear—gives the sense of hearing.

Cells known as sensory cells, which respond to certain types of stimuli, make form the sensory system of cellular organisms. Physical events are transformed into nerve impulses by these sensory receptor-containing cells, which neurons in brain cells subsequently decipher.

Each sense function gets information from the environment and communicates with the brain through the sensory nerve. The brain responds to impulses, helps sense organs respond to stimuli, and connects individuals to their environment. Let's discuss how each sensory organ functions specifically.

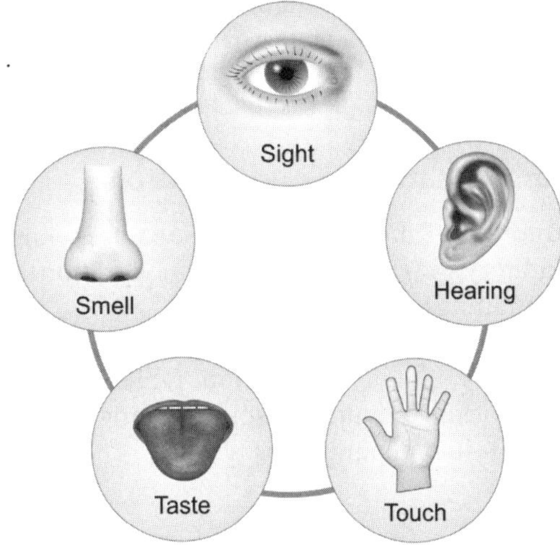

Sensory perception.

Eyes – Sight or Ophthalmoception

These are the visual sense components of our body. These are sensitive to light for images. The amount of pigmentation in our body has an impact on how dark our eyes are. It helps with the perception of sight by helping the user focus on and recognize the light images.

The iris—a colorful area of the eye, controls the pupil's size, breadth, directly affecting how much light enters the eyes. Behind the lens is where the eye's vitreous body is found. The vitreous humor, a gelatinous substance, fills it. The retina is located at the far back in the eyeball, and this material provides the eyeball its shape as well as transmits light there.

This retina contains photoreceptors, which can detect light. There are two distinct cell kinds that perform different functions. These are cones and rods.

Rods: These sensors are found at the edges of the retina and function in low light. Additionally, they assist peripheral vision.

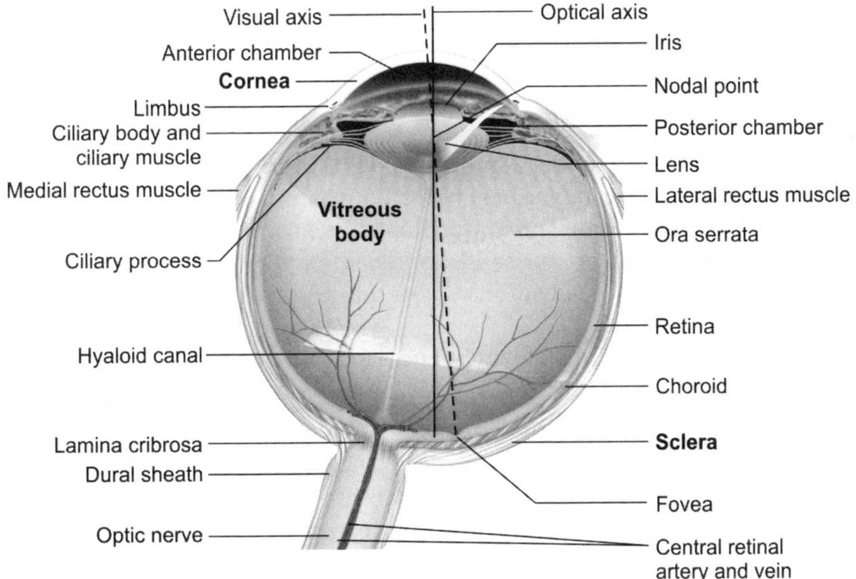

Cones: Under bright light, these retinal sorts of cells are the best at detecting fine details and color. Three distinct types of cones exist for determining the presence of the three primary hues of light—blue, red, or green. Color blindness often develops from the absence of even one of these types of cones.

Ears – Hearing or Audioception

The ears are the auditory sense organs in our body. They improve our capacity for hearing. Our auditory system catches up on air vibrations, which is how we hear sounds. Hearing or hearing captioning are two names for it.

There are three parts of the ear are the middle ear, the inner ear, and the outer ear. Every sound is actually a vibration, which the outer ear conveys to the ear canal and the brain transforms into audible sound. Along with hearing, this sense is essential for preserving the equilibrium of our bodies.

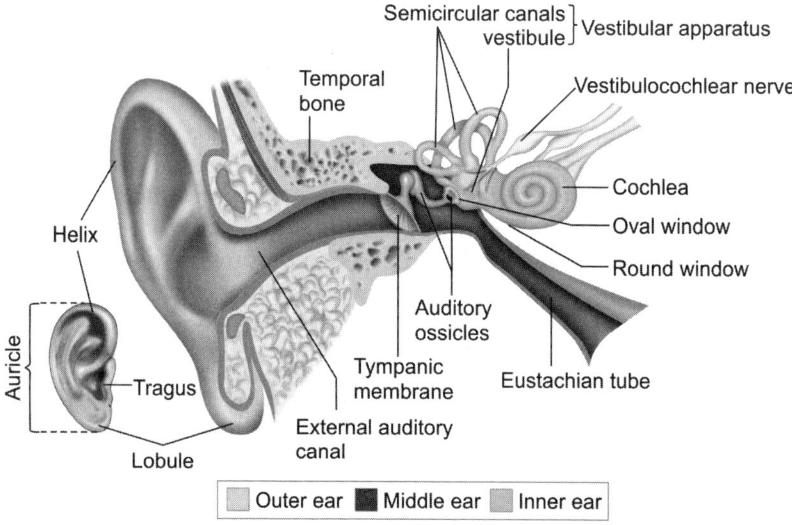

Tongue – Taste or Gustaoception

The tongue helps in forming an understanding of several tastes and sensations. The buds that detect flavors are located on the tongue in between both papillae and help in flavor perception.

The sensations of taste and smell often work together. Anything that a person was not able to smell, they could not taste. The taste sense is often referred to as gustaoception.

Taste buds on the tongue have chemoreceptors that work similarly to those located in the opening in the nose.

There are four distinct kinds of taste buds, and each one can detect various sorts of tastes including sweetness, sourness, bitterness, and saltiness. In contrast, the chemoreceptors of the nose would sense any form of scent.

Nose – Smell or Olfalcoception

The nose serves as the olfactory organ. With the help of our olfactory system, we can recognize different smells. This sensory organ also aids in our experience of taste. Another word for it, is olfaction, which is the sense of smell.

Often, olfactory cells line the upper part of the sinuses. Olfactory cells have olfactory fibers of nerves on one end and cilia on the other end, with the cilia extending into the nasal cavity.

During inhalation, air travels into the nasal cavity. Chemical cells found in the nose have protein receptors and can detect even minute differences in chemicals. These materials stick to the cilia, which then send a nerve signal to the brain. The brain then transforms this impulse into a particular fragrance. Everything we eat when sick tastes bland because our sense of smell is restricted by the mucus that the body produces during a cold.

Skin – Touch or Tactioception

The skin is the largest organ in the human body. It is related to our sense of touch. The tactile sense is often referred to as tactioception.

Universal receptors in the skin allow it to detect touch, temperature, pressure, pain, and other sensations. They might be located anywhere on the skin. Skin receptors that are activated generate an impulse that first goes to the spinal cord and then to the brain.

COMPONENTS OF SENSORY EXPERIENCE

When a person becomes aware of their surroundings and understands informational signals, they have experienced perception. Receiving inputs and generating a nerve impulse is referred to as reception. How a person reacts to a perceived stimuli is called a reaction. The knowledge of sensory inputs via the body's sense processes is referred to as sensation, a broad phrase.

Our bodies use reception, perception, and response to understand stimuli. When a nerve cell a sensory receptor is triggered by a feeling, reception is the initial stage of the sensory process. Mechanical, chemical, or thermal stimulation may cause sensory receptors to become active. We have somatosensation in addition to the five senses. Somatosensation are those that react to stimuli including pain, temperature, pressure, and vibration. Proprioception, the awareness of our joint, bone, and muscles' positions, as well as vestibular sensation, a feeling of spatial direction and balance, are also included.

There are two types of cellular systems that carry out sensory transduction. In one, a neuron uses a receptor for senses, cell, or activity within a cell that is intended to connect to and detect a certain stimulus. When a sensory receptor gets activated, an associated afferent neuron is triggered, which subsequently communicates information about the stimulus to the brain's neurological system. In the second category of sensory transduction, the receptor for sensation is a neuron that responds to events that occur in either the internal or external environment. Since different stimuli may activate free nerve terminals, their receptor specificity is restricted. The pain receptors inside the teeth and gums, for instance, may be activated by pressure, chemical encouragement, or temperature changes.

Reception

Reception includes the activation of the receptors for sensory information by stimuli like chemicals, temperatures, or motion which is the first step of sensation. The receptor may then respond to the inputs after that. The receptor's receptive field is the region of space in which a certain sensitive receptor in order whether it be one that is near the body or far away, may respond to a stimulus. Think for a moment about the distinct receptive fields that each sense has. The body must be in close proximity to a stimulus in order for touch to be felt. For the sense of hearing, a stimulus may be fairly distant (some baleen whales calls may reach great distances). A stimulus for vision may be located at great distances; for instance, the visual system can detect light from stars at great distances.

Sensory Information Coding and Transmission

The four elements of perception that are kept by sensory systems are type of stimulus, location in the field of contact, duration, and relative intensity. As a consequence, the action potentials generated by the afferent axonal of sensory receptors only encode one kind of information, and other perceptual circuits maintain this difference between the senses. For instance, the brain perceives electrical signals in the axons of auditory receptors, which employ a different method to transmit information, as an audio stimulus—a sound.

The power of the stimulus is often conveyed by the frequency of potentials for action produced by the sensory receptors. As a consequence, a strong stimulus will cause a train to create action potentials more quickly, while a weak stimulus would cause a train to produce action potentials more slowly. Another way to encode intensity is by counting the number of activated receptors. A strong stimulus has the ability to activate a lot more receptors than a weak stimulus, which may only activate a limited number of neighboring receptors. The central nervous system (CNS) begins integrating sensory input as soon as it arrives, and the brain keeps processing incoming information.

Perception

Perception is the process through which an individual perceives a stimulus. Perception really occurs higher up in the neurological system, in the cortex, despite being the case that it relies on the activation or nerve cells. Because action potentials form the senses pass via neurons that are specially tuned to that stimulus as they go down a sensory pathway, the brain may be able to distinguish between various sensory inputs. These neurons have been trained to that particular stimulus and form synapses with certain neurons in the circulatory system or spinal cord.

All central nervous system-transmitted sensory impulses, with the sole exception that originate from the olfactory system, are received by the thalamus and the corresponding region of the cortex. Keep in mind that the thalamus in the forebrain serves as a hub and relay of sensory (as well as motor) impulses. A sensory signal is sent from the thalamus of the cerebellum to the area of brain called the cortex located particularly in charge of processing that feeling.

Individuals' reactions to their perceptions of received stimuli are referred to as reactions. Because it is difficult to respond to all of the inputs that are continually being received from our surroundings, the brain decide which experiences are important.

AROUSAL MECHANISM

The brain has to be aware, or arousal, for the subject to receive and comprehend inputs. It is believed that the brainstem's reticular activating system (RAS) mediates the arousal process. The reticular excitatory region (REA) and the reticular inhibitory area (RIA) are the two halves of the RAS. The REA is in charge of awakening and wakefulness. Each individual has an own zone of optimal arousal, or a point at which they feel at ease. The word "sensoristasis" is used to indicate the optimally aroused condition of a person. People must adjust to an upsurge or reduction in sensory stimuli once they leave their comfort zone. The brain becomes inert or worthless in the absence of impulses sent by the RAS and the cerebrum. The brain may change in response to sensory inputs. Certain sensory data is processed immediately, while other sensory input is stored in the memory for later use. For example, a person from a rural area would not be able to hear the loud, frightening traffic noise that someone from a metropolis would.

Arousal is the biological or psychological state of awakening or the sense organs being sufficiently alert. It activates the ascending reticular active system (ARAS), which controls hormone production, immunity, and alertness. This leads to a condition of awareness of the senses, desire, activity, and responsiveness as well as an increase in the heart rate and blood pressure.

Arousal is mediated by several neural systems. The connections from five primary neuronal networks that stretch across the cortex and originate in the brainstem make up the ARAS, which regulates wakefulness. Neurons that produce substances including the amino acid ACE, dopamine, norepinephrine, histamine, and serotonin cause the ARAS to become active. The activity of these neurons increases, causing a rise in mental activity and alertness.

Arousal is essential for managing awareness, attention, alertness, and data processing. Movement, the search for food, the fight-or-flight response, and penile activity (the arousal stage of the sexual response that humans experience cycle, according to Masters and Johnson) are just a few of the behaviors that are dependent on it.

Neurophysiology

Wakefulness is regulated by the ascending reticular drive system, which is composed of the chemical called dopamine, histamine, acetylcholine, norepinephrine and serotonin five primary neurotransmitter routes that arise in the cerebral cortex and establish connections that extend throughout the cerebral cortex. When activated, these systems produce mental activity and attention.

The locus coeruleus serves as the beginning of the noradrenergic system, which ascends into the neocortex, emotional system, or basal forebrain. The bulk of neurons project to the posterior cortex, which is important for alertness and sensory information. Norepinephrine is released when the coeruleus nerve is stimulated, resulting in increased alertness and wakefulness. Acetylcholine floods the cerebral cortex from the neurons' effects on cholinergic neurons throughout the basal forebrain.

The pons and basal forebrain contain the neurons of the acetylcholinergic system. Cortical activity and alertness are produced by stimulating these neurons, as seen by EEG recordings. The cholinergic neurons are activated by all four of the other neurotransmitters.

The substantia nigra is dopaminergic system, another arousal system releases dopamine. The neurons that make up the medial tegmental part of the midbrain originate in the core of the tendons, and are located in the frontal lobe of the limbic system with the prefrontal cortex. The limbic system is essential for managing mood, and the nucleus accumbens acts as a signal for enthusiasm and arousal. The prefrontal cortex (PFC) is a critical part of the pathway that controls motor actions, particularly reward-oriented motions.

Almost majority of the serotonergic neurons in the serotonergic system are born in the raphe nuclei. The limbic system and prefrontal cortex of the brain are both affected by this system. These axons are stimulated, and serotonin is released, which affects mood and movement by enhancing cortical arousal.

The neurons of the histaminergic system are located in the hypothalamic tuberomammillary nucleus. These neurons send signals to the cerebral cortex, thalamus, and basal forebrain, which in turn cause the cerebral cortex to release choline.

Importance

The regulation of awareness, attention, and data processing depends on arousal. It is essential for driving several actions, including movement, nutrition-seeking, the fight-or-flight reaction, and sexual behavior.

Arousal has a role in the recognition, storage, and recall of data throughout the memory process. knowledge that stirs the emotions may improve memory encoding, which will improve knowledge retention and retrieval. By demonstrating that individuals are more likely to encode exciting information than neutral information, arousal is associated to particular focus during the encoding process. Selective encoding of arousing stimuli outperforms neutral encoding in terms of long-term memory performance.

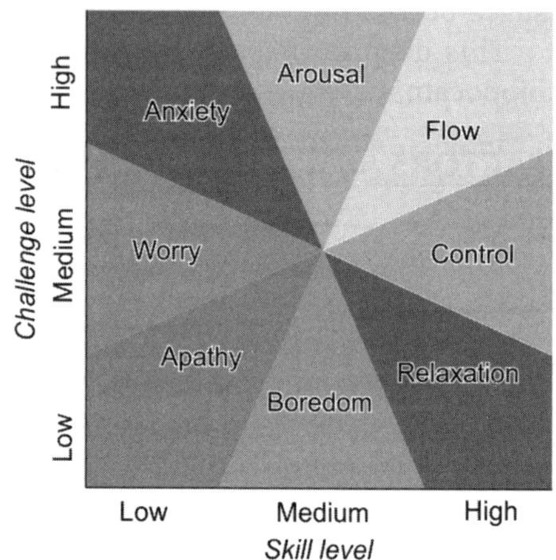

In other words, exposure to stimulating events or information increases the retention and accumulation of knowledge. Information that is stimulating is also recalled or retrieved more vividly and precisely.

Arousal generally enhances memory, however, there are a couple of things to remember. When learning, arousal is more closely linked to retrieval and long-term memory than short-term memory. For instance, one research discovered that participants could recall enticing phrases better one week after learning them than they did only two minutes later. Arousal has various effects on people's memories, according to another research. Eysenck discovered a link between memory and introverts' vs extroverts' arousal. The total number of words recovered by extroverts rose with higher levels of excitement, whereas the number of items recalled by introverts dropped.

Associated Problems

Both anxiety and sadness are linked to altered arousal experiences.

Depression may affect one's degree of arousal by impairing the right hemisphere's ability to operate. Depression has been demonstrated to reduce arousal in that left visual field in women, demonstrating the right hemisphere's effect.

Arousal and sadness interact differently than arousal and anxiety. Arousal perceptions are often aberrant and heightened in people with anxiety disorders. Fear and skewed self-perceptions are then produced by the disorganized feelings of arousal. For instance, someone who is really anxious about taking a test could think that taking the exam would make them sick. The concern of arousing anxiousness and how others may react to this arousal can subsequently raise anxiety levels.

Unusually High Behavioral Arousal

The causes include dementia, rabies and their hemispheric lesions in stroke, acute withdrawal from alcohol or barbiturates, acute encephalitis, head injury causing an unconscious state, partial seizures throughout epilepsy, metabolic diseases of imbalance of electrolyte, intracranial space-occupying lesions, metabolic illnesses of an electrolyte imbalance, and multiple sclerosis.

This disorder has anatomical effects on the frontal lobes, amygdala, limbic system, hippocampus, and temporal lobes.

FACTORS AFFECTING SENSORY FUNCTION

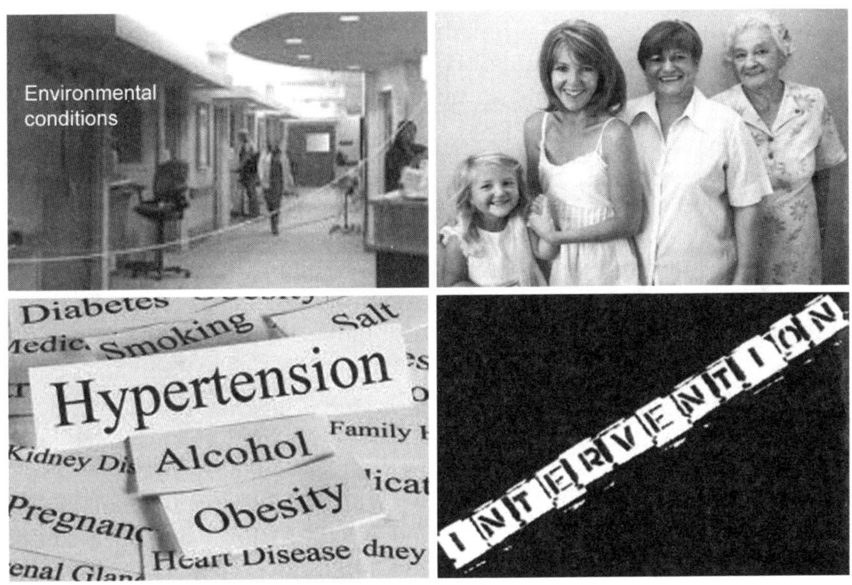

Factors affecting sensory function.

Age: Infants and young children may be at risk for developing hearing and vision impairment due to a variety of genetic, prenatal, and postnatal causes. Early, intensive audio and visual stimulation has the potential to harm visual auditory pathways and change how other sensory organs develop in high-risk newborns. Presbyopia and the need for reading glasses are two visual alterations that happen as people age. Ages 40 to 50 are the typical range for these alterations. The cornea also becomes thicker and flatter, which helps with bending light to the retina. Astigmatism results from these aging changes. Collagen fibers accumulate in the front chamber and pigment is lost to the iris, increasing the risk of hypertension by reducing intraocular fluid absorption.

Other common visual changes brought on by aging include reduced visual fields, lower glare sensitivity, impaired night vision, diminished depth perception, with decreased color discrimination.

At age 30, hearing changes start to occur. Decreased speech understanding, hearing acuity, and pitch discrimination are all effects of aging. Although low-pitched noises are the easiest to hear, background noise makes it challenging to hear conversations. Consonants (z, t, f, g) and high-frequency sounds (s, sh, ph, k) are also challenging to distinguish. Low-pitched vowels are the most easily audible. Speech reception and response are delayed, and speech sounds are distorted. An issue with typical aging-related changes in sensory function is that elderly people with an impairment may sometimes get an incorrect dementia diagnosis.

Around age 50, olfactory and gustatory changes start to occur, including a reduction in the number of senses or sensory cells that line the sinus lining. It's typical to have diminished odor sensitivity and taste discrimination.

After age 60, proprioceptive changes are prevalent and include a rise in problems with coordination, spatial orientation, and balance. The instinctive reaction to defend and brace oneself while falling is slower in older folks, and they are unable to dodge obstacles as rapidly. Due to circulatory disorders and neuropathies, people over 65 endure tactile alterations, including a decline in their sensitivity to discomfort, pressure, and temperature.

Throughout the lifespan, several modifications take place.

Positive Stimuli Fewer People Experience Sensory Deprivation

Amount of stimulation possibly leading to sensory overload: Sensory overload is brought on by an environment with too many stimuli. In a critical health care environment, operations and observations are often stressful. Overstimulation is often an issue for patients who are in pain or who are constrained by casts or traction. Additionally, sensory overload is exacerbated by a room that is close to loud or repeated sounds (such as an elevator, staircase, or nurse's station).

Social engagement increases when family interaction is lacking: Both the number and the quality of social interactions with close friends and family members who are supportive of one another affect sensory function. Whether a patient is hospitalized or residing in a nursing home without visits affects how isolated they feel. This is a frequent issue in hospital critical care units because visiting hours are often limited. For the majority of individuals, being able to talk about worries with close ones is an essential coping tool. Therefore, a patient who lacks meaningful communication experiences emotions of loneliness, anxiety, and sadness. This is often not apparent until there are behavioral changes.

Environmental factors: A person's line of work puts them at risk for peripheral nerve, hearing, and vision changes. People who work in noisy environments (such as factories or airports) run the risk of hearing loss brought on by noise, thus it is important to get their hearing checked. Hazardous noise is often present during both work and leisure activities. Target shooting, hunting, carpentry, and loud music listening are examples of noisy pastimes that impair hearing.

People who work in jobs where exposure to solvents or flying objects is a possibility (such as welders) are at risk for damage to the eyes and should be tested for visual impairments. Persons are also exposed for visual changes when participating in sports and using consumer fireworks. The median nerve is compressed by repeated wrist or finger motions in jobs like heavy assembly line labor, which leads to carpal tunnel syndrome. One of the most frequent industrial or occupational injuries is carpal tunnel syndrome, which affects tactile perception. Numbness, sensation of tingling weakness, and discomfort must all be carefully examined in patients who are at risk of developing carpal tunnel.

A hospitalized patient can at times be at risk having sensory abnormalities as a result of exposure to outside stimuli or a change in sensory input. Patients who are bedridden or who have a long-term handicap are unable to fully appreciate the feelings of unrestricted mobility. Patients secluded in a medical facility or at home due to illnesses like active TB are another group at risk. These individuals reside in secluded rooms and often are unable to engage in typical visitor exchanges.

Developmental Stage

For newborns and young children to grow intellectually, socially and physically, sensory perception is essential. Infants acquire facial recognition skills and bonding relationships that are crucial to later mental growth. When young toddlers hear music, they sing and dance as they start to socialize with others in groups. As they become older, kids have the ability to understand visual and aural cues while getting ready to cross the path of traffic. Adults have a wide range of ingrained reactions to sensory inputs. Therefore, a person if any age is profoundly affected by the unexpected loss or degradation of any sense. Older people are more likely to have reduced sensory function due to age-related physiological changes. Age or chronic sickness may cause a reduction of feeling perception, which often occurs gradually.

Culture

The degree of stimulation that an individual considers usual or "normal" is frequently determined by their culture. Additionally, an individual's desire for and perception of how much stimulation is significant is influenced by the typical levels of stimulation related to factors like ethnicity, religion, and socioeconomic status, for instance. The sudden change in cultural surroundings as immigrants or visitors to a new country experience may also cause cultural shock and sensory overload, especially when there are differences in language, attire, and cultural practices.

Stress

People may feel that their senses are already overstimulated during times of elevated stress and desire to reduce sensory stimulation. For instance, a client who is experiencing physical sickness, discomfort, hospitalization, and diagnostic testing may want only close support individuals to come. Additionally, a client could want the nurse's assistance in minimizing unnecessary stimuli (such as noise). On the other side, while under minimal stress, clients could look for sensory stimulation.

Medications and Illness

A person's awareness of external cues may change as a result of taking certain drugs. For instance, narcotics and sedatives may reduce sensitivity to stimuli. Some antidepressants may also change how stimuli are perceived. Anyone taking many drugs at once may have changes in visual function; older persons are particularly vulnerable to these changes and need to be closely watched. Some drugs may become ototoxic if used in high dosages or for an extended length of time, harming the auditory nerve potentially resulting in permanent hearing loss.

Examples of such medications include aspirin, furosemide (Lasix), the aminoglycosides, and a few chemotherapy drugs. Atherosclerosis is a disorder that restricts blood flow to the cerebral cortex or receptor organs, which decreases awareness and delays responses. Different degrees of paralysis and sensory loss are brought on by several central nervous system illnesses. The kinesthetic sensation may be impacted by inner ear diseases.

Lifestyle and Personality

The kind and amount of stimulus to which a person is used depends on their lifestyle. A client who works for a major firm could be used to a wide variety of stimuli, while a client who works for themselves from home is confronted with fewer, less varied stimuli. Individual personalities also vary in terms of how much and what kind of stimulus they find pleasant. While some individuals prefer a more organized existence with minimal changes, others like the stimulation and excitement that comes with continual change.

Psychiatric Conditions

Autism spectrum disorder (ASD): Neuromolecular and structural changes in the brain's primary sensory regions are the primary causes of sensory symptoms connected to autism. These modifications are often caused by GABAergic (gamma-aminobutyric acid) transmission, which is frequently impacted.

Sensory overload is a symptom of attention-deficit hyperactive disorder (ADHD), which is caused by an inability to block irrelevant sensory external impulses. This happens as a result of defective perceptual ability and information processing impairment. People who have ADHD are less able to filter out distracting motor, sensory and/or cognitive input.

Schizophrenia: The positive symptoms indicate schizophrenia is caused by altered processing of sensory information and perceptual inference. Schizophrenia's pathophysiology is thought to be influenced by faulty cortical plasticity processes and inappropriate serotonin signaling along the sensory pathway. Dysfunctional facial emotion recognition at motion processing are key traits of both ASD and schizophrenia.

In children with sensory processing disorder (SPD), the brain is unable to properly and effectively handle incoming information, which results in inaccurate processing and appraisal of sensory input. Children may have trouble controlling their emotions, paying attention, and changing their behavior.

Sleep Disorders

Delirium brought on by disrupted sleep or sleep loss may impair sensory and perceptual perception. It has been shown that a reduction in rapid eye movement (REM), sleep may contribute to delirium.

Delirium in Intensive Care Unit

Very ill patients treated in intensive care unit (ICU) are more prone to have delirium. Sensational changes and altered perceptions may be caused by host factors, acute diseases, and environmental influences. Some examples of environmental and iatrogenic causes include lack of sleep, loss of feeling, immobility, and social isolation. Patients who are admitted into an ICU are more likely to have delirium if they have trouble getting enough restful sleep. These changes have a negative effect on the quality of care provided to patients.

Causes of disturbed sleep in ICU may be due to:
* Mechanical ventilation and medicine (benzodiazepines used to treat delirium, in particular in older patients, might negatively contribute to delirium).
* Constant exposure to light might throw off the circadian cycle.
* Exposure to noise from machinery, sirens, and interactions between medical professionals and patients.
* Activities related to patient care—vital signs, nursing techniques, imaging, and lab draws.

Prolonged or frequent sleep deprivation can lead to:
* Delirium due to impaired cognitive function
* Prolonged neurocognitive dysfunction
* A decrease in quality of life
* Impaired immune function.

Patients may need to be isolated under certain conditions (such as infection control). A patient's mood will be negatively impacted by contact isolation, increasing the likelihood of sadness, anxiety, aggression and terror. A person may feel as if they lose control when in social isolation as a result of the situation's unpredictability, which will affect their mood. Elderly individuals with neurocognitive issues who are kept in physical isolation are more prone to experience delirium.

Neurological Disorders

Due to altered function of the brain, a number of neurological illnesses and syndromes may manifest with alterations in behavior including cognitive performance. These may be brought by sudden alterations, trauma, metabolic and imbalances in electrolytes, medicines, infections, or vascular abnormalities. Furthermore, hereditary problems, neurodegenerative illnesses, cancers, or structural issues may all these alterations to take place slowly and sneakily.

Alzheimer's condition: Sensory visual abnormalities are a frequent symptom of Alzheimer's disease because of cortical disruptions. The cortical thinning and atrophy caused by the accumulation of neurofibrillary tangles and neuritic plaques over the visual cortex areas is the cause of this. Higher visual talents often suffer. These include simultanagnosia, issues with visual focus and recall, the ability to distinguish structure from emotion, the perception of faces and objects, visual learning, and reading. These patients' quality of life is decreased by visual perception impairment, which also makes it more difficult to assess other cognitive deficiencies.

Parkinson's disease: Patients with Parkinson's disease have poor visuoperception because the lens of the eye and other areas of the visual system gradually lose catecholamine-producing cells. This dopamine deficiency results in specific spatial-temporal abnormalities in the visual nerve cell activity. Dementia is more likely to occur in those who have visuoperceptual impairments.

Patients with epilepsy may experience seizures that affect their five senses. Sensitivity is affected, or sometimes is above average as a consequence. Although interictal functions may also be impacted, ictal perceptual events are rather prevalent. Since epilepsy is an interpersonal disorder, neuronal circuits far from the seizure site may be impacted. This might explain how the underlying epileptic illness is related to the impaired sensory modality. People with temporal lobe epilepsy often have odor bias, recognition difficulties, and memory impairment. This changed emotion is brought on by the limbic system's close relationship to the olfactory system, which is often associated with mesial temporal lobe epilepsy. Processing of sight may be hampered in occipital lobe epilepsy.

Visual Dysfunction

Common causes of visual dysfunction in the elderly are:
* Age-related changes in the optics of the eye
* Diabetic retinopathy
* Glaucoma
* Cataract
* Age-related maculopathy
* Visual hallucinations due to Bonnet syndrome

Visual acuity, contrast sensitivity, color discrimination, motion perception, outer eye sensitivity, temporal awareness, and visual speed processing are all impaired as a result of these dysfunctions.

Hearing Problems

Hearing loss can cause auditory hallucinations, such as Anton's syndrome.

Electrolyte Imbalance

This may result in altered sensorium, particularly in older individuals who may have hyponatremia and hypocalcemia.

Alcohol or Illicit Drug Use

This may result in sensory and perceptual changes as well as cognition problems.

ASSESSMENT OF SENSORY ALTERATIONS

Assessment

Each patient should be carefully evaluated throughout the assessment process, and nurses should critically evaluate findings to make the patient-centered clinical choices necessary for providing safe nursing care.

Through the Patient's Eyes

Consider the person receiving treatment as a full collaborator in the planning, delivery, and evaluation of care while performing an assessment.

Patients often refuse to acknowledge sensory loss. So, the first step is information collection to build a therapeutic relationship with the patient.

Find out what values, preferences, and goals the person has in relation to their sensory impairment. A lot of clients have a clear idea of the kind of treatment they desire to get. Some patients anticipate their carers to be aware of their sensory demands, manage their surroundings correctly, and make necessary adjustments.

Depending on the patient's specific sensory impairment, this entails helping them adapt to an entirely novel mode of life. Assess the patient's understanding of their own ailments and health. Always bear in mind that patients with sensory impairments have generally acquired stronger senses and anticipate their demands, such as those of safety and security, from service providers.

Consider the causes of any current impairment and the variables affecting sensory function before examining a patient who has or at risk for visual change in order to plan your approach. For instance, you may alter your communication strategy and focus the examination on relevant criteria for hearing impairments if your patient possessed a hearing problem.

Gather a history that evaluates the patient's present sensory state as well as how much a sensory impairment impacts lifestyle, psychological adjustment, developmental stage, ability to care for oneself, health-promoting habits, and security of the patient are all taken into consideration. The amount and quality of stimuli present in the patient's surroundings should also be emphasized throughout the examination.

Persons at Risk

Because aging is associated with physiological changes to the sensory organs, older people are considered to be in a high-risk group. However, don't immediately assume that an elderly patient's sensory impairment is related to aging. For instance, adult hearing loss that is sensorineural may be brought on by exposure to excess and sustained loudness or by metabolic, vascular, and other systemic changes. If testing shows substantial hearing issues, some people benefit from an appointment to an auditory or otolaryngologist.

Others who reside in a constrained setting, such as the elderly, are also at risk for changes in their senses. There are certain exceptions, despite the fact that the majority of high-quality nursing homes or facilities provide stimulating group activities, attractive environments, and mealtime interactions. Risk factors for sensory deprivation include being confined to a scooter, having impaired hearing and/or vision, having less energy, and avoiding social interaction. A monotonous setting makes it harder for a person to absorb information and think. A strange and inattentive setting puts critically unwell patients at danger as well. This does not imply that every patient in a hospital has sensory impairments. However, you must carefully evaluate patients who are exposed to ongoing sensory stimulation (such as in an intensive care unit, throughout a lengthy hospital stay, or during many therapy). Examine the patient's surroundings, both in the hospital and at home, and search for any elements that need to be changed for safety or to give greater stimulation.

Sensory Alterations History

The nursing history includes an appraisal of the kind and characteristics of sensory alterations as well as any problem related to an alteration. It is crucial to include the patient's ethnic and cultural background while taking a history since certain alterations are more prevalent in particular cultural groups.

Asking the patient to rate their own perception of a sensory impairment throughout the history is helpful.

Consider the following example: "Rate your sense of listening as excellent, acceptable, adequate, poor, or bad." After that, carefully consider how the patient experiences a sensory loss based on their self-rating. This provides a complete analysis of the effects of the sensory loss on the individual's way of life. A screening instrument like Hearing Handicap Inventory for Elderly-Screening (HHIE-S) is efficient in identifying people with hearing issues who need audiological care. The HHIE-S is a 10-item, 5-minute survey that evaluates how the respondent views the social and emotional consequences of hearing loss. The handicapping impact of hearing impairment increases with HHIE-S score.

Any recent alterations in a patient's conduct may also be seen in their nursing history. The finest sources of this knowledge are often friends or relatives. Ask the following questions to the family:

- Has any family member recently shown any mood fluctuations (such as angry outbursts, anxiety, fear, or irritability)?
- Have you noticed that another family member avoids social gatherings?

Nursing Assessment Questions

Nature of the Problem

- What type of problem are you having with your vision/hearing?
- What have you tried to correct the vision/hearing difficulty?
- Do you use any devices to improve your vision/hearing?

Signs and Symptoms

- Ask a patient with visual alterations: Do you require books with large print or on audiotape? Are you able to prepare a meal or write a check?
- Ask a patient with hearing alterations: What types of sounds or tones do you have difficulty hearing? Do people tell you that they have to "shout" for you to hear them? Do you have a ringing, crackling, or buzzing in your ears?
- Is there pain; sharp, dull, burning, itching?
- Have you noticed any redness, swelling, or drainage? Any signs of infection?

Onset and Duration

- When did you notice the problem? How long has this problem lasted?
- Does it come and go, or is it constant?

Predisposing Factors

- Do you work or participate in any activities that have the potential for vision/hearing injury? If so, how do you protect your hearing and vision?
- Do you have a family history of cataracts, glaucoma, macular degeneration, or hearing loss?
- When was your last vision/hearing examination?

Effect on Patient

- What effect has your vision/hearing problem had on your work, family, or social life?
- Have changes in your vision/hearing affected your feelings of independence?
- How does your vision/hearing problem make you feel about yourself?
- Do you have problems with routine care of glasses, contact lenses, or hearing aids?

Knowledge
- Pathophysiology of specific sensory deficit
- Factors that potentially may alter sensory function
- Effects of sensory deprivation/ overload
- Communication principles use to interact with patients having sensory deficits

Experience
- Caring for patients with sudden and long-term sensory alterations
- Personal experience with temporary or permanent sensory deficit

Assessment
- Patient's health promotion practices
- Nursing history regarding extent of risks for and existing sensory deficits
- Review of factors that affect the patient's sensory function
- Extent of lifestyle and self-care alterations
- Patient's expectations regarding sensory alterations

Standards
- Apply intellectual standards of clarity, precision, accuracy, and depth when assessing the patient's sensory function
- Standards of care from American Academy of Ophthalmology and American Speech-Language-Hearing Association

Attitudes
- Show confidence in your ability to provide a safe level of care
- Use curiosity to clarify and explore the nature of signs and symptoms to rule out cause other than sensory change

Mental Status

When you detect sensory overload or deprivation, a mental state assessment is important. Observing a patient while obtaining his or her history, doing a physical exam, and giving nursing care provides useful information on the patient's main behaviors and mental state. Consider the patient's behavior and outward look, as well as his or her mental health and cognitive functioning.

You may gauge disorientation, changes in problem-solving skills, changed conceptualization, and altered abstract thinking using the Mini-Mental State Examination (MMSE). For instance, a patient with significant sensory impairment may not always be able to maintain attention, carry out a conversation, or recall recent events. Nurse education on the illness process, relevant resources, and assistive technologies is a crucial first step in reducing cognition-related impairment.

Physical Assessment

Use physical assessment procedures to evaluate the ability to see, hear, smell, taste, and the capacity to discern light touch, heat, pain, or position in order to detect sensory deficiencies and the degree of those abnormalities. Summarizes particular evaluation methods for finding sensory deficiencies. If the examination space is private, peaceful, and welcoming for the patient, you will get more accurate results. Moreover, depend on your own observation to spot sensory changes. Patients who have hearing loss may seem uninterested to others, react angrily when talked to improperly, assume others are not talking about them, and answer questions incorrectly, struggle to understand instructions, have monotonous voices, and speak excessively loudly or softly.

Assessment of Sensory Function

Assessment activities	Behavior indicating deficit (children)	Behavior indicating deficit (adults)
Vision		
• Ask patient to read newspaper, magazine, or lettering on menu. • Ask patient to identify colors on color chart or crayons. • Observe patients performing ADLs.	Self-stimulation including eye rubbing, body rocking, sniffing or smelling, arm twirling; hitching (using legs to propel while in sitting position) instead of crawling	Poor coordination, squinting, underreaching or overreaching for objects, persistent repositioning of objects, impaired night vision, accidental falls
Hearing		
• Assess patient's hearing acuity using spoken word and tuning fork tests. • Assess for history of tinnitus. • Observe patient conversing with others. • Inspect ear canal for hardened cerumen. • Observe patient behaviors in a group.		

Alterations in Sensory Perception

Individuals may experience anxiety if they experience a significant shift in the sensory inputs they are accustomed to. For example, people frequently bring stimuli with them from their usual experiences when they visit a healthcare institution, which may differ in terms of number and quality. People may become confused and bewildered by these changes. The potential reactions that can be set off by a variety of triggers are becoming increasingly apparent to nurses. Clients are being offered more privacy, sounds, color, and social interaction issues in order to make the stimuli seem more like those found in a home.

Changes in Sensations

The three most common types of changes in sensory perception are sensory overload, sensory deficits, and loss of sensation.

Sensory Deficits

A sensory deficit is a breakdown in the usual receipt and perception of sensory information. With compromised senses, a person loses their sense of self. In an effort to adjust to the sensory loss, he or she first withdraws by avoiding interaction with others. Until he and she acquires new abilities, it becomes challenging for the individual to engage securely with the surroundings. A person learns to depend on unaffected senses when a deficiency gradually develops or after a significant amount of time has elapsed since the commencement of an acute loss of sensation. To make up for a change, certain sensations could even become sharper. As a case study, a blind person develops a keen hearing sense to make up for their vision loss.

Patients with sensory impairments often alter their behavior in either positive or negative ways. While one patient with a hearing impairment avoids social events out of shame over not comprehending what other individuals are saying, another patient with a hearing impairment pushes the unaffected ears nearer the speaker in order to take in better.

A sensory deficit is a difficulty with the receipt, perception, or both, of one or more senses. The sensory impairments caused by eyesight and hearing loss. When sensory function is progressively diminished, people often acquire habits to make up for it; sometimes, these actions are unconscious.

For instance, a person whose right ear progressively loses hearing may unconsciously tilt their left head towards the direction of the speaker. However, an abrupt impairment of one of the sensations may cause confusion, and it sometimes takes days or weeks for compensatory behavior to emerge. Both sensory loss and sensory excess may be harmful to clients who have sensory deficiencies. People with vision issues, for instance, may not be able to read or view television, or identify nurses by sight, all might result in sensory deprivation. Contrarily, the variety and apprehension of the healthcare environment might cause sensory overload in blind individuals since their homes are often highly ordered. At one time, eyesight problems often make it difficult to move about or interact with people.

Common Sensory Deficits

* ❖ **Visual deficits**
  * ◆ *Presbyopia:* A progressive loss of the lens' capacity to focus or adapt to objects that are close up. Person is unable to clearly observe items in close proximity.
  * ◆ *Cataract:* Cloudy of opaque patches that block light from passing through the lens completely or in part, resulting in glare and visual impairments. Cataracts often appear gradually, without any discomfort, ocular redness, or tears.
    When tear glands don't generate enough tears, dry eyes develop, which may itch, burn, or even impair vision.
  * ◆ *Glaucoma* is a gradually increasing intraocular pressure condition that, if untreated, presses steadily on the optic nerve and produces peripheral vision loss, poor visual acuity, trouble adjusting to darkness, or a halo effect around objects.
  * ◆ *Diabetic retinopathy:* When blood vessels in the retina undergo pathological alterations, it may lead to bleeding, macular edema, and impaired vision or visual loss.
    The condition known as macular degeneration causes the macula, a specific area of the retina that is responsible for central vision, to lose its effectiveness. The first symptoms include difficulty reading, loss or distortion of the center of vision, and displacement of vertical lines.
* ❖ **Hearing deficit:** A frequent progressive hearing problem affecting elderly person is presbycusis.
  Cerumen accumulation is the external auditory canal's buildup of earwax. Conduction deafness is brought on by cerumen that hardens and accumulates in the canal.
* ❖ **Balance deficit:** Disequilibrium and vertigo are frequent conditions in older adults, often brought on by vestibular dysfunction. A shift in head posture often triggers a vertigo or disequilibrium episode.

- ❖ **Taste deficit**
  Xerostomia: A decrease in salivation that causes a dry mouth and heavier mucus. Often hinder the ability to eat, which causes issues with hunger and nutrition.
- ❖ **Neurological deficits**
  Numbness and tingling in the afflicted region, as well as a stumbling stride, are signs of peripheral neuropathy, a disorder in the peripheral nerve system.
  Stroke: Cerebrovascular accident brought on by a blood clot, hemorrhage or emboli that cut off the blood supply to the brain. Alters proprioception and produces pronounced imbalance and lack of coordination. Additionally, the damaged brain area-controlled extremities lose their ability to move and feel. Speech difficulties are among the signs of a stroke that affects the left half of the brain. Left-side symptoms of a stroke in the right hemisphere include visual spatial changes, such as the loss of half of the visual field, or inattention and neglect, particularly to the left side.

Sensory Deprivation

Patients may receive impulses even if they are profoundly asleep because the system for reticular activation in the brainstem transmits all sensory inputs to the cerebral cortex. A person's consciousness must be maintained through sensory input that is both of adequate quality and quantity. Reduced input from the senses (sensory loss from visual or auditory loss), the removal of patterns or meaning and input (e.g., exposure to unusual places), and limiting conditions (e.g., bed rest) that result in monotony and boredom are three forms of sensory deprivation.

The consequences of sensory deprivation are many. Adults may have symptoms that are comparable to those of a psychiatric condition, disorientation, a serious imbalance in electrolytes, or the effects of psychotropic medicines. Therefore, you should constantly be mindful of a patient's current sensory function as well as the caliber of environmental stimuli.

Effects of Sensory Deprivation

Cognitive

- ❖ Reduced capacity to learn
- ❖ Inability to think or problem solve
- ❖ Poor task performance
- ❖ Disorientation
- ❖ Bizarre thinking
- ❖ Increased need for socialization, altered mechanisms of attention

Affective

- ❖ Boredom
- ❖ Restlessness
- ❖ Increased anxiety
- ❖ Emotional lability
- ❖ Panic
- ❖ Increased need for physical stimulation

Perceptual

- ❖ Changes in visual/motor coordination
- ❖ Reduced color perception

* Less tactile accuracy
* Changes in ability to perceive size and shape
* Changes in spatial and time judgment

Sensory Overload

A person who encounters a multitude of sensory stimuli and is unable to willfully or perceptually disregard some of them is said to be experiencing sensory overload. The brain cannot react to or ignore certain cues properly when there is too much sensory input. Due to overload brought on by the abundance of stimuli, a person is no longer able to comprehend their surroundings in a rational manner. Overload inhibits the brain from responding in a meaningful way; the patient's thoughts rush, their concentration wanders, and they become anxious and restless. As a consequence, overload results in a condition resembling sensory deprivation. Deprivation is generalized, while overload is specific. Each person has a different threshold for the stimuli that are required for good function. Environmental overload often affects people more severely at some times than others. The amount of exhaustion, attitude, and mental and physical health that a person can tolerate influences how much sensory overload they can handle.

A patient who is really unwell might quickly get overstimulated. Patients who have ongoing discomfort or whose vital signs are often monitored are at risk. Even if the healthcare provider comforts the patient or gives them a gentle back massage, the combination of many stimuli still results in overload. Because they are focused on greater stress stimuli, some patients may not benefit from nurse involvement. A patient receiving inpatient treatment in a critical-care unit (ICU), where their activity is continual, is another example. Lights are always on. The noises of monitoring devices, staff chats, equipment alerts, and entrance activities of individuals are all audible to patients. The ICU is quite loud, even at night.

It is possible to mistake mood swings or plain confusion for the behavioral changes brought on by sensory overload. Pay alert to signs including racing thoughts, erratic attention, restlessness, and worry. Sometimes ICU patients may repeatedly finger dressings and tubes. An essential component of a patient's treatment is the continual reorientation and management of excessive stimuli.

ALTERATION IN SENSE OF MOTION

Sensations are affected by kinesthetic deficits, such as peripheral neuropathy. Peripheral neuropathy is characterized by pain, burning, buzzing and tingling in the extremities, which impair touch, pressure, especially vibration sensitivity. Position awareness may be compromised, which makes it challenging to coordinate complicated actions like walking, button-fastening, or keeping one's balance when one's eyes are closed. Nerve injury that often develops in people with type 2 diabetes or a vascular condition that leads to peripheral neuropathy. Injuries to the body, infections, autoimmune disorders, vitamin deficiency, renal, liver, and other ailments are all possible causes.

Management

Some of the risk factors that result in weakened and altered sensory as well as perceptual abilities include impaired perception of information, a lack of processing of inputs related to illnesses like hearing or blindness, a loss of taste or smell, or the inability to feel things. These conditions may be brought on by genetics, aging, trauma, or metabolic mechanisms. Reasons include electrolyte depletion and impairments related to sensory stimulation.

Occasionally, independent of location, time, or environmental cues, the client will exhibit the tell-tale signs and symptoms of a subjective and perceptual decline. Other times, despite these variables, the client will exhibit the tell-tale signs and symptoms of a sensory and intellectual loss. Almost all sensory and visual issues tend to get further exacerbated in an odd or unaccustomed environment, such as a hospital room that is foreign to the hospitalized person's daily life. For example, auditory deficits could become more severe in a noisy environment or one that is full of other disruptive stimuli. During the evening hours, visual abnormalities, including poor vision, might also offer hazards, indicators, and indications.

Patients with sensory and perceptual anomalies must be evaluated by nurses, who must then plan their care in line with the patients' particular needs as well as changes in time, place, and other stimuli. In order to minimize sensory overload, it's crucial to safeguard the safety of individuals who are partly or fully blind, therefore certain clients may need to be placed in low-stimulation situations.

Assisting the Client to Develop Strategies for Dealing with Sensory and Thought Disturbances

The safety of the numerous clients who are impacted by cognitive and sensory disruptions is of utmost importance.

Thought disturbance treatments include the following for issues caused by organic brain disorder, dementia, particularly Alzheimer's disease, delirium, other psychiatric symptomatology:

- Providing safety by, utilizing falls risk guidelines for persons who are at risk of falling and storing hazardous cleaning agents in a secure location.
- Constant monitoring of the client's needs
- Maintenance of the client's comfort
- Anticipation the client's requirements and subsequent attention to them
- Provision of a setting free of extraneous stimuli
- Reorientation, the client for time, place, and person when required. Maintaining as much continuity as possible between the client's routines with those who provide nursing care for them; explaining techniques to the client in a way that they understand while using adaptive equipment and aids that can help the client's comprehension, such as depicts and gestures; managing hallucinations alongside a medication like a dopamine antagonist; when necessary, using closed-ended questions that only require an simple yes or no response.

Assessment as well as tracking of vulnerable body parts, especially the feet along with lower extremity about clients with neuropathy due to diabetes and exposed body parts that are susceptible to frost bite, can help treat tactile or kinesthetic impairments because these conditions may not be perceived by the client when their sensory functioning is compromised.

The client will be more able to manage vision-related sensory and perceptual impairments if the nurse and other medical professionals:

- Ensure that a customer with poor vision has and is using lenses for correction, including eyeglasses and other devices like magnifiers, by communicating with them near eye level in their functional range of vision.
- Maintain a clutter-free and organized client environment. Give the client information about the locations of items in the client's immediate and extended environment. Greet the client by name and introduce yourself when entering the client's space. Use Braille and large print

materials for low vision clients. Assist the client with meals by describing items on the dinner plate or meal tray according to the position of a clock's hands, such as 1 o'clock or 3 o'clock.

Foods that are very appealing may be provided so that the client's need to eat is stimulated by their look, which is one way to ease the coping for a client who has a gustatory sensory deficit that impacts their sense of taste. For whatever reason, clients who are mentally handicapped may benefit from the same appealing presentation.

Clients with hearing impairments may manage this deficiency more effectively when the nurse in addition to healthcare professionals:

❖ When appropriate, use written communication rather than oral communication.
❖ Provide the client using assistive devices, such as a hearing aid.
❖ Speak slowly while sitting close to the client's eye level and precisely pronouncing expressions to facilitate lip reading.
❖ Eliminate all unnecessary environmental noises and interruptions when connecting with the client.

Providing Care for a Client Experiencing Visual, Auditory or Cognitive Distortions

Providing Care in a Nonthreatening and Nonjudgmental Manner

Nurses treat patients of all ages with all types of diseases, including both physical and psychological ones. All of this healthcare must be delivered in a way that is encouraging, non-threatening, impartial, kind, sympathetic, and non-judgmental. Since the client is the main focus of care in all nurse-client interactions, nurses must provide for the client's requirements without imposing their own prejudice or judgment.

Providing Reality-based Diversions

Realistic diversions and hobbies might be beneficial for clients who are not goal-oriented.

These reality-based diversions can include talking about the month, morning of the week, the weather to earn the season, reading the newspaper, participating in daily "news of the week" or actual events group sessions, thought therapy, and other activities for both people and groups that match the individual's interests and needs.

Nursing Interventions to Address Sensory Alterations

Sensory alteration	Nursing interventions
Impaired vision	• Ensuring that the patients are able to access their clean, current prescription eyewear or contacts. If necessary, provide magnifying glasses. • Every time you enter the room, identify yourself. • Observe the effects of visual loss on your daily activities. • Make sure the space has enough light. • Provide sunglasses or pull the window curtain to reduce glare. • If necessary, describe the surroundings to the patient. • Don't organize the environment. Keep your area clutter-free, and whenever required, remove hazards such scatter rugs and oxygen tubing. • Verbally describe the location of the goods or meal. • When necessary, provide reading materials with big print. • Apply labels to goods that are used often (for instance, mark medicine bottles with highly contrasting colors). • Encourage and assist in arranging for glaucoma screenings to be performed during annual eye exams.

Contd...

Contd...

Hearing impairment	• Perform regular hearing tests or make arrangements for them. When necessary, help the patient in getting a hearing instrument or other assistive listening equipment. • As required, be sure to use assistive hearing devices properly; maintain battery life and equipment cleanliness. • Prior to speaking, get the patient's attention. • When conversing, stay away from loud surroundings. • Communicate with the patient no further than two to three feet away. • When appropriate, use motions. • Use short, basic phrases rather than slang and simplify language as necessary. • By speaking directly to the patient while facing them in excellent lighting, you may help them lip-read by letting them see your lips. Avoid chewing gum or mints while speaking, and don't glance away from them while you're talking. Speak in a deep, low voice. • In the plan of treatment for individuals with significant hearing impairment, note the preferred form of communication (such as speech, writing, lip-reading, even American sign language).
Impaired sensitivity to odor	• Encourage the patient to visually inspect the pilot lights of their household appliances. • Remind the patient to look for dates on food packaging and on any leftovers in the freezer.
Impaired tactile sensation	• To prevent burns, keep the water heater temperature within a safe range. • Use a thermometer to measure the temperature of the bathwater.
Impaired oral communication	• Allow the patient enough time to speak before responding. Don't use words or phrases that are childish. • For people with expressive aphasia, provide questions that merely call for brief "yes" or "no" responses. • Explain things simply. • As necessary, provide a communication whiteboard or other substitute channels of contact. • Work together with a speech language pathologist to create a communication strategy. • To improve communication, educate the family and caregivers.
Sensory overload	• To prevent disturbing sleep time, schedule and mix nursing activities. • Reduce whenever possible the amount of background noise, such as conversations and sounds from medical equipment, in the room or the corridor outside. • If you can, shut the door to the room.
Sensory deprivation	• Give the patient engaging stimuli, such as the radio, television, books, calendars, pictures of loved ones, and pets. • As necessary, encourage family members or caregivers to participate in meaningful dialogue with persons by providing social engagement.

APHASIA

Aphasia is a disorder that results from damage to the parts of the brain that control language. These brain regions are often located on the left side of most people. Aphasia often manifests slowly as a result of a brain tumor or a degenerative brain disorder, but it may also strike suddenly, commonly after a stroke or other head by coincidence. The illness affects all aspects of language understanding, including reading and writing. Aphasia may co-occur with speech issues related to brain damage, such as dysarthria or speech difficulty.

Aphasia is a language disability caused by damage to a specific area of the brain that controls language expression and interpretation. Aphasia makes it challenging for a person to communicate with others.

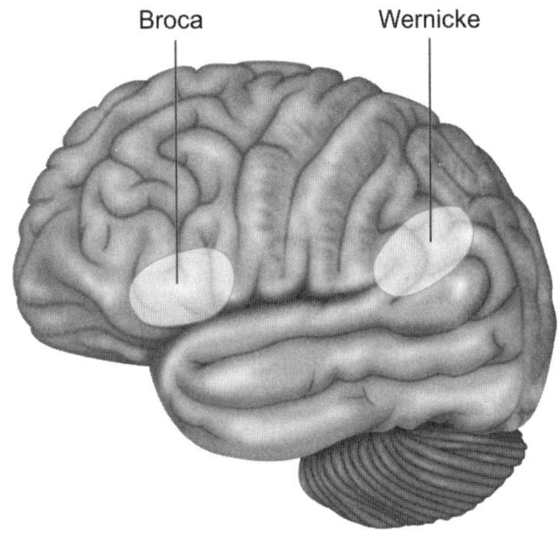

Types of Aphasia

Global Aphasia

This is the most severe kind of aphasia, while it refers to person who have little to no comprehension of spoken language and produce few familiar words. Worldwide aphasia prevents a person from reading or writing. Global aphasia is often present right away after a stroke, and if the damage was not too severe, it may quickly heal. Greater brain injury, however, may lead to severe and long-lasting impairment.

* Severe problems in using words.
* Severe problems in understanding words
* Limited ability to use a few words together.
* An almost non-existent ability to read or write.

Broca's Aphasia ('Non-Fluent Aphasia')

Speech production is significantly reduced by this type of complete aphasia, which is often limited to short utterances of about four words. Patients with Broca's aphasia have limited language access, and their speech synthesis is often challenging and imperfect. The person may read and understand, speech rather well; however their writing abilities could be limited. Speaking is difficult and halting with Broca's aphasia, which is why it's also known as a "non-fluent aphasia."

* Speak in short, incomplete sentences
* Able to convey basic messages but may be missing some words
* Have a limited ability to understand what others say
* Experience frustration because others can't understand them
* Have weakness or paralysis on the right side of the body.

Mixed Non-fluent Aphasia

Patients who talk laboriously and slowly, resembling severe Broca's aphasia, are given this designation. However, they have limited understanding of language and are unable to read or write at greater proficiency than that, unlike people who have Broca's aphasia.

* Have a limited comprehension of speech
* Can only read and write at a very elementary level

Wernicke's Aphasia

('Fluent Aphasia')

Understanding spoken words is challenging with this kind of aphasia, but producing connected speech remains unaffected. As a consequence, Wernicke's aphasia is known regarded as a "fluent aphasia". But the speech is not ordinary. The flow of the sentences is awkward, and extraneous words often obscure the meaning of the jargon. Reading and writing abilities are often seriously compromised.

* Being unable to understand and use language correctly
* Tending to speak in long, complex sentences that are meaningless and include incorrect or nonsense words
* Not realizing that others can't understand them
* Impaired reading and writing.

Anomic Aphasia

This label is given to those who consistently struggle to find the right words to express the very topics they wish to discuss particularly the important nouns and verbs. Their speech is thus full of hazy equivocations and frustrated sentiments while being proficient in grammar and production. They typically read well and have good verbal comprehension. Finding the right words may be challenging in both speech and writing.

* They can understand others' speech well.
* They can read well.
* Their difficulty in finding words is also evident in their writing.

Primary Progressive Aphasia

Language skills gradually deteriorate over time in a neurological disease known as *primary progressive aphasia (PPA)*. PPA is a kind of aphasia that develops from neurodegenerative illnesses like Alzheimer's disease or frontotemporal lobar degeneration, as opposed to other types of aphasia that are brought on by brain damage or stroke. PPA is brought on by the degeneration of speech and language-related brain tissue. Although speech and language issues are often the earliest signs of the illness, other symptoms, such as memory loss, frequently appear later.

Signs of Aphasia

Communication, language comprehension, reading, and writing difficulties may result from aphasia.

Communicating

Client may find that client go through one or several of these experiences:

* The client is having trouble thinking of the phrases they wish to use or is searching for words that are "on the tip of their tongue."
* Client uses the incorrect term. Sometimes, client may use a word with a similar meaning or pronunciation (for example, "fish" instead of "chicken" or "art" instead of "arm") in place of the original word. Sometimes, client may substitute a word (like "radio" for "ball") that is unrelated to the intended meaning or sound.

* Client alters word sounds. For instance, client may substitute "wish dasher" for "dishwasher."
* Client invents new words that are meaningless to other people (either when used alone or in conjunction with actual words, as in the case of the term "thratble").
* The client may repeat words or speeches.
* Client has difficulty forming whole phrases. It can be simpler for client to speak in simple language.

Understanding Spoken or Signed Language

Client may have trouble in doing any or all of the following tasks:
* Calling anything out by name.
* Adhering to instructions.
* Comprehending what the client's partner is saying, particularly if they are speaking quickly if the client is unfamiliar with the subject.
* Acknowledging when there are several discussing subjects or outside distractions.
* Understanding difficult to understand languages. Jokes, puns, irony, and expressions like "better late than never" are a few instances of this kind of language.
* Understanding the significance of words.

Reading and Writing

Client may have trouble in:
* Spelling and stringing words together to make sentences
* Making use of numbers or doing arithmetic
* Reading symbols, forms, books, and computer screens. It could be difficult, for instance, to tell the time, manage money, add or subtract.

Symptoms

Aphasia is a sign of another illness, such as a brain tumor or a stroke.

A person with aphasia may:
* Use terse or incomplete phrases while speaking.
* Speak in sentences that don't make sense.
* Substitute one word for another or one sound for another.
* Speak unrecognizable words.
* Have difficulty finding words.
* Not understand other people's conversation.
* Not understand what they read.
* Write sentences that don't make sense.

Causes

Possible causes for this include:
* Alzheimer's disease.
* Aneurysms.
* Brain surgery.
* Brain tumors (including cancer).
* Cerebral hypoxia (brain damage from lack of oxygen).
* Concussion and traumatic brain injury.
* Dementia and frontotemporal dementia.

- Developmental disorders and congenital problems (conditions that client has problem during fetal development).
- Epilepsy or seizures (especially if these cause permanent brain damage).
- Genetic disorders (conditions client have at birth that client inherited from one or both parents, such as Wilson's disease).
- Inflammation of client's brain (encephalitis) from viral or bacterial infections or autoimmune conditions.
- Migraine (this effect is temporary).
- Radiation therapy or chemotherapy.
- Toxins and poisons (such as carbon monoxide poisoning or heavy metal poisoning).
- Strokes or transient ischemic attacks (TIAs).

Diagnosis

- Blood tests (these can look for anything from immune system problems to toxins and poisons, especially certain metals like copper).
- Computerized tomography (CT) scan.
- Electroencephalogram (EEG).
- Electromyogram.
- Evoked potentials test.
- Genetic testing.
- Magnetic resonance imaging (MRI).
- Positron emission tomography (PET) scan.
- Spinal tap (lumbar puncture).
- X-rays.

Management

The goal of aphasia therapy is to help a person communicate more effectively by teaching them how to use their remaining abilities in language, recovering some of their impaired language skills, and utilizing alternate forms of communication including gestures, drawings, or technology. Individual treatment focuses on the patient's particular needs, while group therapy allows patients the ability to practice new communication techniques in a small-group setting.

Recent developments have made new tools available to people with aphasia. Patients of "virtual" language pathologists may get therapy at home with the convenience and flexibility of obtaining it online. The use of speech-generating software on lightweight gadgets like tablets may be a helpful alternative for those who have trouble speaking.

Patients are increasingly participating in literary organizations, tech groups, art and theater clubs, and other activities. Such interactions help patients restore their self-assurance and confidence in society, in addition to improving their communication skills. In a majority of large cities, there exist stroke clubs, which are neighborhood support groups created by stroke sufferers. These organizations can help an individual and their loved ones adapt for the changes in their lives brought through a stroke and aphasia.

Family involvement is a common part of aphasia treatment since it teaches loved ones the best methods to communicate with the person they are caring for.

Family members are encouraged to:
- To take part in counselling sessions.
- Simplify language by use short, straightforward statements.

* If necessary, repeat the crucial phrases or dot them down on paper to make the meaning clear.
* Continue to speak in a casual way that is suitable for an adult.
* Whenever feasible, reduce distractions like a loud music or TV.
* Participate in talks with the aphasic individual.
* Seek out and appreciate the aphasic person's input, particularly when it comes to family issues.
* Encourage all forms of communication, including sketching, pointing, gesturing, and talking.
* Refrain from modifying the speaker's speech.
* Give the speaker plenty of time to speak.
* Assist the individual in participating outside of the house. Look for support organizations, such clubs for stroke victims.

Tips for Communicating with a person who has Aphasia

These pointers could help to communicate and comprehend people more easily. Give your friends and relatives.

To help client understand, do these things:
* Before you speak, get their attention.
* Maintain a regular vocal volume. Unless the customer requests it, you don't need to speak louder.
* Use language that is straightforward yet mature. You shouldn't "talk down" to him.
* Go slowly.
* Only use brief phrases. Repeat the important phrases you want people to comprehend.
* Use facial expressions, writing, gestures, and visuals. Sometimes, they may be understood more clearly than words.
* When providing straightforward alternatives and ensuring that you get their message, use "yes" and "no" questions. As necessary, repeat their instructions back to them so they can verify your understanding.
* Provide them with options rather than asking them open-ended questions. Instead of asking, "What should we do this afternoon?" try asking, "Do you want some TV or go to the movies?"

To help client to communicate their thoughts, do these things:
* Give them some time.
* Take note of their motions and the client's body language.
* Refrain from finishing your clients' sentences.
* When a client is struggling, ask them to sketch, write, point, or make a gesture.
* Permit them to make errors. They may not always be able to express themselves correctly. The transmission of their messages is what matters.
* Allow them to take care of themselves. They may have to make several attempts. Only assist a client when they request it.
* Eliminating distractions (such turning on the TV or the radio) could improve their ability to speak and comprehend.

Transcranial magnetic stimulation (TMS), which is a noninvasive form of brain stimulation, is one new method that has also shown some promise when it comes to improving certain symptoms of aphasia.

ARTIFICIAL AIRWAY

For a number of individuals who need help keeping their airways open, artificial airways are employed. The insertion of an airway flap is indicated to alleviate blockage, enable lower airway suctioning, enable mechanical breathing and/or avoid aspiration. Endotracheal, tracheotomy, and the procedure tube are examples of artificial airways.

Any patient whose breathing mechanism has been drastically changed may need mechanical ventilation. Any ailment that hinders the patient from sustaining appropriate carbon dioxide (CO) and oxygen (O_2) levels in the circulatory system might result in this change. Patients who are unable to defend their airway may additionally need mechanical breathing.

Airway management is an essential technique for clinicians taking care of individuals in critical situations and emergency medicine. Airway management involves a series of maneuvers and medical procedures used to maintain or restore airway functionality. Airway management may be required in situations of airway obstruction, respiratory distress, or when the individual is under sedation. Depending on the clinical presentation of an individual, basic or advanced forms of airway management may be used.

Basic airway management techniques are non-invasive, whereas advanced airway management techniques are invasive and require specialized medical equipment, such as oropharyngeal airway (OPA), nasopharyngeal airway (NPA) and endotracheal airway (ETA). Bag valve mask ventilation serves as another approach to prevent inadequate ventilation, which can result from impaired breathing or airway obstruction. The most effective and commonly used method of airway management involves the use of rapid sequence intubation (RSI), which involves endotracheal intubation (ETI) and medications to induce unconsciousness and muscle relaxation.

Indications for an Artificial Airway

There are four traditional indications for an artificial airway:
1. Provide ventilatory support.
2. Aid in the removal of secretions.
3. Bypass upper airway obstruction.
4. Prevent aspiration.

Types of airway include:
❖ Oropharyngeal

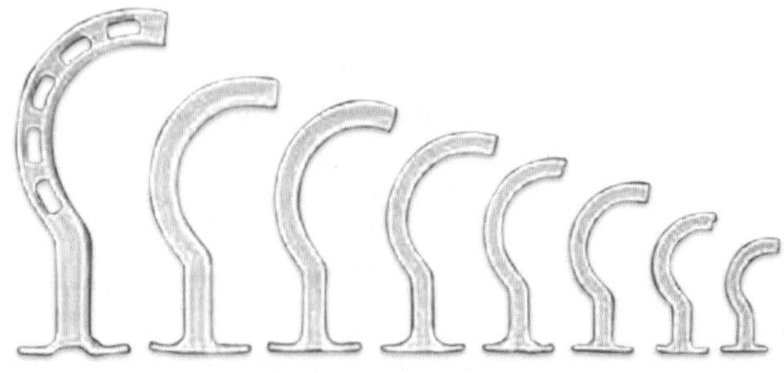

❖ Nasopharyngeal

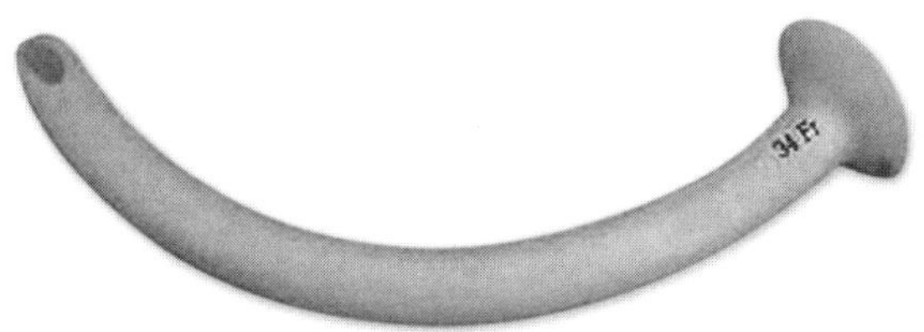

❖ Endotracheal tube

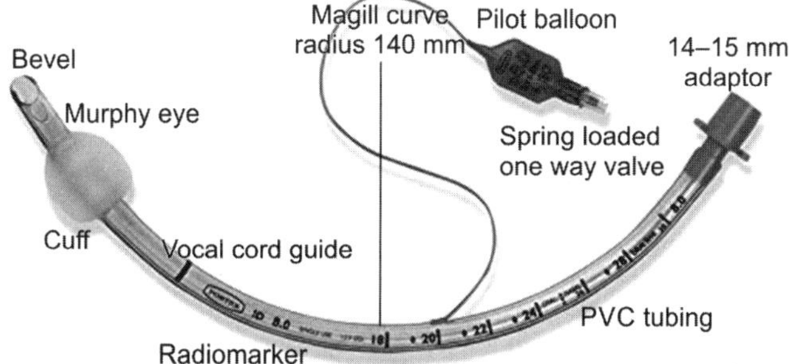

❖ Laryngeal mask airway

Name	Type	Image	Material	Advantages	Disadvantages
LMA Classic	First generation		Silicone	Original design, less pharyngolaryngeal trauma, respiratory problems vs. ETT, rescue device	Low OSP, increased cost with processing
LMA Unique	First generation		Polyvinyl chloride	Disposable form of classical LMA	Low OSP

Contd...

Contd...

Name	Type	Image	Material	Advantages	Disadvantages
LMA FasTrach			Polyvinyl chloride and silicone	Intubating LMA to guide blind, difficult intubation	Bulky, no pediatric sizes, increased cost of processing
LMA Flexible			Polyvinyl chloride and silicone	Wire-reinforced tubing, head and neck procedures	Low OSP, increased cost with processing
LMA ProSeal	Second generation		Silicone	Gastric suction port, built in bite block, high OSP	Bulky, folding of mask can obstruct the gastric port, increased cost of processing
LMA Supreme	Second generation		Polyvinyl chloride	Disposable version of ProSeal LMA	Bulky, folding of mask can obstruct the gastric port

❖ Cricothyroidotomy

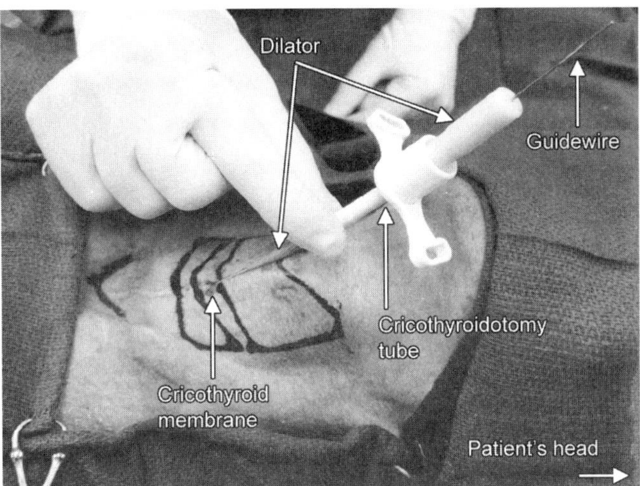

❖ Tracheostomy

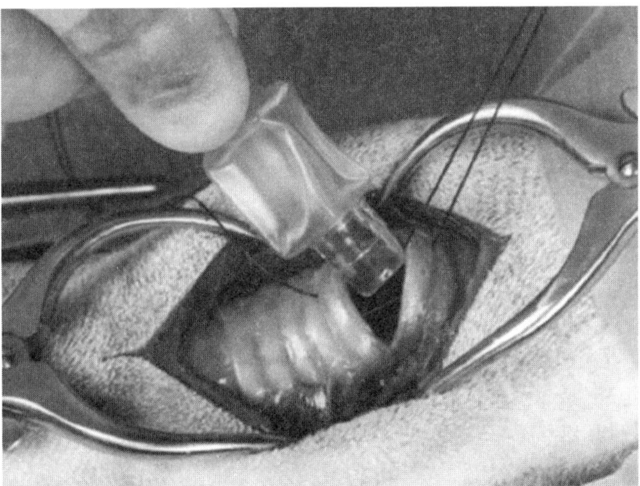

Choice of airway depends on various factors:

❖ Try nasopharyngeal breathing on a patient who has evidence of airway blockage but who is still reasonably aware.

❖ Try oropharyngeal airways for the patient if there is evidence of airway blockage and diminished level of awareness.

❖ Needs an endotracheal tube and intubation if they are unconscious or unable to safeguard the airway.

Background

- Assessment, planning, and procedures to maintain/restore ventilation
  - Essential in critical situations and emergency medicine
- Necessary during airway obstruction, respiratory distress or sedation

Types of artifical airways

Oropharyngeal airway (OPA)

Nasopharyngeal airway (NPA)

Endotracheal airway (ETA) with intubation

Management scenario

Basic
(non-invasive)

- Chest compressions
- Abdominal thrusts
- Back blows
- CPR
- Head-tilt/chin-lift
- Jaw-thrust
- Bag valve mask

Advanced
(Invasive and specialized)

- Laryngeal mask airway (LMA)
- OPAs and NPAs
- ETA with intubation
- Rapid sequence induction (RSI) of anesthesia and intubation
- Cricothyrotomy
- Tracheotomy

Communication

The Importance of Communication

❖ Sharing experiences, events, ideas, and emotions via verbal (sounds, words, sentences) and nonverbal (body language, tone of voice, touch) channels is referred to as communication.

❖ Interaction among humans is made possible via communication. Controlling, sharing emotions, informing, comprehending, envisioning, and maintaining social interactions are just a few of the many purposes fulfil.

❖ For a patient to provide informed consent for their treatment in a medical context, communication is a crucial ability.

❖ Patients who need tracheostomies are severely incapacitated and unwell. Due to the side effects of the medication and the severe nature of their illness, patients may become physically weak and need to be admitted to the intensive care unit (ICU). Despite the fact that this is a short-term circumstance, and many people may recover well, the psychological impacts might endure a long time. The inability to express oneself is among the hardest things for individuals to deal with. Due to the patient's incapacity to engage in goal planning, therapy, and end-of-life choices, communication problems are also linked to a longer stay in the intensive care unit.

❖ If necessary, the patient and/or family members should be told prior to the tracheostomy operation that because air is no longer traveling through the vocal chords, the patient/relatives may not be able to speak while the tracheostomy tube stays place (a patient consent sheet is advised). They should be reassured that, excepting cases where a laryngectomy has been done, it is anticipated that the voice will be back once the tube is withdrawn or otherwise altered, and that, in the meantime, the nursing staff, medical personnel, and family members would offer the patient with alternate communication methods.

❖ Various patient requirements, such as "social interaction, material giving, reassurance, discussion of feelings, advice, and counselling," are met via communication.

❖ The purpose of communication in critically ill patients is in order to assist them maintain a sense of self as well as mental in nature structural, personal, and social integrity

❖ The patient's psychological condition must be taken into account since they could be unable to talk and are often nervous in a hospital setting. As a communication professional, a language and speech therapist's mission and duty is to promote communication and provide fair communication and individual time for every patient. Initial evaluation of the tracheostomized patient often takes place in a critical care environment, thus it is important to examine the patient's medical condition and ensure that the assessment is practical and flexible enough to meet the patient's demands.

Non-verbal Communication

Lip Reading

Request that the patient make louder lip motions. Encourage the use of succinct, comprehensive phrases to help the reader understand the information.

Facial Expression and Gestures

Focus on the patient's body language and facial expressions, which will supplement their "mouthed" words with additional information.

Coded Eye Blink or Hand Gesture

When you ask the patient a question, instruct them to blinked once for "yes" and twice for "no". As an alternative, think about using the patient's hands to clearly indicate "yes" and "no" by giving them the thumbs up or down.

Alphabet Board, Picture Board and Phrase Books

Laminating A4 sheets with the alphabet in bold letters or plain images of necessities (such water, toilet paper) may help them last longer. A list or book of helpful words for the patient (such as "Please call my husband") might be used in addition to these methods. Each patient's communication board may be customized by the speech and language therapist.

Electronic Larynx and Electronic Communication Aids

The speech and language therapist must determine if the patient needs to use one of these tools before providing recommendations on how to utilize it to the patient, their family, caregivers, and other staff members, as required. These aids may not be suited for short-term usage since using them requires the person using them to gain the necessary degree of proficiency.

Verbal Communication

Manipulation of Tracheostomy Tube for Communication

When a patient has a tracheostomy tube in place, at least one of the following techniques may be used to produce voice:

Cuff Deflation

On expiration, air will be able to enter the upper airway thanks to the deflation of the tracheostomy tube's cuff. Air will be guided into the larynx to produce phonation, but some air may leak out via an open tracheostomy, which might result in a weaker voice.

Fenestrated Tracheostomy Tube

By using a fenestrated tracheostomy tube, air may also enter the upper airway during expiration, creating voice. If an inner cannula is not fenestrated, it must be removed. It is necessary for the fenestration to be patent since, in certain cases, it may come in touch with the membrane of the trachea and prevent ventilation. Try to clear the fenestration, the patient's head and shoulders might be adjusted again.

Downsizing of Tracheostomy Tube

The use of a thinner tracheostomy tube will increase the amount of air that passes between tube and tracheal walls during exhalation, but it will also raise the amount of labor required to breathe because of more resistance to air flow. Therefore, the MDT will need to be consulted about this.

Intermittent Finger Occlusion

The tracheostomy tube may often be intermittently blocked with a gloved finger to enable successful voice in many people. The patient must have a fenestrated a breathing tube (with a fenestrated inner cannula) situated if they are unable to tolerate glove deflation before using this procedure.

One-Way Speaking Valve

The use of one-way speaking valves with tracheostomized and ventilator-dependent patients is quite beneficial. The capacity of the patient to withstand cuff deflation determines whether or not a one-way speaking valve should be used.

This particular speaking valve functions in a one-way manner, opening on inspiration to let air enter the airway by the tracheostomy and closing on expiration to force air into the throat and larynx to enable phonation.

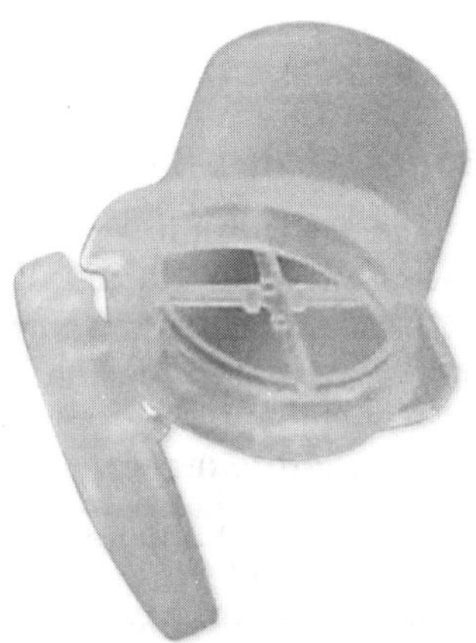

One-way speaking valve.

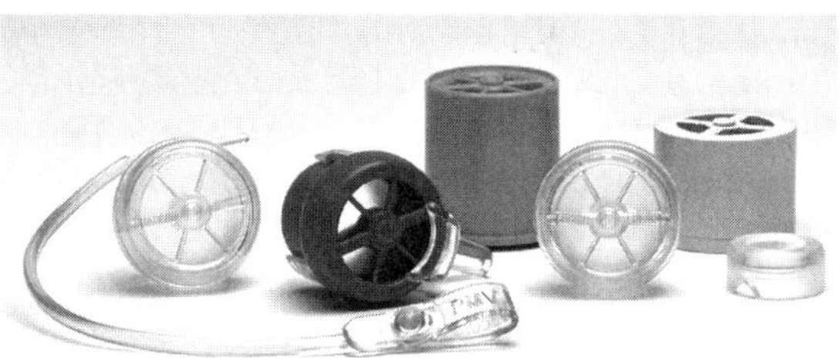

"Passy Muir" tracheostomy and ventilator speaking valves.

For the patient who is ventilator dependent and can tolerate cuff deflation, the "Passy-Muir" valve should be considered.

Talking Tracheostomy Tube

Vocal aid tracheostomy tubes should be used in patients who cannot tolerate cuff deflation (such as ventilated patients). For the purpose of phonation, air is given above the cuff from an outside source. This would enable the tracheostomized patient to speak, however the voice might be faint due to the restricted airflow.

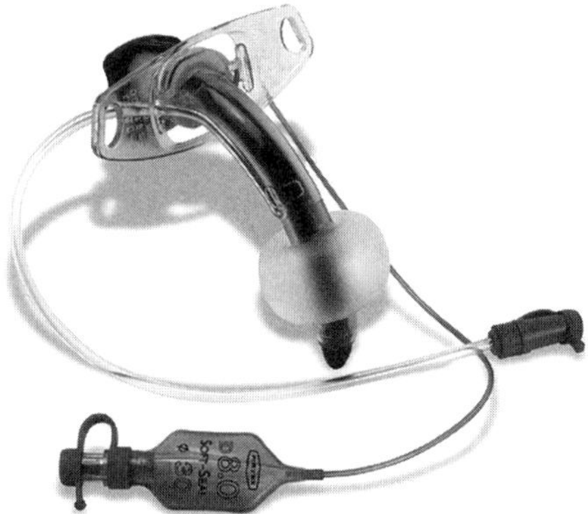

Vocaloid/Suctionaid Blue Line Ultra® tracheostomy tube.

The speech and language therapist is going to able to advise and counsel patients on how to develop the best communication system for them.

I. **Procedure for using a one-way speaking valve—self ventilating patient**

Action

Rationale
- A pulse oximeter must be used to monitor the patient's SpO$_2$ levels.
  To determine the patient's accurate baseline condition.
- The patient must, wherever possible, thoroughly comprehend the method and how it works, therefore explanation is crucial.
  Lowering the patient's anxiety, which may affect the quality of voice output.
- A medical opinion should be acquired before deflating the cuff when employing a non-fenestrated tube and the inner cannula ought to be eliminated if it is not fenestrated.

A voice cannot be created if the cuff is full while employing a non-fenestrated tube because air cannot travel through the vocal chords. The patient's breathing will be hampered.

- In the usual way, insert this over the speaker valve if humidified or fresh air is needed. Maintaining a same setting for the individual being evaluated through the evaluation.
- After inserting the speaking valve, advise that patient to breathe in via the tube attached to their tracheostomy and slowly exhale through their mouth.
  In particular, if the tube that connects to the tracheostomy has been kept in place for a while, the patient won't be used to regular breathing.
- Asking a client to say "ah" or count from "one" to "five" is a trial phonation technique. For the patient, automatic speech like counting is often simpler than spontaneous speech.
- Ask the patient to cough and remove any secretions if they have a "wet" or "gurgly" sounding voice.
  Any secretions that can impede vocal clarity are present.
- Pay close attention to the weaning strategy and communicate with all of the team members about it.

Remove the speaking valve if:

- Respiratory difficulty occurs.
- SpO$_2$ levels decrease.
- The patient becomes fatigued.
- The patient requests it.

Always follow the recommendations provided by the speech and language therapist in the weaning plan, medical records, and nursing notes.

At the conclusion of the trial time, if necessary, remove the mouth valve and re-inflate the tube attached to the tracheostomy cuff following the MOV approach while monitoring cuff pressure.

- The speaking valve should be cleaned, dried, and stored in an appropriately labeled, sealed container in accordance with the manufacturer's instructions.
- Record each step taken in the weaning plan.
- To make sure the diverse team communicates well.

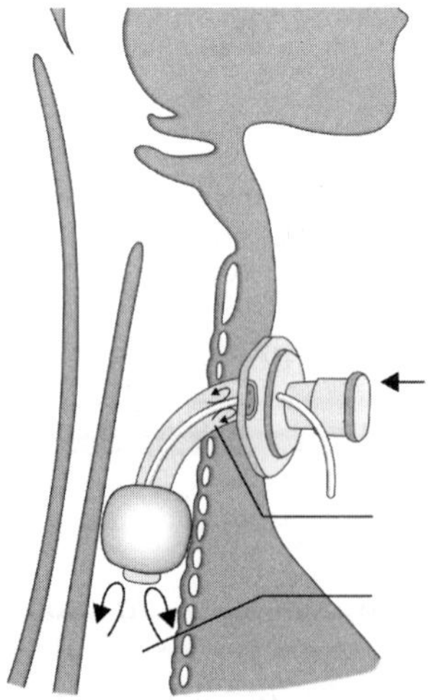

Incorrect speaking valve used in the presence of an inflated cuff preventing exhalation

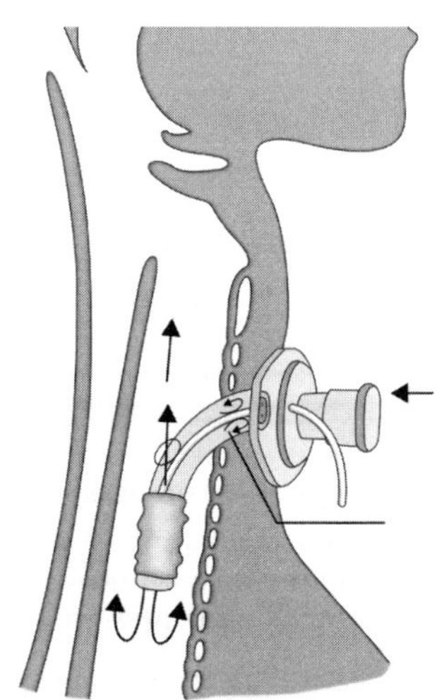

Correct speaking valve with cuff deflated

II. Procedure for using a Passy Muir Speaking Valve inline with ventilator

Action

Rationale

- Obtain medical approval before beginning the operation.
  To guarantee that the patient is safe to endure cuff deflation and ventilator modifications, the patient must be healthy and weaning off mechanical ventilation.
- The patient must, wherever possible, thoroughly comprehend the method and how it works, therefore explanation is crucial.
  Lowering the patient's anxiety, which might affect the quality of voice production.
- Check for signs of decreased airway patency in the patient's history, bronchoscopy findings, and ABGs.
  The patient should ideally be on arterial support of between 15 and 18 cm H_2O with no more than 8 cm H_2O of PEEP.
- Check RR/HR/SpO_2
  To ensure within normal limits for the patient.
- Determine potential changes to ventilation modes and O_2 therapy.
  To allow for air leak within the ventilator system.
- Suction orally and via tracheal tube prior to cuff deflation.

To ensure minimum residual secretions during procedure:

❖ **Cuff deflation procedure**

- Slowly deflate cuff while carrying out synchronous suction. Check for airflow at mouth
- Know your ventilator
- It is best to use the NIV mode on your ventilator while using the Passy Muir valve.

To ensure that cuff deflation is tolerated. Signs of intolerance:

❖ Increased coughing

❖ Increased respiratory rate

❖ Respiratory effort

❖ Need for suction increases

❖ SpO_2 levels decrease
  If signs of intolerance are observed, please remove valve, re-inflate cuff and do not proceed without further reassessment.

❖ Once the patient is tolerating cuff deflation insert the Passy Muir valve into the ventilator circuit as close to the trachea as possible.

❖ Assess patient's ability to phonate.

To ensure supraglottic airflow. Remove the speaking valve if:

❖ Respiratory rate/effort increases

❖ Heart rate rises

❖ SpO_2 levels decrease

❖ Patient experiences distress/discomfort

❖ No supraglottic airflow

❖ Weak/breathy/hoarse voice

❖ Inspiratory/expiratory stridor

❖ The patient requests it

- If the patient's voice sounds "wet" or "gurgly" ask them to cough and clear secretions
- Any secretions present may adversely affect voice clarity

Remove the speaking valve if:

- ❖ Respiratory difficulty occurs
- ❖ SpO_2 levels decrease
- ❖ The patient becomes fatigued
- ❖ The patient requests it

At the conclusion of the trial time, if warranted, remove the articulation valve and, if necessary, re-inflate the tube that connects to the tracheostomy cuff using the minimal occlusion volume (MOV) procedure.

- ❖ Clean, dry, and store the speaking valve in the box given by the manufacturer with the patient's name on it, as directed by the manufacturer.
- ❖ Record each step taken in the weaning strategy.
- ❖ The diverse team's good communication must be ensured.
- ❖ When using this valve, the cuff must first be deflated, as specified by the aquamarine label included in the spoken valve pack, if the first trial is profitable and it is decided to continue using it.

Contradictions for speaking valve use:

- ❖ Inability to tolerate full cuff deflation
- ❖ Airway obstruction
- ❖ Unstable medical/pulmonary status
- ❖ Laryngectomy
- ❖ Severe anxiety/cognitive dysfunction
- ❖ Anarthria
- ❖ Severe tracheal/laryngeal stenosis
- ❖ End stage pulmonary disease.

COMMUNICATION WITH VISUAL IMPAIRMENT

DO's

Ask your patients how they want to receive their medical records, treatment protocols and other information materials. Options include:

- ❖ Large print—at least 18-point true type font such as Arial or Calibri.
- ❖ By email—check what file format is best for the individual. Understand how to create accessible documents, and ensure the content is screen reader and high contrast accessible, especially that all images include descriptive alt text.
- ❖ Audio—a digital file can be provided by email or given on a thumb drive/CD.

Hospitals should have procedures in place to enable patients as well as professionals to ensure everything is done properly since providing medical documents in accessible formats is a legal obligation in many countries.

Independent access to one's own health records safeguards that person's right to privacy and control over their personal data.

Talk about a workable method for marking prescriptions with your patient, and make sure they or someone on your team arranges this with the pharmacist. Options consist of:

- ❖ Attach two rubber bands and tags to a package of twice-daily pill dosage instructions.
- ❖ Use Tacti-mark or an equivalent ink-pen which become tactile when dry to mark the package. This lowers the chance of mistake if indications like elastics or stickers are misplaced.
- ❖ Print the instructions in braille; many blind or vision-impaired patients and parents cannot read braille.

❖ Help the person receive instruction in the competent use of a label-reading tool like Seeing AI. Be aware that using such an app might take time since the phone's camera has to be properly focused on the label. This can't be feasible if medicine has to be taken soon.

❖ Encourage the person to get a grant for a hearing labeler or scanner.

❖ Encourage the person to create an organized system for storing at home to make it easier to find various drugs. Since medicine may be moved even with meticulous monitoring, this shouldn't be the sole way to identify it.

DON'T Leave out visual information from medical consultations or from your descriptions of rooms or objects because you think the person can't use it.

If you would display and explain imaging scans, pictures, or anatomical diagrams to a parent or patient who is seeing, then do the same for the person who is blind. By doing this, you can guarantee that they get the same amount of information as everyone else while also letting them know that this information is included in the patient's medical file. The individual might advocate by requesting that photos or drawings from various time periods be compared in the future.

When describing a medical doll that a blind mother can employ to play alongside her seeing child, be sure to include specifics like "she wears a red shirt" or "blue shoes." The parent may remember that information and use it to widen the kid's play enjoyment beyond the strictly medical focus and help the youngster acquire a sense of color. When explaining the procedure room, bring up the seascape picture on the wall; the parent may then use that information to keep their child amused while waiting for procedures.

I've seen medical experts make gestures toward objects in the room that I shouldn't have been able to see, or they would show my companions items like a picture without explaining it to me. Saying something like, "This is what's inside of your retina," takes just a brief amount of time. The area where we reattached it during surgery is displaying a healthy pink color.

DO Let them feel the equipment beforehand if you can, and explain the technique you will be doing to them. Specify each action you intend to do, the body part it will effect, and if it is going to influence the left or right limb or eyesight. Do not yell, but rather explain sounds and quiet periods.

In order to best promote coping for both mother and kid while treating a child whose parent has visual impairment, ask the parent in advance how they and the kid would want the stages of the process narrated, and by whom. In this circumstance, speaking with *ONE VOICE* and paying close attention to both the child's and the parent's needs is very beneficial.

DON'T be impatient. Show empathy and collaborate with the person to consider their requirements in order to have a good conversation or process. This can seem like a routine, uncomplicated procedure to you, but your patient nor their parent could have a totally different perspective. Every routine medical encounter might be traumatizing after years of distressing conversations and intrusive treatments, particularly if retinoblastoma was discovered when the patient was a young kid. The passing of time will not automatically lessen that dread and worry, but how you interact with the person might have an impact.

It is still challenging to deal with the trauma from treatments. They attempted to place the breathing apparatus on me while I was still somewhat "with it" after surgery a couple of months ago. I managed it after promptly freaking out. I was immediately transported back to my childhood as a child waiting to undergo anesthesia so that my eyes could be examined by a doctor thanks to the scent, the air, and the tightness of the mask. No fun.

DO Possess a high level of empathy! Imagine yourself at a medical facility: wearing a provocative medical gown that exposes your butt, being completely reliant, and having bed baths. People sometimes think that those who are blind or have visual problems are unintelligent or incapable of speaking for themselves.

DON'T When assessing their eyesight, request that they cover their prosthesis eye or attempt reading with it. Giving them such straightforward guidance shows you have not taken the time to learn about their fundamental cancer history. Even while the operation is routine for ophthalmic surgeons, it is crucial for parents and children, and even when an individual has full vision on one more eye, it may still be a highly emotional event decades later. Do not think if the past is over.

Listen to the patient's health files if you haven't got time to read them. If someone tells people they have a prosthetic for the eye, so it don't make matters worse by asking that to cover their viewing eye or take it out so you can check their vision. Both are dreadfully typical occurrences.

DO Always have the patient hear what you put in their health record out loud. Parents and patients who have been sighted may read this booklet and note any mistakes. People who are blind or have reduced eyesight cannot. As a result, when writing, read the piece aloud and respect the other person's freedom to bring up a topic for clarification, debate, or a query.

DON'T Assume that a parent or patient who is blind or vision-impaired cannot handle their own medical care. If allow the person to do each stage of the treatment until they are comfortable if they need to conduct it at home. As you guide them through the process, ask for their assistance in determining any modifications that may be required. It can take a bit more time and patience, but in the long run, it will relieve a lot of tension for everyone.

DO Always explain things to young blind or vision impaired patients. There is no guarantee that parents will tell their children and teenagers the truth about cancer and long-term risks, or that the facts they offer will be accurate or comprehensive. Engaging cancer patients and survivors early on helps clarify our health experience along with medical history and inspires us to be strong, accountable healthcare advocates throughout our lives.

Until I was older and attending appointments by myself, my physicians often spoke to my parents without ever explaining anything to me.

DON'T Inform your patient that since they have retinoblastoma, they shouldn't have children. Regardless of a person's health or impairment, choosing to be parental is a personal decision. The patient should be sent to a geneticist that's knowledgeable in retinoblastoma genetics after you as a medical expert have explained the facts and hazards relevant to the individual's genetic condition. Then you should take a step back.

Do not provide advice on family planning if you are not talking about retinoblastoma genetics and if the individual does not ask for it. Family planning choices are made by the person and the couple, not by the medical staff, the survivor's family, or the partner's friends. Expressing opinions, particularly before the person has accepted the ramifications of the RB1 mutation, may be very damaging psychologically.

Offering Assistance

DO Ask the person if and how they need assistance. Never ask a question of a companion ("does she...") or make conclusions about the person. If the individual is sitting, stay standing or, if it's feasible, take a seat close to them. Never stoop or hunch over to talk. Many teenagers and adults with disabilities find this stooping/crouching stance, which an adult may assume while addressing a kid, to be quite offensive. Sitting next to us sends a subtle message of equality and respect.

If the individual needs help, say hello, introduce yourself, and inquire. The other party will either accept or reject your offer. If assistance is asked, pay attention to their answer and provide it as required. If the request is rejected, don't take it personally; it was made with prudence and respect, so it will probably still be valued.

DON'T Touch canes/guide dogs or distract guide dogs. People who are blind or visually impaired may use a cane or a guide dog as an independence aid to safely navigate their surroundings. Moving it without the individual's awareness or seizing hold of it to "guide" the person puts them at risk for harm and adds needless stress to their life.

Guide dogs are taught to obey their handlers' commands and make choices that will keep them safe. If they are distracted, they can't do this task successfully. No matter how cute and appealing the dog may be, or even if it looks to visitors that the dog is at ease, always ask the person who is handling it before establishing eye contact to, speaking to, or petting their dog. Be careful not to take the handler's "no" personally; they are just trying to keep the working atmosphere conducive for both the dog or themselves.

DO Before you start, always ask the individual how they like to be led and pay close attention while they explain. You might provide guiding help by saying, "Would you like to take my arm?" The individual would often request that you release your arm (just above your elbow). In this situation, let your arm rest comfortably by your side. Follow your normal walking speed.

It is improper and impracticable to take someone's arm without their permission since doing so puts them one step beyond you. You go forward a step by extending your arm. Even if you neglect to mention variations in the landscape, slopes, stairs, etc., the person who are leading will be better equipped to notice them.

Verbal signals with specificity are still extremely valuable. For instance, the fact that a gradient is moving up or down rather than merely that it is approaching. In my research, many individuals confuse terms like "incline/decline," "ascending/descending," etc., and giving the wrong directions may be just as harmful as giving no instructions at all. Simple "up/down" is what I like since I can depend on it.

DON'T Point or say "over there" when giving directions. To make sure you left and right directions are clear, stand facing the identical direction as the individual whom you are guiding. If you want to assist the person turn in the proper way so they may go directly to their destination, you might also offer them to take their arm ("Would you be willing to give my hand so I can point to the correct direction?").

Make your descriptions precise and clear. For example, "The desk is just ahead of you, about 20 walks around, the floor has no trace of obstacles within here and there", or "To get to the stairs, follow the corridor straight on for about 30 meters, past the coffeehouse on the right." Because there is a housekeeping cart inside the coffeehouse, stay on your left of the hallway. Straight ahead, via the double doors. The elevator bank is on your right, and the stairs are immediately on your left.

DO Describe the layout of a room. Navigation may be made simpler and safer, while communication can be improved with a quick explanation of how the decor is set up. For instance, the following may be used to describe a conference room: The room is rectangular and the short wall back us. We find ourselves at the uncovered end of the U-shaped table. There are full-length windows from floor to ceiling along the left side, and another exit door is located halfway down the right wall.

Describe any barriers in a person's path as well (and eliminate them if you can). Be sure to leave enough space around risks and obstructions and to glance both up and below. Inform people if there are any overhangs, such as panels or cabinets, or if there are protruding side mirrors on the automobiles and trees outside. Allow precise directions and allow the other person enough time to reply. The phrase "bend your head low so as to prevent the branch of the tree coming up from your left" is an example.

DON'T Touch or hold someone forcefully when providing assistance. Just tell them verbally what to do. To help them choose a seat, you may say something like, "The back of the chairs is directly in the middle of you, and the seat is directed away from you. Would you mind for me to guide a hand to the upper part of the chair?" Whenever more help is required, extend it. Usually, this is sufficient, and the individual may take a seat by themself.

DO Describe what's happening around you. Recognize that if they can't see what's happening, they will be at a disadvantage. So, discuss what is going on. You may make us feel more at ease in circumstances that are unfamiliar to us (and perhaps to you) by describing what others are doing, how they are wearing, and how they are grouped (in small groups, big groups, standing, etc.).

In order to feel more at ease and integrated when they are in a new (social) environment, sighted persons often mimic the body language and behavior of others. Blind persons may need some covert assistance to learn what to anticipate and how to behave in certain, unfamiliar circumstances.

DON'T In a social environment when everyone is standing, seat the individual at a table without first seeking their choice.

Even though they are near by, a person without sight loss may feel as if they are being "talked down to" due to the height disparity. Describe the situation, who is there, and the available alternatives before letting the individual make a choice. Think about if a few of the group members could eat with the individual at the table.

DO Offer to collect refreshments for the person at events where food and beverages are served. Once you have explained what is available, ask the individual what they have would want you to do. Some guests may want to circle the buffet table alongside you to sample everything, especially if they're following dietary restrictions, while others could want a selection with more precise instructions, such "vegetarian only." Follow their directions and avoid choosing any food items they have expressly requested that you avoid; doing so will make them uncomfortable and agitated and, if they have allergies, might be quite harmful.

DON'T Because you believe it will take an excessive amount of time to describe every alternative, you restrict the choices you provide. Think about your reaction if this had occurred to you. Most individuals are aware of their goals. Give a broad picture by reciting menu headers or summarizing the primary alternatives in a table to assist the person in reducing their selections. On the buffet table, there are three plates of sandwiches—one each of meat, vegetarian, and seafood—along with sausage rolls, crisps, an assortment of cakes, or green leaf salad. For instance: Pastas, salads, and sandwiches are the menu categories.

DO Tell the person when you have items to place near them, especially food or drinks. Let them advise you on the ideal location for the gift so they can find it simply and securely. Keep in mind that the individual may be left-handed and/or have vision in only one eye. Describe the temperature of the plate or cup and the direction the handle is pointing. If there are laptops or other gadgets on the table, it's crucial to let the individual know that you have beverages to set down.

DON'T Totally fill glasses or mugs. Contrast may make it simpler for someone with some eyesight to determine how full a mug is. Black tea and coffee are more visible in a light mug, whereas milky liquids are more visible in a dark cup.

CARE OF UNCONSCIOUS PATIENTS

Being conscious is being aware of oneself and one's surroundings as well as having the capacity to react to outside stimuli.

Syncope: Syncope is the medical term for a transient loss of consciousness followed by a spontaneous return.

Unconsciousness: Reduced attentiveness, the capacity to be awakened, or a lack of awareness of yourself and the surroundings are all examples of impaired consciousness.

A temporary or permanent loss of consciousness accompanied by a disruption in self and environmental awareness.

When a person unexpectedly loses the ability, to react to stimuli and looks to be sleeping, they are said to be unconscious. A person may lose consciousness of himself and their surroundings completely or partially.

A person may faint briefly or lose consciousness for a prolonged amount of time. Shaking or loud sounds have no effect on someone who is unconscious. They could even stop breathing or develop a weak pulse.

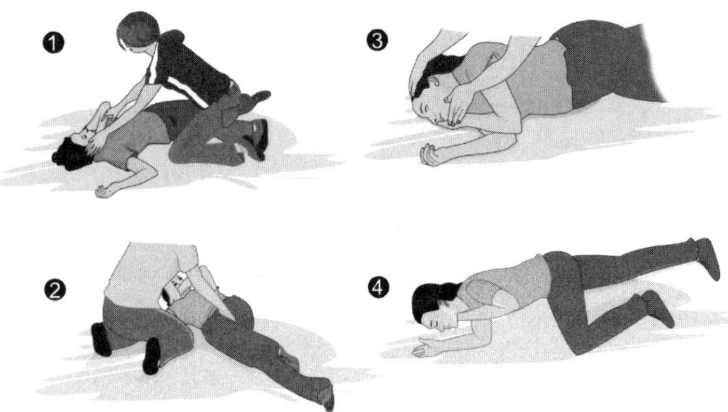

Unconsciousness is a state in which a living individual exhibits a complete, or near-complete, inability to maintain an awareness of self and environment or to respond to any human or environmental stimulus.

Causes of Unconsciousness

The two cerebral hemispheres, the bilateral thalami, or a transient or permanent defect of the reticular stimulating system located inside the brainstem are often what causes unconsciousness. It is possible to distinguish between systemic illness and localized structural pathology in the brain as the reasons of an unconscious patient.

Structural

These factors either directly injure a region or produce indirect harm by compressing nearby tissue or raising intracranial pressure. The global cerebral flow of blood is hampered by elevated intracranial pressure, which may also encourage tissue deformation and brain herniation.

❖ Stroke
❖ Traumatic brain injury (TBI)

- ❖ Intracranial, epidural, subdural hemorrhages
- ❖ Intracranial tumors
- ❖ Inflammation
- ❖ Venous thrombosis
- ❖ Acute hydrocephalus.

Systemic

- ❖ Hypoglycemia
- ❖ Hyperglycemia
- ❖ Hyponatremia
- ❖ Hypernatremia
- ❖ Hypercalcemia
- ❖ Seizures
- ❖ Systemic infections (sepsis)
- ❖ Meningitis
- ❖ Encephalitis
- ❖ Adrenal crisis
- ❖ Pituitary apoplexy with pituitary hormonal insufficiency
- ❖ Endocrine abnormalities
- ❖ Myxedema coma
- ❖ Medication overdose
- ❖ Illicit drug use
- ❖ Neuroleptic malignant syndrome
- ❖ Excessive alcohol intake
- ❖ Hepatic encephalopathy
- ❖ Uremia
- ❖ Heavy metals (lead poisoning)
- ❖ Malaria
- ❖ Fungemia (aspergillosis)
- ❖ Herbicides
- ❖ Gases (carbon monoxide)
- ❖ Anesthesia

Psychiatric

- ❖ Catatonia
- ❖ Severe depression
- ❖ Conversion disorder
- ❖ Malingering

Pathophysiology

The pathophysiology of sleepiness is caused by neuronal dysfunction, which is caused by a decrease in the quantity in glucose or gas reaching the brain. Coma may be brought on by structural lesions involving the nervous system, which may harm the brain's arousal regions directly or inadvertently by secondary damage brought on by intracranial movement, vascular compression, or increased intracranial pressure.

Arousal occurs in the brainstem, namely in the ascending circular stimulating system. The neurons of this system have their beginning in the dorsal, the pons and midbrain, which connect to the thalamus in the brain, then project to a multitude of cortical areas. The process of receiving, integrating, and contextualizing the information received by the brain results in awareness. The reticular activating structure, which enables it to be aware of its environment, receives signals from the spinal cord and brain.

Three major regions of the brain are affected by the many factors that result in an unconscious patient:

Bilateral Hemispheric Damage/Effect

Brain trauma or hypoxic-ischemic injury may cause substantial harm to the bilateral brain's cerebral cortex, which results in the death of neurons and de-innervation of the affected cortical areas. These individuals become incapable of processing stimuli and consciously reacting to them. This group also includes the systemic root causes of coma because they result in an aberrant physiological milieu that impairs neural function. If the underlying systemic issue can be treated, this kind of pattern is often reversible.

Diencephalic (Thalamic) Injury

Therefore, bilateral thalamic injuries may mirror the effects that result from bilateral cortical injury because the thalamus has relay nuclei that route afferent information to the cortex.

Upper Brainstem Injury

The system that activates the reticular retina is located in the midbrain and dorsal pons. This region is susceptible to injuries that impair awareness and cause comatose states.

Clinical Menifestations

The following symptoms may occur after a person has been unconscious:
* Amnesia for (not remembering) events before, during, and even after the period of unconsciousness
* Confusion
* Drowsiness
* Headache
* Inability to speak or move parts of the body (stroke symptoms)
* Lightheadedness
* Loss of bowel or bladder control (incontinence)
* Rapid heartbeat (palpitations)
* Slow heartbeat
* Stupor (severe confusion and weakness)

If the person is unconscious from choking, symptoms may include:
* Inability to speak
* Difficulty breathing
* Noisy breathing or high-pitched sounds while inhaling
* Weak, ineffective coughing
* Bluish skin color

Risk Factors

- ❖ High blood pressure
- ❖ High cholesterol
- ❖ History of stroke
- ❖ Diabetes
- ❖ Heart disease
- ❖ Smoking

Stages of Unconsciousness

- ❖ Clouding of consciousness
- ❖ Confusional state
- ❖ Delirium
- ❖ Lethargy
- ❖ Obtundation
- ❖ Stupor
- ❖ Dementia
- ❖ Hypersomnia
- ❖ Vegetative state
- ❖ Akinetic mutism
- ❖ Locked-in syndrome
- ❖ Coma and brain death.

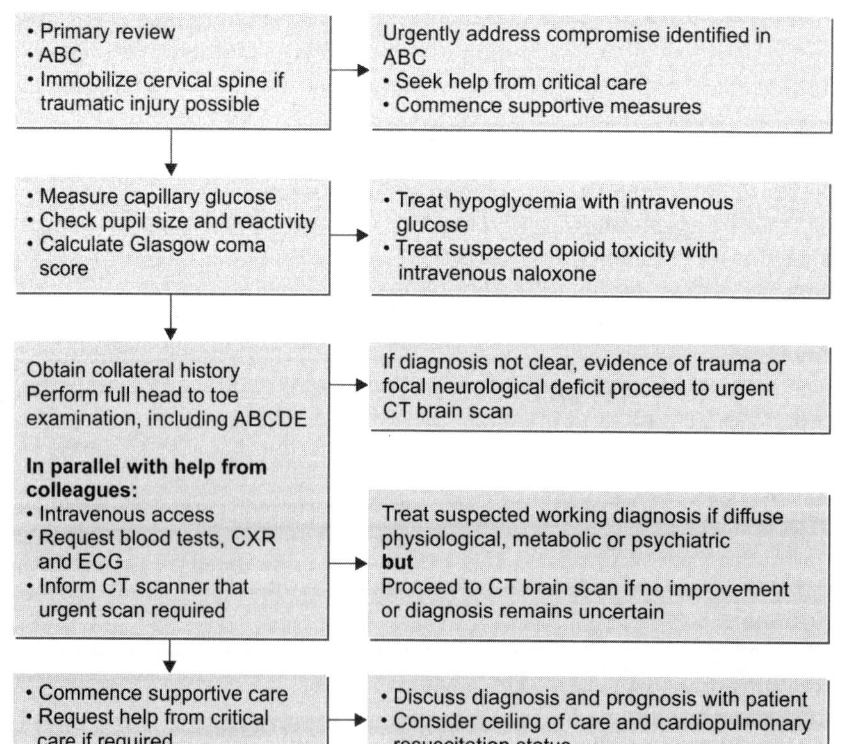

Assessment of Unconcious Patients

General principles of initial assessment and management: The history, examination, investigation, and treatment/management—the four essential elements of care should take place simultaneously.

Teams caring for unconscious patients should use an organized and systematic ABCDE (airway, breathing, circulation, disability, exposure) strategy. Specific therapies as well as supportive care must not be postponed.

History

It is crucial to get a second-hand account from family members or other witnesses, such as paramedics.

Recent health, functional condition, and prior medical history of the patient may provide diagnostic hints as well as help in making choices about follow-up treatment, such admission to a unit for critical care.

Urgent requests for previous medical records must be made, and next of kin must be informed.

From pooled primary-care information, hospital pharmacists may learn about patients' prescription histories. While paramedics are competent at searching the site for evidence like empty medication packets, booze, or a suicide note, bystanders may have seen the patient fall.

Examination

Following the first ABC evaluation, the Glasgow Coma Scale (GCS) should be used to properly gauge and record the patient's degree of consciousness.

Nurses utilize the Glasgow Coma Scale (GCS) to determine a patient's level of consciousness. The level of consciousness (LOC) of our patients may be continuously assessed at the bedside utilizing this approach in conjunction with other clinical observations. Since over 40 years ago, the GCS has been used in medical facilities all around the world.

Utilizing a universal assessment method enables physicians to measure the level of care (LOC) of patients under our care and results in a common comprehension of patients' circumstances.

Behavior	*Response*	*Score*
Eye opening	Spontaneous	4
	To sound	3
	To pressure	2
	None	1
Verbal response	Orientated	5
	Confused	4
	Words	3
	Sounds	2
	None	1

Contd...

Contd...

Behavior	Response	Score
Motor response	Obey commands	6
	Localize to pain	5
	Normal flexion	4
	Abnormal flexion	3
	Extension	2
	None	1

The chart above illustrates the three main components of the GCS: The evaluation of eye opening up, verbal response, and motor reaction.

The pupillary response, vital signs, and limb power are further indicators.

We will be focusing on the three core areas of the GCS:
1. Eyes opening (scored from 1–4)
2. Verbal response (scored from 1–5)
3. Motor response (scored from 1–6)

Behavior	Minimum Score	Maximum Score
Eye opening	1	4
Verbal response	1	5
Motor response	1	6
Total	3	15

An unconscious patient's gaze and gaze patterns cannot be evaluated in their entirety. If there is no chance of a neck injury, the doll's eyes with the oculocephalic reflex might have been checked. Eyes that loiter in the midorbital position and an absence of conjugate eye movement away from the direction the head moves suggest brainstem dysfunction. A fundoscopy should be performed if subarachnoid hemorrhage or posterior reversible encephalopathy syndrome (PRES) with papilledema or subhyaloid hemorrhage are discovered. Examining the pupil may help in diagnosis:

* Small pupils (<2 mm)—opioid toxicity or a pontine lesion
* Midsize pupils (4–6 mm) unresponsive to light—midbrain lesion
* Maximally dilated pupils (>8 mm)—drug toxicity, e.g. anticholinergic overdose
* Mixed and dilated pupil(s)—3rd (oculomotor) nerve lesion from uncal herniation.

Even if the unconscious patient has certain regions that are particularly relevant, a thorough examination must be done. Hepatic encephalopathy may smell musty, whereas organophosphate poisoning could smell like garlic. A comprehensive investigation into other potential causes of unconsciousness ought to go on when the breath indicates alcohol usage. Even in the event of a history or falls or external injuries, a cerebral bleed in older persons, particularly those using anticoagulant medication, is nevertheless quite likely to occur. However, bruising and other signs of mild trauma are often present in elderly patients, which should serve as a warning sign for more severe cerebral disease. The presence of myoclonus or generalized tremor suggests a metabolic etiology. Drug injection sites may be visible on skin examination.

The pattern of breathing should be assessed as well as the respiratory rate.

❖ Kussmaul respiration—deep, labored breathing, indicative of severe metabolic acidosis and commonly associated with diabetic ketoacidosis.

❖ Shallow with an extremely depressed respiratory rate seen in opiate overdose.

❖ Ataxic breathing (Biot's respiration)—groups of quick, shallow inspirations followed by regular or irregular periods of apnea, suggesting a lesion in the lower pons.

❖ Central neurogenic hyperventilation—breathing characterized by deep and rapid breaths at a rate of at least 25 breaths per minute indicating a lesion in the pons or midbrain.

❖ Cheyne-Stokes breathing is seen with many underlying pathologies and is not helpful in making a firm diagnosis.

Investigations

Investigations support diagnosis, severity evaluation, and care monitoring. To rule out hypoglycemia, a bedside capillary test for blood sugar must be completed before contemplating any other investigations. A structural pathology ought to always be taken into consideration if the reason of unconscious is not clear from the first quick examination and urgent brain imaging is necessary. The examination of choice to rule out frequent diseases such intracranial bleeding, stroke, or space-occupying lesions is computed tomography (CT) of the brain. A MR scan may be necessary for further imaging if the CT brain scan results are normal but the diagnosis is still not obvious. When the reason of unconsciousness is still unknown or an internal nerve disease is suspected, a puncture to the lumbar spine should be taken into consideration if there are no medical conditions that would prevent it.

Initial Investigations in an Unconscious Patient

❖ Full blood count
❖ Blood glucose—even if the capillary blood glucose is normal
❖ Urea and electrolytes
❖ Calcium and bone profile
❖ Liver function tests
❖ Clotting screen
❖ Toxicology screen including paracetamol, salicylate and blood alcohol level electrocardiogram (ECG) > chest X-ray
❖ Arterial blood gas—including carbon monoxide concentration
❖ Blood cultures should be taken from patients with fever or suspected sepsis, preferably before the administration of empirical antibiotics
❖ Other microbiology samples should be taken based on the clinical assessment.

In suspected instances of non-convulsive status epilepticus, electroencephalography (EEG) should be carried out. In this situation, persistent seizure activity occurs without any visible motor symptoms. Older patients are more likely to experience it. Clinically, patients exhibit myoclonic twitches, lip-smacking, and an appearance of staring into space.

PUPILLARY RESPONSES

Different sized pupils relate to different types of lesions; pinpoint pupils occur in pontine. While cancers and some overdoses (e.g., opioid, clonidine); fixed mid-sized pupils hit in midbrain lesions; one dilated pupil suggests cranial nerve III compression; examples include intracerebral hemorrhage, polycystic ovarian morphology, aneurysm, or raised ICP. (Parasympathetic nerves reside at the surface sections of the nerve, making them more susceptible to compressive lesions; ptosis and 'down and out' eye placement are less common since the more central motor nerves are not damaged.)

OCULAR DEVIATION AND DYSCONJUGATE GAZE

Dysconjugate Gaze

Dysconjugate gaze is challenging to interpret when dealing with a stuporous or vegetative patient due to the fact that most people experience some exophoria while sleepy for whatever cause.

Tonic Deviance

❖ A lesion, often a stroke, in the same hemisphere and the eye deviation in the frontal lobe. Since Todd's eyes often wander in the other direction following a seizure, away from the source of the "irritative" attention, this may be the result of Todd being paralyzed after the seizure.
❖ On the side whereby the pupils are turned out, there is a pontine lesion. Another side effect of thalamic hemorrhage is "wrong way eyes. "The oculocephalic or oculovestibular reflexes cannot be activated to correct the lateral gaze deviation brought on by a pontine lesion, in comparison with supranuclear lesions (such as frontal lesions). They might thus be recognized clinically.

Skewed Departure

Skew deviation, also known as a vertical split of the ocular axis, may be a sign of a medial continuous fasciculus lesion on the side of the top eye or a pontine or vestibulocerebellar illness on the side of the lower eye.

Additionally, cranial nerve palsies (CN6 is especially vulnerable owing to its lengthy travel) and orbital entrapment from trauma may cause abnormal eye position.

Oculovestibular Reflexes

Oculocephalic Reflex ('Doll's Eye' Reflex)

❖ The patient's eyes should remain open, the C-spine should be unobstructed, and the head should be swiftly moved from side to side while being held still shortly at the end of each revolution. The brainstem (CN3,6,8) is in good condition when the vision rotates in the opposite direction from the direction of head rotation. When the heads are flexed and extended, a similar reaction is seen; a positive lead is a downward deviation of the pupils during extension and an upward deviation during flexion. These vertical responses demonstrate the brainstem's (CN3,4,8) intact status.
❖ The eyes should travel smoothly and conjugately return to their mid-position if the brainstem is still intact. Patients who are in a metabolic coma (caused, for instance, by liver failure) may have heightened rapid oculocephalic reflexes.
❖ Oculovestibular reflex (caloric stimulation)—the head is raised up to 30 degrees above the horizontal position to ensure the angle of the lateral semicircular canal is vertical in nature and that stimuli will result in the maximum response; the tympanum is intact; the outer

canal of the ear is clear; C-spine clearance is not necessary; and iced water is inserted by a small catheter to the external ear canals until one of the following occurs:

- Nystagmus, when the slow wave is directed toward the irrigated ear in an undamaged brainstem.
- Eye-movement deviation

❖ As consciousness fades, the fast component—which was moving in the direction of the non-irrigated ear is eliminated, and the slow period tonically moves away from the eye and moves in the direction of the irrigated ear.

❖ Allow 5 minutes before testing each ear to allow the oculovestibular system to re-adjust.

One method to measure vertical oculovestibular ocular responses is to concurrently irrigate both ears.

❖ If the spinal cord is intact, the eyes will deviate in either a downward or upward direction depending on the temperature.

Limitations

❖ Deep metabolic coma, brainstem encephalitis, and several medications may all simulate brainstem death.

❖ Anticonvulsants that have recently been administered include barbiturates and phenytoin. Similar to phenytoin, vestibulotoxicity from aminoglycosides and tricyclic overdose may lead to bilateral vestibular failure. The effects of a baclofen overdose may mimic brain death.

❖ A blowout fracture that has imprisoned the extraocular muscles is another caution that applies to trauma patients.

Below figure from Posner et al. (2008) illustrates typical results for different lesions:

	Oculocephalic responses				Caloric responses			
	Turn right	Turn left	Tilt back	Tilt forward	Cool water			Warm water
					Right side	Left side	Bilateral	Bilateral
A Brainstem intact (metabolic encephalopathy)								
B Right lateral pontine lesion (gaze paralysis)								
C MLF lesion (bilateral internuclear ophthalmoplegia)								
D Right paramedian pontine lesion (1½ syndrome)								
E Middrain lesion (bilateral)								

Spontaneous Eye Movements

Corneal Reflex

Corneal reflex is of limited use:
- ❖ In coma, loss in the cornea sensation is often an elderly sign. Assessment regular contact lens wearers may have decreased corneal reflexes.
- ❖ Corneal stimulation is traditionally accomplished by stroking a cornea with cotton wool. However, applying a few droplets of pure saline to the eyeball over a height of 10 cm is a less unpleasant option. If someone blinks and the lids roll up, the natural response is still active.
- ❖ The reflex route includes the trigeminal neuron, which is the CN5 nucleus of the spinal column, the lower midline tegmentum, as well as the CN3 and CN7 nuclei, demonstrating that the pons or the middle brain is intact. A CN7 lesion, often known as Bell's phenomenon, occurs when the eye moves up but the lid remains shut.
- ❖ A CN5 lesion exists if the eyelid cannot close and the eye is not pointing upward.

Gag Reflex

- ❖ Sensory = CN9, motor = CN10
- ❖ May be absent in normal people and those accustomed to an endotracheal tube
- ❖ Best assessed using a laryngoscope and a tongue depressor in intubated patients, look for bilateral palatal elevation.

Cough Reflex

- ❖ Mediated by CN10
- ❖ Can be stimulated by a suction catheter down and endotracheal tube.

Motor Responses

Posturing can occur spontaneously or in response to a stimulus:
- ❖ Decorticate posture, which involves adduction of one's arm, internal twisting of the shoulder, pronation. This of one's forearm, and bending of the wrist, is indicative of a lesion above the cerebellum.
- ❖ Decerebrate posture, also known as extension, is characterized by the flexion of the arm, rotated outside of the armpit, supination of the upper arm, extension of the wrist, and extensions of the lower limbs. This posture denotes a lesion that has reached the midbrain.

Assess for:
- ❖ Tone
- ❖ Clonus
- ❖ Deep tendon reflexes
- ❖ Plantar reflexes
- ❖ Involuntary movements (such as subtle signs of seizures and myoclonus). Look for asymmetry.

Signs of the Underlying Cause

- ❖ Consider the neurological findings in regard to the patient's vital signs, any trauma or shock symptoms, chronic or acute illnesses, and/or drug use. Also consider cranial scars, gutters, ICP monitors, and VP shunts. Also consider neck stiffness, track marks, drugs, and toxidromes, a ventilator, and

❖ The fundi should be examined for subhyaloid blood loss, papilledema, and diabetic or hypertensive retinopathy.

MANAGEMENT OF UNCONSCIOUS PATIENT

Immediate Management

❖ Maintenance of airway: clear airway (oropharyngeal suction) if necessary.
❖ Maintenance of breathing:
  ◆ Only neck extended and lateral position if respiration is ok.
  ◆ Mouth to mouth breathing, O_2 inhalation, intubation, tracheostomy if necessary.
❖ Maintenance of circulation: Cardiac pulmonary resuscitation, secure IV channel and start normal saline if appropriate.
❖ If dehydration by vomiting—cholera saline.
❖ If overhydrated—diuretics
❖ Maintain intake/output chart.
❖ BP, if SBP > 240 mm of Hg and DBP >120 mm of Hg then reduce BP, otherwise not necessary, if BP does not comes to normal even after first week then start antihypertensive agents.
❖ Blood glucose maintaining >11.1 mmol/L it reduces by insulin (increased blood glucose-increased infarction).
❖ Carefully move the individual toward you into their side if they are breathing and laying on their back and you do not believe there's a spinal injury. The upper leg should be bent until your knees and hips are at 90 degrees. To keep their nostrils open, gently tilt one's head back. Roll the individual onto his back and start doing CPR if their breathing or pulse cease at any point.
❖ As long as the individual is still breathing, leave them the way you found them if you suspect a spinal injury. If the individual throws up, roll them to their side all at once. As you roll them, support the spine and neck to maintain alignment of the head and body.
❖ Maintain the patient's warmth until emergency assistance comes.
❖ Aim to stop a person from falling if you notice them about to faint. Raise the person's feet by approximately 12 inches (30 cm) and place them level on the ground.
❖ If fainting is likely due to low blood sugar, give the person something sweet to eat or drink only when they become conscious.

If the person is unconscious from choking: Begin CPR. Chest compressions may help dislodge the object.

If you find anything loosely obstructing the airway, attempt to get rid of it. Don't attempt to grab the item if it's stuck in someone's throat. This can force the item farther into the nostrils.

Until emergency aid comes, keep doing CPR and checking to see whether the item has been moved.

General Treatment

❖ First pay attention to airway, breathing, circulation.
❖ Maintenance of **nutrition**—give the patient Ryle's tube feeding 2 hourly. Liquid diet is given the help of 50cc syringe adequate carbohydrate and high protein should be present in diet.
❖ Care of skin—change the posture of the patient 2 hourly. Keep the skin dry and clean.
❖ Care of mouth—antifungal agent is used to prevent candida infection.
❖ Care of eye—chloramphenicol eye drop to prevent exposure keratitis.
❖ Care of bowel—bed pan is used to prevent soiling of cloth.
❖ Care of bladder—catheterization is done.
❖ Control of infection by antibiotic.

Care of Terminally Ill, Death and Dying

UNIT OUTLINE

- Loss
- Grief, bereavement and mourning
- Theories of grief and loss–Kübler-Ross
- Five stages of dying
- The R process model (Rando's)
- Death
- Dying patient's bill of rights
- Care of dying patient
- Physiological changes occurring after death
- Death declaration, certification
- Autopsy
- Embalming
- Last office/death care
- Counseling and supporting grieving relatives
- Placing body in the mortuary
- Releasing body from mortuary
- Overview–medico-legal cases, advance directives, DNI/DNR, organ donation, euthanasia

LEARNING OBJECTIVES

At the end of this unit, the reader will be able to:

- Define terminal illness.
- Describe loss.
- Enumerate sources and factors influencing loss.
- Describe grief and grief cycle.
- List out reactions of grief.
- Classify types of grief.
- Lineout symptoms of grief.
- Explain factors affecting grief and loss.
- Describe bereavement.
- Define mourning.
- Explain Six "R" process by Rando.
- Define dying.
- List down types of dying.
- Recognize signs of impending death.
- Propose bill of rights of dying person.
- Practice care of dying patient.
- Explain end of life care.
- Define changes following death (algor mortis, livor mortis, rigor mortis, Putrefaction, decomposition, mummification).

- ◆ Analyze death declaration and certification.
- ◆ Explain autopsy and types.
- ◆ Define benefits of autopsy.
- ◆ Describe embalming and types.
- ◆ Define last office.
- ◆ Counseling for grieving persons.
- ◆ Interpret guidelines for placing and relieving body from mortuary.
- ◆ Define advance directives.
- ◆ Explain DNR/DNI.
- ◆ Describe organ donation.
- ◆ Identify medico-legal cases.
- ◆ Define ethunasia and types of ethunasia.

INTRODUCTION

A terminal illness is an illness or condition which cannot be cured and is likely to lead to someone's death. It is sometimes called a life-limiting illness.

Examples of some illnesses which can be terminal include:

- ❖ Advanced cancer
- ❖ Dementia (including Alzheimer's)
- ❖ Motor neurone disease (MND)
- ❖ Lung disease
- ❖ Neurological diseases, like Parkinson's
- ❖ Advanced heart disease.

Medicines and treatments people receive at the end of life can control pain and other symptoms, such as constipation, nausea, and shortness of breath. Some people remain at home while receiving these treatments, whereas others enter a hospital or other facility. Either way, services are available to help patients and their families with the medical, psychological, social, and spiritual issues around dying.

Although everyone has individual requirements, the majority of people who are dying have certain concerns.

Dread of desertion and dread of becoming a burden are two of these worries. People who have dread worry about losing their autonomy and their sense of dignity. Here are a few ways caregivers might reassure someone who is experiencing these fears:

- ❖ Keep the individual company. Discuss, watch a movie, read a book, or simply hang out with them.
- ❖ Allow the individual to voice their worries and anxieties about passing away, such as leaving behind family and friends. Prepare yourself to listen.
- ❖ Be open to talking about the person's past.
- ❖ Do not withhold sensitive information. The majority of patients like to participate in conversations on topics that matter to them.
- ❖ Reassure the patient that you will honor advance directives, such as living wills.
- ❖ Ask if there is anything you can do.
- ❖ Respect the person's need for privacy.

❖ Support the person's spirituality.

❖ Let them talk about what has meaning for them, pray with them if they'd like, and arrange visits by spiritual leaders and church members, if appropriate. Keep objects that are meaningful to the person close at hand.

The experience of dying is unique for each individual. One person's experience may not apply to another. Additionally, the existence of any one of the aforementioned symptoms does not always indicate that someone is in danger of passing away. Caregiver and family members may learn more about what to anticipate from an aspect of the medical team. Terminal patients often need a caregiver, who could be a nurse, licensed practical nurse or a family member. Caregivers can help patients receive medications to reduce pain and control symptoms of nausea or vomiting. They can also assist the individual with daily living activities and movement. Caregivers provide assistance with food and psychological support and ensure that the individual is comfortable.

Withdrawal from friends and family: In the later weeks of life, people often turn inward. This does not imply that the patients are always hostile, unhappy, or unloving of their caretakers. It could be brought on by reduced blood flow, decreased brain oxygenation, or mental death planning.

They can stop enjoying things they formerly did, including their favorite TV programs, friends, or pets.

The patient should be informed that the caregivers are there to help. Even if they are unwilling to communicate, the individual may still be awake and able to hear. Giving people permission to "let go" might be beneficial, according to experts. If they want to speak, they may wish to discuss their past triumphs and tragedies or complete unfinished business.

Sleep changes: People may have drowsiness, increased sleep, intermittent sleep, or confusion when they first wake up.

Patients may have insomnia due to worries or fears. They might be asked whether they want to sit within the spot with them when they nod off by caregivers.

As time goes on, patients could sleep more and more. Even if a patient is unconscious, caregivers should still speak to them since the patient could still be able to hear them.

Hard-to-control pain: As the disease progresses, pain management may grow more challenging. Regular administration of pain medicine is crucial.

For guidance on the proper medications and dosages, caregivers should request an appointment with a pain specialist or palliative care physician.

Investigating alternative pain management strategies like massage and relaxation techniques may be beneficial.

Increasing weakness: Over time, weakness and exhaustion will worsen. The patient could have good and terrible days, which means they might need extra assistance with everyday hygiene and mobility.

Caregivers can help patients save energy for the things that are most important to them.

Appetite changes: A person with cancer often has less of a desire for and need for meals as their body gradually slows down. The body's urge to save energy and declining capacity to use meals and liquids correctly lead to the loss of appetite.

The decision of whether and when something to eat or drink should be left up to the patient. Small portions of the patient's favorite meals may be provided by caregivers. They might enjoy milkshakes, sorbet, or pudding since chewing requires energy.

Offer sips of liquids if the patient has no problem in swallowing, and if they can not sit up, use a flexible straw.

Offer ice chips if someone's swallowing becomes difficult. Keep their mouths clean with a gentle, wet towel and their lips moisturized with lip balm.

Awareness: People often experience moments of bewilderment or waking nightmares as they approach death. They can become uncertain about the date, the location, or the identities of loved ones. Patients may be gently reminded of their location and their companions by their caregivers. They need to exude serenity and assurance. However, they shouldn't try to restrain a patient who is upset. In order to assist reduce or reverse considerable agitation, let the medical professionals know if it happens.

Patients may claim to have seen or spoken with deceased relatives. They could discuss traveling, seeing lights, bugs, or other invisible markers of reality. Caregivers may ask the patient to talk more as long as it doesn't disrupt them. Instead of attempting to convince them otherwise, they may allow them to share their dreams and visions.

Incontinence: The pelvic muscles relaxing may lead to a loss of urination nor bowel control. Continue to offer gentle personal care and clean, dry bedding as directed by caregivers. Disposable pads may be placed on the patient's bed and taken off as they get dirty. The volume of urine may also decrease as a result of slowed renal function or reduced fluid intake. It could smell strongly and be dark.

Cycles of slower or quicker breathing may occur. Even though the patient might not be aware of the changes, caregiver should let the medical professional know that they are concerned. Saliva and fluids accumulating in the back of the throat and the upper airway may generate rattling or gurgling noises. The patient is often not in discomfort at this point, despite the fact that it may be quite upsetting for caretakers. If a person's torso is shifted to one side and cushions are positioned under and behind the head, breathing could be made easier. If a patient has trouble breathing because they are out of breath, caregivers may also inquire with the medical staff about utilizing a humidifier or an outside source of oxygen.

As blood flow decreases, skin may take on a cold, blue hue. The patient doesn't feel pain or discomfort because of this. Electric blankets and heating pads should not be used to warm the patient since they might result in burns. However, they could continue to keep the patient wrapped in a thin blanket.

MANAGEMENT

For terminal conditions, there is, by definition, neither a cure nor an effective therapy. However, certain medical procedures, such as those that facilitate breathing or relieve pain, could be necessary regardless.

Some individuals with terminal illnesses quit all debilitating therapies to lessen adverse effects. Others continue aggressive treatment in the hope of an unexpected success. Still others reject conventional medical treatment and pursue unproven treatments such as radical dietary modifications. Patient's choices about different treatments may change over time.

Palliative care is normally offered to terminally ill patients, regardless of their overall disease management style, if it seems likely to help manage symptoms such as pain and improve quality of life. Hospice care, which can be provided at home or in a long-term care facility, additionally provides emotional and spiritual support for the patient and loved ones. Some complementary approaches, such as relaxation therapy, massage, and acupuncture may relieve some symptoms and other causes of suffering.

LOSS

Introduction

Life events that create change in a familiar pattern of existence all can be experienced as loss, and all can trigger behaviors associated with the grieving process.

Anything that is perceived as such by the individual.
- ❖ Throughout our lives, from birth to death, we form attachments and suffer losses.
- ❖ Universal phenomenon
- ❖ Different for different individuals—the separation from loved ones or the giving up of treasured possessions, for whatever reason:
  - ◆ Loss is the fact of no longer having something or having less of it than before. Loss is the feeling of sadness you experience when someone or something you like is taken away from you.
  - ◆ A loss is the disadvantage you suffer when a valuable and useful person or thing leaves or is taken away.
  - ◆ Loss is defined as the experience of parting with an object, person, belief or relationship that one values. The object may be animate or inanimate, a relationship or situation, or even a change or a failure (real or perceived).

Types of Loss

- ❖ Actual loss – Can be recognized by others as well as the person sustaining the loss
- ❖ Perceived loss – Sense of loss felt by the individual but not tangible to others.
- ❖ Physical loss – Loss of a part or aspect of the body, such as loss of an extremity in an accident, scarring from burns.
- ❖ Physiological loss – Emotional loss, such as woman feeling inadequate after menopause and resultant infertility
- ❖ Anticipatory loss – A person displays loss and grief behaviors for a loss that has not yet taken place. It is often seen in families of terminally ill patients.

Categories of Loss

There are four major categories of loss:
1. Loss of aspect of self
2. Loss of significant others
3. Loss of external objects
4. Loss of familiar environment

Factors Influencing a Loss Reaction

Significance of loss:
- ❖ Age of the person
- ❖ Value placed on the lost person

* Degree of change required because of loss
* The person's beliefs and values, culture
* Customs of expression of grief
* Family structure
* Family and social roles
* Spiritual beliefs
* Death rituals
* Gender differences
* Socioeconomic status affects support system available
* Coping skills, previous experiences of loss
* Emotional stability
* Physical health

Sources of Loss

* The loss of an aspect of one self—a body part, a physiologic function or psychologic attribute.
* The loss of an object external to oneself
* Separation from an accustomed environment
* Loss of loved or valued person

GRIEF

Grief is defined as a state of mental or emotional anguish brought on by loss or regret. It is specifically used to describe the grief and loss brought on by the loss of someone you love.

People who are overwhelmed by grief are often described as grief-stricken. This kind of grief is most commonly associated with death, but the word can also be used in the context of other situations involving loss, such as a divorce or the loss of a job.

The related verb grieve means to mourn to feel or express intense grief, especially due to a death or loss.

The sadness experienced after the loss of someone you cherish is specifically referred to as grief. Additionally, it is often used colloquially to denote difficulty or irritation.

A normal response to losing anyone or anything is grief. Grief may be brought on by a material loss, such as passing away, or an interpersonal loss, such as losing a job or a relationship.

The term "grief" first appears in writing about 1,200. Its root is the Latin verb gravare, which means "to burden," derived from the noun gravis, "heavy." The adjective grave, which means "serious," and the word gravity both derive from the same root.

Elisabeth Kübler-Ross, a psychiatrist, created the widely accepted view that there are indeed five phases of mourning. The five phases of mourning, according to Kübler-Ross, are as follows:

Denial (At this point, it might be difficult to accept that what happened really occurred)

Anger (This includes resentment that it occurred to you)

Negotiating (This may entail considering "what if" scenarios and attempting to find a method to change what has already occurred)

Depression (This is the sadness that results from realizing that what has occurred is true and that there is nothing that can be accomplished to alter it)

Acceptance (This phase entails accepting what has occurred and making an effort to move on)

The Grief Cycle

Kübler-Ross (1969, 1975) outlines five phases of loss that a person goes through when they learn they are about to die.

Indeed, a person's life experiences, the schedule of their death with respect to life events, the foreseeable nature of their death depending on health or disease, their point of view, and their evaluation of the value of their own life all have an impact on the process of dying. However, by comprehending these phases, we may better understand and identify some of the psychological experiences of the dying, which will make it easier for us to assist them as they pass away.

When faced with shocking, unfathomable news, denial is frequently the first response. By allowing the news to spread slowly and giving us time to process what is happening, denial, disbelief, or shock shields us. Even when they are aware that the findings are accurate, people who obtain positive tests for fatal illnesses may doubt them, seek second views, or just experience psychological denial.

Fury also gives us the energy to struggle against things and provides structure to an incident that might not otherwise be leaving us in an atmosphere of disbelief. Being furious is more simpler than being unhappy, in suffering, or depressed. It gives us a false feeling of power over the future and the satisfaction of having at least voiced our outrage at how unjust life can be. Anger might be directed towards a specific individual, a medical professional, God, or the whole universe. Being at this stage of grief is not always clear since it might be expressed over things that have nothing connection with our dying.

Negotiating involves considering various ways to make the situation better. If doing so will increase one's life expectancy, one may consciously decide to live more successfully, contribute more of herself to a trigger, or be a better friend, parent, or spouse. When bartering, one could just require to live enough time to see an occasion with relatives or finish a task. If this __, then this—thought pattern may occur at this stage of the mourning process. For instance, "I'll do anything to stop the pain" or "I'll never commit sin ever if my companion is spared." "What if" remarks are a method of negotiation. What if, for instance, we discovered the cancer earlier? alternatively, "What if the incident never happened?" These "what ifs" are a means to discuss the desire for life to resume its previous course.

After such an event, it's appropriate to experience sadness or depression. The full intensity of loss, crying, and losing interest about the natural world are all major aspects of dying. Family members may attempt to soothe their loved one since depression makes other people feel very uncomfortable. In order to minimize depression at this time, psychiatrists are sometimes administered as a component of hospice care. Although seeking assistance may be the best course of action, this form of sadness is not an indication of a mental disorder. It is a fitting reaction to such a tragic loss. A person may become isolated from their regular routines and experience acute grief. It would be strange if you didn't experience any depression right away after losing a loved one. The moment of feeling sad is a critical one in the grieving and healing process. Healthcare practitioners must be able to discern between patients who are depressed and feeling basic grief and those who are experiencing more complicated grief. Learn to see early indications of suicidal thoughts, and if you're unsure, ask. As necessary, make the relevant resources available.

Acceptance requires learning to deal with and incorporate this aspect of life into daily existence. Reaching acceptance does not imply that persons who are dying are at ease or content with their circumstances. It shows that they are managing it, keeping up their plans, and interacting with others as necessary. Some terminally ill people find that once they get to this stage, they enjoy their lives more fully than before. Acceptance need not imply that one is "okay with what has happened." A person might never completely recover after a loss. They may never experience "OK" grief. The stage of acceptance is understanding that this is what they have become and that it is irreversible. Although life cannot continue as it always did so, it can and will continue with acceptance. The roles will change. There will be new partnerships and connections formed. People that are accepting themselves realize that they need to listen to what they want and change. Even though some days may be more difficult than others, someone who has allowed their sorrow the time it needs to heal will start to live again.

According to Kübler-Ross (1969), underlying these five stages, which are concentrated on the acknowledged emotions, there is a sense of hope.

Common Reactions to Grief

There is no one right or incorrect method to grieve after a loss, and there also is no particular length of time that constitutes a "normal" period of mourning. There are several typical grieving responses, even though everyone feels loss differently:

Grief may affect sleep patterns, alter stress hormone levels and health, and result in physical symptoms such as weakness, difficulty breathing, restlessness, and changes to the immune system.

Strong feelings may come to the surface, including depression, loneliness, anxiety, concern, or even hatred and rage. Some people may feel guilty, as if they are betraying the person who has gone away, when they start engaging in activities and relationships again after a time of bereavement.

Mentally, the grieving individual could struggle to accept the loss, have problems focusing or making choices, experience changes with their sense of self, or think that their future has been disturbed. Sometimes they may try to avoid contemplating the loss, and other times they could find it difficult to stop. They can discover that they are going out of their way to keep the person's memories alive. They can be afraid of losing happy recollections of their time spent with the deceased or of forgetting who they were.

Socially, the grieving individual may struggle to form new connections and may suffer loneliness, boredom, social retreat, lack of assurance, emotional sensitivity (or feeling "overemotional").

Grief by and of itself may be normal. It is very normal to feel melancholy after losing anybody or something. As we go through the process of grief, individual could experience a broad range of emotions. Others of these could be medical, while others might be physiological, psychological, or social.

Examples of physical reactions to grief:
- An actual tightness in your chest
- Feeling weak
- Lack of energy
- Nausea
- Heart palpitations
- Restlessness
- Tearfulness
- And many more

Examples of behavioral reactions to grief:

❖ Forgetfulness
❖ Confusion
❖ Dreaming of the person you've lost
❖ Absent-mindedness

Examples of emotional reactions to grief:

❖ Anger
❖ Shock
❖ Denial
❖ Numbness
❖ Loneliness
❖ Relief
❖ Apathy
❖ Irritability
❖ Misplaced anger

Examples of social reactions to grief:

❖ Being unusually dependent on other people
❖ Withdrawing from friends
❖ Relationship difficulties
❖ Avoiding family
❖ Avoiding colleagues
❖ Avoiding friends
❖ Increased substance abuse
❖ Neglecting yourself but caring for others

TYPES OF GRIEF

Grief may seem like such an overwhelming subject because of the magnitude of the suffering. It is crucial to keep in mind that every living thing will eventually feel the pain associated with the typical grieving process.

Anticipatory Grief

Anticipatory sorrow or sorrow may be usual if you are worried about losing a close friend or relative soon. You could try to imagine life without them to psychologically be ready for the upcoming loss. If a loved one has a terminal illness, it could happen often.

When you experience anticipatory grieving, you could make plans for your response and mourning once the memory of your loved one dies away. You could experience grief, extreme dread, or intense feeling for the dying individual.

However, there are certain advantages for anticipating sadness. Many individuals believe they were unable to allocate the time required to say farewell or have difficult discussions about tolerance. Simply taking the time along with space to say "I love you" might be beneficial for your health. All of this may aid in preparing for the time when you start to grieve after suffering a bodily loss.

Complicated Grief

Complicated grief happens when the stages of sorrow are not fully traversed throughout the mourning process. It may last for a long time and get considerably stronger, and it usually has a considerable negative influence on your capacity to operate. You can have increased anxiety and depressive symptoms. When you are experiencing difficult sorrow, it's probable that your feelings and behaviors will last for a very long time without changing much.

A mental health specialist should usually be consulted for assistance with complicated sorrow. Given that complex grieving is one of the most challenging forms of sorrow, it might be helpful to speak with someone who has experience with complicated grief. Understanding that complicated sadness won't go completely on its own is essential.

Chronic Grief

Chronic grief develops when very emotional reactions to loss do not dissipate. You will experience enormous discomfort that only becomes worse as a result of these feelings, which will linger for an extended time. You won't be able to make much, if any of them, progress in healing from your sorrow.

Delayed Grief

Even though your loved one passed away quite some time ago, delayed mourning may develop if you're still having really strong sensations of sadness and desire. It simply means that your emotional reaction, which may endure for years after a loss, did not happen when it should have. Disassociation may be to blame, which happens often when something is too unpleasant for you to experience. Your mind uses blocking as a coping method to hold back many of the thoughts, feelings, and emotions associated with the loss until you're ready to examine and deal with them.

Distorted Grief

A particularly strong or disproportionate response to a loss is known as distorted sorrow. In general, there will usually be a discernible shift in conduct, and self-harming conduct is also normal. Of the most typical emotional signs of misdirected mourning is anger and lash out, both at oneself and at others.

Cumulative Grief

Cumulative sorrow is the term used to describe a second bereavement that happens shortly after (or while you're grieving over) a first loss. This sort of sadness, often referred to as loss overflow or mourning excess, could be lost of the hardest to get over. Losses that keep adding up might make you feel as if "I just can't do this anymore." However, you can go through any sort of grieving, even cumulative, with the correct counseling and assistance.

Exaggerated Grief

Exaggerated sadness involves more powerful emotional responses than are generally seen with other forms of loss. Your feelings and behaviors could stand out more and be more disruptive when they are exaggerated. Self-destructive behavior, aberrant fears, self-harm or suicide ideas, drug or alcohol misuse, and nightmares are just a few possible symptoms. Additionally, heightened grieving may sometimes lead to the emergence of a mental disease.

Secondary Loss

Secondary loss grief may emerge when a passing has an effect on other facets of your life. In the end, you can experience a number of deaths that are all connected to the initial one you experienced.

Masked Grief

Body language or other physical manifestations of masked melancholy may have the tendency to hinder or interfere with regular functioning. However, most of the time you may not be able to recognize these items that are a result of a shortage or perhaps comprehend how they're related to it.

Disenfranchised Grief (Ambiguous)

When you believe that others have not acknowledged your loss, grief may become disenfranchised. This may occur if a culture or community fails to acknowledge your loss. For instance, there may be a tremendous stigma associated with overdosing or committing suicide, and your grieving may be disregarded.

Alternately, maybe the deceased was someone for whom others believe you shouldn't or wouldn't mourn, such as a same-sex lover, a former husband, a member of a gang. If a loss isn't recognized or you lack the sense of heard or understood in how you're feeling and grieving, disenfranchised sadness may result.

It is important to keep in mind that disenfranchised sorrow may also happen when a loss isn't really caused by death but instead results from an injury to the head, drug misuse, or a disorder of the mind that fundamentally changes a relationship.

Traumatic Grief

Traumatized regret is often the result of the effort to process grief when there is extra stress caused by a terrible, unforeseen loss or violent death. Your ability to operate in life on a daily basis may be impacted.

Collective Grief

Collective grief occurs when a disaster hits a broad community or group of people. It often occurs after significant natural catastrophes that might have long-lasting effects and during times of conflict. Other instances of communal grieving include the aftermath of a terrorist attack, the death of a well-known public figure, a mass casualty, or a major catastrophe.

Inhibited Grief

You are exhibiting restrained sorrow if you aren't displaying any overt or evident signs of it. This often continues for a long time and prevents efficient movement through the stages of grief. If you're suffering suppressed grieving, you'll probably ultimately have bodily repercussions as a result of failing to deal with your emotions.

Abbreviated Grief

Short-term replacement of the deceased with an individual or thing fresh in your life might provide abbreviated grieving. In general, being able to rapidly accept the first loss may have an impact on this. Or it can be because there wasn't a deep bond or relationship to the lost individual.

Absent Grief

You are not exhibiting any of the standard grieving symptoms if you are absent from mourning. Perhaps you're acting as if you've gained nothing at all. It often happens after a sudden or unexpected loss and may be brought on by intense shock or complete denial. Even though absent grieving might be natural, it has to be dealt if it lasts for a long time.

Manifestations of Grief

Below is a chart that outlines common physical, emotional, social, behavioral, and spiritual responses to loss. This can be a helpful tool if you know a family member, friend, student, or colleague who is grieving. All reactions below are completely normal, but the individual might benefit from a caring friend, teacher, parent or co-worker reaching out to support.

Physical	*Emotional*	*Social*	*Behavioral*	*Spiritual*
Hyperactive or underactive	Numbness	Overly sensitive	Forgetfulness	Questioning: the reason for
Feelings of unreality	Sadness	Dependent	Slowed thinking	the death; the
Physical distress	Yearning	Withdrawn	Mental confusion	purpose of pain
such as chest pain,	Crying	Avoid others	Trouble	and suffering;
abdominal pain,	Anger	Detached	concentrating	the purpose of
headaches, nausea	Fear	Lack of initiative	Difficulty making	life; the meaning
Decreased immune	Relief	Lack of interest	decisions	of death
system	Irritability	Loss of interest in	Dreams and/or	Anger at a
Unusual clumsiness	Guilt	previously enjoyed	flashbacks	higher power
Change in appetite	Regret	activities	Sense the loved	Sense of
Weight change	Loneliness	Behaving in ways	one's presence	distance from a
Digestive problems	Longing	not normal for you	Wandering	higher power
Fatigue	Anxiety	Relational distress	aimlessly	Sense of
Sleeping problems	Meaninglessness	Loss of interest in	Trying not to	closeness to a
Restlessness	Bitterness	intimacy	talk about loss	higher power
Crying and sighing	Apathy	Preoccupation with	in order to help	Isolation from
Feelings of	Vulnerability	own feelings and	others feel	one's spiritual
emptiness	Abandonment	needs exclusively	comfortable	community
Shortness of breath	Helplessness	Impatience with	around them	Searching for
Tightness in the	Loss of	others grieving the	Needing to retell	a continuing
throat	confidence	same loss due to	the story of the	bond with the
	Lowered self-esteem	different grieving styles	loved one's death	deceased

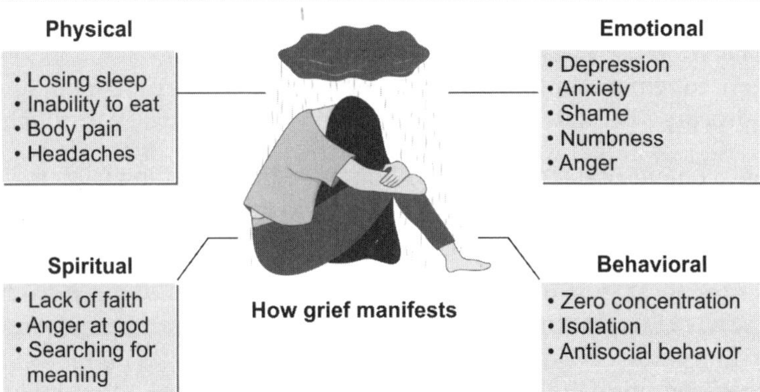

THEORIES OF LOSS AND GRIEF

Losing someone you cherish is a universal feeling. Everyone will experience loss and unfortunate situations at some point in their lives. This event has the potential to change someone's expectations for their life's course.

To attempt to comprehend the complex process of loss and grieving, several ideas and frameworks have been established. Three of these types of structures are examined in this article:

1. Freud's model of bereavement
2. Kübler-Ross grief cycle
3. Bowlby's attachment theory

Freud's Model of Bereavement

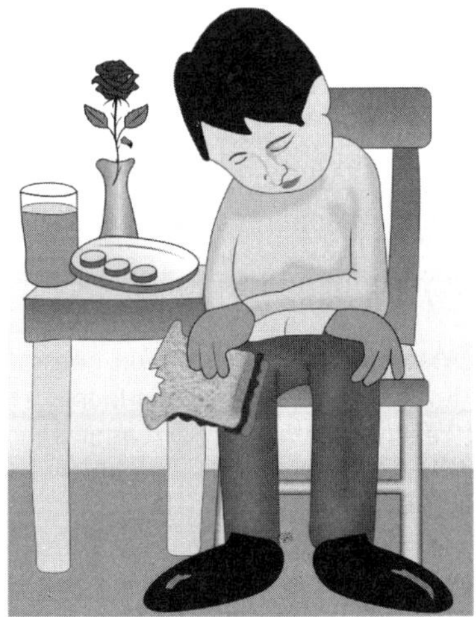

Losing someone you love is a universal feeling. Everyone will experience loss and unfortunate situations at some point in their lives. This event has the potential to change someone's expectations for their life's course.

According to some, melancholia is a serious kind of depression characterized by a complete absence of pleasure in everything or almost anything. One must experience the profound pain of loss, which evokes the affectionate influence of the dead loved one, in order to restore their inner world. Losing a loved one may cause a person to lose their sense of self (Freke, 2004). According to some ideas, a person who passed away a loved one must let go of a lot of attachments needed for a relationship to form while grieving.

The ego is said to adapt the loss when the loss is acknowledged, allowing the bereaved to look for novel ties (Humphrey and Zimpfer, 1998; Susillo, 2005).

Kübler-Ross Grief Cycle

The grieving cycle approach provides an insightful lens for understanding our own and other people's mental responses to calamity and change in how we live. To explain the experience of those who were terminally ill, the model was first developed. It continues to be utilized to refer to the mourning process in a broader sense.

It is important to remember that from the perspective of this paradigm, mourning is not an organized process. It is claimed that most people do not progress through the stages of this framework in a systematic fashion since sorrow is seen to be fluid (Baxter and Diehl, 1998).

Kübler-Ross Five Stages of Grief Cycle

1. **Denial:** Refuse to accept information about the situation, whether consciously or subconsciously, may include facts, understanding, the truth, etc. It is quite natural and acts as a kind of safeguard. It is easy for people to become stuck at this phase while dealing with stressful experiences.
2. **Anger:** There are many ways that anger may manifest. People who are under emotional turmoil may get enraged with themselves as well as with others, especially those close to them. Anger might also be directed against the deceased.
3. **Negotiation:** In the past, people who were close to passing away sometimes sought to negotiate with the "god" they believed in. Even when a decision is a matter of life and death, bartering seldom produces a long-lasting outcome.
4. **Depression:** This stage is characterized by feelings of regret, fear, and uncertainty. This may indicate that the person has at least begun to accept the reality of the loss.
5. **Acceptance:** This level stands for emotional detachment and objectivity. The individual who is grieving is beginning to come to terms with their loss. The bereaved attempt to go on without their daily affairs.

Bowlby's Attachment Theory

Bowlby claims that attachments start to develop in infants and give a person a feeling of security and survival. When these affectionate ties are broken or destroyed, people experience trouble and emotional distress, including concern, crying, and fury (Freeman, 2005).

Grief is often a result of these emotions. According to Bowlby, there are four basic phases of grief: numbness, desire and searching, disorganization, and reorganization.

Feelings of denial that death has happened are characterized as numbing, which gives the bereaved individual momentary comfort from the grief brought on by the loss. There generally follows a brief time of this with emotional outbursts.

As the numbness wears off, yearning and longing entail the realization of the loss. At this stage, the mourning person is likely to feel angry and frustrated as they look for someone to blame.

During the disorganization phase, it's important to recognize the loss's reality and all the chaos it causes. At this stage, it is common for people to evaluate themselves without the dead.

The remodeling phase begins when the bereaved realizes they will live a new life without the departed. As the bereaved strive to move on with their lives, this phase is characterized by incremental adjustments (Freeman, 2005; Worden, 2005).

Bowlby identified four stages in the grief process:
1. Experiencing numbness and denying the loss
2. Emotionally yearning for the lost loved one and pro-testing the permanence of the loss

3. Experiencing cognitive disorganization and emotional despair with difficulty functioning in the everyday world
4. Reorganizing and reintegrating the sense of self to pull life back together.

FACTORS AFFECTING GRIEF AND LOSS

- Current health situation
- Relationship with person who has died/thing which has been lost
- Age of person grieving
- Previous experience of grief
- Cultural background
- Belief system
- Financial situation
- Knowledge around cause of loss/death
- Personality
- Concurrent losses/changes occurring
- Support systems – family/friends/community
- Cause of death (i.e., expected or not expected)
- Expectation of death
- Recognition of loss by others (i.e., disenfranchised grief)
- Social 'acceptability' of cause of death
- Social 'acceptability' of relationship of bereaved to deceased
- Ability to communicate feelings
- Language levels

Each person has their response to grief. There are certain factors that can affect grief responses. Learning about grief responses would help provide support for grief.

- A person's culture and religion are vital parts of their belief system.
- Most people, either directly or indirectly, are influenced by their culture and religion.
- One of the most critical factors that affect grief responses is the culture and religion of a person.
- The loss of a loved one can cause multiple responses from a grieving person.
- The strength of the relationship with a lost one can make it more difficult to grieve.
- However, it is essential each person grieves in their own fashion.
- In cases where the death of a person is expected, it increases the chances of a healthier grief response.
- Expected death can allow people to prepare for their impending loss.
- This is one of the important factors that affect grief responses.

Culture and Religion

- The majority of the time, a person's religion and culture dictate their fundamental views.
- Every area of a person's life is impacted by culture and religion.
- This is just another element that may influence how we react to loss.
- In many cultures, the idea of death may signify different things.
- Most cultures have a specific style of dealing with a person's death.

* The way you typically handle sorrow may have an impact on how you respond to it.
* A person's religious convictions may also be crucial.
* For instance, having faith in an afterlife might ease the pain of losing a loved one.
* Religion may also elicit a powerful, unchangeable sense of remorse.
* Every culture and religion gives an own viewpoint on grieving and related topics.
* Our religious and cultural views may have a big impact on how you react to bereavement.
* It is important to remember that everyone grieves uniquely and in their own way.

Level of Intimacy with the Deceased

* The degree of closeness you had with the deceased was one of the characteristics that influenced your grieving reactions.
* The majority of people do not lament for strangers, after all.
* A person will often grieve more the more intimate the relationship.
* One of the key aspects of grieving is coming to terms with the passing on of someone else in one's own life.
* Naturally, the closer the connection was with the deceased, the harder it was for most individuals to grieve.
* Your life could seem to be missing something.
* It is important to keep in mind the complexity of mourning.
* Although you would imagine that the depth of your sorrow over a loss dictates the degree of closeness, this may not be the case.
* In addition to closeness, there are other elements that affect a person's mourning reaction.
* Losing significant someone in your life, such as a spouse or close friend, may cause difficult grieving reactions.
* Accepting aid from other family members might ease the pain of losing a close friend.
* Finding new methods to stay in touch with the missing person may also be beneficial.

Anticipated Loss

Grieving may be a very difficult process. The likelihood of loss is another element that might influence how people react to sorrow. Your response to an unexpected loss will probably vary from your response to an anticipated death.

There are two types of influences that might influence the mourning process: external and internal. These elements are referred to as grief determinants when they are together.

External Variables

The following outside factors have been identified as influencing a person's mourning reaction after a loss:

* **The location of death:** Accepting a person's death is put off and mourning takes longer when they pass away at a place other than their home;
* **Coincidental losses or fatalities:** Simultaneous losses in loved ones or region cause more difficult grieving and may leave the bereaved with less support;
* **Deaths or losses that occur in fast succession:** If there have been many deaths or damages, the sorrow of one may be disrupted or overwhelmed by the pain of the others;

❖ **The manner of death:** Grieving after a sudden, unexpected, or untimely death might be particularly difficult. If the passing away was additionally traumatic, then this becomes much more challenging;

❖ **Social media:** Communities and families that are close-knit and supportive of one another may be especially beneficial at a time of loss or sorrow.

Internal Elements

The following internal elements are also thought to have an impact on a person's mourning reaction after a loss:

❖ **Associated history:** The ability to express emotions and deal with grief eventually in life is influenced by a child's early relationship with their parents or other caregivers; a child has a secure attachment when they feel protected by them and know they can count on them to come back after an extended period of separation.

❖ **Personal past experiences with loss and death:** If prior losses were challenging to accept and mourn, the most recent loss may bring those losses to the forefront and make them all challenging to do so.

❖ **Age and stage of being a griever:** Grief may be particularly difficult for small children and young adults, as well as those going through life transitions (such as going from infancy to adolescence, becoming parents, beginning retirement, etc.).

❖ **Sensitivity level:** The level of sorrow might increase depending on how close a person was to them (spouse, kid, parent, etc.).

❖ **Emotional complexity:** Due to suppressed emotions or unacknowledged ambivalence in the connection, grieving may grow more complicated the more complicated the relationship was with the departed.

❖ **Social networks:** As previously mentioned, close-knit and supportive families and communities may be very beneficial through a loss or mourning.

- The possibility of a person's passing away is referred to as the expectation of loss.
- For instance, a person's lifespan may have been predicted in medical reports.
- It might be difficult to learn that you will likely lose a loved one.
- Some individuals can cope with loss and their emotions before any loss by preparing for it.
- Some individuals may benefit from a more tranquil mourning experience as a result of this.
- But for other individuals, anticipating the death of a loved one might make their suffering last longer.
- The abrupt loss of a family member is usually quite traumatic for the majority of individuals.
- To say goodbye, they fight.
- This may slow down their mourning process and prolong their sorrow reactions.

Support System

❖ Having a support network is helpful while coping with bereavement.

❖ A system of assistance is essentially a network of individuals who provide help to another person.

❖ Most people's support systems are typically comprised of their friends and family. Support from close companions may be an essential component of any grieving process.

❖ For instance, relatives and close friends may give assistance with dinners or even money.

❖ A strong support network will ease a bereaved person's difficulties.
❖ It may be enticing to withdraw oneself from friends and relatives when one is grieving.
❖ In times of mourning, it could be challenging to accept any help from friends and family.
❖ The person's support network is one of the variables that impacts grieving reactions.
❖ A support system may also consist of consulting a specialist.
❖ To aid in the grieving process, you may want to go to your neighborhood hospital or find a counselor.
❖ This will probably result in an appropriate mourning reaction.

Prior Grief Experience

❖ Most individuals will probably go through sorrow more than once in their lives.
❖ Some individuals become better at controlling their grieving reaction over time.
❖ It is vital to keep in mind that other elements that influence grieving reactions might still alter this response.
❖ Grief might be difficult to handle for someone who has never experienced it before.
❖ It might be hard to comprehend and digest the idea of death.
❖ People who have gone through the mourning process before may be able to comprehend how to do so.
❖ A loss could also bring up memories of previous grieving experiences.
❖ Reliving unpleasant times might result from experiencing many losses in a same way.
❖ This could even happen if the death has nothing to do with a loved one.
❖ A susceptible reaction to sorrow might also result from losing many individuals quickly.
❖ This can result in the loss of two significant pillars of their support network for some individuals.
❖ Losing someone might render it more difficult to deal with the passing of someone you cherish.

The Six "R" model of procedures or behaviors that are crucial to adjusting to a loss is provided by Therese Rando, a clinical psychologist whose practice and study have focused on mourning, anticipatory grieving, and traumatic loss (1984, 1993). Realizing the loss, reacting towards the divorce, remembering and reliving the life of the departed, letting go of attachments and presumptions, readjusting into a new environment, and reinvesting in new pursuits and relationships are all steps in the grieving process.

Causes of Grief

❖ Loss of a job
❖ Loss of a beloved pet
❖ Loss of a friendship
❖ Loss of a personal dream
❖ Loss of a romantic relationship

BEREAVEMENT

The most physically and emotionally devastating event a person may go through is bereavement. When someone dear to us passes away, we all respond differently, and the time it takes for healing and rehabilitation is unique for each of us. There is no fast cure for healing, and although each of us will deal with loss in our own unique ways, there are universal phases of sorrow.

Bereavement is the period of sorrow and grief that follows a loss. The circumstances around the loss and the level of attachment felt for the departed influence how long it takes to heal when a loved one passes away.

Important Terms

- **Bereavement:** It is the condition of having experienced a loss. It is the overall reaction to the loss of a close relationship.
- **Grief:** Grief is defined as severe mental anguish caused by a loss. The usual reaction to a feeling of loss is grief.
- **Mourning:** It is initiated by loss. It involves customs and rituals, that are influenced by socio-cultural and religious beliefs and values.

Counseling Directives for the Bereaved

- Talking on the loss will help make the loss more real.
- Identify and express feelings related to the loss.
- Assist the bereaved in making decisions.
- Promote the growth of new relations and facilitate emotional disengagement.
- Allocate time for mourning while keeping holidays and anniversaries in mind.
- Reassure the bereaved that their behavior is normal and that they are not abnormal because of their feelings.
- Recognize that everyone experiences grief in a different way.
- Provide assistance.
- Analyze personal barriers and coping mechanisms (keep an eye out for issues with drink or other drug usage).
- Recognize abnormal behaviors and recommend therapy.
- Preparing family and relatives after the death has been declared, the family members have been prepared to accept the bad news.

The skill of breaking terrible news:
- Keep it basic.
- Meet on cool ground first.
- Wait for questions.
- Do not argue with denial.
- Do not say any thing that is not true. Family members and relatives may respond to 'bad news' with disbelief, anger or denial. So, being caretaker accept their reaction to this defense mechanism. Additionally, be ready to confront death.

Prepare yourself by:
- As the caregiver, you must ask the family whether they have any traditions or rituals related to death that have special value for them.
- Make the viewing of the dead peaceful for the family.
- Show respect to the deceased.
- If family had not been there when the patient passed away, they could be interested in knowing what happened in the last minutes. Saying to the family, "She was not solitary" or "He looked to be of peace" is a terrific way to soothe them and should be done with caution.

❖ It is best if arrangements can be made for a friend or relatives, to spend the night with the bereaved or take the bereaved to their own home for the night.
❖ As per the social custom, arrangement should be made for the support system who can take initiatives for the funerals and other last rituals.

Emotional Support to Family and Relatives

The family members and relatives might feel shocked or guilty It may only be after the funeral and the guests have left, the family members/relatives experience the full sense of loss and grief. Following the loss of a loved one, receiving expert care from a social worker or health visitor may help shield them from becoming sick. It will be crucial to assist in preserving equilibrium and a feeling of normality during this. You must be able to comfort the family as they go through their loss.

The following actions should be made to help the family and other members:
❖ Active sympathetic listening since grieving families need someone who can listen to them more than other families. You might reply succinctly by saying something like, "I will keep you in my prayers or thoughts."
❖ Allow the family members to cry naturally as they would in a normal situation; this promotes healing.
❖ You should be on occasion quiet to give the family a chance to speak out and ask more inquiries.
❖ Use touch to reassure people. Even while some individuals at this time desire interpersonal contact, others may retreat out of sadness.
❖ The social distance between the living and the dead, must be increased after death, so that they can reestablish their normal activities without paralyzing attachment to the cause.
❖ Participate in the parting rituals.

MOURNING

People go through a time of grief to get over a loss. Culture's beliefs, practices, and rituals having a big influence on grief.

Mourning is the process by which people adapt to a loss. Mourning is greatly influenced by cultural beliefs, practices, and rituals.

Bowlby's attachment theory, published in 1980, serves as the basis for his phases of grief.

Attachment: Is described as an instinctive behavior that the leads in the development of affectional bonds between children and their primary caregiver.

Numbing: May last from a few hours to a week or more and maybe interrupted by period of extremely intense emotion; it is the briefest phase of mourning; the grieving person describes this stage as feeling "stunned or unreal."

Yearning and searching: Arouses emotional outbursts of tearful sobbing and acute distress inmost person; separation anxiety.

Disorganization and despair: Individual may endlessly examine how and why the loss occurred.

Reorganization: May require as much as a year or more, the person beings to accept unaccustomed roles, acquire new skills, and build new relationships.

According to worden's four tasks of mourning (1982)

Task-based mourning theory

- ❖ **Task I:** People who are grieving may be actively engaged by assisting themselves and can receive outside assistance. Accepting the loss's reality is the first task. This entails coming to terms with the fact that that individual or thing is gone and is not coming back.
- ❖ **Task II:** Feel the suffering of loss. People respond with grief, feelings of isolation, desperation, or regret and use their most comfortable and known coping techniques to get through difficult emotions.
- ❖ **Task III:** Adapt to the departed person's absence in the world. People undertaking this work start to assume duties formerly held by the deceased, even some occupations they do not desire, since it takes at least three months for a person to fully comprehend the consequences of loss.
- ❖ **Task IV:** Emotionally relocate the deceased and move on with life. The deceased person is not forgotten but rather takes a different and less prominent place in the survivor's emotional life.

THE SIX 'R' PROCESSES BY RANDO

Therese A Rando promoted the six 'R' processes within three phases of mourning; avoidance phase, confrontation phase and accommodation phase, which are essential in order for there to be a healthy and satisfactory conclusion to grief and mourning.

Avoidance Phase

1. **Recognize the loss:** This is achieved through admitting the death, acknowledging the death by recognizing on a cognitive level that the death has happened, entailing an admitting and dispensation of the reality. This is brought on by the ongoing encounter with the deceased person's absence. A person might start their mourning process by confirming and realizing that the loss is irreparable, which prevents mummification of the dead. This is comparable to Worden's (1983) first obligation of mourning, which states that it takes time to embrace the truth of the loss since it requires both an intellectual and an emotional acceptance. Without this, "the bereaved adult lacks the critical stimuli that causes bereavement" (Rando 1993), hence it is not likely to happen.

   Knowing the factors surrounding a death, how it happened, and the facts surrounding it are all necessary for understanding it. Understanding the reality thoroughly requires determining the what, why, and how of death. If a person is to deal with and adapt to the loss of a loved one, it must make sense. 'The death of a loved one must make logical sense if the mourner is to cope with and readjust well to it' (Rando 1993).

Confrontation Phase

2. **React to the separation:** When the mourner gives themselves permission to feel and express these emotions correctly, healthy grieving may take place. Experiencing the pain of the severance and the nuances of the process of mourning, felt on a physical, behavioral, social, spiritual, psychological, emotional and sexual realm.

   Feel the psychological reactions to the loss, whether they be good, negative, or ambiguous, and then recognize, accept, and express them. This requires actively controlling the spectrum of experienced emotional responses, differentiating each one independently, appreciating their importance in the mind, and looking for opportunities that allow for the appropriate expression of these feelings. Failure to do this 'leaves mourning incomplete and consequently complicated (Rando 1993).

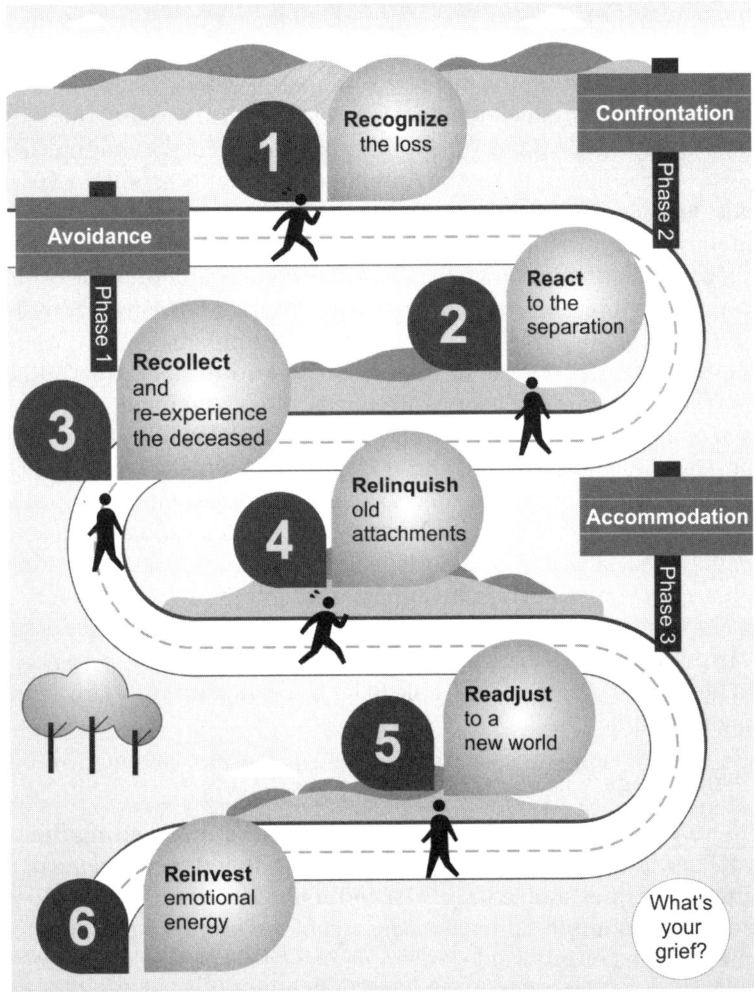

The six 'R's of mourning by Therese A Rando.

Be aware of and express your grief for any secondary losses that may arise from the loss of unmet needs, wants, wishes, desires, deadlines, status, hypotheses, and fantasies—the bereaved's assumptive world "We can begin redefining ourselves once we are aware of the gap than has been created." (Noel 2004). This includes any additional gifts received from the departed, such as fulfillment, acknowledgment, contentment, relating, and fortifying; Rando (1993) identifies this as "the totality of the losses associated with this death."

3. **Recollect and re-experience the deceased and the relationship:** The outcome is a reformation of the relationship from one of company to one of remembrance which is the conclusion comprising the following: Reassessing and realistically remembering all aspects of his bond with the lost the other, including the factors that led to their development in the initial instance, the advantages and disadvantages associated with the relationship or the person, that which was planned and the related thoughts which were attached each of the events related to the deceased. The mourner may then recognize the responses that need

being addressed with the goal to alter and modify the emotional connection and mental commitment to the departed as a consequence of "the creation of an emotionally realistic material image that represents the deceased" (Rando 1993).

Revive and experience the feelings because "the ties linking the mourner to the once deceased must be untied," (Rando 1993). This indicates that the mourner will specifically relive and experience all the interactions, moments, thoughts, emotions, reactions, wishes, expectations, and beliefs that are connected to the relationship to the one who passed away, ultimately resulting in an ongoing diffusion of the emotional force associated with it and a reduction in intensity of affect. In due course there is a renouncing of old attachments and readjustment to progress and acclimatize to a new way of living, without forgetting the past.

4. **Relinquish the old attachments to the deceased and the old assumptive world:** The assumptive world may be seen as organized cognitions that include everything a person thinks, based on prior experiences, to be true regarding themselves and their environment. Philosophical, spiritual, theological, and existential concerns are essential components of the assumption-based universe, and there are two types of assumptions: Specific and Global. Specific presumptions relate specifically to the mourner's expectations and convictions towards the departed, such as "she'll never leave me." While the generalizations apply to life and individuals in general, such as that unpleasant things only happen for certain people. The mourner might be seen as looking for and changing their previous assumptions with alternative hypotheses or beliefs which can reorganize or re-clarify the reality of which they continue to be a part of in order to be able to let go of what was formerly believed to be the whole truth of the situation.

Accommodation Phase

5. **Readjust to move adaptively into the new world without forgetting the old:** The order of this is to; Determine which assumptions should be abandoned, changed, or retained, as well as, if any, which ones should be introduced and the justifications for those additions, in order to revise the assumptive universe. The aim of the bereaved person is to comprehend what they have gained or lost inside, including how they act, think, and feel. In addition to reflecting the new realities created as a direct result of the dead person's death, e.g. I am currently without a "best friend." This allows the individual to start seeing and experiencing oneself in new ways, which is "closely related to achieving success in incorporating a new self-image" (Rando 1993).

Establish a fresh relationship with the deceased before adjusting to "selecting life-promoting so instead of death-denying reminiscences" (Rando 1993, p. 438). To do this, the person gives in to or lets go of desires that the deceased previously satisfied, and she adjoins, surrenders, or adjusts a number of facets of her life as a way to absorb the specific damages that the death brings. The mourner substitutes it with the nonfigurative loving of a lost loved one in addition to giving up the tangible love of someone that is physically there. This process of reestablishing contact with the deceased focuses on "maintaining the dead individual present in memories without interfering with their sorrow or progress in life," according to Rando (1993). This indicates that the ideas, convictions, and lessons of the deceased—learned via a relationship that existed over the past—are being preserved. Worden (2005) refers to this as "relocating."

Adopt new ways of being in the world in order to compensate for and fill the vacuum created by the loved one's absence. The griever alters her desires to reflect the fact that the deceased is no longer there or looks for other means of obtaining her wants. This redefinition is carried out in the hope that the return would be advantageous to the survivor.

Create an alternate identity that includes the loss of the part of the deceased's identity that was formerly tied to us but is now me. This compensation may manifest as the acquisition of new skills, the loss of desires, or a combination of many facets of experience.

6. **Reinvest:** This task enables the mourner to take all of the emotion that was invested in the relation with the departed and reinvest it. This redirection is acceptable because it "can connect people who are in mourning with unknown people, items, and activities... that can provide emotional gratification to compensate for that which was lost' (Rando 1993).

DYING

Death is a process involving the cessation of physiological functions and the determination of death is the final event in that process. At the cellular level, death occurs gradually, and the capacity of different tissues to resist oxygen deprivation varies.

The passing away of a living thing or cell. Death occurs when critical biological processes, such as the heartbeat, breathing on its own, and brain activity, permanently stop. This occurs in both humans and animals.

Death was formerly determined by the cessation of breathing and the heartbeat.

An individual who has sustained either:

1. Irreversible cessation of circulatory and respiratory functions, or
2. Irreversible cessation of all functions of the entire brain, including the brain stem, is dead. According to recognized medical criteria, death must be determined.

Types of Death

1. **Cellular death**
   - Cells no longer functioning or have metabolic activities or aerobic respiration.
   - Different tissue die at different rate; cerebral cortex tolerate only few minutes of
   - Anoxia while connective tissue and muscles may survive longer (for hours).
2. **Somatic death**
   - The individual experiences somatic death when they are irrevocably unconscious, unaware of their surroundings, and unable to respond to sensory inputs or make any voluntary movements.
   - Reflex nervous activity may persist and circulatory and respiratory function continue either spontaneously or with artificial support.

   Somatic death= brain death = vegetative state
3. **Brain death:** Due to its capacities to appropriately oxygenate blood from human beings (lungs) and transmit this blood to all key organs (heart), the heart and lungs are essential for maintaining human life. Therefore, failing to get enough oxygen into the lungs or the heart may result in cardiopulmonary death, in which the heart stops beating because there is no pulse. This may be seen in the brain as a hypoxic condition that causes cerebral edema and a rise in intracranial pressure. Increased cerebral blood flow disturbance brought on by the increase in intracranial pressure may result in necrosis or tissue death. The most frequent

pathway for brain death is the one indicated above, however a rise in intracranial pressure is not always brought on by a cessation of cardiac function. Traumatic brain injuries may subarachnoid hemorrhages may both raise intracranial pressure, which can cause the brain to stop functioning and, ultimately, cause death.

When the brain's oxygen or blood supply is cut off, brain death may result.

This can be caused by:

- Cardiac arrest – when the heart stops beating and the brain is starved of oxygen
- A heart attack – when the blood supply to the heart is suddenly blocked
- A stroke – when the blood supply to the brain is blocked or interrupted
- A blood clot – a blockage in a blood vessel that disturbs or blocks the flow of blood around your body.

Brain death can also be caused by:

- A severe head injury
- A brain hemorrhage
- Infections, such as encephalitis
- A brain tumor

4. **Circulatory death:** Circulatory death happens whenever oxygen delivery and blood circulation to the tissues halt permanently, along with the heart's irreversible cessation of pumping.

Common causes of circulatory death:

- Ischemic heart disease
- Myocardial infarction
- Anomalous coronary origin
- Coronary spasm
- Inherited channelopathies
- Long QT syndrome (LQTS)
- Short QT syndrome (SQTS)
- Brugada syndrome
- Early repolarization syndrome
- Catecholaminergic polymorphic ventricular tachycardia (CPVT)
- Cardiomyopathies
- Alcoholic
- Hypertrophic
- Idiopathic
- Obesity-related
- Fibrotic
- Arrhythmogenic right ventricular cardiomyopathy (ARVC)
- Myocarditis
- Heart failure
- Nonpreserved ejection fraction (EF) systolic heart failure (EF less than 35%)
- Valve disease
- Aortic stenosis
- Congenital diseases
- Tetralogy of Fallot

5. **Signs of impending death**

- Unconsciousness
- Loss of all reflexes

- No reaction to painful stimuli
- Muscular flaccidity
- Cessation of heart beat and respiratory movement
- *Eye signs:*
    ◊ Loss of corneal and light reflexes
    ◊ Mid-dilated position of the pupils
    ◊ Irregular size and shape of the pupils
    ◊ Eyelids usually closed incompletely
    ◊ Tache noire: Two triangles of discoloration, either brown or black, occur at either side of the cornea where the sclera is still visible.

Indicators of Death

1. **Decreasing appetite**
   - Loss of appetite might indicate impending death.
   - As one gets closer to death, they become less active. This shows that their body now uses less energy than it did before. As their hunger steadily declines, they cease to eat and drink as much.

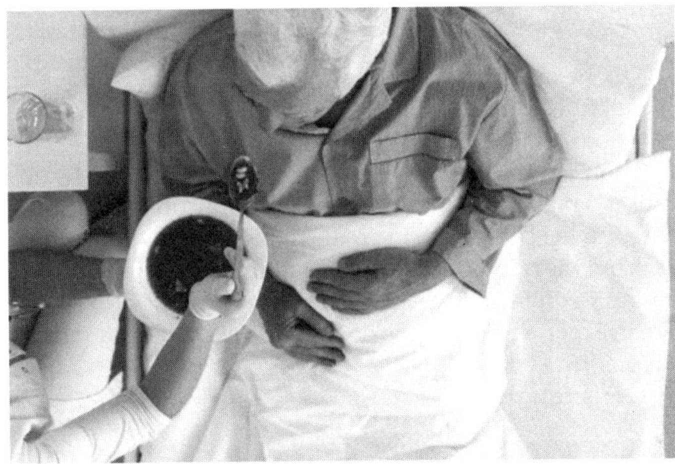

   - Allowing a dying companion to eat when they are hungry is important if the person truly cares for them. Ice pops are a great way to keep children hydrated.
   - A person may completely stop eating a few days before dying. People may keep their lips hydrated with lip balm to reduce pain when this happens.

2. **Increased sleep**
   - In the 2–3 months before a person dies, they may spend less time awake.
   - Their body's metabolism is deteriorating, which is the reason of their lack of wakefulness. A person may fall asleep much more if they lack metabolic energy.
   - Make sure the individual receiving care is comfortable and allow them to sleep if they are drowsy. To assist prevent bedsores; parents should urge their loved one to move or move out of bed when they feel to have energy.

3. **Becoming less social**
   - A dying person may not desire to interact with others as much as they previously did.
   - If a dying person is becoming less social, their loved ones should try not to be offended.
   - It is common for someone to feel uneasy about allowing others to see them weaken. It is advisable to plan visits for while the patient is prepared to see someone.
4. **Changing vital signs:** Vital signs may alter in the following ways when a person nears death:
   - Blood pressure drops
   - Breathing changes
   - Heartbeat becomes irregular
   - Heartbeat may be hard to detect
   - Urine may be brown, tan, or rust-colored

When the kidneys shut down, a person's urine changes in color. It could be upsetting to see these as well as additional alterations in a loved one. However, the modifications are not unpleasant, so it can be helpful for one to attempt not to dwell on them too much.

5. **Modifying toilet habits**
   - A person who is dying could have fewer bowel movements as a result of consuming food and beverages less. They could pass solid waste more sparingly. They could also have less frequent urination.
   - When they stop eating and drinking completely, they may no longer need to use the toilet.
   - Although it might be upsetting to see these changes in someone you cherish, they need to be anticipated. It could be helpful to talk to the doctors about getting the patient a catheter.
6. **Muscle deterioration**
   - A person's muscles may deteriorate in the days leading up to a person's death.
   - The person may not be competent to do the modest chores they were previously able to do due to weak muscles. Some activities, including rolling over in bed or drinking from a cup, may be beyond their ability.
   - If a dying person experiences this, the ones they love should assist them in lifting objects or turning over in bed.
7. **Dropping body temperature**

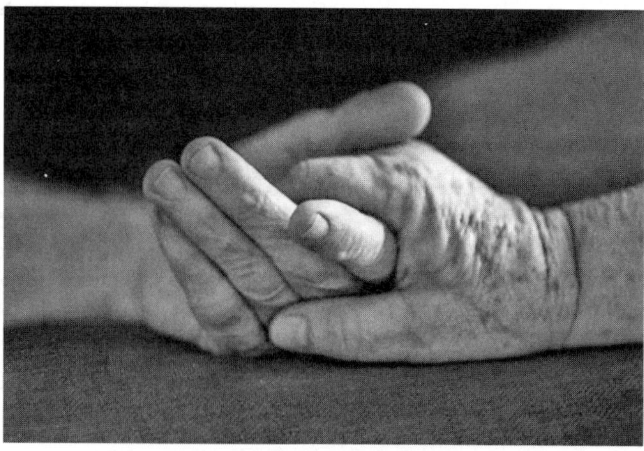

- A drop in body temperature can be a sign that the hands are not getting enough blood flow.
- A person's circulation decreases in the days leading up to death, allowing blood to concentrate on their internal structures. They still have very little blood circulating to their arms, feet, or legs as a result.
- Due to diminished circulation, a dying individual's skin will feel cool to the touch. Additionally, their skin may seem pale or spotted with violet and blue spots.
- The person who is dying may not feel cold themselves. Offering them a blanket is a good idea if a relative or friend thinks they may need one.

8. **Experiencing confusion**
   - The brain of a dying person is still quite active. They could sometimes, nevertheless, become disoriented or incoherent. This could occur if they become unaware of their surroundings.
   - When a loved one is dying, the person caring for them should make an effort to maintain communication. It is crucial to describe the surroundings and introduce each guest.

9. **Change breathing**
   - When someone is dying, they could seem to be having problems during breathing. They might stop breathing altogether, dramatically slow down their respiration, or gasp for air.
   - If a person caring for a loved one notices this, they should try not to worry. This is not usually painful or bothersome when being experienced by the dying person.
   - If someone is worried about this alteration in breathing pattern, it is an excellent decision to seek medical help.

10. **Increasing pain**
    - It may be challenging to accept the inevitable reality that a person's degree of pain may rise as they get closer to passing away.
    - It is never simple to see someone who is in pain or to hear someone who seems to be in suffering.
    - When a loved one is dying, the person caring for them should discuss pain management alternatives with the health care provider. The health care provider may make an effort to provide the dying individual the most comfort possible.

11. **Hallucinations**
    - It is uncommon for someone who is about to pass away to have some hallucinations or distorted visions.
    - Although this may seem concerning, a person caring for a dying loved one should not be alarmed. It is best not to try to correct them about these visions, as doing so may cause additional distress.

How to Cope the Last Few Hours

- ❖ A person's body and organs quit functioning in the hours preceding death. They may desire their loved ones at their side right now.
- ❖ Making a dying loved one as comfortable as possible in those final hours is the responsibility of the person caring for them.
- ❖ It is best to talk to someone who has passed on until they pass away. They often continue to hear what is going on around them.

Other Indicators of Death

If a person in the process of dying is strapped to a cardiac monitor, others around him will be ready to determine when their cardiovascular system has stopped beating and they have passed away.

Other signs of death include:
- Not having a pulse
- Not breathing
- No muscle tension
- Eyes remaining fixed
- Bowel or bladder releasing
- Eyelids partially shut

THE BILL OF RIGHTS FOR DYING PEOPLE

The Dying Person's Bill of Rights gives meaning to a dying person's right to die a good death with dignity. This blueprint offers a checklist for end-of-life preparation. It assists in ensuring that everyone in a position of authority complies as closely possible with the person's last wishes.

A person in the last stages of life has similar requirements to everyone else. The basic requirements for comfort, assistance, and appropriate care for the duration of one's life are the same for all patients, even those who are terminally ill. They have an right to relief from pain, respect from their physicians and carers on their deathbeds, and dignity both in live and in death. The bill for rights sets out the most essential necessities of someone who is dying as their life approaches its end.

Origin

The Dying Person's Bill of Rights was first introduced in 1975 at a workshop sponsored by Southwestern Michigan In-service Education Council entitled The Terminally Ill Patient and the Helping Person. The session was led by Amelia Barbus, a visiting assistant professor of nurse practitioner at Wayne State University. The end-of-life rights of the dying patient are now respected in hospitals and hospices all around the globe as result of this training.

David Kessler, an American expert on death and grieving, included a more comprehensive dying person's bill of rights in his book, The Needs of the Dying. The bill of rights is a set of guidelines that create a roadmap for medical staff, caregivers, and families of the dying to follow in the care and treatment of the patient nearing the end of life.

Purpose of the Dying Person's Bill of Rights

The Dying Person's Bill of Rights has been created in order to safeguard the patient's quality of life, which includes their physical, mental, social, and spiritual welfare. A passing patient, loved ones, and the caregivers should not have to endure any unnecessary pain or suffering in order to get the best end-of-life care possible. Every patient has the fundamental right to pass away peacefully and in accordance with their desires.
- **The right to be treated as a living human being until death:** Dying with dignity means having the right to be treated as a living human being with autonomy for as long as possible. Many patients fear losing their identity and ability to interact with their medical team and family members because of their limitations or incapacities.

- ❖ **The right to maintain a sense of hopefulness:**
  - ◆ Amongst patients facing a terminal illness or their end of life, many remain hopeful for a cure, the discovery of a new medical treatment, or a wonder drug that will save them at the last minute.
  - ◆ Some remain hopeful that, as they transition to death, their final days will be comfortable and that death will be quick and relatively painless. Regardless of how realistic it is, the sense of hope motivates many patients to maintain good spirits and endure anything that might come next.
- ❖ **The right to be cared for by those who maintain a sense of hope:** This patient right ensures that the doctors and caregivers responsible for the patient's care and wellbeing express some of the same hopes and desires as the patient. When the individuals caring for the dying patient mimic the patient's hopes, it softens the blows of impending death.
- ❖ **The right to express feelings and emotions about death:** Remaining free to process grief and express it in ways that resonate with how the patient feels and thinks is integral to patient autonomy. The dying patient has a right to experience their journey without interference from others.
- ❖ **The right to participate in decisions concerning care:** It is essential to respect and allow the dying patient to contribute to the decision-making process regarding their end-of-life care, even when the doctor disagrees with the patient's approach to dying.
- ❖ **The right to expect continuing medical and nursing attention:** A dying person whose aims are no longer to restore health but to find comfort in their final days has the right to continued medical care and attention with clearly defined treatment goals as they near death.
- ❖ **The right not to die alone:** The dying patient has the right to have family, friends, and other loved ones accompany them as they transition to death. Having others present in their final moments contributes to a peaceful end.
- ❖ **The right to be free from pain:** To ensure everyone's on the same page, choosing to live the last days free from pain even if it hastens death is a dying patient's fundamental right that the doctor and family should discuss. Not every doctor or family member will agree with the patient, and it's vital to clarify everyone's position ahead of time.
- ❖ **The right to have questions answered honestly:** Every patient has a right to ask about their condition and know the truth about their diagnosis and prognosis. A doctor needs to feel comfortable discussing the patient's prognosis even when it's not favorable.
- ❖ **The right to hear the truth:** A dying patient may want to know the truth about what to expect in their care and treatment, even when the news is not good. Many patients prefer their doctors to be honest in communicating their condition. Often, a patient's more concerned with how the doctor delivers the message than what they have to say about their situation.
- ❖ **The right to have help from and for family in accepting my death:** Many dying individuals and their families struggle with accepting death. Families tend to fall apart when dealing with the impending death of one of their members. Grief counseling should be available to all family members and the patient.
- ❖ **The right to die in peace and dignity:** Many dying patients have come to terms with their death and are ready to die when the time comes. It's usually their loved ones who want to prolong the patient's life, often without considering that the patient no longer wishes to extend their life.
- ❖ **The right to retain individuality and not be judged for their choices:** Dying is a very sacred and individual process to the terminally ill patient. When someone is nearing death, their

decisions regarding their end of life, their spiritual needs, or any other beliefs need to be respected.

- ❖ **The right to discuss and engage in religious or spiritual experiences:** Spirituality and religion are central to each individual's beliefs. A dying person may have thoughts that don't necessarily align with the rest of the family, doctors, or caregivers. However, every patient has the right to spiritual and religious fulfillment near the end of life.
- ❖ **The right to expect that the sanctity of the human body will be respected after death:** Plans for the disposal or burial of the body after death should consider the patient's wants as much as possible. There are times when the patient cannot communicate their dying wishes, and the family or loved one must decide what best aligns with the patient's wants or desires, whenever known.
- ❖ **The right to be cared for by caring, sensitive, knowledgeable people** who will attempt to understand the person's needs and will be able to gain some satisfaction in helping them face their death.

  The people who care for a dying patient play a unique role in their impending death. They have the power to facilitate a more caring, nurturing, and relaxed final transition for a person facing the end of life.

CARE OF DYING PATIENT

The provision of comfort for the dying, is a great challenge since your own emotional reactions to the dying patient prevent you from carrying out your duties. Every human culture is impacted by death, whether it be anticipated, sad, or unintentional. Biological and societal processes are represented by sickness, aging, dying, and death.

One of the most challenging areas to work in while providing comforts/services in a variety of settings is with clients who are dying. The dying's demands are diverse. Understanding a dying person's needs is crucial.

NEEDS OF DYING PATIENT

- ❖ **Health needs:** It might take a few seconds, hours, days, or weeks to pass away. There is general slowing of body process, weakness and changes in the level of consciousness. He can be totally reliant on others. The individual is allowed to pass away peacefully and honorably. In order to address his bodily needs as he approaches death, the following care must be given:
  - a. **Hearing, speech, and vision**
    - ◊ Vision may be blurred or gradually fails. A darkened room may frighten the person. So, room should be well-lighted but bright light to be avoided. Eye care to be given If the eyes stay open by covering a moistened pad, a protective ointment to avoid injury to eyes'.
    - ◊ Another crucial bodily function is hearing, and even a patient who is unconscious may hear. Always presume that the dead or the unresponsive can hear. Speak with a regular tone and voice, and provide consoling words. Avoid saying anything offensive in relation to the other person.
    - ◊ The dying person has difficulty in speaking. Even though they are mute, they may sometimes comprehend or follow you. Avoid asking the individual questions that need lengthy responses. Use a pen and paper sometimes to instruct or encourage him to write while he so chooses.

b. **Skin, mouth, and nose**
   - ◊ Good oral (mouth) hygiene is crucial for comfort. Mouth care to be given at least twice a day, if patient is taking orally soon after each feed, even simple rinse, is helpful. Even a simple rinse of mouth might be helpful. When death is near, frequent mouth care is provided because mucus collects in the throat.
   - ◊ *Nose:* You should observe the nostrils for increased nasal secretion, crust or any Irritation. If the patient is on oxygen cannula or nasogastric tube a lubricant may be applied to each nostril to avoid any injury.
   - ◊ Skin serves as an indication of body temperature or circulation. When body temperature rising and fall of circulation are signs that death is close by. Touch the skin whether the skin is cold, clammy and observe paleness and bluish discoloration. Therefore, take careful care of skin by giving bath, changing clothes and bed linens, and provide a blanket or light sleeping sheet as needed by patient. Changing positions may help to avoid bed sores.

c. **Elimination:** The client may have incontinence, constipation, or urine retention, which are all issues with elimination. For individuals who are incontinent, absorbent pads may be utilized, and catheters may be necessary for urine retention. If there is constipation, laxatives or enemas may be used, but care must be taken to avoid any negative effects (a doctor's advice is required). When they experience incontinence, a waterproof bed protector is very useful.
   - ◊ **Placement and comfort:** To improve comfort, you should constantly provide appropriate skin care, personal cleanliness, back massages, and dental hygiene.
   - ◊ **Some people could be in excruciating discomfort:** According to the doctor's instructions, you may provide pain medication. Comfort will be enhanced by frequent position changes, proper body alignment, and the use of supporting equipment. Turning the patient needs to be done carefully and slowly. Person with breathing difficulties, usually prefer-semi-Fowler's position.

d. **Maintaining environment:** A person's room should have good lighting and ventilation so that it may be as comfortable as possible. Focusing on the "patient" rather than the "task" or the "routine" would be a significant addition to a therapeutic environment.
   - ◊ In order to use the surroundings to promote the patient's well-being, it is possible to manage and modify noise, odor, cleanliness, safety risks, and bed location.
   - ◊ If at all feasible, move the patient to a quiet place with less environmental stimulation so that he or she may relax and sleep.
   - ◊ Keep orientation cues in the surroundings, such as a clock and a calendar;
   - ◊ Decorate the space with a nice image, such as a landscape.
   - ◊ If the patient would like, they may use the telephone, radio, or television.

Warning Signs of Impending Death

- ❖ A weak pulse.
- ❖ Potentially lower body temperature.
- ❖ A decrease in blood pressure.
- ❖ Labored breathing, which may involve Cheyne strokes (apnea followed by over breathing).
- ❖ Cyanosis of extremities, nail beds and area around the lips, cold extremities, purplish skin.
- ❖ A sensational loss.
- ❖ Death rattle (the sound of secretions in the throat that the individual no longer coughs up).

❖ Potential coma.
❖ The eventual cessation of breathing, blood pressure, and pulse.

Maintain Basic Safety Needs

Uphold fundamental safety requirements; prevent accidents and injuries by doing the following:
❖ **Fire:** Smoking laws, matchboxes, candles, and agarbattis should all be observed.
❖ **Electrical equipment:** They shouldn't be any loose connections, wires, or electrical leaks. Equipment and furnishings with defects. When a patient is out of bed and using a wheel chair, chair, or foot stool, for instance, if those items are not in functioning order and the foot footstool is not in line with the patient's center of gravity, that increases the risk of harm from a fall.
❖ Accessible bedside tables, furniture, equipment, working-area obstructions, and moist floors should all be taken into consideration.
❖ Friends, family friends of his choosing, and significant ones should be stated to remain with the patient in order to help him.
❖ Should be aided when getting out of bed or changing. On the other hand, as you can see, the room is empty.

Nutrition

❖ Small, regular meals of the patient's preferred foods are probably should be provided.
❖ A patient's preferred diet should be taken into account.
❖ Make sure the meal is pleasant and easy to digest.
❖ The patient should be seated or on their back.
❖ Present food that is 'natural' for the individual patient.
❖ Provide a social environment based on the patient's preferences, such as radio, conversation, television, or silence.
❖ Use clean spoons, forks, and other utensils as desired by the patient.
❖ Offer a very tiny quantity to check the temperature of the food and drink first.
❖ Always encourage patients to eat, but never force them to have any type of food.
❖ Feeding someone with dysphasia should be done with the utmost care in terms of quality and time, and swallowing of food or drink should be stopped if the patient gasps or chokes.

Social Needs

The patient is on dying condition whether terminal illness or chronic illness, whether in hospital or at home, to be viewed as having lots of social values. Humans are social creatures that belong to society; therefore they given that feeling that he is still an important member in the family and society through constant contact with him without disturbing his other needs, e.g., rest, sleep, etc.

Efforts to Meet Social Needs

❖ Use the patient's name while speaking to him or use the appropriate pronouns.
❖ Permit one important companion to remain with the patient.
❖ Effective communication must be maintained.
❖ When the individual is conscious but cannot speak, use paper and pen or you can write for the patient to know his desires. You can use slate and pencil also for communication.

* Establish a rapport based on trust by paying attention to the patient.
* Permit family members to help with caring.

Religious Needs

While nutrition, exercise, and medicine all contribute to the healing process, something that is frequently overlooked is the spiritual component!

So let's look at how to satisfy a dying patient's spiritual needs. Even as he approaches death, the patient will still have his own unique spiritual demands. Regardless of the patient's religion or belief system, it is your obligation to be understanding of such demands and to recognize and support their relevance to the patient.

The assistance that they get from the different faiths provides considerable consolation to many terminally and chronically sick people.

* If he so chooses, arrange up a prayer service.
* Keep a holy book of his religion and read if the patient wishes.

Depending on the patient's requests or circumstances, certain religious chants or music may be played specifically in the early morning hours or late at night on the tape recorder.

* Sometimes, use silence.
* Arrange with a priest other senior church member to help, in accordance with the patient's wishes.

Mental Needs

The most crucial thing is to take care of a dying person's emotional needs. He can be saddened by the fact that his existence is ending ahead of time, leaving things undone or unfinished, ambitions unmet, and chances missed. His personality will thus be greatly impacted by all of this.

The following is a list of anxieties experienced throughout the living-to-death period:

* Fear of unknown
* Fear of lonely ness
* Fear of sorrow
* Fear of loss of body
* Fear of loss of self-control
* Fear of loss of identity
* Fear of loss, suffering and pain

When one is sick, there is a sense of isolation from oneself and from others. This is by the fact that others tend to avoid a dying or terminally ill person and leave him alone.

Approaches to Addressing Emotional Requirements

* Make yourself accessible to the person every day.
  Sit down and pay attention. Allow for the expressing of feelings and listen instead of speaking.
* Make yourself accessible to loved ones and close relationships for information, comprehension, dialogue, and support.
* **Apply touch:** When the patient communicates the need for help by verbal and nonverbal cues (such as sobbing or sharing sad memories).
* Give the dying person equal time as they need to spend with their loved ones and family.

END OF LIFE CARE

Definition

End of life care is the term currently used for issued related to death and dying, as well as services provided to address these issues.

Institute of medicine: Defines end of life care as the period of time during which an individual copes with declining health from a terminal illness or from the frailities associated with advanced age even if death is not clearly imminent.

Goals of End of Life Care

1. To enhance life quality.
2. To affirm a person's life.
3. Treats the individual.
4. Provide support for the family

Healthcare Standards for Providing End-of-Life Care

- ❖ Providing appropriate treatment for any primary and secondary symptom, according to the wishes of the patient and surrogate decision maker.
- ❖ Effectively and aggressively managing pain.
- ❖ Addressing sensitive problems like autopsy and organ donation.
- ❖ Honoring the patient's principles, religion, and beliefs.
- ❖ Include the patient or their family in every step of the healing process.
- ❖ Responding the patient's and family's psychological, social, emotional, spiritual, and cultural problems.

Nursing Care for the Elderly

- ❖ Personal hygiene should come first. Oral swabs, soothing ointment, or petroleum jelly are essential.
- ❖ Providing eye care to increase comfort.
- ❖ To stop eye dryness, use artificial tears or optical saline solutions.
- ❖ Anorexia and DHN—a benefit of DHN is decreased lung congestion, which prevents noisy or labored respirations
- ❖ Skin integrity should be monitored carefully to prevent complications. Lotions, repositioning patient, avoid shearing forces, use of lift sheets.
- ❖ Bowel and bladder incontinence—protective pads to prevent decubitus ulcer—avoid use of catheter because of UTI. Constipation should be treated with stool softeners.
- ❖ Visual or auditory hallucinations—family members maybe upset
- ❖ It is believed that the sense of hearing is intact in comatose patient. Encourage family members to "let go" and give the terminal patient permission to die. Appropriate affection should be encouraged and privacy provided.
- ❖ Read a poem, tell a joke, listen to past story sing a song, provide a hug.

Physical Care

- ❖ Use ice cubes or a wet towel dipped in water to moisten the tongue or fruit juice.
- ❖ Use petroleum jelly (vaseline) or balm to keep lips moisturized.

❖ Keep the individual dry and clean; for urine incontinence, use pads or cloths.

❖ Administer drugs for symptom management at the appropriate times.

❖ Do not wait until the signs and symptoms are severe since it will make them harder to manage.

❖ Do not make them eat or drink against their will. It is acceptable if they choose not to eat.

❖ Assist the individual in shifting positions or turning every two hours to avoid pressure sores.

❖ If pain or other symptoms are not under control, get in touch with the home palliative care team (or whomever is offering round-the-clock telephone assistance).

Spiritual and Emotional Support

❖ Let them know they are loved and will be remembered.

❖ Make sure the individual gets the chance to talk about any guilt, concern, or regret they may be experiencing.

❖ If the individual so desires, make interactions with religious or religious authorities.

❖ Take a seat next to them, grasp their hand, and converse with them.

Escalating Pain, Dyspnea, and Agitation

No ceiling dose exists for symptom management in the last hours or days of life (end-of-life phase). The correct dose is the dose that relieves the patient's symptoms.

Titrate the drugs quickly (over a few minutes to hours).

❖ **Loading dose for those using opioids already:** Give a loading dosage of opioids that is 10% of your total dose from the previous 24 hours.

❖ **Patients who are not already using opioids:** Provide the loading dosage through IV or SC as follows: Children's 5 mg of morphine.

❖ **For excessive respiratory secretions:** SC (hyoscine butylbromide), SC (glycopyrrolate), or oral atropine 1% eye drop solution.

Pain Relief at the End of Life

❖ Providing initial and continuous pain level assessments, pain medication delivery, and assessment of the success of the pain management strategy.

❖ When other vital signs like the temperature, pulse, respiration rate, and BP are evaluated, it is important to frequently check the fifth vital sign, or pain.

❖ Pain causes unnecessary suffering at the end of life and hastens death.

❖ It is crucial to provide culturally appropriate assistance in order to deliver effective and comprehensive end-of-life care. Pain is a subjective sensation. The most accurate way to measure pain is by self-report.

❖ Patients with cognitive impairments or who are unable to talk should be attentively watched by nurses for the following symptoms:

- Lack of eating or drinking,
- Grumbling when at rest or while moving,
- Protecting or not moving bodily parts,
- Refusing treatment, and noncooperation with therapeutic procedures,
- Grimacing or strained facial expression.

PREPARE FOR DEATH

❖ Watching the patient decline and the body itself starting to shutdown life process can bring helplessness and anxiety.

❖ The nurse must work to allay the patient's and family's worries.

❖ Questions about an afterlife, unsolved social, emotional, and financial difficulties, as well as acceptance of death, are all quite predominant. The nurse must take care of oneself at this challenging time and acknowledge and accept their emotions.

❖ Older patients want reassurance from their family members that everything is well and that it is okay to let go.

CHANGES FOLLOWING DEATH

❖ Postmortem changes

❖ Death may present with immediate, quick or late symptoms.

Early signs include:

❖ Eye changes

❖ Algor mortis

❖ Livor mortis

❖ Rigor mortis

Immediate signs include:

❖ 1st sign is insensibility (loss of sensation) and loss of voluntary power.

❖ There is stoppage of respiration and circulation.

Late signs include:

❖ Decomposition signs

❖ Putrefaction

❖ Autolysis

❖ Mummification

Early Signs

Eye Movements

A. **Cattle trucking, the Kevorkian Sign, or the railroading phenomenon:** The retinal blood vessels appear segmented or fragmented. It is seen within a few minutes to one hour after death. It can be seen using an ophthalmoscope. It is the earliest eye sign and it is used to determine time since death (TSD). Before the Kevorkian sign, corneal reflexes are lost, and the pupil is dilated.

B. **Flaccidity of the eyeball (Kevorkian sign):** 20 mm Hg is the average intraocular pressure. The intraocular pressure falls to 0 mm Hg two hours after death. It is also used to determine time since death.

C. **Tache Noire Sclerotique:** The term "Tache Noire Sclerotique" refers to two brownish triangular-shaped opacities that occur on each side of the cornea after death if the eyelids are open and dust is present in the environment. It takes place 3–6 hours after the postmortem and is used to establish the time since death.

D. **Corneal changes:** The cornea is normally clear, but after one hour following death, it becomes cloudy. Contrarily, the cornea becomes opaque after six hours.

E. **Vitreous humor changes:** It is the most significant putrefaction-resistant medium in the eye. After putrefaction, there are zero chemical alterations to the vitreous fluid. Being confined within the eyeball, where germs cannot readily reach it, it is the ideal medium for determining the amount of time since death.

So this medium is quite beneficial even in a body that has progressed decomposition. Vitreous potassium levels are the best parameter. The levels of K^+ and hypoxanthine have increased linearly. It correlates linearly with the interval since death. Sturner's Formula and Madea's Formula are two formulae used to determine the amount of time since death.

F. **Algor mortis, or bodily cooling:** Within 15 minutes after death, it is discovered. Body core temperature (BCT) drops as a result. A chemical thermometer called a thermometer is used in postmortem to measure BCT. Perhaps 25–30 cm. It has a temperature range of 0–50°C. The rectum is the ideal location for temperature measurements since its temperature is almost equivalent to BCT.

Other locations include the lower end of the esophagus, outer auditory meatus, nasal spaces, even the innermost layer of the liver. The graph that depicts the link between temperature and postmortem time has the form of an inverted S-curve or sigmoid.

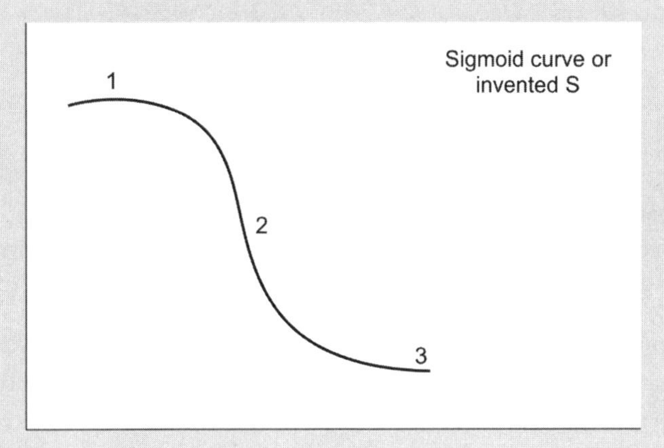

Stage I: Isothermal phase
Stage II: Steep decline
Stage III: Gradual decrease

Algor mortis occurs in three phases:
1st phase: Gradual decrease in BCT
2nd phase: Rapid decrease in BCT
3rd phase: Gradual decrease in BCT. Shape of Algor mortis curve is sigmoid.

Rate of fall of temperature is 0.4–0.7°C/hr that is, in summer it is 0.4°C/hr and in winter it is 0.7°C/hr. Average fall of temperature is 0.5 C/hr. By knowing the rate of fall, we can calculate time since death.

Postmortem Caloricity

Normally, the body becomes cold within 15 mins after death [Algor mortis]. But, if the body remains warm for 1–2 hrs even after death, it is known as postmortem caloricity. Whenever there is increased body core temperature at the time of death, postmortem caloricity is seen.

Increased body core temperature at death is seen in conditions with increased muscle contraction that is tetanus, strychnos nux vomica poisoning exercises, etc. Defective thermoregulation in the body is associated with heat stroke, pontine hemorrhage [have pyrexia, paralysis, pinpoint pupils] and septicemia.

After Death Staining

It is also known as hypostasis, livor mortis, postmortem lividity, vibices, or suggillation. The stain is present on bodily parts that are dependent, or that face the ground but do not contact ground.

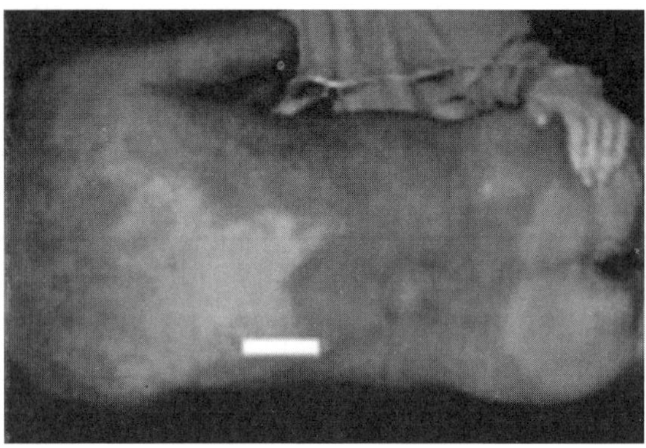

Blood pools in capillaries and venules as a result of gravitational forces, accumulating deoxyhemoglobin, giving the skin a bluish-purple hue. There is Skin discoloration of rete mucosum of the dermis.

Pressure-sensitive areas of the body are devoid of this stain. After 30 minutes, or soon after death, it starts. It is also apparent for two hours after death. Maximum visibility lasts for 6–12 hours, after which fixation takes place.

Secondary lividity occurs when changing the position of the body before 7–8 hours leading to postmortem staining in other areas of the body, it persists till decomposition. Decomposition changes the skin color to green.

Postmortem Staining in Different Positions

* **In the supine position:** The back of the head, back of the neck, back of the chest, back of the leg is stained.
* **In prone position:** The front parts of the body are stained.
* **In hanging position:** The hands and feet are stained, i.e., show glove and stocking pattern.
* **In running water:** There is no postmortem discoloration in running water.

Medical Importance

It helps to determine time since death and determine the position of the body at the time of death and also determine the cause of death (COD).

Color Presentation due to Different causes

* **Toxicity from carbon monoxide:** Cherry-red
* **Cyanide toxicity:** Bright and brick red
* **Hypothermia:** Pink
* **Hydrogen sulfide (H_2S):** Blue-green
* **Opium:** Black

* **Phosphorus or potassium chlorate ($KCLO_3$):** Brown
* **Nitrites, nitrobenzene, and aniline:** Chocolate brown
* **Aniline:** A blue hue
* Chocolate brown color formed due to methemoglobin
* **Clostridium perfringens:** Bronze
* **Methanol toxicity:** Purple

Rigor Mortis or Cadaveric Stiffening or Cadaveric Rigidity

It is sometimes referred to as cadaveric stiffening or cadaveric stiffness. It grants muscular status when a person has passed away. The muscle stiffens occur due to the drop in ATP. Rigor mortis is a widespread condition that affects both voluntary and involuntary muscles, but it is first seen in involuntary muscles.

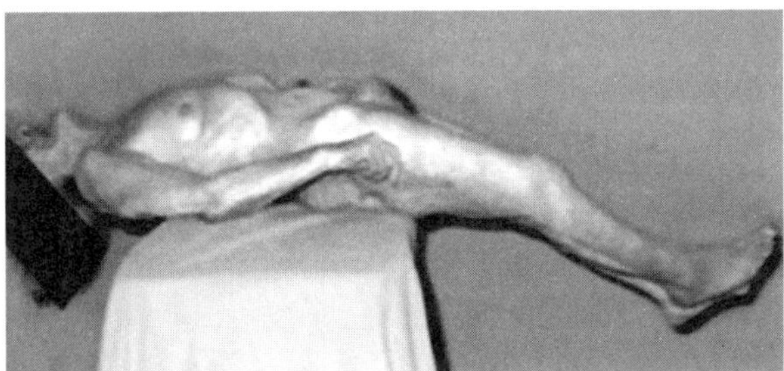

Muscles undergo three stages after death include:
1. Primary relaxation period or the primary flaccidity phase.
2. Mortal rigor.
3. Secondary relaxation phase or the secondary flaccidity phase.

Primary flaccidity occurs during somatic death. Rigor mortis happens when a cellular death occurs. The mechanism for rigor mortis is ATP depletion. Actin-myosin separation takes place in primary flaccidity. Rigor mortis is brought on by a lack of actin-myosin separation.

When disintegration begins in these actin and myosin filaments, it causes separation and secondary flaccidity. When rigor mortis begins, ATP levels drop to 85% of normal. A maximal rigor mortis condition causes ATP levels to drop to 15–30% of normal.

Occurrence of Rigor Mortis in Muscles

It starts one to two hours after death. All muscles, whether voluntary or involuntary, exhibit it. Affected first muscle is the myocardium. The upper eyelid muscle, orbicularis oculi, is the first external muscle to be damaged. The exterior muscles are impacted in the following order:

Eyelid muscles → Neck → Lower jaw → Muscles of face → Muscles of chest → Upper limbs → Abdomen → Lower limbs → Fingers and toes

Rigor mortis disappears in the same order that it appears. It will disappear first from the upper eyelid and last from the fingers and toes.

12th Rule

All bodily muscles experience rigor mortis during the first twelve hours after death.
* It lasts for the following 12 hours in every muscle in the body.
* In the next 12 hours, it disappears from all body muscles.
* Within 36–48 hours after death, rigor mortis emerges and vanishes, assisting in the identification of TSD.

Rigor Mortis in a Fetus

Because the filaments composed of actin and myosin have not yet formed, rigor mortis does not exist in fetuses less than 7 months old. The onset of rigor mortis varies with the seasons. It takes 18–36 hours to appear in the summer, while it takes 24–48 hours to appear in the winter.

Rigor Mortis in Wasting Diseases

In diseases including cholera, TB, cancer, cachexia, and typhoid, the muscle mass is thin with limited ATP storage. In this there is early onset of rigor mortis with short duration.

Rigor Mortis Appears in Violent Death

Instances like a gunshot wound or slit neck cause rigor mortis, which results in a violent death. It has early onset rigor mortis with short duration.

Appearance of Rigor Mortis in Thick Muscle

There is increased ATP storage and it has late onset of rigor mortis.

Causes of muscle stiffening after death:
- Rigor mortis
- Heat stiffening
- Cold stiffening
- Gas stiffening
- Cadaveric spasm

Heat Stiffening

Other names for it include the "boxing attitude," "pugilist attitude," and "fencing attitude." It happens when the ambient temperature is below 65°C. Mechanism involves the coagulation of muscle protein. Heat stiffening persists till decomposition occurs.

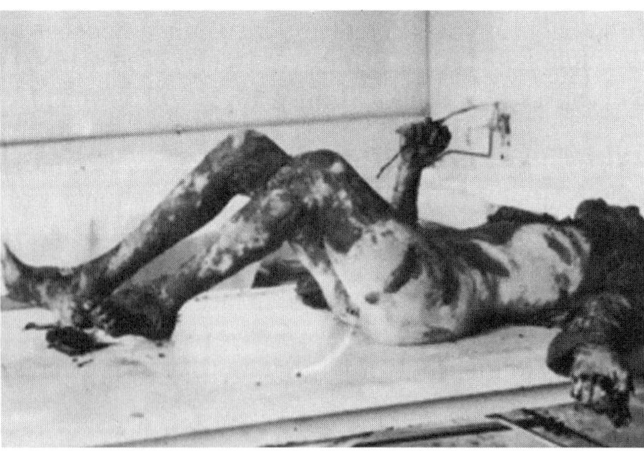

Cold Stiffening

It happens when the outside temperature is below –5°C. Mechanism involves freezing of the body fluid and hardening of the subcutaneous tissue. In warm temperature, cold stiffening disappears. In this normal rigor is present.

Gas Stiffening

This occurs as a result of a significant gas accumulation. It is seen with decomposition. The body produces too much gas during decomposition, and this gas builds up within the body, making the body rigid.

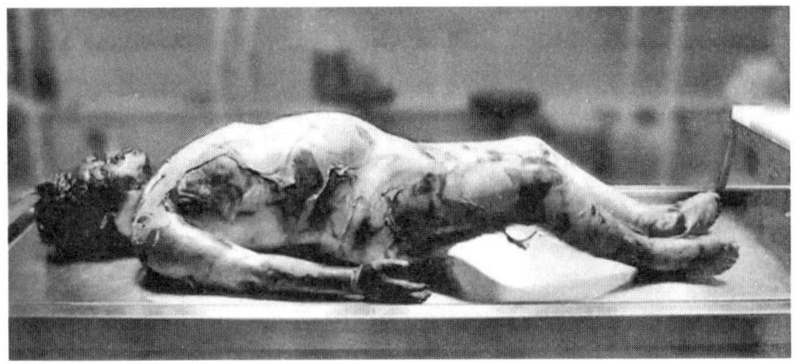

Cadaveric Spasm

It is sometimes referred to as instantaneous rigor or cataleptic stiffness. Mechanism involves ATP depletion. Muscles are permanently tensed and continue to be tight and stiff even after death. It happens right away after death. Primary relaxation is absent whereas secondary relaxation is present. It is an exclusively antemortem event.

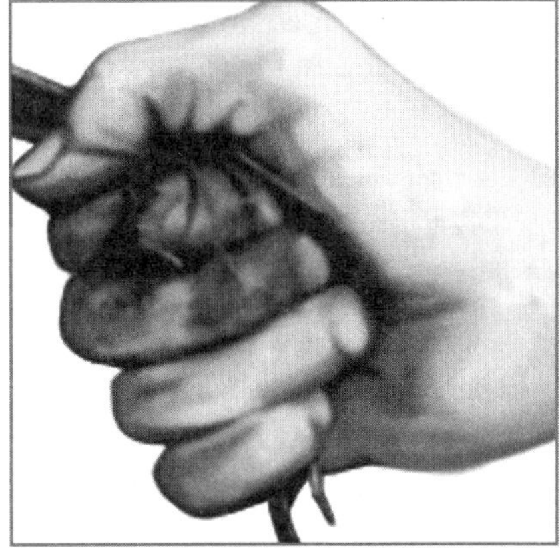

Causes of cadaveric spasm:

- ❖ Asphyxial death
- ❖ Brain injury
- ❖ Cerebral injury
- ❖ Drowning
- ❖ Dinitrocresol poisoning
- ❖ Excitement
- ❖ Fear
- ❖ Firearm, e.g., in suicide

Differences between cadaveric spasm and rigor mortis

	Cadaveric spasm	*Rigor mortis*
Time	Immediately after death	1–2 hours after death
Muscles	Mainly involves voluntary muscles Generally, it involves a short group of muscles, e.g., hand muscles	Involves both voluntary and involuntary muscles
Primary relaxation	Absent	Present
Molecular death	Absent	Present
Electronic stimuli	Response present	Response absent
Importance	Describes the manner of death	Determines TSD

Late Changes

In these changes the body gets decomposed. Decomposition occurs by two mechanisms: autolysis and putrefaction.

- ❖ **Autolysis:** It is a process that is brought on by bodily enzymes causes cell lysis. Autolytic modifications examples:

  Clouding of cornea – 1st external change.

  Changes in brain glandular tissue – 1st internal change.

  Aseptic autolysis involves the mummification of the fetus in intrauterine death.

- ❖ **Putrefaction:** It is stimulated by bacterial activity. Most common bacteria involved is clostridium welchii or clostridium perfringens. Most common enzyme involved is lytic lecithinase.

  Putrefaction occurs in three stages of change:

  1. **Color change:** Reddish-brown staining of the aorta intima is the first internal/overall change of putrefaction. The right iliac fossa's green discoloration is the first visible change.

     ◊ **Mechanism:** Hydrogen sulfide is produced by bacteria. Cecum located beneath the right iliac fossa has maximum bacterial activity. Skin lies superficial to the cecum. Sulphur combines with hemoglobin to form a green color compound. Discoloration begins in the summer within 12–18 hours. Discoloration begins in winter within one to two days.

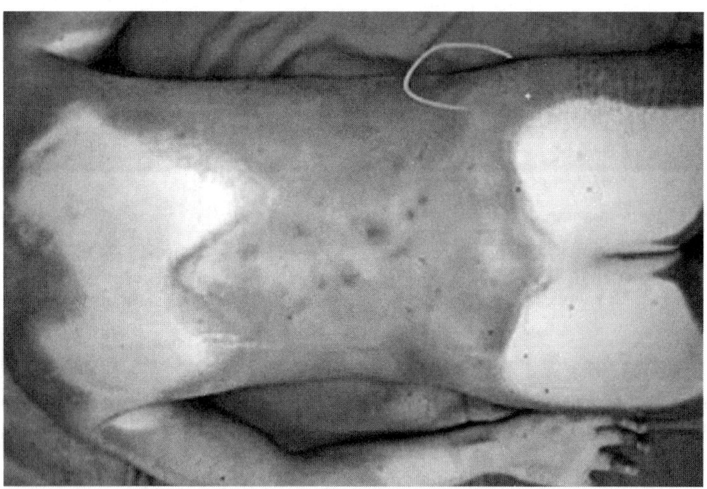

Decomposition—green discoloration of body.

     ◊ **Marbling:** The large superficial veins that are discolored to a greenish-brown tint that corresponds to the vascular channel.

     ◊ **Mechanism:** In the superficial veins, *Clostridium welchii* bacteria produce hydrogen sulfide with the development of green and brown Sulfhemoglobin. It begins in 24 hours and peaks between 36 and 48 hours later. It helps in figuring out TSD. It is seen in the chest, shoulder, belly, and thigh.

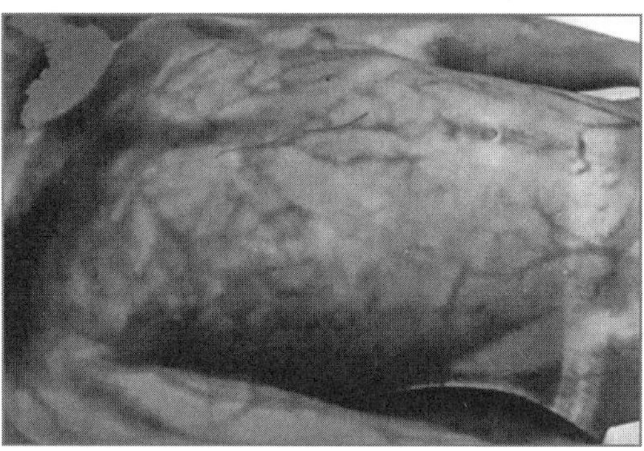

Marbling.

2. **Gas formation:** H_2S is the primary gas produced during decomposition. This gas builds up in the body and stiffens, a condition known as gas stiffening. Gas in the skin at the dermo-epidermal junction causes blister formation.

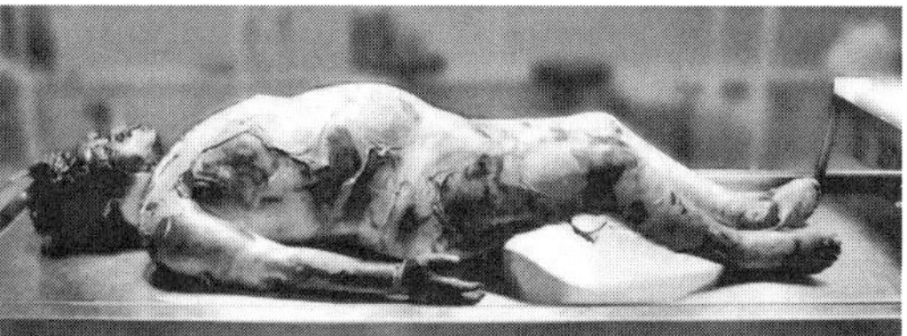

Gas stiffening.

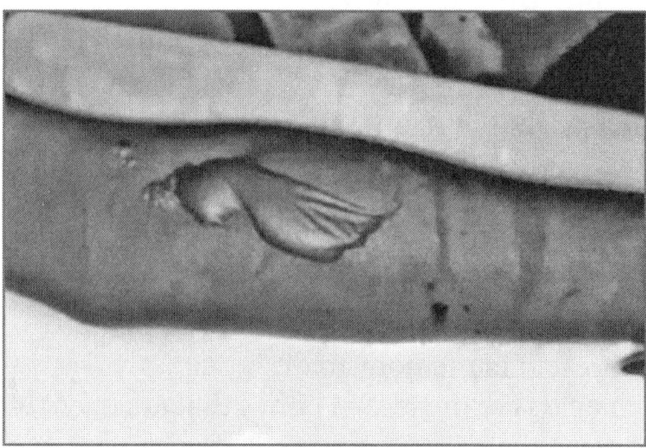

Postmortem blister.

3. **Liquefaction of tissue:** It takes 5–10 days. Loosening of hair/nails, occur in 3–5 days kin around the hands and legs peel off, i.e., degloving/destocking pattern is seen in 5–10 days.
   ◊ **Postmortem purge:** Gas formation during decomposition leads to the expulsion of blood-stained froth and gastric contents from the nose and mouth is seen after 2–3 days.
   ◊ **Postmortem luminescence:** Body emits light after death. Causes of postmortem luminescence are:
   ◊ Bacterial, e.g., photobacteria presence.
   ◊ Fungal, e.g., Armillaria, Ram's bottom.

Casper's Dictum

It is about rate of putrefaction in different medium. Rate of putrefaction is compared b/w 3 imp medium. This formula was proposed by Taylor. It shows the relationship between the rate of decomposition in air, water and soil (earth).

Air > Water > Earth.

Decomposition happens in the air in one week, in the water in two weeks, and in the soil in eight weeks. In air, decomposition happens most quickly.

Putrefaction sequence: 1st organs to decompose are the larynx and trachea due to their direct contact to air.

Followed by (in order):
- Small intestine, stomach, and spleen.
- Lung and liver.
- Uterus, kidney, heart, and brain.
- Muscle, bone, tendon, and skin.
- In females, the nongravid womb is the last organ to decompose.
- In men, the prostate is the very last organ to decompose.
- The overall last organ to decompose is bone/tooth.

Important Points of Putrefaction

- Liver shows gas formation up to 24–36 hours, i.e., foamy liver or honeycomb liver.
- The ideal decomposition temperature ranges from 21 to 38°C.
- At much over 10°C, decomposition begins.
- Poisons prevent putrefaction are:
  - Strychnine
  - Metallic poison, such as thallium, antimony, and arsenic
  - Carbon dioxide
  - Cyanide
  - Carbolic acid
- Proline is the first amino acid to disappear from bones after decomposition.
- Hydroxyproline is the second amino acid that has disappeared.
- Glycine is the last amino acid in the body to disappear.
- Less than seven amino acids are present in bones that are over 100 years old.

Modification of Putrefaction

Grave Wax, or Adipocere, or Saponification

It is often referred to as saponification or grave wax. The body's fat is transformed into fatty acids, which mix with calcium to produce insoluble wax-like compounds called adipocere (SOAP).

When it develops, an adipocere is kept in place for a longer duration. It involves the hydrogenation and hydrolysis of fat. Warm, humid environment, clostridium welchii (lecithinase), and intrinsic lipases (lipases found naturally in the body) are necessary conversion factors. The predominant fatty acid is palmitic acid. Acidic medium Inhibits the multiplication of bacteria (further putrefaction is inhibited), hence the body is preserved, smell of adipocere is ammoniacal.

Appearance of Adipocere

* ❖ Fresh adipocere-greasy and it looks like rancid butter
* ❖ Old adipocere-dry, hard, yellow and brittle
* ❖ Time required for adipocere formation is 3 days to 3 months and it is absent in fetuses of less than 7 months.

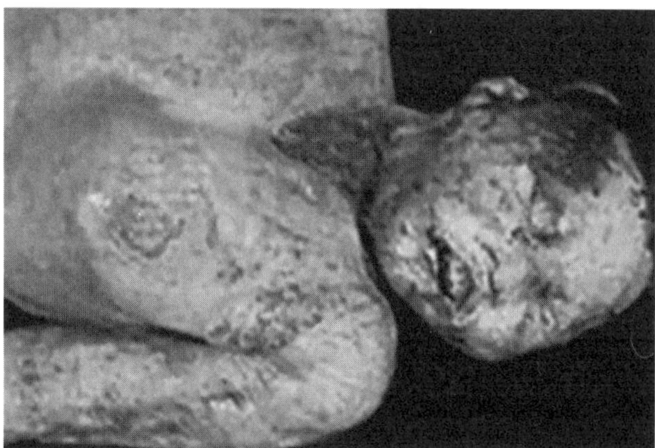

Old adipocere.

Medical Importance

It helps to describe the climate at time of death and determination of time since death and helps in preservation of the dead body for easy identification.

Mummification

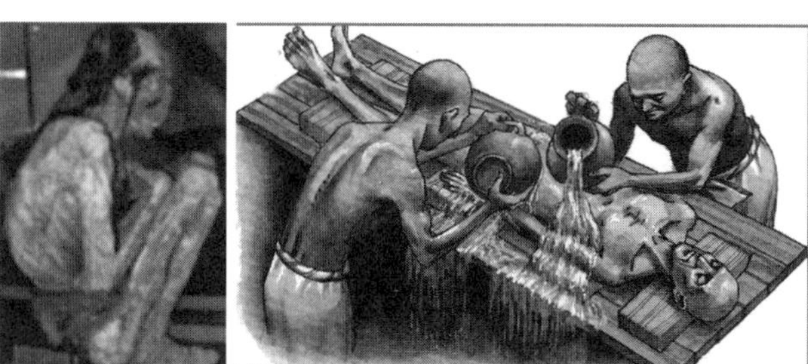

When a body is exposed to dry in hot environment, drying and dehydration take place, which causes mummification. In this process, the body shrinks and loses weight by more than 70%. It has no distinctive fragrance and is odorless. It takes three to twelve months to happen. It is also seen in intrauterine death of fetus, when a fetus dies intrauterinally with its membranes intact and its blood supply is inadequate, mummification may also occur. Mummification is favored by arsenic and antimony. It is a crucial characteristic of intrauterine death.

Medical importance
* ❖ Describes climate at the time of death.
* ❖ Determination of TSD.
* ❖ Identification is comparatively very easy.

Embalming or Tanatopraxia

It is defined as artificial method of preserving the body by injecting antiseptic and preservatives.
Exhumation is lawful digging of the body. Ideal time for embalming is less than 6 hrs after death (very effective).

Composition of embalming fluid

Preservative	Formalin Formaldehyde Methanol
Antiseptic/Germicide	Phenol
Wetting agent	Glycerine Glycerol
Anticoagulant	Sodium citrate
Buffer	Sodium bicarbonate Sodium carbonate Sodium chloride
Vehicle	Water

Ethanol is not a part of embalming fluid.

Embalming Methods

- ❖ Arterial
- ❖ Cavity
- ❖ Surface embalming (not commonly used).
- ❖ Best method is a discontinuous injection and discontinuous drainage.
- ❖ High pressure/low volume method also used.
- ❖ Best vessel is the femoral artery.
- ❖ Embalming is always done after a postmortem or receiving the death certificate.

Antemortem vs Postmortem

	Antemortem	Postmortem
Content	Inflammation Chloride Protein (mainly, albumin)	Gas
Base	Erythematous.	Pale
Redness	Present	Absent
Enzymatic/Vital reaction	Present	Absent

DEATH DECLARATION AND CERTIFICATION

Medical Certification of Death

Accuracy is the most important factor to be considered in the medical death certification. All dates should be indicated by day, month, and year. The time of death should be reported in a 24-hour clock format, military time. For example, if the time of death is 1 PM, it should be recorded as 1,300 on the death certificate.

Part I

The cause of death section in the death certificate should be filled out as specifically as possible. Part I reports the causal events that lead to death and is made up of parts Ia to Id, describes the events that cause death.

Line a lists the "immediate" or "recent" incident that causes death. Lines b through and then progressively list the other requirements. The most remote condition that caused death is referred to as the "underlying" factor in death.

The word "intermediate" or "intermediary" refers to any situations that lie in between both the immediate and underlying causes of mortality. The approximate interval between the onset of each of the events and time of death should be listed in hours, days, weeks, or months.

Part II

All other diseases and injuries that may have contributed to death but did necessarily precipitate the cascade of events leading to death are listed in part II.

Examples of completing a death certificate:

Example 1

Part I
◀◀ Pulmonary edema (2 days) due to or as a consequence of
◀◀ Anasarca (2 months) due to or as a consequence of
◀◀ Chronic renal failure (5 years) due to or as a consequence of

Part II
◀◀ Chronic obstructive pulmonary disease (20 years)
◀◀ The manner of death: natural
◀◀ Autopsy: yes/no

Pulmonary edema is the direct cause of mortality in this instance. The intermediate causes of mortality associated with systemic lupus erythematosus, which is the root cause of death, include anasarca with chronic renal failure. The death certificate has to be quite detailed. Edema must be specific about where it is: pulmonary edema. The reason of death should be described as precisely as possible. It is also preferable to stay away from acronyms and abbreviations.

Example 2

Part I
◀◀ Fat embolism (2 hours) due to or as a consequence of
◀◀ Chronic tissue hypoxia (12 years) due to or as a consequence of
◀◀ Sickle cell anemia (12 years)

Part II
◀◀ Moderate persistent asthma (7 years)
◀◀ The manner of death: natural
◀◀ Autopsy: yes/no

In this case, a fat embolism was the real cause of death. Chronic tissue hypoxia brought on by sickle cell disease is what causes adipose tissue to separate from the bone marrow. The secondary cause of death is this. Sickle cell illness, which is regarded as the main condition cause persistent hypoxia as a result of flawed hemoglobin with restricted oxygen-carrying capacity, is the leading cause of mortality. The death certificate has to state both the reason of death and the manner of death. Cardiopulmonary arrest, (CPA), is often the main cause of death. Since it does not identify the cause of death, it is not advisable to put this diagnosis in a funeral certificate.

Annex 1

Clinical determination of death: two different workflows but a common end point-death

Process for the clinical determination of death

Box 1

Neurological arrest
- Etiology of coma known from clinical assessment or neuroimaging
- Catastrophic structural injury to the CNS

- Hemodynamic stability
- Adequate oxygenation and ventilation
- Absence of severe hydroelectrolytic and acid-base equilibrium alterations
- Absence of hypothermia <35°C
- Absence of severe metabolic and endocrinological alterations
- Absence of toxic substances and their effects
- Absence of clinical significant neuromuscular blockers and neurodepressaent drugs of the CNS

Box 2

Clinical diagnosis
Coma
+
Absence of brain stem reflexes
+
Apnoea

Box 3

Confirmatory testing

Primary supratentorial lesion	Secondary brain damage	Primary infratentorial lesion

and/or

Observation period (according to etiology and age	Instrumental tests (EEG, EP Perfusion)	Instrumental tests (EEG, Perfusion)

Second clinical examination

Box 4

Cardio circulatory arrest
- Unresponsiveness
- Not breathing or only occasional gasps
- Absence of circulation

Cardiopulmonary resuscitation

Failed	Not attempted

Absence of circulation confirmed by the following means:

- Individual has a DNR order, or for other reasons does not meet the criteria for attempting CPR
- Treatment aimed at sustaining life has been withdrawn

Box 5

Clinical diagnosis
Absence of a central pulse on palpation
+
Absence of heart sound on auscultation
+
Absence of breathing
+ absence of pupillary responses to ligh

Box 6

Instrumental tests
(*If indicated*)
Asystole or pulseless electrical activity on a continuous ECG display
and/or
Absence of pulsatile flow with intra-arterial pressure monitoring
and/or
Absence of contractile activity using echocardiography

Wait a minimum of 5 minutes after diagnosis to ensure no spontaneous return of cardiac or respiratory function

Death

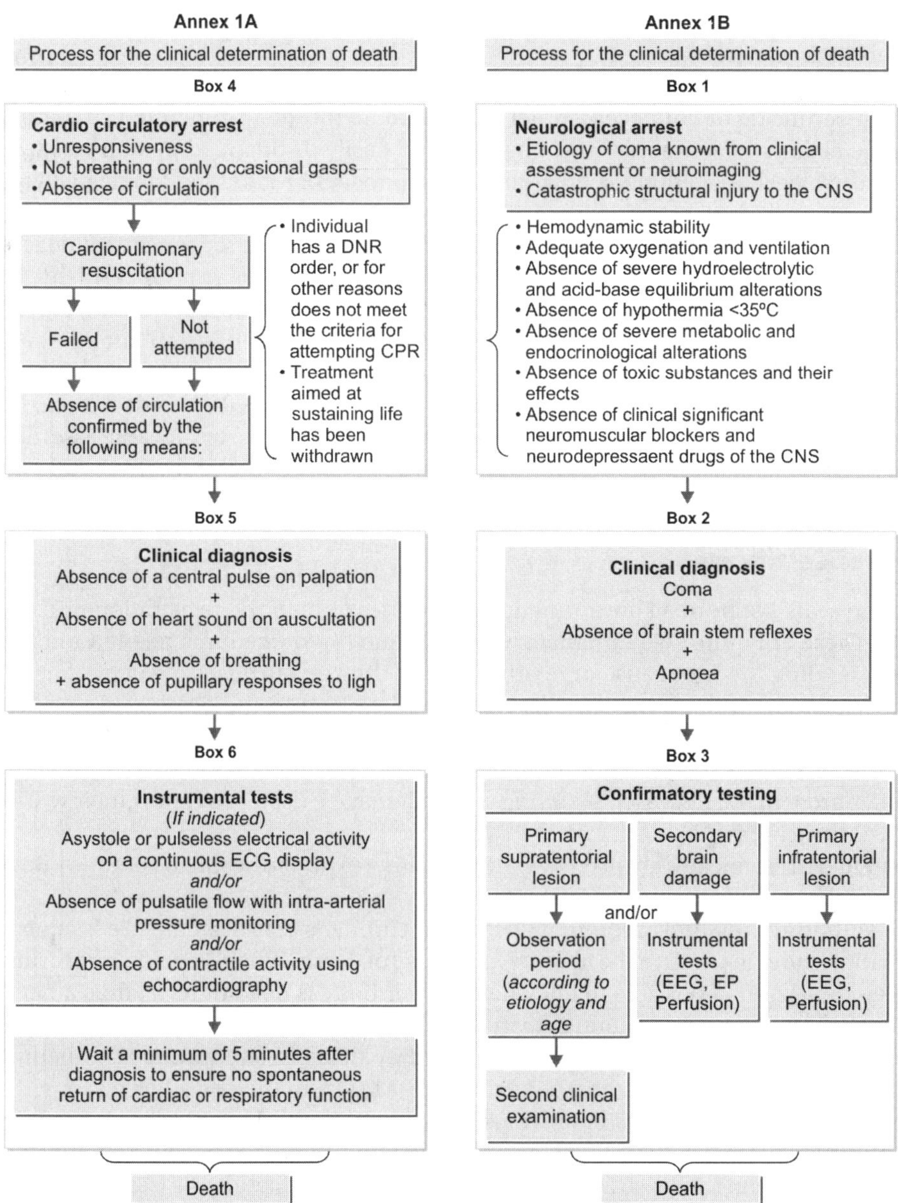

Death Certification

Whether seen from the perspective of the dead person or his or her next of kin, a death record is a significant legal document. This form, once correctly completed, is essential for a number the legal requirements as well as additional duties, but mainly because the cremation or burial passes are obtained from the municipal authorities only on receiving it. With this document, after obtaining the necessary authorization, the funeral rites of the dead may be performed in accordance with his or her faith without delay and without causing any trouble to family members or acquaintances.

The proper registration with the local municipal authorities, mentioning all the details of the death certificate of the deceased person, has to be thoroughly handled so that their life insurance claim and settlement can be processed easily. If the dead person was a salaried employee, all legal obligations, such as gratuities, provident funds, and family pensions, may be paid from their place of employment. The legal heirs might receive the division of property that is both movable and immovable in accordance with the deceased person's final testament or will. The executor of the last will and testament is allowed to acquire certified copies of a certificate of death from the closest municipal authorities before obtaining a probate or inheritance certificate from a civil court. In the instance of a pedestrian fatalities, a lawsuit filed under an individual accident gain insurance coverage can be handled. Another element that is frequently overlooked but must be addressed nonetheless is the deletion of the deceased person's name from the ration card or any extract of an immovable or movable asset, such as a house, apartment, or stock. This will require a certified copy of the properly completed death certificate.

Nature of Certificate

Forms are available from all governmental authorities to help the registration procedure get started. These are quite self-explanatory and outline the procedures needed to be created lawfully. Finding the root cause of death is one of the key purposes of such a form. This is required to assess if there was any illicit activity involved in the death and to rule out an accidental death or murder using the medical examiner's findings.

A death certificate is often required when making burial or cremation arrangements as well as to offer proof of the deceased's passing so that it may be used to support their will or make a life insurance claim.

Lastly, death certificates are used in matters relating to public health to compile information relating to the cause of death and other statistics.

The authorities regularly require a doctor's of coroner's certificate before issuing a death certificate in order to confirm the identity and cause of death. When a person is on artificial life support, it may not be possible to tell whether their body is dead or alive, thus a neurologist must confirm the degree of neural activity and complete the necessary paperwork. A doctor risk losing their ability to practice medicine if they delay in submitting the documents to the government agency noting these data, whether for insurance or other reasons. This was implemented mostly as a result of previous problems with dead people enjoying government perks and even casting votes in elections. For someone who have been pronounced dead in absentia by an inquest or executive decree, death certificates may also be issued. The same way that death certificates are supplied to missing people and victims of major disasters.

Depending on the circumstances, police officers or medical experts such as paramedics may be allowed to sign death certificates. These are exceptional circumstances, not the norm, and they are only permitted when the cause fatality is evident, like in cases of very old age when autopsies are seldom ever done, and there are no indications of foul play. While a doctor's certification is often required for deaths involving children under the threshold of 18, this is not necessarily the case and differs from region to jurisdiction. In certain situations, police are permitted to sign death certificates for infants who suffer from sudden infant death syndrome. Other instances of fatalities being declared by the authorities without a medical examiner present include accidents when there is little prospect of life, such a vehicle wreck where the person has been torn from the body. However, an examination would be performed to confirm that the dead person had no substance of any kind in their system, which might have contributed to the collision.

Four things make to a complete explanation for the cause of death:
1. The immediate cause of death, for example, the heart-stopping,
2. The intermediate causes, which triggered the immediate cause, for examples, a myocardial infarction,
3. The underlying causes, which triggered the chain of events leading to death, e.g., atherosclerosis,
4. Any other diseases and disorders the person might have been suffering from at the time of death, even though not directly connected to the cause the death.

Who is allowed to register a death?
It is important to remember to register a death within 21 days after the actual date of the death. Typically, whoever is in charge of managing this is: Whoever is registering the death should make sure they get it done within 21 days from the actual date that the death occurred. This is usually handled by:
- If the death took place in a home, the head of the household is eligible to register it in the concerned Registrar Office.
- If the individual passed away in a hospital, a person authorized by the medical institution is responsible for recording/registering the death in the respective Registrar Office.
- If the incident were to happen in prison, the jail in-charge can register it with the concerned Registrar Office.
- If death occurs in a public place, the local police in charge of the village are legally obligated to record it.

International Format

The International Classification of Diseases should be referred to when creating a death certificate if it is possible for the purpose of maintaining uniformity and facilitating the faster retrieval of data through the computerization process.

The death certificate that the World Health Organization (WHO) recommends for International use is divided into two parts:

The first part records.
a. The "disease or condition directly leading to the death"
b. The antecedent causes.

For example, the "morbid conditions, if any, that could have given rise to the cause mentioned in (a). Thus, "(a)" must be due to "(b)" which must be due to "(c)", etc. The basic pathological condition is mentioned on the lowermost line, and this is the one that is used for statistical and epidemiological purposes. Symptomatology or method of death, which might include cardio-respiratory failure, asthenia, or suffocation, should not be included in the cause of death unless specifically explained.

The second part contains records.
a. Significant problems that cause death but are unrelated to the illness or condition that caused it. The underlying cause of death is explained as "the disease which initiated the train of morbid events leading directly to death."

Different municipal administrations in India employ international forms, and physicians may access them if they so want. After signing the death certificate, doctors are required to use their rubber stamp. The local authorities provide physicians and hospitals with printed death certificate application forms.

Cause of death		*Approximate interval between onset and death*
I. Disease or condition directly leading to death* *Antecedent causes* Morbid conditions, if any, giving rise to the above cause, stating the underlying condition last	a. ___________ Due to (or as a consequence of) b. ___________ Due to (or as a consequence of) c. ___________ Due to (or as a consequence of)	___________ ___________ ___________
II. Other significant conditions contributing to the death, but not related to the disease or condition causing it	d. ___________ ___________ ___________ ___________	___________ ___________ ___________ ___________
This does not mean the mode of dying, e.g., heart failure, respiratory failure. It means the disease, injury, or complication that caused death		

The death certificate is extremely important since it is the source of mortality statistics. It is essential to establish a uniform, consistent, and standardized method of documenting and categorizing fatalities since it aids in ensuring both national and international comparability. Doctors are not permitted to give out death certificates. According to a recommendation by the Brodrick Committee, doctors are not allowed to issue death certificates, unless they have attended to the deceased at least once in the last seven days preceding the death. The accuracy of a death certificate should be confirmed with "to the best of knowledge and belief" to one of "confidence".

List of Documents Needed to Receive a Death Certificate

❖ Proof of birth of the deceased.
❖ An affidavit with the exact date and time of the death.
❖ A copy of ration card.
❖ The required fee to be paid in court fee stamps.
❖ The person requesting the death certificate must provide documentation proving their relationship to the deceased, their complete address, and a declaration of their nationality.

AUTOPSY

An autopsy (also known to be a postmortem investigation or necropsy), is a examination of the body of a dead person to determine the cause of death, to detect and define the severity of any illnesses they may have had, or to evaluate the effectiveness of any medicinal or surgical interventions. Autopsies are performed by pathologists and medical experts who have received specific training in the diagnosis of disorders via the examination of body fluids and tissues. In academic institutions, autopsies can be done for use in research and teaching. To ascertain if a person's death was caused by an accident, suicide, murder, or a natural disaster, forensic autopsies are conducted. The word autopsy is derived from the Greek word autopsia: "to see with one's own eyes."

An autopsy, sometimes referred to as a postmortem examination, is a specialist diagnostic procedure used to determine the cause and manner of death. The term "cause of death" refers to the medical diagnosis of why a patient passed away. The circumstances of the death are referred to as the manner of death.

Autopsy, also called necropsy, postmortem, or postmortem examination, dissection and examination of a dead body and its organs and structures. To ascertain the cause of death, assess the symptoms of illness, and to determine the growth and causes of disease processes, an autopsy may be conducted.

The inspection of a deceased person's body is known as an autopsy.

An autopsy may be restricted to a specific organ or region of the body.

Autopsies are carried out to ascertain the cause the death, for judicial reasons, for educational and scientific objectives, and more.

The body is opened in a manner that does not interfere with an open casket service.

Postmortem reports are useful for figuring out how, when, and why someone passed away. They aid pathologists in their quest to understand how diseases spread and because it means they'll receive more effective treatment in the future.

Necropsy, also known as a postmortem or postmortem examination, is a procedure where the corpse is dissected after death in order to reveal the essential organs in order to ascertain the cause of passing away or the nature and severity of alterations brought on by illness.

Types of Autopsy

An autopsy, often known at a postmortem, is the medical examination of a body and its internal structures after a person has died. The two distinct types of autopsies are: hospital autopsies and coroner's autopsies.

1. **Coroner's autopsy:** The police or coroner will do a coroner's autopsy if they need information about the cause of death for legal reasons, such as in instances of crime or suspicious deaths.
2. **Hospital autopsy:** A hospital-based (or noncoronial) autopsy might be performed with the immediate family's consent. In this case, the autopsy may reveal the reason of death or

inform the medical profession about the deceased's state of health. Some of the reasons for a hospital autopsy can include:

- The cause of the person's fatal illness may be unknown or uncertain.
- The outcome of an autopsy may be used to assess a treatment's effectiveness.
- If a family member has a hereditary ailment, an autopsy might provide information.
- Medical science can discover more about certain illnesses' prevalences as well as disease processes like atherosclerosis for sudden infant deaths (SIDS).

The Right to Refuse an Autopsy

'Hospital' and 'coronial' mortems follow different regulations regarding refusal rights; both have the ability to decline an autopsy.

A Medical Autopsy

Only the immediate family of the deceased has the authority to accept or refuse a hospital postmortem. They may also choose to consent to an autopsy, but limit the extent of the examination. Additionally, they have the option of taken organs or other body components for later study. Make sure you discuss these issues with hospital staff.

Funeral Autopsy

The senior next of kin may object to the carrying out of a coronial autopsy and the coroner must consider their request to reconsider if the request is made within 48 hours of the senior available next of kin receiving a notification from the coroner.

If the coroner still thinks an autopsy is required, the matter may be carried to the Supreme Court. However, these objections to a coronial postmortem are only valid for a limited period of time.

Need for an Autopsy

Without the consent of the next of kin, a medical examiner may order an autopsy. Deaths that are investigated by the medical examiner or coroner include all suspicious deaths, and, depending upon the jurisdiction, may include deaths of persons not being treated by a physician for a known medical condition, deaths of those who have been under medical care for less than 24 hours, or deaths that occurred during operations or other medical procedures.

In all other cases, including those at colleges or hospitals, getting the next-of-kin's consent is required before an autopsy may be performed. The next-of-kin also has the right to restrict the scope of a deceased person's autopsy, who may decide to, for example, just examine the abdomen or exclude the brain for analysis.

An autopsy is needed in:

- Fire deaths, when the body is changed by fire or the carbon monoxide saturation is below 20%.
- Homicides or any cases in which another person is in anyway a possible factor in the death.
- Apparent suicides that are without clear evidence of intent, such as those without a note.

- ❖ Pilots involved in aircraft crashes.
- ❖ Occupation related deaths.
- ❖ Unwitnessed "accidents."
- ❖ Accidents in which natural disease cannot be ruled out as a factor.
- ❖ Cases where civil litigation may evolve.
- ❖ Deaths of persons in official custody.
- ❖ Sudden, unexpected deaths of children, especially if they are under two years of age.

Procedure

The extent of an autopsy's might vary in-depth investigation or only the examination of one organ, example the heart or brain. Examination of the chest, abdomen, and brain is probably considered by most pathologists as the standard scope of the autopsy. An autopsy has three stages, including:

1. **Complete:** The whole body cavities are examined
2. **Limited:** A single organ such as the heart or brain
3. **Selective:** The chest, abdomen, and brain are examined

When Postmortems are Carried Out

A postmortem examination will be carried out if it's been requested by:

A. **A coroner**—because the cause of death is unknown, or following a sudden, violent or unexpected death
B. **A hospital doctor**—to find out more about an illness or the cause of death, or to further medical research and understanding.
  - There are two different types of postmortem.
  - Coroner's postmortem examination
  - A coroner is a judicial officer responsible for investigating deaths in certain situations.
  - Coroners are usually lawyers or doctors with a minimum of 5 years' experience.
  - In most cases, a doctor or the police refer a death to the coroner.

A death may be referred to the coroner if:

- It is unexpected, such as the sudden death of a baby from sudden infant death syndrome (SIDS)
- It is violent, unnatural or suspicious, such as a suicide or drug overdose
- It is the result of an accident or injury
- It could have been brought about by substances they were exposed to while working (an industrial disease);
- It may have occurred right after or during a medical procedure, e.g., surgery;
- The person was not seen during the last 28 days before they died or any time after they died by a doctor who can issue a medical certificate of cause of death (MCCD), which is a document that allows the death to be registered.
- It may have took place if an person had not been seen in the preceding 14 days for their death or at any point thereafter.
- The cause of death is unknown.
- A coroner's request for a postmortem has as its main objective determining how someone has died or decide whether an inquest is needed.

- An inquest is a legal investigation into the circumstances surrounding a person's death.
- If someone related to you has died and their death has been referred to a coroner, you won't be asked to give consent (permission) for a postmortem to take place.
- This is because anytime a death is suspicious, unexpected, or unnatural, the law requires the coroner to conduct a postmortem.
- A coroner may decide to hold an inquest after a postmortem has been completed. Samples of organs and tissues may need to be retained until after the investigation has finished.
- If the death occurred under dubious circumstances, samples may also need to be kept by authorities as testimonial for a longer period of time.
- Occasionally, samples may need to be kept in storage for a long period of time for more than years.
- If the death occurred in suspicious circumstances, samples may also need to be kept by the police as evidence for a longer period.

Postmortem examination at a hospital

- Hospital doctors may request postmortems to find out further information regarding a patient's illness or reason of death or to additional scientific research.
- In order to discover more about the cause of death, the spouse who survived or family member may sometimes request an inpatient postmortem.
- A hospital may only do a postmortem with consent. Often, someone may have given their permission before dying.
- If this isn't the case, a person close to the deceased can give their consent for a postmortem to take place.
- Hospital postmortems may be limited to particular areas of the body, such as the brain, chest, or abdomen.

When you are asked to consent, this will be discussed with you.

- At the postmortem, only the organs and tissue that you have agreed to given permission will be taken for examination.
- It is advised by the HTA to give at least 24 hours to consider your decision about the postmortem examination.
- You should also be given contact details in case it occurs to change your mind.

What takes place during a postmortem

- A postmortem ought to be carried out as soon as possible after a person passes away typically within two to 3 days of work. In certain cases, it would be possible for it to occur within a day.
- Depending on when the postmortem is planned to take place, you could be able to view the body before it is examined.
- The postmortem is carried out in an examination room that looks like an operating room. The examination room will be licensed and inspected by the HTA.
- During the procedure, the deceased person's body is opened and the organs removed for examination. A diagnosis can sometimes be made by looking at the organs.
- Some organs must be carefully examined at a postmortem. These investigations might take several weeks to complete.

- After the postmortem is finished, the pathologist will return the organs to the body.
- The entrepreneurs you have chosen will be authorized to get the corpse from the mortuary in time for the funeral after, release paperwork have been obtained.

What follows a postmortem

- Following the postmortem, the pathologist write the findings in a report.
- If a postmortem was requested by the coroner, the coroner or coroner's officer will advise you of the cause for death as determined by the pathologist.
- You may get a comprehensive copy of your pathologist's findings from the coroner's office, but there could be a fee.
- Sometimes the report will be shared to a hospital doctor or family doctor so they may discuss to you about it.
- If a physician at the hospital requested the postmortem, you'll have to request the results from the hospital where the postmortem took place. You may be charged a small fee for this.
- You can arrange to discuss the results with the doctor in charge of the deceased person's care while they were in hospital (if applicable), or with your GP.
- The HTA website gives further information about what happens before, during and after the examination.

The Human Tissue Authority

The human tissue authority (HTA) ensures that the use of human tissue is done lawfully, safely, and with appropriate permission.

- It regulates companies that gather, store, and use tissue for research, postmortem examination, instruction, and public display.
- It oversees businesses that collect, preserve, and utilize tissue for analysis, education, and public exhibition.
- All premises where postmortems are carried out must be licensed by the HTA.

Benefits of Autopsies

- **Benefits for families:** The autopsy may benefit families psychologically and emotionally. Uncertainty regarding the cause of an individual's death can delay payment of insurance benefits. Additionally, the autopsy might reveal environmental or hereditary disease triggers, such as bacteria or fungi that could put other family members at risk. The autopsy's disclosure or confirmation of the reason of death brings about psychological closure. If the treatment was successful, an examination may be able to show the family, relieving any guilt that the family may have had and restoring their faith in the caliber of medical care. Lastly, the autopsy is a mechanism that enables the family to participate in medical education and research.
- **Benefits for the clinician and hospital:** The procedure can confirm the accuracy of the clinical diagnoses and the appropriateness of medical care. The autopsy findings can be utilized to educate medical staff, nursing staff, residents, and students thereby contributing to an improved quality of care.

- ❖ **Benefits for society:** The general public enjoys a large number of the advantages of autopsies. The examination of occupational and environmental disorders, as well as the evaluation of new therapeutic measures (drugs, technologies, and surgical procedures), are all aided by the autopsy. It is possible to create reliable mortality statistics using autopsy data derived from death certificates in the absence of autopsy data have repeatedly been shown to be inaccurate. New medical knowledge on existing diseases that is derived from autopsy-based research is clearly important for everyone. Remarkably, new diseases continue to emerge which can only be fully investigated by autopsy.

Role of Nurse

Postmortem care is the delicate management of a deceased patient's body while honoring their religious or cultural beliefs. It may be administered both at home and at a hospital. Health care team personnel should be knowledgeable of the ethics of life and death and attentive to the cultural customs of the patient and relatives as society gets more and more multicultural. Maintaining the integrity of rituals and mourning practices gives families a sense of some familiarity and control in the face of death.

The body undergoes a number of physical changes after death, such as a loss of the elasticity of the skin, a spike in body warmth (algor mortis), the staining of the epithelium with purple pigment (livor mortis), and the body stiffening (rigor mortis). Postmortem care should be provided as soon as possible to prevent tissue damage or disfigurement. To prevent livor mortis of the face, before moving on to other tasks, the top of the bed should be raised and a fresh cushion should be put under the head. A medical staff member ought to showcase the dying individual in a calm way for people who want to see and grief for the patient.

Education

- ❖ Explain to the family, if required, the procedure and logic for postmortem care.
- ❖ Provide developmentally and culturally appropriate education based on the desire for knowledge, readiness to learn, and overall neurologic and psychosocial state.
- ❖ As necessary, provide knowledge on how to protect close ones and others from the patient's infectious diseases. This often includes those patients who were on respiration or contact-related precautions. Inform the family that only close relatives must interact in order to prevent the spread of illness.
- ❖ Encourage questions and answer them as they arise.

Assessment and Preparation

Assessment

- ❖ Hand hygiene should be practiced, and PPE should be worn as directed.
- ❖ Using two identifiers to confirm you have the right patient.
- ❖ Introduce yourself to the family.
- ❖ Ask the practitioner or other designated team member to establish the time of death and determine if the practitioner has requested an autopsy.
- ❖ Check to see if any closest friends or relatives are there and to confirm that they were informed about the death.

- ❖ Identify the patient's surrogate (next of kin or power of attorney).
- ❖ Verify if a patient has given first-person consent, is listed in the donate life registry, or if his or her surrogate has been asked about organ and tissue donation. Verify the signature on the donation request form, and if necessary, notify the organ team of procurement in line per organizations practice.
- ❖ Give your loved ones a quiet space to assemble. Allow him space to reflect and mourn.
- ❖ Ask the family members if there are any specifications for the funeral preparation or viewing (such as the body's position, certain dress, or shaving). Choose whether or not they wish to assist with the body's care or attend.
- ❖ Contact a spiritual care provider consistent with the family's cultural or ask a team member remain with the members of the family who aren't assisting to prepare the corpse.
- ❖ Consult the practitioner's orders for any particular treatment recommendations or directions on how to collect specimens.

Preparation

If at all possible, give the patient's body some privacy. If a patient shares a roommate, inform him or her of the circumstance and relocate the roommate to a temporary place.

Procedure

- ❖ Wear gloves, a face mask, safety glasses, and maintain proper hand hygiene.
- ❖ Gloves, a piece of clothing, a face mask, eye protection, and good hand hygiene are all recommended.
- ❖ Explain the procedure to the family and ensure that they agree to treatment.
- ❖ Assist family members in notifying the news of the death. Notify the morgue or funeral the patient's family has selected to receive their corpse, in accordance with the organization's protocol. Talk about postmortem care arrangements.

Rationale: Following a death, grieving persons have difficulty focusing on details and may need guidance. Being informed increases their sense of control.

- ❖ If tissue or organs are being donated. follow the organization's practice of care of body.
- ❖ Identify and tag the victim's body as per organization regulations.
- ❖ Examine the general condition of the body and note the presence of any type of bandages, tubes than others, or surgical instruments.
- ❖ When an autopsy is being done, indwelling devices should not be removed. Respect family's cultural traditions as well as the organization's policy when it comes to getting ready the body physically.
- ❖ Disconnect and cap the IV lines.

Rationale: The fluids in IV catheters might seep out when they are removed. After embalming, lines are removed by mortuary staff. If the autopsy is planned, it is not recommended to remove tubes and lines.

- ❖ If necessary, remove indwelling devices (such as a urine catheter or endotracheal tube) in accordance with the policies and conditions of the organization.
- ❖ If the patient's dentures are not already in place, place them there. Put the dentures in a denture cups with a label and ensure they are transported to the mortuary with the patient's body if they do not remain stable in the mouth.

Rationale: Dentures give the face a more natural appearance. Jaw muscles relax after death, making it difficult to hold dentures in place. Mortuary staff take out dentures to clean or seal the mouth.

❖ To close the patient's mouth, if culturally acceptable, wrap up a cloth (towel) and place it under the chin.

Rationale: Closing one's lips may less disturbing to family members.

❖ A small cushion should be placed behind the patient's forehead or in another location as appropriate to cultural preferences.

❖ Observe the organization's protocol for holding their hands and feet in place. On the body, simply apply circular gauze bandages. Place the hands on the abdomen in an upward posture.

Rationale: Some organizations require securing appendages to prevent tissue damage when the patient's body is moved. Accumulation of fluid called hypostasis, is a normal postmortem process caused by gravity. The condition is minimized if the affected body part is elevated.

❖ Close the patient's eyes, if culturally acceptable, by gently pulling the eyelids over the eyes.

Rationale: Although certain cultures preferred that the eyelids stay open, others believe that closed eyes give off a calmer, more natural aspect.

❖ Shave patient's facial hair unless cultural traditions forbid it or the patient has a beard.

Rationale: Respecting cultural or religious choices while presenting the patient in his regular appearance are the objectives.

❖ Wash contaminated bodily parts. Instruct family members to put on bathrobes (gown and gloves) and gloves to protect themselves from bodily fluids if they are helping to wash the corpse and provide postmortem care.

Rationale: According to several cultural customs, family members must wash the patient's body.

❖ Remove the dirty dressings, etc., replace them with the clean ones using paper tape or circular gauze bandaging.

Rationale: Removing paper tape causes less skin harm.

❖ Subsequently, place a soft pad beneath the patient's buttocks.

Rationale: When a person passes away, the muscles that makeup the sphincter relax, allowing urine and waste to escape.

❖ Cover the patient's body with a fresh gown.

❖ Brush and comb the patient's hair with caution. Take off any clips, rubber bands, or hairpins.

Rationale: The face and scalp are damaged and discolored by hard items.

❖ Identify which of the patient's belongings are to stay with his or her body and which are to be given to the family.

❖ In accordance with the organization's policies, prepare the patient's corpse and room for a viewing if the family of the deceased asks for.

❖ If preferred, cover the client's body just with a clean sheet up to the chin, leaving the arms free, if desirable.

Rationale: The patient's body has been covered to avoid exposure of any bodily parts.

❖ Take out any extra unneeded healthcare supplies from the room.

Rationale: A quieter, more natural atmosphere is produced by removing medical equipment.

❖ Give the family chairs and soothing lighting.

Rationale: Set a chair beside the bed for any family members who could collapse.

❖ Give the family members water and tissues.

❖ Give the family some private time to observe the patient's body.

❖ Encourage everyone to say goodbye using their customary religious and cultural practices.

Rationale: Compassionate care provides family members an meaningful experience in the early stages of grieving.

❖ Never try to hasten the mourning process.

❖ Do not insist that relatives to see the patient.

❖ Be available to meet issues and respond to inquiries.

❖ As per the organization's protocol, take off gown and bedding after the viewing.

❖ Put the deceased person's corpse in a shroud that provided by the organization.

❖ In accordance with the organization's protocol, attach an identifying label on the exterior of the shroud.

❖ According to the organization's protocol identify a body that might potentially spread an infection to others.

Rationale: The shroud serves as a barrier against potentially contaminated bodily fluids, provides protection against skin injury, and shields the body from becoming exposed. Labeling ensures that the body is identified properly. Marking a body reduces exposure of the morgue and mortuary staff to contamination.

❖ Verify that plans have been made to get the patient's body to the mortuary as soon as possible. If the transfer to graveyard care will take longer than expected, move the patient's body to the morgue.

❖ Wash your hands, take off any protective clothing or gear (PPE), and dispose of every materials.

❖ In the patient's file, note the process.

Monitoring and Care

Observe family members', friends', and significant others' responses to the loss and provide support as needed.

Expected Outcomes

❖ The body has no new skin injury.

❖ Significant others provided the opportunity to express grief.

Unexpected Outcomes

❖ A family person or close friend may immobilized by grief and has difficulty in functioning.

❖ A grieving person is agitated and threatens to strike out or strikes out against others.

❖ On the body, there are visible lacerations, bruises, or abrasions. Skin damage is caused by how the body is prepared or positioned.

Documentation

- ❖ Death timing
- ❖ Description of any resuscitation techniques used, if any
- ❖ Name of the medical expert who certified the death
- ❖ Any special preparation of the body for autopsy or organ and tissue donation
- ❖ Presence or absence of first-person consent, donate life registry, advance directive, or living will
- ❖ Name of person who made the request for organ and tissue donation, if applicable
- ❖ Name of organ donation agency representative, if contacted
- ❖ Name of mortuary
- ❖ Names of family members consulted at the time of death and their relationships to the deceased
- ❖ Personal articles left on the body (e.g., dentures or glasses), jewelry taped to skin, or tubes and lines left in place
- ❖ Appearance and condition of the patient's skin during preparation of the body
- ❖ Actions taken to secure valuables and personal belongings and name of individual who received them
- ❖ Time body was transported and its destination
- ❖ Location of body identification tags
- ❖ Unexpected outcomes and related interventions
- ❖ Education

Pediatric Considerations

- ❖ Make plans for the child's family, especially their parents, to be there for them throughout the dying process and at the time of death, if they wish.
- ❖ After a kid dies, let family members hold the corpse.
- ❖ Make every effort to honor family members' requests per the organization's practice. A picture, an article of clothing, their footprints, and or a lock of hair are examples of the kind of mementos that grieving parents of infants who have died away may want.

Older Adult Considerations

- ❖ Take into account the fact that some elderly persons have small families and close-knit social networks. Members of the medical staff may be the only individuals there while someone is dying.
- ❖ Arrange for someone to be with the person when death is imminent.

Household Care Considerations

- ❖ When making preparations, consider the kind of assistance that surviving family members will need.
- ❖ If a death happens at home, follow the organization's guidelines for body preparation and transfer and for disposing of medications, soiled bandages or linens, and transportable healthcare supplies (such as tubing, needles, and syringes).
- ❖ Educate family members on how to handle and dispose of medical waste in a safe and appropriate manner.

EMBALMING

Embalming is the process of preserving a body by delaying the natural effects of death. Specialized embalming fluids are injected into the body after someone has passed away, helping to give them a more peaceful appearance. The corpse of someone dear to you is preserved as part of a customary burial rite that is practiced all across the globe. This is a popular option for funerals with open caskets or when the family wants to spend extra time with their deceased loved one. The process takes around two hours to complete, including washing and drying the hair and body of the person who has died. The embalmed body is also carefully massaged to relax muscles and joints tensed by rigor mortis.

Embalming just delays the normal course of death; it has no permanent effects. The corpse will typically be preserved for about a week; but factors such as condition of the body and temperature conditions may affect this.

The science and art of embalming involves treating human remains by treating them (in its modern form with chemicals) to forestall decomposition. Usually, this is done to preserve the dead for use in an anthropological laboratory or to make them presentable for the public's exhibition during the course of the burial process. There are three objectives for embalming sanitization, presentation, preservation, and in certain cases restoration are crucial additional factors.

Definition

Embalming is the process of preserving human remains by using chemicals to prevent decomposition for medical research or social purposes (such as funeral services). The long-term preservation of the complete human body is a component of embalming, which has three objectives:

1. **Sanitization:** During the embalming process, the corpse is washing the body using antibacterial and disinfection solutions. This procedure is carried out to prevent possible smells and to delay decomposition caused by bacterial species.
2. **Preservation:** Removal of blood and interstitial fluid and replacement with embalming fluid is necessary for the preservation of the human body during embalming. Although the body will eventually decompose, such chemicals are able to temporarily preserve the body in its most recent condition.
3. **Presentation:** During embalming, the corpse is normally prepared for presentation during funeral ceremonies. The embalmer will stage the body by clothe the corpse, shave the body, fix the hair, and add makeup to give it a more realistic look. They will also massage the limbs to remove any evidence of rigor mortis.

Embalming Process

Throughout history, embalming has been done for a variety of cultural and religious reasons. As a result, the methods and materials have changed throughout time and may differ depending on the locality. Typically, embalming starts with the dead corpse being positioned in the lying position with the head raised (as illustrated below). The procedure is carried out utilizing a variety of instruments, as follows (shown below):

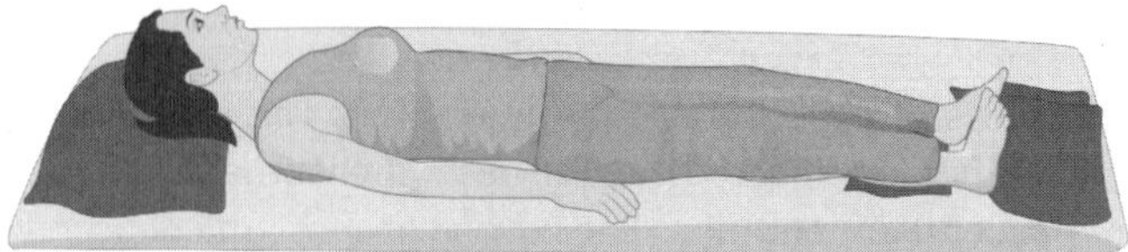

Back lying position.

Step 1: Verification of Death

Verifying that the corpse is really dead is the first stage in the embalming procedure. A lack of a pulse, rigor mortis, clouded eyes, and overall unresponsiveness. Hand and foot badges are used to confirm the deceased's identity.

Step 2: Body Washing and Massage

The person's clothing and other belongings are taken off, and the human being is then cleaned with an antibacterial detergent. Carefully washed orifices (such as the mouth) are used. To treat the rigor mortis symptoms, the limbs are massaged.

Step 3: Setting the Features

The embalmer poses the eyes in a closed position using a specialized eye cap. Either suturing, wiring, or an adhesive is used to close the lips. To get rid of any noticeable stray hairs, the face is shaven.

Step 4: Injection of Embalming Fluid

The embalmer temporarily preserves the body by injecting chemicals into the vessels and peritoneal cavity of the body. Several distinct techniques are available for injecting embalming fluid, as follows:

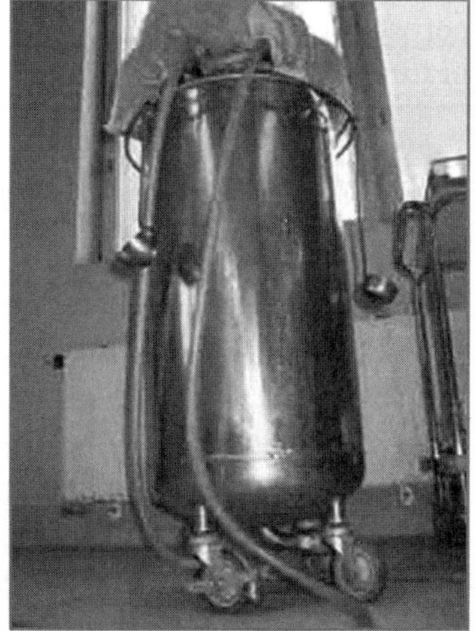

❖ **Arterial embalming:** Arterial embalming involves injecting the embalming fluid into the carotid artery using a centrifugal pump to displace the blood, which drains through the right jugular vein. To guarantee that the formaldehyde fluid is dispersed uniformly throughout the body, any clots that may be present in the veins are massaged out. Even though injecting the cremation fluid normally only requires a single injection site, there are certain circumstances when numerous injection sites are needed to guarantee that the fluid is evenly dispersed. Approximately two gallons of embalming fluid may be stored in an average corpse. Using a specialized device, the fluid is sent into the internal organs which monitor pressure of blood vessels. Although the machine is typically sufficient, a hypodermic needle is occasionally required to inject embalming fluid into locations that may not have been reached.

❖ **Cavity embalming:** Bodily cavity is embalming is performed by making a hole in the abdomen just above the navel. A trocar is placed into the incision and organ contents are aspirated. The peritoneal cavity is then filled with concentrated embalming fluid and closed by suturing or the use of a trocar button.

❖ **Surface embalming:** Surface embalming refers to the process of applying embalming fluid to a dead person's skin in order to preserve any skin damage from a corpse's autopsy, the extraction of organs for donation, or sickness (such as cancer).

Step 5: Cosmetic Application

The embalmer will next use different cosmetics and moisturizers to cover any skin imperfections and give the body a more natural look. The embalmer often asks for a recent picture in order to use makeup in a manner that most closely resembles the departed person. Makeup is used to provide depth and shade to the face and other parts of the body since there isn't enough circulation. Oils and gels are used to style the hair, and powder may be used to mask any offensive odors. The corpse is presented for observation while dressed in formal attire.

Additionally, glutaraldehyde, alcohol, methanol, phenol, water, and dyes may be included in the embalming fluid. The body cavities must also be embalmed after the arterial embalming. A trocar, a sharp surgical device, is introduced into the abdominal cavity after a tiny incision has been cut in the lower abdomen of the dead. The structures in the internal cavity and belly are then pierced and their fluid and gas contents are removed. Chemicals based on formaldehyde are then injected. The corpse is completely embalmed once the incision has been stitched. The corpse is given the necessary quantity of cosmetics once the surgical parts of the resuscitation are finished. Depending on the family's wishes, the hair will be cleaned and set. The person you cherish will put on whatever clothes that have been given to them. The corpse is then dressed and coiffed before being put in a coffin and made ready for a viewing or funeral.

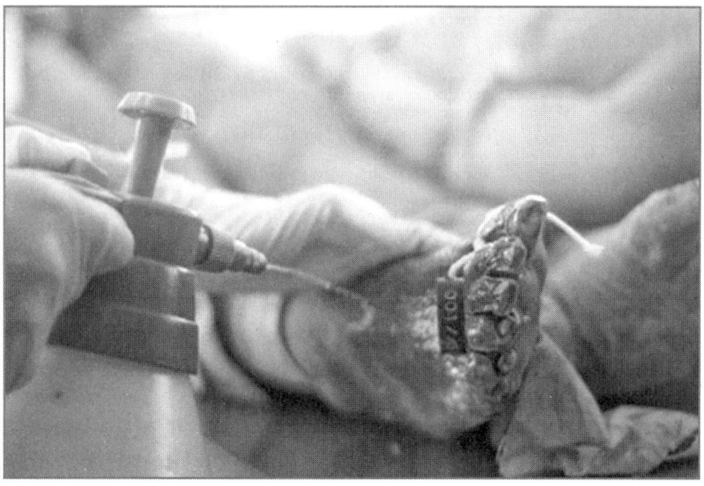

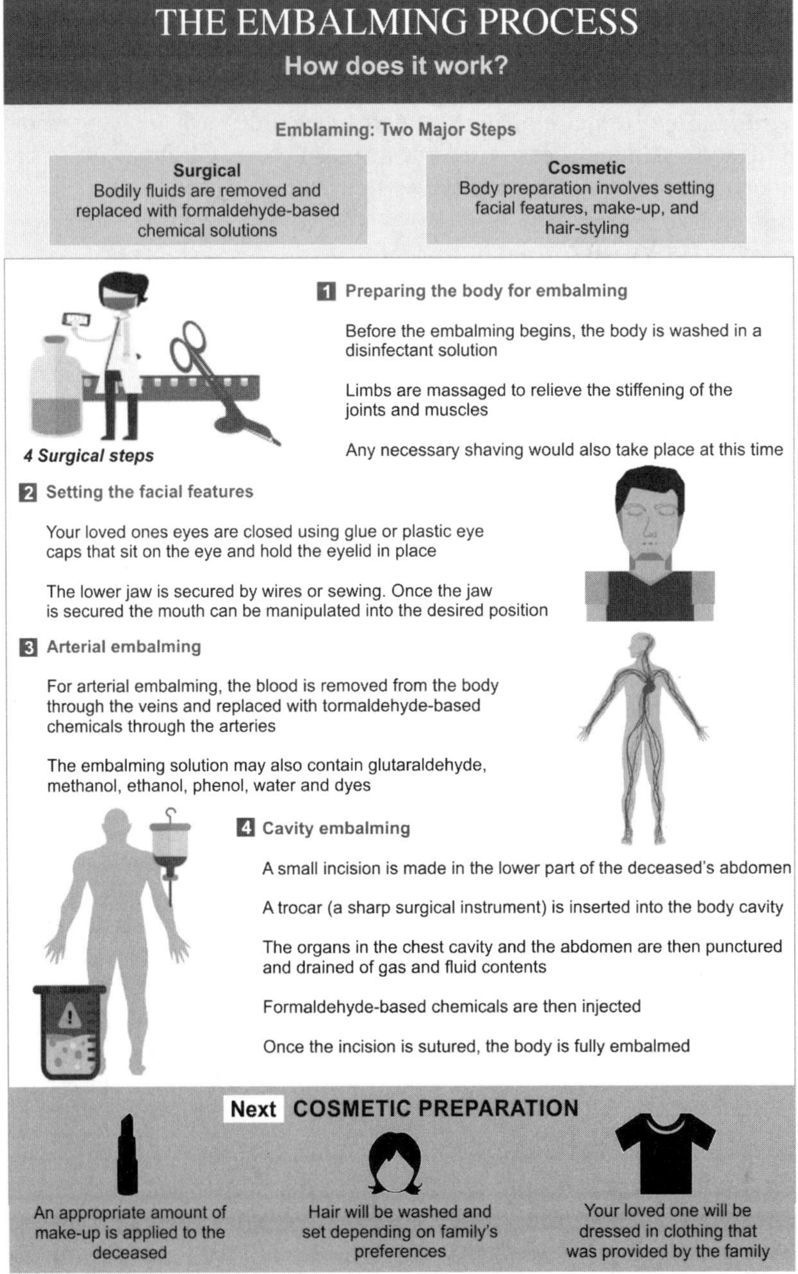

Modern Embalming

In the current method of embalming, the blood is drawn from a vein and replaced with a
fluid that is often based on formalin (a solution of formaldehyde in water) and injected into

a major artery. A trocar, a long, hollow needle, is used to drain the cavity fluid and replace it with preservative. To temporarily prevent the corpse from shriveling and becoming brown, this fluid is likewise based on formalin and is blended with alcohols. This is emulsifiers, and other compounds (such as embalming fluid). Even such meticulously preserved corpses as those of Vladimir Lenin, on display in the Kremlin, need annual renewal treatment since venous embalming is not permanent. Instead, giving the corpse a realistic look during the days when mourners are seeing it is the main goal of embalming. To enhance this, cosmetics and masking pastes are often applied.

LAST OFFICE

Last office is the final service offered as a mark of respect to the dead person before burial or cremation. Otherwise known as laying out there must be sensitivity to the beliefs of the family.

Last offices involves:
- Washing the body
- Closing the eyelids
- Ensuring the jaw remains closed
- Washing hair (if necessary)
- Straightening of arms and legs
- Packing of body orifices (not always necessary)
- Shaving men

The Postdeath Care Process

Following death, there is a process of physical, spiritual, and holistic care, which includes the following:
- Observing ethical or cultural demands of the deceased's family or carers while adhering to legal standards.
- If a local death happens, preparing the patient for transfer to a nearby mortuary or funeral director.
- Giving family members and caregivers the chance to take part in the process and supporting them.
- Preserving the respect and privacy of the departed.
- Ensuring the health and safety of everyone who comes into contact with the deceased.
- Respecting individual choices on the donation of organs and tissue.
- Returning the deceased's personal possessions to their relatives.

The deceased are to be cared for; ensuring that the modesty relating to their body, the sensitivities of any associated people, and the requirements of their culture are considered at all times.

Following a Death Procedure

- Personal care after funeral must be carried out between four and two hours when the person passes away in order to preserve the person's appearance, health, and dignity.
- Before giving care to a deceased patient after death, the named nurse must ensure that the patient has been declared dead by the accompanying physician or a qualified, approved nurse practitioner. The patient's medical file and the nurse's notes provide a confirmation of

death. This must be completed by the doctor or nursing practitioner before any procedure is carried out. Whether a patient dies at home or at a funeral directors, a doctor with a general practice (GP) is often required to certify the demise when it happens in the community. The doctor will often notify the patient's family of the most appropriate course of action. Nurses may confirm the demise of the patient and notify the GP or funeral manager if they are there at the time of the patient's passing and it has been authorized by the family of the patient and GP beforehand of the patient's passing.

❖ The patient identifier bracelet required to be on the deceased's wrist if the death took place in a hospital. If it is not, nursing personnel should check that the identification band has been secured in line with the client's id policy.

Note: If a person is delivered to the mortuary and bereavement services without an identification wristband, a nursing staff employee who was acquainted with the deceased patient must travel to the morgue to formally recognize the patient's passing and apply an identity bracelet. Bereavement services will make an incident report in such cases as well. A dead patient in a community setting who does not have a wristband cannot be handed to the funeral home.

❖ Nursing staff workers are expected to wear gloves and an apron. For further details on appropriate personal protective equipment, such scrubbing, gowning, and gloving.

❖ Light pressure should be used to close the dead patient's eyes for 30 seconds. For corneal or optical donation, the eyes should be covered with gauze soaked in regular saline solution in order to avoid eyes from drying out. The patient's general practitioner, a relative, or an member of the patient's religious group will often do this in the community.

❖ The deceased patient should be placed on their back in compliance to the manual handling policy. The patient's limbs must be straightened as much as possible, and their arms ought to be positioned by their sides. If the patient dies in their own home and it is not possible to lay the body flat due to a medical condition, the funeral professional or a member of their religious group will ensure that the protocol is followed.

❖ Ideally, jewelery should be taken off and according to the directions on the mortuary and bereavement services, property should be given to the family or next of kin if they requests it, property should be delivered to them, with the transfer being documented. If there are no relatives available or no last of kin, all jewelery needs to be left on the deceased patient, but rings must be kept secure. Jewelery must be documented on a property form whether it is removed or remained on the patient's body. The property sheet and the body must be transported to the cemetery or funeral home. When a death occurs in the patient's home, Trust employees will not be involved in any acts or discussions regarding the patient's personal effects, as this is for the family to resolve.

❖ Any surgical incisions that remain unhealed or open wounds that are seeping need to be covered with an uncontaminated, absorbent dressing and secured with a dressing that occludes in order to halt leakage. The funeral director will often do this work at the patient's home.

❖ The removal of gauze and tape is also not advised. Stomas must be covered with a clean bag. Drains must be clamped (bottles must be removed), wounds must be cushioned, and dressings must be used to cover them. It is required to cap intravenous lines and leave them in place. The deceased's lower orifices have to be covered with an incontinence sheet. Leave the catheter in place and plug if one is present.

❖ Noncoroner's cases Hickman lines, IV sites, stitches and clips may be removed by nursing employees and dressed accordingly to prevent any leakage.

❖ Leakages are to be contained, and oral cavity or tracheostomy sites are to be stemmed by suctioning fluids and positioning of the deceased. In accordance with the waste policy's instructions, nasogastric tubes must be suctioned and spigotted. Place an incontinence pad behind and around the head. If leaking continues, get guidance from the mortuary.

❖ The deceased's lower orifices must be covered with an incontinence sheet or pad. Keep the catheter in place if one is present and empty the waste bag. The bottom orifice does not need to be packed.

❖ To get rid of debris and secretions, clean the mouth. Dentures should be cleaned and replaced as soon as is practical after a death. In the event that dentures cannot be fixed, they must be sent to a funeral or cremation director along with the dying individual in an appropriately designated container.

❖ Wash the patient unless requested not to do so for religious/cultural reasons (the patient's relatives may wish to help using this chore).

❖ If there won't be any leaks, the patient may be dressed in their own clean clothes and placed into a shroud before being covered with an overlay of washable material and knotted loosely to allow for safe mobility. If the sheet of paper or tape is overly tight, it might result in disfigurement. A mortuary brown tag should be attached to the front of the deceased patient's sheet and the tag completed (filling in all required fields clearly so it is legible). Never release a dead patient into the custody of the funeral home while they are nude or bring them to the morgue.

❖ If a deceased patient is still bleeding or has any bodily fluids after performing all of the steps mentioned above, the mortuary or funeral director (for community members) should be contacted for advice before placing the remains into a plastic case (the body) bag.

❖ A notification of funeral form must be completed and sent together with medical information about the individual whenever a patient dies away. Then, in accordance with the standard infection control precautions policy, the ward staff arranges for the dead to be taken to the morgue through porters (please ensure that the patient is ready to be moved).

❖ The hospital staff who is primarily responsible for caring for the patient must get in touch with the appointed funeral director to make preparations for the patient's relocation to the funeral home's premises when a local person passes away as expected but has no spouse or next-of-kin to oversee the arrangements.

❖ Within the community, there are no facilities for visiting the dead, and seeing must be organized via the funeral director. Visiting the deceased person after transfer may only be done through bereavement services during office hours.

Responsibilities and obligations of both individuals and groups

1. **Manager of mortuary and bereavement services:** The mortuary and bereavement services manager is responsible for the operational management of this document. This includes ensuring dignity and respect when managing the deceased patient by educating staff workers on the right process to apply so that the dead patients may depart from their unit and the community. The mortuary and grief services manager shall complete an electronic occurrence notification form found that the procedure within the document has not been complied with and work with the appropriate employees to ensure future compliance.

2. **Employees of the mortuary and bereavement services:** Operationally, all parts of this document must be completed by staff members of the funeral and grieving services, who also must help the manager of those services.

3. **Chaplain:** The Chaplain is in charge of aiding the mortuary and funeral staff in both providing grieving individuals with necessary assistance and seeing to any required religious ceremonies.

4. **Nursing employees:** Implementing and completing the operational procedures outlined in this text are the responsibility of nursing staff.

5. **Community managers, ward managers, and matrons:** It is the responsibility of the matrons, wards, and community managers for ensuring that the principles of this document are fully observed and enforced by employees within their departments.
   Clinical coordinators ward clerks must assist in the effective handling of interactions between the general public and trust staff.

6. **Matrons, ward managers, managers for nonclinical services:** Managers, matrons, and ward managers for nonclinical services must ensure that employees within their area are aware of this document; able to implement the document and that any superseded documents are destroyed.

7. **Document author and document implementation lead:** The document author and the document implementation lead are in charge of assessing the need for changes to this document and, if changes are required, resubmitting it for approval or republication. This is due to developing of changes in practice, shifts to the law, updated competent or clinical norms, or local or national directives.

Equipment

* Disposable plastic apron and gloves for staff (consider face protection, i.e., mask and visor where there is a risk from blood and body fluid splashing to face)
* Bowl of warm water, soap, patient's own toilet articles/disposable face cloth
* Razor–patient's own or disposable, comb
* Incontinence pads, wound pads (if necessary)
* Mouth cleaning materials
* Shroud/patient's own nightwear clothing
* 3 clean flat sheets
* Calico bandages, tape
* 2 ID bands (correctly completed) : 1 for wrist 1 for ankle
* Mortuary cards X2
* Linen buggy consider body bag for leakage

Before Commencing Procedure

Requirements

Ensure that verification of expected death by a doctor or approved person has been completed and recorded

When a death has occurred within 24 hours after a procedure, or when a death is unexpected, when the cause of a death is unknown, seek advice from the responsible medical official other medical staff.

Identify if

The nature of death is such that it necessitates, in law, the involvement of the procurator fiscal if an infection is present in the patient or is thought to be present.

The patient has any cultural or religious beliefs which require alternative procedures faith and belief communities manual.

Before attempting to reach the last office, ask the patient and/or a family if they would want to give organs or tissue for transplantation. If so, call the local transplant coordinator and follow their instructions.

- Maintaining the deceased's privacy and dignity while consider the needs of other unit patients and family members. It is necessary to find a room and screened space if a death happens outside the ward area.
- Consider and confirm whether radiation safety procedures are still in effect.
- Consider and confirm if eyeballs are being given for corneal transplantation (if so, tape the eyes gently closed).
- Consider and verify any particular demands made before to death, such as the wearing of clothing or jewelery.

Procedure

After evaluating each of the aforementioned difficulties.

- Get personal protective equipment (PPE) such a plastic apron and gloves, and put them on. Wear face shield if there is a chance of splashing. Remove items needed for last offices from the mortuary bag, if any, and place it beside the bed.
- If a procurator fiscal case, leave all invasive devices in situ–devices should be covered/capped, e.g., urinary catheters, peripheral vascular catheters, central lines. If not, invasive devices should be removed or clamped.
- A pillow should be placed under the dead person's head, and their limbs should be straight. They should be lying flat on the bed.
- A second employee must witness each jewelery removal process. Any property that may have been still on the deceased should be included on the 'notification de death' form. On the card for mortuary notifications, note any jewelery that was left on the body. Jewelery and other valuables should be included in the individual's property book and kept according to local regulations. Tape jewelery to the finger if necessary.

Ensure Adherence to the Patients Religious and/or Cultural Beliefs, by following Guidance

- Place an incontinence pad underneath or on top of the deceased.
  - Gently push on the lower abdomen to express the bladder.
- Wash the corpses with soapy, warm water, dry them off, and then close their eyelids. Ensure that the body is completely free of any blood any bodily fluid leaks.

  About mouth care:
  - Ensure good dental hygiene has performed. Dress the dead in a disposable gown or wear their own clean clothes. If the deceased had dentures, make sure they were in place.
  - Secure identification bracelets on the deceased's opposite ankle and wrist. Both identification bands must include the following information: *Deceased name, CHI number, date of birth, ward.*

- Secure the lower limbs loosely with a bandage at the knees and, ankles.
- Secure with the bandage the lower extremities loosely at the side of the body.
- Attach a second mortuary card with tape on the outer surface of the clothing.
- Wrap the dead carefully in a sheet, leaving adequate amount of sheet to fold over and form a face piece and fasten loosely with tape.
- Instead of using pins, tape the sheet into place.
- At the highest point of the chest, tape a second funerary card to the sheet:
  ◊ A clean bottom sheet should be used and a clean sheet to cover the body.
  ◊ If radiation restrictions are still in force attach a sticker '*risk of ionizing radiation*' to the outside of the shroud (and if a body bag is used to the outside of the body bag).
  ◊ The paper should have a clean bottom and a piece of clean material should cover the body. The corpse should be put in a body bag if it is infectious or contains an alert organism, or if it is likely to become so. Fill out a *mortuary notification card* and fasten it to the outside of the sheet or corpse if a body bag was needed because of a leak or illness.
- ❖ Take off your gloves and your plastic apron, and then put them in a clinical waste bag. Clean your hands. If you need to do any extra cleaning procedure, use clean gloves and an apron.
- ❖ Ensure that all items being sent to the mortuary are recorded on the mortuary card.

Prepare for Transfer

- ❖ Speak with the porters and ask them to take the corpse to the morgue or to whatever arrangements the community has made.
- ❖ If there is a possibility of leakage or infection, the porter or undertaker will put on disposable gloves and apron regardless of whether the body is in a bag or not. After touching the covered corpse, the porters or undertaker would sanitize their hands after taking off their gloves and apron.
- ❖ When transporting the dead from the bed to a trolley, be sure to follow the transporting and handling guidance.
- ❖ Return the funeral backpack to one of the porters, who are going to substitute it with a brand-new pack (where bags have been used).
- ❖ The case records, permission form, and institution summary will accompany the body's corpse at the morgue if the deceased is to undergo a postmortem; see local regulations for further information.
- ❖ The case records, authorization form, and clinical explanation will be brought to the morgue with the corpse if the dead will undergo a postmortem.

Following a Procedure, Aftercare

- ❖ Finish all nursing paperwork.
- ❖ Ensure that the patient's electronic record is handled properly, and return notes to medical records in line with local procedures.
- ❖ If the trolley is contaminated while carrying the corpse, mortuary employees should disinfect the trolley.
- ❖ Relatives may want to see the deceased before it is taken to the morgue. If the deceased has been in the ward for approaching 4 hours the nurse in-charge *must* contact their line manager.
- ❖ We advise family members planning to visit a hospitals burial facility to phone the morgue to make preparations.

Information on Arising the Needs from Religious Beliefs Following a Death in Hospital

Some religious beliefs mandate certain rituals to be followed at the moment of death or specific treatment to be given to the corpse. When it's practical, ward staff members should inquire with the patient (in advance of death) or the patient's family or friends about any last-minute requests or special requirements.

Questions such as these are useful:
* "What is it we need to know to help us to care for your relative/friend at this time?"
* "Is there anything you need to do to help to say goodbye?"
* "Is there anyone you want here with you to support you?"

It is recommended to give the assistance of a healthcare clergy in all dying scenarios, but especially when family or friends are present. In all circumstances of death, it is good practice to offer the support of a healthcare Chaplain.

Buddhism

* Buddhists believe that one's mental condition during death will have an impact on how they are reborn in the afterlife. Therefore, it is crucial to maintain calm and quiet around the sufferer.
* The patient and guests may observe silence, meditation, and chanting.

Christianity

There are several 'denominations' and organizations that makeup Christianity. Needs and behaviors related to religion might differ substantially.

Christian Catholics: The sacrament of the sick, sometimes known as the "last rites," is frequently desired by Roman Catholic patients as well as their visitors. This has to be recorded.
* The dead may get a priest's anointing and blessing after passing away.
* The on-call Roman Catholic priest can be contacted via switchboard.

Patients or visitors may want their priest to be present prior or following death if they are Episcopalian or Anglican. Patients and visitors may ask the priest to be present before or after death, according to the Church of Scotland.

Hinduism

* Friends or relatives may wish to sit with the dying person and stay there till the person passes away.
  There are several funeral rites:
* Since relatives may want to wash the corpse, therefore staff ought to ascertain their wishes.
* Cremation follows a custom; the corpse must be covered in a simple sheet.

Islam

* Visiting the ill and the dying is a religious obligation for family members and friends. The organization of visits will need to be done carefully.
* Family members and friends may pray and recite verses from the Quran.

❖ At the moment of death, prayers will be recited all around the bed.

❖ It is traditional for a Muslim who is about to pass away to lay on one's right side with their back to Makkah (southeast) and their head slightly lifted.

❖ Until the corpse is taken to the mortuary, family members may want to sit with it.

❖ It is the family's and the Muslim community's religious responsibility to prepare for the funeral service (which occurs during the afternoon prayers prayer in the mosque) and to wash the corpse. All Muslim weddings in the city are coordinated by Glasgow Central Mosque (contact information in faith or belief communities manual).

❖ In Islam, burials must occur as quickly as possible after a person passes away. There should be no delays. Every body has to be taken out of the ward and placed in the mortuary.

Judaism

❖ Avoid touching the corpse after death has occurred for 20 minutes,

❖ Do not remove fake teeth or other prosthetics from the corpse (this will be done ritualistically before burial). Drains, tubes, and catheters must be left in place since the fluid they carry is maintained with the corpse during burial because it is regarded to be a part of it. They might have bandages and gauze covering them.

❖ Close the eyes.

❖ Extend the arms out to the side and lie flat with feet together.

❖ Place a simple, white sheet on top of the body.

❖ If there is not a family, inform the Jewish community in area or the Hebrew Burial Society.

❖ After death it is the tradition that the body must be accompanied at all times by a member of the Jewish community.

❖ If it is the Sabbath (from Friday sunset to Saturday sunset) then the family may organize a "watch" over the dead person till after Sabbath, assuming the hospital does not object and does not need the bed (This practice also applies to other special religious days in Judaism).

Sikhism

❖ The dying person may like to hear hymns read aloud or listen to Kirtan, a kind of spiritual music that brings comfort to the soul.

❖ After death has happened, the family is in charge of the funeral services.

❖ Some Sikhs who have undergone baptism carry five religious signs that represent their article of faith on their person all the times (even after death). They are known as 5Ks while their last names start with a "K." The Five K's (Articles of Faith) include the following: Kesh, uncut locks that God gave as a gift and represents spirituality; Kangha, a wooden combs representing purity; Kara, a stainless-steel bracelet signifying restraint and a link towards God; Kirpan, a short sword signifying strength and a dedication to justice and truth; and Kachera, a kind of undergarments signifying moral chastity. The five K's should not be clipped, nor should the beard or hair.

❖ Asking relatives to remove the turban might embarrass them; they may prefer to wash and arrange the body themselves.

COUNSELING AND SUPPORTING GRIEVING RELATIVES

Grief counseling, commonly referred to as mourning therapy, is a kind of therapy designed to assist a person in coping with loss, such as the loss of a spouse, parent, friend, co-worker, or pet.

Losing a loved one may be physically and emotionally painful, which can sometimes make it difficult to cope up. Working with a mental health professional, a therapist, a therapist or a support group to handle emotions is referred to as grief therapy.

Grief therapy may assist with making short-term practical choices, such as funeral preparations, and navigating the following months of a loss. Long-term, it can help you , it can help you accept the loss of loved one and adapt to life without them.

It is a kind of therapy intended to assist individuals in navigating the many phases and emotions associated with grieving a loss. Counseling may assist people in avoiding some of the most severe mourning symptoms and in processing their feelings in a manner that is beneficial.

Types of Grief Counseling

Complicated Grief Therapy

Complicated grief is a state in which sorrow seizes control of you and refuses to release it. You may have disturbing thoughts, disorganized actions, and trouble in controlling your emotions as a consequence, which will make it more difficult for you to adjust to life without someone you love.

Complicated grief therapy (CGT) is a form of psychotherapy that may assist you in overcoming this kind of sadness.

Traumatic Grief Therapy

If you lost someone you care about unexpectedly or if you were there when they passed away (witnessed their death), you can go through severe bereavement.

Traumatic grief therapy may provide you coping mechanisms, help you manage the severity of your sorrow, and lessen the effects of suffering.

Techniques

Grief counseling involves talking about the person you lost, your relationship with them, how they died, how their death has impacted you, and how you're coping with it.

These are some of the techniques that grief counselors or therapists may use:

* **Acceptance and commitment therapy (ACT):** With the aid of ACT, a kind of psychotherapy, accept negative feelings and circumstances so you can begin to focus on healthier patterns that can help you reach your goals.
* **Cognitive behavior therapy (CBT):** CBT is a kind of psychotherapy as well. It involves identifying and changing thought patterns that can negatively influence your behavior.
* **Group therapy:** This form of therapy is carried out in a group setting. It can be comforting to share your feelings with other people who are going through the same thing you are and work toward recovery together.
* **Art therapy:** Art therapy encourages recovery by allowing you to express your feelings in creative ways. People from all ages, even youngsters, who may find it difficult to express their emotions, might benefit from it.
* **Play therapy:** In order to help children and gain insights into a child's thoughts process unresolved emotions and build constructive behavioral patterns, play therapy is often used to obtain insight into their mental and emotional states.
* **Speech therapy:** Speech therapy includes individuals talking about their feelings and expressing their loss. It is one of the more popular counseling techniques. Patients may speak

about their departed loved ones in a secure setting with the support of a grief counselor, which can help them stay connected to the person they've lost. Both individual and group talk therapy are options. Many people find bereavement group counseling helpful in dealing with the symptoms of grief.

Mindfulness

Whether via meditation or another technique, those who adopt awareness remain attentive to the present moment in order get more aware of their feelings and thoughts. The complicated and overpowering feelings of sorrow may be worked through with the use of mindfulness practices.

The following are primary objectives of grief counseling:

Accept the Loss

One of the many important and vital phases of the mourning process is accepting the reality of a loss. Denial is a common response that helps individuals deal with their grief and the pain it causes. However, in order to properly cope with grief and heal, individuals must learn to comprehend their loss.

- ❖ **Managing your pain:** When faced with a loss, the following sadness, many individuals attempt to ignore it and repress their feelings. This just makes their pain worse. An essential part of managing grief is experiencing the pain that comes from it and persevering.
- ❖ **Adjust to life:** People often feel sadness when they lose an individual or thing that played a significant role in their life. It may be very difficult and sometimes seem like a betrayal to adjust to a loss. Many individuals may feel trapped by this logic. After a loss, grief therapy may assist people in reorienting and reorganizing their life.
- ❖ **Maintain a connection:** Maintaining a connection to the lost object is as crucial to the grieving process as acknowledging a loss and adapting to life after it. For instance, when a friend or relative passes away, it may be comforting for the mourning to recall the joy that person offered rather than concentrating just on the sadness of that person's loss.

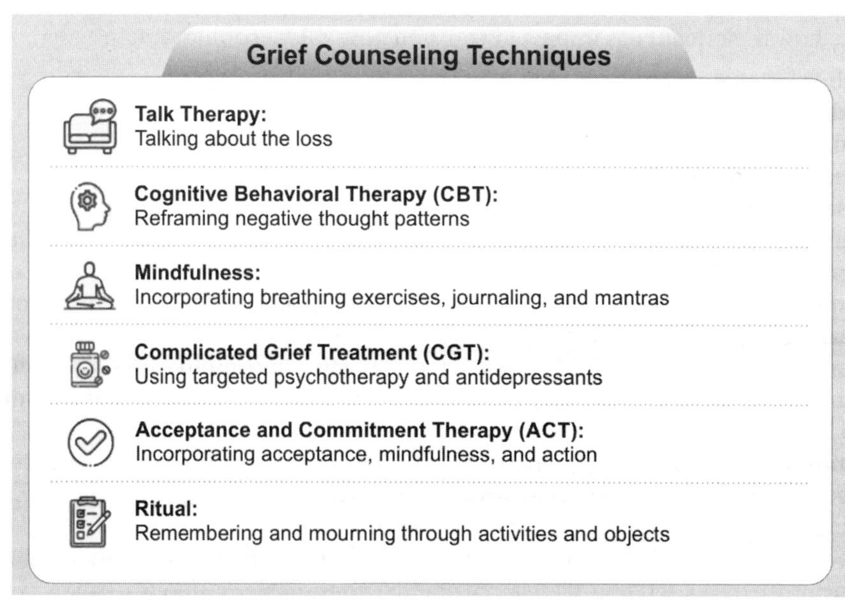

Advantages of Grief Counseling

- You may benefit from grief therapy in a number of ways, including the following:
- Lessening of emotional and physical symptoms.
- Learning coping skills that can help you cope with life without someone you care about.
- Self-awareness grows when you learn to understand your emotions and the causes behind them.
- Accepting your loss entails bringing it into your world and continuing to have a positive relationship with the individual whom you lost while you go on with your life.
- Reduces depression, guilt, and anxiety
  Grief counseling may assist individuals in controlling anxiety and avoiding hopelessness by providing them with the skills to cope with their emotions in a healthy way. Another common sensation among individuals who are mourning is guilt. They could feel guilty for their actions or inactions when the person they loved was still alive or for not expressing their sorrow at the loss of that person. Counseling may be able to overcome these feelings.
- Helps others recognize the grieving process
  Understanding the stages of grief and loss allows individuals to more fully tap into their thoughts and emotions, opening a path to healing. Grief counselors can help patients understand this process.
- Educates people there are different ways to grieve
  People dealing with grief may feel like they're doing it wrong—that they're not sad enough or that they've been grieving too long. But there cannot be a "right" way to mourn; Patients who get counseling are reminded of this and assisted in realizing how different everyone's experiences are.
- Helps people honor the deceased without trauma
  A crucial aspect of the mourning process is letting individuals express what they're feeling and thinking about a departed loved one, therefore it is crucial that they may do so without suffering and more harm. Counseling could offer patients a safe space to talk about the deceased and honor their memory, and it may be a tremendous source of comfort and peace.
- Helps people understand that grief can be caused by different kinds of loss
  Though the passing of a loved one is general cause of mourning, people may grieve for many different reasons losing a beloved pet, getting a divorce, relocating far from friends and family, or receiving a terminal medical diagnosis. Counseling may assist individuals in allowing themselves to mourn such things without feeling weak or self-centered.
- Guides patients back to self-care
  Grief may be a heavy toll on victims, draining them emotionally, psychologically, and physically. Counseling may direct patients toward self-care methods like mindfulness techniques and easy advice like exercising obtaining enough sleep to help them manage and heal.
- Be a good listener
  Take time to listen. Sometimes just listening to somebody who grieves is the finest thing you can do for them. Reassure the individual that discussing their emotions is OK. Even while you cannot take away the grieving person's suffering for their loss, yet can provide them a lot of consolation by just being there to listen.
- Respect the person's way of grieving
  Observe the person's mourning process. Grieving may be done in any way—right or bad. Every person expresses grief differently. However, the pain of loss is shared by all people.

❖ Accept mood swings

Be aware that a person who is mourning will experience emotional ups and down. Grief is often described as an emotional roller coaster. Someone who has just lost a loved one may feel fine one moment and overcome with emotion the next. This is a normal part of the grieving process.

❖ Don't give advice

It is preferable to abstain from advising the grieving individual on what they should or shouldn't do. Such advice is usually well-meaning, but it may make the bereaved person feel worse. Instead, express your understanding of how severe the person's loss is. You may say something like, "This must be a painful time for both you and your family," or "This is undoubtedly a difficult period for you."

❖ Don't try to explain why you lost

Sometimes, words meant to console the bereaved have an exact reverse effect. Avoid saying things like "Let your companion is now in an improved position," "It's God's will," is "At least he or they're not still suffering." Listening them is more positive.

❖ Help out with practical tasks

Assistance with responsibilities like grocery shopping, meal preparation, telephone calls, washing up, child care, and other similar ones could be very appreciated by someone who has recently lost a loved one. Instead of stating, "Let me find out whether there may be anyway you can do to help," offer support with particular tasks you are able to assist with.

❖ Stay connected and available

Grief has no fixed duration. Be patient; grieving people need time to heal. Let the mourning person know that you will keep in touch often. Even if he or she has yet to be prepared to connect or converse with others, just having you there may be comforting.

❖ Talk in a way that is heartfelt

It's usual to struggle to find the right words to say. Sometimes basic language works best. Say something along the lines of, "I'm truly sorry regarding the loss you experienced. How can I help? Regardless of how unsure you may be about the aid you are offering, what matters most is the extent to which you are really concerned and want to help. The bereaved person will likely appreciate your sincere efforts to be supportive.

- Be a good listener. ...
- Respect the person's way of grieving. ...
- Accept mood swings. ...
- Avoid giving advice. ...
- Refrain from trying to explain the loss. ...
- Help out with practical tasks. ...
- Stay connected and available. ...
- Offer words that touch the heart.

PLACING IN AND RELEASING BODY FROM MORTUARY

Custody of MLC Bodies

According to land law, the jurisdictional police are the custodians of dead corpses in all circumstances of fatalities that call for further legal investigations.

❖ In order to preserve the dead corpses while police investigations are on-going, the hospital serves as a facilitator.

❖ Without the involvement of a third party, the Police are directly in charge of the corpse and are responsible for it.

❖ In submitting a request for retention, authorized doctors from AIIMS who use the phrase "allowed to be held in graveyard into the control of police" will take it into consideration.

❖ The prospect of an exchange of dead corpses in this circumstance also arises in the absence of custodial police.

❖ The department offers logistical support for local body relocation, including space, morgue cabinets, and class IV helpers.

❖ In conclusion, it is the duty of the police to keep secure legal possession of all such deceased medical-legal case (MLC) corpses and to provide 24 hour care for them.

MLC Dead Body Preservation Dying Outside AIIMS

The dead body must have a tag or label put to it with a moniker of the investigating station with a FIR or DD number for identification reasons, according to the police personnel who are preserving the corpse.

❖ No dead body will be received and stored in the cold storage without labels or tags for identification.

❖ By filling out a request form, you must ask the officer in charge on duty for permission to preserve the corpse.

❖ To prevent decomposition changes that might make it more difficult to determine the reason and manner of death in cases of unidentifiable remains, the postmortem investigation should be performed as soon as practicable after 72 hours after the death.

Procedure for Release of Dead Bodies of Patients (MLC and Non-MLC) Dying In AIIMS

Whether a patient dies in an MLC situation, the corpse will be transferred to the morgue by law whether it occurs in an inpatient ward, ICU, or emergency.

The sister I/C/senior most sister on duty will hand over the body to the relatives (against receipt in the death register) along with the dead body receipt slip of the patient, against clearance received from the central admission office, if the relatives of the patient want to receive the dead body right away. The ward sister will keep one copy of dead body receipt slip from one of the death report forms before sending the 2 copies of the death report form to the central admission and enquiry office (which is otherwise taken by the mortuary staff along with the dead body shifted to the mortuary).

The process in such circumstances would largely stay the same, i.e., once a patient passes away, his or her attendant goes to the central admission and inquiry office to acquire a dead body receipt sheet with the stamp "Body may be handed over" (after paying bills, etc.).

The patient's attendants will now approach to the ward sister (instead of the morgue) and she will take their signatures accepting the receipt of the dead body in her death register (In place of signatures of mortuary attendant who would have signed if the body was to be taken to mortuary)

The ward sister will keep the dead person's the arrival slip (with stamp from central admission office) in her papers and will give the dead body receipt slip she has on hand from the second copy of the death report form (which is otherwise taken by the mortuary attendant along with the dead body and is given by him to the patient's attendant along with the body) while retaining the dead body receipt slip (with stamp from central admission office) in her records.

In all of these situations, the family must be gently reminded to finish the necessary formalities and remove the patient's corpse within an hour of the death declaration; otherwise the body may be sent to the mortuary. This discretion will remain with the ward sister, who may request the mortuary to take dead body of a non-MLC patient as well.

Preservation of Non-MLC Dead Bodies Dying Outside AIIMS

The AIIMS department of the field of forensic medicine now serves two mortuaries: Main AIIMS and trauma center. The main AIIMS and the trauma center presently cater to the jurisdiction of South and the South-East Delhi with an annual turnover of about 3,000 dead bodies. The department is unable to preserve the remains of non-MLC bodies dying outside AIIMS because of a lack of space in the cool chambers.

In such situations, the families should take a formal permission to the HOD, forensic medicine/mortuary incharge, who will provide permission for the preservation of the corpse, after considering the available space in cold chambers, rationale and need of the relatives.

Transport of Dead Body from Hospital to Mortuary

The nursing personnel on duty should correctly mark the corpse after death, including the deceased's name, father's name, admission number, ward, date and time of death, etc.

The letters 'MLC' should be put on the label prominently in medical-legal cases.

Prior to the corpse being wrapped in impermeable sheets or placed in a plastic bag and sent to the next of kin or a mortuary attendant, the nursing personnel on duty in the hospital should make sure that any drainage sites or surgical operations have been adequately dressed.

The on-duty mortuary attendant is notified that a pick-up or removal from the wards is required.

The hearse van service is provided free of cost to transfer the corpse from the healthcare facility to the mortuary.

The properly wrapped and tagged body will be received by the morgue attendant together with the relevant paperwork, such as a death certificate, in a courteous, sensitive and professional manner.

Intake Procedure and Maintenance of Mortuary Register

The 'death slip' and the corpse will be delivered by the hospital to the mortuary staff.

- The label on the corpse should be compared to the information on the death certificate and should match the ID band to authenticate the identity of the deceased.
- The mortuary employee will record any pertinent information from the death slip into the register and check to see that the information on the corpse's tag matches that on the death slip.

Advance Directive

A legal document that states a person's wishes about receiving medical care in the event that they become incapacitated due to a major illness or accident. An advance directive may also a person (such as a spouse, family, or friend) may be given the power to make medical choices for somebody else when that person is no longer capable of doing so. A living will, a permanent power of attorney for healthcare, and not to resuscitate (DNR) orders are a few examples of advance directives.

The advance directive is intended to advise healthcare team as well as loved ones when they must make these choices on patient's behalf or to designate who will act on their behalf in the event that they are unable to do. The healthcare team may decide to take extra measures or provide emergency treatment in certain medical choices. An advance directive can help patient to think ahead of time about what kind of care they want.

Advance directives only apply to health care decisions and do not affect financial or money matters. The laws around advance directives are different from state to state. Talk to your health care provider (or your lawyer) about filling out your advance directive when you are still healthy, in case you become too ill or are unable to make medical decisions for yourself in the future.

The Patient Self-Determination Act

Everyone is encouraged under the 1990 Patient Self-Determination Act (PSDA) to make choices in advance on the kinds and amounts of medical treatment they wish to accept or reject in the event that they become unable to make decisions due to sickness.

Hospitals, nursing homes, home health agencies, hospice services, and Health Maintenance Organizations (HMOs) are required to comply with the following PSDA requirements:

❖ Providing people with information about their state's legislation regarding their ability to choose their own medical treatment.
❖ To ascertain if they have a power of attorney.
❖ To respect the patient's desires and the advance directive.
❖ Never to treat patients differently depending on whether or not they have completed an advance directive.
❖ Health care facilities cannot require patients to have advance directives: it is the patient's choice.

Advance directives are legal papers that increase a person's ability to make choices about their own health care in cases where they become incapacitated. Advance directives are so named because they express wishes prior to becoming incapacitated. These documents usually address decisions regarding end-of-life care but may also address any aspect of care. Because communicating compassionately and effectively about such end-of-life decisions with patients takes special skill, and training is advisable.

There are two primary types of advanced directives:

❖ **Living will:** Expresses preferences for medical treatment and end-of-life care.
❖ **Durable power of attorney for health care:** Designates a surrogate decision maker.

Power of Attorney

A medical or health care power of attorney is a type of advance directive in which patient choose someone to make decisions on their behalf in making decisions that they are unable to. This directive can additionally be known as a proxy for medical care or a long-term power of lawyer for health care in certain jurisdictions.

Depending on where you live, the person you choose to make decisions on your behalf may be called one of the following:

❖ Health care agent
❖ Health care proxy
❖ Health care surrogate
❖ Health care representative

- ❖ Health care attorney-in-fact
- ❖ Patient advocate

It is crucial to choose the right individual to serve as your health care agent. Even if you hold other legal papers pertaining to the provision of care, not all circumstances can be predicted, and in certain cases, someone may need to make a decisions about your potential care preferences. Choose someone who satisfies the following requirements:

- ❖ Who meets your state's requirements for a health care agent.
- ❖ Is not your doctor or a part of your medical care team.
- ❖ Is willing and able to discuss medical care and end-of-life issues with you.
- ❖ Can be trusted to make decisions that adhere to your wishes and values
- ❖ Able to be relied upon to represent your interests if disputes arise over your treatment
- ❖ The person you specify might be your spouse, another family member, a friend, or a fellow believer. In the event that the individual you selected is unable to perform the task, you can additionally decide one or more backup candidates.

Living Will

- ❖ A living will is a written, legal document that spells out medical treatments you would and would not want to be used to keep you alive, as well as your preferences for other medical decisions, such as pain management or organ donation.
- ❖ Consider your values when you make your requests. Examine how important independence and self-sufficiency are to you and identify any situations that can make you feel as if life doesn't seem worth living. In any circumstance, would you desire medical attention to lengthen your life? In all circumstances? Would you accept medical care if a cure were the only option?
- ❖ In a living will, you should include a number of possible end-of-life care decisions regarding medical care. If you have concerns about one or more of the subsequent medical choices, consult your doctor.
- ❖ The heart may be revived with cardiopulmonary resuscitation (CPR) if it has stopped beating. Determine if and when you would want to be revived using CPR or a machine that shocks the patient's heart with electricity.
- ❖ If you are unable to breathe on your own, mechanical ventilation takes over. Think about if, when, and how soon you would like to be put on an automatic ventilator.
- ❖ Tube feeding delivers nutrition and fluids to the body orally or via a passageway in the stomach. Choose if, when, and how long you are willing to be taken feed in this way.
- ❖ If your kidneys are no longer working, dialysis eliminates waste from your blood and controls fluid levels. Make a decision on it, when, and how long we would want to get this therapy.
- ❖ Many infections may be treated with antibiotics or antiviral drugs. Would you prefer intensive infection treatment if you were at the end of your life, or would you prefer to let illnesses progress naturally?
- ❖ Palliative care, also known as comfort care, refers to a variety of procedures that may be employed to keep you pain-free and comfortable while also honoring your other treatment preferences. This can be having the option to pass away at home, receiving painkillers, being given ice chips to ease oral dryness, and avoiding invasive procedures or examinations.

❖ You may specify in a will the organ and tissue contributions you want to make for transplant. You will briefly remain on life support if your body parts are taken for donation until the surgery is finished. To help your health care agent avoid any confusion, you may want to state in your living will that you understand the need for this temporary intervention.

❖ You might also specify giving your body up for research. For information on how to sign up for a planned gift for research, get in touch with a nearby medical school, university, or donation program.

Do "Not Intubate" and "Not Resuscitate" Orders

You don't need to have an advance directive or living will to have do not resuscitate (DNR) and do not intubate (DNI) orders. Inform your doctor of your wishes in order to create DNR or DNI orders. The instructions will be written down and entered into your medical file.

Even if you already have a living will that includes your preferences regarding resuscitation and intubation, it is still a good idea to establish DNR or DNI orders each time you are admitted to a new hospital or health care facility.

Establishing Advance Directives

❖ Advance directives are required in written. Each state has different forms and requirements for preparing legal papers. Depending on where you live, a form may need to be signed by a witness or notarized. Although it may not be often required, you might seek a lawyer to assist you with this procedure.

❖ The websites of several organizations, including the American Bar Association, AARP, and the Nation's Hospice and Palliative Care Organization, have links to state-specific forms.

❖ To ensure you are filling out the documents properly, go through your advance directive with the doctor and your healthcare agent. After finishing your paperwork, you need to complete the following actions:

  ◆ Keep the originals at a location that is both secure and convenient.
  ◆ Send a copy to your physician.
  ◆ A copy should be given to your health care agent and any substitute agents.
  ◆ Keep a record of who has your advance directives.
  ◆ Share your advance directives and health care preferences with your family and other important persons in your life. By having these conversations now, you help ensure that your family members clearly understand your wishes. Your family members may stay out of dispute and refrain from feeling guilty if they have a clear understanding of your preferences.
  ◆ A copy should always be in your travel bag.

A Review and Modification of Advance Directives

You can change your directives at any time. If you want to make changes, you must create a new form, distribute new copies and destroy all old copies. Specific requirements for changing directives may vary by state.

You should talk about any modifications with the doctor who treats you regularly and confirm that the new directive on your medical record replaces the previous one. The medical records at a hospital or care home also need to be updated with new orders. Discuss the changes you have made with your family, friends, and health care provider as well.

In the following circumstances, consider reviewing your directives and creating new ones:

- ❖ **A new diagnosis:** You could update your living will if you get a terminal diagnosis or one that profoundly affects your life. Discuss with your medical professional the potential choices for care and treatment throughout the anticipated course of the illness.
- ❖ **Change in marital status:** You might need to choose a new healthcare agent if you get married, divorce, separated, or become widowed.
- ❖ **About every ten years:** Your opinions on end-of-life care may change over time. Make sure your directives still represent your current beliefs and intentions by periodically reviewing them.

PHYSICIAN ORDERS FOR LIFE-SUSTAINING TREATMENT

Physician orders for life-sustaining treatment (POLST) is a document that is a part of advance health care planning in several states. The document may also be called provider orders for life-sustaining treatment (POLST) or medical orders for life-sustaining treatment (MOLST).

POLST is designed for those who have previously received a severe disease diagnosis. Your prior directions are not repealed by this form. Instead, it serves as doctor-ordered instructions — not unlike a prescription —, to make sure that you get the care you want in an emergency. Your doctor will fill out the form based on the contents of your advance directives, the discussions you have with your doctor about the likely course of your illness and your treatment preferences.

POLST stays you around always. The paper is displayed next to your bed if you're a patient in a nursing home or medical facility. The paper is publicly placed where it may be readily seen by emergency health care worker or other members of the medical team whether you reside at your place of residence or in a hospital or hospice facility.

In general, a POLST allows your doctor to add information regarding which therapies should not be used, under what circumstances certain treatments may be used, for how long certain treatments may be used, and when medicines should be discontinued. Forms vary by state. Among the topics addressed by a POLST are:

- ❖ Resuscitation
- ❖ Mechanical ventilation
- ❖ Tube feeding
- ❖ Use of antibiotics
- ❖ Requests not to transfer to an emergency room
- ❖ Requests not to be admitted to the hospital
- ❖ Pain management

POLST also indicates what advance directives you have created and who serves as your health care agent. Like advance directives, POLSTs can be canceled or updated.

Duty to Follow Advance Directive

Subject to Section 11, every medical professional in the custody of a mental health facility and the doctor in charge of a patient's treatment are required to suggest or provide treatment to a patient with a mental illness in keeping with his or her legitimate advance directive.

Power to Review, Alter, Modify or Cancel Advance Directive

- ❖ When a mental health professional, a relative, or the person's caretaker decides following an advance directive while providing care for a patient with a mental illness, they must apply

to the relevant Board for a review, alteration, modification, or cancellation of the advance directive.
- After receiving the application either uphold, modify, alter or cancel the advance directive after taking into consideration the following, namely:
  - Whether the advance directive was made by the person out of his own free will and free from force, undue influence or coercion;
  - Whether the person intended the advance directive to apply to the present circumstances, which may be different from those anticipated;
  - Whether the person was sufficiently well informed to make the decision;
  - Whether the person had capacity to make decisions relating to his mental healthcare or treatment when such advanced directive was made;
  - Whether the content of the advance directive is contrary to other laws or constitutional provisions.
- It is the responsibility of the person who drafts the advance directive along with his designated representative to see that it is available when needed to the medical officer at charge of a facility for mental health, a doctor, or a professional in the field of mental health, as the case may be.
- The official guardian has the authority to write an advance directive for a minor, and all advance directive provisions, mutatis mutandis, apply to that minor until he reaches the age of majority.

Review of Advance Directives

- The central authority shall regularly and periodically review the use of advance directives and make recommendations in respect thereof.
- The central authority in its review give specific consideration to the procedure for making an advance directive and also examine whether the existing procedure protects the rights of persons with mental illness.
- The central authority may modify the procedure for making an advance directive or make additional regulations regarding the procedure for advance directive to protect the rights of persons with mental illness.

Liability of Medical Health Professional in Relation to Advance Directive

- A medical practitioner or a mental health professional shall not be held liable for any unforeseen consequences on following a valid advance directive.
- If a mental health care provider or physician does not have a copy of a legal advance directive, he or she cannot be held accountable for failing to abide by it.

Do not Resuscitate/Do not Intubate

A do-not-resuscitate order is a legal document that means a person has decided not to have cardiopulmonary resuscitation attempted on them if their heart or breathing stops. People who choose to have a DNR usually have a terminal illness or other serious medical condition. In most situations, a healthcare provider writes a DNR order after discussing the benefits and risks of CPR with the person, their loved ones or their legal decision-maker.

A do-not-resuscitate order mentioned in a person's medical record by a doctor informs the medical staff that cardiopulmonary resuscitation should not be attempted. Because CPR is not attempted, other resuscitative measures that follow it (such as electric shocks to the heart and artificial respirations by insertion of a breathing tube) will also be avoided. This order has been useful in preventing unnecessary and unwanted invasive treatment at the end of life.

A doctor's medical order known as a "do not resuscitate" order. It urges medical professionals not administer CPR if a patient stops breathing or has a stopped heartbeat.

A DNR order should ideally be established before an emergency arises. A DNR order enables someone to decide whether they want CPR in a dire situation or not.

An order to "Do Not Intubate" allows for the use of cardiac medications and chest compressions but forgoes the insertion of a breathing tube.

Some hospitals employ an AND order, also known as a "Allow Natural Death" order, as a standby to the more common DNR order. An AND request is used to make sure just comfort measures, intended to give great management of pain or additional symptoms, take place, as opposed to a DNR, which merely specifies that no efforts are to be made to revive breathing or cardiac activity if it stops. Resuscitation, artificial nourishment, fluids, and other interventions that prolong the process of death without improving your child's quality of life should be withheld or stopped. Not interfering with the natural process of dying is what is meant by "allowing a natural death." Additionally, it implies that every effort has to be made to ensure that your client's passing occurs in a calm and comforting circumstances, with as many members of your family and friends present as you, the child's parents, and the kid's classmates want.

DNR Order

DNR stands for "do not resuscitate." If your heart stops beating (cardiac arrest), a DNR order means you do not want any lifesaving measures.

The majority of people believe that the primary method of resuscitation is CPR. In reality, there are several treatments and methods.

The essential elements of resuscitation include:

* **Compressions of the chest:** Most people refer to this as CPR. It is a method that keeps the blood moving through the body even when the heart isn't beating by repeatedly applying pressure to the chest.
* **Defibrillation:** This procedure attempts to restart the heartbeat using electricity. Handheld paddles like pads that adhere to the chest may give this electric shock.
* **Drugs used intravenously (IV):** During resuscitation, medical professionals employ a variety of drugs. Some of these are potent drugs that work quickly to restart the heartbeat, such as epinephrine. But when someone gets chest compressions, this is merely one of several IV drugs they could get.
* **Supporting breathing:** During a cardiac arrest, the heart receives the majority of the care. However, it's crucial to maintain carbon dioxide and oxygen flow during resuscitation. This may be done by covering someone's mouth with a mask and inflated bag. It can also be done with intubation.

A DNR order is a legal document signed by you (or someone you elect to make decisions for you) and your healthcare provider. It tells all medical providers that you do not want the above treatments if your heart stops beating.

But, it is important to understand that a DNR order is not a "do-not-treat" order for when you're very sick or dying. It only comes into play when someone has a cardiac arrest.

DNI Order

DNI stands for "do not intubate." Intubation is the process of placing a breathing tube into the airway. It's a small plastic tube that sends in windpipe (trachea). Following that, the breathing tube may be connected to a ventilator, often known as a "life support machine." It is a device that breathes for you, removes carbon dioxide from the air, and distributes oxygen to your lungs. When a person decides against being placed on a ventilator and intubated, they place a DNI order.

Orders give clinicians instructions about the measures a patient wants or does not want; for example, if they lose consciousness, cannot breathe on their own, or face other serious symptoms or complications that could interfere with long-term quality of life.

These decisions and instructions are part of a process called advance care planning. Advance care planning guides the approach to the patient's care, particularly with regard to symptom management and goals of care (comfort care versus aggressive life prolongation).

Working together with the clinician, patients and their families decide whether they want specific treatments, such as:
* Intubation
* Cardiopulmonary resuscitation
* Dialysis
* Artificial (parenteral) nutrition/hydration
* Antibiotics
   DNR and DNI orders are an integral part of advance care planning.

A DNI, as it is known in medicine, denotes a patient's preference not to have a breathing tube put into their trachea via the mouth or nose to get back normal breathing. The tube stays there and is ultimately attached to a compressor to support breathing if the patient's breathing continues to be compromised. When patients fail to take in air on their own on a regular basis, a ventilator maintains oxygen moving between the chambers of the lungs.

A patient can sign a DNI and continue to benefit from oxygen therapy and noninvasive ventilation, such as through BiPAP.

DNR vs. DNI

Typically, a DNR order also includes a DNI order. The general DNR instructs medical staff to refrain from using emergency life-saving techniques on very sick patients if they cease breathing or if their heart stops, including cardiopulmonary resuscitation, chest compressions, breathing tubes, or cardiac medications,

A DNI, however, clearly forbids the insertion of a breathing tube while permitting basic life-saving CPR, compressions on the chest, and drugs.

Why could Patients Choose a DNI?

The majority of hospice patients would rather die naturally than spend a lengthy time on a ventilator. It is not essential to sign a DNI if you have already signed a DNR.

DNI Considerations

When determining whether you want to sign a DNI for oneself or somebody who has given you authority to make choices for them, bear the following factors in mind:

- ❖ What are the short- and long-term risks and benefits of intubation?
- ❖ Will intubation honor a patient's stated goals, wishes, and values for comfort-focused, home-based end-of-life care?
- ❖ Will intubation improve quality of life when a person is towards the end of their life or will it prevent them from having a dignified death?
- ❖ How involved do you want your physician or care team to be in your decision about DNI or DNR? Ask if you need more information about the impact of your options and decision.
- ❖ If you are acting as a patient's healthcare proxy and they have an advanced disease, try to talk to them about their desires for a DNR or DNI while they are still conscious so that you may make the proper choice when the time comes.
- ❖ To ensure that your wishes are considered, recorded, and communicated with others, especially with your delegated decision maker(s) or the hospital and hospice teams, it is important to start conversations about a DNI or DNR early in the course of your sickness (or that of a loved one with whom you are in close contact).

The following are a few motivations for choosing a DNR or DNI order:

- ❖ **Terminal illness:** When the time comes, a person with a terminal illness, such as cancer, may still refuse resuscitation even if they are not actively unwell or in the hospital.
- ❖ **Advanced chronic illness:** Many people with chronic conditions, like heart disease or COPD, know it's more likely that their heart will stop beating or they may stop breathing well. And they want to be proactive about stating their wishes for the end of their life.
- ❖ **Personal choice:** One need not be suffering from a fatal disease to choose this for oneself. For instance, even if they are in excellent health, elderly folks may decide to do this as they age. Additionally, some individuals might do such for religious reasons.

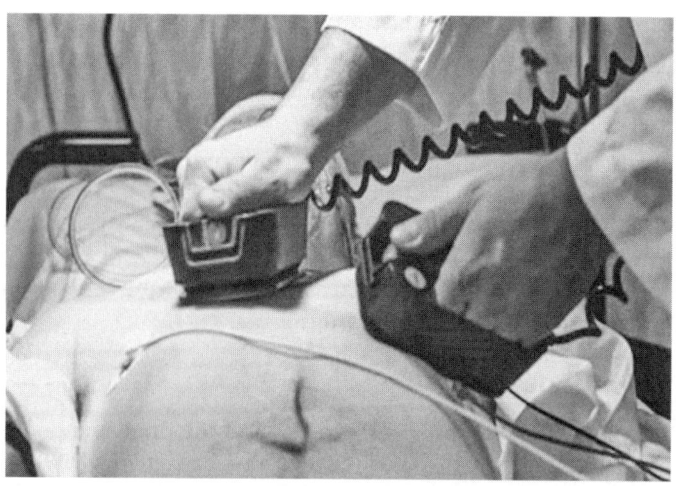

CODE STATUS

All patients will be required to choose their code status for the duration of their stay when they are admitted to a hospital or an outpatient institution (such as a dialysis center or an outpatient surgical center).

When a person's heart stops beating, healthcare professionals may save their life by doing CPR. It's only one of the procedures medical professionals use to attempt to preserve a life.

In the case of a cardiac arrest, a person who has given the order to "do not resuscitate" signifies they are against CPR or other life-saving interventions. An individual who requests a DNI order does not wish to be put on a ventilator.

For those who are suffering from a terminal, life-threatening disease, a DNR and DNI order is often chosen. However, there may be a lot of reasons why someone could choose this. Additionally, DNR and DNI orders can be reversed if someone changes their mind.

❖ **Full code:** defined as full support which includes cardiopulmonary resuscitation, if the patient has no heartbeat and is not breathing.

❖ **DNR:** The patient may desire other life-sustaining procedures but does not want CPR. The patient is not breathing and has no heartbeat.

❖ **Comfort cares only:** Focused end-of-life care is referred to as "COMFORT CARES ONLY." This treatment includes a patient's physical and/or emotional comfort. Adequate pain management is always a part of comfort care. At this stage, cure-related drugs and therapies are stopped. Resuscitation efforts won't be undertaken (DNR) and natural death is permitted. Patients as well as their families will be treated with comfort and respect at all times.

When a patient has heart failure, cardiopulmonary resuscitation, is performed in an effort to restart their heart and give them oxygen. CPR may include actions like external chest compressions and mouth-to-mouth resuscitation. A ventilator may be used to assist air until the individual can breathe on their own during advanced CPR (also known as ALS advanced life support), which may also entail administering an electric shock and/or inserting a tube to open the patient's airway. To control both blood and heart pressure, medication may be necessary. It is crucial to discuss possibilities of recovery or survival with your doctor based on patient's current medical situation.

Do not resuscitate: If a patient's breathing or heartbeat stops, DNR instructs doctors, nurses, and emergency medical workers not to do emergency CPR. Medical workers are instructed not to administer CPR by the DNR. A natural death might occur under DNR.

ORGAN DONATION

The Organ donation (OD) is defined as the process of retrieving or procuring an organ or part of it from a live or deceased person and then, transplanting it into another living person. According to reports, persons may donate 25 different organs and tissues after undergoing medical and psychological screening. One donor's organ donation may save up to eight lives, according to the Organ Procurement and Transplant Network (OPTN, 2015). The most often transplanted tissues are cornea and musculoskeletal grafts, whereas the most frequently transplanted fleshy organs are kidneys, liver, and hearts.

Definition

Organ donation is the donation of biological tissue or an organ of the human body, from a living or dead person to a living recipient in need of a transplantation.

Transplantable organs and tissues are removed in a surgical procedure following a determination, based on the donor's medical and social history, of which are suitable for transplantation. Such procedures are termed allotransplantations, to distinguish them from xenotransplantation, the transfer of animal organs into human bodies.

Types of Donors

There are three kinds of organ donors:

1. **Live donors:** Someone who is willing to donate their organ(s) to someone in need of a transplant is referred to as a live donor. Living donors are often loved ones or close family members for individuals who need a transplant. They must fulfil the relevant medical conditions and consent to the entire range of required medical tests as determined by the circumstances in order to be accepted as prospective donors.
2. **Brain death and cadaveric donors:** Brain death, which is the permanent cessation of cerebral and brain stem function, is shown by the absence of brain currents, normal blood flow to the brain, and neurological activity as determined by the clinical examination of responses. After being considered brain dead, a person's cardiopulmonary function could be artificially maintained for a while, but they are still lifeless. The kidney, liver, circulatory system, lungs, pancreas, gut, cornea, cells, bones, and veins of a patient who has brain death may donate.
3. **Natural decedents who donate:** A person may donate their organs, like the tissue from their eyes, after dying away naturally. There is no minimum age for removal of organs, even from new-borns and early toddlers, according to prior study.

Deceased Donation

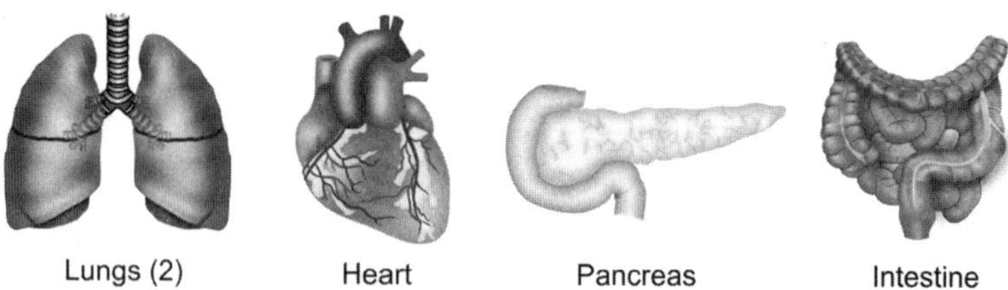

Tissue and Eyes

Tissue donation differs from organ donation in several ways. First off, there is no waiting list for the majority of tissue transplants, as the tissues are always ready for use. Tissue donations may be packaged and kept for a period of five years, but organs must be donated as soon as possible after recovery. People may be helped and cured by donated tissues in a variety of significant ways.

Donated tissues include, for instance:

❖ Bones and tendons may be used to rebuild or repair damaged tissue caused by tumors or wounds. Achilles tendon fractures are a common sports injury that need donor tissue to be healed.
❖ Damaged heart valves are replaced with new ones, which allows the heart to beat again. The valves placed on young kids will truly help them to develop.
❖ Veins and arteries are helpful to patients requiring coronary artery bypass grafting. Patients who suffer from diabetes or other conditions that lower blood flow can receive donated veins to repair ruptured vessels and enhance blood flow.
❖ Burns, cleft palates, and full mastectomy reconstruction may all be treated using skin.
❖ The blind are given sight again via corneas.

Living Donation

A living person may help someone else who needs surgery by giving them a functioning kidney, in addition to a section from their liver, lung, gastrointestinal tract, or pancreas.

There are various factors to think about while allowing for living donation. Blood type and overall health are all taken into account when deciding whether to donate a live organ. Each candidate live donor must go through a complete medical screening that includes blood tests, a physical examination, and a psychological assessment. The decision to accept the live donor is subsequently made by the transplant facility's medical personnel.

CONTRAINDICATIONS

Using OD is definitely not advised if you have viral diseases including hepatitis B/C, HIV, CMV, syphilis, ebola virus, rabies, severe infection/sepsis, active TB, or advanced cancer.

Factors Affecting OD in India

❖ **Sociocultural factors:** The attitude toward OD in Western countries is mostly based on altruistic and humanitarian principles. However, However, in Asian countries such as India, Japan, etc., concepts of religion, morals, and spirituality are entwined with conceptions of life, death, and even life beyond death.
It might be quite difficult to bring up the subject of OD in social or intimate settings in these countries. Additionally, here is no humanitarian tradition and it is frowned upon in Japan to receive someone else's organs. Religious factors may also be obstacles to OD.
❖ **Knowledge, beliefs, and personal values:** Factors accompanying to OD proved that the strongest predictors of OD willingness are knowledge, attitudes and with personal values (including altruism). There is very less public awareness about OD in India. The idea of "brain death" plus the legal implications that come with it are still unclear to Indians. Insufficient knowledge about it has also been noted by healthcare professionals.
❖ **Legal and ethical issues:** Consent, financial assistance for donors and loved ones, and equitable distribution of donated organs are only a few of the factors that have been mentioned in relation to organ transplantation.
In accordance with Indian legislation, as mentioned in subclause (3) clause 9 in chapter II, stated that unrelated live donation has high likelihood to get misused. This is a prime reason why kidney trade still occurs in India.

❖ **Participation of stakeholders' in OD:** The predicted number of cadaveric contributions and the actual number of potential donors are not equal. This could occur as a consequence of the kin of potential donors not abiding by or respecting the choices made by contributors after their passing. In order to raise awareness, a lot of governmental organizations (NGOs), religious leaders, members of civil society, and a variety of interested parties work together.

❖ **Financial issues:** Another obstacle is the incompetency for poor recipients. We often see requests for donations to help poor people requiring organ transplants in magazines, on social media, as well as ads along the highways. Most transplants in India are carried out via social contributions rather than government funding.

Role of Nurses in OD and Transplantation

All nursing professionals should have thorough comprehensive and scientific knowledge about OD. Assessing and monitoring transplant patients, living donors, potential donors, and self-care are all part of this process. Additionally, psychotherapy is provided for both live donors and receivers. All of these things must be done in order to enhance post-transplant quality of life.

The development of a successful transplant program is largely made possible by nurses. They are the primary members of the OD team who provide care to patients through communication, technology, and human resources while providing proper treatment, interaction, education, and research. Nursing professionals must have a good awareness of high ethical standards as well as sufficient resources in order to analyze the social challenges and patient risks related to organ donation and transplantation.

The medical condition of the person at the time of death can determine what organs and tissues can be donated and what cannot be. Organs need to be removed as soon as the person is declared brain-dead. Without the necessary oxygen supply, the organs stop functioning right.

The approximate amount of time between recovering the tissues/organs and transplanting them is:

❖ Lung – 4–6 hours
❖ Heart – 4 hours
❖ Liver – 24 hours
❖ Pancreas – 24 hours
❖ Kidney – 72 hours
❖ Cornea – 14 days
❖ Bones – 5 years
❖ Skin – 5 year
❖ Heart valves–10 years

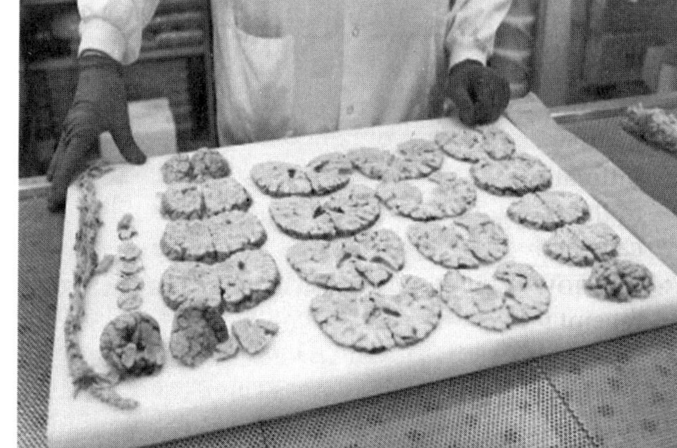

MEDICO-LEGAL CASES

Definition

Medico-legal cases (MLC) are the cases where the doctor feels the requirement of an investigation by law-enforcing agencies, essentially to fix the responsibility regarding the cause of injury.

❖ It may be summarized up by noting that it is a medical case with legal implications or a legal case requiring medical expertise.

❖ A medico-legal case is defined as an instance in which a police investigation is required to identify the party(ies) responsible for the injury or disease.

❖ This medical situation has legal implications for the attending doctor, where the attending doctor, after eliciting history and examining the patient, thinks that some investigation by law enforcement agencies is essential.

❖ Medical expertise may be required in a legal case when a person is brought in by the police for examination.

List of Medico-Legal Cases

❖ Any incidents of burns or injury—the circumstances of which suggest commission of an offense by somebody (irrespective of suspicion of foul play).

❖ All vehicular, factory or other unnatural accident cases specially when there is a likelihood of patient's death or grievous hurt.

❖ Sexual assault incidents that are whether suspect or confirmed.

❖ Whether suspected or confirmed of illegal abortion.

❖ Cases of unconsciousness for unknown or inexplicable reasons.

❖ All cases when poisoning or coma is suspected or shown to have occurred.

❖ All cases referred from court or otherwise for age estimation.

❖ Cases brought dead with improper history creating suspicion of an offense.

❖ Cases of suspected self-infliction of injuries or attempted suicide.

❖ Any other case not falling under the above categories but has legal implications.

REGISTRATION PROCEDURE FOR A MEDICO-LEGAL CASE

Treatment (All Legal Processes Must be Put on Hold Until the Patient is Revived)

❖ Identification (Including whether or not the aforementioned situation is a medico-legal matter)

❖ Intimate to police (He must register the case into the MLC and/or communicate the same to the closest police station, through the telephone or in writing, if it does fall within this category)

❖ Acknowledgement receipt (The police should provide you with an acknowledgment receipt for your future records).

REPORTING OF THE MEDICO-LEGAL CASES

❖ Reports must be generated in three copies and include all pertinent data on the appropriate pro-forma.

❖ When writing, avoid abbreviations and over writing. Correction if any, should be initialed with date and time.

❖ Reports must be sent as quickly as feasible to the authorities.

❖ For 10 years, health records should be stored securely.

❖ Age, sex, father's name, complete address, reporting time, incident date and time, and what brought the individual are all important information.

❖ Fingerprints and identification markers.

❖ The police must be notified of all MLCs in order to collect legal proof.
❖ Inform the prosecutor to record a "dying declaration" if the condition of the patient is terminal.

MEDICO-LEGAL CASE

❖ **Definition of medico-legal case**
  Cases wherever attending doctor after taking history and clinical examination of the patient thinks that some investigation by law enforcing agencies are essential so as to fix the responsibility regarding the case in accordance with the law of land.
❖ **Duty of registered medical practitioner (RMP) in MLC**
  ◆ **To save the life** of a patient and to give primary treatment, is the foremost responsibility.
  ◆ Registered medical practitioner (RMP), i.e., Emergency medical officer (EMO)/assistant emergency medical officer (Asst. EMO) at emergency should decide whether the case is to be registered as MLC or not.
  ◆ **Consent** of family members **NOT** required for registration of a case as MLC.
❖ Workflow for medico-legal cases brought to emergency in AIIMS Bhopal
  ◆ All patients/cases are given hospital registration no. in emergency.
  ◆ From OPD/IPD if a case is medico-legal, information must reach emergency and MLC number is allotted.

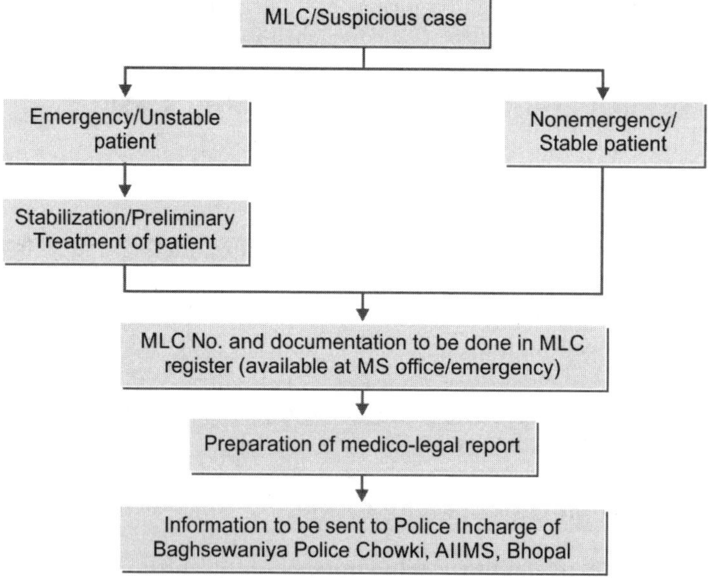

❖ Protocol for filling the medico-legal report (MLR) is as under.
  ◆ *Preliminary*
    ◊ Information to the police should be sent in proper form.
    ◊ Take consent for examination of the patient on the MLR form. If less than 12 years or brought unconscious take the consent of the guardian/accompanying person/police constable.

◊ The preliminary entries should be complete.

◊ Two identification marks have to be noted preferably on accessible parts.

◊ Time and date of examination should be indicated clearly. If the patient is under observation to decide the severity of injury/condition, same should be indicated in medico-legal report.

◊ Take proper history in patient/guardian's own words and document correctly.

◊ In cases of poisoning and other cases, general examination and other signs should be mentioned in detail. Use standard formats wherever possible.

◊ Details of police constable who brought the case should be noted.

- *Examination:* Mention the examination of injuries in detail (type, site, size, shape, color, age of injury, direction, nature, duration). Use diagram wherever necessary.
- *Opinion*
  ◊ Opinion should be crisp and to the point. Articles preserved should be enumerated.

  ◊ Prepare three copies of the document, one copy is kept at emergency room, other as hospital record and the original is given to the police.

GENERAL GUIDELINES

Important guidelines and instructions for dealing with MLC are as following:

❖ If a **MLC, recorded elsewhere (in other hospital) is referred,** it should be treated as MLC but **NO NEW** MLC number should be issued. Treatment should continue in old MLC number. Neither a new MLR should be prepared nor is it needed to inform the police.

❖ If a case is brought several days after the incident, it should be reported and findings to be noted regarding the present condition of the patient.

❖ MLC can be written and signed by (EMO)/Asst. EMO/Faculty. Wherever possible, faculty member should sign along with SR/JR if the report is prepared by them. This will facilitate court, procedure when SR/JR are not available at AIIMS Bhopal and cannot be contacted. In such cases the faculty may be required to give evidence in the court.

❖ All treatment papers, investigation reports, etc., to be labeled as MLC and record should be maintained for future medico-legal use (same may be required by court for the case).

❖ When medico-legal case is to be discharged from hospital, police should be informed and information should also be sent to the emergency to make an entry in medico-legal register.

❖ Belongings of the medico-legal cases should be handed over to the police officer and proper receipt must be obtained in every case.

❖ If a medico-legal case is not admitted, entry shall be made in the MLC register.

❖ Consent for emergency surgery, when no attendant is available can be given by the Medical Superintendent of the hospital.

❖ If (EMO)/(Asst. EMO) in emergency does not register a case as MLC but the treating doctor thinks that the case is a MLC then it should be recorded as MLC and can be considered as MLC at any point of time, even if missed initially.

❖ In case of taking away a patient or body of a medico-legal case forcibly by the attendant, the medical officer should record the same on the file of the patient and police station/post of the area and security staff should be informed immediately.

❖ X-rays, blood reports, microbiological, pathological investigations, etc., in medico-legal case should be labeled as MLC and kept along with other documents of the case.

RECORD KEEPING

- ❖ Always prepare three copies of the medico-legal report, one is kept as hospital record, other is kept in the office of the Medical Superintendent and the original is given to police after getting proper receipt.
- ❖ Hospital records or file of MLC should be kept as confidential in record section till judgment by the court of law pertaining to the case has been issued (for practical purposes, no time limit).
- ❖ If medico-legal report has already been issued, then duplicate medico-legal report should not be issued unless specifically requested by the police in writing or by the order of the court.

DEATH IN MEDICO-LEGAL CASE

- ❖ Whenever there is a death in a medico-legal case, the police officer should be informed. Death certificate should not be issued in medico-legal cases and body must be sent for medico-legal autopsy after filling the appropriate format.
- ❖ All cases brought dead to the institution: In all the cases brought dead, police is informed and body is sent to mortuary of AIIMS Bhopal after filling the appropriate form.
- ❖ Cause of death certification in cases other than MLC can only be issued by emergency medical officer (EMO)/assistant EMO/treating doctor who has attended the case within 7 days and is sure about the cause of death.

MEDICO-LEGAL AUTOPSY IN MLC

- ❖ Autopsy is done in the mortuary complex of AIIMS Bhopal by the Department of Forensic Medicine and Toxicology.
- ❖ Autopsy is conducted Monday to Friday from 10 AM to 5 PM.
- ❖ Timing on Saturday, Sunday and on all holidays is from 10 AM to 2 PM
- ❖ Cold storage facility in the event of death in medico-legal case is available in the mortuary. Any case for autopsy, if brought to mortuary beyond working hours can be kept in cold storage.

DYING DECLARATION

- ❖ In case of impending death in MLC, the medical officer should immediately ask the police officer on duty in writing to call a magistrate. If there is no time to call a magistrate, the dying declaration should be recorded by the doctor himself in the presence of another doctor or staff member.
- ❖ The primary duty of a doctor in dying declaration is to ascertain and document compos mentis (alert mental state) of the patient at the beginning and at the end of the statement.

SPECIFIC CASES

(Important points to be remembered)
- ❖ **Rape/Sexual assault cases (suspect and survivor)**
  - ◆ Be polite to the suspect and victim.
  - ◆ Always take consent. In case of suspect, medical examination can be done even if he declines to give consent.
  - ◆ Take a detailed history and document it in person's own words.

- Examine them properly and fill the prescribed form for suspect and survivor.
- Always provide information regarding psychiatric counseling to the victim.
- All male and female registered medical practitioners are eligible to examine the victim.
- Always examine the victim in presence of female attendees. Victim can have a female acquaintance/relative with her if she wants.
- In case of children, sedative or analgesic may be needed for examining genitalia in painful condition.
- Do not delay the examination. Exact time of commencement and completion must be noted in the report.
- Never attempt to undress the victim for examination. Convince her to undress herself.
- Never pass judgmental remark or comments that might appear unsympathetic.
- Denying examination of the rape victim is unlawful.
- **Following instructions to be followed depending on the circumstances**
  ◊ Take history whether she has taken bath and changed the clothes.
  ◊ With cotton swab collect vaginal secretion from posterior fornix and prepare 4 slides.
  ◊ Place loose pubic hair in a labeled envelope.
  ◊ Obtain fingernail scrapings.
  ◊ Preserve garments for seminal and blood stain.
  ◊ Collect blood sample (15 mL).
  ◊ If age estimation required then refer to the Department of Forensic Medicine.
  ◊ If clothes are to be preserved and sealed, always provide proper clothing or inform the relatives to bring one set of clothes.
  ◊ *Note:* Staining of vaginal smear, examination of slide and opinion in sexual assault cases, is being given by Department of Forensic Medicine and Toxicology. The slide can be prepared, dried and forwarded to Department of Forensic Medicine for needful.
  ◊ Treatment of victim should be given when needed.

❖ **Fire arm injuries**
  - Bullets, lead shots, etc., recovered from the wounds or body in fire arm injury should be air dried then put in a bottle(s), padded with cotton, documented sealed and handed over to the police.
  - Always try to mention about the entry and exit wound.
  - Always take X-ray of the track or whole body.
  - Never pick the bullet using a metal/toothed forceps, rather use fingers or rubber tipped forceps.
  - Never wash the bullet.

❖ **Criminal abortion**
  - Give proper treatment.
  - Always perform examination of clothes and take blood sample.
  - Proper history and documentation.
  - If patient dies, send for medico-legal autopsy.
  - Preserve the remains of product of conception (POC) for chemical analysis and DNA analysis if required.
  - Clothes are recorded and preserved
  - If she refuses to make a statement, the doctor should not pursue the matter. He must consult a senior professional colleague.

❖ **Burns:**
- Proper history and documentation
- Give primary treatment.
- Extent and degree of the burns to be noted.
- Make a proper sketch showing areas involved and state in percentage.
- Inflammable agents on the body/cloth are recorded and preserved.
- Dying declaration if required should be taken especially in young married females.

❖ **Hanging/Strangulation**
- Ligature mark—describe its position, nature, width, direction and extent whether complete or incomplete.
- Ligature material in-situ should be cut away from the knot so as not to disturb the knot. Then the cut ends and knot have to be secured with threads separately.
- Ligature material should be preserved.
- Examination of ligature material in respect of its nature, position, type of knot, circumference of loop, length of short and long free ends, foreign bodies and stains.

❖ **Poisoning**
- Give primary treatment. Take proper history.
- History of substance consumed, amount consumed, when, where and number of people consumed.
- **Proper documentation of history, treatment and articles sealed**
- Send properly sealed, labeled samples of vomitus/stomach wash and blood sample to the police and make record wherever possible.
- Never allow the entry of unauthorized person near the victim in a case of homicidal poisoning.

❖ **Injury cases**
- Give primary treatment.
- Examine and record all injuries properly.
- Proper documentation.
- Opinion should include injury by type of weapon (sharp/blunt) , manner (Self-inflicted, homicidal, accidental) and duration of injury.

EUTHANASIA

Introduction

Many definitions state that euthanasia is the painless demise of a person who could have a terminal illness when the person's death is in the best goal of the person. The term could make people think of a variety of things, such as killing the elderly, the sick, or those who aren't making a good contribution to society.

When someone kills someone or fails to save someone from dying only because they may have a close relationship with that person, including being a caregiver or a relative, it is to be considered an act.

The word "euthanasia" has taken from the Greek terms "eu" for "good" and "thanatos" for "death." Nowadays, it frequently refers to the deliberate execution of a person who is seen as unworthy of life by himself nor others. Sometimes euthanasia is referred to as "mercy killing," which could apply to either intentional death by medical professionals or to intentional killing by family or friends acting in an apparently "merciful" way. There are several words used to describe euthanasia, including assisted suicide, vengeance killing, either active or passive euthanasia, coercive or planned euthanasia, and many more. Greek origins give this expression the meaning of "good death." Greeks had the view that if a person felt their life was no longer important, they should either commit suicide or have a dignified demise. Greek society recognized that it was morally acceptable for someone to beg for help in dying.

A classic example of euthanasia of Socrates, who agreed to drink the hemlock (poison), knows fully well it would bring about his death.

Types of Euthanasia

Euthanasia is broadly divided into three main types:
1. Voluntary
2. Involuntary
3. Nonvoluntary

1. Voluntary euthanasia occurs at the request of the person who expresses a desire to die. The person may do so:
   - By refusing medical treatment
   - Asking for medical treatment or life support to be withdrawn or switched off
   - Refusing to eat
   - Simply deciding to die
   - Asking for help with dying

   As a result, when discussing voluntary dying, a wide range of circumstances can be considered, such as instances in which one individual kills themselves in private without anyone knowing, where the second person knows about it but does nothing to prevent it, or the cases in which the act of suicide is assisted, as well as those cases in which the killing is carried out by another because they are not able to do so by themselves.

   Involuntary euthanasia occurs when the person killed is capable of consenting to his or her own death, but does not do so, either because they are not asked, or because that person is asked and yet decides to go on living. In an active involuntary case of euthanasia, where the person has not waived or cannot waive the duty of noninterference, then any reasons for killing that person must demonstrate that the circumstances favored overruling the duty of noninterference.

2. Involuntary euthanasia occurs when the person killed is capable of consenting to their own death but does not, either because they are not asked, or because they are not asked but continue to choose to live. In the case of active involuntary euthanasia, where the person has not waived the obligation of non-intervention or cannot waive it, it must be shown that all the reasons for killing that person are circumstances favoring the cancellation of the obligation of non-intervention.

   It is apparent that there are no specific criteria or rules which state what duty of care and noninterference involve.

3. Nonvoluntary euthanasia occurs when the person is not in a position to make a meaningful choice between living and dying and an appropriate person takes the decision on their behalf. This can happen due to a number of reasons:
   - The person is in coma
   - The person is too young (child)
   - The person is senile
   - The person is mentally challenged or brain damaged or mentally disturbed.

Think of the challenges in situations when someone might need a life support system. The challenge in this situation is determining when to turn the machine off. When a child is healthy but has a significant mental disability, the parents may come to the conclusion that it might be better for the child to die since they would either be unable to care for it or the child's life would be significantly affected. All of these difficulties undoubtedly show how responsible parents must be for raising their children, but there are also no easy fixes in this case.

To distinguish between killing and letting someone die, whether in an active or passive manner, voluntary/involuntary/nonvoluntary behavior, etc., are distinctions that help in comprehending the differences. These distinctions don't explain the different types of euthanasia.

Voluntary euthanasia is illegal in the United States and most parts of the world.

Countries that allow it include:
- Belgium
- The Netherlands
- Luxembourg
- Canada
- Colombia
- Involuntary euthanasia is illegal worldwide.

UNIT

12

Self-Concept

LEARNING OBJECTIVES

At the end of this unit, the reader will be able to:
- Define self-concept.
- Explain components of self-content.
- Enumerate factors affecting self-concept.
- Nursing management.

INTRODUCTION

The capacity to function and health state are both influenced by one's perception of themselves. In terms of the mental, emotional, intellectual in nature, and functional parts, everyone has both good and negative self-perceptions. These evolve with time. Self-concept, or one's view of oneself, is what contributes to individuality.

COMPONENTS OF SELF-CONCEPT

❖ Identity
❖ Body image
❖ Self-esteem
❖ Role performance

Identity

❖ A person begins to develop identity during childhood and constantly reinforces and modifies it throughout life.
❖ Identity may include a person's name, gender, ethnic identity, family status, occupation, and roles.
❖ A sense of personal identity is what sets one person apart as a unique individual.

Body Image

Body image is variable because it may be impacted by changes to the structure or function of the body, including those that naturally occur throughout growth and development. Body image refers to beliefs about one's physical traits, appearance, and performance.

Self-Esteem

People will determine their level of self-esteem based on the attainment of the qualities they value most (for instance, physical characteristics, social successes). Self-esteem is a person's overall perception of their own value and worth, or how they see themselves.

Role Performance

Expected actions vary depending on the position. People often play many roles at once, including parent, sibling, friend, husband, and student nurse. A collection of anticipated actions that are influenced by social, cultural, and family conventions is referred to as a role.

FACTORS AFFECTING SELF-CONCEPT

- Altered health status
- Experience
- Developmental considerations
- Culture
- Internal and external resources
- History of success and failure
- Crisis or life stressors
- Aging, illness, or trauma

NURSING MANAGEMENT

- **Assessment**
  - Assess the client's strengths to be used as a foundation on which to build therapeutic interventions.
  - Maintain appropriate relationships
  - Care for self in order to meet basic needs
  - Adapt to stressors in a positive manner
- **Nursing diagnoses disturbed body image parental role conflict**
  - Disturbed personal identity
  - Ineffective role performance
  - Chronic low self-esteem
  - Situational low self-esteem
- **Nursing diagnoses disturbed personal identity anxiety social isolation**
  - Hopelessness
  - Powerlessness
- **Implementation initiate therapeutic interaction**
  - Support healthy defense mechanisms
  - Ensure satisfaction of needs
  - Physical needs
  - Psychosocial needs

❖ **Helping patients maintain sense of self**
- Communicate worth with looks, speech, and judicious touch.
- Acknowledge patient status, role, and individuality.
- Speak to patient respectfully.
- Offer simple explanations for procedures.
- Move patient's body respectfully if necessary.
- Respect patient's privacy and sensibilities.
- Acknowledge and allow expression of negative feelings.
- Help patients recognize strengths and explore alternatives.

Sexuality

Unit Outline

- Sexual development throughout life
- Sexual health
- Sexual orientation
- Factors affecting sexuality
- Prevention of STIs, unwanted pregnancy, avoiding sexual harassment and abuse
- Dealing with inappropriate sexual behavior

LEARNING OBJECTIVES

At the end of this unit, the reader will be able to:
- Define sexuality.
- Schedule sexual development.
- Define Freud's stages of development.
- Explain sexual health.
- Describe sexual orientation.
- Explain prevention of STDs.

INTRODUCTION

Sexuality is one of the most important aspects of life. Every cell and fiber of a person's body is sexual. Sexuality permeates the psychological and spiritual areas of a person's life. One of the sad lessons of human history is that sexuality which should have brightened and cheered up lives of people often becomes, instead, a curse. We often see people's lives being disoriented because of the inability to deal with sexuality meaningfully. A person's relationships with others in his/her life are disrupted and distorted because of the inability to exercise sexuality honestly and meaningfully. Sexuality which plays a decisive role in the formation of a family, if not understood and exercised properly, can destroy families, and the intimate relationship that should exist between members of a family. In this unit, you are introduced to a discussion on the healthy way of handling sexuality

SEXUAL DEVELOPMENT

Development starts even before birth and continues throughout the life span.

A variety of influences have an impact on this development:

❖ Psychological influences

- ❖ Hormonal influences
- ❖ Genetic influences

Before birth:
- ❖ The human sexual response cycle begins.
- ❖ The male fetus achieves erections in utero—and some males are even born with erections.
- ❖ The female sexual response cycle is functional before birth.

6 months–1 year:
- ❖ Genital self-exploration and masturbation occur for both sexes.
- ❖ When babies can touch their bodies, they begin to explore their genitals.

By 2 years of age:
- ❖ Aware of their biological sex
- ❖ Show an understanding of sexual identity.

At 3–5 years of age:
- ❖ Understand how females and males should act as well as gender roles
- ❖ Ask questions like where babies come from.

At 5–12 years:
- ❖ Begin to show romantic interest.
- ❖ The first signs of sexual orientation (preference toward males or females or both) characterize this phase.

At ages 8–13 years:
- ❖ The first physical signs of puberty
- ❖ Begin slightly earlier for girls than boys

Girls: First menstruation between ages 9 and 16 years
- ❖ **Boys:** 11–18 years-onset of sperm production.
- ❖ Pubertal milestones depend on the child's nutritional status and may be delayed if nutritional status is severely compromised.

After Puberty

First Sexual Intercourse

- ❖ Varies greatly by culture
- ❖ Mid to later adolescence is fairly common across cultures

First Childbirth

- ❖ Many factors determine when and whether a person has a first child
- ❖ First childbirth also varies by community and individual

Menopause

- ❖ **Female:** Mid 30s–50s
- ❖ Physiological changes are end of ovulation, menstruation, and the capacity to reproduce
- ❖ **Male:** Climacteric occurs at 45–65 years of age
- ❖ Decrease in testosterone production.

Freud's Five Stages of Development

In essence Freud used the term sexuality to refer to the erotic life of the individual. According to him, sexuality is not a matter for adults alone but also infantile. It is all-pervasive and covers all those activities and sensations that are pleasurable and afford sensual gratification. Freud noted that infants were capable of erotic activity from birth onward. The earliest manifestations of infantile sexuality arise in relation to bodily functions such as feeding and elimination of body wastes. Of all the concepts of Freud, the concepts he advanced with regard to the erotic life of infants and young children aroused severe criticism from different corners.

The concept of psychosexual stages of development, as envisioned by Sigmund Freud is the central element in his sexual drive theory. For him, the sex drive is the most important motivating force in man, including children and even infants. Man's capacity for orgasm or sexuality is neurologically present from birth. Sexuality, for Freud, is not only intercourse, but all pleasurable sensation from the skin. At different times in our lives, different parts of our skin give us greatest pleasure. For example, an infant finds greatest pleasure in sucking, especially at the breast. Freud had the making of psychosexual stages of development in man with regard to pleasurable sensation. Each stage is characterized by the erogenous zone that is the source of the libidinal drive during that stage. These stages are, in order: oral, anal, phallic, latency and genital.

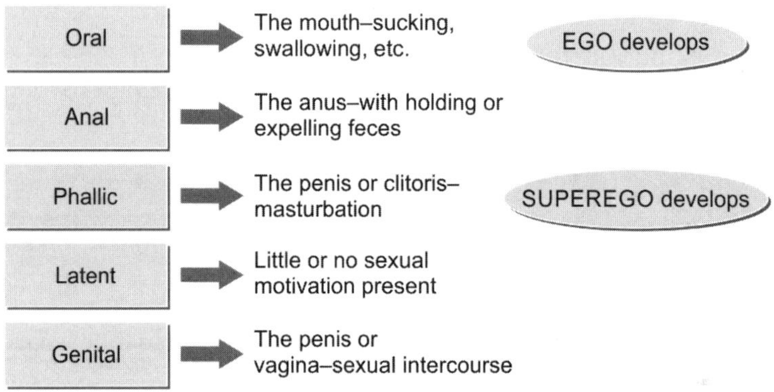

The first stage of psychosexual development is the Oral stage. This stage lasts from the beginning of one's life till (about) the 18th month. During this stage the gratifying activities are nursling, eating, as well as mouth movement, including sucking, gumming biting and swallowing. Here, the mothers' breast is the only source of food and drink, which also represents her love. In this stage, the gratification of needs will lead to the formation of independence and trust.

The second stage is called Anal stage, which lasts from about 18th month till three or four years old. In this stage, the focus of drive energy moves from the upper digestive tract to the lower end and the anus. The gratifying activities are bowel movement and the withholding of such movement. In this stage, children are taught when, where and how excretion is appropriate by the society. Thus, children discover their own ability to control and adjust such movements.

The third stage is called phallic stage, which lasts from three or four years till the fifth or sixth year. Here the gratification is focused on the genital fondling, but not in the form of adult sexuality, since the children are physically immature. Children become increasingly aware of their body and are curious about the bodies of other children. This is probably the most challenging stage in a person's psychosexual development. The key event at this stage, according to Freud, is the child's feeling of attraction toward the parent of the opposite sex, together with envy and fear of the same-sex parent.

The fourth stage of psychosexual development is the Latent stage. This stage lasts from five or six years old till puberty. During this stage, sexual feelings are suppressed in children and for the sake of other aspects of life, like learning, hobbies, adjusting to the social environment outside home, forming beliefs and values, developing same-sex friendship, etc. Problems however might occur during this stage on account of the inability of the child (ego) to redirect the drive energy to activities accepted by the social environment.

The fifth and last stage of psychosexual development is called Genital stage, which starts from puberty onwards until development stops, which is ideally when adulthood starts. The gratifying activities during this stage are masturbation and heterosexual relationships. This stage is marked by a renewed sexual interest and desire without any fixation. It includes the formation of love relationships and families, or acceptance of responsibilities associated with adulthood. If people experience difficulties at this stage, it is because the damage was done in the early stages.

SEXUAL HEALTH

In terms of sexuality, sexual health refers to a condition of physical, mental, and social well-being. It necessitates an upbeat and courteous mindset toward sexuality and romantic relationships in addition to the opportunity for satisfying and secure sexual encounters free from compulsion, bias, and violence.

Sexual Health Concerns Related to Body Integrity and to Sexual Safety

❖ The need for health-promoting practices for the early detection of sexual issues (such as routine health screenings, breast and testicular self-examinations, and so on).
❖ The desire to be free from all types of sexual compulsion and violence, including rape, abuse, and harassment.
❖ The desire to be free from bodily mutilations, such as female genital cutting need to be immune from acquiring or spreading STIs, including HIV.
❖ The need to lessen the sexual effects of mental or physical limitations. Reduce the negative effects of healthcare and surgical disorders or treatments on sexual life.

Sexual Health Concerns Related to Eroticism

❖ The need for understanding how the body affects sexual response and pleasure.
❖ There is a need to acknowledge the importance of sexual pleasure experienced throughout life in secure and responsible ways while adhering to a set of moral principles that respects the rights of others.
❖ Need to encourage the practice of voluntary non-exploitative, honest, mutually enjoyable relationships.
❖ Need to promote sexual activity conducted in a safe and responsible way.

Sexual Health Concerns Related to Gender

❖ Need for gender equality.
❖ Need for freedom from all forms of discrimination based on gender.
❖ Need for respect and acceptance of gender differences.

Sexual Health Concerns Related to Sexual Orientation

❖ Need for freedom from discrimination based on sexual orientation.
❖ Need for freedom to express sexual orientation in safe and responsible manners within a values framework that is respectful of the rights of others.

SEXUAL ORIENTATION

The physical and hormonal modifications of puberty throughout the adolescent years generally cause individuals to start experiencing an increase in feelings of sex. It's normal to have questions and perhaps worries about new sexual sensations. Many individuals need some time to come to terms with who they are as well as who they're becoming. Gaining a deeper knowledge of their individual sexual sensations and the people they are drawn to is one aspect of this.

Emotional, Social and Physical Aspects of Sexual Orientation

A person's attraction to another person, whether it be romantic or sexual. The many varieties of sexual orientation include:

Heterosexual: A heterosexual person is attracted to people of the opposite sex romantically and physically. Male heterosexuals are drawn to females, while female heterosexuals are drawn to males. Heterosexuals are sometimes referred to as "straight."

Others who identify as gay are attracted to others of the same sex romantically and physically: Lesbian refers to women who are drawn to other women, whereas **homosexual** refers to men who are drawn to other men. (The word "gay" is utilized on occasion to refer to homosexual people of any sex.)

Bisexual: Those who identify as bisexual have both romantic and physically drawn to individuals of both sexes.

Asexual: Although asexual individuals might not be drawn to having sex, they nonetheless experience emotional closeness to other individuals.

Sexual orientation refers to the people you have a connection to and feel emotionally, sexually, and romantically. Compared to gender identity, it is distinct. Gender identification refers to who you are—a man, female, genderqueer, etc.—rather than to whom you are attracted. As a result, being transgender—feeling as if the gender that identify with is quite different from the sex you were assigned—is distinct from being gay, lesbian, even bisexual. What you desire to be with determines your sexual orientation. Gender identity is a personal matter.

There are a bunch of identities associated with sexual orientation:
❖ People who are attracted to someone of different gender, such as males or women who are attracted to men, may identify as straight or heterosexual.
❖ The terms "gay" or "homosexual" are often used by persons who are attracted to other individuals of the same gender. Lesbian may be preferred by gay women.
❖ People who are drawn in both men and women often identify as bisexuals.
❖ Pansexual or queer individuals are those who find attraction in many various gender identities (male, female, transgender, genderqueer, intersex, etc.).
❖ People who are unclear about what gender they are may describe themselves as inquisitive or unsure.
❖ Those who don't feel any sexual desire toward someone often identify as asexual.

PREVENTION OF SEXUALLY TRANSMITTED DISEASES

There are various strategies to prevent or lower the risk of contracting sexually transmitted illnesses (STIs) or STDs.

* **Abstain:** The best strategy to prevent STIs is to refrain from having sex.
* **Stay with one uninfected partner:** Being in a long-term monogamous relationship where both partners exclusively have sex with other people and neither is infected is another effective approach to prevent STIs.
* **Wait and test:** Delay vaginal and anal sex with new person until both of you have had STI testing. Although less dangerous, oral intercourse requires the use of a dental dam or latex condom to avoid direct skin-to-skin contact between the genital and mouth mucosal membranes.
* **Get vaccinated:** Certain STIs may be avoided by being vaccinated ahead of schedule, before sexual contact. Hepatitis A, B, and the human papillomavirus (HPV) may all be prevented with vaccines.
* **Use condoms and dental dams consistently and correctly:** For every sexual act, whether oral, vaginal, or anal, use a fresh latex barrier or dental dam. Never use a lubricant that contains oil, such as petroleum jelly.
* **Do not drink alcohol or use drugs:** You are more prone to take risks with sexuality while intoxicated.
* **Communicate:** Prior to any kind of intense sex. Talk to your spouse about engaging in safer sex. Make sure you are clear about the actions that are and are not acceptable.
* **Consider male circumcision:** Male circumcision may help prevent the spread of genital HPV and genital herpes. There is evidence that male circumcision might help lower a man's chance of contracting HIV from a woman she has contracted the virus (heterosexual transmission) by as much as 50%.
* **Consider pre-exposure prophylaxis:** Emtricitabine plus tenofovir alafenamide (Descovy) and Emtricitabine plus tenofovir disoproxil fumarate (Truvada) have been authorized for use by the Food and Drug Administration (FDA) to lower the risk of sexually transmitted HIV infection in those who are at extremely high risk.

PREVENTION OF UNWANTED PREGNANCY

Unintended pregnancy, defined as mistimed or unplanned pregnancy, is associated with significant personal and societal costs.

The Role of Nurses in Primary Prevention of Unintended Pregnancy

* Nurses have a long history of providing sexual and reproductive wellness services to many economically disadvantaged and underserved individuals.
* Additionally, nurses can provide information and guidance regarding implantable devices (such as subcutaneous or intrauterine), as well as changes to lifestyles aimed at enhancing general and reproductive health. Nursing professionals are in an ideal position to begin primary prevention methods, such as communicating women in dialogue about a lifelong sexually active plan, like tactics to avoid unplanned or mistimed being pregnant.

Nurses as Providers of Secondary Prevention of Unintended Pregnancy

Secondary prevention involves evaluating an untimely or unwanted pregnancy, advising on alternatives particular to the stage within the pregnancy, supporting the woman's decision to keep the pregnancy or have it terminated, and referring or providing the necessary resources. Coordination of treatment and avoiding more unplanned pregnancies.

Nurses Providing Tertiary Prevention of Unintended Pregnancy

The nurse's first emphasis is on assessing the pregnancy's state, which includes figuring out the gestational age and identifying whether the pregnancy was unwanted. A midwife or nurse would next review the alternatives available, including options for disposal as well as pregnancy extension with the purpose of adoption and/or birth with the intention of parenting, if the pregnancy is untimely or unwanted and the gestation period is later in the first trimester.

PREVENTION OF SEXUAL HARASSMENT

Preventative measures are the most powerful tool against sexual harassment. Harassment doesn't just stop happening. In fact, it's more probable that if the issue is not resolved, the harassment will become worse and be harder to stop as time passes.

- ❖ Anti-harassment rules outline what constitutes harassment, inform all workers that it will not be permitted, and specify how both employers and staff members should react to harassment events. Additionally, anti-harassment guidelines should provide a thorough procedure for filing complaints of sexual harassment by staff members.
- ❖ Consistently educate and enlighten all staff members about harassment. In order to break the taboo if silence that often surrounds situations of sexual harassment, the dissemination of knowledge, open dialogue, and advice are especially crucial.
- ❖ Work with workers, management, and union representatives to create a harassment policy.
- ❖ Show that you mean it by ensuring that the policy embraces everyone, including executives and supervisors.
- ❖ Ensure that every manager are aware of their responsibility to maintain a harassment-free workplace.
- ❖ Ensure that all employees, both new and long-term, have familiar with the policy and the procedures to earn dealing with harassment.
- ❖ Provide safety and assistance for workers who believe they are being tormented by disciplining harassers appropriately. Quickly investigate and respond to any allegations of harassment.
- ❖ Take steps to remove offensive joking, posters, graffiti, emails, and images from the workplace.
- ❖ To make sure the policy and education/information programs are still useful for your workplace, monitor and adjust them often.

PREVENTION OF SEXUAL ABUSE

Sexual abuse is a significant issue on an individual, family, and social level and may have long-lasting, even life-long, effects. As a result, many forms of prevention constitute a public health concern. To effectively prevent the sexual misconduct of kids, preventative efforts should engage both adults and minors. In addition to changing societal norms, institutions, and values, it is important to reform and revise relevant laws, attitudes, and structures so that perpetrators of abuse are exposed everywhere.

❖ Save women and kids from dangerous or violent situations, and then help them recover in a secure temporary or permanent refuge.

❖ Help disadvantaged women become socially and economically secure by offering them financial assistance or job training.

❖ Offer legal counsel to assist victims of physical or sexual abuse in understanding their rights and starting the legal procedure to seek redress.

❖ Offer psychological rehabilitation and therapy.

❖ Prevention efforts are focused largely on adults and only secondarily on children and adolescents; as a result, adults have primary responsibility for safeguarding minors from sexual abuse.

❖ Preventive actions are carried out at frequent, brief, and regular intervals.

❖ Prevention strategies use language that is suitable; it's crucial to provide the target audience concise information that is clear, precise, and thorough without placing an unreasonable demand on them.

❖ Relevant inquiries in the case of youngsters include if and how much sex education they have received.

❖ Boys and girls are seen are potential victims on an equal footing.

❖ A team with members of both genders implements prevention activities.

❖ Preventive measures address the daily challenges faced by a particular target group, which implies that in addition to gender and language, other factors such as culture, religion, politics, status, and the legal system of the relevant state are also taken into consideration.

UNIT

Stress and Adaptation: Introductory Concepts

14

LEARNING OBJECTIVES

At the end of this unit, the reader will be able to:
- Define stress.
- Explain concepts of stress.
- Layout models of stress: GAS, LAS.
- Enumerate causes of stress.
- Classify types of stress.
- Categories sources of stress.
- Outline symptoms of stress.
- Define stress management.
- Describe adaptive coping strategies.
- Explain role of nurse in stress management.

INTRODUCTION

No matter how powerful, successful, happy, or wealthy you may be, stress and worry are a part of everyday life. Mild stress may be energizing, inspiring, and perhaps even pleasant. Selye used the term "stress" in 1956 to refer to the strain that an individual feels in reaction to demands of daily life. These demands are referred to as stressors.

TERMINOLOGIES

Stress: A state of mental or emotional strain or suspense.

Stressors: Any agent that causes stress to an organism.

Stress is a universal experience. Stress is a natural aspect of life. A common term used to describe a variety of psychological (mental) and physical (bodily) stresses that individuals encounter or feel throughout their lives is stress. The body's response to any modification that necessitates adaptation or response is stress. Physical, intellectual, and emotional reactions are produced by the body in response to these changes. The stress of everyday living is common. Stress may be brought on by your surroundings, body, and thoughts.

Varies twentieth century researchers have contributed to several different concepts of stress.

DEFINITION

* Stress is defined as the body's response to situations that pose demands, constraints or opportunities.
* Stress is defined as "a state of psychological and physiological imbalance resulting from the disparity between situational demand and the individual's ability and motivation to meet those needs.
* Stress may be defined as real or interpretated threat to the physiological or psychological or behavioral response.
* Stress is a process of adjusting to or dealing with circumstances that disrupt or threaten to disrupt a person's physical or psychological functioning.
* Stress is a physical or emotional state always present in a person as a result of living. Stress can be positive or negative:
  * Stress is good when the situation offers an opportunity to a person to gain something. It acts as a motivator for highest performance.
  * Stress is negative when a person faces social, physical, organizational and emotional problems.
  Factors that are responsible for causing stress are called stressors.

Concepts of Stress

The basic concepts of stress and adaptation are stress, stressors, adaptation and homeostasis.
* **Stress:** The major sources of stress in our society arise from interpersonal relationships and performance demands rather than from actual physical threats. Stress has an impact on a person's whole being, including their physical, emotional, intellectual, social, and spiritual aspects. The way that stress is perceived and how we react to it vary greatly from people to person and even within the same person over time.
* **Stressors:** Stressors may be internal (such as sickness or fear) or external (such as noise or a cold environment). Depending on how a person reacts to change, stressors may have either beneficial or negative impacts.
* **Adaptation:** A change that occurs as a result of a stressor's reaction is called adaptation. It is continuing process as a person strives to maintain balance in his/her internal and external environments.
* **Homeostasis:** The human body continually interacts with a changing environment. The environment includes the exterior environment those around our bodies and the interior environment, which contains the systems that control how our bodies work, various physiologic mechanisms within the body respond to internal changes to maintain relative constancy in internal environment called homeostasis.

Stress Models

* **Stimulus-based model:** Stress is described in this model as a stimulus, a life event, or a collection of conditions that elicits physiologic or psychological responses and may make a person more susceptible to disease.

❖ **Transaction-based model:** It is based on Lazarus's (1966) states that individual differences are not considered by stimulus theory or response theory. It includes a collection of cognitive, emotional, and adaptive reactions that arises out of person environment transactions. As the person and environment are inseparable, each affects and is affected by other.

❖ **Response-based model:** It consists of mainly two responses:
1. **Local adaptation syndrome:** It is the body's localized reaction to stress. The local adaption syndrome might be pathological or traumatic. For instance, inflammatory reactions to stress in response to a trauma or injury
2. **General adaptation syndrome:** It describes body's general response to stress. It consists of three stages:
   a. **The alarm reaction:** This occurs when a person detects a particular stressor, and a number of defense systems are triggered. The body gets ready to either face off the stressful circumstance or flee from it when its autonomous nervous system starts the flight and flight response.
   b. **Resistance:** The body attempts to adapt to stressor, after perceiving the threat. Vital signs and hormone levels return to normal. If the stress can be managed or confirmed to small area the body regains homeostasis.
   c. **Exhaustion:** This is what happens when the adaptive mechanisms are exhausted. Without protection against the stressor, the body must either rest or mount its defense to go back to normal, or it would exhaust itself completely and die.

❖ **Stress adaptation model:** The concept is known as the Stuart stress adaption model since it was presented by Gail Stuart. It unifies all of the facets of patient care—biological, sociocultural, psychological, environmental, legal and ethical into a single framework of practice.
   • The Stuart stress adaptation model's first assumption is the nature is organized as a societal hierarchy, going from the simplest unit to the most complex. Nothing exist in isolation since every level is a component of the one above it. As a result, every person is a member of their family, their friends, their community, their society, and the larger ecosystem, through which information and knowledge go to different levels.
   • The model's second underlying assumption is that health care is delivered in a psychological, physiological, sociocultural, environmental, and morally-responsible framework. For the nurse to give holistic nursing care, she or he must understand each of them.
   • The model's third assumption is that there are two separate continuums of health/illness, and adaptation/maladaptation:
     1. The health/illness continuum comes from a medical world view
     2. The adaptation/maladaptation continuum comes from a nursing world view.

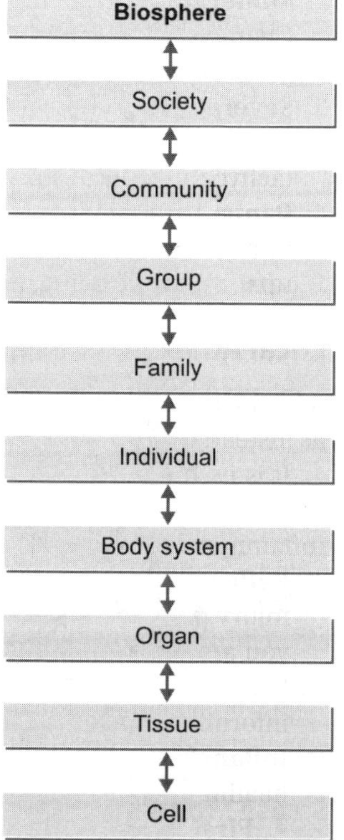

This suggests that a patient with an ailment who has received a medical diagnosis may be handling it well. A person without an illness, however, could have adaptive coping mechanisms.

* The fourth presumption stipulates that the model incorporates all three stages of prevention includes the primary, secondary, and tertiary levels of prevention by describing four stages of psychiatric treatment: crisis, acute, maintenance and health promotion. The model offers a treatment objective, the main area of nursing evaluation, the kind of treatments, and anticipated nursing care outcomes for each step of therapy.
* The fifth assumption is based on the nursing process and professional standards of care. Every stage of the procedure is crucial, and the nurse is entirely responsible for everything nursing care implemented.

Psychological Response to Stress

Stress may cause a range of emotional reactions, including despair and rage. The most typical reaction is anxiousness.

Anxiety: It is vague, uneasy feeling of discomfort or dread accompanied by autonomic response.

The four levels are:
1. **Mild:** Present in everyday life. An increase in questioning and restlessness are its symptoms.
2. **Moderate:** Limits a person's range of perception and focus on immediate concerns. Characterized by tremors, a quavering voice, stiff muscles, a modest rise in breathing and pulse, and other symptoms.
3. **Severe:** Makes someone feel out of control, frightful, and terrified. Characterized by vocal communication difficulties, anxiety, shaking, poor motor coordination, sweating, tachycardia, dyspnea, and palpitations, as well as chest discomfort or pressure
4. **Panic:** A condition of anxiety. Here, a little amount of anxiety has positive effect. For instance, minor anxiety encourages a student to carry out the needed reading for a test that is coming up.

Local Adaptation Response

It is a localized response to stress that only affects a small portion of the body (tissues, organs), as instead of the whole body.

It is essentially a short-term adaptive response which primarily is homeostatic. The two most common stress responses that influence nursing care are reflex pain response and the inflammatory response:
1. **Reflex pain response:** It is the central nervous system's reaction to pain. It functions as an injury prevention system to stop injuries and is quick and automated. For instance, when you are set to walk into a bathtub filled with dangerously hot water, your skin detects the heat and promptly alerts your spinal cord. The motor nerve receives a message at this point informing it that the water around it is excessively hot and unsafe.
2. **Inflammatory response:** It can be a local reaction to an illness or wound. It promotes wound healing and aids in the localization and control of infection. There are three phases:
   * **First phase:** Initially, vasoconstriction is used to stop bleeding. Histamines are recognized, capillary permeability rises, and blood flow to WBCs in the region is boosted. The blood flow then returns to normal, but WBCs are still present to aid in infection resistance.

- **Second phase:** Exudates are produced from the wound and consist of fluids, cells, and inflammatory by products. The location and severity of the wound determine how much exudate is present.
- **Third phase:** Damaged cells are repaired by regeneration (replacement with identical cells) or formation of scar tissue.

Unconscious Mechanisms to Reduce Stress and Anxiety

Coping mechanisms: They are behaviors used to reduce stress and anxiety like
- Crying, laughing, sleeping and cursing
- Physical activity and exercise
- Smoking and drinking

CAUSES OF STRESS

Major Causes of Stress at Work or in Organization

Career concern: An employee may get stressed if he believes he is very much behind in the corporate ladder. He could feel stressed if it looks like there are no prospects for him to progress himself. Therefore, unmet professional expectations are a major cause of stress.

Role ambiguity: It happens when the individual is working and is unsure about his duties. His duties and obligations are unclear. The worker is unsure about his responsibilities. It causes tension and confusion in the brains of the workers.

Rotating work shifts: Individuals who work several shifts may experience stress. Employees could be required to perform the night shift after a few days or the day shift. That might make it difficult for the employee to get used to the new timings, which could have an impact on both their personal and family lives.

Role conflict: It happens when individuals have various expectations of the person filling a certain function. It may also happen when a person's employment falls short of expectations or whether a job requires them to act in a way that goes against their moral principles.

Occupational demands: Certain occupations need more effort than others. Risky and dangerous jobs are more stressful. According to research, stressful jobs need continual attention to machinery, uncomfortable physical circumstances, decision-making, etc.

Lack of participation in decision-making: Many seasoned workers believe that they should be involved in decisions that influence their careers. In practice, managers seldom ever consult with the affected workers before making a decision. That creates a sense of neglect, which may cause stress.

Work overload: Stress comes from having an excessive workload since it puts one under so much strain.

Poor working conditions: Employees could experience unpleasant working circumstances. It would include poor lighting and ventilation, unclean restrooms, a lot of dust and noise, the presence of dangerous gases and fumes, insufficient safety precautions, etc. All of these uncomfortable circumstances lead to physiological and psychological imbalance in people, which leads to stress.

Lack of group cohesiveness: Every group has its cohesion, even though the levels of cohesiveness vary greatly. When there is disunity within a work group, people get stressed. In groups, there is distrust, envy, frequent fighting, etc., and this causes stress in the workers.

Interpersonal and intergroup conflict: These conflicts between two or more people or groups result from disparities in perceptions, attitudes, values, and beliefs. Members of the group may experience stress as a result of these disputes.

Organizational changes: When changes occur, people have to adapt to those changes, and this may cause stress. Stress is higher when changes are significant or unusual like transfer or adoption of new technology.

Lack of social support: People are better able to handle the impacts of stress when they feel like they have the support and companionship of others at work. When there isn't this type of social support, employees are under higher stress.

Main Causes of Stress Outside Work or Organization

Life changes: Stress may be caused by changes in one's life. Changes in life might come slowly or quickly. Growing older is a gradual life change, but a loved one's death or an accident are sudden life changes. Unexpected life changes may be very stressful and challenging to handle.

Frustration: Another source of stress is frustration. It develops as a result of inhibited goal-directed behavior. Management should make an effort to break down obstacles and support people in achieving their goal.

Racial, caste, and religious conflicts: Employees who live in communities where racial, caste, and religious inequalities often lead to interpersonal clashes experience more stress. The lower castes and members of minorities are more stressed when it comes to religion, particularly in India.

Technological changes: Employees in technological industries always worry about losing their employment or having to learn new technologies when there is any developments in such sectors. It could lead to stress.

Career changes: A person is under pressure to handle additional tasks when they abruptly change jobs. Stress may also be brought on by under- or over-promotion, demotion, and transfers.

TYPES OF STRESS

* **Distress:** Stress due to an excess of adaptive demands placed upon us. The demands are so great that they lead to bodily and mental damage, e.g., death of a loved one.
* **Eustress:** The optimal amount of stress, which helps to promote health and growth, e.g., praise from a teacher for a well written assignments.
* **Neutral stress:** In this type, subject neither feels good nor bad about stress. Equilibrium or homeostasis is maintained.

SOURCES OF STRESS

There are many sources of stress are broadly classified as:
* **Internal stressors:** They originate within a person, e.g., cancer, feeling of depression
* **External stressors:** It originates outside the individual, e.g., moving to another city, a death in family.
* **Developmental stressors:** It occurs at predictable times throughout an individual's life, e.g., child—beginning of school.
* **Situational stressors:** They are unpredictable and occur at any time during life. It may be positive or negative, e.g., death of family member, marriage/divorce.

OTHER SOURCES

- ❖ **Environmental stressors:** Noise, pollution, traffic.
- ❖ **Physiological stressors:** Illness, injuries.
- ❖ **Social stressors:** Financial problem, work demand.
- ❖ Change of any kind, e.g., fear of new, fear of rejection.
- ❖ Interpersonal issues.
- ❖ **System issues:** Lack of leadership, lack of team work, confused communication.

STRESS WARNING SIGNS AND SYMPTOMS

Cognitive Symptoms

- ❖ Memory problems
- ❖ Inability to concentrate
- ❖ Poor judgement
- ❖ Seeing only the negative
- ❖ Anxious and racing thoughts
- ❖ Constant worrying

Emotional Symptoms

- ❖ Moodiness
- ❖ Irritability or short temper
- ❖ Inability to relax
- ❖ Sense of loneliness and isolation
- ❖ Depression or unhappiness

Physical Symptoms

- ❖ Ache and pain
- ❖ Diarrhea and constipation
- ❖ Nausea and dizziness
- ❖ Chest pain, rapid heartbeat

Behavioral Symptoms

- ❖ Eating more or less
- ❖ Sleeping too much or too little
- ❖ Isolating yourself from others
- ❖ Using alcohol, cigarettes or drugs to relax

Types of Stressors

- ❖ **Physiological stressors:**
  - ◆ Chemical agents
  - ◆ Physical agents
  - ◆ Infectious agent
  - ◆ Nutrition imbalances
  - ◆ Genetic or immune disorders

- ❖ **Psychological stressors:**
  - ◆ Accidents can cause stress for the victim, the person who caused the accident and the families of both.
  - ◆ Stressful experiences of family members and friends.
  - ◆ Fear of aggression or mutilation from others such as murder, rape, terrorist and attacks.
  - ◆ Events that we see on TV such as war, earthquake, violence.
  - ◆ Developmental and life events.
  - ◆ Rapid changes in our world, including economic and political structures and technology.

STRESS MANAGEMENT

Stress management strategies may be categorized into:
- ❖ Individual strategies
- ❖ Organizational strategies

Individual strategies to cope with stress includes:
- ❖ Muscle relaxation
- ❖ Biofeedback
- ❖ Cognitive restructuring
- ❖ Time management

Organizational strategies:
- ❖ Improvements in the physical environment
- ❖ Job redesign to remove stress
- ❖ Changes in workloads and deadlines
- ❖ Changes in work schedule
- ❖ Greater level of employee participation
- ❖ Workshops dealing with role clarity and role analysis
- ❖ Career counseling
- ❖ Team building

Workplace skills:
- ❖ Delegate
- ❖ Anticipate problems
- ❖ Be assertive
- ❖ Be decisive
- ❖ Organize
- ❖ Balance work and personal life

ADAPTIVE COPING STRATEGIES

Coping Mechanisms used at Higher Levels of Anxiety

- ❖ **Task oriented reactions:** Conscious thinking of the stress situation and then acting to solve problems reduce conflicts or satisfy needs.
- ❖ **Attack behavior:** It occurs when a person attempts to overcome obstacles to satisfy a need. It may be constructive or destructive.
- ❖ **Withdrawal behavior:** Physical withdrawal from the threat or emotional reactions such as admitting defeat, feeling guilty etc.
- ❖ **Compromise behavior:** It involves substitution of goals to fulfill one's need partially. Usually it's constructive.

Defense Mechanisms

- ❖ Compensation
- ❖ Denial
- ❖ Introjections
- ❖ Projection
- ❖ Rationalization
- ❖ Reaction formation
- ❖ Regression
- ❖ Repression
- ❖ Sublimation
- ❖ Undoing
- ❖ Displacement

Coping: Dealing with issues or challenging circumstances is a common definition of coping. A coping mechanism is a natural or learned method of reacting to a changing environment or particular circumstance.

Types of Coping

- ❖ **Problem focused coping:** It refers to efforts to improve a situation by making changes or taking some action.
- ❖ **Emotion focused coping:** It includes ideas and deeds that alleviate emotional pain. Even when nothing changes, the individual often feels better.

Coping can also be classified as:

- ❖ **Short-term coping:** It briefly lowers tension to a manageable level, but it is an unproductive method of dealing with reality like in daydreaming.
- ❖ **Long-term coping:** It is constructive and realistic. For instance, discussing difficulties with others.
- ❖ **Adaptive coping:** It helps a person to deal with a stressful event and minimizes distress associated with them.
- ❖ **Maladaptive coping:** It can result in unnecessary distress for a person and others associated with person or stressful events.

Stress Management Strategies

- ❖ **Take a breath:** If you're feeling stressed, try taking a few minute to relax and breathe deeply. Inhale air via your nose, and then expel it through your mouth. Try to inhale enough air to cause your navel to rise and fall. Count each exhale slowly.
- ❖ **Practice specific relaxation techniques:** Self-hypnosis, meditation, and deep muscle relaxation all have as good as effects. In this state both body and mind are at a rest and outside world is screened out for a time period. The practice of this for a regular basis provides calming and relaxing feeling that seems to have lasting effect for many people.
- ❖ **Manage time:** Put the most important ones first also completes them first. If you are assigned a really unpleasant task to do, do it ASAP in the next day and then move on. Your day will be much less stressful after that. Make time for both work and recreation.
- ❖ **Connect with others:** An excellent strategy for overcoming emotions of sadness, boredom, and loneliness is to participate in activities with other people.

- ❖ **Talk it out:** Describe your feelings. Suppressed emotions make stress and frustration worse. By speaking with a someone that would assist you organize your ideas, you may focus on problem-solving. Consider writing down your thoughts and feelings as well. You could have a better understanding of the problem and a new perspective if you write out your concerns.
- ❖ **Take a minute vacation:** Imagine a calm rural scene to help you get out of a tense circumstance. When you can, close the eyes for a moment and picture a tranquil setting. Take into account every detail of the setting you have chosen, including the pleasant sounds, smells, and temperature. You may also change how you think by relaxing with some quiet music or reading a good book.
- ❖ **Monitor your physical comfort:** Put on casual attire. If it's too hot, go somewhere colder. If the chair is comfortable, keep it. If your computer makes your eyes sore, get a new one. Avoid waiting until pain is a major problem.
- ❖ **Get physical:** When you're feeling tense, agitated, or disturbed, exercise or other types of physical activity may help you unwind. Running, walking, and swimming are all fantastic options for certain people, while dance, etc., is preferred by others. You could find that playing with kids, detailing your car, or doing yard chores all help you unwind. You may do exercises for 20 minutes every single day to decompress.
- ❖ **Take of your body:** A balanced diet and proper sleep nourish both your body and mind. Limit the amount of sugar and coffee you consume. Spend some time each morning eating breakfast. Stress is better handled by bodies in greater health. Increase your fruit and vegetable intake. Make time to indulge your interests and pastimes. Be mindful of your body.
- ❖ **Laugh:** Keep your sense of humor, which includes being able to laugh at oneself.
- ❖ **Know your limits:** Remember that there are many circumstances everyday that are in addition to all your control. Recognize your limits. If the situation is unavoidable or cannot be changed at this time, don't fight it. Learn to accept everything as it is until you are in a position to make changes.
- ❖ **Think positively:** Transform a negative viewpoint into a positive one. Put a stop to whatever negative thoughts you may have.
- ❖ **Clarify your values and develop a sense of life meaning:** By articulating your values and figuring out what you actually want from life, you may feel better regarding yourself, have that sense of satisfaction and centering yourself that helps you deal with life's challenges, and feel happier about yourself. As an alternate to confrontation, think about compromise or cooperation. If both parties make a reciprocal compromise, it could be simpler and more enjoyable.
- ❖ **Have a good cry:** Having an emotional outpouring may relieve stress and prevent physical negative effects including a headache as trying to keep it all within.
- ❖ **Avoid self-medication:** Alcohol or other drugs cannot relieve stress. Considering the fact that their existence could seem to mask or disguise problems. Because it modifies your thinking, makes it more difficult for you to make judgments, and has an adverse effect on other cognitive processes, long-term alcohol use actually increases stress rather than decreasing it.
- ❖ **Look for the pieces of gold around you:** Positive or enjoyable feelings or experiences are priceless. These can seem like small accomplishments, but when added together, they may often offer you a big boost of vigor or morale and inspire you to begin living a new, happier lifestyle.

- Relaxation technique
- Meditation
- Interpersonal communication with caring others
- Problem solving
- Use of healthy coping mechanism like music therapy, physical exercise, etc.
- Progressive muscle relaxation
- Creativity

STEPS TO MANAGING STRESS

Step 1: Identify if you are stressed.
Step 2: Identify the stressors.
Step 3: Identify the reason for the stressor.
Step 4: Select an appropriate stress management strategy and apply it.
Step 5: Evaluate.

ROLE OF NURSE IN STRESS MANAGEMENT

- Raise client awareness of any current or prospective health issues.
- Remind them that their health problems can become worse once they refrain from making any lifestyle changes.
- Identify all available resources to assist the client in the transition process.
Teach about various coping techniques to ease the amount if stress occurs.

Assessment of the Person

Check the person for the characteristics listed below. These people are quite likely to have stress-related ailments.
- Rigid and self-punishing and moral standards.
- High and unrealistic expectations.
- Too much dependence on others for love and affection and approval
- Inability to master change or learn new ways of dealing with frustration.
- Easily prone to extreme emotional responses of fear, anxiety and depression.
- Type personality persons.
- In addition the stressful events like birth, deaths, marriages, divorces, retirement, etc., can predispose to stress related illness.

Assessment of the Family

- Evaluate how the family views the issue and if they are supportive of the client's coping strategies.
- Evaluation of the environment.
- Highly stressful jobs; unfavorable environmental factors such excessive lightning, temperature, etc.

Interventions

- They seek to reduce stress in either the short- or long-term. A nurse may help a patient identify the issue, consider possible solutions, and accept his feelings with feeling guilty or fearful.

❖ Acute stress-related disorders often need patients to change their lives and social contacts. First and foremost, the nurse must help the client understand the significance of change in light of previous changes.

❖ Some clients show resistance to necessary modifications. Increasing client knowledge of any present or upcoming health concerns is one of them.

❖ Assisting him in comprehending that his health condition can become worse if he fails to bring about any changes in his life.

❖ A list of all available materials to support the client throughout their experience change and engage in treatment.

❖ When the client discovers the degree of his health problems and is told that a shift is required, he often feels frightened, despondent, and furious.

❖ The client is asked to talk about the setbacks that resulted from the behavior adjustment.

❖ Families need to be well-informed on the nature of the disease and how to help the client cope with stress. It's important to inform the client's family about various options, like yoga, meditation, and relaxation techniques. These techniques could be quite beneficial in helping individuals cope with difficult life situations.

❖ The nurse must continually remember that their role is only that of change facilitators as their clients have obligations and rights related to change.

DIVERSIONAL THERAPY FOR STRESS

Methods of Diversional Therapies

01 Play therapy
Psychotherapy that helps the child to express his or her emotions through play

02 Dance therapy
Psychotherapeutic use of movement

03 Music therapy
Therapeutic tool for the restoration, maintenance

04 Rehabilitation therapy
Techniques of tension through out the body, and a calm and peaceful state of mind

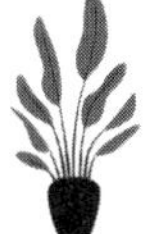

Meditation

Meditation is a kind of self-discipline that helps one achieve inner peace and harmony by focusing uncritically on one thing at a time. Medical meditation—a coming together of meditation and yoga—balances and regenerates spiritual and physical energies, thus forging a healing alliances in which the spirit nurtures body and mind. Nurses can provide the time necessary for meditation. Nurses too could benefit from a mediation practice and could experience a brief meditation during breaks from patient care activities.

Physical Exercise

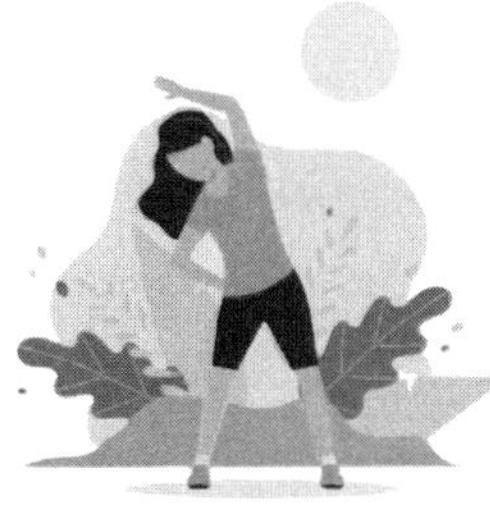

Regular exercise is the most effective method of relieving stress. Aerobic exercises strengthen cardiovascular system and increase the body's ability to use oxygen more efficiently. To achieve the benefit of exercise they must be performed regularly for at least 30 minutes per day.

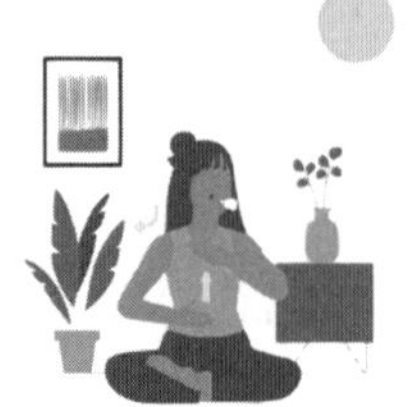

Deep Breathing Exercise

Tension is released when the lungs are allowed to breath in as much oxygen and possible. Breathing exercise have been found to be effective to reducing anxiety, depression, irritability tension and fatigue.

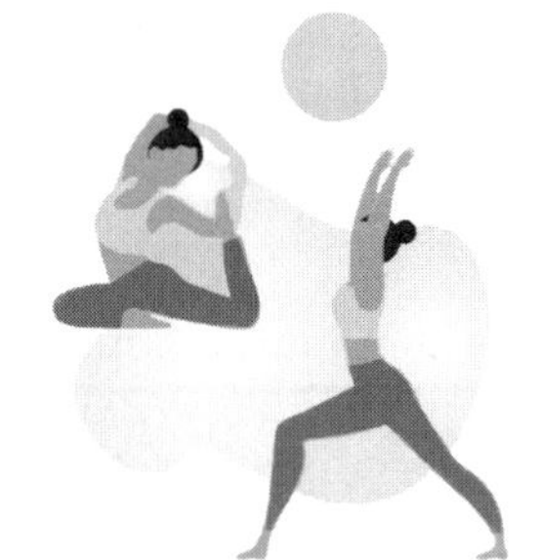

Yoga

Yoga uses combination of physical postures breathing techniques and meditation to promote relaxation and enhance the flow of vital energy called prana. It is essential for a nurse to have baseline information and awareness of yoga which is purely Indian in origin.

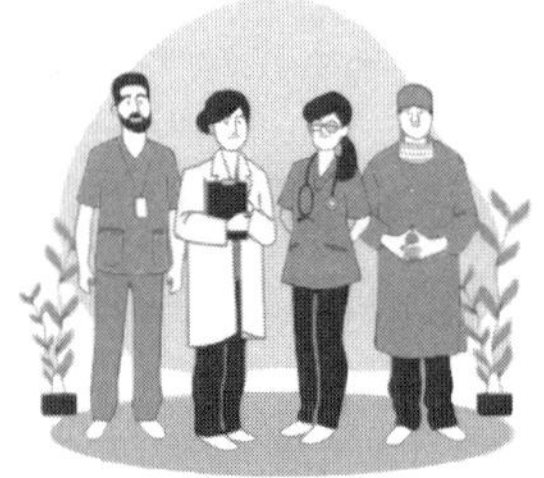

03
Music Therapy

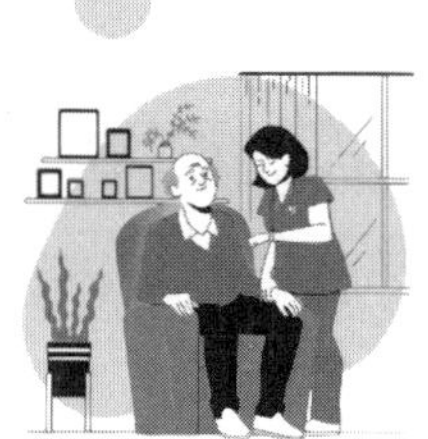

04
Relaxation Therapy

Diversional therapy "is a client centered practice that recognizes that leisure and recreational experiences are the right of all individuals." Diversional therapists promote the involvement in leisure, recreation and play by reducing barriers to their client's participation and providing opportunities where the individual may choose to participate and perform their occupation. Ideally these recreational activities promote self-esteem and personal fulfilment, through an emphasis on holistic care; providing physical, psychological, social, intellectual and spiritual/cultural/temporal support.

Diversional therapists work in a wide variety of settings, such as rehabilitation and hospital units, justice centers, community centers, day and respite services, aged care residential facilities, ethnic specific services, palliative care units and outreach programs, mental health services, specialist organizations, private practice and consultancy and management.

The diversional therapist works with a client to achieve positive health outcomes by incorporating leisure programs into their lifestyles. He or she assists decision-making and participation when developing and managing these programs. These are often quite diverse and can range from:

❖ Games, outings, gardening, computers, gentle exercise, music, arts and crafts.
❖ Individual emotional and social support.
❖ Sensory enrichment, activities like massage and aromatherapy, pet therapy.
❖ Environmental enrichment activities like role play, modelling.

❖ Discussion groups, education sessions like grooming, beauty care, cooking
❖ Social, cultural and spiritual activities.

Diversional therapy is not intended for social or entertainment purposes alone. As an unknown author once said *"Recreation's purpose is not to kill time, but to make time live; not to keep people occupied, but to keep them refreshed; not to offer an escape from life, but to provide a discovery of life."*

<table>
<tr><td>

Concepts of Cultural Diversity and Spirituality

</td><td>

UNIT

15

</td></tr>
</table>

LEARNING OBJECTIVES

At the end of this unit, the reader will be able to:
- Introduce cultural diversity.
- Explain importance of cultural diversity in education.
- Analyze cultural concepts.
- Define transcultural nursing.
- Describe spirituality.

INTRODUCTION TO CULTURAL DIVERSITY

Systemic changes to the health services all across the world are new challenges, nurses now confront. This subject may not have ever been more important than it is right now. Numerous cultural, racial, and other forms of minorities may be found all throughout the world. The consumers the nurse will serve come from a diverse range of cultures, so you should be prepared to offer them with outstanding care in a variety of hues. The location's varied ethnic population is due to this reason why it is imperative that any explanations given during patient treatment prevent bringing up any relevant difficulties. When delivering comprehensive medical care, it is important to take into account the various cultural backgrounds of individuals. Nurses need to be adaptable to different needs and requirements. Culture, or the common ideas, habits, and way of life of a community, becomes both a defining quality and a tactic for surviving and being accepted by others. To truly comprehend a culture, you must be conversant with its characteristics. Our history in the twenty-first century has been shaped by our participation in the European Union. The freedom of activity, establishment, but employment for EU members has increased thanks to multiculturalism, and if we take a closer look, we find that practically all European nations have replaced their prevailing monoculture with diversity. Despite the diversity of the cultural and ethnic groups represented, it is obvious that only just a hardly any of these groups are affected by multiculturalism. The rising diversity of the population offers a significant opportunity to advance civilization in many areas, including healthcare. Fairness in healthcare is crucial for promoting positive health outcomes. Diversity throughout medicine is crucial because of the close relationships nurses have with their patients and the sensitive nature of the care they provide. A nursing workforce that reflects the population it serves can only strengthen healthcare. If you're a practicing or aspiring nurse thinking about obtaining a PhD in nursing practice, you may be particularly interested in studying about the relevance and benefits of diversity in a nursing, as well as accompanying statistics and activities.

Although there has been an increase in diversity in nursing over the last several decades, there are still many improvements that may be made. As the hospital patient population becomes increasingly culturally diverse, all healthcare personnel must treat and work with patients with respect. Respectful communication helps to greatly reduce racial and ethnic differences. Recently, health organizations have started to develop policies that address how to deal problems caused by cultural differences. One solution to the problem is to provide more didactic courses that deal with this kind of challenge. In terms of providing racial and ethnic minority groups with evidence-based healthcare, institutional curriculum should comply to the requirements of competent care. The most important factor in the situation of the students is to educate and prepare them for a comprehension of culture and tolerance.

IMPORTANCE OF CULTURAL DIVERSITY IN EDUCATION

The emergence of cultural differences in education is also key issue. Based on the need should schools of thought be respectful of cultural variety, students have the opportunity to attend excellent colleges and universities anywhere in the world. Students will be far more ready to make contributions to transcultural healthcare during their future work if they are taught the best strategies for negotiating cultural differences. As a consequence of learning this knowledge, their confidence, background, and commitment to patient care will all rise (Budhai, 2021). Following are the most frequent cultural differences in the classroom:

- ❖ **Ways of knowing:** How do students from different cultures get the information they need? In many cultures, the textbook or magazine is the primary source of lexical knowledge, and libraries provide students the most convenient access to these resources. Although, some students opt to study from sources beyond academic ones, the Internet is the primary information source in various nations.
- ❖ **Problem-solving techniques:** Various cultural components are used in the solutions to each problem. The selected response is heavily influenced by the concepts, preferences, and specific values.
- ❖ **Techniques for nonverbal communication:** It is vital for teachers to be knowledgeable about the nonverbal communication characteristics shown by students from different cultural backgrounds. Some students can see making eye contact with the teacher as rude. For Korean pupils, for example, the smile is often one of uncertainty, confusion, or premature judgments rather than one of joy.

CULTURAL DIVERSITY

The idea of cultural diversity recognizes and explains the variances in culture that exist between diverse racial, ethnic, the religious groups along with the existence, cohabitation, the interactions of multiple cultures in the same area. Cultural diversity allows us to experience a wide range of cultural expressions that have been modified or impacted by ways of life in other places a consequence of numerous other factors. Cultural diversity is the acceptance and cooperation of the characteristics of one or more ethnicities within a certain geographical area.

Causes of Cultural Diversity

Cultural diversity began as a slow process that progressed at an unstoppable pace with the passage of time and the development of human activities. For example, cultural diversity stems from the process of invasions, battles, and conquests of new territories in which people of different backgrounds met. Today's ubiquity of cultural diversity has made it possible to develop novel understandings. Nations with a diverse range of cultures include Australia, China, and the United States, whereas we have many of them across Europe, including England, France, and Germany. On the other hand, via a range of techniques, governmental and economic activities have further encouraged cultural diversity. Opportunities for scientific cooperation and other types of personal development have shifted as a result of industrial and technological innovation, just as the hunt for better jobs has been spurred by these developments. Finally, the movement toward globalization is a significant factor in the diversity of cultures. This phenomenon has changed the flow of information, transportation, and international interactions as well as cultural, economic, and political institutions.

CULTURAL CONCEPT

For many people, culture is a way for life. Your culture includes the things you consume, the clothes you wear, the language you speak, and the divinity you worship. In the most basic sense, culture may be thought of as the manifestation of our way of thinking and doing. It also includes information that we have acquired from society at a whole. Culture encompasses all of humanity's accomplishments as members of social institutions. Culture encompasses everything from philosophy and religion to science and poetry to sculpture and architecture. Culture encompasses a person's viewpoint on a broad variety of problems as well as their practices, traditions, festivals, and lifestyles.

Culture is said to be a human-created environment since both material and immaterial components of group life are passed down from a generation to the next. Psychologists believe that implicit and explicit habits that individuals learn throughout their lives make up culture. These include the particular achievements of human communities, including their manifestation as objects, and they may be communicated via symbols. The finer concepts that exist in common within a society and are both historically produced and selected with their related values make up the fundamental basis of culture. The word "culture," as it is now more often used, refers to historically preserved symbolic significance patterns that humans utilize in order to interact, reproduce, and progress their worldviews.

Our nature or the way you behave and think are reflected in our culture. It may be found in our literary works, religious rituals, and hobbies and pastimes. Material culture and non-material culture are the two categories. Examples of items that are a component of the material world and connected to the material aspects of our life are clothing, food, and household products. Ideas, values, views, and beliefs are some examples of non-material culture.

Cultural variations exist across nations as well as between different locations. Its growth is based on a long-standing procedure that takes place at the regional, local, or national levels.

For example, we greet each other differently than those in the West and have distinct clothing, food habits, social and religious customs, and interests. Or, to put it differently, each country's cultural traditions help to define its people.

Culture may be described as follows:

* **Cultural practices as acquired habits:** Even while learning accounts for the majority of behavior, culture is not biological. We do not inherit it from our parents. Learning culture often happens by mistake. We get knowledge about society via our family, friends, schools, and the media. Enculturation occurs when someone learns a new culture. Although everyone has basic biological requirements including those for food, sleep, and sex, how we meet those needs differs between cultures.

* **A culture is a way of life:** Cultural aspects may be found in the thoughts or actions of the individuals that make up a society. The way people behave and think is referred to as their culture. We are limited to seeing human conduct; we are unable to observe civilization as a whole. Cultural behavior is the term used to describe this sort of predetermined, programmed behavior.

* **Culture being shared:** We may behave in manners that are socially acceptable and predict how others will behave because we share our traditions with others in our society. Cultures are widespread, yet this does not imply because they're uniform. Here, the several cultural domains present in every civilization are in-depth examined.

* The term "culture" merely denotes a person's "style of life" or "design for a living." A culture is, in the words of Kluckhohn and Kelly, "a historically constructed system of explicit as well as implicit standards for life as a whole which tends to have been shared by everybody or especially intended members of a group."

* Culture is made composed of a people's ideas and habits, and it is idealistic. It is the result of a group's chosen social norms and behavioral habits. The term "culture" refers to the ideals and traditions that members of a society embrace and strive to preserve on a social, intellectual, and aesthetic level.

* Culture refers to a style of doing; it is societal, not personal. Culture is the result of the systematic interactions between humans and their ancestors.

* A person's established or conventional views are referred to as their legacy, while their whole societal legacy is referred to as their culture. Culture is passed down via the generations. It is a complex fusion of historically important components from the past.

* **Fulfil some needs:** Behaviors make up a culture. Every single behavior has been developed to satisfy a particular need. the requirements of society, ethics, and biology.

* A system of organization is culture. Integration of social systems results in culture. The family system, the religious framework, the system of schools, the economic system, the system of nature, plus the political system are a few examples of social systems.

* Cultures interact and change; in other words, they are dynamic. Since most civilizations have developed means of communication, ideas or symbols are exchanged. All civilizations undergo change through time; if they didn't, it would be challenging for them to adapt to their surroundings. Because cultures are interconnected, it is likely that if one element of the network changed, so would the whole system.

* Adoption may change a culture. Cultures may evolve and adapt through time and from one place to another. Culture is malleable and may evolve. It changes and develops with time.

* **Varieties:** Varieties refers to the concept that things change depending on the culture. Culture, which varies from civilization to civilization and from society to society, is impacted

by both material and intangible cultural traits. For instance, there are differences between urban and rural populations.

- ❖ **Culture as transmissible:** Culture is transmissible in the sense that it is passed on from a generation to the next. The main way that culture is expressed is via language. Culture may be transmitted effectively via both imitation and instruction.
- ❖ **Cultures are super-organic:** Culture has been referred to be super-organic a numerous occasions. According to this, "culture" is preferable than "natural." The term "super-organic" is useful for discussing occurrences that may be very different from a cultural standpoint. A tree, for example, may represent several things to different individuals, including a scientist doing study on it, an elderly person seeking relief from the sun on a hot day in the summer, a farmer harvesting fruit from it, or an automobile colliding with it.
- ❖ Man creates and uses symbols as a way of communication. He has the option of using metaphors as well. Symbols, the cornerstone of culture, are the primary means of cultural communication.
- ❖ **Culture changes throughout time:** Cultures does not emerge suddenly or immediately. Ideas, creative works, morals, and knowledge steadily accumulate throughout time to create culture.
- ❖ Culture affects how an individual's character develops; a child's personality is shaped by the culture in which she or he is reared.

Transcultural nursing is how professional nursing interacts with the concept of culture. It is founded on ethnography and nursing and supported by nursing research, philosophy, and practice. The primary areas of this specific cognitive specialty in nursing include global cultures, comparison cultural care, health, or nursing phenomena. In 1955, it was acknowledged as a subject of inquiry and application. It is a body of knowledge, in the words of Madeleine Leininger, who founded transcultural nurses, that helps in giving nursing care that is suitable for the patient's culture. It is an important field of study as well as practice focused on the traditions of individuals or teams of interchangeable cultures and similar cultural principles of compassion. In a world whose people and nations are intertwined, cross-cultural nursing, according to MEDLINE, is a specialization of nursing that focuses on the requirement for nursing professionals to have a worldwide perspective. Its primary goal is to educate nursing students about global and cross-cultural issues. It involves worldwide medical organizations, nursing overseas, global health issues, and education on cultural diversity.

Goals

The goals of bilingual nursing are to provide racially suitable medical treatment as well as generally applicable and culturally relevant nursing techniques for the well-being and health of individuals or help them as they deal with challenging life circumstances, illness, or death in methods that are significant to their culture.

Founder

The first licensed nurse who earned a PhD in archaeology was Madeleine Leininger. She established and developed the field of transcultural nursing. In 1966, Leininger pioneered transcultural nursing education at the University of Colorado. In 1998, the American Academy of Nursing named Leininger a Living Legend. Leininger edited the Journal of Transcultural Nursing, the official publication of the Transcultural Nursing Society, from 1989 to 1995. She published works on the topic of transcultural nursing.

History

Leininger's idea of the diversity and universality of cultural care served as the inspiration for transcultural nursing. The transcultural nursing field was created between 1955 and 1975. In 1975, Leininger used the "sunrise model" concept to enhance the specialty. Between 1975 and 1983, the area was expanded. It has been acknowledged as a nursing specialty on a worldwide level since 1983. After being officially created as a nursing program at the University of Colorado in 1966, transcultural nursing diplomas or track programs were offered as masters and PhD courses in the early 1970s.

Transcultural Nurses

Registered nurses who specialize in transcultural nursing are known as transcultural nurses. Transcultural nurses often take on roles as physicians, generalists, and consultants in order to explore the linked elements of care provided in variously structured settings from a nursing perspective. They are nurses who provide knowledgeable, competent, and secure care to patients from a variety of cultural backgrounds.

Cultural Competence (CC) is a procedure, according to Campinha-Bacote, that strives to provide medical professionals the ability and availability to work effectively within the cultural context of the family, the individual, or the community. Several elements must be included into this process that constitute the philosophical underpinning of our actions. Professionals are required by CC to assume responsibility for representing persons who are disadvantaged due of their ethnic and empowering people to make decisions about their health. Along with fighting for people's right to receive fair treatment and without prejudice due to their history, additionally asks for promoting equality and people's sense of value. The commitment to helping the underserved exceeds ethnicity and entails taking measures to protect those who are disadvantaged due to their beliefs in a particular religion, positioning of sexuality, education, identity, voice, race, income level, political beliefs, or any other aspect of diversity. It must reject the widely held idea that cultural competence primarily pertains to racial and/or religious diversity and adopt a far broader approach. The American Nursing Association's Panel of Experts on Intercultural Competency (2007) provided the following definition of cultural competence:

- ❖ Health practitioners may provide appropriate cultural support when working with individuals who are culturally competent because they have knowledge, awareness, and skills about a number of ethnic groups.
- ❖ Gaining cultural competence is a lifetime process that involves understanding and accepting differences as well as avoiding imposing one's own viewpoints unreasonably on others.
- ❖ Cultural competence is the ability to ask the appropriate questions by having a working understanding of both fundamental cultural norms in addition to cultural specific facts. As a result, cultural competence is a powerful way to lessen unconscious bias, which is extremely prevalent in most people.

LARRY PURNELL'S MODEL OF CULTURAL COMPETENCE

This middle-range theory was created by Larry Purnell in 1991. Based on his experience dealing with nursing learners during his hospital rotation, Purnell created a thorough clinical assessment technique in 1989. He saw the need of creating an educational structure that could help both teachers and learners to gain knowledge of both the cultures you represent and the cultures of the customers they provide services. Purnell cited evidence of the increased need for cultural competence among North American health professionals to support his claim that people should be handled as individuals irrespective of their socioeconomic status (as well as their uniqueness). It was clear that significant health disparities impacted a wide range of cultural groups. In order to provide better service, improve health outcomes, and contain rising spending on health care, professionals and institutions should be aware of the cultural beliefs, attitudes, and practices of the people they serve.

The following five major concepts form the foundation of Purnell's model:

1. Every individual is a biopsychosocial being with a distinct sense of self, beliefs, and ideals that may affect how they wish to be treated. This person is continuously reacting to their environment.
2. A family is defined as at least two individuals who are emotionally connected but don't necessarily share blood or geographically related.
3. A community is made up of a group of people who have a common hobby and live in the same area. It also includes the physical, social, and symbolic characteristics that help the people in the community form bonds with one another.
4. Our global society is made up of a huge range of people from diverse backgrounds of culture and ethnicity because of how interconnected the world is now.
5. Health is a state of fitness that is determined by a person or a tribe, and it often involves spiritual, biopsychosocial, and societal implications that interact the family life and the national, local, and worldwide social systems. Purnell's model is also vital to bear in mind since it is based on a series of assumptions that give the model meaning: All health professionals should be familiar with cultural diversity and concepts related to the meta-paradigm of global society, belonging, relatives, the individual in question, and health. One culture is not better than another; rather, they are only different from one another. Fundamental similarities exist across all civilizations. Each culture varies both in and between itself. A culture may change over time. The primary and secondary characteristics of a culture determine how far it diverges from the dominant culture. Patients who actively participate in their care and have a voice in the plans, activities, and goals that influence their health will have better medical results. The way that individuals regard themselves and respond to medical care is significantly influenced by culture. Families and individuals come from a variety of cultural origins. Every individual has an obligation to be respected for their uniqueness and cultural background. Nurses need both broad as well as particular training in cultural awareness to provide careful and competent care. Through examination, planning, and action, nurses may effectively enhance the care of patients from a specific culture. Understanding different societies is a lifelong process that occurs primarily via interaction with them.

Raising one's awareness of many cultures might lessen prejudice. In order to be effective, health care must show a clear understanding of the values, beliefs, beliefs, and worldviews of varied populations as well as of individual acculturation models. Depending on an individual's culture, race, and ethnicity, different therapies may be required. Nurses are becoming better at understanding their own culture as well as the cultures of other professionals, groups, and organizations. In order to offer treatment that is culturally competent, the paradigm advanced by Purnell (2014) demands for a full understanding of 12 domains:

1. General information, such as possessions, present residence, reason for migration, political leanings, degree of education, and occupation.
2. Nonverbal language-related communication, dialects, parallel language variation (voice volume, tone), and temporality as it pertains to past, present, and prospective future orientation.
3. **Family structure and roles:** Who is in charge of the home, what gender roles are prevalent, who makes up the larger family, and how tolerant are non-traditional identities and childless unions, and divorce?
4. The autonomy and culture that exist at work.
5. **Biocultural ecology:** Alterations in drug metabolism, biological variations, skin color, and medical issues.
6. Risky sexual behavior, not getting adequate exercise, lacking a seat belt or helmet, and using tobacco products are all examples of high-risk health behaviors.
7. **Nutrition:** This group of topics includes what constitutes food, common foods and traditions, nutritional deficiencies, and dietary practices that promote health.
8. Pregnancy and related practices, such as forbidden, prescribed, and taboo conduct in connection with pregnancy, childbirth, and the puerperium. Additionally included in this category are culturally approved and unapproved reproductive practices.
9. Death rites, include rituals related to death and euthanasia, funeral traditions, and grieving practices.
10. **Spirituality:** Officially held religious beliefs on affiliation, faith, and prayer use, as well as traditions that give life meaning and serve as individual sources of strength.
11. **Health care habits:** Ways to health-related attitudes and behaviors, cultural reactions to health and sickness, people's practices, self-reliance, barriers to getting treatment, rehabilitation, and the use of blood offerings, including donations of organs.
12. **Medical professionals:** Gender, conventional health status, and biological health status.

SPIRITUALITY

Sometimes it is difficult to define spirituality. Although it has been studied by the whole human race to be a composite of the three fundamental qualities of people (i.e., body, mind, and spirit), there is substantial disagreement over its origin, purpose, or even relevance. However, when taken in its broadest sense, spirituality mostly focuses on how we approach life's uncertainties and how we recognize and respond to the holy. According to several psychologists:

- Spirituality is a quality that all individuals are born with. This viewpoint holds that human spirituality is a search for purpose in life or an endeavor to understand and relate to the unknowns of the universe.
- Weaver and Cotrell, who make a similar claim, that spirituality "refers to concerns of greater significance that call for releasing the urges to the heart in search for purposes with personal meaning."
- Others describe it as "an individual's involvement in and contact with an essentials intangible characteristics aspect that comprises the universe" or "a relationship with something sacred" (Beck and Walters).
- Some people refer to the soul or spirit as the "vital principle or animating spirit believed to reside with living organisms" (Zinn) or "the very source of energy" that is inside each person.

According to Danesh, learning about human spirituality enables individuals to tap from a bigger well of strength and energy, which changes how we see ourselves. What is considered to be the core of spirituality is the exploration of our relationships with others, ourselves, nature, a higher power, as well as the meaning of our lives. It is possible to do simultaneous searches at all of these sites. Relationships with the Universal Mind, God, Goddess, Creator, Great Spirit, etc., may or may not be included in this. It does include looking for a link to or understanding of the vital or non-material, as opposed to the concrete or material. Theism, the belief that and naturalism are the three main belief systems in terms of human spirituality (Copan). Naturalists believe that spirituality and ideas of what is holy develop spontaneously in people's thoughts and disappear with the passing of the human body (Mas Low). Pantheists believe that everything in the universe is either a mirror of God or an image of His essence (Levine). Theists believe that God created a non-material mind that is intended to outlive the death of the human body and is the source of humanity's spirituality (Collins).

Numerous faiths, belief systems, and philosophical viewpoints have emerged, multiplied, and perished throughout human history. Though the underlying motivation for each of these structures is definitely influenced by a variety of unique cultural and psychological reasons, a common belief that man is not entire or complete in his naturally occurring human condition permeates almost all of them. This view is accompanied with the notion that man must go through some kind of completion process or self-definition discipline. As long as it falls within the realm of human potential, such a process is often understood by its proponents as the fundamental reason for man's existence. Through it, man is said to gain or grow that which is fundamental and universal, rather than just what is incidental and local. By doing this, he defines who he really is by being his most authentic self. The process frequently referred to as one of "salvation," or being raised to the level of a higher reality from the state of spiritual dead. Such redemption ideas, spiritual ideologies, and spiritual exercises have mostly come from the revealed faiths. In the past, it would seem that all of the revealed faiths have agreed to some extent that the cosmos has an objectively true spiritual component and that such spiritual element of existence is, for humans, the most basic and significant feature of reality. However, the revealed faiths also seem to have a disconcerting degree of divergence in their distinct understandings of the precise nature of this dimension and how man should connect to it, at least on the surface. In addition, the majority of ancient religious belief systems seem to have crystallized into strict social norms and dogmatic attitudes of thinking and belief, which seem irreconcilable with the contemporary ethos of fast social and intellectual change. Modern civilization is changing mostly due to a highly effective, potent, and well-established science that has little to no connection to well-established religion. Science is founded firmly on the notion that truth is relative along with progressive, that what is beneficial and efficient in the field of concepts and strategies today might become obsolete and unproductive tomorrow, in contrast to religions, which, for the majority, keep pursuing harder and harder on their mutually divergent assertions that each possesses an absolute and unchanging truth that admits no compromise. Thus, whereas science thrives on change, traditional religion has learned to despise and dread it. Even if technological advances and science have greatly expanded man's ability to control and manage his physical surroundings, they have not yet provided him with the feeling of completeness he has long sought. In modern civilization, there is a strong feeling of unfinishedness and a conscious desire for transcendence, or connection to a profound spiritual reality. In fact, there has seldom been a period in history or a civilization when the feeling of spiritual inadequacy has been as intense as it is now in industrialized, high-tech, Western culture. However, if a modern man looks to religion for guidance, he too often encounters dogmatism that his thinking cannot accept or mindless emotionalism that is not deserving of embrace. From a contemporary vantage point, each of the main religions of the world appears as a framework that, while largely successful in meeting the spiritual along with social needs of a particular people or the culture during a prior historical era, is no longer sufficient to meet those needs for humanity in the current crucial historical era. Thus, when it comes to the most important spiritual issues, contemporary man is in a very difficult situation. On the contrary hand, the very effective science he has produced helps to amplify his religious and moral wants, needs that science by itself cannot satiate. On the other side, the majority of traditional religious practices, viewpoints, and ideas suddenly seem outmoded and unimportant.

Development of Human Spirituality

There are several perspectives on how spiritual growth happens, just as there are in all other spheres of human development. As a result, some people reach their seventieth year of life with an experienced age of seventeen, while others reach their seventieth year of life closer to one hundred and seventy. The bravery to carry out one's objectives and the desire to take conscious charge of one's life are some of the most crucial characteristics of a well-developed adult. Early childhood has to be addressed in order to promote the formation of these traits (Erikson). Various models of spiritual growth have been drawn from various religious traditions (Wilson). It might be difficult, but not impossible, to distinguish between the procedure of spiritual growth and any particular religious development. Public schools may employ the general descriptions of spiritual (or religious) growth that have been created by a number of studies. Fowler's description is perhaps the best-known. He used the word "faith," which he described as "a person's way of seeing him- or oneself in relation to another against a background of mutual significance and purpose".

Activities for Spiritual Development

Without a doubt, if we see the person as a whole, the growth of the human soul is a crucial problem that has to be handled. The idea put out by Götz and Palmer is to begin with the teacher's spiritual growth. One cannot teach something one has not learned, just as with every other topic. What step in this procedure should educators take first? An investigation of one's growth of faith, as outlined by Fowler, may be one strategy. Another option might be to think about the areas of spiritual growth that Hay and Nye characterized as including "self, others, nature, and God/Creator" or the components of spirituality that Hamilton and Jackson defined as including "self-awareness, interconnectedness, or a relationship with some higher power." These are quite difficult undertakings that almost certainly call for some guidance from an experienced mentor or at the very least participation in a study class. This implies that in order to meet the needs of creating and executing a curriculum for spiritual growth, educators will need to undergo some specific training. Institutions that educate teachers should think about include a course on spiritual growth in their preservice teacher training curriculum. School districts must provide inservice in-struction for teachers who are currently on the job via seminars or conference attendance.

UNIT

Introduction to Nursing Theories

16

Unit Outline

- Meaning and definition
- Purposes, types of theories
- Overview of selected nursing theories—Nightingale, Orem, Roy
- Use of theories in nursing practice

LEARNING OBJECTIVES

At the end of this unit, the reader will be able to:

- Introduction to nursing theories.
- Development of nursing theories.
- Understanding the work of nurse theorists.
- Nursing theorist.
- Application of theory in nursing process.
- Theories and nursing research.
- Nightingale environmental theory.
- Theory of interpersonal relations.
- Application of interpersonal theory in nursing practice.
- Virgenia Henderson's need theory.
- Faye Glenn Abdellah's theory.
- Imogene King: Theory of goal attainment.
- Betty Neuman's theory.
- Application of Betty Neuman theory in nursing practice.
- Dorothea Orem's theory.
- Application of Orem's theory in nursing practice.
- Jean Watson's philosophy of nursing.
- The Roy's adaptation model.
- Application of Roy's adaptation model in nursing practice.
- Johnson's bahavior system model.
- Levine's four conservation principles.
- Health promotion model.
- Transcultural nursing.
- Helping and human relationship theory.
- Martha Rogers' science of unitary human beings.
- Theories based on interactive process.
- Orlando's nursing process theory.
- Theories used in community health nursing.
- Application of Suchman's stages of illness model.

INTRODUCTION

Nursing has made phenomenal achievement in the last century that has lead to the recognition of nursing as an academic discipline and a profession. A move towards theory-based practice has made contemporary nursing more meaningful and significant by shifting nursing's focus from vocation to an organized profession. The need for knowledge-base to guide professional nursing practice had been realized in the first half of the twentieth century and many theoretical works have been contributed by nurses ever since, first with the goal of making nursing a recognized profession and later with the goal of delivering care to patients as professionals.

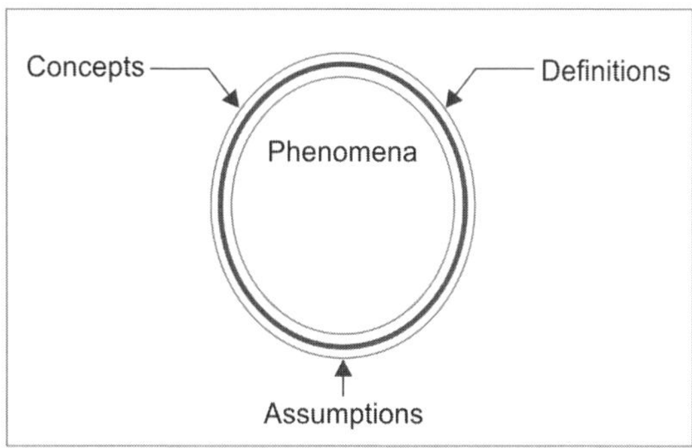

Component of theory.

A theory is a group of related concepts that propose action that guide practice. A **nursing theory** is a set of concepts, definitions, relationships, and assumptions or propositions derived from nursing models or from other disciplines and project a purposive, systematic view of phenomena by designing specific inter-relationships among concepts for the purposes of describing, explaining, predicting, and/or prescribing..

Based on the knowledge structure levels the theoretical works in nursing can be studied under the following headings:

- Metaparadigm (Person, Environment, Health and Nursing)—(Most abstract)
- Nursing philosophies.
- Conceptual models and grand theories.
- Nursing theories and middle range theories (Least abstract).

NURSING PHILOSOPHIES

Nursing philosophies theory and key emphasis.	
Theory	**Key emphasis**
Florence Nightingale's Legacy of caring	Focuses on nursing and the patient environment relationship

Ernestine Wiedenbach: The helping art of clinical nursing	• Helping process meets needs through the art of individualizing care
	• Nurses should identify patients 'need-for-help' by:
	  ➢ Observation
	  ➢ Understanding client behavior
	  ➢ Identifying cause of discomfort
	  ➢ Determining if clients can resolve problems or have a need for help

Contd...

Contd...

Theory	Key emphasis
Virginia Henderson's Definition of Nursing	• Patients require help towards achieving independence • Derived a definition of nursing • Identified 14 basic human needs on which nursing care is based
Faye G Abedellah's Typology of Twenty One Nursing Problems	Patient's problems determine nursing care
Lydia E Hall: Care, Cure, Core Model	Nursing care is person directed towards self love
Jean Watson's Philosophy and Science of Caring	• Caring is moral ideal: Mind-body—soul engagement with one and other • Caring is a universal, social phenomenon that is only effective when practiced interpersonally considering humanistic aspects and caring
Patricia Benner's Primacy of Caring	• Caring is central to the essence of nursing. It sets up what matters, enabling connection and concern. It creates possibility for mutual helpfulness • Caring creates—possibilities of coping possibilities for connecting with and concern for others, possibilities for giving and receiving help • Described systematically five stages of skill acquisition in nursing practice—novice, advanced beginner, competent, proficient and expert

CONCEPTUAL MODELS AND GRAND THEORIES

Nursing conceptual model and grand theories.	

Dorothea E. Orem's: Self-care deficit theory in nursing	• Self-care maintains wholeness.
	• Three theories:
	  1. Theory of Self-care
	  2. Theory of Self-care Deficit
	  3. Theory of Nursing Systems
	• Wholly compensatory (doing for the patient)
	• Partly compensatory (helping the patient do for himself or herself)
	• Supportive-educative (helping patient to learn self-care and emphasizing on the importance of nurses' role

Myra Estrin Levine's: The conservation model	• Holism is maintained by conserving integrity
	• Proposed that the nurses use the principles of conservation of:
	  1. Client energy
	  2. Personal integrity
	  3. Structural integrity
	  4. Social integrity
	  5. A conceptual model with three nursing theories—
	  6. Conservation
	  7. Redundancy
	  8. Therapeutic intention

Martha E. Roger's: Science of unitary human beings	• Person environment are energy fields that evolve negentropically • Martha proposed that nursing was a basic scientific discipline • Nursing is using knowledge for human betterment • The unique focus of nursing is on the unitary or irreducible human being and the environment (both are energy fields) rather than health and illness

Contd...

Contd...

Dorothy E Johnson's: Behavioral system model	• Individuals maintain stability and balance through adjustments and adaptation to the forces that impinges them • Individual as a behavioral system is composed of seven subsystems. • Attachment, or the affiliative subsystems—is the corner stone of social organizations • Behavioral system also includes the subsystems of dependency, achievement, aggressive, ingestive-eliminative and sexual • Disturbances in these causes nursing problems
Sister Callista: Roy's Adaptation model	• Stimuli disrupt an adaptive system • The individual is a biopsychosocial adaptive system within an environment • The individual and the environment provide three classes of stimuli, the focal, residual and contextual • Through two adaptive mechanisms, regulator and cognator, an individual demonstrates adaptive responses or ineffective responses requiring nursing interventions
Betty Neuman's: Health care systems model	• Reconstitution is a status of adaptation to stressors • A conceptual model with two theories "optimal patient stability and prevention as intervention" • Neuman's model includes intrapersonal, interpersonal and extrapersonal stressors • Nursing is concerned with the whole person • Nursing actions (primary, secondary, and tertiary levels of prevention) focuses on the variables affecting the client's response to stressors
Imogene King's: Goal attainment theory	• Transactions provide a frame of reference toward goal setting • A conceptual model of nursing from which theory of goal attainment is derived • From her major concepts (interaction, perception, communication, transaction, role, stress, growth and development) derived goal attainment theory • Perceptions, judgments and actions of the patient and the nurse lead to reaction, interaction, and transaction (Process of nursing)
Nancy Roper, WW Logan and AJ Tierney: A model for nursing based on a model of living	• Individuality in living • A conceptual model of nursing from which theory of goal attainment is derived. • Living is an amalgam of activities of living (ALs) • Most individuals experience significant life events which can affect ALs causing actual and potential problems • This affects dependence—independence continuum which is bi-directional. • Nursing helps to maintain the individuality of person by preventing potential problems, solving actual problems and helping to cope

Hildegard E. Peplau: Psychodynamic nursing theory	• Interpersonal process is maturing force for personality
	• Stressed the importance of nurses' ability to understand own behavior to help others identify perceived difficulties
	• The four phases of nurse-patient relationships are:
	  1. Orientation
	  2. Identification
	  3. Exploitations
	  4. Resolution

Contd...

Contd...

	• The six nursing roles are: 1. Stranger 2. Resource person 3. Teacher 4. Leader 5. Surrogate 6. Counselor

Ida Jean Orlando's: Nursing process theory	• Interpersonal process alleviates distress
	• Nurses must stay connected to patients and assure that patients get what they need, focused on patient's verbal and nonverbal expressions of need and nurse's reactions to patient's behavior to alleviate distress
	• Elements of nursing situation:
	  ➢ Patient
	  ➢ Nurse reactions
	  ➢ Nursing actions

Joyce Travelbee's: Human to human relationship model	• Therapeutic human relationships
	• Nursing is accomplished through human-to-human relationships that began with: The original encounter and then progressed through stages of
	  ➢ Emerging identities
	  ➢ Developing feelings of empathy and sympathy, until the nurse and patient attained rapport in the final stage

Kathryn E. Barnard's: Parent child interaction model	• Growth and development of children and mother–infant relationships • Individual characteristics of each member influence the parent–infant system and adaptive behavior modifies those characteristics to meet the needs of the system
Ramona T Mercer's: Maternal role attainment	• Parenting and maternal role attainment in diverse populations • A complex theory to explain the factors impacting the development of maternal role overtime.
Katharine Kolcaba's: Theory of comfort	• Comfort is desirable holistic outcome of care • These needs include physical, psycho spiritual, social and environmental needs. • Health care needs are needs for comfort, arising from stressful healthcare situations that cannot be met by recipients' traditional support system • Comfort measures include those nursing interventions designed to address the specific comfort needs
Madeleine Leininger's: Transcultural nursing, culture-care theory	• Caring is universal and varies transculturally • Major concepts include care, caring, culture, cultural values and cultural variations • Caring serves to ameliorate or improve human conditions and life base • Care is the essence and the dominant, distinctive and unifying feature of nursing
Rosemarie Rizzo Parse's: Theory of human becoming	• Indivisible beings and environment co-create health • A theory of nursing derived from Roger's conceptual model • Clients are open, mutual and in constant interaction with environment • The nurse assists the client in interaction with the environment and co creating health

Contd...

Contd...

Nola J. Pender's: The health promotion model	• Promoting optimum health supersedes disease prevention. • Identifies cognitive, perceptual factors in clients which are modified by demographical and biological characteristics, interpersonal influences, situational and behavioral factors that help predict in health promoting behavior

Conclusion

The conceptual and theoretical nursing models help to provide knowledge to improve practice, guide research and curriculum and identify the goals of nursing practice. The state of art and science of nursing theory is one of continuing growth. Using the internet the nurses of the world can share ideas and knowledge, carrying on the work begun by nursing theorists and continue the growth and development of new nursing knowledge. It is important the nursing knowledge is learnt, used, and applied in the theory-based practice for the profession and the continued development of nursing and academic discipline.

DEVELOPMENT OF NURSING THEORIES

Introduction

Kerlinger views theories as a set of interrelated concepts that give a systematic view of a phenomenon (an observable fact or event) that is explanatory and predictive in nature. Theories are composed of concepts, definitions, models, propositions and are based on assumptions. They are derived through two principal methods: (1) Deductive reasoning (2) Inductive reasoning. Nursing theorists use both of these methods.

Theories for Professional Nursing

❖ Theory is "a creative and rigorous structuring of ideas that projects a tentative, purposeful, and systematic view of phenomena".
❖ A theory makes it possible to "organize the relationship among the concepts to describe, explain, predict, and control practice".

Definition

❖ Concepts are basically vehicles of thought that involve images. Concepts are words that describe objects, properties, or events and are basic components of theory.
❖ Types:
  ◆ Empirical concepts
  ◆ Inferential concepts
  ◆ Abstract concepts
❖ Models are representations of the interaction among and between the concepts showing patterns.
❖ Propositions are statements that explain the relationship between the concepts.
❖ Process is a series of actions, changes or functions intended to bring about a desired result. During a process one takes systemic and continuous steps to meet a goal and uses both assessments and feedback to direct actions to the goal.
❖ A particular theory or conceptual framework directs how these actions are carried out. The delivery of nursing care within the nursing process is directed by the way specific

conceptual frameworks and theories define the person (patient), the environment, health and nursing.

❖ The terms 'model' and 'theory' are often wrongly used interchangeably, which further confounds matters.

❖ In nursing, models are often designed by theory authors to depict the beliefs in their theory (Lancaster and Lancaster 1981).

❖ They provide an overview of the thinking behind the theory and may demonstrate how theory can be introduced into practice, e.g., through specific methods of assessment.

❖ Models are useful as they allow the concepts in nursing theory to be successfully applied to nursing practice (Lancaster and Lancaster 1981).

❖ Their main limitation is that they are only as accurate or useful as the underlying theory.

IMPORTANCE OF NURSING THEORIES

❖ Nursing theory aims to describe, predict and explain the phenomenon of nursing (Chinn and Jacobs 1978).

❖ It should provide the foundations of nursing practice, help to generate further knowledge and indicate in which direction nursing should develop in the future (Brown 1964).

❖ Theory is important because it helps us to decide what we know and what we need to know (Parsons 1949).

❖ It helps to distinguish what should form the basis of practice by explicitly describing nursing.

❖ The benefits of having a defined body of theory in nursing include better patient care, enhanced professional status for nurses, improved communication between nurses, and guidance for research and education (Nolan 1996). In addition, because the main exponent of nursing—caring—cannot be measured, it is vital to have the theory to analyze and explain what nurses do.

❖ As medicine tries to make a move towards adopting a more multidisciplinary approach to healthcare, nursing continues to strive to establish a unique body of knowledge.

❖ This can be seen as an attempt by the nursing profession to maintain its professional boundaries.

THE CHARACTERISTICS OF THEORIES

❖ Interrelating concepts in such a way as to create a different way of looking at a particular phenomenon.

❖ Logical in nature

❖ Generalizable

❖ Bases for hypotheses that can be tested.

❖ Increasing the general body of knowledge within the discipline through the research implemented to validate them.

❖ Used by the practitioners to guide and improve their practice.

❖ Consistent with other validated theories, laws, and principles but will leave open unanswered questions that need to be investigated.

BASIC PROCESSES IN THE DEVELOPMENT OF NURSING THEORIES

Nursing theories are often based on and influenced by broadly applicable processes and theories. Following theories are basic to many nursing concepts.

General System Theory

It describes how to break whole things into parts and then to learn how the parts work together in "systems." These concepts may be applied to different kinds of systems, e.g., molecules in chemistry, cultures in sociology, and organs in anatomy and health in nursing.

Adaptation Theory

- It defines adaptation as the adjustment of living matter to other living things and to environmental conditions.
- Adaptation is a continuously occurring process that effects change and involves interaction and response.
- Human adaptation occurs on three levels:
  1. The internal (self)
  2. The social (others) and
  3. The physical (biochemical reactions)

Developmental Theory

- It outlines the process of growth and development of humans as orderly and predictable, beginning with conception and ending with death.
- The progress and behaviors of an individual within each stage are unique.
- The growth and development of an individual is influenced by heredity, temperament, emotional, and physical environment, life experiences and health status.

COMMON CONCEPTS IN NURSING THEORIES

Four concepts common in nursing theory that influence and determine nursing practice are:
1. The person (patient).
2. The environment
3. Health
4. Nursing (goals, roles, functions)
   Each of these concepts is usually defined and described by a nursing theorist, often uniquely; although these concepts are common to all nursing theories. Of the four concepts, the most important is that of the person. The focus of nursing, regardless of definition or theory, is the person.

HISTORICAL PERSPECTIVES AND KEY CONCEPTS

- **Nightingale (1860):** To facilitate "the body's reparative processes" by manipulating client's environment.
- **Peplau 1952:** Nursing is; therapeutic interpersonal process.
- **Henderson 1955:** The needs often called Henderson's 14 basic needs.
- **Abdellah 1960:** The nursing theory developed by Faye Abdellah et al (1960) emphasizes delivering nursing care for the whole person to meet the physical, emotional, intellectual, social, and spiritual needs of the client and family.
- **Orlando 1962:** To Ida Orlando (1960), the client is an individual; with a need; that, when met, diminishes distress, increases adequacy, or enhances well-being.

- ❖ **Johnson's Theory 1968:** Dorothy Johnson's theory of nursing 1968 focuses on how the client adapts to illness and how actual or potential stress can affect the ability to adapt. The goal of nursing to reduce stress so that; the client can move more easily through recovery.
- ❖ **Rogers 1970:** To maintain and promote health, prevent illness, and care for and rehabilitate ill and disabled client through "humanistic science of nursing."
- ❖ **Orem 1971:** This is self-care deficit theory. Nursing care becomes necessary when client is unable to fulfill biological, psychological, developmental, or social needs.
- ❖ **King 1971:** To use communication to help client reestablish positive adaptation to environment.
- ❖ **Neuman 1972:** Stress reduction is goal of system model of nursing practice.
- ❖ **Roy 1979:** This adaptation model is based on the physiological, psychological, sociological and dependence-independence adaptive modes.
- ❖ **Watson's Theory 1979:** Watson's philosophy of caring 1979 attempts to define the outcome of nursing activity in regard to the; humanistic aspects of life

CLASSIFICATION OF NURSING THEORIES

Depending on Function

Descriptive	To identify the properties and workings of a discipline
Explanatory	To examine how properties relate and thus affect the discipline
Predictive	To calculate relationships between properties and how they occur
Prescriptive	To identify under which conditions relationships occur

Depending on the Generalizability of their Principles

- ❖ **Metatheory:** The theory of theory. Identifies specific phenomena through abstract concepts.
- ❖ **Grand theory:** It provides a conceptual framework under which the key concepts and principles of the discipline can be identified.
- ❖ **Middle range theory:** It is more precise and only analyses a particular situation with a limited number of variables.
- ❖ **Practice theory:** It explores one particular situation found in nursing. It identifies explicit goals and details how these goals will be achieved.

BASED ON THE PHILOSOPHICAL UNDERPINNINGS OF THE THEORIES

- ❖ "Needs "theories.
- ❖ "Interaction" theories
- ❖ "Outcome "theories
- ❖ Humanistic theories

"Needs" Theories

- ❖ These theories are based around helping individuals to fulfill their physical and mental needs. The basis of these theories is well-illustrated in Roper, Logan and Tierney's Model of Nursing (1980).
- ❖ Needs theories have been criticized for relying too much on the medical model of health and placing the patient in an overtly dependent position.

"Interaction" Theories

- As described by Peplau (1988), these theories revolve around the relationships nurses form with patients.
- Such theories have been criticized for largely ignoring the medical model of health and not attending to basic physical needs.

"Outcome" Theories

- These portray the nurse as the changing force, who enables individuals to adapt to or cope with ill health (Roy 1980).
- Outcome theories have been criticized as too abstract and difficult to implement in practice (Aggleton and Chalmers 1988).

"Humanistic" Theories

- Humanistic theories developed in response to the psychoanalytic thought that a person's destiny was determined early in life.
- Humanistic theories emphasize a person's capacity for self-actualization.
- Humanists believe that the person contains within himself the potential for healthy and creative growth.
- Carl Rogers developed a person-centered model of psychotherapy that emphasizes the uniqueness of the individual.
- The major contribution that Rogers added to nursing practice is the understanding that each client is a unique individual, so, person-centered approach now practice in nursing.

MODELS OF NURSING

- Until fairly recently, nursing science was derived principally from social, biologic, and medical science theories. However, from the 1950s to the present, an increasing number of nursing theorists have developed models of nursing that provide bases for the development of nursing theories and nursing knowledge.
- A model, as an abstraction of reality, provides a way to visualize reality to simplify thinking.
- A conceptual model shows how various concepts are interrelated and applies theories to predict or evaluate consequences of alternative actions.
- According to Fawcett (2000): A conceptual model "gives direction to the search for relevant questions about the phenomena of central interest to a discipline and suggests solutions to practical problems".
- Four concepts are generally considered central to the discipline of nursing: the person who receives nursing care (the patient or client); the environment (society); nursing (goals, roles, functions); and health. These four concepts form a metaparadigm of nursing.
- The term metaparadigm comes from the Greek prefix "meta," which means more comprehensive or transcending, and the word Greek word "paradigm," which means a philosophical or theoretical framework of a discipline upon which all theories, laws, and generalizations are formulated (Merriam-Webster's Collegiate Dictionary, 1994).

GROWTH AND STABILITY MODELS OF CHANGE

- There are two major differences in philosophical beliefs, or world views, about the nature of change.

* "The world view of change uses the growth metaphor, and the persistence view focuses on stability" (Fawcett).
* Within the change world view, change and growth are continual and desirable, "progress is valued, and realization of one's potential is emphasized" (Fawcett).
* Persistence is endurance in time.
* Persistence world view emphasizes equilibrium and balance.

CATEGORIES OF CONCEPTUAL MODELS

Ten conceptual models of nursing have been classified according to two criteria:
* The world view of change reflected by the model (growth or stability); and
* The major theoretical conceptual classification with which the model seems most consistent (systems, stress/adaptation, caring, or growth/development).

SYSTEMS THEORY AS A FRAMEWORK

* Systems theory is concerned with changes caused by interactions among all the factors (variables).
* General systems theory is emphasized.
    * A system is defined as "a whole with interrelated parts, in which the parts have a function and the system as a totality has a function" (Auger).
    * A general systems approach allows for consideration of the subsystems levels of the human being, as a total human being, and as a social creature who networks himself with others in hierarchically arranged human systems of increasing complexity. Thus, the human being, from the level of the individual to the level of society, can be conceptualized as the client and becomes the target system for nursing intervention (Sills and Hall).

An Example of Systems Interaction

* Input (Diet teaching)
* Throughput (Assimilation of information)
* Output (Food intake)
* Feedback (Weight record, Hb estimation etc.)
* Two nursing models based on systems theory:
    * Imogene King's systems interaction model, and
    * Betty Neuman's health care systems model.

Major Concepts as Defined in King's Model

Person (human being)	A personal system that interacts with interpersonal and social systems
Environment	A context "within which human beings grow, develop, and perform daily activities"
Health	"A dynamic life experiences of a human being, which implies continuous adjustment to stressors in the internal and external environment through optimum use of one's resources to achieve maximum potential for daily living"
Nursing	A process of human interaction

Imogene King's Systems Interaction Model

* In interaction model, the purpose of nursing is to help people attain, maintain, or restore health. King's model conceptualizes three levels of dynamic interacting systems:

1. Individuals are called "personal systems."
2. Groups (two or more persons) form "interpersonal systems."
3. Society is composed of "social systems."

❖ As the person interacts with the environment, he or she must continuously adjust to stressors in the internal and external environment (King, 1981).

❖ Health assumes achievement of maximum potential for daily living and an ability to function in social roles. It is the "dynamic life experiences of a human being, which implies continuous adjustment to stressors in the internal and external environment through optimum use of one's resources to achieve maximum potential for daily living" (King, 1981).

❖ "Illness is a deviation from normal, that is, an imbalance in a person's biological structure or in his psychological makeup, or a conflict in a person's social relationships" (King, 1989).

❖ "The goal of nursing is to help individuals and groups attain, maintain, and restore health."

❖ **Stress:** "A dynamic state whereby a human being interacts with the environment to maintain balance for growth, development, and performance."

Betty Neuman's Health Care Systems Model

Betty Neuman specifies that the purpose of nursing is to facilitate optimal client system stability.

❖ **Normal line of defense:** An adaptational level of health considered normal for an individual

❖ **Lines of resistance:** Protection factors activated when stressors have penetrated the normal line of defense.

❖ Neuman's model, organized around stress reduction, is concerned primarily with how stress and the reactions to stress affect the development and maintenance of health.

❖ The person is a composite of physiologic, psychological, sociocultural, developmental, and spiritual variables considered simultaneously.

❖ "Ideally the five variables function harmoniously or are stable in relation to internal and external environmental stressor influences" (Neuman, 2002).

❖ A person is constantly affected by stressors from the internal, external, or created environment.

❖ Stressors are tension-producing stimuli that have the potential to disturb a person's equilibrium or normal line of defense. This normal line of defense is the person's "usual steady state." It is the way in which an individual usually deals with stressors.

❖ Stressors may be of three types:
1. **Intrapersonal:** Forces arising from within the person.
2. **Interpersonal:** Forces arising between persons.
3. **Extrapersonal:** Forces arising from outside the person.

❖ Resistance to stressors is provided by a flexible line of defense, a dynamic protective buffer made up of all variables affecting a person at any given moment the person's resistance to any given stressor or stressors.

❖ If the flexible line of defense is no longer able to protect the person against a stressor, the stressor breaks through, disturbs the person's equilibrium, and triggers a reaction. The reaction may lead toward restoration of balance or toward death.

❖ Neuman intends for the nurse to "assist clients to retain, attain, or maintain optimal system stability" (Neuman, 1996).

❖ Thus, health (wellness) seems to be related to dynamic equilibrium of the normal line of defense, where stressors are successfully overcome or avoided by the flexible line of defense.

❖ Neuman defines illness as "a state of insufficiency with disrupting needs unsatisfied" (Neuman, 2002).

❖ Illness appears to be a separate state when a stressor breaks through the normal line of defense and causes a reaction with the person's lines of resistance.

Stress/Adaptation Theory as a Framework

❖ In contrast to systems theory, stress and adaptation theories view change caused by person–environment interaction in terms of cause and effect.

❖ The person must adjust to environmental changes to avoid disturbing a balanced existence. Adaptation theory provides a way to understand both how the balance is maintained and the possible effects of disturbed equilibrium.

❖ This theory has been widely applied to explain, predict, and control biologic (physiologic and psychological) phenomenon.

A Unique Body of Knowledge

❖ The drive for a unique body of knowledge is based on the assumption that 'borrowed' knowledge is less worthy. However, nurse education is based on theory borrowed from other disciplines, such as sociology and psychology.

❖ It has been argued that applying knowledge from different disciplines only serves to dilute nursing practice.

❖ Nevertheless, as the occupation is focused on humans, perhaps it is inevitable that nursing uses knowledge from other social sciences.

❖ It has been argued that no knowledge is exclusive, and because of nursing's diverse nature it is impossible for it to have a unique body of knowledge and one unified body of theory (Castledine 1994, Levine 1995).

CRITICISMS OF NURSING THEORIES

To understand why nursing theory is generally neglected on the wards it is necessary to take a closer look at the main criticisms of nursing theory and the role that nurses play in contributing to its lack of prevalence in practice.

Use of Language

Scott (1994) states that the crucial ingredients of nursing theory should be accessibility and clarity. However, one of the main criticisms of nursing theory is its use of overtly complex language (Kenny 1993). It is important that the language used in the development of nursing theory be used consistently.

Not Part of Everyday Practice

Despite theory and practice being viewed as inseparable concepts, a theory-practice gap still exists in nursing (Upton 1999). Yet despite the availability of a vast amount of literature on the subject, nursing theory still means very little to most practicing nurses. Perhaps this is because the majority of nursing theory is developed by and for nursing academics (Lathlean 1994). It has been recognized that traditionally nurses are used to 'speaking with their hands' (Levine 1995). Therefore, many nurses have not had the training or experience to deal with the abstract concepts presented by nursing theory. This makes it difficult for the majority of nurses to understand and apply theory to practice (Miller 1985).

Conclusion

Littlejohn (2002) comments that, irrespective of nursing theories nurses will continue to exhibit a caring response to the 'sick and troubled'. If this is true, perhaps nurses are 'nursing' without the knowledge of theories and theory is irrelevant. However, theory and practice are related, and if nursing is to continue to develop, the concept of theory must be addressed. If nursing theory does not drive the development of nursing, it will continue to develop in the footsteps of other disciplines such as medicine.

UNDERSTANDING THE WORK OF NURSE THEORISTS

Theories of Nursing

* Theory is "an internally consistent group of relational statements (concepts, definitions and propositions) that present a systematic view about a phenomenon and which is useful for description, explanation, prediction and control."
* Theories are road maps that provide a framework for selecting and organizing information:
  * What to ask
  * What to observe
  * What to focus on
  * What to think about
* Nursing theory is an organized and systematic articulation of a set of statements related to questions in the discipline of nursing.

Uses of Theory

Theory is used to:
* Describe
* Explain
* Predict
* Prescribe

Uses of Nursing Theory

* Define relationships among the variables of a given field of inquiry
* Guide research, practice and communication
* Allow the prediction of the consequences of care
* Allow the prediction of a range of patient responses

Levels of Theory

There are four levels of theory:
1. Metatheory
2. Grand theory
3. Middle range theory
4. Practice theory

Types of Theory

In Nursing there are four types of theories:
1. Needs
2. Interaction
3. Outcome
4. Humanistic

Practice Value of Theory

- Enhances understanding and explanation for events
- Influence our behavior
- Makes to think differently about a problem or a situation
- Helps to try new approaches or altering behavior
- We can gain a new perspective of events
- Basis for challenge of its speculative tenets or propositions
- Challenges subsequent discovery of new ideas or knowledge that might explain and predict events not yet understood.

PURPOSES OF NURSING THEORIES

In Practice

- Assist nurses to describe, explain, and predict everyday experiences.
- Serve to guide assessment, intervention, and evaluation of nursing care.
- Provide a rationale for collecting reliable and valid data about the health status of clients, which are essential for effective decision making and implementation.
- Help to establish criteria to measure the quality of nursing care.
- Help build a common nursing terminology to use in communicating with other health professionals. Ideas are developed and words defined.
- Enhance autonomy (independence and self-governance) of nursing by defining its own independent functions.

In Education

- Provide a general focus for curriculum design.
- Guide curricular decision making.

In Research

- Offer a framework for generating knowledge and new ideas.
- Assist in discovering knowledge gaps in specific field of study.
- Offer a systematic approach to identify questions for study, select variables, interpret findings, and validate nursing interventions.

Approaches to Developing Nursing Theory

- Borrowing conceptual frameworks from other disciplines.
- Inductively looking at nursing practice to discover theories/concepts to explain phenomena.
- Deductively looking for the compatibility of a general nursing theory with nursing practice.

Questions from Practicing Nurse about Using Nursing Theory

Practice

* ❖ Does this theory reflect nursing practice as I know it?
* ❖ Will it support what I believe to be excellent nursing practice?
* ❖ Can this theory be considered in relation to a wide range of nursing situation?

Personal Interests, Abilities and Experiences

* ❖ What will it be like to think about nursing theory in nursing practice?
* ❖ Will my work with nursing theory be worth the effort?

The Germ Theory

* ❖ Explains the phenomenon of disease transmission.
* ❖ Means of speculative explanation and prediction of certain observable events.
* ❖ Allows us to effectively function to prevent transmission of communicable disease.
* ❖ Viable basis upon which to make decisions about how to prevent certain illnesses.
* ❖ There are phenomena we do not understand that are related to germ transmission.
* ❖ Example—the communicability of cancer.

Nursing Practice

All experiences and events a practicing nurse encounters in the process of providing nursing care.

Events

* ❖ Some may be experienced by the client
* ❖ Others by the nurse
* ❖ Some may be observed in the environment
* ❖ May be observed in the nurse-client interaction.
* ❖ In situations of daily work or living,

...............but as long as they are observable during the process of providing direct nursing care, they are considered part of nursing practice.

Approaches to Inter-relationships between Practice and Theory

* ❖ How nursing practice contributes to the process of theory development?
* ❖ How theory contributes to nursing practice?

Contribution of Practice to Theory Development

* ❖ Theory development within nursing occurs in the context of practice.
* ❖ Two activities contribute significantly to the overall process of developing theory in nursing:
  1. Concept analysis and **(Flowchart 1)**
  2. Practical validation of theory.

Flowchart 1: Concept analysis.

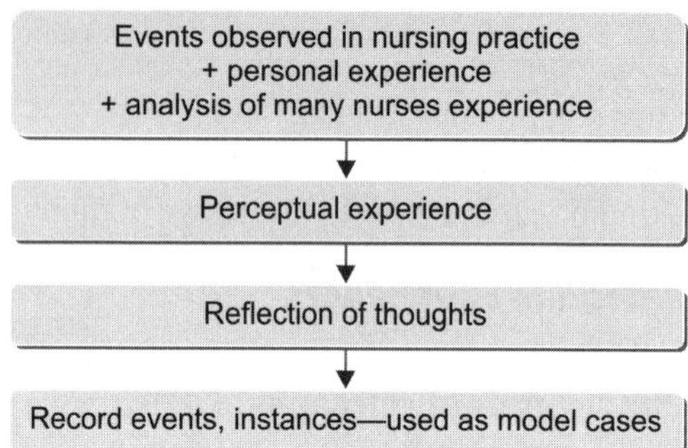

Concept Analysis

- ❖ Identify and verify abstract concepts
- ❖ "What events in practice can be linked with abstract concept x?"
- ❖ Application of theory in practice
- ❖ Nursing process operation of analysis of assessment data.
- ❖ Used as scientific rationale supporting judgments in nursing care plans.

Concepts

- ❖ Concepts may be:
  a. Readily observable, or concrete, ideas such as thermometer, rash, and lesion;
  b. Indirectly observable, or inferential, ideas such as pain and temperature; or
  c. Nonobservable or abstract, ideas such as equilibrium, adaptation, stress, and powerlessness.
- ❖ Nursing theories address and specify relationships among four major abstract concepts referred to as the metaparadigm of nursing.
- ❖ Four concepts are considered to be central to nursing:
- ❖ Person or client, the recipient of nursing care (includes individuals, families, groups, and communities).
- ❖ Environment, the internal and external surroundings that affect the client. This includes people in the physical environment, such as families, friends, and significant others.
- ❖ Health, the degree of wellness or well-being that the client experiences.
- ❖ Nursing, the attributes, characteristics, and actions of the nurse providing care on behalf of, or in conjunction with, the client.

Nightingale's Environmental Theory

Nightingale's environmental theory is "the act of utilizing the environment of the patient to assist him in his recovery." She linked health with five environmental factors:

1. Pure or fresh air
2. Pure water
3. Efficient drainage
4. Cleanliness
5. Light, especially direct sunlight

Deficiencies in these five factors produced lack of health or illness.

Peplau's Interpersonal Relations Model

Nurses enter into a personal relationship with an individual when a felt need is present.

Henderson's Definition of Nursing

Henderson conceptualized the nurse's role as assisting sick or well individuals to gain independence in meeting 14 fundamental needs (Henderson):

- Breathing normally
- Eating and drinking adequately
- Eliminating body wastes
- Moving and maintaining a desirable position
- Sleeping and resting
- Selecting suitable clothes
- Maintaining body temperature within normal range by adjusting clothing and modifying the environment.
- Keeping the body clean and well groomed to protect the integument.
- Avoiding dangers in the environment and avoiding injuring others
- Communicating with others in expressing emotions, needs, fears, or opinions
- Worshipping according to one's faith
- Working in such a way that one feels a sense of accomplishment.
- Playing or participating in various forms of recreation.
- Learning, discovering, or satisfying the curiosity that leads to normal development and health, and using available health facilities

Roger's Science of Unitary Human Beings

- She states that humans are dynamic energy fields in continuous exchange with environmental fields, both of which are infinite.
- Nurses applying Roger's theory in practice (a) focus on the person's wholeness, (b) seek to promote symphonic interaction between the two energy fields (human and environment) to strengthen the coherence and integrity of the person (c) coordinate the human field with the rhythmicity of the environmental field, and (d) direct and redirect patterns of interaction between the two energy fields to promote maximum health potential.

Orem's General Theory of Nursing

Orem's self-care deficit theory explains not only when nursing is needed but also how people can be assisted through five methods of helping: acting or doing for, guiding, teaching, supporting, and providing an environment that promotes the individual's abilities to meet current and future demands.

King's Goal Attainment Theory

King's theory offers insight into nurses' interactions with individuals and groups within the environment. It highlights the importance of client's participation in decision that influence care and focuses on both the process of nurse-client interaction and the outcomes of care.

Neuman's Systems Model

- ❖ The model is based on the individual's relationship to stress, the reaction to it, and reconstitution factors that are dynamic in nature.
- ❖ Betty Neuman's model of nursing is applicable to a variety of nursing practice settings involving individuals, families, groups, and communities.

Roy's Adaptation Model

Roy focuses on the individual as a biopsychosocial adaptive system that employs a feedback cycle of input (stimuli), throughput (control processes), and output (behaviors or adaptive responses).

Watson's Human Caring Theory

- ❖ Jean Watson (1979) believes the practice of caring is central to nursing; it is the unifying focus for practice.
- ❖ Nursing interventions related to human care are referred to as carative factors.
- ❖ Watson's theory of human caring has receiving worldwide recognition and is a major force in redefining nursing as a caring-healing health model.

Parse's Human Becoming Theory

Parse's model of human becoming emphasizes how individuals choose and bear responsibility for patterns of personal health.

Leininger's Cultural Care Diversity and Universality Theory

She emphasizes that human caring, although a universal phenomenon, varies among cultures in its expressions, processes, and patterns; it is largely culturally derived.

Orem's General Theory of Nursing

Assessing

Involves collecting data about the client's capacities (knowledge, skills, and motivation) to perform universal, developmental, and health-deviation self-care requisites. Determine self-care deficits.

Diagnosing

Stated in terms of the client's limitations for maintaining self-care (a deficit in self-care agency).

Planning

Involves considering and designing, with the client's participation, an appropriate nursing system (wholly compensatory, partially compensatory, supportive-educative, or a mix) that will help the client achieve an optimal level of self, care.

Implementing

Assisting the patient

Evaluating

Determining the client's level of achievement.

NURSING THEORISTS

Definitions

- ❖ **Theory:** A set of related statements that describes or explains phenomena in a systematic way.
- ❖ **Concept:** A mental idea of a phenomenon.
- ❖ **Construct:** A phenomena that cannot be observed and must be inferred.
- ❖ **Proposition:** A statement of relationship between concepts.
- ❖ **Conceptual model:** It made up of concepts and propositions.

Nursing Theorists

- ❖ Florence Nightingale
- ❖ Hildegard Peplau
- ❖ Virginia Henderson
- ❖ Fay Abdella
- ❖ Ida Jean Orlando
- ❖ Dorothy Johnson
- ❖ Martha Rogers
- ❖ Dorothea Orem
- ❖ Imogene King
- ❖ Betty Neuman
- ❖ Sister Calista Roy
- ❖ Jean Watson
- ❖ Rosemary Rizzo Parse
- ❖ Madeleine Leininger
- ❖ Patricia Benner

CONCEPTS IN THE NURSING

Metaparadigm

- ❖ **Person**
  - ◆ Recipient of care, including physical, spiritual, psychological, and sociocultural components.
  - ◆ Individual, family, or community.
- ❖ **Environment:** All internal and external conditions, circumstances, and influences affecting the person.
- ❖ **Health:** Degree of wellness or illness experienced by the person.
- ❖ **Nursing:** Actions, characteristics and attributes of person giving care.

Florence Nightingale: Environmental Theory

- ❖ First nursing theorist
- ❖ Unsanitary conditions posed health hazard (Notes on Nursing, 1859)

- ❖ Five components of environment:
  - ◆ Ventilation, light, warmth, effluvia, noise.
- ❖ External influences can prevent, suppress or contribute to disease or death.

Nightingale's Concepts

- ❖ **Person**
  - ◆ Patient who is acted on by nurse
  - ◆ Affected by environment
  - ◆ Has reparative powers
- ❖ **Environment:** Foundation of theory. Included everything, physical, psychological, and social.
- ❖ **Health**
  - ◆ Maintaining well-being by using a person's powers
  - ◆ Maintained by control of environment
- ❖ **Nursing:** Provided fresh air, warmth, cleanliness, good diet, quiet to facilitate person's reparative process

Hildegard Peplau: Interpersonal Relations Model

- ❖ Based on psychodynamic nursing
- ❖ Using an understanding of one's own behavior to help others identify their difficulties
- ❖ Applies principles of human relations
- ❖ Patient has a felt need

Peplau's Concepts

- ❖ **Person**
  - ◆ An individual; a developing organism who tries to reduce anxiety caused by needs
  - ◆ Lives in instable equilibrium
- ❖ **Environment:** Not defined
- ❖ **Health:** Implies forward movement of the personality and human processes toward creative, constructive, productive, personal, and community living.
- ❖ **Nursing**
  - ◆ A significant, therapeutic, interpersonal process that functions cooperatively with others to make health possible.
  - ◆ Involves problem-solving

Virginia Henderson: The Nature of Nursing

The unique function of the nurse is to assist the individual, sick or well, in the performance of those activities contributing to health or its recovery (or to peaceful death) that he would perform unaided if he had the necessary strength, will, or knowledge. And to do this in such a way as to help him gain independence as rapidly as possible. She must in a sense, get inside the skin of each of her patients in order to know what he needs.

Fay Abdella: Topology of 21 Nursing Problems

- ❖ A list of 21 nursing problems
- ❖ Condition presented or faced by the patient or family.

* Problems are in three categories
  * Physical, social and emotional
* The nurse must be a good problem solver.

Abdella's Concepts

* **Nursing**
  * A helping profession
  * A comprehensive service to meet patient's needs
  * Increases or restores self-help ability
  * Uses 21 problems to guide nursing care
* **Health**
  * Excludes illness
  * No unmet needs and no actual or anticipated impairments
* **Person**
  * One who has physical, emotional, or social needs
  * The recipient of nursing care.
* **Environment**
  * Did not discuss much
  * Includes room, home, and community

Ida Jean Orland: Deliberative Nursing Process

* The deliberative nursing process is set in motion by the patient's behavior.
* All behavior may represent a cry for help. Patient's behavior can be verbal or nonverbal.
* The nurse reacts to patient's behavior and forms basis for determining nurse's acts.
* Perception, thought, feeling
* Nurses' actions should be deliberative, rather than automatic.
* Deliberative actions explore the meaning and relevance of an action.

Dorothy Johnson: Behavioral Systems Model

* The person is a behavioral system comprised of a set of organized, interactive, interdependent, and integrated subsystems.
* Constancy is maintained through biological, psychological, and sociological factors.
* A steady state is maintained through adjusting and adapting to internal and external forces.

Johnson's 7 Subsystems

* Affiliative subsystem
  * Social bonds
* Dependency
  * Helping or nurturing
* Ingestive
  * Food intake
* Eliminative
  * Excretion
* Sexual
  * Procreation and gratification

- ❖ Aggressive
  - Self-protection and preservation
- ❖ Achievement
  - Efforts to gain mastery and control

Johnson's Concepts

- ❖ **Person:** A behavioral system comprised of subsystems constantly trying to maintain a steady state.
- ❖ **Environment:** Not specifically defined but does say there is an internal and external environment.
- ❖ **Health:** Balance and stability.
- ❖ **Nursing:** External regulatory force that is indicated only when there is instability.

Martha Rogers: Unitary Human Beings

- ❖ **Energy fields**
  - Fundamental unity of things that are unique, dynamic, open, and infinite.
  - Unitary man and environmental field
- ❖ **Universe of open systems:** Energy fields are open, infinite, and interactive.
- ❖ **Pattern:**
  - Characteristic of energy field
  - A wave that changes, becomes complex and diverse
- ❖ **Pandimensionality:** A nonlinear domain with out time or space.

Roger's Definitions

- ❖ **Integrality:** Continuous and mutual interaction between man and environment.
- ❖ **Resonancy:** Continuous change longer to shorter wave patterns in human and environmental fields
- ❖ **Helicy**
  - Continuous, probabilistic, increasing diversity of the human and environmental fields.
  - Characterized by nonrepeating rhythmicity
  - Change

Dorothea Orem: Self-care Model

- ❖ Self-care comprises those activities performed independently by an individual to promote and maintain person well-being.
- ❖ Self-care agency is the individual's ability to perform self-care activities.
- ❖ Self-care deficit occurs when the person cannot carry out self-care.
- ❖ The nurse then meets the self-care needs by acting or doing for; guiding, teaching, supporting or providing the environment to promote patient's ability.
- ❖ Wholly compensatory nursing system: Patient dependent.
- ❖ Partially compensatory: Patient can meet some needs but needs nursing assistance.
- ❖ Supportive educative: Patient can meet self-care requisites, but needs assistance with decision making or knowledge.

Imogene King: Goal Attainment Theory

- Open systems framework
- Human beings are open systems in constant interaction with the environment
- **Personal system:** Individual; perception, self-growth, development, time space, body image.
- **Interpersonal:** Socialization; interaction, communication and transaction.
- **Society:** Family, religious groups, schools, work, peers.
- The nurse and patient mutually communicate, establish goals and take action to attain goals.
- Each individual brings a different set of values, ideas, attitudes, perceptions to exchange.

Betty Neuman: Health Care Systems Model

- The person is a complete system, with interrelated parts.
- Maintains balance and harmony between internal and external environment by adjusting to stress and defending against tension-producing stimuli.
- Focuses on stress and stress reduction
- Primarily concerned with effects of stress on health
- Stressors are any forces that alter the system's stability
- Flexible lines of resistance
  - Surround basic core
  - Internal factors that help defend against stressors
- Normal line of resistance
  - Normal adaptation state
- Flexible line of defense
  - Protective barrier, changing, affected by variables
- Wellness is equilibrium
- Nursing interventions are activates to:
  - Strengthen flexible lines of defense
  - Strengthen resistance to stressors
  - Maintain adaptation

Sister Calista Roy: Adaptation Model

- Five interrelated essential elements:
  1. *Patiency:* The person receiving care
  2. *Goal of nursing:* Adapting to change
  3. *Health:* Being and becoming a whole person
  4. *Environment*
  5. *Direction of nursing activities:* Facilitating adaptation
- The person is an open adaptive system with input (stimuli), who adapts by processes or control mechanisms (throughput).
- The output can be either adaptive responses or ineffective responses.

Jean Watson: Philosophy and Science of Caring

- Caring can be demonstrated and practiced
- Caring consists of carative factors
- Caring promotes growth
- A caring environment accepts a person as he is and looks to what the person may become.

* A caring environment offers development of potential
* Caring promotes health better than curing
* Caring is central to nursing

Watson's 10 Carative Factors

* Forming humanistic—altruistic value system
* Instilling faith—hope
* Cultivating sensitivity to self and others
* Developing helping—trust relationship
* Promoting expression of feelings
* Using problem—solving for decision making
* Promoting teaching—learning
* Promoting supportive environment
* Assisting with gratification of human needs
* Allowing for existential—phenomenological forces

Watson's Concepts

* **Person:** Human being to be valued, cared for, respected, nurtured, understood and assisted.
* **Environment:** Society.
* **Health:** Complete physical, mental and social well-being and functioning.
* **Nursing:** Concerned with promoting and restoring health, preventing illness.

Rosemary Parse: Human Becoming Theory

Human becoming theory includes:
* **Totality paradigm:** Man is a combination of biological, psychological, sociological and spiritual factors
* **Simultaneity paradigm:** Man is a unitary being in continuous, mutual interaction with environment
* Originally Man-Living-Health Theory

Parse's Three Principles

* **Meaning**
  * Man's reality is given meaning through lived experiences
  * Man and environment cocreate
* **Rhythmicity**
  * Man and environment cocreate (imaging, valuing, languaging) in rhythmical patterns
* **Cotranscendence**
  * Refers to reaching out and beyond the limits that a person sets
  * One constantly transforms
* **Person:** Open being who is more than and different from the sum of the parts
* **Environment**
  * Everything in the person and his experiences
  * Inseparable, complimentary to and evolving with
* **Health:** Open process of being and becoming involves synthesis of values.
* **Nursing:** A human science and art that uses an abstract body of knowledge to serve people.

Madeleine Leininger: Culture Care Diversity and Universality

* Based on transcultural nursing, whose goal is to provide care congruent with cultural values, beliefs, and practices.
* Sunrise model consists of four levels that provide a base of knowledge for delivering cultural congruent care:
  * Modes of nursing action
  * *Cultural care preservation:* Help maintain or preserve health, recover from illness, or face death.
  * *Cultural care accommodation:* Help adapt to or negotiate for a beneficial health status, or face death.
  * *Cultural care re-patterning:* Help restructure or change lifestyles that are culturally meaningful.

Patricia Benner: From Novice to Expert

* Described five levels of nursing experience and developed exemplars and paradigm cases to illustrate each level
* Levels reflect:
  * Movement from reliance on past abstract principles to the use of past concrete experience as paradigms.
  * Change in perception of situation as a complete whole in which certain parts are relevant
    * Novice
    * Advanced beginner
    * Competent
    * Proficient
    * Expert

IMPORTANCE OF THEORETICAL FRAMEWORKS

* Foundation of any profession is the development of a specialized body of knowledge. Theories should be developed in nursing, not borrow theories form other disciplines.
* Responsibility of nurses to know and understand theorists.
* Critically analyze theoretical frameworks

APPLICATION OF THEORY IN NURSING PROCESS

Introduction

Theories are a set of interrelated concepts that give a systematic view of a phenomenon (an observable fact or event) that is explanatory and predictive in nature. Theories are composed of concepts, definitions, models, propositions and are based on assumptions. They are derived through two principal methods; deductive reasoning and inductive reasoning.

Objectives

* To assess the patient condition by the various methods explained by the nursing theory.
* To identify the needs of the patient.
* To demonstrate an effective communication and interaction with the patient.
* To select a theory for the application according to the need of the patient.

❖ To apply the theory to solve the identified problems of the patient.

❖ To evaluate the extent to which the process was fruitful.

Definition

Nursing theory is an organized and systematic articulation of a set of statements related to questions in the discipline of nursing. A nursing theory is a set of concepts, definitions, relationships, and assumptions or propositions derived from nursing models or from other disciplines and project a purposive, systematic view of phenomena by designing specific inter-relationships among concepts for the purposes of describing, explaining, predicting, and/or prescribing.

Importance of Nursing Theories

❖ Nursing theory aims to describe, predict and explain the phenomenon of nursing.

❖ It should provide the foundations of nursing practice, help to generate further knowledge and indicate in which direction nursing should develop in the future.

❖ Theory is important because it helps us to decide what we know and what we need to know.

❖ It helps to distinguish what should form the basis of practice by explicitly describing nursing.

❖ The benefits of having a defined body of theory in nursing include better patient care, enhanced professional status for nurses, improved communication between nurses, and guidance for research and education.

❖ The main exponent of nursing-caring-cannot be measured, it is vital to have the theory to analyze and explain what nurses do.

❖ As medicine tries to make a move towards adopting a more multidisciplinary approach to healthcare, nursing continues to strive to establish a unique body of knowledge.

❖ This can be seen as an attempt by the nursing profession to maintain its professional boundaries.

Characteristics of Theories

❖ Interrelating concepts in such a way as to create a different way of looking at a particular phenomenon.

❖ Logical in nature.

❖ Generalizable.

❖ Bases for hypotheses that can be tested.

❖ Increasing the general body of knowledge within the discipline through the research implemented to validate them.

❖ Used by the practitioners to guide and improve their practice.

❖ Consistent with other validated theories, laws, and principles but will leave open unanswered questions that need to be investigated.

Purposes of Theory in Practice

❖ Assist nurses to describe, explain, and predict everyday experiences.

❖ Serve to guide assessment, intervention, and evaluation of nursing care.

❖ Provide a rationale for collecting reliable and valid data about the health status of clients, which are essential for effective decision making and implementation.

* Help to establish criteria to measure the quality of nursing care.
* Help build a common nursing terminology to use in communicating with other health professionals. Ideas are developed and words defined.
* Enhance autonomy (independence and self-governance) of nursing by defining its own independent functions.

If theory is expected to benefit practice, it must be developed co-operatively with people who practice nursing. People who do research and develop theories think differently about theory when they perceive the reality of practice. Theories do not provide the same type of procedural guidelines for practice as do situation-specific principles and procedures or rules. Procedural rules or principles help to standardize nursing practice and can also be useful in achieving minimum goals of quality of care. Theory is ought to improve the nursing practice. One of the most common ways theory has been organized in practice is in the nursing process of analyzing assessment data.

THEORIES AND NURSING RESEARCH

Introduction

* **Research:** Process of inquiry
* **Theory:** Product of knowledge
* **Science:** Result of the relationship between research and theory.
* To effectively build knowledge to research process should be developed within some theoretical structure that facilities analysis and interpretation of findings.
* Relationship between theory and research in nursing is not well understood. It may be give to the relative youth of the discipline and debates over philosophical world views (empiricism, constructivism, etc.)

Need to Link Theory and Research

* Research without theory results in discreet information or data which does not add to the accumulated knowledge of the discipline.
* Theory guides the research process, forms the research questions, aids in design, analysis and interpretation.
* It enables the scientist to weave the facts together.

Theories from Nursing or other Disciplines?

* Nursing science is blend of knowledge that is unique to nursing and knowledge that is borrowed from other disciplines.
* Debate is whether the use of borrowed theory has hindered the development of the discipline.
* It has contributed to problems connecting research and theory in nursing.

Historical Overview of Research and Theory in Nursing

* Florence Nightingale supported her theoretical propositions through research, as statistical data and prepared graphs were used to depict the impact of nursing care on the health of British soldiers.

- ❖ Afterwards, for almost century reports of nursing research were rare.
- ❖ Research and theory developed separately in nursing.
- ❖ Between 1928 and 1959 only 2 out of 152 studies reported a theoretical basis for the research design.
- ❖ In 1970's growing number of nurse theorists were seeking researchers to test their models in research and clinical application.
- ❖ Grand nursing theories are still not widely used. In 1990's borrowed theories were used more.
- ❖ Now the focus of research and theory have moved more towards middle range theories.

Purpose of Theory in Research

- ❖ To identify meaningful and relevant areas for study.
- ❖ To propose plausible approaches to health problems.
- ❖ To develop or refine theories.
- ❖ Define the concepts and proposed relationships between concepts.
- ❖ To interpret research findings.
- ❖ To develop clinical practice protocols.
- ❖ Generate nursing diagnosis.

Types of Theory and Corresponding Research

Type of theory	Type of research
• Descriptive • Explanatory • Predictive	• Descriptive or explanatory • Co-relational • Experimental

How Theory is used in Research

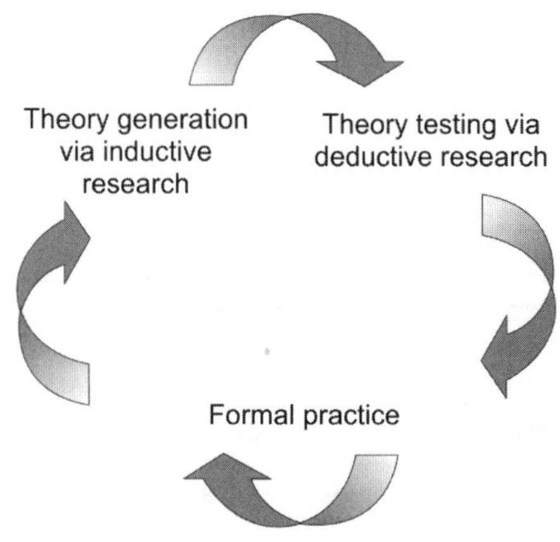

Theories used in research.

Causal Theory of Planned Behavior

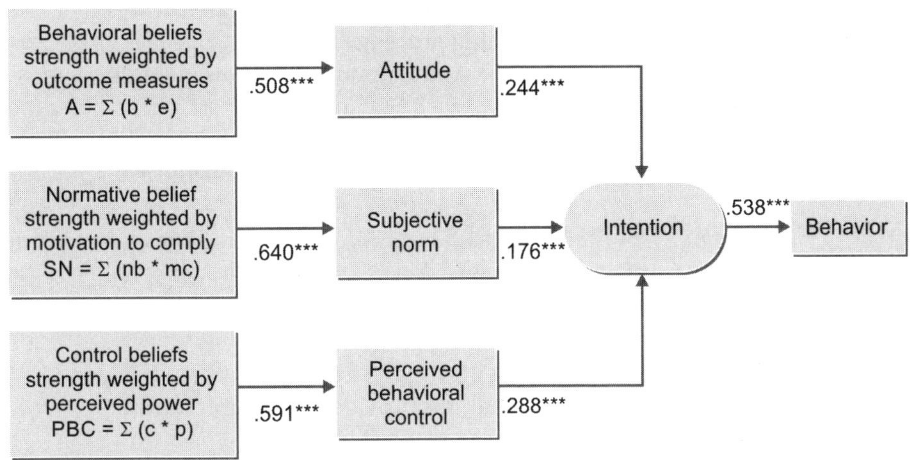

Causal theory of planned behavior.

Theory Generating Research

❖ It is designed to develop and describe relationships between and among phenomena without imposing preconceived notations.
❖ It is inductive and includes field observations and phenomenology.
❖ During the theory generating process, the researcher moves by logical thought from fact to theory by means of a proposition stated as an empirical generalization.

Grounded Theory Research

❖ Inductive research technique developed by Glazer and Strauss (1967).
❖ Grounded theory provides a way to describe what is happening and understanding the process of why it happens.
❖ **Methodology:** The researcher observes, collects data, organizes data and forms theory from the data at the same time.
❖ Data may be collected by interview, observation, records or a combination of these techniques.
❖ Data are coded in preparation for analysis.
❖ **Category development:** Categories are identified and named.
❖ **Category saturation:** Comparison of similar characteristics in each of the categories.
❖ **Concept development:** Defines the categories.
❖ **Search for additional categories:** Continues to examine the data for additional categories.
❖ **Category reduction:** Higher order categories are selected.
❖ **Linking of categories:** The researcher seeks to understand relationships among categories.
❖ Selective sampling of the literature.
❖ **Emergence of the core variable:** Central theme is focus of the theory.
❖ Concept modification and integration – Explaining the phenomenal.

Theory Testing Research

* In theory testing research, theoretical statements are translated into questions and hypothesis. It requires a deductive reasoning process.
* The interpretation determines whether the study supports are contradicts the propositional statement.
* If a conceptual model is used as a theoretical framework for research it is not theory testing.
* Theory testing requires detailed examination of theoretical relationships.

Theory as a Conceptual Framework

* Problem being investigated is fit into an existing theoretical framework, which guides the study and enriches the value of its findings.
* The conceptual definitions are drawn from the framework.
* The data collection instrument is congruent with the framework.
* Findings are interpreted in light of explanations provided by the framework.
* Implications are based on the explanatory power of a framework.

A Typology of Research

* Testing
* Analyzing
* Experimentation
* Deducting
* Deductive research
* Quantitative research
* The scientific method
* Theory/hypothesis testing
* Assaying
* Refining
* Interpreting
* Reflecting
* Inducing
* Inductive research
* Qualitative research
* Phenomenological research
* Theory generation
* 'Divining'; 'heuristic' research

Guidelines for Writing about a Research Study's Theoretical Framework

In the study's problem statement:
* Introduce the framework
* Briefly explain why it is a good fit for the research problem area
* At the end of the literature review
* Thoroughly describe the framework and explain its application to the present study.
* Describe how the framework has been used in studies about similar problems.
* In the study's methodology section.

❖ Explain how the framework is being operationalized in the study's design.
❖ Explain how data collection methods (such as questionnaire items) reflect the concepts in the framework.
❖ In the study's discussion section
❖ Describe how study findings are consistent (or inconsistent) with the framework.
❖ Offer suggestions for practice and further research that are congruent with the framework's concepts and propositions.

Conclusion

The relationship between research and theory is undeniable, and it is important to recognize the impact of this relationships on the development of nursing knowledge. So interface theory and research by generating theories, testing the theories and by using it as a conceptual framework that drives the study.

NIGHTINGALE'S ENVIRONMENTAL THEORY

Introduction

Nightingale was born in 1820 in Florence, Italy. Her greatest achievement was the establishment of the **concept of formal preparation for the practice of nursing;** the profession of nursing started with her commitment to the care of the sick.

She is considered the first nursing theorist, although her writings differ in form, tone, terminology and style from those of contemporary theorists. Miss nightingale fame spread rapidly after she and a group of devoted women cared for the sick during the Crimean war.

Nightingale's Environmental Theory of Nursing

The core concept that is most reflective of Nightingale's writings is that of the foundation of night theory is environment. It is understandable that she, having witnessed in the early 1850s the filth, vermin and death within an enormous barracks hospital, would focus so heavily on improving the environment to assist soldiers to merely survive. Through such an emphasis, the death rate went from staggering 42 per 100 to a low of 22 per 1,000.

This success gave her a strong data base on which to view nursing in her own unique way.

The environment is viewed as all the external conditions and influences affecting the life and development of an organism and capable of preventing, suppressing or contributing to disease or death.

Her goal was to help the patient retain his own vitality by meeting his basic needs through control of the environment.

At this point it is helpful to think of a patient who has had surgery, such as an appendectomy, and relate what Nightingale proposes. Medicine is seen as functioning to remove the diseased part, whereas nursing places the patient in an environment in which nature can assist postoperative patients to reach their optimum health conditions. This approach to nursing is as valid today as it was over 100 years ago, in spite of the fact that both in home and in hospitals the environment today is more sophisticated in structure.

Nightingale described five major components of a positive or health fuel environment:
1. Ventilation, especially with increased fresh air, provided without drafts, is of primary importance, corrupt, stagnant and musty air breeds disease. An outlet is needed for impure air.

2. Light, refers to sunlight for the most part, and is secondary. Beds should be placed in such a position as to allow the patient to see out the window, the sky and sunlight.
3. Warmth, noise and effluvia (smell) are seen as areas in which attention must be given in order to provide a positive environment.
    - *WNoise:* Intermittent sudden noise causes greater excitement them continuous noise, especially during the patient's first sleep. The more the patient sleeps peacefully, the greater his ability to sleep will be.
    - *Effluvia (smell):* Care is needed to get rid of noxious body odor caused by disease.

Situation

Mrs Anderson, a public health nurse has just visited Mrs Rose, an 80-year-old arthritis patient who lives alone in a small rural community. Since Mrs Rose has difficulty ambulating, her neighbors visit her often to assist her in any way they can. One of these neighbors requested Mrs Anderson visit to assess the situation.

On entering Mrs Rose's home, Mrs Anderson was made aware of the lack of fresh air, the darkness in the environment caused by old dusty drapes covering the windows and a draft in the bedroom. Mrs Rose was found sitting in an old chair that provided little or no view of the world around her.

After her visit, Mrs Anderson contacted Mrs Rose's neighbors to set up a plan to improve her environment. The drapes were to be removed and replaced by simple curtains that would let the morning sun enter the home. The windows were to be opened in keeping with the weather during specific periods of the day, with care given to reduce drafts. Mrs Rose's favorite chair was to be placed in such a way that she could look out the window to watch the neighbors coming and going.

This example is not to be viewed as offering a complete assessment of Mrs Rose, but out point out how nightingale's basic environmental concept, interrelated with the nursing process, can give as specific directions.

Nightingale discussed three types of environment:
1. Physical environment
2. Psychological
3. Social environment

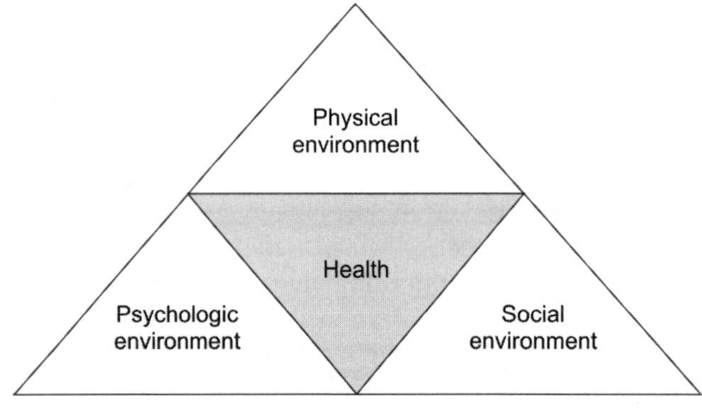

Types of environment.

Physical Environment

Consists of physical elements where the patient is being treated, such as ventilation, warmth, cleanliness, light, noise and drainage.

These basic factor affect one's approach to all other aspects of the environment. Cleanliness is an encompassing notion related to all aspects of the physical environment in which the patient is found. The walls and entire room should not be dusty, smoky or have a close odor.

A patient's bed must be clean, aired, warm, dry and free from odor. One should provide an environment in which the patient can be easily cared for by others or self. The width, height and placement of the bed should facilitate the activities of the patient. The bed should be placed in the best lighted spot, away from sudden noises and the odor of drainage. The position of the patient on the bed should be viewed in the context of the supporting ventilation.

Psychological Environment

The effect of the mind on the body was fairly will accepted in Nightingale's time. Nightingale recognize that a negative environment could cause physical stress, thereby affecting the emotional climate. Therefore, emphasis is placed on offering the patient a variety of activities to keep his mind stimulated. The view of sunlight, the attractiveness of the food and the offering the patient to survive emotionally. Boredom is viewed as painful.

Communication with the patient is viewed in the context of the total environment. Communication should not be hurried or allow for interruptions. When speaking with patients, it is important to sit down in front of them, unless other activities such as eating are occurring.

The place one communicates with the physician and family about the patient is in the context of the environment of the patient. Outside the patient's rooms or within their hearing distance is viewed as inappropriate.

Social Environment

- ❖ Involves collecting data illness and disease prevention.
- ❖ Includes such components of the physical environment as clean air, water and proper drainage.
- ❖ Consists of a person's home or hospital room, as well as the total community that affects the patient's specific environment.

Nightingale's Theory and the Four Major Concepts

The environment affects the human condition, with nursing having the role of affecting that environment, so that health/disease becomes a reparative process.

Each of the major concepts imparts on the others. Nursing functions to influence the human environment to affect health. The individual is affected by the environment and by the nurse who influences his/her health. Society/environment has an impact on the nurse and on the health of the individual. Health is a process affected by nursing and by environment and human conditions.

The following list reflects Nightingale view of the major concepts:

1. **Human or individual**
   - Referred to by Nightingale as the 'patient' in most of her writings.
   - Person is a human being acted upon by a nurse or affected by the environment.
   - Nightingale envisioned the person as comprising physical, intellectual, emotional, social and spiritual components.
   - Person has reparative powers to deal with disease; recovery is within the patient's power as long as a safe environment for recuperation exists.

2. **Nursing**
   - Is a discipline distinct from medicine focusing on the person experiencing a reparative process rather than on the disease of an anatomical structure or the person's physiology.
   - Nightingale believed nursing to be a spiritual calling. The saw nursing as the "science of environmental management."
   - Aims to provide fresh air, light, warmth, cleanliness, quiet and a proper diet.

3. **Environment:** Defined as anything that can be manipulated to place a patient in the best possible condition for nature to act. Involve those external conditions that affect life and development of the individual. The focus is on ventilated, warmth, odors, noise and light.
   - Serves as the foundation of night theory.
   - Includes everything form person's food to a nurses verbal and nonverbal interactions in the person.

4. **Health:**
   - Is maintained by controlling environmental factors to prevent disease; health and disease are the focus of the nurse, who helps a person through the healing process.
   - Nightingale wrote "Health is not to be well, but to be able to use well every power we have."
   - Form this statement, we can infer that she believed in prevention and health promotion to nursing patients from illness to health.

Nightingale's Work and the Characteristics of a Theory

Nightingale theory of nursing has its strength and weakness in relation to the characteristics of a sound theory.

- Theories can interrelate concepts in such a way as to create a different way of looking at a particular phenomenon:
  - As mentioned earlier, the four major concepts are not explicit in Nightingale's theory and yet they do offer nursing a specific way of looking at a particular phenomenon.
  - The theory offer a prediction in relation to the outcomes of nursing care. Creating a positive environment will allow humans to become healthy. Yet we know today that although the human environment in critical in relation to health, other variables such as genetics are also very significant.
- **Theories must be logical in nature:** The relationship between each of the concepts is logical and consistent with similar assumptions. The assumption that the environment affects humans is consistent within Nightingale's explanation of the purpose and goal of nursing and the meaning of health.
- Theories should be relatively simple yet generalizable:
  Nightingale's theory, although limited, has a lot of generalizability. It can be utilized in any environment such as hospitals, nursing homes, schools, the individual's home, or wherever

human beings may be found. The ideas are also basically simple to apply and easy to measure in terms of outcomes.

❖ Theories can be the bases for hypothesis that can be tested.
❖ Theories contribute to and assist in increasing the general body of knowledge within the discipline through the research implemented to validate them.
❖ Theories can be utilized by the practitioners to guide and improve their practice.
❖ Theories must be consistent with other validated theories, laws and principles but will leave open unanswered questions that need to be investigated.

Due to their similarity, these last four characteristics will be discussed together as they relate to Nightingale's theory. In spite of the simplicity and generalizability of her theory. Nursing has not yet adequately incorporated much of it into practice or research.

For example, in a way, her theory has been researched by scientists such as environmentalists. That is, we are increasingly becoming aware of how environmental pollution affects our health in a negative way. From a broad perspective this theory should give validity. However, we have not yet adequately validated the theory within the context for the healthcare and nursing environment.

Research questions that can lead to hypothesis need to be tested within clinical nursing. For instance, what effect does the hospital environment have on the pace of the healing process? Do the nurses have the authority to impact on the patient's environment adequately? Do sudden, frequent environmental changes affect patient's perceptions of their reparative process? These are only a few of the many possible questions that can be used to guide research. The answers to these questions could well be used to develop guidelines for nursing education and practice.

THEORY OF INTERPERSONAL RELATIONS

Hildegard Peplau was a nursing theorist who published the theory of interpersonal relations in 1952.

Introduction

❖ Born in Reading, Pennsylvania (1909)
❖ Graduated from a diploma program in Pottstown, Pennsylvania in 1931.
❖ Done BA in interpersonal psychology from Bennington College in 1943.
❖ MA in psychiatric nursing from Columbia University New York in 1947.
❖ EdD in curriculum development in 1953.
❖ Professor Emeritus from Rutgers University.
❖ Started first Post-Baccalaureate program in nursing.
❖ Published Interpersonal Relations in Nursing in 1952.
❖ 1968:Interpersonal techniques—the crux of psychiatric nursing.
❖ Worked as executive director and president of ANA.
❖ Worked with WHO, NIMH and nurse corps.
❖ Died in 1999.

Psychodynamic Nursing

❖ Understanding of ones own behavior
❖ To help others identify felt difficulties
❖ To apply principles of human relations to the problems that arise at all levels of experience.

* In her book she discussed the phases of interpersonal process, roles in nursing situations and methods for studying nursing as an interpersonal process.
* According to Peplau, nursing is therapeutic in that it is a healing art, assisting an individual who is sick or in need of healthcare.
* Nursing is an interpersonal process because it involves interaction between two or more individuals with a common goal.
* The attainment of goal is achieved through the use of a series of steps following a series of pattern.
* The nurse and patient work together so both become mature and knowledgeable in the process.

Definitions

* **Person:** A developing organism that tries to reduce anxiety caused by needs
* **Environment:** Existing forces outside the organism and in the context of culture
* **Health:** A word symbol that implies forward movement of personality and other ongoing human processes in the direction of creative, constructive, productive, personal and community living.
* **Nursing:** A significant therapeutic interpersonal process. It functions cooperatively with other human process that make health possible for individuals in communities.

Roles of Nurse

* **Stranger:** Receives the client in the same way one meets a stranger in other life situations provides an accepting climate that builds trust.
* **Teacher:** Who imparts knowledge in reference to a need or interest.
* **Resource person:** One who provides a specific needed information that aids in the understanding of a problem or new situation.
* **Counselors:** Helps to understand and integrate the meaning of current life circumstances, provides guidance and encouragement to make changes.
* **Surrogate:** Helps to clarify domains of dependence interdependence and independence and acts on clients behalf as an advocate.
* **Leader:** Helps client assume maximum responsibility for meeting treatment goals in a mutually satisfying way.

Additional roles include:

* Technical expert
* Consultant
* Health teacher
* Tutor
* Socializing agent
* Safety agent
* Manager of environment
* Mediator
* Administrator
* Recorder observer
* Researcher

Theory of Interpersonal Relations

* Middle range descriptive classification theory.
* Influenced by Harry Stack Sullivan's theory of interpersonal relations (1953).
* Also influenced by Percival Symonds, Abraham Maslow's and Neal Elger Miller.
* Identified four sequential phases in the interpersonal relationship:
  1. Orientation
  2. Identification
  3. Exploitation
  4. Resolution

Orientation Phase

* Problem defining phase
* Starts when client meets nurse as stranger
* Defining problem and deciding type of service needed
* Client seeks assistance, conveys needs, asks questions, shares preconceptions and expectations of past experiences.
* Nurse responds, explains roles to client, helps to identify problems and to use available resources and services.

Factors Influencing Orientation Phase

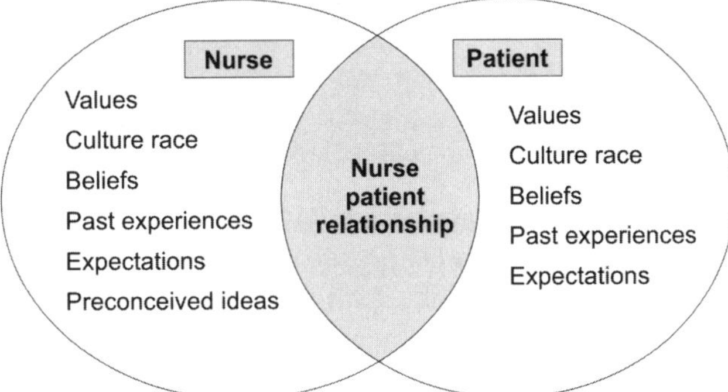

Nurse-patient relationship in orientation phase.

Identification Phase

* Selection of appropriate professional assistance.
* Patient begins to have a feeling of belonging and a capability of dealing with the problem which decreases the feeling of helplessness and hopelessness.

Exploitation Phase

* Use of professional assistance for problem solving alternatives.
* Advantages of services are used is based on the needs and interests of the patients.
* Individual feels as an integral part of the helping environment.
* They may make minor requests or attention getting techniques.
* The principles of interview techniques must be used in order to explore, understand and adequately deal with the underlying problem.
* Patient may fluctuates on independence

❖ Nurse must be aware about the various phases of communication.

❖ Nurse aids the patient in exploiting all avenues of help and progress is made towards the final step.

Resolution Phase

❖ Termination of professional relationship

❖ The patients needs have already been met by the collaborative effect of patient and nurse.

❖ Now they need to terminate their therapeutic relationship and dissolve the links between them.

❖ Sometimes may be difficult for both as psychological dependence persists.

❖ Patient drifts away and breaks bond with nurse and healthier emotional balance is demonstrated and both becomes mature individuals.

Interpersonal Theory and Nursing Process

❖ Both are sequential and focus on therapeutic relationship.

❖ Both use problem solving techniques for the nurse and patient to collaborate on, with the end purpose of meeting the patients needs.

❖ Both use observation communication and recording as basic tools utilized by nursing.

Interpersonal theory and nursing process.	
Assessment • Data collection and analysis (continuous) • May not be a felt need	**Orientation** • Noncontinuous data collection • Felt need • Define needs
Nursing diagnosis • Planning • Mutually set goals	**Identification** Interdependent goal setting
Implementation • Plans initiated towards achievement of mutually set goals • May be accomplished by patient, nurse or family	**Exploitation** • Patient actively seeking and drawing help • Patient initiated
Evaluation • Based on mutually expected behaviors • May led to termination and initiation of new plans	**Resolution** • Occurs after other phases are completed successfully • Leads to termination

Peplau's Work and Characteristics of a Theory

❖ Theories can interrelate concepts in such a way as to create a different way of looking at a particular phenomenon.

    ◆ Four phases interrelate the different components of each phase.

    ◆ The nurse patient interaction can apply to the concepts of human being, health, environment and nursing.

❖ Theories must be logical in nature

    ◆ Provides a logical systematic way of viewing nursing situations

    ◆ Key concepts such as anxiety, tension, goals, and frustration are indicated with explicit relationships among them and progressive phases

❖ Theories should be relatively simple yet generalizable

    ◆ It provides simplicity in regard to the natural progression of the NP relationship.

    ◆ Leads to adaptability in any nurse patient relationship.

    ◆ The basic nature of nursing still considered an interpersonal process.

❖ Theories can be the bases for hypothesis that can be tested.
  ◆ Has generated testable hypotheses.
  ◆ Theories contribute to and assist in increasing the general body of knowledge within the discipline through the research implemented to validate them.
  ◆ In 1950's two third of the nursing research concentrated on N-P relationship.
❖ Theories can be utilized by practitioners to guide and improve their practice.
  ◆ Peplau's anxiety continuum is still used in anxiety patients.
❖ Theories must be consistent with other validated theories, laws, and principles but will leave open unanswered questions that need to be investigated.
  ◆ Consistent with various theories

Limitations

❖ Intra family dynamics, personal space considerations and community social service resources are considered less.
❖ Health promotion and maintenance were less emphasized.
❖ Cannot be used in a patient who doesn't have a felt need, e.g., with drawn patients, unconscious patients.
❖ Some areas are not specific enough to generate hypothesis.

Research Based on Peplau's Theory

❖ **Hays (1961):** Phases and steps of experimental teaching to patients of a concept of anxiety: Findings revealed that when taught by the experimental method, the patients were able to apply the concept of anxiety after the group was terminated.
❖ **Burd SF:** Develop and test a nursing intervention framework for working with anxious patients: Students developed competency in beginning interpersonal relationship.

APPLICATION OF INTERPERSONAL THEORY IN NURSING PRACTICE

Introduction

Peplau's theory focuses on the interpersonal processes and therapeutic relationship that develops between the nurse and client. The interpersonal focus of Peplau's theory requires that the nurse attend to the interpersonal processes that occur between the nurse and client. Interpersonal process is maturing force for personality. Interpersonal processes include the nurse-client relationship, communication, pattern integration and the roles of the nurse. Psychodynamic nursing is being able to understand one's own behavior to help others identify felt difficulties and to apply principles of human relations to the problems that arise at all levels of experience. This theory stressed the importance of nurses' ability to understand own behavior to help others identify perceived difficulties.

The four phases of nurse-patient relationships are:
1. **Orientation:** During this phase, the individual has a *felt need* and seeks professional assistance. The nurse helps the individual to recognize and understand his/her problem and determine the need for help.
2. **Identification:** The patient identifies with those who can help him/her. The nurse permits exploration of feelings to aid the patient in undergoing illness as an experience that reorients feelings and strengthens positive forces in the personality and provides needed satisfaction.

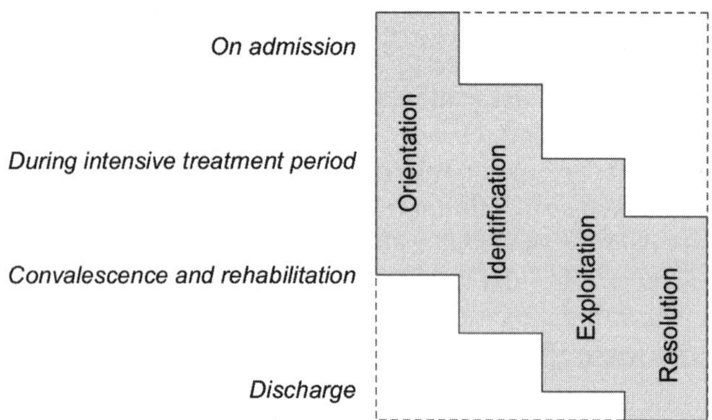

Overlapping phases in Nurse-Patient relationship.

3. **Exploitation:** During this phase, the patient attempts to derive full value from what he/she is offered through the relationship. The nurse can project new goals to be achieved through personal effort and power shifts from the nurse to the patient as the patient delays gratification to achieve the newly formed goals.
4. **Resolution:** The patient gradually puts aside old goals and adopts new goals. This is a process in which the patient frees himself from identification with the nurse.

Peplau's Theory and Nursing Process

Peplau defines nursing process as a deliberate intellectual activity that guides the professional practice of nursing in providing care in an orderly, systematic manner.

Peplau explains four phases such as:
* **Orientation:** Nurse and patient come together as strangers; meeting initiated by patient who expresses a "felt need"; work together to recognize, clarify and define facts related to need.
* **Identification:** Patient participates in goal setting; has feeling of belonging and selectively responds to those who can meet his or her needs.
* **Exploitation:** Patient actively seeks and draws knowledge and expertise of those who can help.
* **Resolution:** Occurs after other phases are completed successfully. This leads to termination of the relationship.

In nursing process, the orientation phase parallels with assessment phase where both the patient and nurse are strangers; meeting initiated by patient who expresses a felt need. Conjointly, the nurse and patient work together, clarifies and gathers important information. Based on this assessment the nursing diagnoses are formulated, outcome and goal set. The interventions are planned, carried out and evaluation done based on mutually established expected behaviors.

Peplau's Theory Application Nursing Process

The nursing process for Mrs JL based on Peplau's theory is as follows:

Mrs JL

27 years

Diagnosis: Intervertebral disc prolapse.

Peplau's theory application and nursing process.

Assessment (orientation phase)	Nursing diagnosis	Planning (identification phase)	Implementation (exploitation phase)	Evaluation (resolution phase)
• Mrs JL is on pelvic traction and she is restricted to bed • The need for bed rest and restriction was discussed	Impaired physical mobility related to the presence of pelvic traction	*Goal setting was done along with patient:* • Patient will have improved physical mobility as evidenced by participating in self-care within the limits • Provide active and passive exercises to all the extremities to improve the muscle tone and strength. • Make the patient to perform the breathing exercises which will strengthen the respiratory muscle • Massage the upper and lower extremities which help to improve the circulation • Provide articles near to the patient and encourage doing activities within limits • Provide positive reinforcement for even a small improvement to increase the frequency of the desired activity.	• Carried out plans mutually agreed upon. • Provided active and passive exercises to all the extremities • Made the patient to perform breathing exercises • Massaged the upper and lower extremities • Provided article within the reach of the patient • Provided positive reinforcement to the patient	• Mrs JL was free to express problems regarding difficulty in mobilizing • She expressed satisfaction when able to move without difficulty
• Mrs JL expresses pain in the low back region • Regarding pain, discussion was made to assess the severity and the type and duration of pain. Also the measures to reduce pain were discussed	Pain related to the degenerative changes in the lumbar region	*Goal setting was done along with patient:* • Mrs JL will have reduction in pain as evidenced by her verbalization of reduction in pain responses • Provide nonpharmacological measures for pain relief such as diversional activity which diverts the patients mind • Give the client a neutral position • Always use back support while turning the patient that reduces the strain on the back	• Carried out plans mutually agreed upon • Provided nonpharmacological measures like diversion, massaging, and pelvic traction • Provided supine position to the client • Supported the back during position change • Used pillows to support the back	• Mrs JL was free to express problems of pain • Expressed that she got slight relief from pain

Contd...

Contd...

Assessment (orientation phase)	Nursing diagnosis	Planning (identification phase)	Implementation (exploitation phase)	Evaluation (resolution phase)
		• Support the areas with extra pillow to allow the normal alignment and to prevent strain • Administer analgesics as prescribed by the physician • Provide pelvic traction to the patient	• Administered Tablet Hifenac P and Capsule Myoril 4 mg as prescribed • Given pelvic traction and explained the need for traction	
• Mrs JL expresses that she need assistance to get down from bed. • Regarding self-care discussion was done and discussed regarding the measures to solve the problems	Self-care deficit related to the presence of pelvic traction	*Goal setting was done along with patient:* • Client will achieve and maintain self-care activities with assistance of caregiver or within her limits • Keep all the articles within the reach of the patient • Provide a call bell to the patient to call in any emergency • Frequently visit the patient and enquire for any needs • Assist the patient in doing herself-care activities • Remove the weight of the traction as needed by the patient	• Carried out plans mutually agreed upon • Kept the articles within the reach of the client • Frequently visited the patient and enquired for any needs • Assisted the client in doing herself-care activities • Removed the weight as and when needed	• Mrs JL was free to express problems of self-care • She used to call for the needs and all her needs were met appropriately • She achieved and maintained self-care activities within her limits
• Mrs JL is enquiring about the disease condition, its outcome and need for surgery • Discussed with the client regarding the disease process and the findings in the client	Anxiety related to hospital admission as evidenced by verbalization and client and family appearing withdrawn	*Goal setting was done along with patient:* • Client will have reduced feeling of anxiety as evidenced by asking fewer questions • Teach the family and client regarding the disease process • Explain in simple understandable language of the client • Allow and encourage the client and family to ask questions. Allow the client and family to verbalize anxiety	• Carried out plans mutually agreed upon • Taught the family regarding the disease process in simple Kannada • Allowed the client and family members to ask questions • She and her husband expressed their anxiety	• Mrs JL was free to express problems of self-care • She asked her doubts regarding the illness and the diagnostic procedures • She verbalized that her anxiety has reduced to some extent

Contd...

Contd...

Assessment (orientation phase)	Nursing diagnosis	Planning (identification phase)	Implementation (exploitation phase)	Evaluation (resolution phase)
		• Stress that frequent assessment are routine and do not necessarily imply a deteriorating condition • Allow the family members to visit the client frequently	• Allowed the family members to frequently visit the client	
• Mrs JL is enquiring about the disease condition, its outcome and need for surgery • Discussed with the client regarding the disease process and the need for follow up	Deficient knowledge related to the treatment measures to be continued even after the discharge	*Goal setting was done along with patient:* • Patient will acquire adequate knowledge regarding the treatment and home care • Explain the treatment measures to the patient and their benefits • Explain to the client the signs of aggravation of illness • Use simple and understandable terms • Clarify all the doubts of the patient of importance • Repeat the information whenever necessary to reinforce learning	• Carried out plans mutually agreed upon. • Explained treatment measures and the need for follow up • Explained regarding the signs of aggravation of disease • Used simple and understandable terms for explaining • Clarified her doubts • Repeated the information	• Mrs. JL was free to express problems of self-care. • She expressed acquisition of knowledge regarding the disease and the signs of aggravation of illness

Summary

- ❖ **Orientation phase:**
  - ◆ Client is initially reluctant to talk due to pain.
  - ◆ Client is expressing that while standing she is having much pain.
  - ◆ Client expressed without movement and supine position gave her relief from pain.
- ❖ **Identification:**
  - ◆ The client participates and interdependent with the nurse.
  - ◆ Expresses the need for measure to get relief from pain.
  - ◆ Expresses need for improving the mobility.
  - ◆ Expresses need to know more about prognosis, discharge and home care and follow up.
- ❖ **Exploitation:**
  - ◆ Client explains that she gets relief of pain when lying down supine.
  - ◆ Cooperates and participates actively in performing exercises.
  - ◆ Client mobilizes changes position and cooperates during position changes.
- ❖ **Resolution:**
  - ◆ Client expressed that pain has reduced a lot and she is able to tolerate it now.
  - ◆ She has agreed upon to continue the exercises at home.
  - ◆ She also expressed that she would come for regular follow up after discharge.

Evaluation of the Theory of Interpersonal Relations by Peplau

With the help of the theory of interpersonal relations, the client's needs could be assessed. It helped her to achieve them within her limits. This theory application helped in providing comprehensive care to the client.

VIRGINIA HENDERSON'S NEED THEORY

"Nursing theories mirror different realities, throughout their development; they reflected the interests of nurses of that time."

Introduction

- ❖ "The Nightingale of Modern Nursing"
- ❖ Born in Kansas City, Missouri, in 1897 and is the 5th child of a family of 8th children but spent her formative years in Virginia
- ❖ Received a Diploma in Nursing from the Army School of Nursing at Walter Reed Hospital, Washington, D.C. in 1921.
- ❖ Worked at the Henry Street Visiting Nurse Service for 2 years after graduation.
- ❖ In 1923, she accepted a position teaching nursing at the Norfolk Protestant Hospital in Virginia, where she remained for several years.
- ❖ In 1929, Henderson determined that she needed more education and entered Teachers College at Columbia University where she earned her; Bachelor's Degree in 1932, Master's Degree in 1934.
- ❖ Subsequently, she joined Columbia as a member of the faculty, where she remained until 1948 (Herrmann,1998)

* Since 1953, she has been a research associate at Yale University School of Nursing.
* Died: March 19, 1996.

Achievements

* Is the recipient of numerous recognitions for her outstanding contributions to nursing?
* Virginia Henderson was a well known nursing educator and a prolific author.
* She has received honorary doctoral degrees from the:
  * Catholic University of America
  * Pace University
  * University of Rochester
  * University of Western Ontario
  * Yale University
* Her stature as a nurse, teacher, author, researcher, and consumer health advocate warranted an obituary in the New York Times, Friday March 22, 1996.
* In 1985, Miss Henderson was honored at the Annual Meeting of the Nursing and Allied Health Section of the Medical Library Association.

Contribution

* In 1937 Henderson and others created a basic nursing curriculum for the National League for Nursing in which education was "patient centered and organized around nursing problems rather than medical diagnoses" (Henderson,1991)
* In 1939, she revised: Harmer's classic textbook of nursing for its 4th edition, and later wrote the 5th; edition, incorporating her personal definition of nursing (Henderson,1991)
* Although she was retired, she was a frequent visitor to nursing schools well into her nineties.
* O'Malley (1996) states that Henderson is known as the modern-day mother of nursing. Her work influenced the nursing profession in America and throughout the world.
* The founding members of ICIRN (Interagency Council on Information Resources for Nursing) and a passionate advocate for the use and sharing of health information resources.
* In 1978, the fundamental concept of nursing was revisited by Virginia Henderson from Yale University School of Nursing (USA). She argued that nurses needed to be prepared for their role by receiving the broadest understanding of humanity and the world in which they lived.

Publications

* 1956 (with B. Harmer): Textbook for the principles and practices of Nursing.
* 1966: The Nature of Nursing. A Definition and its Implication for Practice, Research and Education
* 1991: The Nature of Nursing Reflections after 20 years

Analysis of Nursing Theory

* Images of Nursing, 1950–1970
* The First School of Thought: Needs

❖ This school of thought includes theories that reflect an image of nursing as meeting the needs of clients and were developed in response to such questions as:
  ◆ What do nurses do?
  ◆ What are their functions?
  ◆ What roles do nurses play?
❖ Answers to these questions focused on a number of theorist describing functions and roles of nurses.
❖ Conceptualizing functions led theorists to consider nursing client in terms of a hierarchy of needs. When any of these needs are unmet and when a person is unable to fulfill his own needs, the care provided by nurses is required.
❖ Nurses then provide the necessary functions and play those roles that could help patients meet their needs.

School of Thought in Nursing Theories (1950–1970)

Need theorists	*Interaction theorists*	*Outcome theorists*
• Abdellah • Henderson • Orem	• King • Orlando • Peterson and Zderad • Paplau • Travelbee • Wiedenbach	• Johnson • Levine • Rogers • Roy

Analysis of Nursing Theories According to 1st School

Focus	*Problems*
Human being	• A set of needs or problems • A developmental being
Patient	Need deficit
Orientation	Illness, disease
Role of nurse	• Dependent on medical practice • Beginnings of independent functions • Fulfill needs requisites
Decision making	Primarily healthcare professional

Henderson's Theory Background

❖ Henderson's concept of nursing was derived form her practice and education therefore, her work is inductive.
❖ She called her definition of nursing her "concept" (Henderson1991).
❖ Although her major clinical experiences were in medical-surgical hospitals, she worked as a visiting nurse in New York City. This experience enlarges Henderson's view to recognize the importance of increasing the patient's independence so that progress after hospitalization would not be delayed (Henderson,1991).
❖ Virginia Henderson defined nursing as "assisting individuals to gain independence in relation to the performance of activities contributing to health or its recovery" (Henderson, 1966, p. 15).

❖ She was one of the first nurses to point out that nursing does not consist of merely following physician's orders.

❖ She categorized nursing activities into 14 components, based on human needs.

❖ She described the nurse's role as *substitutive* (doing for the person), *supplementary* (helping the person), *complementary* (working with the person), with the goal of helping the person become as independent as possible.

❖ Her famous definition of nursing was one of the first statements clearly delineating nursing from medicine:

"The unique function of the nurse is to assist the individual, sick or well, in the performance of those activities contributing to health or its recovery (or to peaceful death) that he would perform unaided if he had the necessary strength, will or knowledge. And to do this in such a way as to help him gain independence as rapidly as possible" (Henderson, 1966).

Development of Henderson's Definition of Nursing

Two events are the basis for Henderson's development of a definition of nursing.

1. First, she participated in the revision of a nursing textbook.
2. Second, she was concerned that many states had no provision for nursing licensure to ensure safe and competent care for the consumer.

In the revision she recognized the need to be clear about the functions of the nurse and she believed that this textbook serves as a main learning source for nursing practice should present a sound and definitive description of nursing.

❖ Furthermore, the principles and practice or nursing must be built upon and derived from the definition of the profession.

❖ Although official statements on the nursing function were published by the ANA in 1932 and 1937, Henderson viewed these statements as nonspecific and unsatisfactory definitions of nursing practice.

❖ Then in 1955, the earlier ANA definition was modified.

❖ Henderson's focus on individual care is evident in that she stressed assisting individuals with essential activities to maintain health, to recover, or to achieve peaceful death.

❖ She proposed 14 components of basic nursing care to augment her definition.

❖ In 1955, Henderson's first definition of nursing was published in Bertha Harmer's revised nursing textbook.

Fourteen Components

1. Breathe normally.
2. Eat and drink adequately.
3. Eliminate body wastes.
4. Move and maintain desirable postures.
5. Sleep and rest.
6. Select suitable clothes-dress and undress.
7. Maintain body temperature within normal range by adjusting clothing and modifying environment
8. Keep the body clean and well groomed and protect the integument
9. Avoid dangers in the environment and avoid injuring others.

10. Communicate with others in expressing emotions, needs, fears, or opinions.
11. Worship according to one's faith.
12. Work in such a way that there is a sense of accomplishment.
13. Play or participate in various forms of recreation.
14. Learn, discover, or satisfy the curiosity that leads to normal development and health and use the available health facilities.

Assumptions

The major assumption of the theory is that:

- ❖ Nurses care for patients until patient can care for themselves once again.
- ❖ Patients desire to return to health, but this assumption is not explicitly stated.
- ❖ Nurses are willing to serve and that "nurses will devote themselves to the patient day and night"
- ❖ A final assumption is that nurses should be educated at the university level in both arts and sciences.

Henderson's Theory and the Four Major Concepts

Individual

- ❖ Have basic needs that are component of health.
- ❖ Requiring assistance to achieve health and independence or a peaceful death.
- ❖ Mind and body are inseparable and interrelated.
- ❖ Considers the biological, psychological, sociological, and spiritual components.
- ❖ The theory presents the patient as a sum of parts with biopsychosocial needs, and the patient is neither client nor consumer.

Environment

- ❖ Settings in which an individual learns unique pattern for living.
- ❖ All external conditions and influences that affect life and development.
- ❖ Individuals in relation to families
- ❖ Minimally discusses the impact of the community on the individual and family.
- ❖ Supports tasks of private and public agencies
- ❖ Society wants and expects nurses to act for individuals who are unable to function independently.
- ❖ In return she expects society to contribute to nursing education.
- ❖ Basic nursing care involves providing conditions under which the patient can perform the 14 activities unaided

Health

- ❖ Definition based on individual's ability to function independently as outlined in the 14 components.
- ❖ Nurses need to stress promotion of health and prevention and cure of disease.
- ❖ Good health is a challenge.

❖ Affected by age, cultural background, physical, and intellectual capacities, and emotional balance

❖ Is the individual's ability to meet these needs independently?

Nursing

❖ Temporarily assisting an individual who lacks the necessary strength, will and knowledge to satisfy 1 or more of 14 basic needs.

❖ Assists and supports the individual in life activities and the attainment of independence.

❖ Nurse serves to make patient "complete" "whole", or "independent."

❖ **Henderson's classic definition of nursing:** *"I say that the nurse does for others what they would do for themselves if they had the strength, the will, and the knowledge. But I go on to say that the nurse makes the patient independent of him or her as soon as possible."*

❖ The nurse is expected to carry out physician's therapeutic plan.

❖ Individualized care is the result of the nurse's creativity in planning for care.

❖ Use nursing research

❖ Categorized:
- Nursing: Nursing care
- Non nursing: Ordering supplies, cleanliness and serving food.

❖ In the Nature of Nursing "that the nurse is and should be legally, an independent practitioner and able to make independent judgments as long as s/he is not diagnosing, prescribing treatment for disease, or making a prognosis, for these are the physicians function."

❖ "Nurse should have knowledge to practice individualized and human care and should be a scientific problem solver."

❖ In the Nature of Nursing:
- Nurse role is, to get inside the patient's skin and supplement his strength will or knowledge according to his needs."
- And nurse has responsibility to assess the needs of the individual patient, help individual meet their health need, and or provide an environment in which the individual can perform activity unaided.

Henderson's Classic Definition of Nursing

"I say that the nurse does for others what they would do for themselves if they had the strength, the will, and the knowledge. But I go on to say that the nurse makes the patient independent of him or her as soon as possible."

Henderson's and Nursing Process

❖ Henderson views the nursing process as "really the application of the logical approach to the solution of a problem. The steps are those of the scientific method."

❖ "Nursing process stresses the science of nursing rather than the mixture of science and art on which it seems effective health care service of any kind is based."

Summarization of the stages of the nursing process as applied to Henderson's definition of nursing and to the 14 components of basic nursing care.

Nursing process	Henderson's 14 components and definition of nursing
Nursing assessment	Henderson's 14 components Analysis: Compare data to knowledge base of health and disease.
Nursing diagnosis	Identify individual's ability to meet own needs with or without assistance, taking into consideration strength, will or knowledge.
Nursing plan	• Document how the nurse can assist the individual, sick or well. • Assist the sick or well individual in to performance of activities in meeting human needs to maintain health, recover from illness, or to aid in peaceful death.
Nursing implementation	• Implementation based on the physiological principles, age, cultural background, emotional balance, and physical and intellectual capacities. • Carry out treatment prescribed by the physician.
Nursing evaluation	• Use the acceptable definition of; nursing and appropriate laws related to the practice of nursing. • The quality of care is drastically affected by the preparation and native ability of the nursing personnel rather that the amount of hours of care. • Successful outcomes of nursing care are based on the speed with which or degree to which the patient performs independently the activities of daily living.

14 Components of Virginia Henderson's Nursing Need Theory

1. Breathe normally
2. Eat and drink adequately
3. Eliminate body wastes
4. Move and maintain desirable postures
5. Sleep and rest
6. Select suitable clothes; dress and undress
7. Maintain body temperature within a normal range by adjusting clothing and modifying the environment
8. Keep the body clear and well groomed and protect the integument
9. Avoid dangers in the environment and avoid injuring others
10. Communicate with others in expressing emotions, needs, fears, or opinions
11. Worship according to one's faith
12. Work in such a way that there is a sense of accomplishment
13. Play or participate in various forms of recreation
14. Learn, discover, or satisfy the curiosity that leads to normal development and health, and use the available health facilities

Comparison with Maslow's Hierarchy of Need

Maslow's	Henderson
Physiological needs	• Breathe normally • Eat and drink adequately • Eliminate by all avenues of elimination • Move and maintain desirable posture • Sleep and rest • Select suitable clothing • Maintain body temperature • Keep body clean and well groomed and protect the integument
Safety needs	Avoid environmental dangers and avoid injuring others
Belongingness and love needs	• Communicate with others • Worship according to faith
Esteem needs	• Work at something providing a sense of accomplishment • Play or participate in various forms of recreation • Learn, discover, or satisfy curiosity
Self-actualization needs	

Characteristic of Henderson's Theory

❖ Theories can interrelate concepts in such a way as to create a different way of looking at a particular phenomenon.

❖ Concepts of fundamental human needs, biophysiology, culture, and interaction, communication and is borrowed from other discipline, e.g., Maslow's hierarchy of human needs; concept of interaction-communication, i.e., nurse-patient relationship

❖ Theories must be logical in nature.

❖ Her definition and components are logical and the 14 components are a guide for the individual and nurse in reaching the chosen goal.

❖ Theories should be relatively simple yet generalizable.

❖ Her work can be applied to the health of individuals of all ages.

❖ Theories can be the bases for hypotheses that can be tested.

❖ Her definition of nursing cannot be viewed as theory; therefore, it is impossible to generate testable hypotheses.

❖ However some questions to investigate the definition of nursing and the 14 components may be useful.

❖ Is the sequence of the 14 components followed by nurses in the USA and the other countries?

❖ What priorities are evident in the use of the basic nursing functions?

❖ Theories contribute to and assist in increasing the general body of knowledge within the discipline through the research implemented to validate them.

❖ Her ideas of nursing practice are well accepted throughout the world as a basis for nursing care.

❖ However, the impact of the definition and components has not been established through research.

❖ Theories can be utilized by practitioners to guide and improve their practice.

- ❖ Ideally the nurse would improve nursing practice by using her definition and 14 components to improve the health of individuals and thus reduce illness.
- ❖ Theories must be consistent with other validated theories, laws, and principles but will leave open unanswered questions that need to be investigated.

Philosophical Aims

The philosophy reflected in Henderson's theory is an integrated approach to scientific study that would capitalize on nursing's richness and complexity, and not to separate the art from the science, the "doing" of nursing from the "knowing", the psychological from the physical and the theory from clinical care.

Values and Beliefs

- ❖ Henderson believed nursing as primarily complementing the patient by supplying what he needs in knowledge, will or strength to perform his daily activities and to carry out the treatment prescribed for him by the physician.
- ❖ She strongly believed in ***"getting inside the skin"*** of her patients in order to know what he or she needs. The nurse should be the substitute for the patient, helper to the patient and partner with the patient. Like she said... ***"The nurse is temporarily the consciousness of the unconscious, the love of life for the suicidal, the leg of the amputee, the eyes of the newly blind, a means of locomotion for the infant and the knowledge and confidence for the young mother..."***
- ❖ Henderson stated that "Thorndike's fundamental needs of man" (Henderson, 1991, p.16) had an influence on her beliefs.

Value in Extending Nursing Science

- ❖ From an historical standpoint, her concept of nursing enhanced nursing science this has been particularly important in the area of nursing education.
- ❖ Her contributions to nursing literature extended from the 1930s through the 1990s and has had an impact on nursing research by strengthening the focus on nursing practice and confirming the value of tested interventions in assisting individuals to regain health.

Usefulness

- ❖ Nursing education has been deeply affected by Henderson's clear vision of the functions of nurses.
- ❖ The principles of Henderson's theory were published in the major nursing textbooks used from the 1930s through the 1960s, and the principles embodied by the 14 activities are still important in evaluating nursing care in the 21st century.
- ❖ Others concepts that Henderson (1966) proposed have been used in nursing education from the 1930s until the present O'Malley, 1996.

Testability

- ❖ Henderson supported nursing research, but believed that it should be clinical research (O'Malley, 1996). Much of the research before her time had been on educational processes and on the profession of nursing itself, rather than on; the practice and outcomes of nursing, and she worked to change that.

❖ Each of the 14 activities can be the basis for research. Although the statements are not.

❖ Written in testable terms, they may be reformulated into researchable questions. Further, the theory can guide research in any aspect of the individual's care needs.

Limitations

❖ Lack of conceptual linkage between physiological and other human characteristics.

❖ No concept of the holistic nature of human being.

❖ If the assumption is made that the 14 components prioritized, the relationship among the components is unclear.

❖ Lacks inter-relate of factors and the influence of nursing care.

❖ Assisting the individual in the dying process she contends that the nurse helps, but there is little explanation of what the nurse does.

❖ "Peaceful death" is curious and significant nursing role.

Summary

❖ Background
❖ Achievements
❖ Publications
❖ Analysis of nursing theories
❖ Development of Henderson's definition of nursing
❖ Fourteen components
❖ Major four concepts
❖ Nursing process with Henderson's theory
❖ Comparison with Maslow's hierarchy need
❖ Assumptions
❖ Usefulness
❖ Testability
❖ Characteristics
❖ Limitation

Conclusion

In conclusion, Henderson provides the essence of what she believes is a definition of nursing. She didn't intend to develop a theory of nursing but rather she attempted to define the unique focus of nursing. Her emphasis on basic human needs as the central focus of nursing practice has led to further theory development regarding the needs of the person and how nursing can assist in meeting those needs. Her definition of nursing and the 14 components of basic nursing care are uncomplicated and self-explanatory.

FAYE GLENN ABDELLAH'S THEORY

Introduction

❖ Faye Glenn Abdellah, pioneer nursing researcher, helped transform nursing theory, nursing care and nursing education

❖ Birth:1919

- ❖ Dr Abdellah worked as Deputy Surgeon General
- ❖ Former Chief Nurse Officer for the US Public Health Service, Department of Health and human services, Washington, DC
- ❖ She has been a leader in nursing research and has over one hundred publications related to nursing care, education for advanced practice in nursing and nursing research.
- ❖ In 1960, influenced by the desire to promote client-centered comprehensive nursing care, Abdellah described nursing as a service to individuals, to families, and, therefore to, to society.
- ❖ According to her, nursing is based on an art and science that mold the attitudes, intellectual competencies, and technical skills of the individual nurse into the desire and ability to help people, sick or well, cope with their health needs.
- ❖ As a comprehensive service, nursing includes
  - ◆ Recognizing the nursing problems of the patient
  - ◆ Deciding the appropriate course of action to take in terms of relevant nursing principles
  - ◆ Providing continuous care of the individuals total needs
  - ◆ Providing continuous care to relieve pain and discomfort and provide immediate security for the individual
  - ◆ Adjusting the total nursing care plan to meet the patient's individual needs
  - ◆ Helping the individual to become more self-directing in attaining or maintaining a healthy state of mind and body
  - ◆ Instructing nursing personnel and family to help the individual do for himself that which he can within his limitations
  - ◆ Helping the individual to adjust to his limitations and emotional problems
  - ◆ Working with allied health professions in planning for optimum health on local, state, national and international levels
  - ◆ Carrying out continuous evaluation and research to improve nursing techniques and to develop new techniques to meet the health needs of people
  - ◆ These original premises have undergone an evolutionary process. As result, in 1973, the item 3, - "providing continuous care of the individual's total health needs" was eliminated.
  - ◆ From these premises, Abdellah's theory was derived.

Philosophical Underpinnings of the Theory

- ❖ Abdellah's patient-centered approach to nursing was developed inductively from her practice and is considered a human needs theory.
- ❖ The theory was created to assist with nursing education and is most applicable to the education of nurses.
- ❖ Although it was intended to guide care of those in the hospital, it also has relevance for nursing care in community settings.

Major Assumptions, Concepts and Relationships

- ❖ The language of Abdellah's framework is readable and clear.
- ❖ Consistent with the decade in which she was writing, she uses the term 'she' for nurses, 'he' for doctors and patients, and refers to the object of nursing as 'patient' rather than client or consumer.
- ❖ She referred to nursing diagnosis during a time when nurses were taught that diagnosis was not a nurses' prerogative.

❖ Assumptions were related to:
  ◆ Change and anticipated changes that affect nursing
  ◆ The need to appreciate the interconnectedness of social enterprises and social problems
  ◆ The impact of problems such as poverty, racism, pollution, education, and so forth on health care delivery
  ◆ Changing nursing education
  ◆ Continuing education for professional nurses
  ◆ Development of nursing leaders from under reserved groups
❖ Abdellah and colleagues developed a list of 21 nursing problems.
❖ They also identified 10 steps to identify the client's problems.
❖ 11 nursing skills to be used in developing a treatment typology.

10 Steps to Identify the Client's Problems

1. Learn to know the patient.
2. Sort out relevant and significant data.
3. Make generalizations about available data in relation to similar nursing problems presented by other patients.
4. Identify the therapeutic plan.
5. Test generalizations with the patient and make additional generalizations.
6. Validate the patient's conclusions about his nursing problems.
7. Continue to observe and evaluate the patient over a period of time to identify any attitudes and clues affecting his behavior.
8. Explore the patient's and family's reaction to the therapeutic plan and involve them in the plan.
9. Identify how the nurses feels about the patient's nursing problems.
10. Discuss and develop a comprehensive nursing care plan.

Eleven Nursing Skills

1. Observation of health status
2. Skills of communication
3. Application of knowledge
4. Teaching of patients and families
5. Planning and organization of work
6. Use of resource materials
7. Use of personnel resources
8. Problem-solving
9. Direction of work of others
10. Therapeutic use of the self
11. Nursing procedures

The Twenty One Nursing Problems

Three major categories:
1. Physical, sociological, and emotional needs of clients
2. Types of interpersonal relationships between the nurse and patient
3. Common elements of client care

Basic to All Patients

1. To maintain good hygiene and physical comfort
2. To promote optimal activity: Exercise, rest and sleep
3. To promote safety through the prevention of accidents, injury, or other trauma and through the prevention of the spread of infection
4. To maintain good body mechanics and prevent and correct deformities

Sustenal Care Needs

5. To facilitate the maintenance of a supply of oxygen to all body cells
6. To facilitate the maintenance of nutrition of all body cells
7. To facilitate the maintenance of elimination
8. To facilitate the maintenance of fluid and electrolyte balance
9. To recognize the physiological responses of the body to disease conditions
10. To facilitate the maintenance of regulatory mechanisms and functions
11. To facilitate the maintenance of sensory function

Remedial Care Needs

12. To identify and accept positive and negative expressions, feelings, and reactions
13. To identify and accept the interrelatedness of emotions and organic illness
14. To facilitate the maintenance of effective verbal and non verbal communication
15. To promote the development of productive interpersonal relationships
16. To facilitate progress toward achievement of personal spiritual goals
17. To create and/or maintain a therapeutic environment
18. To facilitate awareness of self as an individual with varying physical, emotional, and developmental needs

Restorative Care Needs

19. To accept the optimum possible goals in the light of limitations, physical and emotional
20. To use community resources as an aid in resolving problems arising from illness
21. To understand the role of social problems as influencing factors in the case of illness

Abdellah's 21 problems are actually a model describing the "arenas" or concerns of nursing, rather than a theory describing relationships among phenomena. In this way, the theory distinguished the practice of nursing, with a focus on the 21 nursing problems, from the practice of medicine, with a focus on disease and cure.

Abdellah's Theory and Nursing

Although Abdellah's writings are not specific as to a theoretical statement, such a statement can be derived by using her three major concepts of health, nursing problems, and problem solving. Abdellah's theory would state that nursing is the use of the problem solving approach with key nursing problems related to health needs of people. Such a statement maintains problem solving as the vehicle for the nursing problems as the client is moved toward health—the outcome

Nursing

According to Abdellah, nursing is based on an art and science that mold the attitudes, intellectual competencies, and technical skills of the individual nurse into the desire and ability to help people, sick or well, cope with their health needs.

Health

Health is a dynamic pattern of functioning whereby there is a continued interaction with internal and external forces that results in the optimum use of necessary resources that serve to minimize vulnerabilities.

Nursing Problems

❖ Nursing problem presented by a client is a condition faced by the client or client's family that the nurse through the performance of professional functions can assist them to meet. The problem can be either an overt or covert nursing problem.

❖ An overt nursing problem is an apparent condition faced by the patient or family, which the nurse can assist him or them to meet through the performance of her professional functions.

❖ The covert nursing problem is a concealed or hidden condition faced, by the patient or family, which the nurse can assist him or them to meet through the performance of her professional functions.

❖ In her attempt to bring nursing practice into its proper relationship with restorative and preventive measures for meeting total client needs, she seems to swing the pendulum to the opposite pole, from the disease orientation to nursing orientation, while leaving the client somewhere in the middle.

Problem Solving

The problem solving process involves identifying the problem, selecting pertinent data, formulating hypothesis, testing hypothesis through the collection of data, and revising hypothesis where necessary on the basis of conclusions obtained from the data.

Comparison with Other Theories

Maslow	Henderson	Abdellah
Physiological needs	1. Breathe normally 2. Eat and drink adequately 3. Eliminate by all avenues of elimination 4. Move and maintain desirable posture 5. Sleep and rest 6. Select suitable clothing 7. Maintain body temperature 8. Keep body clean and well groomed and protect the integument	1. To facilitate the maintenance of a supply of oxygen to all body cells 2. To facilitate the maintenance of nutrition of all body cells 3. To facilitate the maintenance of fluid and electrolyte balance 4. To facilitate the maintenance of elimination 5. To maintain good body mechanics and prevent and correct deformities 6. To promote optimal activity: exercise, rest and sleep 7. To facilitate the maintenance of regulatory mechanisms and functions 8. To maintain good hygiene and physical comfort

Contd...

Contd...

Maslow	Henderson	Abdellah
Safety needs	9. Avoid environmental dangers and avoid injuring others	9. To promote safety through the prevention of accidents, injury, or other trauma and through the prevention of the spread of infection 10. To facilitate the maintenance of sensory function
Belongingness and love needs	10. Communicate with others 11. Worship according to faith	11. To facilitate the maintenance of effective verbal and non verbal communication 12. To promote the development of productive interpersonal relationships 13. To facilitate progress toward achievement of personal spiritual goals
Esteem needs	12. Work at something providing a sense of accomplishment 13. Play or participate in various forms of recreation 14. Learn, discover, or satisfy curiosity	14. To accept the optimum possible goals in the light of limitations, physical and emotional 15. To recognize the physiological responses of the body to disease conditions 16. To identify and accept positive and negative expressions, feelings, and reactions 17. To identify and accept the interrelatedness of emotions and organic illness 18. To create and/or maintain a therapeutic environment 19. To facilitate awareness of self as an individual with varying physical, emotional, and developmental needs 20. To use community resources as an aid in resolving problems arising from illness 21. To understand the role of social problems as influencing factors in the case of illness
Self-actualization needs		

Abdellah's Theory and the Four Major Concepts

Nursing

- ❖ Nursing is a helping profession. In Abdellah's model, nursing care is doing something to or for the person or providing information to the person with the goals of meeting needs, increasing or restoring self-help ability, or alleviating impairment.
- ❖ Nursing is broadly grouped into the 21 problem areas to guide care and promote use of nursing judgment.
- ❖ She considers nursing to be comprehensive service that is based on art and science and aims to help people, sick or well, cope with their health needs.

Person

- ❖ Abdellah describes people as having physical, emotional, and sociological needs. These needs may overt, consisting of largely physical needs, or covert, such as emotional and social needs.

❖ Patient is described as the only justification for the existence of nursing.
❖ Individuals (and families) are the recipients of nursing.
❖ Health, or achieving of it, is the purpose of nursing services.

Health

❖ In Patient-Centered Approaches to Nursing, Abdellah describes health as a state mutually exclusive of illness.
❖ Although Abdellah does not give a definition of health, she speaks to "total health needs" and "a healthy state of mind and body" in her description of nursing as a comprehensive service.

Society/Environment

❖ Society is included in "planning for optimum health on local, state, national, and international levels". However, as she further delineated her ideas, the focus of nursing service is clearly the individual.
❖ The environment is the home or community from which patient comes.

Abdellah's Work and Characteristics of a Theory

Characteristic 1

❖ Abdellah's theory has interrelated the concepts of health, nursing problems, and problem solving as she attempts to create a different way of viewing nursing phenomenon.
❖ The result was the statement that nursing is the use of problem solving approach with key nursing problems related to health needs of people.

Characteristic 2

Problem solving is an activity that is inherently logical in nature.

Characteristic 3

Framework seems to focus quite heavily on nursing practice and individuals. This somewhat limit the ability to generalize although the problem-solving approach is readily generalizable to clients with specific health needs and specific nursing problems.

Characteristic 4

One of the most important questions that arise when considering her work is the role of client within the framework. This question could generate hypothesis for testing and thus demonstrates the ability of Abdellah's work to generate hypothesis for testing.

Characteristic 5

The results of testing such hypothesis would contribute to the general body of nursing knowledge.

Characteristic 6

Abdellah's problem solving approach can easily be used by practitioners to guide various activities within their practice. This is true when considering nursing practice that deals with clients who have specific needs and specific nursing problems.

Characteristic 7

Although consistency with other theories exist, many questions remain unanswered.

Use of Twenty one Problems in the Nursing Process

Assessment Phase

- ❖ Nursing problems provide guidelines for the collection of data.
- ❖ A principle underlying the problem solving approach is that for each identified problem, pertinent data are collected.
- ❖ The overt or covert nature of the problems necessitates a direct or indirect approach, respectively.

Nursing Diagnosis

- ❖ The results of data collection would determine the client's specific overt or covert problems.
- ❖ These specific problems would be grouped under one or more of the broader nursing problems.
- ❖ This step is consistent with that involved in nursing diagnosis.

Planning Phase

- ❖ The statements of nursing problems most closely resemble goal statements. Therefore, once the problem has been diagnosed, the goals have been established.
- ❖ Given that these problems are called nursing problems, then it becomes reasonable to conclude that these goals are basically nursing goals.

Implementation

Using the goals as the framework, a plan is developed and appropriate nursing interventions are determined.

Evaluation

- ❖ According to the American Nurses' Association Standards of Nursing Practice, the plan is evaluated in terms of the client's progress or lack of progress toward the achievement of the stated goals.
- ❖ This would be extremely difficult if not impossible to do for Abdellah's nursing problem approach since it has been determined that the goals are nursing goals, not the client goals.
- ❖ Thus, the most appropriate evaluation would be the nurse progress or lack of progress toward the achievement of the stated goals.

An Illustration of the Implementation of Abdellah's Framework in Ryan's Care

Consider a case of Ryan who experienced severe crushing chest pain 'shortness of breath, tachycardia and profuse diaphoresis:

- ❖ Stage of illness is basic to care
- ❖ Selected Abdellah nursing problem
- ❖ To maintain good hygiene and personal comfort
- ❖ Classification and approach

* Overt problem of pain: Direct and indirect method
* Selected nursing interventions
* Administer oxygen
* Elevate headrest
* Reposition client
* Administer prescribed analgesic
* Remain with client
* Criterion measure-Amount of pain

Concept of Progressive Patient Care

* Progressive patient care (PPC) is defined as better patient care through the organization of hospital facilities, services and staff around the changing medical and nursing needs of the patient
* PPC is tailoring of hospital services to meet patients needs.
* PPC is caring for the right patient in the right bed with the right services at the right time.
* PPC is systematic classification of patients based on their medical needs.

Elements of PPC

* **Intensive care:** Critically and seriously ill patients requiring highly skilled nursing care, close and frequent if not constant, nursing observation are assigned to the ICU. One patient in an ICU requires at least three nurses to observe him in 24 hours.
* **Intermediate care:** Patients assigned to this unit are both the moderately ill and those for whom the treatment can only be palliative.
* **Self-care:** Ambulatory patients who are convalescing or require diagnosis or therapy may be cared for in this unit.
* **Long-term care unit:** This unit will provide services to certain patients now cared for in the general hospital, in nursing homes, or in their own homes and who would benefit by care in a hospital environment to achieve its maximum potential.
* **Home care:** This program makes it possible to extend needed services to the patient after he leaves the hospital and returns to his home in the community.

Benefits of PPC

Patient

* Better attention
* Better adjustment
* Minimized problems
* Life-saving care
* Constant medical and nursing care

Physician

* Assuring best nursing care
* Drugs and equipment's at hand
* Orders carried out effectively
* Better clinical an team service

Hospital

❖ Effective and efficient use of staff
❖ Improved public image

Nursing Personnel

❖ Individual skills can be used
❖ More time with patient
❖ Helping patient and family to solve problems
❖ Job satisfaction
❖ In-service education

Community

❖ Continuity with hospital services
❖ Minimize the need of hospitalization

Implications of PPC for Nursing Education

❖ Many nurse educators feel that the PPC hospital where all five phases of care are available can provide clinical experience in which the nurse can learn to solve basic nursing problems in meeting patients' needs.
❖ The three month assignment of professional nurses may no longer be realistic in such a setting.

Organization of Hospital and Community Services Based on Patients Needs

❖ In the intensive care unit, the critically ill patients are concentrated regardless of diagnosis.
❖ These patients are under the constant audio-visual observation of the nurse, with life saving techniques and equipment immediately available.
❖ In the intermediate care unit there are concentrated patients requiring a moderate amount of nursing care, not of an emergency nature, who are ambulatory for short periods, and who are beginning to participate in the planning of their own care.
❖ The self-care unit provides for patients who are physically self-sufficient and require diagnostic and convalescent care in hotel-type accommodations. This unit serves as a link between the hospital and the home.
❖ In the long-term care unit are concentrated patients requiring prolonged care. The grouping of such patients will permit staffing patterns that are less costly.
❖ Home care, the fifth element of progressive patient care, extends hospital services into the home to assist the physician in the care of his patients.

Usefulness

❖ The patient centered approach was constructed to be useful to nursing practice, with impetus for it being nursing education.
❖ Abdellah's publications on nursing education began with her dissertation; her interest in education for nurses continues into the present.
❖ Abdellah has also published on nursing, nursing research, and public policy related to nursing in several international publications. She has been a strong advocate for improving nursing practice through nursing research.

Value in Extending Nursing Science

- ❖ It helped to bring structure and organization to what was often a disorganized collection of lectures and experiences.
- ❖ She categorized nursing problems based on the individual's needs and developed a typology of nursing treatment and nursing skills.

Nursing Research

She has been a leader in nursing research and has over one hundred publications related to nursing care, education for advanced practice in nursing and nursing research.

Limitations

- ❖ Very strong nursing centered orientation.
- ❖ Little emphasis on what the client is to achieve.
- ❖ Her framework is inconsistent with the concept of holism.
- ❖ Potential problems might be overlooked.

Summary

- ❖ Using Abdellah's concepts of health, nursing problems, and problem solving, the theoretical statement of nursing that can be derived is the use of the problem solving approach with key nursing problems related to health needs of people.
- ❖ From this framework, 21 nursing problems were developed.

Conclusion

- ❖ Abdellah's theory provides a basis for determining and organizing nursing care. The problems also provide a basis for organizing appropriate nursing strategies.
- ❖ It is anticipated that by solving the nursing problems, the client would be moved toward health. The nurse's philosophical frame of reference would determine whether this theory and the 21 nursing problems could be implemented in practice.

IMOGENE KING: THEORY OF GOAL ATTAINMENT

Introduction of Theorist

- ❖ Born in 1923
- ❖ Completed her Bachelor in Science of Nursing from St. Louis University in 1948
- ❖ Completed her Master of Science of Nursing from St. Louis University in 1957
- ❖ Completed her Doctorate from Teacher's college, Columbia University

King's Conceptual Framework

It includes:
- ❖ Several basic assumptions
- ❖ Three interacting systems
- ❖ Several concepts relevant for each system

Basic Assumptions

- ❖ Nursing focus is the care of human being.
- ❖ Nursing goal is the health care of individuals and groups.
- ❖ Human beings are open systems interacting constantly with their environment.
- ❖ Interacting systems:
    - ◆ Personal system
    - ◆ Interpersonal system
    - ◆ Social system
- ❖ Concepts are given for each system

Concepts for Personal System

- ❖ Perception
- ❖ Self
- ❖ Growth and development
- ❖ Body image
- ❖ Space
- ❖ Time

Concepts for Interpersonal System

- ❖ Interaction
- ❖ Communication
- ❖ Transaction
- ❖ Role
- ❖ Stress

Concepts for Social System

- ❖ Organization
- ❖ Authority
- ❖ Power
- ❖ Status
- ❖ Decision making

Major Theses of King's Conceptual Framework

- ❖ Each human being perceives the world as a total person in making transactions with individuals and things in environment.
- ❖ Transaction represents a life situation in which perceiver and thing perceived are encountered and in which person enters the situation as an active participant and each is changed in the process of these experiences.

King's Theory of Goal Attainment

- ❖ Theory of goal attainment was first introduced by Imogene King in the early 1960's.
- ❖ Theory describes a dynamic, interpersonal relationship in which a person grows and develops to attain certain life goals.
- ❖ Factors which affects the attainment of goal are: roles, stress, space and time.

Propositions of King's Theory

From the theory of goal attainment king developed predictive propositions, which includes:

* If perceptual interaction accuracy is present in nurse-client interactions, transaction will occur.
* If nurse and client make transaction, goal will be attained.
* If goal are attained, satisfaction will occur.
* If transactions are made in nurse-client interactions, growth and development will be enhanced.
* If role expectations and role performance as perceived by nurse and client are congruent, transaction will occur.
* If role conflict is experienced by nurse or client or both, stress in nurse-client interaction will occur.
* If nurse with special knowledge skill communicate appropriate information to client, mutual goal setting and goal attainment will occur.

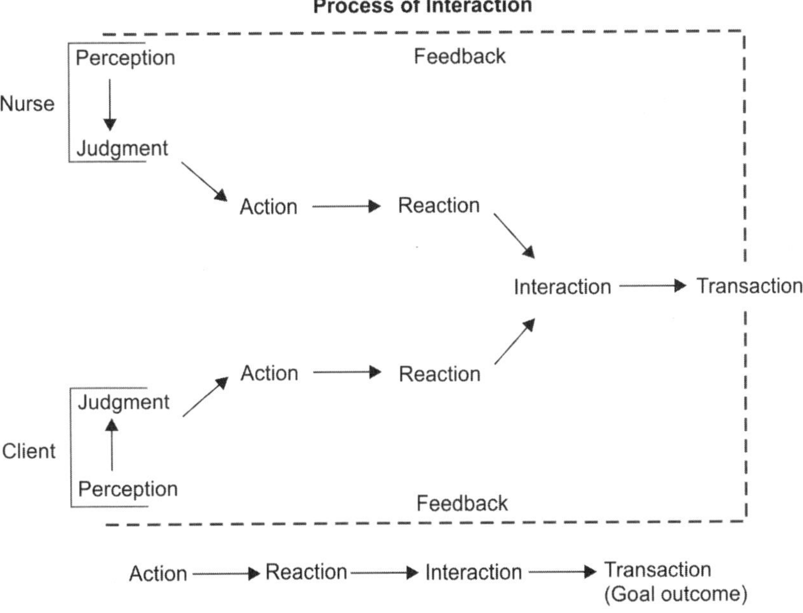

Imogene King's theory of goal attainment.

Major Concepts of King's Theory

* **Human being/person** is social being who are rational and sentient. Person has ability to:
  * Perceive
  * Think
  * Feel
  * Choose
  * Set goals
  * Select means to achieve goals and to make decision

According to King, human being has three fundamental needs:

1. The need for the health information that is unable at the time when it is needed and can be used.
2. The need for care that seek to prevent illness, and
3. The need for care when human beings are unable to help themselves.

❖ **Health:** According to King, health involves dynamic life experiences of a human being, which implies continuous adjustment to stressors in the internal and external environment through optimum use of one's resources to achieve maximum potential for daily living.

❖ **Environment:** It is the background for human interactions. It involves:

- *Internal environment:* It transforms energy to enable person to adjust to continuous external environmental changes.
- *External environment:* It involves formal and informal organizations. Nurse is a part of the patient's environment.

Nursing: It is defined as "A process of action, reaction and interaction by which nurse and client share information about their perception in nursing situation" and " a process of human interactions between nurse and client whereby each perceives the other and the situation, and through communication, they set goals, explore means, and agree on means to achieve goals."

- **Action:** Is defined as a sequence of behaviors involving mental and physical action.
- **Reaction:** Not specified, but might be considered as included in the sequence of behaviors described in action.
- In addition king discussed:
  ◊ Goal
  ◊ Domain
  ◊ Functions of professional nurse
- **Goal of nurse:** "To help individuals to maintain their health so they can function in their roles."
- **Domain of nurse:** "includes promoting, maintaining, and restoring health, and caring for the sick, injured and dying".
- **Function of professional nurse:** "To interpret information in nursing process to plan, implement and evaluate nursing care".

King said in her theory, "A professional nurse, with special knowledge and skills, and a client in need of nursing, with knowledge of self and perception of personal problems, meet as strangers in natural environment. They interact mutually, identify problems, establish and achieve goals.

Nursing process and theory of goal attainment.	
Nursing process method	**Nursing process theory**
A system of oriented actions	A system of oriented concepts
Assessment	Perception, communication and interaction of nurse and client
Planning	• Decision making about the goals • Be agree on the means to attain the goals
Implementation	Transaction made
Evaluation	Goal attained

Application of Imogene King's Theory of Goal Attainment

Objectives

- To assess the patient condition by the various methods explained by the nursing theory
- To identify the needs of the patient
- To demonstrate an effective communication and interaction with the patient.
- To select a theory for the application according to the need of the patient.
- To apply the theory to solve the identified problems of the patient.
- To evaluate the extent to which the process was fruitful.

Introduction

King's theory offers insight into nurses' interactions with individuals and groups within the environment. It highlights the importance of client's participation in decision that influences care and focuses on both the process of nurse-client interaction and the outcomes of care. Mr. Sy (74 years) was admitted in L3 ward of...Hospital, for a herniorrhaphy on... for his left indirect inguinal hernia and was expecting discharge from hospital... the theory of goal attainment was used in his nursing process.

Major Concepts and Definitions

1. **Interaction**
   - A process of perception and communication
   - Between person and environment
   - Between person and person
   - Represented by verbal and nonverbal behaviors
   - Goal-directed
   - Each individual brings different knowledge, needs, goals, past experiences and perceptions, which influence interaction
2. **Communication**
   - Information from person to person
   - Directly or indirectly
   - Information component of interaction
3. **Perception:** Each persons representation of reality
4. **Transaction:** Purposeful interaction leading to goal attainment
5. **Role:**
   - A set of behaviors expected of persons occupying a position in a social system
   - Rules that define rights and obligations in a position
6. **Stress:**
   - Dynamic state
   - Human being interacts with the environment
7. **Growth and development:**
   - Continuous changes in individuals
   - At cellular, molecular and behavioral levels of activities
   - Helps individuals move towards maturity

8. **Time:**
   - Sequence of events
   - Moving onwards to the future
9. **Space:**
   - Existing in all directions
   - Same everywhere
   - Immediate environment (nurse and client interaction)

Major Assumptions

Nursing

- Observable behavior
- In health care system in society
- Goal to help individuals maintain health
- Interpersonal process of action; reaction, interaction and transaction

Person

- Social being
- Sentient being
- Rational being
- Perceiving being
- Controlling being
- Purposeful being
- Action-oriented being
- Time-oriented being

Health

- Dynamic state in the life cycle
- Continuous adaptation to stress
- To achieve maximum potential for daily living
- Function of nurse, patient, physicians, family and other interactions

Environment

- Open system
- Constantly changing
- Influences adjustment to life and health

Dynamic Interacting Systems

Personal System

Concepts

- Perception
- Self

- Body image
- Growth and development
- Time
- Space

Interpersonal System

Concepts

- Interaction
- Transaction
- Communication
- Role
- Stress

Social System

Concepts

- Organization
- Authority
- Power
- Status
- Decision making

Assumptions

- Perceptions, goals, needs and values of the nurses and client influence interaction process.
- Individuals have the right to knowledge about themselves and to participate in decisions that influence their life, health and community services.
- Health professionals have the responsibility that helps individuals to make informed decisions about their health care.
- Individuals have the right to accept or reject health care.
- Goals of health professionals and recipients of health care may not be congruent.

Propositions of King's Theory

From the theory of goal attainment king developed predictive propositions, which includes:

- If perceptual interaction accuracy is present in nurse-client interactions, transaction will occur
- If nurse and client make transaction, goal will be attained
- If goal are attained, satisfaction will occur
- Proposition content
- If transactions are made in nurse-client interactions, growth and development will be enhanced
- If role expectations and role performance as perceived by nurse and client are congruent, transaction will occur
- If role conflict is experienced by nurse or client or both, stress in nurse-client interaction will occur

❖ If nurse with special knowledge skill communicate appropriate information to client, mutual goal setting and goal attainment will occur.

Theory of Goal Attainment and Nursing Process

Assumptions

Basic assumption of goal attainment theory is that nurse and client communicate information, set goal mutually and then act to attain those goals, is also the basic assumption of nursing process.

Assessment

❖ King indicates that assessment occur during interaction. The nurse brings special knowledge and skills whereas client brings knowledge of self and perception of problems of concern, to this interaction.

❖ During assessment nurse collects data regarding client (his/her growth and development, perception of self and current health status, roles, etc.)

❖ Perception is the base for collection and interpretation of data.

❖ Communication is required to verify accuracy of perception, for interaction and transaction.

The first process in nursing process is nurse meets the patient and communicates and interacts with him. Assessment is conducted by gathering data about the patient based on relevant concepts.

Mr. Sy is 74 years married, got admitted in L3 ward of...Hospital on 27/03/08 with a diagnosis of indirect inguinal hernia underwent herniorrhaphy with prolene mesh done on 30/03/08. The following areas were addressed to for gathering data.

What is the patient's perception of the situation?	Patient says • "I have undergone surgery for hernia". "The wound is getting healed, I have no other problem" • "I have pain in the area of surgery when moving" • "I'm taking medicines for hypertension for the last 7 years from here" • "I have vision problem to my left eye. I had undergone a surgery for my right eye about 10 years back".
What are my perceptions of the situation?	• Patient underwent herniorrhaphy operation on 30th March for indirect inguinal hernia which he kept untreated for 35 years. • Patient has health maintenance related problems. • Patient is at risk of developing infection. • Patient has pain related to surgical incision. • Patient may develop hypertension related complications in future.
What other information do I need to assist this patient to achieve health?	**History** **Identification details** Mr. Sy is 74 years married, male, studied up to 7th Std is doing Business, a practicing Muslim, got admitted in L3 ward of...Hospital on 27/03/08 with a diagnosis of indirect inguinal hernia underwent herniorrhaphy with prolene mesh done on 30/03/08. **Present history of illness** • Abdominal swelling for 35 years with difficulty in activities and occasional abdominal pain. He has hypertension for seven years.

Contd...

Contd...

- The swelling remained stable with uncomplicated progress, getting increasing size when standing for long and reducible on applying pressure
- No history of severe pain but increasing size for the last few years
- Relived after pressing the swelling back to position and on taking rest and applying pressure

Past health history

Patient underwent cataract surgery about 10 years back
- On treatment for hypertension
- No other significant illness

Family history
- Patient's next elder brother and next younger brother had inguinal hernia and were operated
- Elder brother underwent three surgeries for hernia

Socioeconomic status

High economic status > ₹ 20,000/- per month

Lifestyle
- Nonvegetarian
- No habit of smoking or alcoholism
- Aware about healthcare facilities

Physical examination
- Alert, conscious and oriented
- Moderately built, adequate nourishment, with BMI of 22
- Vital signs—normal except BP 140/90 mm Hg
- General head-to-foot examination reveals normal finding except for the vision difficulty of the right eye and healing surgical wound on th left inguinal region.
- Subjective problems
- Pain at the surgical wound site
- Lack of bowel movement for 2 days
- Review of relevant systems

Gastrointestinal (GI) system

Inspection: Healing wound, no infection, no redness, no swelling

Auscultation: Normal bowel sounds

Palpation: No pain at the site, Normal abdominal organs

Percussion: No dull sound suggesting fluid collection or ascites

Genitourinary system

Inspection: Testicles in position, no infection, no swelling or enlargement

Palpation: No c/o pain, no prostate enlargement

Percussion: No fluid collection in scrotum

Contd...

Contd...

	Auscultation: Normal Bowel sounds **Laboratory investigations:** • FBS: 91 mg/dL • Na (130–143 mEq/dL)–134 mEq/dL • K$^+$ (3.5–5 mg/dL)–3.5 mEq/dL • Urea (8–35 mg/dL)–29 mg/dL • Cr (0.6–1.6 mg/dL)–<1 mg/dL **Other investigations:** • Electrocardiogram • Anterior fascicular block • Left atrial enlargement • Normal axis
What does this information means to this situation?	• Patient neglected a health problem for 35 years • Patient has acute pain at the site of surgical wound • Patient has family history of inguinal hernia and risk for recurrence • Patient has a risk for recurrence due to constipation • Patient has risk for infection due to inadequate knowledge and age • Patient is at risk of developing complications of hypertension • Patient requires education regarding health maintenance
What conclusion (judgement) does this patient make?	• Patient requires management for his pain • Patient understands the need taking care of health risks and agrees to work on these aspects
What conclusions (judgement) do I make? **Nursing diagnosis** The data collected by assessment are used to make nursing diagnosis in nursing process. According to King in process of attaining goal, the nurse identifies the problems, concerns and disturbances about which person seek help.	Based on the assessment following nursing diagnoses were formulated, i.e., the clinical judgement about the patient's actual and potential problems. 1. Acute pain related to surgical incision 2. Risk for infection related to surgical incision 3. Risk for constipation related to bed rest, pain medication and NPO or soft diet 4. Deficient knowledge regarding the treatment and home care 5. Ineffective health maintenance

Planning

❖ After diagnosis, planning for interventions to solve those problems is done.

❖ In goal attainment planning is represented by setting goals and making decisions about and being agreed on the means to achieve goals.

❖ This part of transaction and client's participation is encouraged in making decision on the means to achieve the goals.

Identifying the goals and planning to achieve these goals (this step is congruent with planning in the traditional nursing process)	

What goals do I think will serve the patient's best interest?	1. The client will experience improved comfort, as evidenced by:
	  ➢ A decrease in the rating of the pain
	  ➢ The ability to rest and sleep comfortably
	2. The client will be free of infection as evidenced by normal temperature, normal vital signs.
	3. The client will have improved bowel elimination, as evidenced by:
	  ➢ Elimination of stool without straining
	4. Client will acquire adequate knowledge regarding the treatment and home care.
	5. Client will attend to health problems promptly

What are the patient's goals?	Patient's goals are: • Freedom from pain • Rapid healing • Adequate bowel movement • Acquiring adequate knowledge regarding his health problems
Are the patient's goals and professional goals are congruent?	Yes
What are the priority goals?	• Relief of pain • Freedom from infection • Adequate bowel movement • Improvement knowledge aspect of health conditions • Prompt attendance to health problems
What does the patient perceives as the best way to achieve goals?	• Working with the health professionals • Gaining knowledge • Disclosing adequate information regarding health problems
Is the patient willing to work towards the goals?	Yes
What do I perceive to be the best way to achieve the goals?	**Goal 1:** • Assess the characteristics of pain • Administration of prescribed medicine • Monitor the responses to drug therapy • Provide calm, efficient manner that reassures the client and minimizes anxiety • Provide a comfortable position as per client's requests. **Goal 2:** • Monitor vital signs • Administer antibiotics as advised • Use aseptic techniques while changing dressing • Kept the surgical wound site clean • Report surgeon regarding early signs of infection

Contd...

Contd...

	Goal 3: • Ensure that the client has adequate bulk in diet and adequate fluid intake • Instruct the client on prevention of straining and avoiding Valsalva maneuver • Consult treating physician regarding medications. **Goal 4:** • Explain the treatment measures to the patient and their benefits in a simple understandable language. • Explain demonstrate about the home care. • Clarify the doubts of the patient as the patient may present with some matters of importance. • Repeat the information whenever necessary to reinforce learning. **Goal 5:** Health education given about the following: • Restriction of heavy weight lifting (more than 20 kg) for 6 months • Further management which may be necessary • Diet control for his hypertension • Rehabilitation measures to promote better living • For regular examination of the site for recurrence of hernia
Are the goals short-term or long-term?	Goals are both short-term and long-term
What modifications required based on mutuality?	• Pain is tolerable to the patient and requires no SOS medication • Constipation is not that severe enough to take medication • Other interventions are mutually acceptable.

Implementations

- ❖ In nursing process implementation involves the actual activities to achieve the goals.
- ❖ This step results in transactions being made.
- ❖ Transactions occur as a result of perceiving the other person and the situation, making judgments about those perceptions, and taking some actions in response.
- ❖ Reactions to action lead to transactions that reflect a shared view and commitment

This step reflects implementation in the traditional nursing process.

Am I doing what the patient and I have agreed upon?	Yes
How am I carrying out the actions?	On a mutually acceptable manner in accordance with the goals set.
When do I carry out the action?	• According to priority, a few interventions require immediate attention. • Other interventions are carried out during the period of hospitalization till 5th April.
Why am I carrying out the action?	Patient's condition demands nursing car.
Is it reasonable to think that the identified goals will be reached by carrying out the action?	Yes

Evaluation

- ❖ It involves to finding out weather goals are achieved or not.
- ❖ In King's description evaluation speaks about attainment of goal and effectiveness of nursing care.

Are my actions helping the patient achieve mutually defined goals?	Yes
How well are goals being met?	• Short-term goals are met before discharge from hospital • Long-term goals are expected to be met, because the patient is motivated to continue home care.
What actions are not working?	
What is patient's response to my actions?	Patient is satisfied with my actions
Are other factors hindering goal achievement?	Patient's age is a hindering factor in goal achievement regarding health maintenance.
How should the plan be changed to achieve goals?	• Health teaching can be modified according to developmental stage. • Involvement of family member in care of the patient.

BETTY NEUMANN'S SYSTEM MODEL

Introduction

- ❖ Betty Neumann's system model provides a comprehensive flexible holistic and system based perspective for nursing.
- ❖ It focuses attention on the response of the client system to actual or potential environmental stressors.
- ❖ And the use of primary, secondary and tertiary nursing prevention intervention for retention, attainment, and maintenance of optimal client system wellness.

History and Background of the Theorist

- ❖ Betty Neumann was born in 1924, in Lowel, Ohio.
- ❖ She completed BS in nursing in 1957 and MS in Mental Health Public health consultation, from UCLA in 1966. She holds a PhD in clinical psychology.
- ❖ She was a pioneer in the community mental health movement in the late 1960s.
- ❖ Betty Neumann began developing her health system model while a lecturer in community health nursing at University of California, Los Angeles.
- ❖ The models was initially developed in response to graduate nursing students expression of a need for course content that would expose them to breadth of nursing problems prior to focusing on specific nursing problem areas.
- ❖ The model was published in 1972 as "A Model for Teaching Total Person Approach to Patient Problems" in Nursing Research.
- ❖ It was refined and subsequently published in the first edition of Conceptual Models for Nursing Practice, 1974, and in the second edition in 1980.

Development of the Model

❖ Neumann's model was influenced by a variety of sources.
❖ The philosophy writers deChardin and cornu (on wholeness in system).
❖ Von Bertalanffy, and Lazlo on general system theory.
❖ Selye on stress theory.
❖ Lazarus on stress and coping.

Basic Assumptions

❖ Each client system is unique, a composite of factors and characteristics within a given range of responses contained within a basic structure.
❖ Many known, unknown, and universal stressors exist. Each differ in it's potential for disturbing a client's usual stability level or normal LOD.
❖ The particular inter-relationships of client variables at any point in time can affect the degree to which a client is protected by the flexible LOD against possible reaction to stressors.
❖ Each client/client system has evolved a normal range of responses to the environment that is referred to as a normal LOD. The normal LOD can be used as a standard from which to measure health deviation.
❖ When the flexible LOD is no longer capable of protecting the client/client system against an environmental stressor, the stressor breaks through the normal LOD.
❖ The client whether in a state of wellness or illness, is a dynamic composite of the inter-relationships of the variables. Wellness is on a continuum of available energy to support the system in an optimal state of system stability.
❖ Implicit within each client system are internal resistance factors known as LOR, which function to stabilize and realign the client to the usual wellness state.
❖ Primary prevention relates to GK, " that is applied in client assessment and intervention, in identification and reduction of possible or actual risk factors."
❖ Secondary prevention relates to symptomatology following a reaction to stressor, appropriate ranking of intervention priorities and treatment to reduce their noxious effects.
❖ Tertiary prevention relates to adjustive processes taking place as reconstitution begins and maintenance factors move the back in circular manner toward primary prevention.
❖ The client as a system is in dynamic, constant energy exchange with the environment.

Concepts

❖ **Content:** The variables of the person in interaction with the internal and external environment comprise the whole client system.
❖ **Basic structure/central core:** Common client survival factors in unique individual characteristics representing basic system energy resources.
❖ The basic structure or central core, is made up of the basic survival factors that are common to the species (Neumann, 2002).
❖ **These factors include:** Normal temperature range, genetic structure, response pattern, organ strength or weakness, ego structure.
❖ Stability or homeostasis occurs when the amount of energy that is available exceeds that being used by the system.

- A homeostatic body system is constantly in a dynamic process of input, output, feedback, and compensation, which leads to a state of balance.
- **Degree to reaction:** The amount of system instability resulting from stressor invasion of the normal LOD.
- **Entropy:** A process of energy depletion and disorganization moving the system toward illness or possible death.
- **Flexible LOD:** A protective, accordion like mechanism that surrounds and protects the normal LOD from invasion by stressors.
- **Normal LOD:** It represents what the client has become over time, or the usual state of wellness. It is considered dynamic because it can expand or contract over time.
- **LOR:** The series of concentric circles that surrounds the basic structure.
- Protection factors activated when stressors have penetrated the normal LOD, causing a reaction symptomatology, e.g., mobilization of WBC and activation of immune system mechanism.
- **Input-output:** The matter, energy, and information exchanged between client and environment that is entering or leaving the system at any point in time.
- **Negentropy:** A process of energy conservation that increase organization and complexity, moving the system toward stability or a higher degree of wellness.
- **Open system:** A system in which there is continuous flow of input and process, output and feedback. It is a system of organized complexity where all elements are in interaction.
- **Prevention as intervention:** Interventions modes for nursing action and determinants for entry of both client and nurse into health care system.
- **Reconstitution:** The return and maintenance of system stability, following treatment for stressor reaction, which may result in a higher or lower level of wellness.
- **Stability:** A state of balance of harmony requiring energy exchanges as the client adequately copes with stressors to retain, attain, or maintain an optimal level of health thus preserving system integrity.
- **Stressors:** Environmental factors, intra (emotion, feeling), inter (role expectation), and extrapersonal (job or finance pressure) in nature, that have potential for disrupting system stability.
- A stressor is any phenomenon that might penetrate both the F and N LOD, resulting either a positive or negative outcome.
- **Wellness/Illness:** Wellness is the condition in which all system parts and subparts are in harmony with the whole system of the client.
  - Illness is a state of insufficiency with disrupting needs unsatisfied (Neumann, 2002).
  - Illness is an excessive expenditure of energy... when more energy is used by the system in its state of disorganization than is built and stored; the outcome may be death (Neumann, 2002).

Prevention

According to Neumann's model, prevention is the primary nursing intervention. Prevention focuses on keeping stressors and the stress response from having a detrimental effect on the body.

Primary Prevention

- Primary prevention occurs before the system reacts to a stressor. On the one hand, it strengthens the person (primary the flexible LOD) to enable him to better deal with stressors

❖ On the other hand manipulates the environment to reduce or weaken stressors.
❖ Primary prevention includes health promotion and maintenance of wellness.

Secondary Prevention

❖ Secondary prevention occurs after the system reacts to a stressor and is provided in terms of existing system.
❖ Secondary prevention focuses on preventing damage to the central core by strengthening the internal lines of resistance and/or removing the stressor.

Tertiary Prevention

❖ Tertiary prevention occurs after the system has been treated through secondary prevention strategies.
❖ Tertiary prevention offers support to the client and attempts to add energy to the system or reduce energy needed in order to facilitate reconstitution.

Four Major Concepts

Person

❖ The focus of the Neumann model is based on the philosophy that each human being is a total person as a client system and the person is a layered multidimensional being.
❖ Each layer consists of five person variable or subsystems:
    1. **Physiological:** Refer of the physicochemical structure and function of the body.
    2. **Psychological:** Refers to mental processes and emotions.
    3. **Sociocultural:** Refers to relationships; and social/cultural expectations and activities.
    4. **Spiritual:** Refers to the influence of spiritual beliefs.
    5. **Developmental:** Refers to those processes related to development over the lifespan.

Environment

❖ The environment is seen to be the totality of the internal and external forces which surround a person and with which they interact at any given time.
❖ These forces include the intrapersonal, interpersonal and extrapersonal stressors which can affect the person's normal line of defense and so can affect the stability of the system.
    • The *internal environment* exists within the client system.
    • The *external environment* exists outside the client system.
    • Neumann also identified a *created environment* which is an environment that is created and developed unconsciously by the client and is symbolic of system wholeness.

Health

❖ Neumann sees health as being equated with wellness. She defines health/wellness as "the condition in which all parts and subparts (variables) are in harmony with the whole of the client (Neumann, 1995)".
❖ The client system moves toward illness and death when more energy is needed than is available. The client system moved toward wellness when more energy is available than is needed.

Nursing

- Neumann sees nursing as a unique profession that is concerned with all of the variables which influence the response a person might have to a stressor.
- The person is seen as a whole, and it is the task of nursing to address the whole person.
- Neumann defines nursing as "action which assist individuals, families and groups to maintain a maximum level of wellness, and the primary aim is stability of the patient/client system, through nursing interventions to reduce stressors."
- Neumann states that, because the nurse's perception will influence the care given, then not only must the patient/client's perception be assessed, but so must those of the caregiver (nurse).
- The role of the nurse is seen in terms of degree of reaction to stressors, and the use of primary, secondary and tertiary interventions.

Stages of Nursing Process (By Neumann)

Nursing Diagnosis

- It depends on acquisition of appropriate database; the diagnosis identifies, assesses, classifies, and evaluates the dynamic interaction of the five variables.
- Variances from wellness (needs and problems) are determined by correlations and constraints through synthesis of theory and database.
- Broad hypothetical interventions are determined, i.e., maintain flexible line of defense.

Nursing Goals

These must be negotiated with the patient and take account of patient's and nurse's perceptions of variance from wellness.

Nursing Outcomes

- Nursing intervention using one or more preventive modes.
- Confirmation of prescriptive change or reformulation of nursing goals.
- Short-term goal outcomes influence determination of intermediate and long-term goals.
- A client outcome validates nursing process.

Neumann's System Model Format

Neumann's nursing process format designates the following categories of data about the client system as the major areas of assessment.

Assessment

- Potential and actual stressors.
- Condition and strength of basic structure factors and energy sources.
- Characteristics of flexible and normal line of defenses, lines of resistance, degree of reaction and potential for reconstitution.
- Interaction between client and environment.
- Life process and coping factors (past, present and future) actual and potential stressors (internal and external) for optimal wellness external.
- Perceptual difference between care giver and the client.

Nursing Diagnosis

- ❖ The data collected are then interpreted to condition and formulate the nursing diagnosis.
- ❖ Health seeking behaviors.
- ❖ Activity intolerance.
- ❖ Ineffective coping.
- ❖ Ineffective thermoregulation.

Goal

In Neumann's systems model, the goal is to keep the client system stable.

Planning

Planning is focused on strengthening the lines of defense and resistance.

Implementation

The goal of stabilizing the client system is achieved through three modes of prevention:
1. **Primary prevention:** Actions taken to retain stability
2. **Secondary prevention:** Actions taken to attain stability
3. **Tertiary prevention:** Actions taken to maintain stability

Evaluation

The nursing process is evaluated to determine whether equilibrium is restored and a steady state maintained.

Acceptance by the Nursing Community

- ❖ Neumann's model has been described as a grand nursing theory by walker and Avant.
- ❖ Grand theories can provide a comprehensive perspective for nursing practice, education, and research and Neumann's model does.

Practice

- ❖ The Neumann systems model has been applied and adapted to various specialties include: family therapy, public health, rehabilitation, and hospital nursing.
- ❖ The subspecialties include: pulmonary, renal, critical care, and hospital medical units. One of the model's strengths is that it can be used in a variety of settings.
- ❖ Using this conceptual model permits comparison of a nurse's interpretation of a problem with that of the patient, so the patient and nurse do not work on two separate problems.
- ❖ The role of the nurse in the model is to work with the patient to move him as far as possible along a continuum toward wellness.
- ❖ Because this model requires individual interaction with the total health care system, it is indicative of the futuristic direction the nursing profession is taking.
- ❖ The patient is being relabeled as a consumer with individual needs and wants.

Education

❖ The model has also been widely accepted in academic circles.
❖ It has often been selected as a curriculum guide for a conceptual framework oriented more toward wellness than toward a medical model and has been used at various levels of nursing education.
❖ In the associate degree program at Indiana University.
❖ One of the objectives for nursing graduate is to demonstrate ability to use the Neumann health care system in nursing practice. This helps prepare the students for developing a frame of reference centered on holistic care.
❖ At northwestern State University in Shreveport, Louisiana, the faculty determined that a systems model approach was preferred for their master's program because of the universality framework.
❖ Acceptance by the nursing community for education therefore is evident.

Research

❖ A study was published by Riehl and Roy to test the usefulness of the Neumann model in nursing practice.
❖ There were two major objectives of the study.
  1. To test the model/assessment' tool for its usefulness as a unifying method of collecting and analyzing data for identifying client problems.
  2. To test the assessment tool for its usefulness in the identification of congruence between the client's perception of stressors and the care giver's perception of client stressors.
❖ Results indicated that the model can help categorize data for assessing and planning care and for guiding decision making.
❖ Neumann's model can easily generate nursing research.
❖ It does this by providing a framework to develop goals for desired outcomes. Acceptance by the nursing community for research applying this model is in the beginning stages and positive.

Characteristics of Neumann's Theory

❖ **Theories connect the interrelated concepts in such a way as to create a different way of looking at a particular phenomenon:**
  ◆ The Neumann model represents a focus on nursing interest in the total person approach to the interaction of environment and health.
  ◆ The interrelationships between the concepts of person, health, nursing and society/environment are repeatedly mentioned throughout the Neumann model and are considered to be basically adequate according to the criteria.
❖ **Theories must be logical in nature:**
  ◆ Neumann's model in general presents itself as logically consistent.
  ◆ There is a logical sequence in the process of nursing wherein emphasis on the importance of accurate data assessment is basic to the sequential steps of the nursing process.
❖ **Theories should be relatively simple yet generalizable:**
  ◆ Neumann's model is fairly simple and straightforward in approach.
  ◆ The terms used are easily identifiable and for the most part have definitions that are broadly accepted.
  ◆ The multiple use of the model in varied nursing situations (practice, curriculum, and administration) is testimony in itself to its broad applicability.

- The potential use of this model by other health care disciplines also attests to its generalizability for use ion practice.
- One drawback in relation to simplicity is the diagrammed model since it presents over 35 variables and tends to be awesome to the viewer.

❖ **Theories can be the bases for hypotheses that can be tested.**
  - Neuman's model, due to its high level and breadth of abstraction, lends itself to theory development.
  - One are for future consideration as a beginning testable theory might be the concept of prevention as intervention, subsequent to basis concept refinement in the Neuman model.

❖ **Theories contribute to and assist in increasing the general body of knowledge within the discipline through the research implemented to validate them.**
  - The model has provided clear, comprehensive guidelines for nursing education and practice in a variety of settings; this is its primary contribution to nursing knowledge.
  - The concept within the guidelines is clearly explicated and many applications of the theory have been published, little research explicitly derived from this model has been published to date.

❖ **Theories can be utilized by the practitioner to guide and improve their practice.**
  - One of the most significant attributes of the Neumann model is the assessment/intervention instrument together with comprehensive guidelines for its use with the nursing process.
  - These guidelines have provided a practical resource for many nursing practitioners and have been used extensively in a variety of setting in nursing practice, education and administration.

❖ **Theories must be consistent with other validated theories, laws and principles but will leave open unanswered questions that need to be investigated.**
  In general, there is no direct conflict with other theories. There is, however, a lack of specificity in systems concepts such as "boundaries" which are indirectly addressed throughout the model.

Research Articles

❖ **Using the Neuman Systems Model for Best Practices—Sharon A DeWan, Pearl N Ume-Nwagbo, Nursing Science Quarterly, Vol 19, No 1, 31-35 (2006).**
  - The purpose of this study was to present two case studies based upon Neuman systems model; one case is directed toward family care, and the other demonstrates care with an individual. Theory-based exemplars serve as teaching tools for students and practicing nurses.
  - These case studies illustrate how nurses' actions, directed by Neuman's wholistic principles, integrate evidence-based practice and generate high quality care.

❖ **Melton L, Secrest J, Chien A, Andersen B. "A community needs assessment for a SANE program using Neuman's model"** J Am Acad Nurse Pract. 2001 Apr;13(4):178-86.
  - The purpose of the study was to present guidelines for a community needs assessment for a sexual assault nurse examiner (SANE) program using Neuman's systems model.
  - Sexual assault is a problem faced by almost every community. A thorough community assessment is an important first step in establishing programs that adequately meet a community's needs.
  - Guidelines for conducting such an assessment related to implementation of a SANE program are rare, and guidelines using a nursing model were not found in the literature.

APPLICATION OF BETTY NEUMAN'S SYSTEMS MODEL

Objectives

- To assess the patient condition by the various methods explained by the nursing theory
- To identify the needs of the patient
- To demonstrate an effective communication and interaction with the patient
- To select a theory for the application according to the need of the patient
- To apply the theory to solve the identified problems of the patient
- To evaluate the extent to which the process was fruitful.

Introduction

System Model: Betty Neuman

A theory is a group of related concepts that propose action that guide practice. A nursing theory is a set of concepts, definitions, relationships, and assumptions or propositions derived from nursing models or from other disciplines and project a purposive, systematic view of phenomena by designing specific inter-relationships among concepts for the purposes of describing, explaining, predicting, and/or prescribing.

The Neuman's system model has two major components, i.e., stress and reaction to stress. The client in the Neuman's system model is viewed as an open system in which repeated cycles of input, process, output and feedback constitute a dynamic organizational pattern. The client may be an individual, a group, a family, a community or an aggregate. In the development towards growth and development open system continuously become more differentiated and elaborate or complex. As they become more complex, the internal conditions of regulation become more complex. Exchange with the environment are reciprocal, both the client and the environment may be affected either positively or negatively by the other.

The system may adjust to the environment to itself. The ideal is to achieve optimal stability. As an open system the client, the client system has propensity to seek or maintain a balance among the various factors, both within and outside the system, that seek to disrupt it. Neuman seeks these forces as stressors and views them as capable of having either positive or negative effects. Reaction to the stressors may be possible or actual with identifiable responses and symptoms.

Major Concepts

- **Person variables:** Each layer, or concentric circle, of the Neuman model is made up of the five person variables. Ideally, each of the person variables should be considered simultaneously and comprehensively.
  1. Physiological—refers to the physicochemical structure and function of the body.
  2. Psychological—refers to mental processes and emotions.
  3. Sociocultural—refers to relationships; and social/cultural expectations and activities.
  4. Spiritual—refers to the influence of spiritual beliefs.
  5. Developmental—refers to those processes related to development over the lifespan.
- **Central core:** The basic structure, or central core, is made up of the basic survival factors that are common to the species (Neuman, 1995, in George, 1996). These factors include: system variables, genetic features, and the strengths and weaknesses of the system parts. Examples

of these may include: hair color, body temperature regulation ability, functioning of body systems, cognitive ability, physical strength, and value systems. The person's system is an open system and therefore is dynamic and constantly changing and evolving. Stability, or homeostasis, occurs when the amount of energy that is available exceeds that being used by the system. A homeostatic body system is constantly in a dynamic process of input, output, feedback, and compensation, which leads to a state of balance.

❖ **Flexible lines of defense:** The flexible line of defense is the outer barrier or cushion to the normal line of defense, the line of resistance, and the core structure. If the flexible line of defense fails to provide adequate protection to the normal line of defense, the lines of resistance become activated. The flexible line of defense acts as a cushion and is described as accordion-like as it expands away from or contracts closer to the normal line of defense. The flexible line of defense is dynamic and can be changed/altered in a relatively short period of time.

❖ **Normal line of defense:** The normal line of defense represents system stability over time. It is considered to be the usual level of stability in the system. The normal line of defense can change over time in response to coping or responding to the environment. An example is skin, which is stable and fairly constant, but can thicken into a callus over time.

❖ **Lines of resistance:** The lines of resistance protect the basic structure and become activated when environmental stressors invade the normal line of defense. Example: activation of the immune response after invasion of microorganisms. If the lines of resistance are effective, the system can reconstitute and if the lines of resistance are not effective, the resulting energy loss can result in death.

❖ **Reconstitution:** Reconstitution is the increase in energy that occurs in relation to the degree of reaction to the stressor. Reconstitution begins at any point following initiation of treatment for invasion of stressors. Reconstitution may expand the normal line of defense beyond its previous level, stabilize the system at a lower level, or return it to the level that existed before the illness.

❖ **Stressors:** The Neuman systems model looks at the impact of stressors on health and addresses stress and the reduction of stress (in the form of stressors). Stressors are capable of having either a positive or negative effect on the client system. A stressor is any environmental force which can potentially affect the stability of the system. They may be:
  ◆ *Intrapersonal*—occur within person, e.g., emotions and feelings
  ◆ *Interpersonal*—occur between individuals, e.g., role expectations
  ◆ *Extrapersonal*—occur outside the individual, e.g., job or finance pressures
  The person has a certain degree of reaction to any given stressor at any given time. The nature of the reaction depends in part on the strength of the lines of resistance and defense. By means of primary, secondary and tertiary interventions, the person (or the nurse) attempts to restore or maintain the stability of the system.

❖ **Prevention:** As defined by Neuman's model, prevention is the primary nursing intervention. Prevention focuses on keeping stressors and the stress response from having a detrimental effect on the body.
  ◆ *Primary:* Primary prevention occurs before the system reacts to a stressor. On the one hand, it strengthens the person (primarily the flexible line of defense) to enable him to better deal with stressors, and on the other hand manipulates the environment to reduce or weaken stressors. Primary prevention includes health promotion and maintenance of wellness.

- ◆ **Secondary:** Secondary prevention occurs after the system reacts to a stressor and is provided in terms of existing systems. Secondary prevention focuses on preventing damage to the central core by strengthening the internal lines of resistance and/or removing the stressor.
- ◆ **Tertiary:** Tertiary prevention occurs after the system has been treated through secondary prevention strategies. Tertiary prevention offers support to the client and attempts to add energy to the system or reduce energy needed in order to facilitate reconstitution.

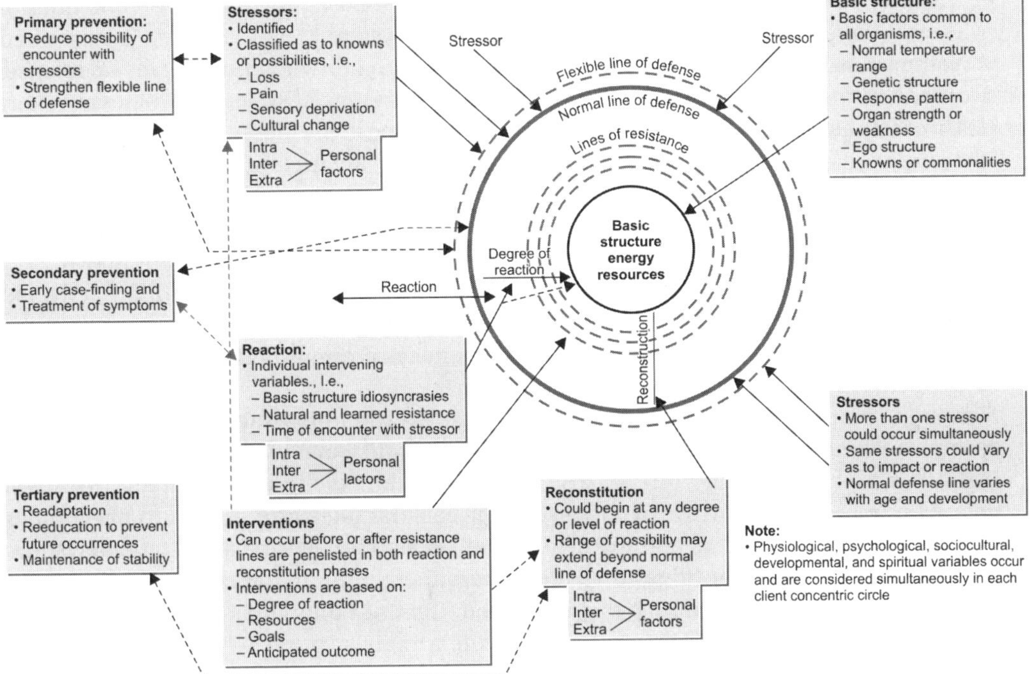

Nursing Metaparadigm

❖ **Person:** The person is a layered multidimensional being. Each layer consists of five person variables or subsystems:
1. Physical/physiological
2. Psychological
3. Sociocultural
4. Developmental
5. Spiritual

The layers, usually represented by concentric circle, consist of the central core, lines of resistance, lines of normal defense, and lines of flexible defense. The basic core structure is comprised of survival mechanisms including: organ function, temperature control, genetic structure, response patterns, ego, and what Neuman terms 'knowns and commonalities'. Lines of resistance and two lines of defense protect this core. The person may in fact be an individual, a family, a group, or a community in Neuman's model. The person, with a core of basic structures, is seen as being in constant, dynamic interaction with the environment. Around the basic core structures are lines of defense and resistance (shown diagrammatically as concentric circles, with the lines of resistance nearer to the core. The person is seen as being in a state of constant change and-as an open system-in reciprocal interaction with the environment (i.e., affecting, and being affected by it).

- ❖ **The environment:** The environment is seen to be the totality of the internal and external forces which surround a person and with which they interact at any given time. These forces include the intrapersonal, interpersonal and extrapersonal stressors which can affect the person's normal line of defense and so can affect the stability of the system.
  - ◆ The *internal environment* exists within the client system.
  - ◆ The *external environment* exists outside the client system.
  - ◆ Neuman also identified a ***created environment*** which is an environment that is created and developed unconsciously by the client and is symbolic of system wholeness.
- ❖ **Health:** Neuman sees health as being equated with wellness. She defines health/wellness as "the condition in which all parts and subparts (variables) are in harmony with the whole of the client (Neuman, 1995)". As the person is in a constant interaction with the environment, the state of wellness (and by implication any other state) is in dynamic equilibrium, rather than in any kind of steady state. Neuman proposes a wellness-illness continuum, with the person's position on that continuum being influenced by their interaction with the variables and the stressors they encounter. The client system moves toward illness and death when more energy is needed than is available. The client system moves toward wellness when more energy is available than is needed.
- ❖ **Nursing:** Neuman sees nursing as a unique profession that is concerned with all of the variables which influence the response a person might have to a stressor. The person is seen as a whole, and it is the task of nursing to address the whole person. Neuman defines nursing as actions which assist individuals, families and groups to maintain a maximum level of wellness, and the primary aim is stability of the patient/client system, through nursing interventions to reduce stressors. Neuman states that, because the nurse's perception will influence the care given, then not only must the patient/client's perceptions be assessed, but so must those of the caregiver (nurse). The role of the nurse is seen in terms of degrees of reaction to stressors, and the use of primary, secondary and tertiary interventions.

Neuman envisions a three-stage nursing process:

1. **Nursing diagnosis:** Based of necessity in a thorough assessment, and with consideration given to five variables in three stressor areas.
2. **Nursing goals:** These must be negotiated with the patient, and take account of patient's and nurse's perceptions of variance from wellness.
3. **Nursing outcomes**: Considered in relation to five variables, and achieved through primary, secondary and tertiary interventions.

Nursing Process Based on System Model

Assessment: Neuman's first step of nursing process parallels the assessment and nursing diagnosis of the six-phase nursing process. Using system model in the assessment phase of nursing process the nurse focuses on obtaining a comprehensive client database to determine the existing state of wellness and actual or potential reaction to environmental stressors.

Nursing diagnosis: The synthesis of data with theory also provides the basis for nursing diagnosis. The nursing diagnostic statement should reflect the entire client condition.

Outcome identification and planning: It involves negotiation between the care giver and the client or recipient of care. The overall goal of the care giver is to guide the client to conserve energy and to use energy as a force to move beyond the present.

Implementation: Nursing actions are based on the synthesis of a comprehensive data base about the client and the theory that are appropriate to the client's and caregiver's perception and possibilities for functional competence in the environment. According to this step the evaluation confirms that the anticipated or prescribed change has occurred. Immediate and long-range goals are structured in relation to the short term goals.

Evaluation: Evaluation is the anticipated or prescribed change has occurred. If it is not met the goals are reformed.

Assessment

Patient Profile

- ❖ **Name:** Mr AM
- ❖ **Age:** 66 years
- ❖ **Sex:** Male
- ❖ **Marital status:** Married
- ❖ **Referral source:** Referred from------- Medical College, -------

Stressors as Perceived by Client

(Information collected from the patient and his wife)

1. **Major stress area, or areas of health concern:**
   - ◆ Patient was suffering from severe abdominal pain, nausea, vomiting, yellowish discolorations of eye, palm, and urine, reduced appetite and gross weight loss (8 kg with in 4 months)
   - ◆ Patient is been diagnosed to have Periampullary carcinoma one week back.
   - ◆ Patient underwent operative procedure, i.e., Whipple's procedure—Pancreato duodenectomy on 27/3/08.
   - ◆ Psychologically disturbed about his disease condition—anticipating it as a life threatening condition. Patient is in depressive mood and does not interacting.
   - ◆ Patient is disturbed by the thoughts that he became a burden to his children with so many serious illnesses which made them to stay with him at hospital.
   - ◆ Patient has pitting type of edema over the ankle region, and it is more during the evening and will not be relieved by elevation of the affected extremities.
   - ◆ He had developed BPH few months back (January 2008) and underwent surgery TURP on January 17. Still he has mild difficulty in initiating the stream of urine.
   - ◆ Patient is a known case of Diabetes since last 28 years and for the last 4 years he is on Inj. H. Insulin (4U-0-0). It is adding up his distress regarding his health.
2. **Lifestyle patterns:**
   - ◆ Patient is a retired school teacher
   - ◆ Cares for wife and other family members

- Living with his son and his family
- Active in church
- Participates in community group meeting, i.e., local politics
- Has a supportive spouse and family
- Taking mixed diet
- No habits of smoking or drinking
- Spends leisure time by reading newspaper, watching TV, spending time with family members and relatives

3. **Have you experienced a similar problem?**
   - The fatigue is similar to that of previous hospitalization (after the surgery of the BPH)
   - Severity of pain was somewhat similar in the previous time of surgery, i.e., TURP
   - Was psychologically disturbed during the previous surgery, i.e., TURP
   - What helped then—family members psychological support helped him to overcome the crisis situation

4. **Anticipation of the future:**
   - Concerns about the healthy and speedy recovery
   - Anticipation of changes in the lifestyle and food habits
   - Anticipating about the demands of modified lifestyle
   - Anticipating the needs of future follow-up

5. **What doing to help himself?**
   - Talking to his friends and relatives
   - Reading the religious materials, i.e., reading the Bible
   - Instillation of positive thoughts, i.e., planning about the activities to be resume after discharge, spending time with grandchildren, going to the church, return back to the social interactions, etc.
   - Avoiding the negative thoughts, i.e., diverts the attentions from the pain or difficulties, try to eliminate the disturbing thoughts about the disease and surgery, etc.
   - Trying to accept the reality, etc.

6. **What is expected of others?**
   - Family members visiting the patient and spending some time with him will help to a great extent to relieve his tension.
   - Convey a warm and accepting behavior towards him.
   - Family members will help him to meet his own personal needs as much as possible.
   - Involve the patient also in taking decisions about his own care, treatment, follow-up, etc.

Stressors as Perceived by the Care Giver

1. **Major stress areas;**
   - Persistent fatigue
   - Massive weight loss, i.e. (8 kg of body weight within 4 months)
   - History of BPH and its surgery
   - Persistence of urinary symptoms (difficulty in initiating the stream of urine) and edema of the lower extremities
   - Persistent disease—chronic hypertensive since last 28 years
   - Depressive ideations and negative thoughts

2. **Present circumstances differ from the usual pattern of living:**
    - Hospitalization
    - Acute pain (before the surgery patient had pain because of the underlying pathology and after the surgery pain is present at the surgical site)
    - Nausea and vomiting which was present before the surgery and is still persisting after the surgery also
    - Anticipatory anxiety concerns the recovery and prognosis of the disease
    - Negative thoughts that he has become a burden to his children
    - Anticipatory anxiety concerning the restrictions after the surgery and the lifestyle modifications which are to be followed.

3. **Clients past experience with the similar situations:**
    - Patient verbalized that the severity of pain, nausea, fatigue, etc. was similar to that of patient's previous surgery. Counter checked with the family members that what they observed.
    - Psychologically disturbed previously also before the surgery (collected from the patient and counter checked with the relatives).
    - Client perceived that the present disease condition is much more severe than the previous condition. He thinks it is a serious form of cancer and the recovery is very poor. So patient is psychologically depressed.

4. **Future anticipations:**
    - Client is capable of handling the situation—will need support and encouragement to do so.
    - He has the plans to go back home and to resume the activities which he was doing prior to the hospitalization.
    - He also planned in his mind about the future follow-up, i.e., continuation of chemotherapy

5. **What client can do to help himself?**
    - Patient is using his own coping strategies to adjust to the situations.
    - He is spending time to read religious books and also spends time in talking with others.
    - He is trying to clarify his own doubts in an attempt to eliminate doubts and to instill hope.
    - He sets his major goal, i.e., a healthy and speedy recovery.

6. **Client's expectations of family, friends and caregivers:**
    - He sees the health care providers as a source pf information.
    - He tries to consider them as a significant member who can help to overcome the stress.
    - He seeks both psychological and physical support from the care givers, friends and family members.
    - He sees the family members as helping hands and feels relaxed when they are with him.

Evaluation/summary of impressions: There are no apparent discrepancies identified between patients perception and the care givers perceptions.

Intrapersonal Factors

1. **Physical examination and investigations:**
    - **Height:** 162 cm
    - **Weight:** 42 kg
    - **TPR:** 37oC, 74 b/m, 14 breaths per min
    - **BP:** 130/78 mm of Hg

- **Eye:** Vision is normal, on examination the appearance of eye is normal. Conjunctiva is pale in appearance. Pupils reacting to the light.
- **Ear:** Appearance of ears normal. No wax deposition. Pinna is normal in appearance and hearing ability is also normal.
- **Respiratory system:** Respiratory rate is normal, no abnormal sounds on auscultation. Respiratory rate is 16 breaths per min.
- **Cardiovascular system:** Heart rate is 76 per min on auscultation no abnormalities detected. Edema is present over the left ankle which is non pitting in nature.
- **GIT:** Patient has the complaints of reduced appetite, nausea; vomiting, etc., food intake is very less. Mouth—on examination is normal. Bowel sounds are reduced. Abdomen could not be palpated because of the presence of the surgical incision. Bowel habits are not regular after the hospitalization.
- **Extremities:** Range of motion of the extremities are normal. Edema is present over the left ankle which is non pitting in nature. Because of weakness and fatigue he is not able to walk without support.
- **Integumentary system:** Extremities are mild yellowish in color. No cyanosis. Capillary refill is normal.
- **Genitor urinary system:** Patient has difficulty in initiating the urine stream. No complaints of painful micturition or difficulty in passing urine.
- **Self-acre activities:** Perform some of his activities, for getting up from the bed he needs some other person's support. To walk also he needs a support. He do his personal care activities with the support from the others.
- **Immunizations:** It has been told that he has taken the immunizations at the specific periods itself and he also had taken hepatitis immunization around 8 years back.
- **Sleep:** He said that sleep is reduced because of the pain and other difficulties. Sleep is reduced after the hospitalization because of the noisy environment.
- **Diet and nutrition:** Patient is taking mixed diet, but the food intake is less when compared to previous food intake because of the nausea and vomiting. Usually he takes food three times a day.
- **Habits:** Patient does not have the habit of drinking or smoking.
- **Other complaints:** Patient has the complaints of pain fatigue, loss of appetite, dizziness, difficulty in urination, etc.

2. **Psycho-socio cultural:**
   - Anxious about his condition
   - Depressive mood
   - Patient is a retired teacher and he is Christian by religion
   - Studied up to BA
   - Married and has four children (two sons and two daughters)
   - Congenial home environment and good relationship with wife and children
   - Is active in the social activities at his native place and also actively involved in the religious activities too
   - Good and congenial relationship with the neighbors
   - Has some good and close friends at his place and he actively interact with them. They also very supportive to him
   - Good social support system is present from the family as well as from the neighborhood

3. **Developmental factors:**
   - Patient confidently says that he had been worked for 32 years as a teacher and he was a very good teacher for students and was a good coworker for the friends.
   - He told that he could manage the official and house hold activities very well
   - He was very active after the retirement and once he go back also he will resume the activities
4. **Spiritual belief system:**
   - Patient is Christian by religion.
   - He believes in got and used to go to church and also an active member in the religious activities.
   - He has a personal Bible and he used to read it min of two times a day and also whenever he is worried or tensed he used to pray or read Bible.
   - He has a good social support system present which helps him to keep his mind active.

Interpersonal Factors

- Has supportive family and friends
- Good social interaction with others
- Good social support system is present
- Active in the agricultural works at home after the retirement
- Active in the religious activities.
- Good interpersonal relationship with wife and the children
- Good social adjustment present

Extrapersonal Factors

- All the health care facilities are present at his place.
- All communication facilities, travel and transport facilities, etc., are present at his own place.
- His house at a village which is not much far from the city and the facilities are available at the place.
- Financially they are stable and are able to meet the treatment expenses.

Summary

- **Physiological:** Thin body built pallor of extremities, yellowish discoloration of the mucus membrane and sclera of eye. Nausea, vomiting, reduced appetite, reduced urinary out put. Diagnosed to have periampullary carcinoma.
- **Psycho-socio cultural factors:** Patient is anxious abut his condition. Depressive mood. Not interacting much with others. Good support system is present.
- **Developmental:** No developmental abnormalities. Appropriate to the age.
- **Spiritual:** Patient's belief system has a positive contribution to his recovery and adjustment.

Clinical Features

- Pain abdomen since 4 days
- Discoloration of urine
- Complaints of vomiting

- Fatigue
- Reduced appetite
- On and off fever
- Yellowish discoloration of eye, palms and nails
- Complaints of weight loss
- Edema over the left leg

Investigations

Investigations	Values
Hemoglobin (13–19 g/dL)	6.9
HCT (40–50%)	21.9
WBC (4,000–11,000 cells/cumm)	12,200
Neutrophil (40–75%)	77.2
Lymphocyte (25–45%)	10.5
Monocyte (2–10%)	4.5
Eosinophil (0–10%)	2.6
Basophil (0–2%)	.2
Platelet (150,000–400,000 cells/cumm)	345,000
ESR (0–10 mm/hr)	86
RBS (60–150 mg/dL)	148
Pus C/S	—
USG	USG shows mild diffuse cell growth at the Ampulla of Vater which suggests peri ampullary carcinoma of Grade I without metastasis and gross spread
Urea (8–35 mg/dL)	28
Creatinine (0.6–1.6 mg/dL)	1.8
Sodium (130–143 mEq/L)	136
Potassium (3.5–5 mEq/L)	4
PT (patient) (11.4–15.6 sec)	12.3
APTT—patient (24–32.4 sec)	26.4
Blood group	A+
HIV	Negative
HCV	Negative
HBsAg	Negative
Urine Protein (negative)	Negative
Urine WBC (0–5 cells/hpf)	Nil
RBC (nil)	Nil

Therapeutic Management

<table>
<tr><td>

Initial treatment:
Patient got admitted to—Medical college for 3 days and the symptoms not relieved. So they asked for discharge and came to—this hospital There treated with
- Inj Tramazac IV SOS
- IV fluids—DNS

Treatment at this hospital...
Preoperative period
- Tab Clovipas 75 mg 0-1-0
- Tab Monotrate 1-0-1
- Tab Metalor XL 1-0-0
- Inj H Insulin S/C 6-0-6U
- Inj Tramazac 50 mg IV Q8H
- Inj Emset 4 mg Q8H
- Tab Pantodac 40 mg 1-0-0
- Cap beneficiale 0-1-0
- Syp Aristozyme 1-1-1
- K bind I sachet TID

Surgical management
Patient underwent Whipple's procedure (pancreatoduodenectomy)

</td><td>

Postoperative period (immediate postoperative)
- Inj Pethedine 1 mg SOS
- Inj Phenargan SOS
- Inj Pantodac 40 mg IV OD
- Inj Clexane 0.3 mL S/C OD
- Inj Vorth P 40 mg IM Q12H
- Inj calcium Gluconate 10 mL over 10 min
- IV fluids—DNS

Late postoperative period after 3 days of surgery
- Inj H Insulin S/C 6-0-6U
- Tab Pantodac 40 mg 1-0-0
- Cap beneficiale 0-1-0
- Tab Clovipas 75 mg 0-1-0
- Tab Monotrate 1-0-1
- Tab Metalor XL 1-0-0

Other instructions
- Incentive spirometry
- Steam inhalation
- Early ambulation
- Diabetic diet

</td></tr>
</table>

Nursing Process

I. **Nursing Diagnosis**

Acute pain related to the presence of surgical wound on abdomen secondary to periampullary carcinoma

Desired outcome/goal: Patient will get relief from pain as evidenced by a reduction in the pain scale score and verbalization

Nursing action		
Primary prevention	*Secondary prevention*	*Tertiary prevention*
• Assess severity of pain by using a pain scale • Check the surgical site for any signs of infection or complications • Support the areas with extra pillow to allow the normal alignment and to prevent strain • Handle the area gently. Avoid unnecessary handling as this will affect the healing process • Clean the area around the incision and do surgical dressing at the site of incision to prevent any form of infections	• Teach the patient about the relaxation techniques and make him to do it • Encourage the patient to divert his mind from pain and to engage in pleasurable activities like taking with others • Do not allow the patient to do strenuous activities. And explain to the patient why those activities are contraindicated	• Educate the client about the importance of cleanliness and encourage him to maintain good personal hygiene • Involve the family members in the care of patient • Encourage relatives to be with the client in order provide a psychological well-being to patient

Contd...

Contd...

Primary prevention	Secondary prevention	Tertiary prevention
• Provide non-pharmacological measures for pain relief such as diversional activity which diverts the patient's mind. • Administer the pain medications as per the prescription by the pain clinics to relieve the severity of pain. • Keep the patient's body clean in order to avoid infection	• Involve the patient in making decisions about his own care and provide a positive psychological support • Provide the primary preventive care whenever necessary	• Educate the family members about the pain management measures • Provide the primary and secondary preventive measures to the client whenever necessary

Evaluation: Patient verbalized that the pain got reduced and the pain scale score also was zero. His facial expression also reveals that he got relief from pain.

II. Nursing Diagnosis

Activity intolerance related to fatigue secondary to pain at the surgery site, and dietary restrictions

Outcome/goals: Client will develop appropriate levels of activity free from excess fatigue, as evidenced by normal vital signs and verbalized understanding of the benefits of gradual increase in activity and exercise.

Nursing action		
Primary prevention	**Secondary prevention**	**Tertiary prevention**
• Adequately oxygenate the client • Instruct the client to avoid the activities which causes extreme fatigue • Provide the necessary articles near the patient's bed side. • Assist the patient in early ambulation • Monitor client's response to the activities in order to reduce discomforts • Provide nutritious diet to the client • Avoid psychological distress to the client. Tell the family members to be with him. • Schedule rest periods because it helps to alleviate fatigue	• Instruct the client to avoid the activities which causes extreme fatigue • Advice the client to perform exercises to strengthen the extremities and promote activities • Tell the client to avoid the activities such as straining at stool, etc. • Teach the client about the importance of early ambulation and assist the patient in early ambulation • Teach the mobility exercises appropriate for the patient to improve the circulation	• Encourage the client to do the mobility exercises • Tell the family members to provide nutritious diet in a frequent intervals • Teach the patient and the family about the importance of psychological well-being in recovery • Provide the primary and secondary level care if necessary

Evaluation: Patient verbalized that his activity level improved. He is able to do some of his activities with assistance. Fatigue relieved and patient looks much more active and interactive.

III. Nursing Diagnosis

Impaired physical mobility related to presence of dressing, pain at the site of surgical incision

Outcomes/goals: Patient will have improved physical mobility as evidenced by walking with minimum support and doing the activities in limit.

Nursing action		
Primary prevention	*Secondary prevention*	*Tertiary prevention*
• Provide active and passive exercises to all the extremities to improve the muscle tone and strength • Make the patient to perform the breathing exercises which will strengthen the respiratory muscle • Massage the upper and lower extremities which help to improve the circulation • Provide articles near to the patient and encourage doing activities within limits which promote a feeling of well-being.	• Provide positive reinforcement for even a small improvement to increase the frequency of the desired activity • Teach the mobility exercises appropriate for the patient to improve the circulation and to prevent contractures • Mobilize the patient and encourage him to do so whenever possible • Motivate the client to involve in his own care activities • Provide primary preventive measures whenever necessary	• Educate and reeducate the client and family about the patients care and recovery • Support the patient, and family towards the attainment of the goals • Coordinate the care activities with the family members and other disciplines like physiotherapy • Teach the importance of psychological well-being which influence indirectly the physical recovery • Provide primary preventive measures whenever necessary

Evaluation: Patient's physical activity improved and he is able to move from bed with support. Patient started doing the active and passive exercises and he verbalized improvement.

Conclusion

The Neuman's system model when applied in nursing practice helped in identifying the interpersonal, intrapersonal and extrapersonal stressors of Mr. AM from various aspects. This was helpful to provide care in a comprehensive manner. The application of this theory revealed how well the primary, secondary and tertiary prevention interventions could be used for solving the problems in the client.

DOROTHEA OREM'S THEORY

Introduction

❖ One of America's foremost nursing theorists.

❖ Dorothea Orem earned her Bachelor of science in nursing education in 1939 and Master of science in nursing in 1945

❖ During her professional career, she worked as a staff nurse, private duty nurse, nurse educator and administrator and nurse consultant

❖ Received honorary Doctor of Science degree in 1976

❖ Dorothea Orem as a member of a curriculum subcommittee at Catholic University, recognized the need to continue in developing a conceptualization of nursing.

❖ Published first formal articulation of her ideas in ***Nursing: Concepts of Practice*** in 1971. second in 1980, and finally in 1995.

Development of Theory

- ❖ 1949–1957 Orem worked for the Division of Hospital and Institutional Services of the Indiana State Board of Health. Her goal was to upgrade the quality of nursing in general hospitals throughout the state. During this time she developed her definition of nursing practice.
- ❖ 1958–1960 US Department of Health, Education and Welfare where she help publish "Guidelines for Developing Curricula for the Education of Practical Nurses" in 1959.
- ❖ 1959 Orem subsequently served as acting dean of the school of Nursing and as an assistant professor of nursing education at CUA. She continued to develop her concept of nursing and self-care during this time.
- ❖ **Orem's nursing:** Concept of practice was first published in 1971 and subsequently in 1980, 1985, 1991, 1995, and 2001.
- ❖ Continues to develop her theory after her retirement in 1984.

Definitions of Domain Concepts

- ❖ **Nursing** is art, a helping service, and a technology.
- ❖ Actions deliberately selected and performed by nurses to help individuals or groups under their care to maintain or change conditions in themselves or their environments.
- ❖ Encompasses the patient's perspective of health condition, the physician's perspective, and the nursing perspective.
- ❖ **Goal of nursing:** To render the patient or members of his family capable of meeting the patient's self-care needs:
  - ◆ To maintain a state of health.
  - ◆ To regain normal or near normal state of health in the event of disease or injury.
  - ◆ To stabilize, control, or minimize the effects of chronic poor health or disability.
- ❖ **Health:** Health and healthy are terms used to describe living things ... it is when they are structurally and functionally whole or sound ... wholeness or integrity..includes that which makes a person human,...operating in conjunction with physiological and psychophysiological mechanisms and a material structure and in relation to and interacting with other human beings.
- ❖ **Environment:** Environment components are environmental factors, environmental elements, conditions, and developmental environment.
- ❖ **Human being:** Has the capacity to reflect, symbolize and use symbols:
  - ◆ Conceptualized as a total being with universal, developmental needs and capable of continuous self-care.
  - ◆ A unity that can function biologically, symbolically and socially.
- ❖ **Nursing client:** A human being who has "health related/health derived limitations that render him incapable of continuous self-care or dependent care or limitations that result in ineffective/incomplete care.
  - ◆ A human being is the focus of nursing only when a self-care requisites exceed self-care capabilities.
- ❖ **Nursing problem:** Deficits in universal, developmental, and health derived or health related conditions.
- ❖ **Nursing process:** A system to determine (1) why a person is under care (2) a plan for care, (3) the implementation of care.
- ❖ **Nursing therapeutics:** Deliberate, systematic and purposeful action.

Orem's General Theory of Nursing

Orem's general theory of nursing in three related parts:
1. Theory of self-care
2. Theory of self-care deficit
3. Theory of nursing systems

Theory of Self-care

Includes:
- **Self-care:** Practice of activities that individual initiates and perform on their own behalf in maintaining life, health and well-being.
- **Self-care agency:** Is a human ability which is "the ability for engaging in self-care." Conditioned by age developmental state, life experience sociocultural orientation health and available resources.
- **Therapeutic self-care demand:** "Totality of self-care actions to be performed for some duration in order to meet self-care requisites by using valid methods and related sets of operations and actions":
  - Self-care requisites-action directed towards provision of self-care
  - Three categories of self-care requisites are:
    1. Universal
    2. Developmental
    3. Health deviation

Universal Self-care Requisites

- Associated with life processes and the maintenance of the integrity of human structure and functioning
- Common to all, ADL
- Identifies these requisites as:
  - Maintenance of sufficient intake of air, water, food
  - Provision of care associated with elimination process
  - Balance between activity and rest, between solitude and social interaction
  - Prevention of hazards to human life well-being and
  - Promotion of human functioning

Developmental Self-care Requisites

Associated with developmental processes/derived from a condition or associated with an event, e.g., adjusting to a new job and adjusting to body changes.

Health Deviation Self-care

Required in conditions of illness, injury, or disease. These include:
- Seeking and securing appropriate medical assistance
- Being aware of and attending to the effects and results of pathologic conditions
- Effectively carrying out medically prescribed measures
- Modifying self-concepts in accepting oneself as being in a particular state of health and in specific forms of health care
- Learning to live with effects of pathologic conditions

Theory of Self-care Deficit

❖ Specifies when nursing is needed
❖ Nursing is required when an adult (or in the case of a dependent, the parent) is incapable or limited in the provision of continuous effective self-care

Orem Identifies Five Methods of Helping

❖ Acting for and doing for others
❖ Guiding others
❖ Supporting another
❖ Providing an environment promoting personal development in relation to meet future demands
❖ Teaching another

Theory of Nursing Systems

❖ Describes how the patient's self-care needs will be met by the nurse, the patient, or both.
❖ Identifies three classifications of nursing system to meet the self-care requisites of the patient:
  1. Wholly compensatory system
  2. Partly compensatory system
  3. Supportive-educative system
❖ Design and elements of nursing system define
❖ Scope of nursing responsibility in health care situations
❖ General and specific roles of nurses and patients
❖ Reasons for nurses' relationship with patients and
❖ The kinds of actions to be performed and the performance patterns and nurses' and patients' actions in regulating patients' self-care agency and in meeting their self-care demand
❖ Orem recognized that specialized technologies are usually developed by members of the health profession
❖ A technology is systematized information about a process or a method for affecting some desired result through deliberate practical endeavor, with or without use of materials or instruments

Categories of Technologies

Social or Interpersonal

❖ Communication adjusted to age, health status
❖ Maintaining interpersonal, intragroup or intergroup relations for coordination of efforts
❖ Maintaining therapeutic relationship in light of psychosocial modes of functioning in health and disease
❖ Giving human assistance adapted to human needs, action abilities and limitations
❖ Regulatory technologies
❖ Maintaining and promoting life processes
❖ Regulating psycho physiological modes of functioning in health and disease

❖ Promoting human growth and development
❖ Regulating position and movement in space

Orem's Theory and Nursing Process

❖ Orem's approach to the nursing process presents a method to determine the self-care deficits and then to define the roles of person or nurse to meet the self-care demands.
❖ The steps within the approach are considered to be the technical component of the nursing process.
❖ Orem emphasizes that the technological component "must be coordinated with interpersonal and social processes within nursing situations

Comparison of Orem's Nursing Process and the Nursing Process

Nursing Process

❖ Assessment
❖ Nursing diagnosis
❖ Plans with scientific rationale
❖ Implementation
❖ evaluation

Orem's Nursing Process

❖ Diagnosis and prescription; determine why nursing is needed. Analyze and interpret—make judgment regarding care
❖ Design of a nursing system and plan for delivery of care
❖ Production and management of nursing systems
  ◆ **Step 1—collect data in six areas:**
    ◊ The person's health status
    ◊ The physician's perspective of the person's health status
    ◊ The person's perspective of his or her health
    ◊ The health goals within the context of life history, lifestyle, and health status
    ◊ The person's requirements for self-care
    ◊ The person's capacity to perform self-care
  ◆ **Step 2**
    ◊ Nurse designs a system that is wholly or partly compensatory or supportive-educative.
    ◊ The two actions are:
      1. Bringing out a good organization of the components of patients' therapeutic self-care demands
      2. Selection of combination of ways of helping that will be effective and efficient in compensating for/overcoming patient's self-care deficits
  ◆ **Step 3**
    ◊ Nurse assists the patient or family in self-care matters to achieve identified and described health and health related results. Collecting evidence in evaluating results achieved against results specified in the nursing system design
    ◊ Actions are directed by etiology component of nursing diagnosis
    ◊ Evaluation

Orem's Work and the Characteristics of a Theory

* Theories can interrelate concepts in such a way as to create a different way of looking at a particular phenomenon
* Theories must be logical in nature
* Theories must be relatively simple yet generalizable
* Theories are the basis for hypothesis that can be tested
* Theories contribute to and assist in increasing the general body of knowledge within the discipline through the research implemented to validate them
* Theories can be used by the practitioners to guide and improve their practice
* Theories must be consistent with other validated theories, laws and principles

Theory Testing

* Orem's theory has been used as the basis for the development of research instruments to assist researchers in using the theory
* A self-care questionnaire was developed and tested by Moore (1995) for the special purpose of measuring the self-care practice of children and adolescents
* The theory has been used as a conceptual framework in associated degree programs (Fenner 1979) also in many nursing schools

Strengths

* Provides a comprehensive base to nursing practice
* It has utility for professional nursing in the areas of nursing practice nursing curricula, nursing education administration, and nursing research
* Specifies when nursing is needed
* Also includes continuing education as part of the professional component of nursing education
* Her self-care approach is contemporary with the concepts of health promotion and health maintenance
* Expanded her focus of individual self-care to include multiperson units

Limitations

* In general system theory a system is viewed as a single whole thing while Orem defines a system as a single whole, thing
* Health is often viewed as dynamic and ever changing. Orem's visual presentation of the boxed nursing systems implies three static conditions of health
* Appears that the theory is illness oriented rather with no indication of its use in wellness settings

APPLICATION OF OREM'S SELF-CARE DEFICIT THEORY IN NURSING PRACTICE

Introduction

* The history of professional nursing begins with Florence nightingale.
* Later in last century nursing began with a strong emphasis on practice.

❖ Following that came the curriculum era which addressed the questions about what the nursing students should study in order to achieve the required standard of nursing.

❖ As more and more nurses began to pursue higher degrees in nursing, there emerged the research era.

❖ Later graduate education and masters education was given much importance.

❖ The development of the theory era was a natural outgrowth of the research era.

❖ With an increased number of researches it became obvious that the research without theory produced isolated information; however research and theory produced the nursing sciences.

❖ Within the contemporary phase there is an emphasis on theory use and theory-based nursing practice and lead to the continued development of the theories.

Objectives

❖ To assess the patient condition by the various methods explained by the nursing theory

❖ To identify the needs of the patient

❖ To demonstrate an effective communication and interaction with the patient.

❖ To select a theory for the application according to the need of the patient

❖ To apply the theory to solve the identified problems of the patient

❖ To evaluate the extent to which the process was fruitful.

Areas	Patient details
• Name	• Mrs X
• Age	• 56 years
• Sex	• Female
• Education	• No formal education
• Occupation	• Household
• Marital status	• Married
• Religion	• Hindu
• Diagnosis	• Rheumatoid arthritis
• Theory applied	• Orem's theory of self-care deficit

Orem's Theory of Self-care Deficit

❖ The self-care deficit theory proposed by Orem is a combination of three theories, i.e., theory of self-care, theory of self-care deficit and the theory of nursing systems.

❖ In the theory of self-care, she explains self-care as the activities carried out by the individual to maintain their own health.

❖ The **self-care agency** is the acquired ability to perform the self-care and this will be affected by the **basic conditioning factors** such as age, gender, health care system, family system etc.

❖ Therapeutic self-care demand is the totality of the self-care measures required.

❖ The self-care is carried out to fulfill the **self-care requisites**.

❖ There are mainly 3 types of self-care requisites such as universal, developmental and health deviation self-care requisites.

❖ Whenever there is an inadequacy of any of these self-care requisite, the person will be in need of self-care or will have a **deficit in self-care**.

❖ The deficit is identified by the nurse through the thorough assessment of the patient.

❖ Once the need is identified, the nurse has to select required nursing systems to provide care: wholly compensatory, partly compensatory or supportive and educative system.

- ❖ The care will be provided according to the degree of deficit the patient is presenting with.
- ❖ Once the care is provided, the nursing activities and the use of the nursing systems are to be evaluated to get an idea about whether the mutually planned goals are met or not.
- ❖ Thus the theory could be successfully applied into the nursing practice.

For example Mrs X (A patient) ...

- ❖ She came to the hospital with complaints of pain over all the joints, stiffness which is more in the morning and reduces by the activities.
- ❖ She has these complaints since 5 years and has taken treatment from local hospital.
- ❖ The symptoms were not reducing and came to—MC, Hospital for further management.
- ❖ Patient was able to do the ADL by herself but the way she performed and the posture she used was making her prone to develop the complications of the disease.
- ❖ She also was malnourished and was not having awareness about the deficiencies and effects.

Data Collection According to Orem's Theory of Self-care Deficit

1. **Basic conditioning factors:**

Age	56 years
Gender	Female
Health state	Disability due to health condition, therapeutic self-care demand
Development state	Ego integrity vs despair
Sociocultural orientation	No formal education, Indian, Hindu
Health care system	Institutional health care
Family system	Married, husband working
Patterns of living	At home with partner
Environment	Rural area, items for ADL not in easy reach, no special precautions to prevent injuries
Resources	Husband, daughter, sister's son

2. **Universal self-care requisites:**

Air	Breaths without difficulty, no pallor cyanosis
Water	• Fluid intake is sufficient. Edema present over ankles • Turgor normal for the age
Food	• Hb—9.6 g%, BMI = 14. Food intake is not adequate or the diet is not nutritious
Elimination	• Voids and eliminates bowel without difficulty
Activity/rest	• Frequent rest is required due to pain • Pain not completely relieved • Activity level has come down • Deformity of the joint secondary to the disease process and use of the joints
Social interaction	• Communicates well with neighbors and calls the daughter by phone Need for medical care is communicated to the daughter
Prevention of hazards	• Need instruction on care of joints and prevention of falls. Need instruction on improvement of nutritional status. Prefer to walk bare foot
Promotion of normalcy	• Has good relation with daughter

3. Developmental self-care requisites:

Maintenance of developmental environment	Able to feed self, Difficult to perform the dressing, toileting, etc.
Prevention/management of the conditions threatening the normal development	Feels that the problems are due to her own behaviors and discusses the problems with husband and daughter

4. Health deviation self-care requisites:

Adherence to medical regimen	Reports the problems to the physician when in the hospital. Cooperates with the medication, not much aware about the use and side effects of medicines
Awareness of potential problem associated with the regimen	• Not aware about the actual disease process. • Not compliant with the diet and prevention of hazards. Not aware about the side effects of the medications
Modification of self-image to incorporates changes in health status	• Has adapted to limitation in mobility. • The adoption of new ways for activities leads to deformities and progression of the disease
Adjustment of lifestyle to accommodate changes in the health status and medical regimen	• Adjusted with the deformities • Pain tolerance not achieved

5. Medical problem and plan:

- **Physician's perspective of the condition**: Diagnosed with rheumatoid arthritis and is on the following medications:
  - ◊ T. Valus SR OD
  - ◊ T. Pan 40 mg OD
  - ◊ T. Tramazac 50 mg OD
  - ◊ T. Recofix Forte BD
  - ◊ T. Shelcal BD
  - ◊ Syp. Heamup 2 tsp TID
- **Medical diagnosis:** Rheumatoid arthritis
- **Medical treatment:** Medication and physical therapy.

Areas and priority according to Orem's theory of self-care deficit. Important for prioritizing the nursing diagnosis:

- Air
- Water
- Food
- Elimination
- Activity/Rest
- Solitude/Interaction
- Prevention of hazards
- Promotion of normalcy
- Maintain a developmental environment
- Prevent or manage the developmental threats
- Maintenance of health status
- Awareness and management of the disease process
- Adherence to the medical regimen

- Awareness of potential problem
- Modify self-image
- Adjust lifestyle to accommodate health status changes and MR

Nursing Care Plan According to Orem's Theory of Self-care Deficit

Nursing diagnosis (diagnostic operations)	Outcome and plan (Prescriptive operations)	Implementation (control operations)	Evaluation (regulatory operations)
Based on self-care deficits	• Outcome • Nursing goal and objectives • Design of nursing system • Appropriate method of helping	Nurse—patient actions to: • Promote patient as self-care agent • Meet self-care needs • Decrease the self-care deficit	• Effectiveness of the nurse patient action to: ➢ Promote patient as self-care agent ➢ Meet self-care needs ➢ Decrease the self-care deficit • Effectiveness of the selected nursing system to meet the needs

Thus in the patient Mrs X the areas that need assistance were:

- Air
- Water
- Food
- Elimination
- Activity/Rest (2)
- Solitude/Interaction
- Prevention of hazards (2)
- Promotion of normalcy
- Maintain a developmental environment
- Prevent or manage the developmental threats
- Maintenance of health status
- Awareness and management of the disease process
- Adherence to the medical regimen
- Awareness of potential problem
- Modify self-image
- Adjust lifestyle to accommodate health status changes and medical regimen

Applying the Orem's Theory of Self-Care Deficit, a Nursing Care Plan for Mrs X Could be Prepared as Follows:

I. **Therapeutic self-care demand:** Deficient area—food

   Adequacy of self-care agency: Inadequate

Nursing Diagnosis

Inability to maintain the ideal nutrition related to inadequate intake and knowledge deficit.

Outcomes and Plan

- **Outcome:**
  Improved nutrition
  Maintenance of a balanced diet with adequate iron supplementation.

- **Nursing goals and objectives**
  Goal: To achieve optimal levels of nutrition.
  Objectives: Mrs X will:
  ◊ State the importance of maintaining a balanced diet.
  ◊ List the food items rich in iron that are available in the locality.
- **Design of the nursing system:** Supportive educative
- **Method of helping:**
  ◊ Guidance
  ◊ Support
  ◊ Teaching
  ◊ Providing developmental environment

  Implementation: Mutually planned and identified the objectives and the patient were made to understand about the required changes in the behavior to have the requisites met.

  Evaluation:
  ◊ Mrs X understood the importance of maintaining an optimum nutrition.
  ◊ She told that she will select the iron rich diet for her food.
  ◊ She listed the foods that are rich in iron and that are locally available.
  ◊ The self-care deficit in terms of food will be decreased with the initiation of the nutritional intake.
  ◊ The supportive educative system was useful for Mrs X

II. **Therapeutic self-care demand:** Deficient area—Activity
   Adequacy of self-care agency: Inadequate

   Nursing Diagnosis
   Self-care deficit: dressing, toileting related to restricted joint movement, secondary to the inflammatory process in the joints.

   Outcomes and Plan
   - **Outcome:**
     ◊ Improved self-care
     ◊ Maintain the ability to perform the toileting and dressing with modification as required.
   - **Nursing goals and objectives**
     Goal: to achieve optimal levels of ability for self-care.

     Objectives: Mrs X will:
     ◊ Perform the dressing activities within limitations
     ◊ Utilize the alternative measures available for improving the toileting
     ◊ Perform the other activities of daily living with minimal assistance.
   - **Design of the nursing system:** Partly compensatory
   - **Method of helping:**
     Guidance: Assess the various hindering factors for self-care and how to tackle them.
     Support: Provide all the articles needed for self-care, near to the patient and ask the family members also to give the articles near to her.
     ◊ Provide passive exercises and make to perform active exercises so as to promote the mobility of the joint.
     ◊ Make the patient use commodes or stools to perform toileting and insist on avoidance of squatting position

◊ Provide assistance whenever needed for the self-care activities
◊ Provide encouragement and positive reinforcement for minor improvement in the activity level.
◊ Initiate the pain relieving measures always before the patient go for any of the activities of daily living
◊ Make the patient to use loose fitting clothes which will be easy to wear and remove.

Teaching: Teach the family members the limitation in the activity level the patient has and the cooperation required.

Promoting a developmental environment: Teach the family and help them to practice how to help the patient according to her needs.

Implementation: Mutually planned and identified the objectives and the patient was made to understand about the required changes in the behavior to have the requisites met.

Evaluation:

- Patient was performing some of the activities and she practiced toileting using a commode in the hospital.
- She verbalized an improved comfort and self-care ability.
- She performed the dressing activities with minimal assistance
- Patient verbalized that she will perform the activities as instructed to get her ADL done.
- The partly compensatory system was useful for Mrs X

III. **Therapeutic self-care demand:** Deficient area—Pain control.

Adequacy of self-care agency: Inadequate

Nursing Diagnosis

Ineffective pain control related to lack of utilization of pain relief measures

Outcomes and Plan

- **Outcome:**
  ◊ Improved pain self control
  ◊ Achieve and maintain a reduction in the pain
- **Nursing Goals and objectives**

  Goal: to achieve reduction in the pain.

  Objectives: Mrs X will:
  ◊ Describe the total plan of pharmacological and non pharmacological pain relief
  ◊ Demonstrate a reduction in the pain behaviors
  ◊ Verbalize a reduction in the pain scale score from 7–4
- **Design of the nursing system:** supportive educative
- **Method of helping:**

  Guidance
  ◊ Explore the past experience of pain and methods used to manage them.
  ◊ Ask the client to report the intensity, location, severity, associated and aggravating factors.

  Support:
  ◊ Provide rest to the joints and avoid excessive manipulations
  ◊ provide hot and cold application to have better mobility.
  ◊ Encourage exercises to the joints by immersing in the warm water.

◊ Administer T. Ultracet and Tab Diclofenac as prescribed.

◊ Provide diversion and psychological support to the patient

Teaching: Teach the non-pharmacological method to the patient once the pain is a little reduced.

Providing the developmental environment:

◊ Discuss with the patient the necessity to maintain a pain diary with all information regarding episodes of pain and refer to that periodically

◊ Enquire from the health team, the need for opioid analgesics or other analgesics and get a prescription for the patient.

Implementation

____

____

Evaluation:

♦ Patient still has pain over the joints and she agreed that she will use the measures for pain relief that is told to her.

♦ The pain scale score was 6 after the measures were provided to the patient.

♦ She demonstrated slight reduction in the pain behaviors.

♦ The supportive educative system was useful for Mrs X

IV. **Therapeutic self-care demand:** Deficient area—prevention of hazards.

Adequacy of self-care agency: Inadequate

Nursing Diagnosis

Potential for fall and fractures related to rheumatoid arthritis.

Outcomes and Plan

♦ **Outcome:** Absence of falls and injury to the patient

♦ **Nursing goals and objectives:**

Goal: Prevent the falls and injury and to maintain a good body mechanics.

Objectives: Mrs X will:

◊ Remain free from injury as evidenced by:

◊ Absence of signs and symptoms of fall or injury

◊ Explaining the methods to prevent the injury

♦ **Design of the nursing system:** Supportive educative

♦ **Method of helping:**

Support

◊ Never leave the client alone in the unit

◊ Assess the patients gait, activities and the mental status for any confusion or disorientation

◊ Encourage the patient to use supportive devices as required.

◊ Provide a safe environment in the hospital by avoiding sharp objects or wooden objects on the way and slippery floor.

◊ Involve the family members in providing and maintaining a safe environment in the home

◊ Involve the family members to provide support to the patient whenever necessary

◊ Plan a balanced diet for the patient with a mutual interaction

Implementation

____

____

Evaluation

- Patient remained free from injury as evidenced by absence of signs and symptoms.
- Patient explained the various measures that they will take to prevent the injury.
- The supportive educative system was useful for Mrs X

V. **Therapeutic self-care demand:** Deficient area—prevention of hazards.
Adequacy of self-care agency: Inadequate

Nursing diagnosis:
Potential for impaired skin integrity related to edema secondary to renal cysts.

Outcomes and Plan

- **Outcome:** Maintenance of normal skin integrity.
- **Nursing goals and objectives:**
  Goal: Maintain the skin integrity and take measures to prevent skin impairment.
  Objectives: Mrs X will:
  ◊ Maintain a normal skin integrity
  ◊ List the measures to prevent the loss of skin integrity
  ◊ Identify the measures to relieve edema.
- **Design of the nursing system:** supportive educative
- **Method of helping:**
  Support
  ◊ Assess the skin regularly for any excoriation or loss of integrity or color changes. Keep the skin clean always.
  ◊ Avoid stress or pressure over the area of edema by providing extra cushions or padding.
  ◊ Monitor the lab values as well as the patient for any signs and symptoms of renal failure.
  ◊ Encourage the patient to use slippers while walking and that should not be tight fitting.
  ◊ Assess the edema for its degree, pitting or non pitting and continue the assessment daily.
  ◊ Provide a leg end elevated position or elevation of the leg on a pillow if no cardiac abnormalities are identified.
  ◊ Explain the patient the need for taking care of the edematous parts.
  ◊ Explain the patient to report the symptoms like decreased urine output, palpitations, increased edema etc. to the health team.

Implementation

____

____

Evaluation

- Patient remained free from impaired skin integrity
- She listed the measures to prevent the loss of skin integrity
- She identified the measures to relieve edema.
- The supportive educative system was useful for Mrs. x

VI. **Therapeutic self-care demand:** Deficient area—awareness of the disease process and management.

Adequacy of self-care agency: Inadequate

Nursing Diagnosis

Potential for complications related to rheumatoid arthritis secondary to knowledge deficit.

Outcomes and Plan

- **Outcome:** Absence of complications and improved awareness about the disease process.
- **Nursing goals and objectives:**
  Goal: Improve the knowledge of the patient about the disease process and the complications.
  Objectives: Mrs X will:
  ◊ Verbalize the various complication and their preventions
  ◊ Verbalize the changes occurring with the disease process and the treatment available
  ◊ Describe the actions and side effects of the medications which she is using
- **Design of the nursing system:** Supportive educative
- **Methods of helping:**
  ◊ Guidance
  ◊ Teaching
  ◊ Promoting a developmental environment

Implementation

Evaluation

- Patient got adequate information regarding the disease
- She verbalized what she understood about the disease and its management.
- Patient has cleared her doubts regarding the medication actions and the side effect
- The supportive educative system was useful for Mrs X

Evaluation of the Application of Self-care Deficit Theory

The theory of self-care deficit when applied could identify the self-care requisites of Mrs X from various aspects. This was helpful to provide care in a comprehensive manner. Patient was very cooperative. the application of this theory revealed how well the supportive and educative and partly compensatory system could be used for solving the problems in a patient with rheumatoid arthritis.

JEAN WATSON'S PHILOSOPHY OF NURSING

Introduction

- ❖ **Born:** West Virginia
- ❖ **Educated:** BSN, University of Colorado, 1964, MS, University of Colorado, 1966, PhD, University of Colorado, 1973
- ❖ Dr Jean Watson is Distinguished Professor of Nursing and holds an endowed Chair in Caring Science at the University of Colorado Health Sciences Center.

- ❖ She is founder of the original Center for Human Caring in Colorado and is a Fellow of the American Academy of Nursing. She previously served as Dean of Nursing at the University Health Sciences Center and is a Past President of the National League for Nursing
- ❖ Dr Watson has earned undergraduate and graduate degrees in nursing and psychiatric-mental health nursing and holds her PhD in educational psychology and counseling.
- ❖ She is a widely published author and recipient of several awards and honors, including an international Kellogg Fellowship in Australia, a Fulbright Research Award in Sweden and six (6) Honorary Doctoral Degrees, including 3 International Honorary Doctorates (Sweden, United Kingdom, Quebec, Canada).
- ❖ Her research has been in the area of human caring and loss.
- ❖ The foundation of Jean Watson's theory of nursing was published in 1979 in nursing: "The philosophy and science of caring"
- ❖ In 1988, her theory was published in "nursing: human science and human care".
- ❖ Watson believes that the main focus in nursing is on carative factors. She believes that for nurses to develop humanistic philosophies and value system, a strong liberal arts background is necessary.
- ❖ This philosophy and value system provide a solid foundation for the science of caring. A humanistic value system thus under grids her construction of the science of caring.
  - ◆ She asserts that the caring stance that nursing has always held is being threatened by the tasks and technology demands of the curative factors.

The Seven Assumptions

Watson proposes seven assumptions about the science of caring. The basic assumptions are:
- ❖ Caring can be effectively demonstrated and practiced only interpersonally.
- ❖ Caring consists of carative factors that result in the satisfaction of certain human needs.
- ❖ Effective caring promotes health and individual or family growth.
- ❖ Caring responses accept person not only as he or she is now but as what he or she may become.
- ❖ A caring environment is one that offers the development of potential while allowing the person to choose the best action for himself or herself at a given point in time.
- ❖ Caring is more "healthgenic" than is curing. A science of caring is complementary to the science of curing.
- ❖ The practice of caring is central to nursing.

The Ten Primary Carative Factors

The structure for the science of caring is built upon ten carative factors. These are:
1. The formation of a humanistic- altruistic system of values.
2. The installation of faith-hope.
3. The cultivation of sensitivity to one's self and to others.
4. The development of a helping-trust relationship
5. The promotion and acceptance of the expression of positive and negative feelings.
6. The systematic use of the scientific problem-solving method for decision making
7. The promotion of interpersonal teaching-learning.
8. The provision for a supportive, protective and/or corrective mental, physical, sociocultural and spiritual environment.
9. Assistance with the gratification of human needs.

10. The allowance for existential-phenomenological forces.

The first three carative factors form the "philosophical foundation" for the science of caring. The remaining seven carative factors spring from the foundation laid by these first three.

1. **The formation of a humanistic-altruistic system of values**
   - Begins developmentally at an early age with values shared with the parents.
   - Mediated through ones own life experiences, the learning one gains and exposure to the humanities.
   - Is perceived as necessary to the nurse's own maturation which then promotes altruistic behavior towards others.

2. **Faith-hope**
   - Is essential to both the carative and the curative processes.
   - When modern science has nothing further to offer the person, the nurse can continue to use faith-hope to provide a sense of well-being through beliefs which are meaningful to the individual.

3. **Cultivation of sensitivity to oneself and to others**
   - Explores the need of the nurse to begin to feel an emotion as it presents itself.
   - Development of one's own feeling is needed to interact genuinely and sensitively with others.

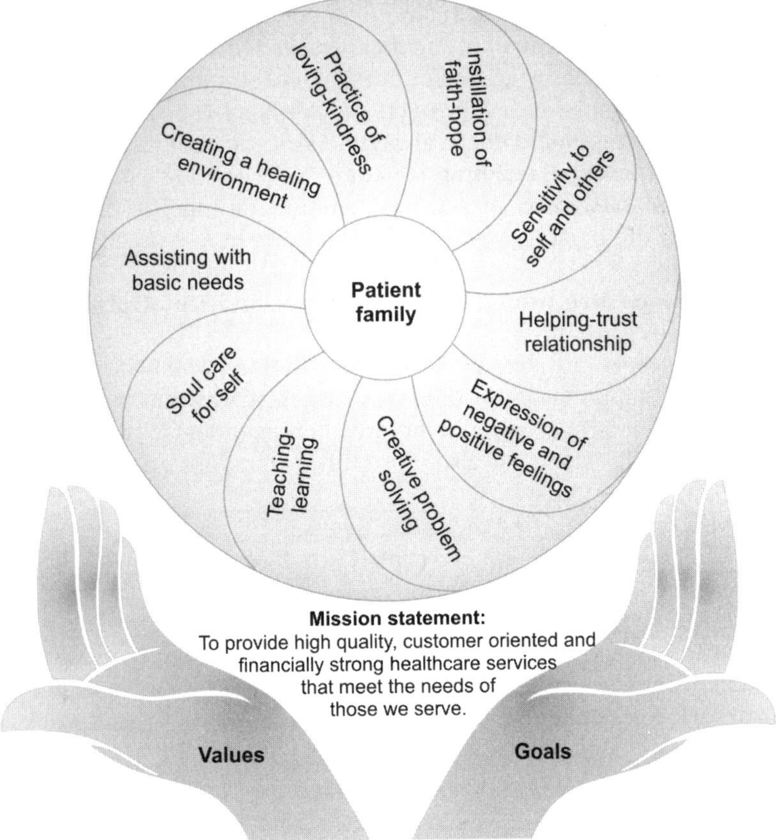

Factors of Watson theory.

- Striving to become sensitive, makes the nurse more authentic, which encourages self-growth and self-actualization, in both the nurse and those with whom the nurse interacts.
- The nurses promote health and higher-level functioning only when they form person to person relationship.

4. **Establishing a helping-trust relationship**
   - Strongest tool is the mode of communication, which establishes rapport and caring.
   - She has defined the characteristics needed to in the helping-trust relationship. These are:
     ◊ *Congruence*
     ◊ *Empathy*
     ◊ *Warmth*
   - Communication includes verbal, nonverbal and listening in a manner which connotes empathetic understanding.

5. **The expression of feelings, both positive and negative**
   - According to Watson, **"feelings alter thoughts and behavior, and they need to be considered and allowed for in a caring relationship".**
   - According to her such expression improves one's level of awareness.
   - Awareness of the feelings helps to understand the behavior it engenders.

6. **The systematic use of the scientific problem-solving method for decision making**
   - According to Watson, the scientific problem-solving method is the only method that allows for control and prediction, and that permits self-correction.
   - She also values the relative nature of nursing and supports the need to examine and develop the other methods of knowing to provide an holistic perspective.
   - The science of caring should not be always neutral and objective.

7. **Promotion of interpersonal teaching-learning**
   - The caring nurse must focus on the learning process as much as the teaching process.
   - Understanding the person's perception of the situation assist the nurse to prepare a cognitive plan.

8. **Provision for a supportive, protective and/or corrective mental, physical, sociocultural and spiritual environment**
   - Watson divides these into eternal and internal variables, which the nurse manipulates in order to provide support and protection for the person's mental and physical well-being.
   - The external and internal environments are interdependent.
   - Watson suggests that the nurse also must provide comfort, privacy and safety as a part of this carative factor.

9. **Assistance with the gratification of human needs**
   - It is grounded in a hierarchy of need similar to that of the Maslow's.
   - She has created a hierarchy which she believes is relevant to the science of caring in nursing.
   - According to her each need is equally important for quality nursing care and the promotion of optimal health. All the needs deserve to be attended to and valued.

   Watson's ordering of needs
   - Lower order needs (biophysical needs)
     ◊ *The need for food and fluid*
     ◊ *The need for elimination*
     ◊ *The need for ventilation*

- Lower order needs (psychophysical needs)
  - ◊ *The need for activity-inactivity*
  - ◊ *The need for sexuality*
- Watson's ordering of needs
  - ◊ *Higher order needs (psychosocial needs)*
  - ◊ *The need for achievement*
  - ◊ *The need for affiliation*
  - ◊ *Higher order need (intrapersonal-interpersonal need)*
  - ◊ *The need for self-actualization*
- Research findings have established a correlation between emotional distress and illness. According to Watson, the current thinking of holistic care emphasizes that:
  - ◊ *Factors of the etiological component interact and produce change through complex neuro-physiological and neuro-chemical pathways*
  - ◊ *Each psychological function has a physiological correlate*
  - ◊ *Each physiological component has a psychological correlate*

  Example: Bulimia, anorexia and gastrointestinal ulcers are a just few of the disorders that indicate a complex interaction between the physiological and psychological.

10. **Allowance for existential-phenomenological forces**
    - Phenomenology is a way of understanding people from the way things appear to them, from their frame of reference.
    - Existential psychology is the study of human existence using phenomenological analysis.
    - This factor helps the nurse to reconcile and mediate the incongruity of viewing the person holistically while at the same time attending to the hierarchical ordering of needs.
    - Thus the nurse assists the person to find the strength or courage to confront life or death.

Watson's Theory and the Four Major Concepts

1. **Human being:** She adopts a view of the human being as: "..... a valued person in and of him or herself to be cared for, respected, nurtured, understood and assisted; in general a philosophical view of a person as a fully functional integrated self. He, human is viewed as greater than and different from, the sum of his or her parts".
2. **Health:** Watson believes that there are other factors that are needed to be included in the WHO definition of health. She adds the following three elements:
   a. A high level of overall physical, mental and social functioning
   b. A general adaptive-maintenance level of daily functioning
   c. The absence of illness (or the presence of efforts that leads its absence)
3. **Environment/society:** According to Watson caring (and nursing) has existed in every society. A caring attitude is not transmitted from generation to generation. It is transmitted by the culture of the profession as a unique way of coping with its environment.
4. **Nursing**
   - According to Watson " nursing is concerned with promoting health, preventing illness, caring for the sick and restoring health".
   - It focuses on health promotion and treatment of disease. She believes that holistic health care is central to the practice of caring in nursing.
   - She defines nursing as.....
     "A human science of persons and human health-illness experiences that are mediated by professional, personal, scientific, esthetic and ethical human transactions".

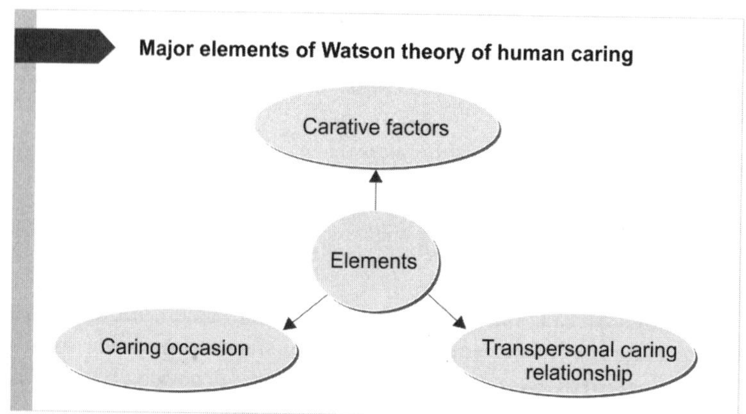

Watson's Theory and Nursing Process

Watson points out that nursing process contains the same steps as the scientific research process. They both try to solve a problem. Both provide a framework for decision making. Watson elaborates the nursing processes as:

1. **Assessment**
   - Involves observation, identification and review of the problem; use of applicable knowledge in literature.
   - Also includes conceptual knowledge for the formulation and conceptualization of framework.
   - Includes the formulation of hypothesis; defining variables that will be examined in solving the problem.
2. **Plan:** It helps to determine how variables would be examined or measured; includes a conceptual approach or design for problem solving. It determines what data would be collected and how on whom.
3. **Intervention**
   - It is the direct action and implementation of the plan.
   - It includes the collection of the data.
4. **Evaluation**
   - Analysis of the data as well as the examination of the effects of interventions based on the data. Includes the interpretation of the results, the degree to which positive outcome has occurred and whether the result can be generalized.
   - It may also generate additional hypothesis or may even lead to the generation of a nursing theory.

Watson's Work and the Characteristic of a Theory

- According to Watson, "a theory is an imaginative grouping of knowledge, ideas and experiences that are represented symbolically and seek to illuminate a given phenomenon"
- She views nursing as, "....both a human science and an art and as such it cannot be considered qualitatively continuous with traditional, reductionistic, scientific methodology".
- She suggests that nursing might want to develop its own science that would not be related to the traditional sciences but rather would develop its own concepts, relationships and methodology.

❖ Theories can interrelate concepts in such a way as to create a different way of looking at a particular phenomenon

❖ The basic assumptions for the science of caring in nursing and the ten carative factors that form the structure for that concept is unique in Watson's theory.

❖ She describes caring in both philosophical and scientific terms.

❖ Watson also indicates that needs are interrelated.

❖ The science of caring suggests that the nurse recognize and assist with each of the interrelated needs in order to reach the highest order need of self-actualization.

Theories Must be Logical in Nature

❖ Watson's work is logical in that the factors are based on broad assumptions which provide a supportive framework.

❖ With these carative factors she delineates nursing from other professions

❖ These carative factors are logically derived from the assumptions and related to he hierarchy of needs.

Theories should be Relatively Simple yet Generalizable

❖ The theory is relatively simple as it does not use theories from other disciplines that are familiar to nursing.

❖ The theory is simple relatively but the fact that it de-emphasizes the pathophysiological for the psychosocial diminishes its ability to be generalizable.

❖ She discusses this in the preface of her book when she speaks of the "trim" and the "core" of nursing.

❖ She defines trim as the clinical focus, the procedure and the techniques.

❖ The core of the nursing is that which is intrinsic to the nurse-client interaction that produces a therapeutic result. Core mechanisms are the carative factors.

Theories can be the Basis for Hypotheses that can be Tested

❖ Watson's theory is based on phenomenological studies that generally ask questions rather than state hypotheses. Its purpose is to describe the phenomena, to analyze and to gain an understanding.

❖ Theories contribute to and assist in increasing the general body within the discipline through research implemented to validate them

❖ According to Watson the best method to test this theory is through field study.

❖ An example is her work in the area of loss and caring that took place in Cundeelee, Western Australia and involved a tribe of aborigines.

Theories can be Utilized by Practitioners to Guide and Improve their Practice

❖ Watson's work can be used to guide and improve practice.

❖ It can provide the nurse with the most satisfying aspects of practice and can provide the client with the holistic care so necessary for human growth and development.

❖ Theories must be consistent with other validated theories, laws and principles but will leave open unanswered questions that need to be investigated.

❖ Watson's work is supported by the theoretical work of numerous humanists, philosophers, developmentalists and psychologists.

❖ She clearly designates the theories of stress, development, communication, teaching-learning, humanistic psychology and existential phenomenology which provide the foundation for the science of caring.

Strengths

❖ Besides assisting in providing the quality of care that client ought to receive, it also provides the soul satisfying care for which many nurses enter the profession. As the science of caring ranges from the biophysical through the intrapersonal, each nurse becomes an active coparticipant in the client's struggle towards self-actualization.

❖ The client is placed in the context of the family, the community and the culture.

❖ It places the client as the focus of practice rather than the technology.

Limitations

❖ Given the acuity of illness that leads to hospitalization, the short length stay, and the increasing complex technology, such quality of care may be deemed impossible to give in the hospital.

❖ While Watson acknowledges the need for biophysical base to nursing, this area receives little attention in her writings.

❖ The ten caratiive factors primarily delineate the psychosocial needs of the person.

❖ While the carative factors have a sound foundation based on other disciplines, they need further research in nursing to demonstrate their application to practice.

Research Related to Watson's Theory

❖ Saint Joseph Hospital in Orange, California has selected Jean Watson's theory of human caring as the framework base for nursing practice.

❖ The effectiveness of Watson's Caring Model on the quality of life and blood pressure of patients with hypertension. J Adv Nurs. 2003 Jan;41(2):130-9.

❖ This study demonstrated a relationship between care given according to Watson's Caring model and increased quality of life of the patients with hypertension. Further, in those patients for whom the caring model was practiced, there was a relationship between the Caring model and a decrease in patient's blood pressure. The Watson Caring Model is recommended as a guide to nursing patients with hypertension, as one means of decreasing blood pressure and increase in quality of life.

❖ Martin, LS (1991). Using Watson's theory to explore the dimensions of adult polycystic kidney disease. ANNA Journal, 18, 403-406.

❖ Mullaney, JAB (2000). The lived experience of using Watson's actual caring occasions to treat depressed women. Journal of Holistic Nursing, 18(2), 129-142.

Conclusion

❖ Watson provides many useful concepts for the practice of nursing.

❖ She ties together many theories commonly used in nursing education and does so in a manner helpful to practitioners of the art and science of nursing.

❖ The detailed descriptions of the carative factors can give guidance to those who wish to employ them in practice or research.

❖ Using her theory can add a dimension to practice that is both satisfying and challenging.

THE ROY'S ADAPTATION MODEL

Introduction

- Sr Callista Roy, a prominent nurse theorist, writer, lecturer, researcher and teacher.
- Professor and Nurse Theorist at the Boston College of Nursing in Chestnut Hill.
- Born at Los Angeles on October 14, 1939 as the 2nd child of Mr and Mrs Fabien Roy.
- She earned a Bachelor of Arts with a major in nursing from Mount St Mary's College, Los Angeles in 1963.
- A master's degree program in pediatric nursing at the University of California, Los Angeles in 1966.
- She also earned a master's and PhD in Sociology in 1973 and 1977, respectively.
- Sr Callista had the significant opportunity of working with Dorothy E Johnson.
- Johnson's work with focusing knowledge for the discipline of nursing convinced Sr Callista of the importance of describing the nature of nursing as a service to society and prompted her to begin developing her model with the goal of nursing being to promote adaptation.
- She joined the faculty of Mount St Mary's College in 1966, teaching both pediatric and maternity nursing.
- She organized course content according to a view of person and family as adaptive systems.
- She introduced her ideas about 'Adaptation Nursing' as the basis for an integrated nursing curriculum.
- Goal of nursing to direct nursing education, practice and research.
- Model as a basis of curriculum impetus for growth—Mount St Mary's College.
- 1970—The model was implemented in Mount St Mary's School.
- 1971—She was made chair of the nursing department at the college.

Influencing Factors

- Family
- Education
- Religious background
- Mentors
- Clinical experience

Theory Description

- The central questions of Roy's theory are:
  - Who is the focus of nursing care?
  - What is the target of nursing care?
  - When is nursing care indicated?
- Roy's first ideas appeared in a graduate paper written at UCLA in 1964.
- Published these ideas in *"Nursing outlook"* in 1970.
- Subsequently different components of her framework crystallized during 1970s, '80s, and '90s.
- Over the years she identified assumptions on which her theory is based.

Explicit Assumptions (Roy 1989; Roy and Andrews 1991)

- The person is a bio-psycho-social being.
- The person is in constant interaction with a changing environment.

- To cope with a changing world, person uses both innate and acquired mechanisms which are biological, psychological and social in origin.
- Health and illness are inevitable dimensions of the person's life.
- To respond positively to environmental changes, the person must adapt.
- The person's adaptation is a function of the stimulus he is exposed to and his adaptation level.
- The person's adaptation level is such that it comprises a zone indicating the range of stimulation that will lead to a positive response.
- The person has four modes of adaptation: physiologic needs, self-concept, role function and inter-dependence.
- "Nursing accepts the humanistic approach of valuing other persons' opinions, and view points". Interpersonal relations are an integral part of nursing.
- There is a dynamic objective for existence with ultimate goal of achieving dignity and integrity.

Implicit Assumptions

- A person can be reduced to parts for study and care.
- Nursing is based on causality.
- Patient's values and opinions are to be considered and respected.
- A state of adaptation frees an individual's energy to respond to other stimuli.

Roy Adaptation Model Concepts: Early and Revised

- Adaptation—goal of nursing
- Person—adaptive system
- Environment—stimuli
- Health—outcome of adaptation
- Nursing—promoting adaptation and health

Concepts of Adaptation

- Responding positively to environmental changes
- The process and outcome of individuals and groups who use conscious awareness, self reflection and choice to create human and environmental integration

Concepts of Person

- Bio-psycho-social being in constant interaction with a changing environment
- Uses innate and acquired mechanisms to adapt
- An adaptive system described as a whole comprised of parts
- Functions as a unity for some purpose
- Includes people as individuals or in groups-families, organizations, communities, and society as a whole

Concepts of Environment

- Focal—internal or external and immediately confronting the person
- Contextual—all stimuli present in the situation that contribute to effect of focal stimulus
- Residual—a factor whose effects in the current situation are unclear
- All conditions, circumstances, and influences surrounding and affecting the development and behavior of persons and groups with particular consideration of mutuality of person and earth resources, including focal, contextual and residual stimuli

Concepts of Health

* Inevitable dimension of person's life
* Represented by a health-illness continuum
* A state and a process of being and becoming integrated and whole

Concepts of Nursing

* To promote adaptation in the four adaptive modes.
* To promote adaptation for individuals and groups in the four adaptive modes, thus contributing to health, quality of life, and dying with dignity by assessing behaviors and factors that influence adaptive abilities and by intervening to enhance environmental interactions.

Concepts of Subsystems

* **Cognator subsystem:** A major coping process involving four cognitive-emotive channels: perceptual and information processing, learning, judgment and emotion.
* **Regulator subsystem:** S basic type of adaptive process that responds automatically through neural, chemical, and endocrine coping channels.

Relationships

* Derived four adaptive modes
* Five hundred samples of patient behavior
* What was the patient doing?
* What did the patient look like when needing nursing care?

Adaptive Modes

* Physiologic needs
* Self-concept
* Role function
* Interdependence

Adaptive Mode Categories

* Tested in practice for 10 years
* Criteria of significance, usefulness, and completeness were met.

Sample Proposition and Hypothesis for Practice

* Self-concept mode: Increased quality of social experience leads to increased feelings of adequacy.
* Providing support for new mothers can lead to positive parenting.

Theory Development

Derived Theory

* Ninety-one propositions
* Described relationships between and among regulator and cognator and four adaptive modes.
* Twelve generic propositions

Questions Raised by 21st Century Changes

❖ How can ethics and public policy keep pace with developments in science?
❖ How can nurses focus on human needs not machines?
❖ How can nurses contribute to creating meaning and purpose in a global society?

Scientific Assumptions for the 21st Century

❖ Systems of matter and energy progress to higher levels of complex self-organization.
❖ Consciousness and meaning are constitutive of person and environment integration.
❖ Awareness of self and environment is rooted in thinking and feeling.
❖ Human decisions are accountable for the integration of creative processes.
❖ Thinking and feeling mediate human action.
❖ System relationships include acceptance, protection, and fostering of interdependence.
❖ Persons and the earth have common patterns and integral relations.
❖ Person and environment transformations are created in human consciousness.
❖ Integration of human and environment meanings results in adaptation.

Philosophical Assumptions

❖ Persons have mutual relationships with the world and God.
❖ Human meaning is rooted in an omega point convergence of the universe.
❖ God is intimately revealed in the diversity of creation and is the common destiny of creation.
❖ Persons use human creative abilities of awareness, enlightenment, and faith.
❖ Persons are accountable for the processes of deriving, sustaining, and transforming the universe.

Adaptation and Groups

Includes relating persons, partners, families, organizations, communities, nations, and society as a whole

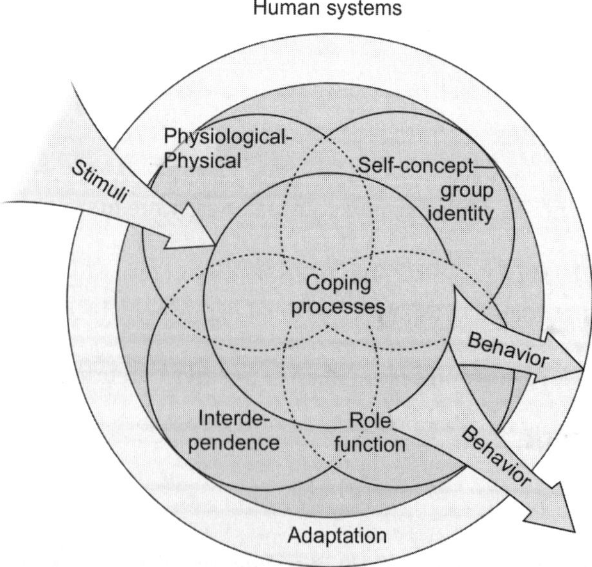

Roy adaptation model.

Adaptive Modes

- ❖ Persons
  - ◆ Physiologic
  - ◆ Self-concept
  - ◆ Role function
  - ◆ Interdependence
- ❖ Groups
  - ◆ Physical
  - ◆ Group identity
  - ◆ Role function
  - ◆ Interdependence

Role Function Mode

- ❖ Underlying need of social integrity
- ❖ The need to know who one is in relation to others so that one can act
- ❖ The need for role clarity of all participants in group

Adaptation Level

- ❖ A zone within which stimulation will lead to a positive or adaptive response
- ❖ Adaptive mode processes described on three levels:
  - ◆ Integrated
  - ◆ Compensatory
  - ◆ Compromised

Integrated Life Processes

- ❖ Adaptation level where the structures and functions of the life processes work to meet needs
- ❖ Examples of integrated adaptation:
  - ◆ Stable process of breathing and ventilation
  - ◆ Effective processes for moral-ethical-spiritual growth

Compensatory Processes

- ❖ Adaptation level where the cognator and regulator are activated by a challenge to the life processes.
- ❖ Compensatory adaptation examples:
  - ◆ Grieving as a growth process, higher levels of adaptation and transcendence
  - ◆ Role transition, growth in a new role

Compromised Processes

- ❖ Adaptation level resulting from inadequate integrated and compensatory life processes
- ❖ Adaptation problem
- ❖ Compromised adaptation examples:
  - ◆ Hypoxia
  - ◆ Unresolved loss
  - ◆ Stigma
  - ◆ Abusive relationships

The Nursing Process

- ❖ RAM offers guidelines to nurses in developing the nursing process.
- ❖ The elements:
  - ◆ First level assessment
  - ◆ Second level assessment
  - ◆ Diagnosis
  - ◆ Goal setting
  - ◆ Intervention
  - ◆ Evaluation

Usefulness of Adaptation Model

- ❖ Scientific knowledge for practice
- ❖ Clinical assessment and intervention
- ❖ Research variables
- ❖ To guide nursing practice
- ❖ To organize nursing education
- ❖ Curricular framework for various nursing colleges

Characteristics of the Theory

- ❖ Theories can interrelates concept in such a way as to present a new view of looking at a particular phenomenon.
- ❖ Theories must be logical in nature
- ❖ Theories should be relatively simple yet generalizable
- ❖ Theories can be the basis for the hypotheses that can be tested
- ❖ Theories contribute to and assist in increasing the general body of knowledge of a discipline through the research implemented to validate them.
- ❖ Theories can be utilized by the practitioners to guide and improve their practice.
- ❖ Theories must be consistent with other validated theories, laws and principles but will leave open unanswered questions that need to be investigated.

Testability

- ❖ RAM is testable
- ❖ BBARNS (1999) reported that 163 studies have been conducted using this model.
- ❖ RAM is complete and comprehensive.
- ❖ It explains the reality of client, so nursing interventions can be specifically targeted.

Summary

- ❖ Five elements-person, goal of nursing, nursing activities, health and environment.
- ❖ Persons are viewed as living adaptive systems whose behaviors may be classified as adaptive responses or ineffective responses.
- ❖ These behaviors are derived from regulator and cognator mechanisms.
- ❖ These mechanisms work within four adaptive modes.
- ❖ The goal of nursing is to promote adaptive responses in relation to four adaptive modes, using information about person's adaptation level, and various stimuli.

❖ Nursing activities involve manipulation of these stimuli to promote adaptive responses.
❖ Health is a process of becoming integrated and able to meet goals of survival, growth, reproduction, and mastery.
❖ The environment consists of person's internal and external stimuli.

APPLICATION OF ROY'S ADAPTATION MODEL IN NURSING PRACTICE

Introduction

❖ Born at Los Angeles on October 14, 1939 as the 2nd child of Mr and Mrs Fabien Roy
❖ At age 14 she began working at a large general hospital, first as a pantry girl, then as a maid, and finally as a nurse's aid.
❖ She entered the Sisters of Saint Joseph of Carondelet.
❖ She earned a Bachelor of Arts with a major in nursing from Mount St Mary's College, Los Angeles in 1963.
❖ A master's degree program in pediatric nursing at the University of California, Los Angeles in 1966.
❖ She also earned a master's and PhD in Sociology in 1973 and 1977, respectively
❖ Sr Callista had the significant opportunity of working with Dorothy E Johnson
❖ Johnson's work with focusing knowledge for the discipline of nursing convinced Sr Callista of the importance of describing the nature of nursing as a service to society and prompted her to begin developing her model with the goal of nursing being to promote adaptation.

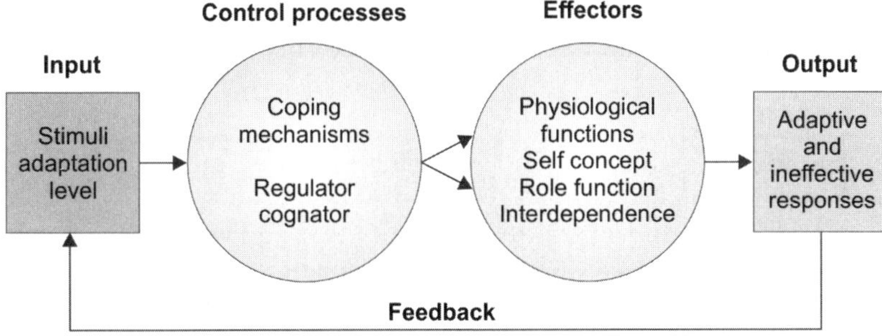

Sister Callista Roy (1984), Introduction to Nursing: An Adaptation Model (2nd ed)

Assumptions of Roy's Adaptation Model

Scientific

❖ Systems of matter and energy progress to higher levels of complex self-organization.
❖ Consciousness and meaning are constitutive of person and environment integration.
❖ Awareness of self and environment is rooted in thinking and feeling.
❖ Humans by their decisions are accountable for the integration of creative processes.
❖ Thinking and feeling mediate human action.
❖ System relationships include acceptance, protection, and fostering of interdependence.
❖ Persons and the earth have common patterns and integral relationships.
❖ Persons and environment transformations are crated in human consciousness.
❖ Integration of human and environment meanings results in adaptation.

Philosophical

- Persons have mutual relationships with the world and God.
- Human meaning is rooted in an omega point convergence of the universe.
- God is intimately revealed in the diversity of creation and is the common destiny of creation.
- Persons use human creative abilities of awareness, enlightenment, and faith.
- Persons are accountable for the processes of deriving, sustaining, and transforming the universe.

Persons and Relating Persons

- An adaptive system with coping processes
- Described as a whole comprised of parts
- Functions as a unity for some purpose
- Includes people as individuals or in groups (families, organizations, communities, nations, and society as a whole).
- An adaptive system with cognator and regulator subsystems acting to maintain adaptation in the four adaptive modes: physiologic-physical, self-concept-group identity, role function, and interdependence.

Environment

- All conditions, circumstances, and influences surrounding and affecting the development and behavior of persons and groups with particular consideration of mutuality of person and earth resources.
- Three kinds of stimuli: Focal, contextual, and residual
- Significant stimuli in all human adaptation include stage of development, family, and culture.

Health and Adaptation

- **Health:** A state and process of being and becoming integrated and whole that reflects person and environmental mutuality.
- **Adaptation:** The process and outcome whereby thinking and feeling persons, as individuals and in groups, use conscious awareness and choice to create human and environmental integration.
- **Adaptive responses:** Responses that promotes integrity in terms of the goals of the human system, that is, survival, growth, reproduction, mastery, and personal and environmental transformation.
- **Ineffective responses:** Responses that do not contribute to integrity in terms of the goals of the human system.
- Adaptation levels represent the condition of the life processes described on three different levels: Integrated, compensatory, and compromised.

Nursing

- Nursing is the science and practice that expands adaptive abilities and enhances person and environment transformation.
- Nursing goals are to promote adaptation for individuals and groups in the four adaptive modes, thus contributing to health, quality of life, and dying with dignity.
- This is done by assessing behavior and factors that influence adaptive abilities and by intervening to expand those abilities and to enhance environmental interactions.

Roy Adaptation Model (RAM)–Terms

System: A set of parts connected to function as a whole for some purpose.

Stimulus: Something that provokes a response, point of interaction for the human system and the environment.
- ❖ **Focal stimuli:** Internal or external stimulus immediately affecting the system.
- ❖ **Contextual Stimulus:** All other stimulus present in the situation.
- ❖ **Residual Stimulus:** Environmental factor, that effects on the situation that are unclear.

Regulator subsystem: Automatic response to stimulus (neural, chemical, and endocrine).

Cognator subsystem: Responds through four cognitive-emotive channels (perceptual and information processing, learning, judgment, and emotion).

Behavior: Internal or external actions and reactions under specific circumstances.

Physiologic-Physical Mode

- ❖ Behavior pertaining to the physical aspect of the human system
- ❖ Physical and chemical processes
- ❖ Nurse must be knowledgeable about normal processes
- ❖ Five needs (oxygenation, nutrition, elimination, activity and rest, and protection)

Self-Concept-Group Identity Mode

The composite of beliefs and feelings held about oneself at a given time. Focus on the psychological and spiritual aspects of the human system. Need to know who one is, so that one can exist with a state of unity, meaning, and purposefulness of two modes (physical self, and personal self).

Role Function Mode

Set of expectations about how a person occupying one position behaves toward a occupying another position. Basic need-social integrity, the need to know who one is in relation to others.

Interdependence Mode

Behavior pertaining to interdependent relationships of individuals and groups. Focus on the close relationships of people and their purpose. Each relationship exists for some reason. Involves the willingness and ability to give to others and accept from others. Balance results in feelings of being valued and supported by others. Basic need-feeling of security in relationships
- ❖ **Adaptive responses:** Promote the integrity of the human system.
- ❖ **Ineffective responses:** Neither promote not contribute to the integrity of the human system
- ❖ **Copping process:** Innate or acquired ways innate or of interacting with the changing of environment.

Nursing Process

- ❖ A problem-solving approach for gathering data, identifying the capacities and needs of the human adaptive system, selecting and implementing approaches for nursing care, and evaluation the outcome of care provided.
  - ♦ **Assessment of behavior:** The first step of the nursing process which involves gathering data about the behavior of the person as an adaptive system in each of the adaptive modes.

- **Assessment of stimuli:** The second step of the nursing process which involves the identification of internal and external stimuli that are influencing the person's adaptive behaviors. Stimuli are classified as: (1) Focal—those most immediately confronting the person; (2) Contextual—all other stimuli present that are affecting the situation and (3) Residual—those stimuli whose effect on the situation is unclear.
- **Nursing diagnosis:** Step three of the nursing process which involves the formulation of statements that interpret data about the adaptation status of the person, including the behavior and most relevant stimuli.
- **Goal setting:** The fourth step of the nursing process which involves the establishment of clear statements of the behavioral outcomes for nursing care.
- **Intervention:** The fifth step of the nursing process which involves the determination of how best to assist the person in attaining the established goals.
- **Evaluation:** The sixth and final step of the nursing process which involves judging the effectiveness of the nursing intervention in relation to the behavior after the nursing intervention in comparison with the goal established.

Demographic Data

• Name	• Mr NR
• Age	• 53 years
• Sex	• Male
• IP number	• ——
• Education	• Degree
• Occupation	• Bank clerk
• Marital status	• Married
• Religion	• Hindu
• Informants	• Patient and wife
• Date of admission	• 21/01/08

First Level Assessment

Physiologic-Physical Mode

Oxygenation

Stable process of ventilation and stable process of gas exchange. RR = 18 BPM. Chest normal in shape. Chest expansion normal on either side. Apex beat felt on left 5th intercostal space mid-clavicular line. Air entry equal bilaterally. Apex beat felt-normal rhythm, depth and rate. Dorsalis pedis pulsation of affected limp is not palpable. All other pulsations are normal in rate, depth, tension with regular rhythm. No abnormal heart sounds. BP: Normotensive. Peripheral pulses felt: Normal rate and rhythm, no clubbing or cyanosis.

Nutrition

He is on diabetic diet (1,500 kcal). Nonvegetarian. Recently his weight reduced markedly (10 kg/6 month). He has stable digestive process. He has complaints of anorexia and not taking adequate food. No abdominal distension. Soft on palpation. No tenderness. No visible peristaltic movements. Bowel sounds heard. Percussion revealed dullness over hepatic area. Oral mucosa is normal. No difficulty to swallow food.

Elimination

No signs of infections, no pain during micturition or defecation. Normal bladder pattern. Using urinal for micturition. Stool is hard and he complaints of constipation.

Activity and Rest

Taking adequate rest. Sleep pattern disturbed at night due unfamiliar surrounding. Not following any peculiar relaxation measure. Like movies and reading. No regular pattern of exercise. Walking from home to office during morning and evening. Now, activity reduced due to amputated wound. Mobility impaired. Walking with crutches. Pain from joints present. No paralysis. ROM is limited in the left leg due to wound. No contractures present. No swelling over the joints. Patient need assistance for doing the activities.

Protection

Left lower fore foot is amputated. Black discoloration present over the area. No redness, discharge or other signs of infection. Normothermic. Wound healing better now. Walking with the use of left leg is not possible. Using crutches. Pain form knee and hip joint present while walking. Dorsalis pedis pulsation, not present over the left leg. Right leg is normal in length and size. Several papules present over the foot. All peripheral pulses are present with normal rate, rhythm and depth over right leg.

Senses

No pain sensation from the wound site. Relatively, reduced touch and pain sensation in the lower periphery; because of neuropathy. Using spectacle for reading. Gustatory, olfaction, and auditory senses are normal.

Fluids and Electrolytes

Drinks approximately 2,000 mL of water. Stable intake output ratio. Serum electrolyte values are within normal limit. No signs of acidosis or alkalosis. Blood glucose elevated.

Neurological Function

He is conscious and oriented. He is anxious about the disease condition. Like to go home as early as possible. Showing signs of stress. Touch and pain sensation decreased in lower extremity. Thinking and memory are intact.

Endocrine Function

He is on insulin. No signs and symptoms of endocrine disorders, except elevated blood sugar value. No enlarged glands.

Self-Concept Mode

Physical Self

He is anxious about changes in body image, but accepting treatment and coping with the situation. He deprived of sexual activity after amputation.

Belongs to a nuclear family. Five members. Stays along with wife and three children. Good relationship with the neighbors. Good interaction with friends. Moderately active in local social activities

Personal Self

Self-esteem disturbed because of financial burden and hospitalization. He believes in God and worshiping Hindu culture.

Role Performance Mode

He was the earning member in the family. His role shift is not compensated. His son doesn't have any work. His role clarity is not achieved.

Interdependence Mode

He has good relationship with the neighbors. Good interaction with the friends relatives. But he believes, no one is capable of helping him at this moment. He says "all are under financial constrains." He was moderately active in local social activities.

Second Level Assessment

Focal Stimulus

Nonhealing wound after amputation of great and second toe of left leg-4 week. A wound first found on the junction between first and second toe-4 month back. The wound was nonhealing and gradually increased in size with pus collected over the area.

He first showed in a local (—) hospital. From there, they referred to—medical college, where he was admitted for 1 month and 4 days. During hospital stay great and second toe amputated. But surgical wound turned to nonhealing with pus and black color. So, the physician suggested for below knee amputation. That made them come to—Hospital,—. He underwent a plastic surgery 3 weeks before.

Contextual Stimuli

Known case DM for past 10 years. Was on oral hypoglycemic agent for initial 2 years, but switched to insulin and using it for 8 years now. Not wearing footwear in house and premises.

Residual Stimuli

He had TB attack 10 years back, and took complete course of treatment. Previously, he admitted in—hospital for leg pain about 4 years back. Mother's brother had DM. Mother had history of PTB. He is a graduate in humanities, no special knowledge on health matters.

Conclusion

Mr NR who was suffering with diabetes mellitus for past 10 years. Diabetic foot ulcer and recent amputation made his life more stressful. Nursing care of this patient based on Roy's adaptation model provided had a dramatic change in his condition. Wound started healing and he planned to discharge on 25th April. He studied how to use crutches and mobilized at least twice in a day. Patient's anxiety reduced to a great extends by proper explanation and reassurance. He gained good knowledge on various aspects of diabetic foot ulcer for the future self-care activities.

Nursing Care Plan

Assessment of behavior	Assessment of stimuli	Nursing diagnosis	Goal	Intervention	Evaluation
Ineffective protection and sense in physical-physiological mode (No pain sensation from the wound site)	**Focal stimuli:** Nonhealing wound after amputation of great and second toe of left leg-4 weeks	**Impaired skin integrity related to fragility of the skin secondary to vascular insufficiency**	**Long-term objective:** 1. Amputated area will be completely healed by 20/5/08 2. Skin will remain intact with no ongoing ulcerations **Short-Term Objective:** 1. Size of wound decreases to 1 x 1 cm within 24/4/08 2. No signs of infection over the wound within 1-week 3. Normal WBC values within 1-week 4. Presence of healthy granular tissues in the wound site within 1-week	• Maintain the wound area clean as contamination affects the healing process • Follow sterile technique while providing cares to prevent infection and delay in healing • Perform wound dressing with betadine which promote healing and growth of new tissue • Do not move the affected area frequently as it affects the granulation tissue formation • Monitor for signs and symptoms of infection or delay in healing • Administer the antibiotics and vitamin C supplementation which will promote the healing process	**Short-term goal:** **Met:** Size of wound decreased to less than 1 x 1 centimeters WBC values became normal on 24/4/08 **Long-term goal:** **Partially met:** Skin partially intact with no ulcerations. • Continue plan Reassess goal and interventions **Unmet:** Not achieved complete healing of amputated area. • Continue plan • Reassess goal and interventions
Impaired activity in physical-physiological mode	**Focal stimuli:** During hospital stay great and second toe amputated. But surgical wound turned to nonhealing with pus and black color.	**Impaired physical mobility related to amputation of the left forefoot and presence of unhealed wound**	**Long-term objective:** Patient will attain maximum possible physical mobility within 6 months **Short-term objective:** 1. Correct use of crutches within 22/4/08 2. Walking with minimum support 22/4/08	• Assess the level of restriction of movement • Provide active and passive exercises to all the extremities to improve the muscle tone and strength • Make the patient to perform the ROM exercises to lower extremities which will strengthen the muscle	**Short-term goal:** **Met:** Used crutches correctly on 22/4/08 he is self-motivated in doing minor excesses **Partially met:** Walking with minimum support

Contd...

Contd...

Assessment of behavior	Assessment of stimuli	Nursing diagnosis	Goal	Intervention	Evaluation
			• He will be self-motivated in activities 20/4/08	• Massage the upper and lower extremities which help to improve the circulation • Provide articles near to the patient and encourage performing activities within limits which promote a feeling of wellbeing • Provide positive reinforcement for even a small improvement to increase the frequency of the desired activity • Measures for pain relief should be taken before the activities are initiated as pain can hinder with the activity	**Long-term goal:** **Unmet:** Not attained maximum possible physical mobility: • Continue plan • Reassess goal and interventions
Alteration in physical self in self-concept mode (He is anxious about changes in body image) *Change in role performance mode* (He was the earning member in the family. His role shift is not compensate)	**Contextual stimuli:** Known case DM for past 10 years and on treatment with insulin for 8 years. **Residual stimuli:** No special knowledge in health matters	**Anxiety related to hospital admission and unknown outcome of the disease and financial constrains**	**Long-term objective:** The client will remain free from anxiety **Short-term objective:** • Demonstrating appropriate range effective coping in the treatment • Being able to rest and • Asking fewer questions	• Allow and encourage the client and family to ask questions. Bring up common concerns • Allow the client and family to verbalize anxiety • Stress that frequent assessment is routine and do not necessarily imply a deteriorating condition • Repeat information as necessary because of the reduced attention span of the client and family • Provide comfortable quiet environment for the client and family	**Short-term goal:** **Met:** Demonstrated appropriate range effective coping with treatment • He is able to rest quietly **Long-term goal:** **Unmet:** Client not completely remained free from anxiety due to financial constrains: Continue plan Reassess goal and interventions

Contd...

Contd...

Assessment of behavior	Assessment of stimuli	Nursing diagnosis	Goal	Intervention	Evaluation
—	**Contextual stimuli:** Known case DM for past 10 years and on treatment with insulin for 8 years **Residual stimuli:** No special knowledge in health matters	**Deficient knowledge regarding the foot care, wound care, diabetic diet, and need of follow up care**	**Long-term objective:** Patient will acquire adequate knowledge regarding the foot care, wound care, diabetic diet, and need of follow up care and practice in their day-to-day life **Short-term objective:** • Verbalization and demonstration of foot care • Strictly following diabetic diet plan • Demonstration of wound care	• Explain the treatment measures to the patient and their benefits in a simple understandable language • Explain about the home care. Include the points like care of wounds, nutrition, activity etc. • Clear the doubts of the patient as the patient may present with some matters of importance • Repeat the information whenever necessary to reinforce learning	**Short-term goal:** **Met:** Verbalization and demonstration of foot care. Strictly following diabetic diet plan: **Unmet:** Demonstration of wound care **Long-term goal:** **Unmet:** Not completely acquired and practiced the required knowledge. • Continue plan • Reassess goal and interventions

JOHNSON'S BEHAVIOR SYSTEM MODEL

Introduction

* Dorothy E Johnson was born August 21, 1919, in Savannah, Georgia.
* BSN from Vanderbilt University in Nashville, Tennessee, in 1942; and her MPH from Harvard University in Boston in 1948.
* From 1949 until her retirement in 1978 she was an assistant professor of pediatric nursing, an associate professor of nursing, and a professor of nursing at the University of California in Los Angeles.
* Dorothy Johnson has had an influence on nursing through her publications since the 1950s. Throughout her career, Johnson has stressed the importance of research-based knowledge about the effect of nursing care on clients.

Johnson's Behavior System Model

* In 1968 Dorothy first proposed her model of nursing care as fostering of "the efficient and effective behavioral functioning in the patient to prevent illness."
* She also stated that nursing was "concerned with man as an integrated whole and this is the specific knowledge of order we require."
* In 1980 Johnson published her conceptualization of "behavioral system of model for nursing" this is the first work of Dorothy that explicates her definitions of the behavioral system model.

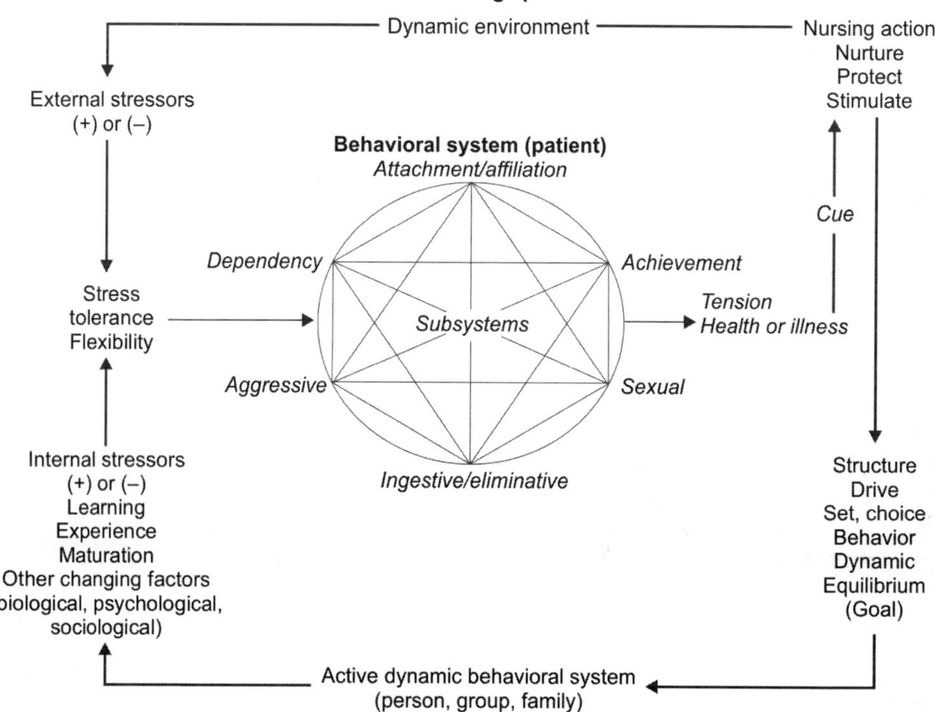

Johnson's behavioral system model. (Conceptualized by Jude A Magers, Indianapolis).

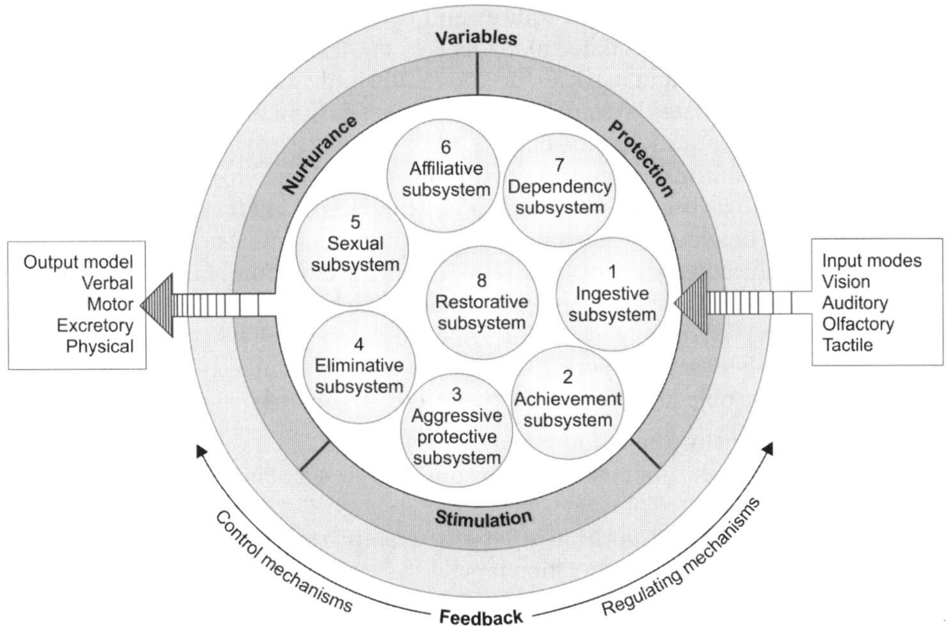

Johnson's behavioral system model. (From Reihl JP and Roy Sr C: Conceptual models for nursing, ed 2, New York, 1980, Appleton-Century-Crofts, p 227).

Definition of Nursing

She defined nursing as "an external regulatory force which acts to preserve the organization and integration of the patients behaviors at an optimum level under those conditions in which the behaviors constitutes a threat to the physical or social health, or in which illness is found."

Based on this definition there are four goals of nursing are to assist the patient:
1. Whose behavior commensurate with social demands?
2. Who is able to modify his behavior in ways that it supports biological imperatives?
3. Who is able to benefit to the fullest extent during illness from the physicians knowledge and skill?
4. Whose behavior does not give evidence of unnecessary trauma as a consequence of illness?

Assumptions of Behavioral System Model

There are several layers of assumptions that Johnson makes in the development of conceptualization of the behavioral system model (Johnson was influenced by Buckley, Chin and Rapport) there are four assumptions of system:
1. First assumption states that there is "organization, interaction, interdependency and integration of the parts and elements of behaviors that go to make up the system."
2. A system "tends to achieve a balance among the various forces operating within and upon it, and that man strive continually to maintain a behavioral system balance and steady state by more or less automatic adjustments and adaptations to the natural forces impinging upon him."

3. A behavioral system, which both requires and results in some degree of regularity and constancy in behavior, is essential to man that is to say, it is functionally significant in that it serves a useful purpose, both in social life and for the individual.
4. The final assumption states "system balance reflects adjustments and adaptations that are successful in some way and to some degree."
   - **The integration of these assumptions provides** the behavioral system with the pattern of action to form "an organized and integrated functional unit that determines and limits the interaction between the person and his environment and establishes the relation of the person to the objects, events and situations in his environment.
   - **The integration of these assumptions provides** the behavioral system with the pattern of action to form "an organized and integrated functional unit that determines and limits the interaction between the person and his environment and establishes the relation of the person to the objects, events and situations in his environment."

Assumptions about structure and function of each subsystem:
- "From the form the behavior takes and the consequences it achieves can be inferred what "drive" has been stimulated or what "goal" is being sought?"
- Each individual has a "predisposition to act with reference to the goal, in certain ways rather than the other ways". This predisposition is called as "set."
- Each subsystem has a repertoire of choices or "scope of action."
- The fourth assumption is that it produce "observable outcome" that is the individual's behavior.

Each subsystem has three functional requirements:
1. System must be "protected" from noxious influences with which system cannot cope."
2. Each subsystem must be "nurtured" through the input of appropriate supplies from the environment.
3. Each subsystem must be "stimulated" for use to enhance growth and prevent stagnation.

Johnson believes each individual has patterned, purposeful, repetitive ways of acting that comprise a behavioral system specific to that individual. These actions and behaviors form an organized and integrated functional unit that determines and limits the interaction between the person and his environment and establishes the relationship of the person to the objects event situations in the environment. These behaviors are "orderly, purposeful and predictable and sufficiently stable and recurrent to be amenable to description and explanation."

Johnson's Behavioral Subsystem

- **Attachment or affiliative subsystem:** "Social inclusion intimacy and the formation and attachment of a strong social bond."
- **Dependency subsystem:** "Approval, attention or recognition and physical assistance."
- **Ingestive subsystem:** "The emphasis is on the meaning and structures of the social events surrounding the occasion when the food is eaten."
- **Eliminative subsystem:** "Human cultures have defined different socially acceptable behaviors for excretion of waste, but the existence of such a pattern remains different from culture to culture."
- **Sexual subsystem:** "Both biological and social factor affect the behavior in the sexual subsystem."

6. **Aggressive subsystem:** "It relates to the behaviors concerned with protection and self-preservation Johnson views aggressive subsystem as one that generates defensive response from the individual when life or territory is being threatened."
7. **Achievement subsystem:** "Provokes behavior that attempt to control the environment intellectual, physical, creative, mechanical and social skills achievement are some of the areas that Johnson recognizes."

Representation of Johnson's Model

Goal—Set—Choice of Behavior—Behavior
- Affiliation
- Dependency
- Sexuality
- Aggression
- Elimination
- Ingestion
- Achievement

The Four Major Concepts

1. Johnson views *"human being"* as having two major systems, the biological system and the behavioral system. It is role of the medicine to focus on biological system where as *Nursling's focus is the behavioral system.*
2. *"Society"* relates to the environment on which the individual exists. According to Johnson an individual's behavior is influenced by the events in the environment.
3. *"Health"* is a purposeful adaptive response, physically mentally, emotionally, and socially to internal and external stimuli in order to maintain stability and comfort.
4. *"Nursing"* has a primary goal that is to foster equilibrium within the individual. She stated that nursing is concerned with the organized and integrated whole, but that the major focus is on maintaining a balance in the behavior system when illness occurs in an individual.

Nursing Process

Assessment

Grubbs developed an assessment tool based on Johnson's seven subsystems plus a subsystem she labeled as restorative which focused on activities of daily living. An assessment based on behavioral model does not easily permit the nurse to gather detailed information about the biological systems:
- Affiliation
- Dependency
- Sexuality
- Aggression
- Elimination
- Ingestion
- Achievement
- Restorative

Diagnosis

Diagnosis tends to be general to the system than specific to the problem. Grubb has proposed four categories of nursing diagnosis derived from Johnson's behavioral system model:

1. Insufficiency
2. Discrepancy
3. Incompatibility
4. Dominance

Planning and Implementation

Implementation of the nursing care related to the diagnosis may be difficult because of lack of clients input in to the plan. The plan will focus on nurses actions to modify clients behavior, these plan than have a goal, to bring about homeostasis in a subsystem, based on nursing assessment of the individuals drive, set behavior, repertoire, and observable behavior. The plan may include protection, nurturance or stimulation of the identified subsystem.

Evaluation

Evaluation is based on the attainment of a goal of balance in the identified subsystems. If the baseline data are available for an individual, the nurse may have goal for the individual to return to the baseline behavior. If the alterations in the behavior that are planned do occur, the nurse should be able to observe the return to the previous behavior patterns. Johnson's behavioral model with the nursing process is a nurse centered activity, with the nurse determining the clients needs and state behavior appropriate for that need.

Situation

John Smith, 6 weeks brought into the clinic for a routine check-up. He presents with no weight gain since his check up at the age of 2 weeks. His mother stated she feeds him but he does not seem to eat much. He sleeps 4–5 hours between the feedings. His mother holds him in her arms without trunk-to-trunk contact. As the assessment is made the nurse notes that Mrs Smith never looks at Johnny and never speaks to him. She stated he was a planned baby but that she never realized how much work a baby could be. She says, her mother told her she was not a good mother because John is not gaining weight like he should. She states she had not called the nurse when she knew John was not gaining weight because she thought nurse would think she was a bad mother just like her own mother thought she was a bad mother.

Assessment

- Affiliative subsystem between mother and John.
- Dependency subsystem between mother and John.
- Affiliative subsystem between Mrs Smith and her mother.
- Insufficiency ingestion subsystem.

Diagnosis

- Insufficient development of the affiliative subsystem.
- Insufficient development of the dependency subsystem.

Planning and Implementation

- ❖ Increasing mother's awareness of the baby's clues.
- ❖ Assisting her to talk with the baby.
- ❖ Teach her to bring a bond between her and the baby by touch, pat and cuddles etc.

Evaluation

- ❖ Johnny's weight gain or weight loss will be carefully assessed.
- ❖ The infant interaction could be reassessed, using the nursing child assessment feeding scale.
- ❖ The interaction of Mrs Smith with her mother.

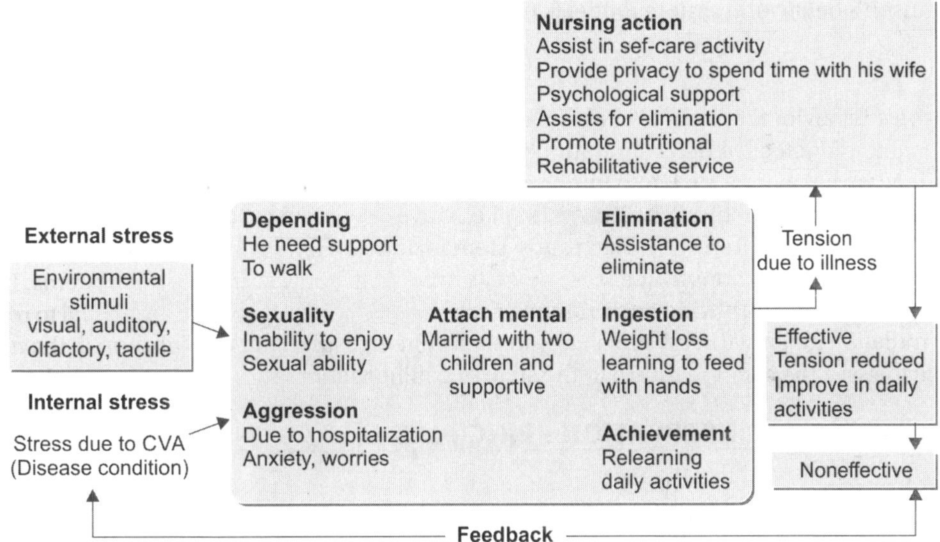

Cerebrovascular accident patient.

Johnson's and Characteristics of a Theory

- ❖ Interrelate concepts to create a different way of viewing a phenomenon.
- ❖ Theories must be logical in nature.
- ❖ Theories must be simple yet generalizable
- ❖ Theories can be bases of hypothesis that can be tested.
- ❖ Theories contribute to and assist in increasing the body of knowledge within the discipline through the research implemented to validate them.
- ❖ Theories can be utilized by practitioners to guide and improve their practice.
- ❖ Theories must be consistent with other validated theories, laws and principles but will leave unanswered questions that need to be investigated.

Limitation

- ❖ Johnson does not clearly interrelate her concepts of subsystems comprising the behavioral system model.
- ❖ The definition of concept is so abstract that they are difficult to use.

- It is difficult to test Johnson's model by development of hypothesis.
- The focus on the behavioral system makes it difficult for nurses to work with physically impaired individual to use this theory.
- The model is very individual oriented so the nurses working with the group have difficulty in its implementation.
- The model is very individually oriented so the family of the client is only considered as an environment.
- Johnson does not define the expected outcomes when one of the system is affected by the nursing implementation an implicit expectation is made that all human in all cultures will attain same outcome—homeostasis.
- Johnson's behavioral system model is not flexible.

Summary

Johnson's behavioral system model is a model of nursing care that advocates the fostering of efficient and effective behavioral functioning in the patient to prevent illness. The patient is defined as behavioral system composed of seven behavioral subsystems. Each subsystem composed of four structural characteristics, i.e., drives, set, choices and observable behavior. Three functional requirement of each subsystem includes:

1. Protection from noxious influences
2. Provision for the nurturing environment, and
3. Stimulation for growth. Any imbalance in each system results in disequilibrium. It is nursing role to assist the client to return to the state of equilibrium.

LEVINE'S FOUR CONSERVATION PRINCIPLES

Introduction

- Born in Chicago, raised with a sister and a brother with whom she shared a close loving relationship.
- Also, very fond of her father who was often ill and frequently hospitalized with GI problem. This was the reason of choosing nursing as a career.
- Also called as renaissance women-highly principled, remarkable and committed to patient's quality of care.
- Died in 1996

Educational Achievement

- **Diploma in nursing:** Cook County SON, Chicago, 1944
- **BSN:** University of Chicago, 1949
- **MSN:** Wayne State University, Detroit, 1962
- **Publication:** An Introduction to Clinical Nursing, 1969, 1973 and 1989
- Received honorary doctorate from Loyola University in 1992

Achievements

- Clinical experience in OT technique and oncology nursing
- Civilian nurse at the Gardiner general hospital
- Director of nursing at Drexel home in Chicago

* Clinical instructor at Bryan memorial hospital in Lincoln, Nebraska
* Administrative supervisor at University of Chicago
* Chairperson of clinical nursing at Cook County SON
* Visiting professor at Tel Aviv University in Israel

Conservational Model

* **Goal:** To promote adaptation and maintain wholeness using the principles of conservation.
* Model guides the nurse to focus on the influences and responses at the organismic level.
* Nurse accomplishes the goal of model through the conservation of energy, structure and personal and social integrity.

Adaptation

* Every individual has a unique range of adaptive responses.
* The responses will vary by heredity, age, gender or challenges of illness experiences.
* Example: The response to weakness of cardiac muscle is an increased heart rate, dilation of ventricle and thickening of myocardial muscle.
* While the responses are same, the timing and manifestation of organismic responses will be unique for each individual pulse rate.
* An ongoing process of change in which patient maintains his integrity within the realities of environment.
* Achieved through the "frugal, economic, contained and controlled use of environmental resources by individual in his or her best interest."

Wholeness

* Exist when the interaction or constant adaptations to the environment permits the assurance of integrity.
* Promoted by use of conservation principle.

Conservation

* The product of adaptation
* "Keeping together" of the life systems or the wholeness of the individual
* Achieving a balance of energy supply and demand that is with in the unique biological realities of the individual.

Nursing's Paradigm

Person

* A holistic being who constantly strives to preserve wholeness and integrity.
* A unique individual in unity and integrity, feeling, believing, thinking and whole system of system.

Environment

* Competes the wholeness of person
* Internal
* Homeorhesis

- ❖ External
- ❖ Preconceptual
- ❖ Operational
- ❖ Conceptual

Internal Environment

- ❖ **Homeostasis:** A state of energy sparing that also provide the necessary baselines for a multitude of synchronized physiological and psychological factors.
- ❖ A state of conservation
- ❖ **Homeorhesis:** A stabilized flow rather than a static state.
- ❖ Emphasis the fluidity of change within a space-time continuum.
- ❖ Describe the pattern of adaptation, which permit the individual's body to sustain its well-being with the vast changes which encroach upon it from the environment.

External Environment

- ❖ **Preconceptual:** Aspect of the world that individual are able to intercept.
- ❖ **Operational:** Elements that may physically affects individuals but not perceived by hem: radiation, micro-organism and pollution.
- ❖ **Conceptual:** Part of person's environment including cultural patterns characterized by spiritual existence, ideas, values, beliefs and tradition.

Person and Environment

- ❖ Adaptation
- ❖ Organismic response
- ❖ Conservation

Adaptation

Historicity: Adaptations are grounded in history and await the challenges to which they respond.

Specificity: Individual responses and their adaptive pattern varies on the base of specific genetic structure.

Redundancy: Safe and fail options available to the individual to ensure continued adaptation.

Organismic Response

- ❖ A change in behavior of an individual during an attempt to adapt to the environment.
- ❖ Help individual to protect and maintain their integrity.
- ❖ They co-exist
- ❖ They are four types
  1. *Flight or fight:* An instantaneous response to real or imagined threat, most primitive response.
  2. *Inflammatory:* Response intended to provide for structural integrity and the promotion of healing.

3. *Stress:* Response developed over time and influenced by each stressful experience encountered by person.
4. *Perceptual:* Involves gathering information from the environment and converting it into a meaning experience.

Nine Models of Guided Assessment

1. Vital's signs
2. Body movement and positioning
3. Ministration of personal hygiene needs
4. Pressure gradient system in nursing interventions
5. Nursing determination in provision of nutritional needs
6. Pressure gradient system in nursing
7. Local application of heat and cold
8. Administration of medicine
9. Establishing an aseptic environment

Assumption

- The nurse creates an environment in which healing could occur
- A human being is more than the sum of the part
- Human being respond in a predictable way
- Human beings are unique in their responses
- Human being know and appraise objects, condition and situation
- Human being sense, reflects, reason and understand
- Human being action are self-determined even when emotional
- Human being are capable of prolonging reflection through such strategists raising questions.
- Human being make decision through prioritizing course of action
- Human being must be aware and able to contemplate objects, condition and situation
- Human being are agents who act deliberately to attain goal
- Adaptive changes involve the whole individual
- A human being has unity in his response to the environment
- Every person possesses a unique adaptive ability based on one's life experience which creates a unique message.
- There is an order and continuity to life change is not random
- A human being respond organismically in an ever changing manner
- A theory of nursing must recognized the importance of detail of care for a single patient with in an empiric framework that successfully describe the requirement of the all patient.
- A human being is a social animal
- A human being is an constant interaction with an ever changing society
- Change is inevitable in life
- Nursing needs existing and emerging demands of self-care and dependent care
- Nursing is associated with condition of regulation of exercise or development of capabilities of providing care.

Levine's Work and Characteristics of Theory

- Theories can interrelate concepts in such a way as to create a different way of looking at a particular phenomenon.

* The concept of illness adaptation, using interventions, and the evaluation of nursing interventions are interrelated. They are combined to look at nursing care in a different way (more comprehensive view incorporating total patient care) from previous time.
* Theories must be logical in nature.
* Levine's idea about nursing care are organized in such a way as to be sequential and logical. They can be used to explain the consequences of nursing action.
* Theories should be relatively simple yet generalizable.
* Levine's theory is easy to use.
* It is major elements are easily comprehensible and the relationship have the potential for being complex but are easily manageable.
* Certain isolated aspect of the theory are the generalizable, i.e., those related to the conservational principles.
* Theories can be the bases for hypotheses that can be tested.
* Levine's idea can be tested.
* Hypothesis can be derived from them.
* The principle of conservation are specific enough to be testable.
* Levine's work and characteristics of theory.
* Theories contribute to and assist in increasing the general body of knowledge within the discipline through the research implemented to validate them.
* Since Levine's idea have not yet been widely researched, it is hard o determine the contribution to the general body of knowledge with in the discipline.
* Theories can be utilized by the practitioner to guide and improve their practice.
* Paula E Crawford-Gamble: Successfully applied Levine's theory to the female patient undergoing surgery for the traumatic amputation of the fingers .
* These ideas lend themselves to use in practice particularly in acute care setting.
* Theories must be consistent with other validated theories, laws and principles but will leave open unanswered questions that need to be investigated.
* Levine's ideas seem to be consistent with other theories, laws and principles particularly those from the humanities and sciences.

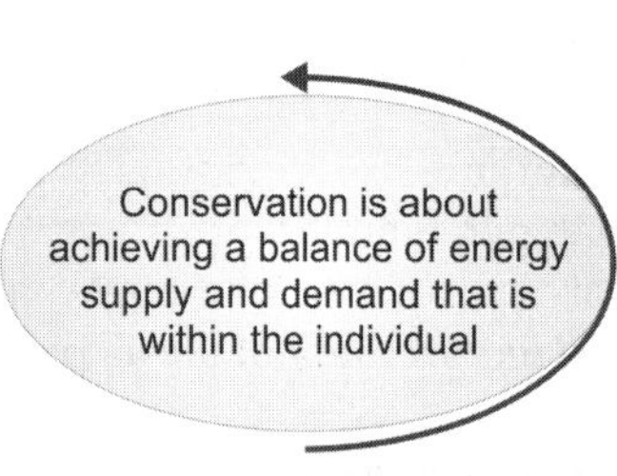

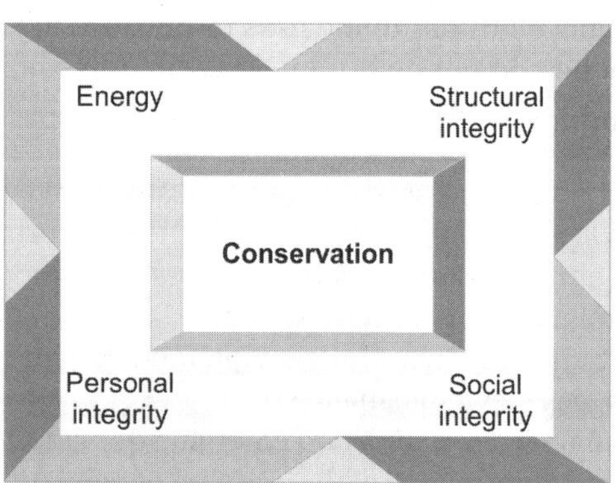

Conservational Principle

* Conservation of energy
* Conservation of structural integrity
* Conservation of personal integrity
* Conservation of social integrity

1. **Conservation of energy**
   - Refers to balancing energy input and output to avoid excessive fatigue
   - Includes adequate rest, nutrition and exercise
     Examples:
     ◊ Availability of adequate rest
     ◊ Maintenance of adequate nutrition
2. **Conservation of structural integrity**
   Refers to maintaining or restoring the structure of body preventing physical breakdown and promoting healing

   Examples
   - Assist patient in ROM exercise
   - Maintenance of patient's personal hygiene

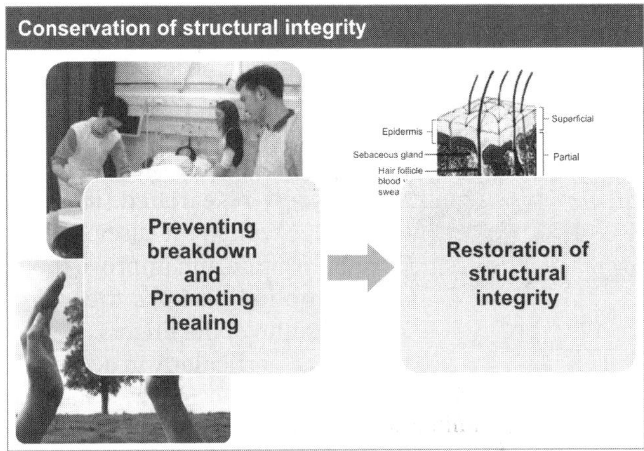

3. **Conservation of personal integrity**
   Recognizes the individual as one who strives for recognition, respect, self-awareness, selfhood and self-determination.

   Example: Recognize and protect patient's space needs

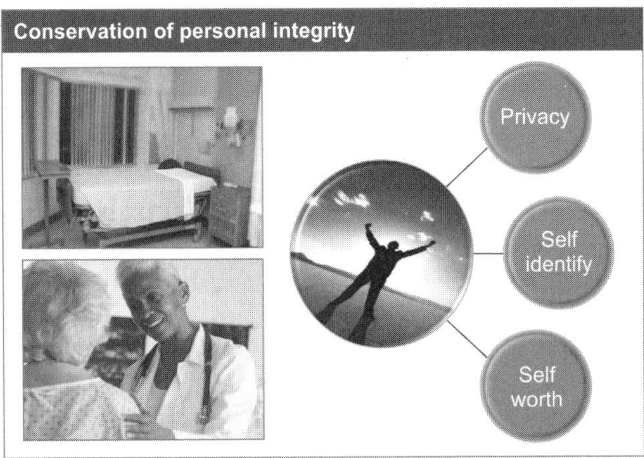

4. **Conservation of social integrity**

An individual is recognized as someone who resides with in a family, a community, a religious group, an ethnic group, a political system and a nation.

Examples:

- Position patient in bed to foster social interaction with other patients
- Avoid sensory deprivation
- Promote patient's use of newspaper, magazines, radio, TV
- Provide support and assistance to family

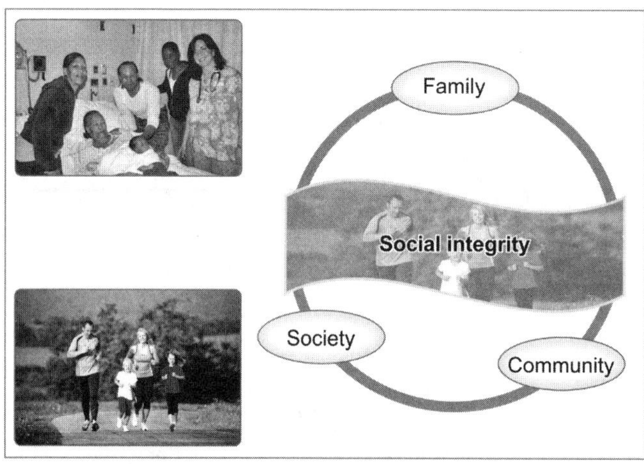

Health

- ❖ Health is a wholeness and successful adaptation.
- ❖ It is not merely healing of an afflicted part, it is return to daily activities, selfhood and the ability of the individual to pursue once more his or her own interest without constraints.
- ❖ **Disease:** It is unregulated and undisciplined change and must be stopped or death will ensue.

Nursing

- ❖ "Nursing is a profession as well as an academic discipline, always practiced and studied in concert with all of the disciplines that together from the health sciences".
- ❖ The human interaction relying on communication, rooted in the organic dependency of the individual human being in his relationships with other human beings.
- ❖ Nursing involves engaging in "human interactions."

Goal of Nursing

- ❖ To promote wholeness, realizing that every individual requires a unique and separate cluster of activities.
- ❖ The individual integrity is his abiding concern and it is the nurse's responsibility to assist him to defend and to seek its realization.

Nursing Process

- ❖ Assessment
- ❖ Trophicognosis

- ❖ Hypothesis
- ❖ Interventions
- ❖ Evaluation

Assessment

- ❖ Collection of provocative facts through observation and interview of challenges to the internal and external environment using four conservation principles.
- ❖ Nurses observes patient for organismic responses to illness, reads medical reports. talks to patient and family.
- ❖ Assesses factors which challenges the individual.

Trophicognosis

- ❖ Nursing diagnosis gives provocative facts meaning.
- ❖ A nursing care judgment arrived at through the use of the scientific process.
- ❖ Judgment is made about patient's needs for assistance.

Hypothesis

- ❖ Planning
- ❖ Nurse proposes hypothesis about the problems and the solutions which becomes the plan of care.
- ❖ Goal is to maintain wholeness and promoting adaptation.

Interventions

- ❖ Testing the hypothesis
- ❖ Interventions are designed based on the conservation principles
- ❖ Mutually acceptable
- ❖ Goal is to maintain wholeness and promoting adaptation

Evaluation

- ❖ Observation of organismic response to interventions
- ❖ It is assessing whether hypothesis is supported or not supported
- ❖ If not supported, plan is revised, new hypothesis is proposed

Conservational Models

Conservational model provides the basis for development of two theories:
1. Theory of redundancy
2. Theory of therapeutic intention

Theory of Redundancy

- ❖ Untested, speculative theory that redefined aging and everything else that has to do with human life.
- ❖ Aging is diminished availability of redundant system necessary for effective maintenance of physical and social well being.

Theory of Therapeutic Intention

- ❖ **Goal:** To seek a way of organizing nursing interventions out of the biological realities which the nurse has to confront.
- ❖ Therapeutic regimens should support the following goals:
  - ◆ Facilitate healing through natural response to disease
  - ◆ Provide support for a failing auto regulatory portion of the integrated system
  - ◆ Restore individual integrity and well being
- ❖ Provide supportive measure to ensures comfort
- ❖ Balance a toxic risk against the threat of disease
- ❖ Manipulate diet and activity to correct metabolic imbalance and stimulate physiological process.
- ❖ Reinforce usual response to create a therapeutic changes.

Uses

- ❖ Critical, acute or long-term care unit
- ❖ Neonates, infant and young children, pregnant young adult and elderly care unit.
- ❖ Primary healthcare
- ❖ OT
- ❖ Community setting

Utility of Theory

- ❖ Nursing research
- ❖ Nursing education
- ❖ Nursing administration
- ❖ Nursing practice

Nursing Research

- ❖ Principles of conservation have been used for data collection in various researches.
- ❖ Conservational model was used by Hanson et al. in their study of incidence and prevalence of pressure ulcers in hospice patient.
- ❖ Newport used principle of conservation of energy and social integrity for comparing the body temperature of infant's who had been placed on mother's chest immediately after birth with those who were placed in warmer.

Nursing Education

- ❖ Conservational model was used as guidelines for curriculum development.
- ❖ It was used to develop nursing undergraduate program at Allentown College of St Francis DeSales, Pennsylvania.
- ❖ Used in nursing education program sponsored by Kupat Holim in Israel.

Nursing Administration

- ❖ Taylor described an assessment guide for data collection of neurological patients which forms basis for development of comprehensive nursing care plan and thus evaluate nursing care.

- McCall developed an assessment tool for data collection on the basis of four conservational principles to identify nursing care needs of epileptic patients.
- Family assessment tool was designed by Lynn-Mchale and Smith for families of patient in critical care setting.

Nursing Practice

- Conservational model has been used for nursing practice in different settings.
- Bayley discussed the care of a severely burned teenagers on the basis of four conservational principles and discussed patient's perceptual, operational and conceptual environment.
- Pond used conservation model for guiding the nursing care of homeless at a clinic, shelters or streets.

Nursing Process According to Levine's Model

Mrs Mona, a wife of an abusive husband, underwent a radical hysterectomy. Post operatively has pain, weight loss, nausea and inability to empty bladder. Patient has history of smoking and stays in house which is less than sanitary.

Assessment

- **Challenges to the internal environment:** Weight loss, nausea, loss of reproductive ability.
- **Challenges to the external environment:** Abusive husband, insanitary condition in home.
- **Energy conservation:** Weight loss, nausea, pain.
- **Structural integrity:** Threatened by surgical procedure, inability to pass urine.
- **Personal integrity:** Not able to give birth to more children.
- **Social integrity:** Strained relationship with husband.

Trophicognosis

- Inadequate nutritional status
- Pain
- Potential for wound and bladder infection
- Need to learn self-catheterization
- Decreased self-worth
- Potential for abuse

Hypothesis

- Nutritional consultation
- Teaching and return demonstration of urinary self-catheterization
- Care of surgical wound
- Exploring concern regarding hysterectomy

Interventions

Energy Conservation

- Provide medication for pain and nausea
- Allowing rest period

Structural Integrity

* Administrating antibiotic for wound
* Teaching self-catheterization

Personal integrity: Exploring her feeling about uterus removal while respecting her privacy.

Social Integrity

* Assess potential abuse form husband
* Support to the family

Organismic Response

* Controlled pain
* Abdominal wound healing
* Improved appetite, weight gain
* Clean urinary self-catheterization
* Assistance from husband

Critiquing the Theory

* She values the holistic approach to all individual, well or sick
* Values patient's participation in nursing care
* Comprehensive content in depth
* Provides direction of nursing research, education, administration and practice
* Logically congruent
* Shows high regard to adjunctive disciplines to develop theoretical basis for nursing.

Limitation

* Limited attention can be focused on health promotion and illness prevention.
* Nurse has the responsibility for determining the patient ability to participate in the care, and if the perception of nurse and patient about the patient ability to participate in care don't match, this mismatch will be an area of conflict.

The major limitation is the focus on individual in an illness state and on the dependency of patient.

Index